MASTERING

Medical-Surgical Nursing

MASTERING
Medical-Surgical Nursing

SPRINGHOUSE CORPORATION
Springhouse, Pennsylvania

Staff

Senior Publisher
Matthew Cahill

Clinical Manager
Judith Schilling McCann, RN, MSN

Art Director
John Hubbard

Senior Editor
H. Nancy Holmes

Clinical Editors
Maryann Foley, RN, BSN (project manager);
Joanne Bartelmo, RN, MSN, CCRN; Pamela Kovach, RN;
Karen E. Michael, RN, MSN; Carla Roy, RN, BSN;
Beverly Tscheschlog, RN

Editors
Marcia Andrews, Doris Weinstock, Patricia A. Wittig

Copy Editors
Cynthia C. Breuninger (manager), Karen C. Comerford,
Stacey A. Follin, Janet Hodgson, Brenna H. Mayer,
Pamela Wingrod

Designers
Arlene Putterman (associate art director),
Linda Franklin (project manager), Joseph John Clark,
Donald Knauss, Mary Ludwicki, Jeffrey Sklarow

Illustrator
Jacalyn Bove Facciolo

Typography
Diane Paluba (manager), Joyce Rossi Biletz,
Phyllis Marron, Valerie Rosenberger

Manufacturing
Deborah Meiris (director), Pat Dorshaw (manager),
T.A. Landis, Otto Mezei

Production Coordinator
Margaret Rastiello

Editorial Assistants
Beverly Lane, Mary Madden

Indexer
Dorothy Hoffman

The clinical procedures described and recommended in this publication are based on currently accepted clinical theory and practice and on consultation with medical and nursing authorities. Nevertheless, they cannot be considered absolute and universal recommendations. For individual application, recommendations must be considered in light of the patient's clinical condition and, before administration of new or infrequently used drugs, in light of the latest package-insert information. The authors and the publisher disclaim responsibility for any adverse effects resulting directly or indirectly from the suggested procedures, from any undetected errors, or from the reader's misunderstanding of the text.

Printed in the United States of America.

MMSN-010997

 A member of the Reed Elsevier plc group

Library of Congress Cataloging-in-Publication Data
p.cm.
Includes index.
1. Nursing.   2. Surgical nursing.   I. Springhouse Corporation.
[DNLM: 1. Perioperative Nursing.   2. Nursing Process.
WY 161M423 1997]
RT41.M418   1997
610.73—dc21
DNLM/DLC
ISBN 0-87434-909-5 (alk. paper)   CIP   97-22241

Contents

◆◆◆   **v**

Consultants

Mary Ann Ascani, *RN, MSN, OCN*
Director of Oncology Services
Easton Hospital
Easton, Pa.

Sandra H. Clark, *RN, MSN*
Assistant Professor
Armstrong Atlantic State University
Savannah, Ga.

Mary R. Figlear, *RN, MEd, MSN, CRNA*
Faculty Emeritus
St. Luke's School of Nursing
Bethlehem, Pa.

Ellie Z. Franges, *RN, MSN, CCRN, CNRN*
Director Neuroscience Services
Sacred Heart Hospital
Allentown, Pa.

Sandra Smith Huddleston, *RN, PhD, CCRN*
Associate Professor
Berea (Ky.) College

Christine A. Kogel, *RN, ASN*
Clinical Nurse Coordinator—Kidney Stone Clinic
University Hospital
Denver

Tamara Luedtke, *RN, MSN, CCRN*
Nurse Manager, Critical Care Unit
Hendrick Medical Center
Abilene, Tex.

Margaret Massoni, *RN, MS, CS*
Assistant Professor
The College of Staten Island (N.Y.)

Chris Platt Moldovanyi, *RN, MSN*
Nurse Consultant
Middleburg Hts., Ohio

Nancy V. Runta, *RN,C, BSN, CCRN*
Medical-Surgical Staff Development Educator
North Penn Hospital
Lansdale, Pa.

Sheila M. Sparks, *RN, DNSc, CS*
Assistant Professor, School of Nursing
Georgetown University
Washington, D.C.

Bonnie Zauderer, *RN, MS, CNS*
Assistant Professor of Clinical Nursing
University of Texas, Houston
School of Nursing

Joan Zieja, *RN, MPH*
Assistant Professor of Nursing
Holy Family College
Philadelphia

Foreword ||||||||||||||||||||||||||||||||||||||||||||||||||||||||||||||||||||||||||||||||||||||

The movement toward cost-effective managed care coupled with advances in treatment has produced a growing demand for nurses with expanded medical-surgical skills. More than ever are needed medical-surgical nurses who can care for a diverse patient population in a variety of inpatient and outpatient settings. In every setting, nurses must function more independently and care for more acutely ill patients than at any time in the past, using advanced assessment, critical thinking, and therapeutic skills. *Mastering Medical-Surgical Nursing* is specifically designed to meet the wide-ranging needs of medical-surgical nurses practicing in a rapidly changing health care environment.

Focus on collaborative management

This all-encompassing reference incorporates the newest insights into the causes of illnesses, the latest advances in technology, and the most recent developments in the clinical care of patients with medical and surgical disorders. But one of the book's real strengths is its collaborative approach to patient care. Its 16 chapters provide a comprehensive, single-volume reference that emphasizes collegiality and expanded nursing responsibilities. Nursing assessment and diagnosis, medical diagnosis and treatment, planning of care, expected patient outcomes, nursing interventions, patient teaching, and discharge planning are integrated throughout the text.

Mastering Medical-Surgical Nursing is divided into two parts. The overview chapters in Part I highlight general concepts essential to practicing medical-surgical nursing. Chapter 1 covers such topics as the health-illness continuum, the nurse's role in health promotion, today's health care delivery system, and current issues and trends affecting medical-surgical nursing practice. Chapter 2 examines the components of the nursing process and relates them to the scientific method and problem-solving skills.

Part II presents information related directly to the clinical care of patients with specific disorders. Chapter 3 emphasizes collaborative teamwork through each phase of the perioperative experience—preoperative, intraoperative, and postoperative.

Body systems approach

Succeeding chapters, each on a specific body system, begin by reviewing the system's anatomy and physiology. Then each delves into disorders, highlighting key assessment and nursing actions.

Of particular note in chapters 4 and 5 are the discussions of coronary artery disease, myocardial infarction, heart failure, lung cancer, pneumonia, adult respiratory distress syndrome, and the new dangers of tuberculosis. Chapters 6 and 7 focus on common GI and neurologic disorders, including current thinking on peptic ulcer disease, hepatitis, cirrhosis, Alzheimer's disease, and meningitis. Chapters 8, 9, and 10—on eye and ear, renal, and endocrine disorders, respectively—take into account recent advances in assessing and managing sensory disorders, urinary tract infection, and incontinence and the newly released guidelines for diabetes mellitus, among others.

Chapters 11 and 12 examine reproductive and breast disorders. A highlight is the detailed coverage of current women's health issues, such as mammography, sexually transmitted diseases, and rape trauma. Chapters 13 and 14 cover musculoskeletal and hematologic disorders. Breakthroughs in performing arthroscopic surgery, understanding anemias, and managing bone marrow transplantation stand out among the topics included. Chapters 15 and 16 address immunologic and skin disorders. These chapters represent the most updated understanding of the relationship between immune function and immune-mediated disorders and between host defense mechanisms and the skin. They also provide current guidelines for human immunodeficiency virus infection and pressure ulcers.

Clinical paths and practice guidelines

Several recurring features enhance the text and promote understanding, such as the clinical paths and clinical practice guidelines.

Multidisciplinary care guides for major medical and surgical disorders, the clinical paths designate collaborative care activities and desired outcomes for each day of patient care. Because of managed care, clinical paths are now used by most health care agencies to standardize care, reduce costs, and improve quality of care. Any deviation is documented as a variance, and then evaluated for its potential to improve care and for incorporation into the path.

Concise information in the clinical practice guidelines focuses on recommendations for one or more aspects of a disorder, test, or procedure as established by the Agency for Health Care Policy and Research of the U.S. Department of Health and Human Services. Based on scientific evidence, the guidelines cover pain, urinary incontinence, pressure ulcer care, cataracts, benign prostatic hyperplasia, heart failure, and more.

"Discharge ready" sidebars list criteria a patient must meet before discharge from acute care. For example, criteria for discharge after GI obstruction might include vital signs within normal limits for the patient, fluid and electrolyte levels returning to normal, regular bowel patterns, and no evidence of pulmonary complications. This information is extremely helpful in planning for the intense patient teaching and advanced home care needs that reflect shortened hospital stays.

"Healthy living" items list actions the patient can take to promote health and prevent specific illness, including alternative therapies and insights. From acute care to community-based settings, medical-surgical nurses today are well placed to teach health promotion; these sidebars provide them with content that patients need to maintain wellness.

At the back, the helpful appendices review the very latest CDC infection-control recommendations and supply the full list of NANDA nursing diagnoses. And a large section of completed documentation samples covers myriad charting forms and styles.

Truly, *Mastering Medical-Surgical Nursing* will be of great value to nurses caring for any patient with a medical or surgical condition. Nurses who work in acute care settings as well as nurses in subacute care, skilled care, long-term care, community care, and home care will find this book extremely valuable. Student nurses, advanced practice nurses, and nurses continuing their education will also find this book to be a worthy supplement to their basic and specialty care texts. It's a winner.

Joyce K. Keithley, RN, DNSc, FAAN
Practitioner-Teacher and Professor
Department of Medical-Surgical Nursing
Rush University College of Nursing
Chicago

Part I

Overview of Medical-Surgical Nursing

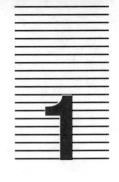

Health care and medical-surgical nursing

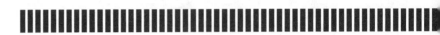

As the year 2000 approaches, nurses are assuming an increasingly significant role in the health care industry, gaining power and influence, and achieving greater control over their professional lives. This is the time for nurses to reaffirm their commitment to excellence in clinical care.

To keep pace with growing demands made on the health care system, nurses must develop new skills and refine existing ones. For example, as hospitals make greater use of noninvasive technology and bedside monitoring equipment, nurses will be expected to demonstrate full familiarity with arterial blood gas analysis, cardiac output measurement, electrocardiogram interpretation, and other diagnostic and monitoring techniques. Similarly, patient teaching will assume greater importance because effective teaching promotes compliance, and compliance in turn reduces hospital readmissions.

Profound changes in hospital care and a new emphasis on alternative settings have changed the nature of nursing practice. The average patient is older, with more complicated health problems, and the average hospital stay is shorter, making long-term care facilities an increasingly common alternative to prolonged hospitalization. Furthermore, as health care delivery shifts from the hospital to the community, the demand increases for highly skilled nurses both in and out of the hospital setting.

The health-illness continuum

How people view themselves—as individuals and as part of the environment—affects the way health is defined. Many people view health as a continuum, with wellness—the highest level of function—at one end and illness and death at the other. All people are somewhere on this continuum and, as their health status changes, their location on the continuum also changes.

HEALTH DEFINED
Throughout history, the focus and expression of health have changed depending on the knowledge and beliefs of the time. Some people regarded health and disease as reward or punishment for their actions. Others considered health as soundness or wholeness of the body.

Today, although *health* is a commonly used term, definitions abound. No single definition is universally accepted. A common one describes health as a disease-free state, but this presents an either-or situation—a person is either healthy or ill.

The World Health Organization calls health "a state of complete physical, mental, and social well-being and not merely the absence of disease or infirmity." This definition doesn't allow for degrees of health or illness. It also fails to reflect the concept of health as dynamic and constantly changing.

Sociologists view health as a condition that allows for the pursuit and enjoyment of desired cultural values. These include the ability to carry out activities of daily living, such as going to work and performing household chores.

Many people view health as a level of wellness. According to this definition, a person is striving to attain his full potential.

FACTORS AFFECTING HEALTH
One of nursing's primary functions is to assist patients in reaching an optimal level of wellness. When assessing a patient, the nurse must be aware of factors that affect the person's health status and plan to tailor interventions accordingly. Such factors include the following:

- genetics (biological and genetic makeup that causes illness and chronic conditions)
- cognitive abilities (which affect a person's view of health and ability to seek out resources)
- demographic factors, such as age and sex (certain diseases are more prevalent in a certain age-group or sex)
- geographic locale (which predisposes a person to certain conditions)
- culture (which determines a person's perception of health, the motivation to seek care, and the types of health practices performed)
- lifestyle and environment (such as diet, level of activity, and exposure to toxins)
- health beliefs and practices (which can affect health positively or negatively)
- previous health experiences (which influence reactions to illness and the decision to seek care)
- spirituality (which affects a person's view of illness and health care)
- support systems (which affect the degree to which a person adapts and copes with a situation).

ILLNESS DEFINED

Illness may be defined as a sickness or deviation from a healthy state. It's considered a broader concept than disease. Disease commonly refers to a specific biological or psychological problem that's supported by clinical manifestations and results in a body system or organ malfunction.

Illness, on the other hand, includes the perceptions and responses of the patient and those around him to being unwell. It encompasses how the patient interprets the source and importance of the disease, how the disease affects his behavior and relationships with others, and how he tries to remedy the problem. Another significant component is the meaning that a person attaches to the experience of being ill.

TYPES OF ILLNESS

Illness may be acute or chronic. Acute illness usually refers to a disease or condition that has a relatively abrupt onset, high intensity, and short duration. If no complications occur, most acute illnesses end in a full recovery and the person returns to the previous or a similar level of functioning.

Chronic illness refers to a condition that typically has a slower onset, less intensity, and a longer duration than an acute illness. The goal is to help the patient regain and maintain the highest possible level of health, although some patients fail to return to their previous level of functioning.

EFFECTS OF ILLNESS

When a person experiences an illness, one or more changes occur that signal its presence. These may include:

- changes in body appearance or function
- unusual body emissions
- sensory changes
- uncomfortable physical manifestations
- changes in emotional status
- changes in relationships.

Most people experience a mild form of some of these changes in their daily lives. However, when the changes are severe enough to interfere with usual daily activities, the person is usually considered ill.

People's reactions to feeling ill vary. Some people seek action immediately, others take no action, and still others seek counteraction.

EFFECTS OF ILLNESS ON FAMILY

The presence of illness in a family can have a dramatic effect on the functioning of the family as a unit. The type of effect depends on the following factors:

- which member is ill
- the seriousness and duration of the illness
- the family's social and cultural customs (each member's role in the family and the tasks specific to that role).

The types of role change that occur also vary, depending on the family member affected. For example, if the affected member is the primary breadwinner, other members may need to seek employment to supplement the family income. As the primary breadwinner assumes a dependent role, the rest of the family must adjust to new roles. If the affected family member is a working single parent, serious economic and child care problems may result. That person must depend on support systems for help or face additional stress.

Health promotion

The recent trend toward health promotion removes illness as the primary focus of health care. Health promotion refers to activities that are directed toward developing a person's resources to maintain or enhance well-being as a protection from illness. It's based on the principles of self-responsibility, nutritional awareness, stress reduction and management, and physical activity. Reversing the emphasis from curing the disease to promoting health provides a more positive direction for health care.

HEALTHY PEOPLE 2000 GUIDELINES

In 1991, the U.S. Department of Health and Human Services published a set of national health objectives for the year 2000. These objectives identify specific healthy behavior practices with the expectation that by the year 2000, people will be healthier and practicing healthier lifestyles. (See *Healthy People 2000: Selected objectives*.)

CONSUMER AWARENESS AND EDUCATION

Because of increased media coverage of health, wellness, and health promotion in recent years, consumer awareness about health and illness has risen noticeably. The result has been a public outcry for information and a tremendous response by health care professionals and agencies. Information about nutrition, exercise, stress management, and routine health examination is now available in a wide variety of settings. Health promotion programs once limited to

hospital settings have now moved into community settings, such as schools, churches, and community centers, and the workplace is quickly becoming an important site for such programs.

Health care delivery system

Health care encompasses three aspects: prevention of illness, promotion and maintenance of health, and restoration of health when illness occurs. Traditionally, health care has been delivered primarily through acute care hospital and doctor services. A patient who becomes acutely ill, is a victim of trauma, or experiences an exacerbation of a chronic illness needs acute care in a hospital setting. This type of care is high-cost care that relies on advanced technology and the expertise of highly trained caregivers to stabilize the patient and prepare him for the eventual transition to a less costly health care setting.

Driven by financial pressures and social changes, today's health care system is evolving from a hospital-based system to an interconnecting web of facilities and services designed to care for patients in the most cost-effective way. Duties of nurses and other health care providers are changing drastically as the focus shifts from traditional acute care settings to new and not-so-new alternative settings, such as subacute care, outpatient services, home health care, hospice care, nurse-managed clinics, and assisted living and long-term care facilities.

Medical-surgical nursing practice

Medical-surgical nursing is the care of adults in health and illness. It's based on knowledge derived from the arts and sciences and further enhanced by knowledge from nursing. The focus of medical-surgical nursing is the adult patient's response to actual or potential alterations in health.

SCOPE OF PRACTICE

Medical-surgical nursing is one of many specialties in nursing, yet its scope is much broader than such specialties as cardiovascular or orthopedic nursing. In 1991, the Academy of Medical-Surgical Nurses was created as the first specialty organization for this group.

Medical-surgical nurses assume diverse roles and, with them, varied responsibilities. They may work in any health care setting, but most are employed by acute care facilities.

The focus of medical-surgical nursing is on adult patients with acute or chronic illness. Such patients range from age 18 to over age 100, and their health problems are usually complex. To care for this wide range of patients, medical-surgical nurses need a broad knowledge of the biological, psychological, and social sciences. Because the typical medical-surgical patient is older than age 65, these nurses also need a strong background in gerontology.

ROLES AND FUNCTIONS
Health care today reflects changes in the populations requiring nursing care and a philosophical shift toward health promotion rather than illness care. The roles of the medical-surgical nurse have broadened and expanded in response to these changes. (See *Major roles of the medical-surgical nurse*, page 6.)

PRACTICE SETTINGS
Nurses working in medical-surgical nursing provide health care in a variety of settings. These include hospitals, long-term care facilities, and community health care settings.

HOSPITALS
The majority of nurses practice in hospitals. Because of the different specialty areas within this acute care setting, hospitals offer numerous medical-surgical opportunities.

LONG-TERM CARE FACILITIES
Another large practice setting for nurses is the long-term care facility, or free-standing nursing home. These facilities provide long-term nursing care to patients who are typically older than age 65, although the age range is now expanding to include younger patients with chronic and disabling conditions.

A major change in long-term care is the acuity level of the patients. Largely as a result of earlier patient discharges from hospitals, many long-term care facilities have specialty or subacute units for patients with such conditions as dementia, head trauma, or spinal cord injury.

COMMUNITY HEALTH CARE SETTINGS
Community health care settings represent a growing practice arena for nursing. They include schools, doctors' offices, industrial centers, public health departments, visiting nurse organizations, health maintenance organizations, and other ambulatory care centers. These settings offer a wide variety of services, including family planning, substance abuse interventions, preventive care, and home health care. Nurses in such settings have much responsibility and influence. In some cases, because a doctor isn't readily available, the nurse determines the patient's health care needs initially and on an ongoing basis.

Increased emphasis on health promotion and maintenance has led to growth in the number of community health care settings; soon they may outnumber acute care facilities. Also, early patient discharge from hospital to home has created a greater need for nurses in home care.

Related issues and trends

Health care is a vast and complicated system, affected by and reflecting changes in society. Trends and issues now facing medical-surgical nurses are ones that will shape the philosophy and provision of care in the next century.

POPULATION CHANGES
Over the last decade, the demographic profile of those requiring nursing care has changed dramatically. Over half of the patients admitted to acute care facilities are over age 75, and almost half admitted to critical care units are over age 65. As projected by the U.S. Census Bureau, hospital services to the elderly by the year 2000 will have increased by almost 40% from 1987 levels. In addition to the increasing number of elderly patients, other population changes are occurring. The number of people infected with human immunodeficiency virus is also rising rapidly. And the number of medically indigent patients has almost doubled with the increasing number of homeless people. All of these factors impact greatly on nursing care.

CHANGES IN HEALTH CARE DELIVERY
Issues and trends affecting the method of delivery for health care include:
■ reforms in cost and reimbursement of doctor services, with reimbursement for an amount considered equitable
■ changes in health care financing through expanded Medicaid coverage, universal health insurance, mandated employers' insurance, and a national health plan addressing the problem of uncompensated care
■ increased support for ambulatory services as a means of cost control
■ increased government intervention in quality assurance necessary for accreditation
■ decrease in the health of the population as a result of illiteracy, violence, drug use, poverty, and unemployment.

Major roles of the medical-surgical nurse

Medical-surgical nurses today are caregivers, as always, but they are also educators, advocates, leaders and managers, change agents, and researchers. The nurse assumes these roles to promote health, prevent illness, and facilitate coping with disability or death for any patient in any health care setting.

Caregiver

Nurses have always been caregivers, but the activities this role encompasses have changed dramatically in this century. Increased education of nurses, research in and development of nursing knowledge, and the recognition that nurses are autonomous and informed professionals have caused a shift from the once dependent role to one of independence and collaboration.

The nurse independently makes assessments and plans and implements patient care based on nursing knowledge and skills. The nurse also collaborates with other members of the health care team to implement and evaluate care.

Educator

With the greater emphasis on health promotion and illness prevention, the nurse's role as educator has become increasingly important. The nurse assesses learning needs, plans and implements teaching strategies to meet those needs, and evaluates the effectiveness of the teaching. To be an effective educator, the nurse must have effective interpersonal skills and be familiar with principles of adult learning.

Teaching is also a major part of discharge planning. Along with teaching come responsibilities for making referrals, identifying community and personal resources, and arranging for necessary equipment and supplies for home care.

Advocate

Many patients are entering the health care system unprepared to make independent decisions. The nurse as advocate actively promotes the patient's rights to autonomy and free choice, thus speaking for the patient, mediating between the patient and other people, and protecting the patient's right to self-determination.

The basis for the advocate role is the patient's right to choose treatment options without coercion. The nurse accepts and respects a patient's decision, even if it differs from the decision the nurse would make.

Leader and manager

All nurses practice leadership and manage time, people, resources, and the environment in which they provide care. They carry out these tasks by directing, delegating, and coordinating activities.

A variety of health care team members, including the nurse, provide patient care. Although the doctor is usually considered the head of the team, the nurse plays an important role in coordinating the efforts of all team members to meet the patient's goals and may conduct team conferences to facilitate communication among team members.

Change agent

The nurse's role as change agent involves planning and implementing a system to change patients' health-related behaviors. For example, in the work setting, the nurse assesses health behaviors to identify those that need altering. A vital factor in this process is assessing the patient's readiness to change. If the patient isn't ready, he won't comply with the change and the nurse will be ineffective in this role.

In the community, the nurse serves as a role model and assists consumers in bringing about changes to improve the environment, work conditions, or other factors that affect health. Nurses also work together to bring about change through legislation, such as shaping and supporting bills to mandate the use of car safety seats and motorcycle helmets.

Researcher

Nurses have always identified problems in patient care but, although they've developed interventions to meet specific needs, many of their activities have not been conducted within a scientific framework or communicated to other nurses through nursing literature. This situation is changing as more and more nurses recognize the importance of their role as researcher and the special vantage point that their role as caregiver affords them.

The primary tasks of nursing research are to promote growth of the science of nursing and to develop nursing theories to serve as a scientific basis for nursing practice. Every nurse has a responsibility to become involved in nursing research and to apply research findings in nursing practice.

Although not all nurses are trained in research methods, each nurse can participate by remaining alert for nursing problems and asking questions about care practices. Many nurses who give direct care identify such problems, which then serve as a basis for research investigation. Nurses can promote nursing care by incorporating research findings into their practice and by communicating the research to others.

ADVANCED PRACTICE ROLE

Professional nursing is adapting to meet changing health care needs and expectations. One method is the advanced practice role, which has developed in response to the need for improved distribution of health care services and decreased cost. The nurse who functions in an advanced practice role provides direct care to patients through independent practice, interdependent practice, or practice within a health agency. This new nursing role has compelled state nursing associations to more clearly define the practice of nursing. Nurse practice acts have been amended to give nurses authority to perform functions that were previously restricted to the practice of medicine.

The advanced practice role requires expert skills in interviewing, observation, physical assessment and examination, data gathering, and the latest clinical techniques. It also requires an understanding of behavioral patterns and an ability to promote problem-solving skills for individuals, families, and groups. In addition, the nurse must be skilled in decision making, evaluating outcomes of care, and implementing measures to promote cost containment and reduction.

HEALTH CARE REFORM

Over the years, health care has become increasingly expensive, insurance premiums have climbed, and businesses have been less inclined to offer health benefits or have cut back on the scope of these benefits. Many people today have less health care coverage than before or no coverage at all. The current system provides consistent services only to those who are able to pay, have health insurance, or qualify for health care through government programs. Solutions are being sought to provide low-cost health care to all, and the debate is ongoing.

Current market forces are causing major changes in the way health care is delivered, paid for, and evaluated. The market approach to health care reform is controlled primarily by insurance companies, health maintenance organizations, and other financial organizations. This approach is finance- and outcome-oriented. The financial orientation monitors patient care aspects, such as length of stay, readmission rates, complications, and patient satisfaction. The outcome orientation examines morbidity, mortality, clinical outcomes, access to care, human resources, regulatory reporting, and customer service.

Capitation is now touted as the way to help ensure the most cost-effective care. In this method, a health care institution receives a fixed dollar amount for each patient, corresponding to the patient's diagnosis and the mandated length of stay for that diagnosis regardless of how long the patient actually stays. Additional reimbursement is possible only if a complication occurs that requires a new or additional diagnosis and added length of stay. Thus, capitation demands that health care institutions constantly evaluate care and seek ways to streamline and improve care delivery to reduce length of stay.

COMPUTERIZATION

Use of computerized records has helped speed record-keeping and allowed nurses to spend more time with patients. Institutions are using computers in numerous timesaving ways, such as for ordering supplies and services, storing and providing immediate access to diagnostic test results, developing and implementing patient acuity classification systems to determine staffing need, documenting nursing assessments and care, and developing individualized plans of care. More and more institutions are placing computers at the patient's bedside to decrease the time required for documentation and to minimize the potential for documentation errors. However, the use of computers has raised some concerns. Computerized decision making for nursing plans of care is based solely on scientific fact and thus negates the humanistic, caring aspect of nursing. The potential exists for nurses to interact more with the computer than with the patient. And access to records from multiple sources, including insurance companies, employers, and the government, threatens confidentiality of patient health care information.

Selected readings

Beare, P.G., and Myers, J.L. *Principles and Practice of Adult Health Nursing,* 2nd ed. St. Louis: Mosby–Year Book, Inc., 1994.

Cronenwett, L.R. "Molding the Future of Advanced Practice Nursing," *Nursing Outlook* 43(3):112-18, May-June 1995.

Douglass, L.M. *The Effective Nurse: Leader and Manager,* 5th ed. St. Louis: Mosby–Year Book, Inc., 1996.

Ellis, J.R., and Hartley, C.L. *Nursing in Today's World: Challenges, Issues, and Trends,* 5th ed. Philadelphia: Lippincott-Raven Pubs., 1995.

Kelly, L.Y., and Joel, L.A. *Dimensions of Professional Nursing,* 7th ed. New York: McGraw-Hill Book Co., 1995.

Hutchinson, D. "A Nurse's Guide to the Internet," *RN* 60(1): 46-51, January 1997.

Ignatavicius, D.D., et al., eds. *Medical-Surgical Nursing: A Nursing Process Approach,* 2nd ed. Philadelphia: W.B. Saunders Co., 1995.

Illustrated Manual of Nursing Practice, 2nd ed. Springhouse, Pa.: Springhouse Corp., 1994.

Monahan, F.D., et al. *Nursing Care of Adults.* Philadelphia: W.B. Saunders Co., 1994.

Nurse's Pocket Companion, Patient-Focused Care Edition. Springhouse, Pa.: Springhouse Corp., 1996.

Phipps, W.J., et al. *Medical Surgical Nursing: Concepts and Clinical Practice,* 5th ed. St. Louis: Mosby–Year Book, Inc. 1995.

Polaski, A.L., and Tatro, S.E. *Luckmann's Core Principles and Practice of Medical-Surgical Nursing.* Philadelphia: W.B. Saunders Co., 1996.

Taylor, C., et al. *Fundamentals of Nursing: The Art and Science of Nursing Care,* 3rd ed. Philadelphia: Lippincott-Raven Pubs., 1997.

U.S. Department of Health and Human Services. *Healthy People 2000: National Health Promotion and Disease Prevention Objectives.* Boston: Jones and Bartlett, 1991.

Ventura, M.J., "Workload, UAPs, and You—A New Survey," *RN* 59(9):41-47, September 1996.

Zerwekh, J., and Claborn, J. *Nursing Today: Transition and Trends.* Philadelphia: W.B. Saunders Co., 1994.

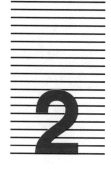

The nursing process

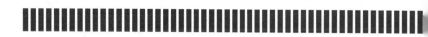

The cornerstone of clinical nursing, the nursing process is a systematic method for taking independent nursing action. Its phases, as defined in the American Nurses' Association (ANA) Standards of Care (1991), include:
■ assessing the patient's problems
■ forming a diagnostic statement (nursing diagnosis)
■ identifying expected outcomes
■ creating a plan of care to achieve expected outcomes
■ implementing the plan or assigning others to handle it
■ evaluating the plan's effectiveness.
These phases are dynamic and flexible; they often overlap.

Becoming familiar with this process has many benefits. It allows you, the nurse, to apply your knowledge and skills in an organized, goal-oriented manner. It also enables you to communicate about professional topics with colleagues from all clinical specialties and practice settings.

Growing recognition of the nursing process is an important development in the struggle for greater professional autonomy. By clearly defining problems that a nurse may treat independently, the nursing process has helped to dispel the notion that nursing practice is based solely on carrying out doctors' orders. Despite recent advances, nursing is still in an early state of professional evolution. In the years ahead, researchers and expert practitioners will continue to develop a body of knowledge specific to the field. A strong foundation in the nursing process will enable you to better assimilate emerging concepts and to incorporate these concepts into your practice.

The ANA's six-step nursing process echoes the scientific method and the similar problem-solving method. (See *Nursing approach to problem solving,* page 10.) Used properly, it promotes critical thinking—the

analysis of information gathered by observation, experience, and communication to guide action. In carrying out the nursing process, you need to be open-minded, creative, and responsive to changes in your patients and in the health care environment.

Assessment

The vital first phase in the nursing process, assessment consists of data collection (patient history, physical examination findings, and laboratory study results). The effectiveness of the other nursing process phases—nursing diagnosis formation, outcome identification, planning, implementation, and evaluation—depends on the quality of the assessment data.

A properly recorded initial assessment provides:
■ a way to communicate patient information to other caregivers
■ a method of documenting initial baseline data
■ a foundation on which to build an effective plan of care.

DATA COLLECTION
The information you collect in taking your patient's history, performing a physical examination, and analyzing laboratory test results serves as your assessment database. You can't collect or use *all* the information that exists about your patient. To limit your database to facts that will help most in assessing your patient, ask yourself these questions: What data do I want to collect? How should I collect the information? How should I organize it to make care planning decisions?

The well-defined database for a patient may begin with admission signs and symptoms, chief complaint, or medical diagnosis. It also may center on the type of patient care given in a specific nursing unit, such as

Nursing approach to problem solving

Dynamic and flexible, the phases of the nursing process resemble the steps that many other professions rely on to identify and correct problems. Here's how the nursing process phases correspond to the standard scientific and critical thinking methods.

Nursing process	Scientific method	Critical thinking
ASSESSMENT ■ Collect and analyze subjective and objective data about the patient's health problem.	■ Recognize that a problem exists. ■ Learn about the problem by obtaining facts.	■ Collect the data.
DIAGNOSIS ■ State the health problems.	■ State the nature of the problem.	■ State the problem.
PLANNING ■ Identify expected outcomes. ■ Write a plan of care that includes the nursing interventions designed to achieve expected outcomes.	■ Think of and select ways to achieve goals and solve the problem.	■ Formulate the hypothesis.
IMPLEMENTATION ■ Put the plan of care into action. ■ Document the actions taken and their results.	■ Act on ways to solve the problem.	■ Test the hypothesis.
EVALUATION ■ Critically examine the results achieved. ■ Review and revise the plan of care as needed.	■ Decide if the actions taken have effectively solved the problem.	■ Analyze and evaluate.

the intensive care unit or the emergency department (ED). For example, you wouldn't ask a trauma victim in the ED if she has a family history of breast cancer, nor would you perform a routine breast examination on her. You would, however, do these types of assessment during a comprehensive health checkup in an ambulatory care setting.

The assessment data that you collect and analyze fall into two important categories: subjective and objective. Subjective data include the patient's history and embody a personal perspective. Although the patient is your most important source of information, he's also the most subjective source, and the information he provides must be interpreted carefully.

Objective data about your patient's health status or about the pathologic processes that may be related to his illness or injury come from the physical examination, which involves inspection, palpation, percussion, and auscultation. This information helps you interpret the patient's history more accurately because it provides a basis for comparison. Use it to validate and amplify the historical data. However, don't allow the physical examination to assume undue importance.

The most objective form of assessment data, laboratory test results provide another source for interpreting your history and physical examination findings. The advanced technology used in laboratory tests enables you to assess anatomic, physiologic, and chemical processes that neither your senses nor your patient's are capable of measuring. For example, if your patient complains of feeling tired (patient history) and you observe conjunctival pallor (physical examination), check his hemoglobin level and hematocrit (laboratory data) to obtain more information about his condition.

You need both subjective and objective data for comprehensive patient assessment. They validate each other and together provide more data than either could provide alone.

HEALTH HISTORY
The health history portion of the assessment consists of the subjective data you collect from the patient.

You'll use your interviewing skills to help the patient describe biological, social, and psychological responses to the particular anatomic, physiologic, and chemical processes involved in his illness or injury. In addition, the patient may recall events in his own life or in relatives' lives that may indicate an increased risk for certain pathologic processes.

INTERVIEW

The information for the health history is gathered from an interview with the patient. A complete health history provides the following information about a patient:
- biographical data
- chief complaint (or concern)
- history of present illness (or current health status)
- current prescription and over-the-counter medications
- past history
- family history
- psychosocial history
- activities of daily living (ADLs)
- review of systems.

This orderly format is helpful when taking a patient's history. However, you may need to modify it based on the patient's chief complaint or concern. For example, the health history of a patient with a localized allergic reaction will be much shorter than that of a patient who complains vaguely of mental confusion and severe headaches.

If your patient has a chief complaint, use information from the health history to decide if his problems stem from physiologic causes or psychophysiologic maladaptation and how your nursing interventions may help. The depth of such a history depends on the patient's cooperation and your skill in asking insightful questions.

A patient who requests a complete physical checkup may not even have a chief complaint. Such a patient's health history would be comprehensive, with detailed information about lifestyle, self-image, family and other interpersonal relationships, and degree of satisfaction with current health status.

Review of systems. When interviewing the patient, use this review of systems as a guide.

General: overall state of health, ability to carry out ADLs, weight changes, fatigue, exercise tolerance, fever, night sweats, repeated infections

Skin: changes in color, pigmentation, temperature, moisture, or hair distribution; eruptions; pruritus; scaling; bruising; bleeding; dryness; excessive oiliness; growths; moles; scars; rashes; scalp lesions; brittle, soft, or abnormally formed nails; cyanotic nail beds; pressure ulcers

Head: trauma, lumps, alopecia, headaches

Eyes: nearsightedness, farsightedness, glaucoma, cataracts, blurred vision, double vision, tearing, burning, itching, photophobia, pain, inflammation, swelling, color blindness, injuries, use of glasses or contact lenses, date of last eye examination

Ears: deafness, tinnitus, vertigo, discharge, pain, tenderness behind the ears, mastoiditis, otitis or other ear infections, earaches, ear surgery

Nose: sinusitis, discharge, colds, or coryza more than four times a year; rhinitis; trauma; sneezing; loss of sense of smell; obstruction; breathing problems; epistaxis

Mouth and throat: changes in tongue color, sores on tongue, dental caries, tooth loss, toothaches, bleeding gums, lesions, loss of taste, hoarseness, sore throats (streptococcal), tonsillitis, voice changes, dysphagia, date of last dental checkup, use of dentures, bridges, or dental appliances

Neck: pain, stiffness, swelling, limited movement

Breasts: changes in development or lactation pattern, trauma, lumps, pain, nipple discharge, gynecomastia, changes in contour or in nipples, history of breast cancer, knowledge of breast self-examination

Cardiovascular: palpitations, tachycardia, or other rhythm irregularities; chest pain; dyspnea on exertion; orthopnea; cyanosis; edema; ascites; intermittent claudication; cold extremities; phlebitis; hypertension; orthostatic hypotension; rheumatic fever; recent electrocardiogram

Respiratory: dyspnea, shortness of breath, pain, wheezing, paroxysmal nocturnal dyspnea, orthopnea (number of pillows used), cough, sputum, hemoptysis, night sweats, emphysema, pleurisy, bronchitis, tuberculosis (contacts), pneumonia, asthma, upper respiratory tract infections, recent chest X-ray and tuberculin skin test results

Gastrointestinal: changes in appetite or weight, dysphagia, nausea, vomiting, heartburn, eructation, flatulence, abdominal pain, colic, hematemesis, jaundice (pain, fever, intensity, duration, color of urine), stools (color, frequency, consistency, odor, use of laxatives), hemorrhoids, rectal bleeding, changes in bowel habits

Renal, genitourinary: urine color, polyuria, oliguria, nocturia (number of times per night), dysuria, frequency, urgency, problem with stream, dribbling, pyuria, retention, passage of stones or gravel, venereal disease (discharge), infections, perineal rashes and irritations, protein or sugar in urine (now or in past)

Reproductive: male—lesions, impotence, prostate problems, use of contraceptives; *female*—irregular bleeding; discharge; pruritus; pain on intercourse; protrusions; dysmenorrhea; vaginal infections; number of pregnancies, delivery dates, complications, abortions; onset, regularity, and amount of flow during menarche; last normal period; use of contraceptives; date of menopause; last Papanicolaou test

Neurologic: headaches, seizures, fainting spells, dizziness, tremors, twitches, aphasia, loss of sensation, weakness, paralysis, numbness, tingling, balance problems

Psychiatric: changes in mood, anxiety, depression, inability to concentrate, phobias, suicidal or homicidal thoughts, hallucinations, delusions

Musculoskeletal: muscle pain; muscle strength; joint swelling, redness, or pain; back problems; injuries (such as broken bones, pulled tendons); gait problems; weakness; paralysis; deformities; limited motion; contractures, atrophy

Hematopoietic: anemia (type, degree, treatment, response), bleeding, fatigue, bruising, petechiae, ecchymoses, current anticoagulant therapy

Endocrine, metabolic: polyuria, polydipsia, polyphagia, thyroid problem, heat or cold intolerance, excessive sweating, changes in hair distribution and amount, nervousness, swollen neck (goiter), moon face, buffalo hump

Your patient's health history becomes part of the permanent written record, a subjective database with which you and other health care professionals can monitor the patient's progress. Remember that history data must be specific and precise. Avoid generalities; instead, gather pertinent, concise, detailed information that can help determine the direction and sequence of the physical examination—the next phase in your patient assessment.

PHYSICAL EXAMINATION

During the physical examination, you obtain objective data that usually confirm or rule out suspicions raised during the health history interview.

EXAMINATION TECHNIQUES

You use four basic techniques to perform a physical examination: inspection, palpation, percussion, and auscultation (IPPA). These skills require you to use your senses of sight, hearing, touch, and smell—all necessary for an accurate appraisal of the structures and functions of body systems. In addition, you may use specialized equipment, such as an ophthalmoscope or otoscope. Learning to use IPPA skills effectively will make you less likely to overlook something important during the physical examination. In addition, each of the four IPPA techniques collects data that validate and amplify data collected through the other IPPA techniques.

Accurate and complete physical assessments depend on two interrelated elements. One is the critical act of sensory perception, by which you receive and perceive external stimuli during the physical examination. The other element is the conceptual, or cognitive, process by which you relate these stimuli to your knowledge base. This two-step process gives meaning to your assessment data.

EXAMINATION METHODS

You need to develop a system for assessing patients that identifies their problem areas in priority order. By performing physical assessments systematically and efficiently instead of in a random or indiscriminate manner, you'll save time and identify priority problems quickly. The most commonly used methods are the head-to-toe and major-body-systems methods.

Using the head-to-toe method, you systematically assess your patient—as the name suggests—beginning at the head and working toward the toes. Examine all parts of one body region before progressing to the next region, and proceed from left to right within each region so that you can make symmetrical comparisons.

The major-body-systems method involves systematically assessing your patient by examining all body systems in priority order or in a predesignated sequence.

Both the head-to-toe and the major-body-systems methods are systematic and provide a logical, organized framework for collecting physical assessment data. They also provide the same information; therefore, neither is more correct than the other. So choose the method (or a variation of it) that works best for you and is appropriate for your patient population.

To decide which method to use, first determine whether the patient's condition is life-threatening. Identifying the priority problems of a patient suffering from a life-threatening illness or injury—for example, myocardial infarction, severe trauma, or GI hemorrhage—is essential to preserve his life and function and to prevent compounded damage.

Next, identify the patient population to which the patient belongs, and take the common characteristics of that population into account in choosing an examination method. For example, elderly or debilitated patients tire easily; for a patient in either category, you'd select a method that requires minimal position changes. Also, you'd probably defer parts of the examination to avoid tiring your patient.

Regardless of the examination method you use, try to view your patient as an integrated whole rather than as a collection of parts. Remember, the integrity of a body region may reflect adequate functioning of many body systems, both inside and outside this particular region. For example, the integrity of the chest region may provide important clues about the functioning of the cardiovascular and respiratory systems. Similarly, the integrity of a body system may reflect adequate functioning of many body regions and of the various systems within these regions. For example, the integrity of the GI system reflects the functioning of the head, chest, and abdominal regions.

The chief complaint. You may want to plan your physical examination around your patient's chief complaint or concern. To do this, begin by examining the body system or region that corresponds to the chief complaint. This allows you to identify priority problems promptly and reassures your patient that you're paying attention to his primary reason for seeking health care.

Consider the following example: Your 65-year-old patient is an active, well-nourished woman who appears younger than her chronological age. She complains of having difficulty breathing on exertion; she also has a dry, frequent, painful cough and intermittent chills that have persisted for 3 days. First, you'd record her vital signs: temperature, 103° F (39.4° C); pulse rate, 106 beats/minute; respiratory rate, 29 to 30 breaths/minute; blood pressure, 128/82 mm Hg.

Because your patient's chief complaints are difficulty breathing, a cough, and chills, your physical examination would initially focus on her respiratory system. You'd examine the patency of her airways, observe the color of her lips and extremities, and systematically palpate her lung fields for symmetry of expansion, crepitus, increased or decreased fremitus, and areas of tenderness. Then after auscultating her lung fields for abnormal or adventitious sounds (such as crackles, rhonchi, pleural friction rub, or wheezing), you'd percuss her lung fields for increased or decreased resonance.

Next, you'd examine the patient's cardiovascular system, looking for further clues to the cause of her signs and symptoms. You'd inspect her neck veins for distention and her extremities for edema, venous engorgement, and pigmented areas. Then you'd palpate her chest to see if you could feel the heart's apical impulse at the fifth intercostal space, in the midclavicular line. You'd also palpate for a precordial heave and for valvular thrills. After determining her apical pulse rate, you'd auscultate for any abnormal heart sounds.

At this point in the examination, you'd probably be aware of your patient's level of consciousness, motor ability, and ability to use her muscles and joints. You probably wouldn't need to perform a more thorough musculoskeletal or neurologic examination. You would, however, proceed with an examination of her GI, genitourinary, and integumentary systems, modifying the examination sequence depending on your findings and the patient's tolerance. If her signs and symptoms worsened during the examination, you'd interrupt the procedure to report her condition to her doctor. Then you'd plan to come back and finish the examination after her condition had stabilized.

Documentation tips

Keep these rules in mind as you document your initial assessment.

■ Always document your findings as soon as possible after you take the health history and perform the physical examination.
■ Always document your assessment away from the patient's bedside. Jot down only key points while you're with the patient.
■ Always answer every question on the assessment form if you're using one. If a question doesn't apply to your patient, write "N/A" or "not applicable" in the space.
■ Always focus your questions on areas that relate to the patient's chief complaint or reason for visit. Record information that has significance and will help you build a plan of care.
■ If you delegate the job of filling out the first section of the form to another nurse or an aide, remember that you must review the information gathered and validate it if you're not sure it's correct.
■ Always accept accountability for your assessment by signing your name to the areas you've completed.
■ Always directly quote the patient or family member who gave you the information if you fear that summarizing will make it lose some of its meaning.
■ Always write or print legibly in ink.
■ Always be concise, specific, and exact when you describe your physical findings.
■ Always go back to the patient's bedside to clarify or validate information that seems incomplete.

DOCUMENTATION

Remember that the assessment information you record will be used by others who are involved in caring for your patient. It could even be used as a legal document in a liability case, a malpractice suit, or an insurance disability claim. With these considerations in mind, record history data thoroughly, clearly, precisely, and in an organized fashion. (See *Documentation tips*.)

Some hospitals provide patient questionnaires or computerized checklists. (See *Using an assessment checklist*, page 14.) These forms make history taking easier, but they're not always available; you must know how to take a comprehensive health history without them. Although some examiners don't like to use a printed form and prefer to work with a blank paper, these forms simplify comprehensive data collection and documentation by providing a concise format for outlining and recording information. They

Using an assessment checklist

To make sure you cover all key points during your health history interview, you may use an assessment checklist such as the one shown below. Though the format of the guide may vary from one institution to another, all include the same key elements.

☑ *Reason for health care visit or chief complaint:* As patient sees it.

☑ *Duration of this problem:* As patient recalls it. Has it affected patient's lifestyle?

☑ *Other illnesses and previous experience with health care provider or hospitalization:* Reason? When? Results? Impressions of previous hospitalizations? Problems encountered? Effect of this illness or hospitalization on self? Family? Child care? Employment? Finances?

☑ *Observation of patient's condition:* Level of consciousness? Well nourished? Healthy? Color? Skin turgor? Senses? Headaches? Cough? Syncope? Nausea? Seizures? Edema? Lumps? Bruises or bleeding? Inflammation? Integrity of skin? Pressure areas? Temperature? Range of motion? Unusual sensations? Paralysis? Odors? Discharges? Pain?

☑ *Mental and emotional status:* Cooperative? Understanding? Anxious? Language? Expectations? Feelings about illness? State of consciousness? Mood? Self-image? Reaction to stress? Rapport with interviewer and staff? Compatibility with roommate?

☑ *Review of systems:* Neurologic; eye, ear, nose, and throat; respiratory; cardiovascular; GI; genitourinary; skin; reproductive; musculoskeletal; and so forth.

☑ *Allergies:* Food? Drugs? Type of reaction?

☑ *Medication:* Dosage? Why taken? When taken? Last dose? Does he have it with him? Any others taken occasionally? Recently? Why? Ask about over-the-counter drugs, cough preparations, and use of alcohol or illegal drugs.

☑ *Adaptive equipment or prostheses:* Pacemaker? Intermittent positive-pressure breathing unit? Tracheostomy tube? Drainage tubes? Feeding tube? Catheter? Ostomy appliance? Breast form? Hearing aid? Glasses or contacts? Dentures? Cane? Walker? Brace? False eye? Prosthetic leg? Does the patient have the device with him? Need anything?

☑ *Hygiene patterns:* Dentures? Gums? Teeth? Bath or shower? When?

☑ *Rest and sleep patterns:* Usual times? Aids? Difficulties?

☑ *Activity status:* Self-care? Ambulatory? Aids? Daily exercise?

☑ *Bladder and bowel patterns:* Continent? Frequency? Nocturia? Characteristics of stool and urine? Discharge? Pain? Ostomy? Appliances? Who cares for these? Laxatives? Medications?

☑ *Meals and diet:* Feeds self? Diet restrictions (therapeutic and cultural or preferential)? Frequency? Snacks? Allergies? Dislikes? Fad diets? Usual dietary intake?

☑ *Health practices:* Breast self-examination? Physical examination? Papanicolaou smear? Testicular self-examination? Digital rectal examination? Smoking? Electrocardiogram? Annual chest X-ray? Practices related to other conditions, such as glaucoma testing, urine testing, weight control?

☑ *Lifestyle:* Parent? Family? Number of children? Residence? Occupation? Recreation? Diversion? Interests? Financial status? Religion? Education? Ethnic background? Living environment?

☑ *Typical day profile:* Have patient describe.

☑ *Informant:* From whom did you obtain this information? Patient? Family? Old records? Ambulance driver?

---

also remind you to include all essential assessment data.

If taking notes for documentation seems to make your patient anxious, explain the importance of keeping an accurate written record. Inform him that your findings are crucial to arriving at a nursing diagnosis and, ultimately, to developing a sound nursing plan of care.

When documenting, describe exactly what you've inspected, palpated, percussed, or auscultated. Also document what you *don't* find—the absence of symptoms that other history data indicate could be present. For example, if a patient reports pain and burning in his abdomen, ask him if he has experienced nausea and vomiting or noticed blood in his stools. Record the presence *or* absence of these symptoms.

Don't use general terms, such as *normal, abnormal, good,* or *poor.* Instead, be specific. Don't be satisfied with inadequate answers, such as "a lot" or "a little." These words mean different things to different people and must be explained to be meaningful. Continue your questioning until you're satisfied that you've recorded sufficient detail.

To facilitate accurate and concise recording of your patient's answers, familiarize yourself with standard history data abbreviations.

Nursing diagnosis

According to the North American Nursing Diagnosis Association (NANDA), the nursing diagnosis is a "clinical judgment about individual, family, or community responses to actual or potential health problems/life processes." It's the basis for selecting nursing interventions to achieve outcomes for which the nurse is accountable, and it must be supported by clinical information obtained during patient assessment. (See *Nursing diagnosis and the nursing process.*) You perform this step so that you can develop your plan of care.

Each nursing diagnosis describes a patient problem that a nurse can legally manage. Though the identification of problems commonly overlaps in nursing and medicine, the approach to treatment clearly differs. Medicine focuses on curing disease; nursing focuses on holistic care that includes cure and comfort. Nurses can independently diagnose and treat the patient's response to illness, certain health problems, and the need for patient education. Nurses care for, comfort, and counsel patients and their families until they're physically and emotionally ready to provide self-care.

ANALYSIS OF DATA
The nursing diagnosis expresses your professional judgment of the patient's clinical status, response to treatment, and nursing care needs. In addition to identifying the patient's needs in coping with the effects of illness, you also consider what type of assistance he requires to grow and develop to the fullest extent possible.

Arriving at a nursing diagnosis involves organizing the patient's history, physical examination, and laboratory data into clusters and interpreting what the clusters reveal about your patient's ability to meet basic needs. Each nursing diagnosis and its cluster of signs and symptoms indicates an actual or potential (risk for) health problem that you can identify—and that your care can resolve.

Creating your nursing diagnosis is a logical extension of collecting assessment data. In your patient assessment, you asked each history question, performed each physical examination technique, and considered each laboratory test result because it provided evidence of how your patient could be helped by your care or because the data could affect nursing care.

PATIENT HEALTH PROBLEMS
To develop the nursing diagnosis, use the assessment data you've collected to develop a problem list. Less formal in structure than a fully developed nursing diagnosis, this list describes your patient's problems or

Nursing diagnosis and the nursing process

When first described, the nursing process included only assessment, planning, implementation, and evaluation. However, during the past 25 years, several important events have helped to establish diagnosis as a distinct part of the nursing process.

■ In 1973, the American Nurses' Association Standards of Nursing Practice mentioned nursing diagnosis as a separate and definable act performed by a registered nurse. The 1991 revised standards continue to list nursing diagnosis as a distinct step in the nursing process.
■ Individual states have passed nurse practice acts that list diagnosis as part of the nurse's legal responsibility.
■ In 1973, the North American Nursing Diagnosis Association (NANDA) began a formal effort to classify nursing diagnoses. NANDA continues to meet biennially to review proposed new nursing diagnoses and examine applications of nursing diagnoses in clinical practice, education, and research. Their most recent meeting was held in April 1996, in Pittsburgh. NANDA publishes *Nursing Diagnoses: Definitions and Classification*, the official list of nursing diagnoses, definitions, defining characteristics, and taxonomy.
■ In 1991, the Joint Commission on Accreditation of Healthcare Organizations (JCAHO) incorporated the concept of nursing diagnosis into its revised standards for nursing care. The JCAHO now requires that each patient's care be based on nursing diagnoses that have been made by a registered nurse.

needs. Generating such a list is easy if you use a conceptual model or an accepted set of criterion norms. Examples of such norms include normal physical and psychological development, Maslow's hierarchy of needs, and Gordon's functional health patterns.

You can identify the patient's problems and needs with such simple phrases as "poor circulation," "high fever," or "poor hydration." Next, prioritize the problems on the list and then develop the working nursing diagnosis.

NURSING DIAGNOSIS STATEMENTS
By remembering these basic guidelines, you can ensure that your diagnostic statement is correct:
■ Use proper terminology that reflects the patient's *nursing* needs.
■ Make your statement concise so that it's easily understood by other health team members.
■ Use the most precise words possible.
■ Use a problem-cause format, stating the problem and its related cause.

■ Whenever possible, use terminology recommended by NANDA.

NANDA diagnostic headings, when combined with suspected etiology, provide a clear picture of the patient's needs. Thus, for clarity in charting, start with one of the NANDA labels as a heading for the diagnostic statement. The label can reflect an actual problem or risk response, or it may be related to wellness. Consider this sample diagnosis:

Heading: Impaired physical mobility

Etiology: Related to pain and discomfort following surgery

Signs and symptoms: "I can't walk without help." Patient has not ambulated since surgery on (give date and time). Range of motion limited to 10 degrees flexion in the right hip. Patient can't walk 3' (1 m) from the bed to the chair without the help of two nurses.

This format links the patient's problem to the etiology without stating a direct cause-and-effect relationship (which may be hard to prove). Remember to state only the patient's problems and the probable origin. Omit references to possible solutions. (Your solutions will derive from your nursing diagnosis, but they aren't part of it.)

One major pitfall in developing a nursing diagnosis is writing one that nursing interventions can't treat. Errors can also occur when nurses take shortcuts in the nursing process, either by omitting or hurrying through assessment or by basing the diagnosis on inaccurate assessment data.

Keep in mind that a nursing diagnosis is a statement of a health problem that a nurse is licensed to treat—a problem for which you'll assume responsibility for therapeutic decisions and accountability for the outcomes. A nursing diagnosis is *not:*

■ a diagnostic test ("schedule for cardiac angiography")

■ a piece of equipment ("set up intermittent suction apparatus")

■ a problem with equipment ("the patient has trouble using a commode")

■ a nurse's problem with a patient ("Mr. Jones is a difficult patient; he's rude and won't take his medication")

■ a nursing goal ("encourage fluids up to 2 qt [2 L] per day")

■ a nursing need ("I have to get through to the family that they must accept their father's dying")

■ a medical diagnosis ("cervical cancer") or treatment ("catheterize after each voiding for residual urine").

The following tips and examples should make the distinctions clear:

■ Don't state a need instead of a problem.

Incorrect: Fluid replacement related to fever

Correct: Fluid volume deficit related to fever

■ Don't reverse the two parts of the statement.

Incorrect: Lack of understanding related to noncompliance with diabetic diet

Correct: Noncompliance with diabetic diet related to lack of understanding

■ Don't identify an untreatable condition instead of the actual problem it indicates (which can be treated).

Incorrect: Inability to speak related to laryngectomy

Correct: Social isolation related to inability to speak because of laryngectomy

■ Don't write a legally inadvisable statement.

Incorrect: Red sacrum related to improper positioning

Correct: Impaired skin integrity related to immobility

■ Don't identify as unhealthful a response that would be appropriate or culturally acceptable.

Incorrect: Anger related to terminal illness

Correct: Ineffective management of therapeutic regimen related to anger over terminal illness

■ Don't make a tautological statement (one in which both parts of the statement say the same thing).

Incorrect: Pain related to alteration in comfort

Correct: Pain related to postoperative abdominal distention and anxiety

■ Don't identify a nursing problem instead of a patient problem.

Incorrect: Difficulty suctioning related to thick secretions

Correct: Ineffective airway clearance related to thick tracheal secretions.

Outcome identification and planning

The nursing plan of care is a written plan of action designed to help you deliver quality patient care. It usually forms a permanent part of the patient's health record and is used by other members of the nursing team.

Planning involves the following stages:

■ assigning priorities to the nursing diagnoses

■ identifying expected outcomes (goals)

■ selecting appropriate nursing actions (interventions) to accomplish identified expected outcomes

■ documenting the nursing diagnoses, expected outcomes, nursing interventions, and evaluations on the plan of care.

PRIORITY SETTING

Any time you develop more than one nursing diagnosis for your patient, you must assign priorities to them and begin your plan of care with those that have the highest priority. High-priority nursing diagnoses involve the patient's most urgent needs (such as emergency or immediate physical needs). Intermediate-priority diagnoses involve nonemergency needs, and low-priority diagnoses involve needs that don't directly relate to the patient's specific illness or prognosis.

Just as you prioritize your nursing diagnoses, you must set priorities for collaborative problems. For example, if your patient needs whirlpool treatments by the physical therapy department and nebulizer treatment from a respiratory therapist, you are responsible for coordinating these activities. Respiratory therapy should always have a higher priority than physical therapy. With careful planning and attention to the patient's response to treatments, all members of the health care team should be able to carry out their respective actions for the patient's benefit.

OUTCOME IDENTIFICATION

Expected outcomes are measurable, patient-focused goals that are derived from the patient's nursing diagnoses. These goals may be short- or long-term. Short-term goals include those of immediate concern that can be achieved quickly. Long-term goals take more time to achieve and usually involve prevention, patient teaching, and rehabilitation.

In many cases, you can identify expected outcomes by converting the nursing diagnosis into a positive statement. For instance, for the nursing diagnosis "impaired physical mobility related to a fracture of the right hip," the expected outcome might be, "The patient will ambulate independently before discharge."

When writing the plan of care, state expected outcomes in terms of the patient's behavior—for example, "The patient will correctly demonstrate turning, coughing, and deep breathing." The expected outcomes will serve as the basis for evaluating the effectiveness of your nursing interventions.

Keep in mind that each expected outcome must be stated in measurable terms. If possible, consult with the patient and family when establishing expected outcomes. As the patient progresses, expected outcomes should be increasingly directed toward planning for discharge and follow-up care.

When developing expected outcomes in your plan of care, always start with a specific action verb that focuses on the patient's behavior. By describing how your patient should look, walk, eat, drink, turn, cough, speak, or stand, for example, you give a clear picture by which to evaluate his progress. Avoid starting expected outcome statements with *allow, let, enable,* or similar verbs. Such words focus attention on your own and other health team members' behavior instead of on the patient's.

You should also identify a target time or date by which each expected outcome should be accomplished. Make sure that target dates are realistic. Be flexible enough to adjust the date if your patient needs more time to respond to your interventions.

CLINICAL PATHS

A clinical path is a predetermined outline of patient care for a specific episode of care. Health-team members collaborate in determining the activities, diagnostic tests, target dates for consultations, and other related actions that need to be accomplished during hospitalization for a particular problem. For example, a clinical path for a patient who is admitted with a fracture of the femur would include diagnostic tests, operative or nonoperative plan, dates for consultation with physical therapy, and a day-by-day summary of who needs to see the patient and what goals need to be met along the way.

Outcomes for collaborative problems should be stated on the clinical path you're using for your patient. Each clinical path should state the key events that need to occur at a particular time. For example, on a clinical path for care of a patient having total knee replacement surgery, you may find the following expected outcomes for day 1: *The patient will have normal temperature and dry and intact dressings, will void within 12 hours of surgery, and will ambulate to chair using crutches.*

Because clinical paths are interdisciplinary in nature, they usually minimize system problems (such as not having a timely response to a consultation) and provide the patient with the benefit of coordinated care. One of the disadvantages is that combining nursing activities with all the rest may not allow proper credit for those patient outcomes for which nursing was responsible.

NURSING INTERVENTION SELECTION

You must develop one or more nursing interventions for each of the expected outcomes identified for your patient. For example, if one expected outcome reads, "The patient will transfer to chair with assistance," the appropriate nursing interventions include placing the wheelchair facing the foot of the bed and assisting the patient to stand and pivot into the chair. If another expected outcome statement reads, "The patient will express feelings related to recent injury," appropriate interventions might include spending time with the patient each shift, conveying an open and nonjudgmental attitude, and asking open-ended questions.

Reviewing the second part of the nursing diagnosis statement (the part describing etiologic factors) may help guide your choice of nursing interventions. For example, for the nursing diagnosis "risk for injury, related to inadequate blood glucose levels," you'd determine the best nursing interventions for maintaining an adequate blood glucose level—typically, observing the patient for evidence of hypoglycemia and providing an appropriate diet.

Try to think creatively during this step in the nursing process. This is an opportunity to describe exactly what you and your patient would like to have happen and to establish the criteria against which you'll judge further nursing actions.

Nursing interventions for collaborative problems include patient care. For example, you might note an unusual amount of drainage from a surgical site. Your role as a nurse would include gathering all relevant assessment data (vital signs, characteristics of the drainage, and so on), implementing emergency measures such as applying a pressure dressing, and notifying the doctor. After notifying the doctor, you'd complete any orders written by him, such as changing dressings, administering medication, and providing fluid and blood replacement. Your knowledge base of normal physiology and pathophysiology provides you with a framework to identify when you need to call on other members of the health care team to manage a patient problem.

The planning phase culminates when you write the plan of care and document the nursing diagnoses, expected outcomes, nursing interventions, and evaluations for expected outcomes. Write your plan in concise, specific terms so that other health team members can follow it. Keep in mind that because the patient's problems and needs will change, you'll have to review your plan of care frequently and modify it when necessary.

BENEFITS OF WRITING A PLAN OF CARE

To provide quality care for each patient, you must plan and direct that care. Writing a plan of care lets you document the scientific method you've used throughout the nursing process. On the plan of care, you summarize the patient's problems and needs (as nursing diagnoses) and identify appropriate nursing interventions and expected outcomes. A plan of care that's well conceived and properly written helps decrease the risk of incomplete or incorrect care by:

- giving direction
- providing continuity of care
- establishing communication between you and nurses on other shifts, you and health care team members in other departments, and you and your patient
- serving as a key for patient care assignments.

Giving direction. A written plan of care gives direction by showing colleagues the goals you've set for your patient and giving clear instructions for helping to achieve them. It also makes clear exactly what to document on the patient's progress notes. For instance, it lists what observations to make and how often, what nursing measures to take and how to implement them, and what to teach the patient and family before discharge.

Providing continuity. A written plan of care identifies the patient's needs to each hospital shift and tells what must be done to meet those needs, eliminating the confusion that can exist between shifts. And if your patient is discharged from the hospital to another health care facility, your plan of care can help ease this transition.

Establishing communication. By soliciting your patient's input as you develop the plan of care, you build a rapport that lets the patient know you value his opinions and feelings. And by reviewing the plan of care with other health-team members and with other nurses during change-of-shift reports, you can regularly evaluate your patient's response or lack of response to the nursing care and medical regimen.

Guiding patient care assignments. If you're a team leader, a clear plan of care can help you identify and delegate specific routines or duties described in each nursing intervention—not all of them need your professional attention.

DOCUMENTATION

Care-planning formats vary from one facility to another. For example, you may write your plan of care on a Kardex or another type of form. Your facility may require you to write a traditional plan of care from scratch, or you may be allowed to customize a standardized plan of care to meet the needs of each patient. Some facilities are adopting newer documentation tools, such as protocols, which give specific sequential instructions for treating patients with particular problems. However, nearly all care-planning formats include space in which to document the nursing diagnoses, expected outcomes, and nursing interventions. In many facilities, you may also document assessment data and discharge planning on the plan of care.

No matter which format you use, be sure to write the plan of care in ink (and sign it), even though you may have to make revisions if your nursing interventions don't work. Remember—your patient's plan of care becomes part of the permanent record and shouldn't be erased or destroyed. If you write it in pencil—so you can erase to revise—you make it seem unimportant. The information must remain intact, enabling you and other health-team members to readily refer to nursing interventions used in the past. (See *Guidelines for writing the plan of care.*)

Be specific when writing your plan of care. By listing specific problems, specific expected outcomes, specific nursing interventions, and specific evaluations for expected outcomes, you leave no doubt as to what needs to be done by other health-team members. When listing nursing interventions, for instance, be sure to include when the action should be implemented, who should be involved in each aspect of

Guidelines for writing the plan of care

Keeping these tips in mind will help you write a plan of care that's both accurate and useful.

- Your patient's plan of care is a part of the permanent record. Write it in ink and sign your name.
- Be specific; don't use vague terms or generalities.
- Be alert for abbreviations that have more than one meaning; don't use them.
- Take time to review all your assessment data *before* you select an approach for each problem. (*Note:* If you can't complete the initial assessment, immediately note "insufficient data base" on your records.)
- Write down a specific expected outcome for each problem you identify, and record a target date for its completion.
- Avoid setting an initial goal that's too ambitious to be achieved. For example, for a newly admitted patient with cerebrovascular accident, the outcome "Patient will ambulate with assistance" would not be appropriate as an initial goal; several patient outcomes would need to be achieved before this goal could be addressed.

- Consider the following three phases of patient care when writing nursing interventions: what observations to make and how often; what nursing measures to do and how to do them; and what to teach the patient and family before discharge.
- Make each nursing intervention specific.
- Make sure nursing interventions match staff capabilities and resources. Combine what's necessary to correct or modify the problem with what's reasonably possible in your setting.
- Be creative when you write your patient's plan of care; include a drawing or an innovative procedure if either will make your directions clearer or more specific.
- Don't overlook any of the patient's problems or concerns. Include them on the plan of care so that they won't be forgotten.
- Make sure your plan of care is implemented correctly.
- Evaluate the results of your plan of care, and discontinue any nursing diagnoses that have been resolved. Select new approaches, if necessary, for problems that have not been resolved.

implementation, and the frequency, quantity, and method to be used. Specify dates and times, when appropriate. List target dates for each expected outcome.

You'll need to update and modify your plan of care as problems (or priorities) change or resolve, as new assessment information becomes available, and as you evaluate the patient's responses to nursing interventions.

If your nursing interventions have resolved the problem on which you've based the nursing diagnosis, write "discontinued" next to the diagnostic statement on the plan of care, and list the date on which you discontinued the interventions. If your nursing interventions haven't resolved the problem by the target date, reevaluate your plan and do one of the following:

- Extend the target date and continue the intervention until the patient responds as expected.
- Discontinue the intervention and select a new one that will achieve the expected outcome.

Implementation

During this phase, you put your plan of care into action. Implementation encompasses all nursing interventions aimed at solving the patient's nursing prob-

lems and meeting health care needs. Be sure to incorporate these elements into the implementation stage:

- *Reassessment.* Although it may be brief or narrowly focused, reassessment should confirm that the planned interventions remain appropriate.
- *Reviewing and modifying the plan of care.* Never static, an appropriate plan of care changes with the patient's condition. As necessary, update the plan of care's assessment, nursing diagnoses, implementation, and evaluation sections. Date the revisions.
- *Seeking assistance.* Determine whether you need help from other staff members or additional information before you can intervene. While you coordinate implementation, you also seek help from other caregivers, the patient, and the patient's family.

NURSING INTERVENTIONS

Implementation involves some or all of the following actions:

- assessing and monitoring (for example, recording vital signs)
- therapeutic interventions (for example, giving medications)
- supporting his respiratory and elimination functions
- providing food and fluids
- providing skin care
- making the patient more comfortable and helping him with ADLs

- managing the environment (for example, controlling noise to ensure a good night's sleep)
- teaching, counseling, and giving emotional support
- referring the patient to appropriate agencies or services.

These nursing actions can be classified as one of three types: independent, dependent, or interdependent. Independent nursing actions fall within the realm of nursing practice and don't require a doctor's direction or supervision. Most nursing actions required by the patient's plan of care are independent interventions.

Dependent nursing actions are based on written or oral instruction from another professional, such as a doctor or nurse-practitioner. Dependent actions include administering medication, inserting indwelling urinary catheters, and obtaining specimens for laboratory tests.

Interdependent actions are performed in collaboration with other professionals. These include such actions as following a protocol and carrying out standing orders.

CLINICAL PRACTICE GUIDELINES

The Agency for Health Care Policy and Research (AHCPR) is a federal agency charged with enhancing "the quality, appropriateness, and effectiveness of health care services and access to those services." Agency members formulate clinical practice guidelines after a panel of experts reviews research literature and conducts consensus-building conferences on selected health topics. These guidelines are intended to assist practitioners in providing competent, standardized care for specific clinical conditions. Among the guidelines developed by the AHCPR are those for performing cataract surgery, preventing and treating pressure ulcers, and treating urinary incontinence, benign prostatic hyperplasia, depression, acute pain, chronic pain, and otitis media.

Different formats are available to meet the needs of practitioners and consumers. The AHCPR's *Clinical Practice Guidelines* presents recommendations with brief supporting information, tables and figures, and pertinent references. The *Quick Reference Guide for Clinicians,* a distilled version of the guidelines, contains summary points for quick reference. A consumer version of *Clinical Practice Guidelines* is available in English and Spanish to help the public become informed consumers capable of making decisions about their health care.

COLLABORATIVE MANAGEMENT

In today's health care environment, collaboration among members of the interdisciplinary health care team—through communication, consultation, and referral—is essential to achieve patient outcomes that require the expertise of others. Collaborative problems are the health care needs listed on an interdisciplinary patient progress note, clinical path, or other record that combines more than one discipline's actions.

These integrated records provide a means of communication for multiple providers and can serve to show the "whole" picture of services provided and patient responses. For example, the doctor may focus on a surgical procedure, use of a particular drug, or application of a cast to treat a patient's problem. The physical therapist may focus on an exercise regimen, application of moist heat, or whirlpool therapy for the same patient. The social worker may investigate the patient's resources and support systems and assist with obtaining outpatient services. The nurse may assist the patient in maintaining independence in self-care activities, educate him about drug adverse effects, and monitor the condition of the cast.

DOCUMENTATION

All of the collaborative actions performed and the responses to them need to be recorded on the patient record. Implementation isn't complete until you've documented each intervention, the time it occurred, the patient's response, and all other pertinent information. Make sure each entry relates to a nursing diagnosis. Remember that only documented actions are considered during evaluation of care or quality assurance monitoring. Thorough documentation also offers you a way to take rightful credit for your contribution in helping a patient achieve the highest possible level of wellness.

Forms used for documentation vary among facilities. They may include progress notes, flow charts, and plans of care. They may also include clinical paths, which are written by interdisciplinary health care team members to present the expected combined outcomes and key events that occur for a specific procedure, operation, or medical diagnosis. In this system, the case manager is usually a registered nurse who assumes responsibility for ensuring that the patient achieves outcomes at predesignated times; she also coordinates treatments, patient teaching, ordering of equipment and supplies, consultations, and discharge planning. Regardless of the type of form used, the information must be complete and accurate.

Evaluation

In this phase of the nursing process, you assess the effectiveness of your plan of care by answering such questions as the following:

- How has the patient progressed in terms of the plan of care's projected outcomes?
- Does the patient have new needs?
- Does the plan of care need revision?

Evaluation also helps you determine whether the patient received high-quality care from the nursing staff. Your health care facility, in turn, bases its nursing quality assurance system on nursing evaluations.

STEPS IN THE EVALUATION PROCESS

Include the patient, family members, and other health care professionals in the evaluation. Then follow these steps:

- *Select evaluation criteria.* The plan of care's projected outcomes—the desired effects of nursing interventions—form the basis for evaluation.
- *Compare the patient's response to the evaluation criteria.* Did the patient respond as expected? If not, the plan of care may need revision.
- *Analyze your findings.* If your plan wasn't effective, determine why. You may conclude, for example, that a nursing diagnosis wasn't precise enough to direct care.
- *Modify the plan of care.* Make revisions (for example, reword the nursing diagnosis) and implement the new plan of care.
- *Reevaluate.* Like all steps in the nursing process, evaluation is ongoing. Continue to assess, plan, implement, and evaluate for as long as you care for the patient.

When evaluating your patient's care, collect information from all available sources—for example, the patient's medical record, family members, other caregivers, and the patient. Also include your own observations.

During the evaluation process, ask yourself these questions:

- Has the patient's condition improved, deteriorated, or stayed the same?
- Were the nursing diagnoses accurate?
- Have the patient's nursing needs been met?
- Did the patient meet the plan of care's outcome criteria?
- Which nursing interventions should I revise or discontinue?
- Why did the patient fail to meet some goals (if applicable)?
- Should I reorder priorities? Revise goals and outcome criteria?

DOCUMENTATION

After you've provided the care outlined in your plan, you must record your evaluation of the patient's response. Among the items you'll document are physical findings and results of treatments, referrals made, the patient's expression of relief or lack of relief of symptoms, your observations of the family's interactions with the patient, and a summary of goal achievement. For example, if your patient has a feeding self-care deficit with outcomes to maintain weight at 130 lb (50 kg), to exhibit no evidence of aspiration, to consume meals when fed, and to demonstrate correct use of assistive feeding devices, you'd need to document the following evaluation: patient's weight, food intake, use of assistive devices, and breath sounds. You could then make a summary statement, for example: "Feeding self-care deficit exists; continue plan outlined; reevaluate status in 1 week."

Evaluation of patient responses can lead to three main outcomes:

- The patient's problem is resolved and no further nursing intervention is needed.
- The patient is making progress but hasn't achieved all of the goals.
- The patient's condition has changed, creating a need for reassessment and planning to meet the current situation.

If the patient's problem is resolved, you can discontinue the interventions listed on the plan (noting "discontinued"). If the patient is making progress, you'll indicate the need to continue the plan. If the patient's condition changes, your revised plan will be based on assessment data and will reflect new interventions and goals to resolve the problem.

A final evaluation of patient status is written in the discharge summary. This summary must be comprehensive, addressing each patient problem and its current status. The discharge summary should provide the basis for providing follow-up care.

CONTINUOUS QUALITY IMPROVEMENT

Sometimes called *quality assurance* or *total quality management*, continuous quality improvement is a standardized system that sets standards and provides a way for a health care facility to measure the care provided. It's a way of assessing quality and taking measures to improve clinical practice if standards aren't met.

Nursing units develop standards of care that are evaluated through audits or monitors at regular intervals. Data are collected through use of an audit tool designed to evaluate structure, process, or outcome. Today, the focus is on outcomes of care. However, an evaluation of structure (resources, equipment, supplies) or process (procedure and policies) may reveal correctable problems. The outcome audit evaluates the patient's response to care provided. This information is used in analyzing whether or not standards have been met. If not, a corrective action plan is carried out and a repeat audit is done at a specified time.

Selected references

Bergstrom, N., et al. *Treatment of Pressure Ulcers.* Clinical Practice Guideline No. 15 (AHCPR Publication No. 95-0652). Rockville, Md.: U.S. Department of Health and Human Services, Public Health Service, Agency for Health Care Policy and Research, 1994.

McCloskey, J.C., and Bulechek, G.M. *Nursing Interventions Classification,* 2nd ed. St. Louis: Mosby–Year Book, 1996.

Nursing Diagnoses: Definitions and Classification 1997-1998. Philadelphia: North American Nursing Diagnosis Association, 1996.

Paul, R.W. *Critical Thinking: How to Prepare Students for a Rapidly Changing World.* Santa Rosa, Calif.: Foundation for Critical Thinking, 1993.

Rubenfeld, M.G., and Sheffer, B.K. *Critical Thinking in Nursing: An Interactive Approach.* Philadelphia: Lippincott-Raven Pubs., 1995.

Sparks, S.M., and Taylor, C.M. *Nursing Diagnosis Reference Manual,* 4th ed. Springhouse, Pa.: Springhouse Corp., 1998.

Standards of Clinical Nursing Practice. Washington, D.C.: American Nurses Association, 1991.

Part II

Medical-Surgical Disorders

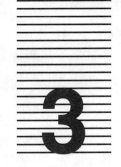

Perioperative care

Despite technological advances that have made operations quicker, safer, and more effective, surgery remains one of the most stressful experiences a patient can undergo. Before the patient enters the operating room, you'll need to fully address his psychological as well as physiologic needs. A surgical patient who's prepared through careful teaching will experience less pain and fewer postoperative complications and have a shorter hospitalization.

Overview of surgery

Surgery refers to an invasive medical procedure performed to diagnose or treat an illness, injury, or deformity. Although a doctor performs this medical treatment, the nurse plays a crucial role in caring for the patient and family before, during, and after surgery. Collaboration with all members of the health care team helps prevent complications and promote optimal patient recovery.

CATEGORIES OF SURGERY
Surgical procedures can be categorized by their purpose, degree of risk or extent, and urgency. (See *Classification of surgeries*.)

SURGICAL SETTINGS
Any procedure classified as surgery takes place in the operating room. The procedure may be done on either an inpatient or an outpatient basis.

INPATIENT SURGERY
With inpatient surgery, the patient is admitted to the hospital 1 or more days before the scheduled procedure or, more commonly in recent years, the patient is admitted early on the morning of surgery. Follow-

ing the procedure, the patient usually remains in the hospital for 1 or more additional days. The average length of stay after major surgery, although shortened in recent years, usually ranges from 4 to 6 days.

OUTPATIENT SURGERY
Thanks to significant advances in surgical techniques and anesthesia, many surgical procedures that once required a hospital stay can now take place on an outpatient basis in an ambulatory center. These centers may be part of a hospital or located in an independent care facility. The surgical procedures performed are usually elective procedures of short duration (15 to 90 minutes) that produce minimal postoperative nausea, vomiting, and pain and present minimal risk for postoperative complications.

Patients undergoing outpatient surgery are carefully screened to ensure that they're in general good health. Any existing chronic medical conditions must be well controlled and pose little risk for postoperative complications. Patients must be capable of understanding and following preoperative and postoperative instructions.

Any preoperative assessments, teaching, and diagnostic testing are completed before the day of surgery. Depending on the type of surgery, patients may need another person present to help them get home and to assist with self-care measures in the immediate postoperative period.

PHASES OF SURGERY
Surgery can be divided into three separate phases: preoperative, intraoperative, and postoperative. In larger institutions, different nurses may provide care during each of these phases. In smaller institutions, one nurse may provide care through all three phases. (See *Phases of surgery*, page 26.)

24 ◆◆◆

Classification of surgeries

	Classification	Function	Examples
PURPOSE	Diagnostic	Reach or confirm a diagnosis	Lymph node biopsy, colonoscopy
	Ablative	Remove diseased tissue, organ, or limb	Amputation, cholecystectomy
	Constructive	Build congenitally absent tissue or organ	Cleft palate repair
	Reconstructive	Rebuild damaged tissue or organ	Postmastectomy breast reconstruction, total hip replacement
	Palliative	Relieve disease symptoms (noncurative)	Bowel resection in patient with terminal cancer
	Transplant	Replace tissue or organ to restore function	Bone marrow or liver transplant
RISK FACTOR	Minor	Minimal physical trauma with minimal risk	Incision and drainage of cyst, myringotomy
	Major	Extensive physical trauma or serious risk	Total abdominal hysterectomy, colon resection, pneumonectomy
URGENCY	Elective	Suggested; delay won't harm patient	Bunionectomy, cataract extraction, cosmetic surgery
	Urgent	Needed within 1 to 2 days	Fractured hip, heart bypass, complete arterial occlusion
	Emergency	Needed immediately	Bowel obstruction, life-threatening trauma, severe postpartal hemorrhage, ruptured aneurysm

Preoperative collaborative care

The patient undergoing surgery receives care from many different members of the health care team. The goal is to place the patient in the best possible health status before, during, and after the surgery.

PATIENT EVALUATION

A thorough preoperative assessment helps to systematically identify risk factors, identify and correct problems before surgery, and establish a baseline for intraoperative and postoperative comparisons. When you're performing this assessment, focus on problem areas suggested by the patient's history and on any body system that will be directly affected by surgery.

HISTORY

A complete nursing history should include the following points:
- chief complaint or reason for the surgery, in the patient's own words
- existing and past medical problems, injuries, and surgeries
- allergies to foods and drugs, including reactions
- current medications, including when the patient last took them
- smoking history
- mobility impairment
- communication limitations
- psychosocial aspects, such as the patient's perception of the surgery and availability of support systems.

PHYSICAL EXAMINATION

A thorough physical examination is essential to a successful surgical outcome. You'll perform a complete review of systems, with special emphasis on the body area planned for surgery and the cardiac, respiratory, GI, genitourinary (GU), and nervous systems.

Assessing the cardiovascular system. Begin by inspecting the chest for any abnormal pulsations. Then auscultate at the fifth intercostal space over the left midclavicular line. If you can't hear an apical pulse, ask the patient to turn onto his left side; the heart

Phases of surgery

Phase	Description	Typical activities
PREOPERATIVE	Begins with the decision for surgery and ends when the patient is transferred to the operating room; aims to prepare patient for surgery	Preoperative patient teaching, skin preparation, medication administration
INTRAOPERATIVE	Begins when the patient is placed on the operating room bed and ends when he is transferred to the postanesthesia care unit (PACU); aims to protect the patient during surgery	Surgical asepsis, minimizing traffic flow, maintaining patient safety
POSTOPERATIVE	Begins when the patient is admitted to the PACU and ends when surgery-related nursing care is no longer required; aims to alleviate the patient's pain and nausea and support the patient until normal physiologic responses return	Monitoring fluid intake and output, assessing cardiac and respiratory function, meeting nutritional and activity needs, providing guidance and return to functional level

may shift closer to the chest wall. Note the rate and quality of the apical pulse.

Next, auscultate for heart sounds. If you hear murmurs, suspect valvular insufficiency or stenosis. Remember that murmurs you hear on the right side of the heart are more likely to change with respiration than left-sided murmurs.

Palpate for radial and pedal pulses bilaterally, and note any differences in quality, rate, or rhythm. Check for extremity coolness or edema. Compare blood pressure bilaterally, using a cuff with a bladder whose width is 40% of the circumference of the extremity to be used and whose length is 80% of the circumference. A difference greater than 15 mm Hg in systolic or diastolic pressure may indicate unilateral arterial compression or obstruction. Remember that preoperative anxiety may spuriously elevate systolic pressure.

Assessing the chest and lungs. First, inspect the patient's chest for scars suggesting previous surgery. Next, assess his respiratory rate and pattern. A patient with questionable pulmonary status may require an alternative to inhalation anesthesia such as a spinal block.

Check for asymmetrical chest expansion and use of accessory muscles. Auscultate the lungs for diminished breath sounds and crackles or rhonchi. Differentiate crackles from rhonchi by asking the patient to cough; crackles will not clear with coughing.

Now check for circumoral and nail-bed pallor, which may indicate recent hypoxia. Clubbing of the fingers, a barrel chest, and cyanotic earlobes indicate chronic hypoxia and hypercapnia, common symptoms in patients with chronic obstructive pulmonary disease (COPD). Be sure to chart any shortness of breath or cough (noting with or without sputum).

Ask the patient whether he smokes. If he does, ask how many packs per day and whether he's recently quit or cut down in anticipation of surgery. His doctor should have advised him to stop 4 to 6 weeks before surgery. If the patient still smokes, urge him to stop immediately.

Assessing the GI system. Inspect abdominal contour and symmetry, and auscultate for bowel sounds in each quadrant. (To avoid stimulating peristalsis, always auscultate before palpating.) Then palpate the abdomen for any tenderness or distention, and percuss for air and fluid.

Chart fluid intake. Also, assess the patency and function of any ostomy, the adequacy of the appliance, and the condition of the peristomal skin.

Assessing the GU system. First, palpate above the symphysis pubis for any bladder distention. Then obtain a urine sample for urinalysis and, if you notice a foul odor, for cultures. If indicated, monitor urine output and try to correlate any excess or deficit with blood urea nitrogen or creatinine levels. If urine output falls, first assess catheter patency and urinary drainage system patency, if applicable. Compare intake and output over the last several days as well as daily body weights. Also check for pedal edema; its presence along with bibasilar crackles may signal impending congestive heart failure.

Assessing neurologic function. Begin by evaluating the patient's orientation to person, place, and time. However, recognize that anxiety may make him slightly disoriented. Note whether his pupils are uniform in size and shape.

Assess the patient's gross motor function (for example, how he walks) and fine motor function (how he writes). Look for any neurologic changes such as slurred speech. Inform the doctor of any behavioral changes, from lethargy to agitation, which may herald increased intracranial pressure.

DIAGNOSTIC TESTING

Laboratory and diagnostic tests are performed prior to surgery to provide baseline data and to detect problems that may place the patient at additional risk after surgery. Because of the trend toward shorter hospital stays, many diagnostic tests for elective surgery may be performed within a week of the surgery in an outpatient setting such as a preadmission clinic.

Tests usually include a complete blood count, electrolyte and coagulation studies, and urinalysis. In addition, a chest X-ray is typically performed to provide baseline information about the heart and lungs. An electrocardiogram (ECG) is routine for patients who are receiving general anesthesia, are over age 40, or have cardiovascular disease. The ECG evaluates the patient's cardiac status and any new or preexisting cardiac conditions.

Other laboratory tests, such as pulmonary function tests, blood typing and crossmatching, and blood chemistry studies, may be performed as the history and physical examination findings indicate.

PHYSIOLOGIC PREPARATION

To ready the patient for surgery, a member of the anesthesia team evaluates the patient to determine the best choice of anesthetic. In addition, you may have to perform skin and bowel preparation and administer drugs.

ANESTHESIA EVALUATION

Preoperatively, a member of the anesthesia team sees every patient who's scheduled for anesthesia. Preferably, this is the person who'll administer the anesthetic, unless this proves impractical (for example, in an emergency). Properly conducted, the preanesthesia visit enables the examiner to establish rapport and provide emotional support while assessing the patient's emotional and physical status. It also helps calm the patient, an important function because anxiety can stimulate catecholamine production, leading to hypertension and arrhythmias.

The preanesthesia evaluation includes discussion of alternative anesthetic techniques when feasible, a review of the risks and benefits of these techniques, instruction on the importance of compliance with presurgery restrictions on food and fluids, and verification that the patient understands the anesthesia plans. Patients with specific religious practices or beliefs, such as Jehovah's Witnesses, receive counseling about options if they refuse blood transfusions.

The American Society of Anesthesiologists (ASA) has developed a numerical system of classifying a patient's preoperative physical status. The higher the assigned number, the higher the patient's risk under anesthesia. An "E" beside the status designation denotes emergency surgery. Knowledge of the ASA classification helps nurses anticipate and prepare for perioperative complications that may arise. (See *Physical status classification for anesthesia*, page 28.)

SKIN PREPARATION

Rendering the skin as free as possible from microorganisms reduces the risk of infection at the incision site. The procedure for preoperative skin preparation is determined by hospital policy, surgeon preference, surgical site and type, and the time element. Skin preparation can involve a bath, shower, or local skin scrub with an antiseptic detergent solution. However, it doesn't duplicate or replace the full sterile preparation that immediately precedes surgery.

When doing preoperative skin preparation, always prepare an area much larger than the expected incision site to minimize the number of microorganisms in adjacent areas and to allow surgical draping of the patient without contamination. When preparing a large area, wash body hair in small sections, beginning with the expected incision site. This keeps your work area moist and avoids chilling the patient. After you've finished all sections, rinse and dry the entire preparation area.

Remove hair only if it interferes with the surgery. It should be removed as close to the time of surgery as possible and in an area outside the room where surgery will be performed. Sterilize or dispose of all articles used for hair removal. Shaving is the least desirable method of hair removal. If you use a depilatory cream, perform a skin patch test first to determine sensitivity. Any locks of hair that you remove are regarded as personal property and should be returned to the patient.

Avoid shaving facial or neck hair on women and children unless ordered. Never shave eyebrows because this disrupts normal hair growth and the new growth may prove unsightly. Scalp shaving usually takes place in the operating room, but if you're required to prepare the patient's scalp, retain all hair in a plastic or paper bag with the patient's possessions.

Removing hair with a depilatory cream produces clean, intact skin without risking cuts or abrasions, but it can cause skin irritation or rash, especially in the groin. If possible, cut long hairs with scissors before applying the cream because removal of remaining hair requires less cream. Then, use a glove to ap-

Physical status classification for anesthesia

The following chart from the American Society of Anesthesiologists' *Relative Value Guide* (1990) gives physical status descriptions for patients undergoing anesthesia.

Status	Description
P1	Normal, healthy patient
P2	Patient with mild systemic disease, such as heart disease that only slightly limits physical activity, essential hypertension, diabetes mellitus, anemia, extremes of age, morbid obesity, or chronic bronchitis
P3	Patient with severe systemic disease, such as heart disease or chronic obstructive pulmonary disease, that limits activity; poorly controlled essential hypertension; diabetes mellitus with vascular complications; angina pectoris; or history of myocardial infarction
P4	Patient with severe systemic disease that's a constant threat to life, such as congestive heart failure, persistent angina pectoris, or advanced pulmonary, renal, or hepatic dysfunction
P5	Moribund patient who isn't expected to survive without the operation, such as one with uncontrolled hemorrhage from a ruptured abdominal aneurysm, cerebral trauma, or pulmonary embolus
P6	Patient declared brain-dead whose organs are being removed for donation

ply the cream; after about 10 minutes, remove the cream with moist gauze sponges. Next, wash the area with antiseptic soap solution, rinse, and pat dry.

BOWEL PREPARATION

The extent of preparation depends on the type and site of surgery. For example, a patient scheduled for several days of postoperative bed rest who hasn't had a recent bowel movement may receive a mild laxative or enema. A patient slated for GI, pelvic, perianal, or rectal surgery may undergo more extensive intestinal preparation. Preoperative enemas or an intestinal lavage with an oral solution, such as GoLYTELY, helps empty the intestine, thereby minimizing injury to the colon and improving visualization of the operative site.

Expect to perform extensive intestinal preparation for patients undergoing elective colon surgery. During surgical opening of the colon, escaping bacteria may invade adjacent tissue, leading to infection. Perform mechanical preparation and administer antimicrobial agents as ordered. Mechanical bowel preparation removes gross stool; oral antimicrobials suppress potent microflora without causing overgrowth of resistant strains.

If enemas are ordered until the bowel is clear and the third enema still hasn't removed all stool, notify the doctor. Repeated enemas may cause fluid and electrolyte imbalances, especially in elderly patients and those who are allowed nothing by mouth and haven't received I.V. fluids.

PREOPERATIVE DRUGS

The doctor may order preoperative or preanesthesia drugs for various reasons: to ease anxiety, to permit a smoother induction of anesthesia, to decrease the amount of anesthesia needed, to create amnesia for the events preceding surgery, or to minimize the flow of pharyngeal and respiratory secretions. The patient may receive anticholinergics (vagolytic or drying agents), sedatives, antianxiety drugs, narcotic analgesics, neuroleptanalgesic agents, and histamine$_2$-receptor antagonists.

Expect to administer ordered drugs 45 to 75 minutes before induction of anesthesia. If the operating room scheduled time is delayed, the person responsible for administering the anesthesia may choose to administer the preoperative drug I.V. in the operating room holding area. Teach the patient about ordered drugs and the effect they'll have on the patient. (See *Common preoperative drugs.*)

PSYCHOSOCIAL PREPARATION

Because depression and anxiety can significantly interfere with recovery from surgery, set aside plenty of time to allow the patient to discuss his feelings about the impending surgery. Give him the option of seeing a clergyman. Show understanding if he displays regressive behavior, regardless of his age. Expect some anxiety. If the patient seems inappropriately relaxed or unconcerned, consider that he's suppressing his fears. Such a patient may cope poorly with surgical stress.

Common preoperative drugs

Drug	Usual adult dosage	Desired effects	Adverse reactions
ANTICHOLINERGICS			
ATROPINE SULFATE	0.4 mg S.C. or I.M.	■ Decreases oral, respiratory, and gastric secretions, thus facilitating intubation ■ Prevents laryngospasm ■ Prevents reflex bradycardia	■ Excessive dryness of the mouth; tachycardia, flushing; depressed sweating ■ Increased intraocular pressure, blurred vision, dilated pupils ■ Urine retention ■ Arrhythmia and hypotension possible
GLYCOPYRROLATE Robinul	0.0044 mg/kg I.M.	■ Decreases oral, respiratory, and gastric secretions, thus facilitating intubation; some doctors feel that glycopyrrolate decreases oral secretions more effectively than atropine ■ Prevents laryngospasm ■ Prevents reflex bradycardia	■ Excessive dryness of the mouth; tachycardia, flushing ■ Increased intraocular pressure, blurred vision, dilated pupils ■ Urine retention
SCOPOLAMINE HYDROBROMIDE	0.3 to 0.65 mg S.C. or I.M.	■ Decreases oral, respiratory, and gastric secretions, thus facilitating intubation ■ Prevents laryngospasm ■ Prevents reflex bradycardia ■ Produces drowsiness and sedation (more so than atropine)	■ Excessive dryness of the mouth; tachycardia, flushing ■ Increased intraocular pressure, blurred vision, dilated pupils ■ Urine retention ■ Excessive drowsiness
ANTIANXIETY DRUGS			
DIAZEPAM Valium	10 mg I.M. (preferred) or I.V.	■ Provides sedation and amnesia ■ Reduces anxiety and apprehension ■ Provides skeletal muscle relaxation	■ Excessive sedation ■ Preoperative or postoperative nausea and vomiting ■ Local tissue irritation (with I.V. administration) ■ Hypotension and respiratory depression
HYDROXYZINE HYDROCHLORIDE Vistaril	25 to 100 mg I.M.	■ Reduces anxiety ■ Provides antiemetic effect ■ Acts as antihistamine	■ Drowsiness and dry mouth ■ Dizziness ■ Local discomfort at injection site
MIDAZOLAM HYDROCHLORIDE Versed	0.07 to 0.08 mg/kg I.M. (about 5 mg)	■ Provides sedation and amnesia (quick acting and short duration used for conscious sedation) ■ Reduces anxiety and apprehension	■ Respiratory depression (with high doses) ■ Hypotension
HISTAMINE$_2$-RECEPTOR ANTAGONISTS			
CIMETIDINE Tagamet	300 mg I.M. or I.V.	■ Decreases gastric acidity and volume	■ Decreased clearance of diazepam, lidocaine, propranolol, and other drugs ■ Hypotension and arrhythmia with rapid administration
RANITIDINE Zantac	50 mg I.M. or I.V.	■ Decreases gastric acidity and volume	■ Decreased clearance of diazepam, lidocaine, propranolol, and other drugs ■ Confusion, blurred vision, elevated liver enzymes

(continued)

Common preoperative drugs *(continued)*

Drug	Usual adult dosage	Desired effects	Adverse reactions
NARCOTICS			
MEPERIDINE HYDROCHLORIDE Demerol	50 to 100 mg I.M. or S.C.	■ Reduces anxiety, promotes relaxation ■ Minimizes perception of pain ■ Decreases amount of anesthetic needed ■ Produces sedation	■ Depressed respiration, circulation, and gastric motility ■ Dizziness, tachycardia, and sweating ■ Hypotension, restlessness, and excitement ■ Preoperative or postoperative nausea and vomiting
MORPHINE SULFATE Duramorph	5 to 10 mg I.M. or S.C.	■ Decreases amount of anesthetic needed ■ Produces sedation ■ Reduces anxiety, promotes relaxation ■ Minimizes perception of pain	■ Hypotension, restlessness, and excitement ■ Preoperative or postoperative nausea and vomiting ■ Depressed respiration, circulation, and gastric motility ■ Dizziness, tachycardia, and sweating
SEDATIVE-HYPNOTICS			
PENTOBARBITAL SODIUM Nembutal	150 to 200 mg I.M.	■ Reduces anxiety ■ Promotes sleep and relaxation	■ Confusion or excitement, especially in the elderly or in patients with severe pain
TRANQUILIZERS			
PROMETHAZINE Phenergan	25 to 50 mg I.M. or I.V. Not to be given S.C.	■ Reduces anxiety ■ Provides antiemetic effect ■ Reduces antihistamine effect	■ Postoperative hypotension ■ Blurred vision, dry mouth

Encourage the patient to draw support from his family or friends. If possible, allow them to visit with the patient preoperatively. Also, include them in your nursing plan of care.

INFORMED CONSENT

Informed consent implies that the patient has been given basic information about the surgery in language he can understand and that he agrees to the surgery. Obtaining the patient's consent for elective or urgent surgery is a legal requirement that must be met before the patient undergoes the procedure. It can be waived in emergencies, when the patient is in danger of losing life or limb.

The surgeon is responsible for obtaining informed consent, but most hospitals require the nurse to verify that informed consent has been given before transporting the patient to the operating room. Most commonly, informed consent is documented on a special form and the nurse witnesses the patient's signature on this document. In addition, the surgeon may also document it in the progress notes.

Nursing responsibilities associated with informed consent include:
■ witnessing the patient's signature on the form only after the surgeon has discussed the procedure with the patient

■ informing the surgeon of anything that the patient doesn't understand
■ ensuring that consent forms are accurately completed, witnessed, dated, and signed by the responsible parties
■ withholding preoperative sedation until the patient's signature has been obtained (the validity of informed consent can be challenged if the patient signs the form after being sedated)
■ alerting the surgeon if the patient has been sedated before consent is obtained and carefully documenting events that follow because of the increased possibility of litigation.

PATIENT EDUCATION

Teaching can help the patient cope with the physical and psychological stress of surgery. With shorter hospital stays and same-day surgeries on the rise, preadmission and preoperative teaching has become more important than ever. Nurses must structure their teaching to fit a limited time period.

ASSESSING LEARNING NEEDS

Expect some patients to have many questions, while others may want to know as little as possible. Most will want to know how long they must wait before returning to normal activities. The doctor will usually answer most questions, but you should evaluate the patient's understanding and dispel any lingering doubts or misconceptions. Be sure to adapt your teaching to fit the patient's age and level of understanding.

DISCUSSING DIAGNOSTIC TESTS
Provide explanations of chest X-rays, blood and urine studies, ECG, and other preoperative tests for the patient and his family. Explain that test results will determine readiness for surgery.

CALMING FEARS ABOUT ANESTHESIA
Tell the patient the name of his anesthesiologist, and explain that this person is responsible for his care until he leaves the postanesthesia room. The patient can expect a visit from the anesthesiologist before surgery; during this visit he will have the opportunity to ask questions. Encourage the patient to jot down his questions beforehand.

Your patient may be reluctant to admit his fears. He may fear awakening in the middle of the operation or never awakening at all. Assure your patient that the anesthesiologist will monitor his condition carefully throughout surgery and will provide just the right amount of anesthetic.

DISCUSSING DIET AND FAMILY VISITS
Explain the importance of eating nutritious meals prior to surgery. Address any restriction that may be necessary. Foods and fluids are usually withheld for 6 to 8 hours before surgery to decrease gastric contents. Noncompliance with preoperative restrictions on food and fluids may necessitate cancellation of elective surgery because of the markedly increased risk of gastroesophageal reflux aspiration, which can result in aspiration pneumonitis, respiratory arrest, or death. Make sure the patient understands that he can't eat or drink anything after the specified time. Remind the family, too.

Show the patient's family where they can wait during the operation. If they want to visit preoperatively, tell them to arrive 2 hours before the scheduled surgery.

REVIEWING OPERATING ROOM PROCEDURE
Warn the patient that he may have to wait a short time in the holding area. Explain that the doctors and nurses will wear surgical dress and that even though they'll be observing him closely, they may not talk to him a great deal. This will vary, depending on whether or not he has received preoperative medication. Explain that minimal conversation helps the medication to take effect.

When discussing transfer procedures and techniques, describe sensations the patient will experience. Tell him that he'll be taken to the operating room on a stretcher and transferred from the stretcher to the operating table. For his own safety, he'll be held securely to the table with soft restraints. The operating room nurses will check his vital signs frequently.

Alert the patient that the operating room may feel cool and that electrodes may be put on his chest to monitor his heart rate during surgery.

Describe the drowsy floating sensation he'll feel as the anesthetic takes effect. Tell him it's important that he relax at this time.

EXPLAINING I.V. TUBES AND DRAINS
Describe the site and technique to be used for I.V. therapy. Tell the patient when the I.V. will be started (before or after he goes to the operating room). Explain that fluids and nutrients given during surgery help prevent postoperative complications.

Inform the patient about the possibility of tube or drain insertion prior to or during the surgical procedure. Explain the rationale for the device and the expected length of time that it may be in place.

PREPARING THE PATIENT FOR RECOVERY
Briefly describe the sensations that the patient will experience when the anesthetic wears off. Tell him that the postanesthesia room nurse will call his name and then ask him to answer questions and follow simple commands, such as taking deep breaths and wiggling his toes. He may feel pain at the surgical site, but the nurse will try to minimize it. Describe the oxygen delivery device, such as a nasal cannula, that he'll need after surgery. Explain that some anesthetics may temporarily distort vision, but these distortions will disappear upon recovery.

Tell the patient that once he's recovered from the anesthesia, he'll return to his room. He'll be able to see his family but will probably feel drowsy and wish to nap.

Make sure he's aware that you'll be checking the surgical site and taking his blood pressure and pulse rate frequently. That way, he won't be alarmed by these routine precautions.

CONTROLLING PAIN
The patient may be anxious about how much pain he'll feel after surgery. You can help reduce his anxiety by advising him of pain-control measures that you'll be using. If he's having patient-controlled analgesia (PCA), tell him how to use it and arrange for him to see the device before he goes to surgery. Also, be sure to explain the device to the patient's family; ask them not to push the button for the patient but to let him do it himself.

Briefly explain that pain stems from stimulation of nerve endings in the skin as well as from tissue swelling and organ manipulation. Postoperative pain

Using a preoperative checklist

Before a patient leaves the nursing unit for surgery, all preoperative procedures must be completed. The nurse can use a checklist like the one shown below to avoid overlooking important details. As each procedure is completed, the nurse or other health care professional responsible for the procedure checks it off by initialing the list. An operating room nurse in the holding area double-checks each item on the checklist before the patient enters the operating room.

Patient's name　*Marian Welsch*

Room　*403A*　**Date**　*7/21/97*

ID band		v	*LKJD*
History and physical		v	*LK*
Doctors' consultations		v	*LK*
Consent form		v	*LK*
Blood-typing and crossmatching		v	*LK*
Complete blood count		v	*LK*
Urinalysis		v	*LK*
Chest X-ray		v	*LK*
Electrocardiogram		v	*LK*
Special tests		*Upper GI*	*LK*
NPO as ordered		v	*LK*
Skin preparation	*LK*	v *11/21*	*6 a.m.*
Vital signs	*LK*	v *130/84–76–18*	*T-98*
Dentures removed		v *none*	*LK*
Prostheses removed		v *none*	*LK*
Jewelry removed		v *none*	*LK*
Makeup, nail polish removed		v *ring taped*	*LK*
Voided		v	*LK JD*
Preanesthetic medication ordered		v *none*	*LK JD*

Drugs and dosages　*Demerol 50 mg. I.M.,*
Atropine 0.4 mg. I.M.

Time medicated　*8:15 a.m.*

By whom　*Joyce Dobler, GN*

Unit nurse　*Linda Krantz, R.N.*

Operating room nurse

---

typically lasts for 24 to 48 hours but may last longer with extensive surgery.

Explain that the doctor will order pain medication to be given according to the patient's needs. Instruct the patient to describe pain in terms of its quality, severity, and location. Encourage him to let you know as soon as he feels any pain, instead of waiting until it becomes intense, because early treatment makes controlling pain easier. Discuss the type of medication he'll receive, how it works, and the route of administration—whether by I.M.injection, I.V. (as in PCA), or orally (once the patient resumes eating, usually 48 hours postoperatively).

Describe measures you'll take to relieve pain and promote patient comfort, such as repositioning, diversionary activities, and splinting.

PERFORMING POSTOPERATIVE EXERCISES

Teach the patient preoperatively the techniques that promote early mobility and ambulation and help prevent complications. Early mobility and ambulation increase the rate and depth of deep breathing, preventing atelectasis and hypostatic pneumonia. Circulation improves as a result of early mobility, thus increasing cerebral oxygenation, making the patient feel more alert and helping prevent thrombophlebitis from venous stasis.

Early ambulation hastens peristalsis, which usually slows to a halt during surgery from the effects of the general anesthetic. Ambulation helps diminish postoperative constipation and abdominal distention, increases metabolism, and prevents loss of muscle tone.

Deep breathing and sustained maximal inspiration prevent atelectasis. Teach the patient deep-breathing exercises. The patient with congested lungs may need to practice coughing as well. Make it clear that he will repeat these maneuvers after surgery.

Demonstrate the use of an incentive spirometer, and explain to the patient that this device will provide feedback when he's doing deep-breathing exercises. Also explain how performing simple leg exercises, such as alternately contracting the calf muscles, prevents venous pooling.

TRANSFER TO THE SURGICAL SUITE

Many institutions require that the nurse complete a preoperative checklist before transferring the patient to the surgical suite. (See *Using a preoperative checklist.*) In addition to the checklist, be sure to follow these important steps:

■ Verify that the patient has adhered to fluid and food restrictions or has had nothing by mouth since midnight.

■ Make sure that a valid informed consent form has been signed and is on the patient's chart.

■ Make sure the results of ordered diagnostic tests appear on the chart. If the patient has diabetes, fasting blood glucose levels are reported to the internist, who then decides on the need for insulin and the amount to be given.

■ Have the patient remove jewelry, makeup, and nail polish.

■ Ask the patient to shower with antimicrobial soap, if ordered, and to perform mouth care. Warn against swallowing water.

■ Instruct the patient to remove any dentures or partial plates. Note on the chart if he has dental crowns, caps, or braces. Also have him remove contact lenses, glasses, or prostheses (such as an artificial eye). You may remove his hearing aid to ensure that it doesn't become lost. However, if the patient wishes to keep his hearing aid in place, inform operating room and postanesthesia room staff.

■ Have the patient void and put on a surgical cap and gown.

■ Take and record his vital signs.

■ Administer preoperative medication.

Intraoperative collaborative care

The intraoperative period begins with transfer of the patient to the operating room bed and ends with his admission to the postanesthesia care unit (PACU). In the operating room, all of the surgical team members play a vital role in the overall success of the procedure. The surgeon and anesthesiologist maintain primary roles, but the nurses collaborating with the doctors are responsible for maintaining the safety of the patient and the environment and providing physiologic monitoring and psychological support.

SURGICAL TEAM
Because of the complexity of the intraoperative environment, members of the surgical team must function as a coordinated unit. The surgeon, surgical assistant, anesthesiologist or certified registered nurse anesthetists, circulating nurse, and scrub nurse or operating room technician constitute the surgical team, with each member providing specialized skills.

The surgeon is the head of the team and is responsible for all medical actions and judgments. The surgical assistant works closely with the surgeon during the operation and performs such duties as exposing the operative site, retracting nearby tissue, sponging or suctioning the wound, ligating bleeding vessels, and suturing or assisting with suturing the wound.

The anesthesiologist or certified registered nurse anesthetist evaluates the patient preoperatively, administers the anesthetic and other required medications, transfuses blood or other blood products, infuses I.V. fluids, and continuously monitors the patient's

physiologic status. The anesthesiologist alerts the surgeon to any problems that develop, treats them as they arise, and supervises the patient's recovery in the PACU.

The circulating nurse coordinates and manages a wide range of activities before, during, and after the surgery. This team member oversees the physical aspects of the operating room itself, assists with transferring and positioning the patient, prepares the patient's skin, and counts all sponges and instruments. The circulating nurse assists all other team members and documents intraoperative activities.

The scrub nurse or operating room technician is primarily involved with technical skills, manual dexterity, and mechanical aspects of the particular surgery. The scrub nurse handles sutures, instruments, and other equipment immediately adjacent to the sterile field.

The nurse's role in surgery continues to evolve to improve patient care, and nurses have begun to specialize within this area. Specialty surgical teams have developed in response to the demands of increasingly complex surgeries.

ANESTHESIA
Anesthesia, an artificially induced state of partial or total loss of sensation, may occur with or without loss of consciousness. The purpose of anesthesia is to produce muscle relaxation, block transmission of pain impulses, suppress reflexes, and cause loss of consciousness.

The anesthesiologist, in consultation with the surgeon and the patient, makes the decision on the type of anesthesia. The choice of anesthetic depends on the following:

■ patient's age and physical condition
■ type, location, and duration of the surgery
■ degree of technical intricacy of the surgery
■ patient's previous anesthetic history
■ anesthesiologist's personal preference, expertise, and judgment.

GENERAL ANESTHESIA
General anesthesia suspends sensation in the entire body. It causes loss of consciousness, generalized loss of sensation, skeletal muscle relaxation, and reduction of reflexes.

Although some general anesthetics are given I.V., most are inhaled. That's because inhaled anesthetics are excreted more rapidly and their effects are more quickly reversed than nonvolatile drugs administered by other routes. Inhalation anesthetics include gases and halogenated volatile liquids. I.V. anesthetics include barbiturates and benzodiazepines. (See *Common general anesthetics*, pages 34 to 36.)

(Text continues on page 36.)

Common general anesthetics

Drug	Indications	Advantages	Disadvantages	Nursing considerations
INHALATION AGENTS				
ENFLURANE **Ethrane**	■ Used for maintenance of anesthesia ■ Occasionally used for induction of anesthesia	■ Allows for rapid induction and recovery ■ Is nonirritating and eliminates secretions ■ Causes bronchodilation ■ Provides good muscle relaxation ■ Allows cardiac rhythm to remain stable	■ Causes myocardial depression ■ Lowers seizure threshold ■ Increases hypotension as depth of anesthesia increases ■ May cause shivering during emergence ■ May cause circulatory or respiratory depression, depending on the dose ■ Has slightly irritating odor	■ Monitor for decreased heart and respiratory rates and hypotension. ■ Shivering may lead to increased oxygen consumption.
HALOTHANE **Fluothane**	■ Used for maintenance of general anesthesia	■ Is easy to administer ■ Allows for rapid, smooth induction and recovery ■ Has relatively pleasant, nonirritating odor ■ Depresses salivary and bronchial secretions ■ Causes bronchodilation ■ Easily suppresses pharyngeal and laryngeal reflexes	■ May cause myocardial depression, leading to arrhythmias ■ Sensitizes heart to action of catecholamine ■ May cause circulatory or respiratory depression, depending on the dose ■ Has no analgesic property ■ Provides poor muscle relaxation	■ Watch for arrhythmias, hypotension, and respiratory depression. ■ Body temperature may fall and patient may shiver after prolonged use, which increases oxygen consumption.
ISOFLURANE **Forane**	■ Used for maintenance of general anesthesia ■ Occasionally used for induction of general anesthesia	■ Allows for rapid induction and recovery ■ Causes bronchodilation ■ Allows for extremely stable cardiac rhythm ■ Provides good muscle relaxation	■ Depending on dose, may cause circulatory or respiratory depression ■ Potentiates the action of nondepolarizing muscular relaxants ■ May cause shivering ■ Tends to lower blood pressure as depth of anesthesia increases; pulse remains somewhat elevated ■ Has slightly offensive odor	■ Watch for respiratory depression and hypotension. ■ Shivering may lead to increased oxygen consumption.
NITROUS OXIDE	■ Used for maintenance of general anesthesia ■ May provide an adjunct for induction of general anesthesia ■ Used for induction and maintenance of balanced anesthesia	■ Has little effect on heart rate, myocardial contractility, respiration, blood pressure, liver, kidneys, or metabolism in absence of hypoxia ■ Produces excellent anesthesia ■ Allows for rapid induction ■ Doesn't increase capillary bleeding ■ Doesn't sensitize myocardium to epinephrine	■ May cause hypoxia with excessive amounts ■ Provides no muscle relaxation; procedures requiring muscle relaxation need addition of a neuromuscular blocker	■ Monitor for signs of hypoxia.

Common general anesthetics *(continued)*

Drug	Indications	Advantages	Disadvantages	Nursing considerations
I.V. BARBITURATES				
THIOPENTAL Pentothal	■ Primarily used in induction of general anesthesia	■ Rapid, smooth, and pleasant induction; quick recovery ■ Infrequently causes complications ■ Doesn't sensitize autonomic tissues of heart to catecholamines	■ Is associated with airway obstruction, respiratory depression, and laryngospasm, possibly leading to hypoxia ■ Provides no muscle relaxation and little analgesia ■ May cause cardiovascular depression, especially in hypovolemic or debilitated patients	■ Watch for signs and symptoms of hypoxia, airway obstruction, and cardiovascular and respiratory depression.
I.V. BENZODIAZEPINES				
DIAZEPAM Valium	■ Used for induction of general anesthesia ■ Used to induce amnesia during balanced anesthesia	■ Affects the cardiovascular system only minimally ■ Acts as a potent anticonvulsant Produces amnesia ■ Potentiates action of meperidine and barbiturates; decreasing amount required. ■ Decreased skeletal muscle spasticity	■ May cause irritation when injected into a peripheral vein ■ Has a long elimination half-life	■ Monitor vital signs.
MIDAZOLAM Versed	■ Used for induction of general anesthesia ■ Used for amnesia during balanced anesthesia	■ Affects the cardiovascular system minimally ■ Acts as a potent anticonvulsant ■ Produces amnesia	■ Can cause respiratory depression	■ Monitor vital signs and respiratory rate and volume.
I.V. NONBARBITURATE DRUGS				
KETAMINE Ketalar	■ Used for induction when a barbiturate is contraindicated ■ Sole anesthetic agent for short diagnostic and surgical procedures not requiring skeletal muscle relaxation	■ Produces a dissociative state of consciousness ■ Produces rapid anesthesia and profound analgesia ■ Doesn't irritate veins or tissues ■ Suppresses laryngeal and pharyngeal reflexes, a patent airway can be maintained without endotracheal intubation	■ May cause unpleasant dreams, hallucinations, and delirium during emergcence ■ Increases heart rate, blood pressure, and intraocular pressure ■ Preserves muscle tone, leading to poor relaxation during surgery	■ Protect patient from visual, tactile, and auditory stimuli during recovery. ■ Monitor vital signs.
PROPOFOL Diprivan	■ Used for induction of general anesthesia; useful in short procedures and outpatient surgery ■ Used for sedation with regional anesthesia	■ Allows for rapid, smooth induction ■ Causes less vomiting ■ Allows patients to awaken rapidly, responsive and oriented	■ Can cause hypotension ■ Can cause pain if injected into small veins ■ May cause clonic or myoclonic movements on emergence ■ May interact with benzodiazepines, increasing propofol's effects ■ Does not cause prolonged analgesia	■ Monitor for hypotension. ■ Prepare for rapid emergence.

(continued)

Common general anesthetics *(continued)*

Drug	Indications	Advantages	Disadvantages	Nursing considerations
I.V. TRANQUILIZER **DROPERIDOL** **Inapsine**	■ Used for induction and maintenance of anesthesia as an adjunct to general or regional anesthesia	■ Allows for rapid, smooth induction and recovery ■ Produces sleepiness and mental detachment for several hours	■ Because it's a peripheral vasodilator, may cause hypotension	■ Monitor for increased pulse rate and hypotension.
NARCOTICS **FENTANYL** **Sublimaze**	■ Used preoperatively for minor and major surgery, urologic procedures, and gastroscopy ■ Used as an adjunct to regional anesthesia and for induction and maintenance of general anesthesia	■ Allows for rapid, smooth induction and recovery ■ Doesn't cause histamine release ■ Minimally affects cardiovascular system ■ Can be reversed by narcotic antagonist (naloxone)	■ May cause respiratory depression, euphoria, bradycardia, bronchoconstriction, nausea, vomiting, and miosis ■ May cause skeletal-muscle and chest-wall rigidity	■ Observe for respiratory depression. ■ Watch for nausea and vomiting; if vomiting occurs, position the patient to prevent aspiration. ■ Monitor blood pressure. ■ Decrease postoperative narcotics to one-third to one-fourth the usual dose.
NEUROLEPTICS **DROPERIDOL** **AND FENTANYL** **Innovar**	■ Used for short procedures during which the patient must remain conscious ■ Used as a premedication and as an adjunct for induction and maintenance of general anesthesia	■ Produces somnolence and psychological indifference to the environment without total unconsciousness ■ Allows for rapid short induction and recovery ■ Eliminates voluntary movement ■ Makes it possible to use less analgesia postoperatively ■ Produces satisfactory amnesia	■ May cause respiratory depression, extrapyramidal symptoms, apnea, laryngospasm, bronchospasm, bradycardia, and hallucinations	■ Closely monitor vital signs. ■ Decrease postoperative narcotic dose to one-third to one-fourth of usual dose for first 8 hours.

REGIONAL ANESTHESIA

Regional anesthesia suspends sensation in a selected part of the body. The doctor achieves a local anesthetic effect by administering the appropriate drug on or near the nerve or nerve pathway between the site of the painful stimuli and the central nervous system. Regional anesthetics can be applied topically or be injected (nerve infiltration or epidural or spinal administration). The patient remains awake throughout the procedure and retains control of his airway. However, if the patient is anxious about remaining awake, make it clear to him that he'll be heavily sedated and won't remember what happens. Commonly used agents include procaine, lidocaine, and bupivacaine.

NEUROMUSCULAR BLOCKERS

Neuromuscular blockers are anesthesia adjuncts that produce muscle relaxation, thereby decreasing the dosage of general anesthetic needed. Furthermore, they facilitate endotracheal intubation and prevent laryngospasm. Note, however, that neuromuscular blockers have no effect on consciousness and don't produce analgesia. Because they paralyze the facial and eyelid muscles, the patient may appear to be asleep. Nevertheless, he is awake, can hear, and can feel pain.

Neuromuscular blockers are either nondepolarizing (competitive) or depolarizing. Nondepolarizing agents include atracurium, gallamine, metocurine, pancuronium, tubocurarine, and vecuronium. Depolarizing agents include succinylcholine. (See *Common neuromuscular blockers.*)

BALANCED ANESTHESIA

A combination of narcotics, sedative-hypnotics, nitrous oxide, and muscle relaxants can be used to achieve what's called balanced anesthesia. Drug selection and dosage depend on the planned procedure, the patient's condition, and the patient's response to the medications.

Common neuromuscular blockers

Drug	Adverse reactions	Nursing considerations
NONDEPOLARIZING NEUROMUSCULAR BLOCKERS		
ATRACURIUM Tracrium	■ Slight hypotension in a few patients	■ Acts for 20 to 25 minutes ■ May cause slight histamine release ■ Won't accumulate with repeated doses ■ Is useful in underlying hepatic, renal, and cardiac disease
GALLAMINE Flaxedil	■ Tachycardia, hypertension ■ Allergic reaction (in patients sensitive to iodine) ■ Decrease in respiratory minute volume	■ Acts for 15 to 20 minutes ■ Should be avoided in patients with cardiac disease; tachycardia occurs regularly after doses of 0.5 mg/kg ■ Doesn't cause bronchospasm ■ Will accumulate; don't administer to patients with impaired renal function or myasthenia gravis
METOCURINE Metubine	■ Hypotension ■ Bronchospasm	■ Acts for 35 to 60 minutes ■ May cause histamine release
PANCURONIUM Pavulon	■ Tachycardia, hypertension ■ Transient rashes, burning sensation at injection site	■ Acts for 35 to 45 minutes ■ Is five times more potent than curare ■ Doesn't cause ganglion blockage or (usually) hypotension; has vagolytic action that increases heart rate
TUBOCURARINE CHLORIDE	■ Hypotension ■ Bronchospasm	■ Acts for 25 to 90 minutes with single dose or multiple single doses; may last 24 hours ■ Causes histamine release; in higher doses, causes sympathetic ganglion blockade ■ May have prolonged action in elderly or debilitated patients and in those with renal or liver disease
VECURONIUM Norcuron	■ Minimal and transient cardiovascular effects ■ Skeletal muscle weakness or paralysis, respiratory insufficiency, respiratory paralysis, prolonged, dose-related apnea	■ Acts for 25 to 40 minutes ■ Probably is mostly metabolized in liver ■ Has a short duration of action and causes fewer cardiovascular effects than other nondepolarizing neuromuscular blockers
DEPOLARIZING NEUROMUSCULAR BLOCKERS		
SUCCINYLCHOLINE (SUXAMETHONIUM) Anectine, Quelicin, Sucostrin	■ Respiratory depression ■ Bradycardia ■ Excessive salivation ■ Hypotension ■ Hypertension ■ Arrhythmias ■ Tachycardia ■ Increased intraocular and intragastric pressure ■ Fasciculations ■ Muscle pain ■ Malignant hyperthermia	■ Acts for 0.5 to 10 minutes ■ Is mostly metabolized in plasma by pseudocholinesterase; contraindicated in patients with a deficiency of plasma cholinesterase due to a genetic variant defect, liver disease, uremia, or malnutrition ■ Should be used cautiously in patients with glaucoma or penetrating wounds of the eye or in those undergoing eye surgery ■ Should be used cautiously in patients with cardiovascular, hepatic, pulmonary, metabolic, or renal disorders and in patients with burns, severe trauma, spinal cord injuries, and muscular dystrophies; may cause sudden hyperkalemia and consequent cardiac arrest ■ In pregnant patients who also receive magnesium sulfate, may cause increased neuromuscular blockade because of decreased pseudocholinesterase levels

Advantages of balanced anesthesia include rapid induction, minimal cardiac depression, and decreased nausea, pain, and other adverse postoperative effects. Besides producing sleep and analgesia, balanced anesthesia eliminates certain reflexes and provides good muscle relaxation.

A schedule for balanced anesthesia might include:
- premedication with a sedative, a narcotic analgesic (meperidine, morphine, fentanyl), and a parasympathetic inhibitor (atropine)
- induction with an ultra-short-acting barbiturate anesthetic (thiopental)
- maintenance of general anesthesia with an anesthetic gas (nitrous oxide), possibly in conjunction with an I.V. barbiturate or narcotic analgesic (fentanyl or sufentanil)
- induction of muscle relaxation with a curare-type drug as a neuromuscular blocking agent.

CONSCIOUS SEDATION
Conscious sedation is drug-induced partial sedation that still allows the patient to respond appropriately to verbal and nonverbal stimuli and to maintain a patent airway independently with the protective reflexes intact. By contrast, deep sedation produces arousable sleep, but the protective reflexes are somewhat compromised.

Conscious sedation serves as an adjunct to regional and local anesthesia and during the induction phase of some anesthetics. It's also used during diagnostic tests, such as endoscopy or cardiac catheterization, and in specialized and acute care units to manage anxiety and pain. The agents used most commonly to produce sedation and amnesia are midazolam and diazepam; to produce sedation and analgesia, morphine, meperidine, and fentanyl.

Most conscious sedation is administered I.V. For any other route, a venous access device must be in place. Reversing agents, such as flumazenil and naloxone; emergency equipment; and personnel who can provide advanced life support should be readily available. Registered nurses who administer and monitor conscious sedation should understand their health care facility's policy and clinical practice guidelines for administering conscious sedation and should complete an educational program to demonstrate competency in this procedure.

PATIENT PREPARATION AND CARE
Operating room responsibilities are divided among all members of the surgical team. Typically, the scrub nurse scrubs before the operation, sets up the sterile table, prepares sutures and special equipment, and helps the surgeon and his assistants throughout the operation. The circulating nurse manages the operating room and monitors cleanliness, humidity, lighting, and equipment safety. In addition, this nurse co-ordinates the activities of operating room personnel and monitors aseptic practices.

Other nursing responsibilities during the intraoperative period may include positioning the patient, preparing the incision site, draping the patient, monitoring the patient, managing skin closures, and transferring the patient to the PACU.

PATIENT POSITIONING
Factors that determine proper patient positioning include the type of surgery being performed and coexisting medical problems. The patient's position should:
- provide optimum exposure to the operative site
- allow the anesthesiologist access for induction and for administration of I.V. fluids or drugs
- promote circulatory and respiratory function
- avoid undue pressure on any body part
- allow for draping that will assure the patient's privacy and dignity.

Every surgical position is a variation of one of three basic positions: dorsal (supine), prone, or lateral. Special operating room tables and attachments will allow you to modify the patient's position.

SITE PREPARATION
Before the incision, prepare the skin of the operative site and surrounding area with an antimicrobial agent. This removes superficial flora, soil, and debris, thereby reducing the risk of wound contamination. Immediately before surgery, apply a preoperative skin preparation to keep the deeper resident flora from contaminating the skin surface. Consider the condition of the skin at the incision site, the proximity of mucous membranes, and the nature of the proposed surgery. You may also need to remove hair.

Prepare an area large enough to protect against wound contamination by inadvertent movement of drapes during the procedure. The prepared area should be able to accommodate an extension of the incision, the need for additional incisions, and all drain sites.

PATIENT DRAPING
By establishing a sterile field around the surgical site, patient draping prevents the passage of microorganisms between nonsterile and sterile areas. Sterile drapes cover all unprepared areas of the patient; only the incision site remains exposed.

PATIENT MONITORING
Throughout the intraoperative phase, all body systems are monitored continuously. The circulating nurse is responsible for documenting intraoperative nursing activities, medication and blood administration, placement of drains and catheters, and the length of the procedure. The circulating nurse also

Suture methods

The illustrations below show the different types of common suturing methods that can be used to close a wound.

Plain interrupted suture
The doctor sews individual sutures, each with a separate piece of thread tied independently. Half of the thread length crosses under the suture line and the other half appears above the skin surface.

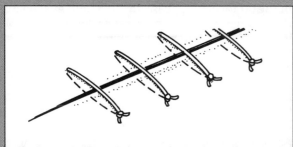

Plain continuous suture
Also called a continuous running suture, this series of connected stitches has a knot tied at the beginning and end of the suture.

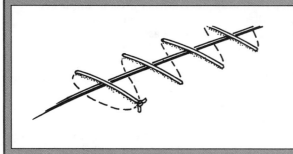

Mattress interrupted suture
This term describes independent stitches tunneling completely under the incision line, except for a tiny portion visible on the skin surface at each side of the wound.

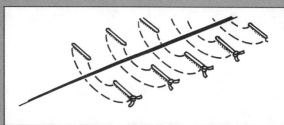

Mattress continuous suture
This series of connected mattress stitches has a knot only at its beginning and end.

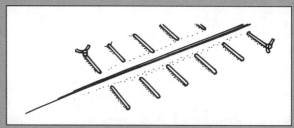

Blanket continuous suture
Here the doctor sews a series of looped stitches, tying a knot only at the beginning and end of the series.

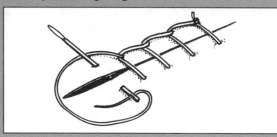

formulates a plan of care based on the physiologic and psychosocial condition of the patient.

SKIN CLOSURES
The type of suture material used to close a wound varies according to the suturing method. (See *Suture methods*.)

Nonabsorbable sutures are commonly used to close the skin surface, providing strength and immobility with minimal tissue irritation. Nonabsorbable suture materials include silk, cotton, stainless steel, and dermal synthetics such as nylon.

Absorbable sutures are commonly used when removing the sutures is undesirable, for example, in underlying tissue layers. Absorbable materials include:
- chromic catgut, which is natural catgut treated with chromium trioxide for strength and prolonged absorption time
- plain catgut, which is absorbed faster than chromic catgut and tends to cause more tissue irritation
- synthetics such as polyglycolic acid, which are replacing catgut because they're stronger, more durable, and less irritating.

Obtaining background information

When working in the postanesthesia care unit, after you assess the patient's respiratory and cardiovascular status, be sure to obtain the following information from members of the surgical team:

■ patient's name, age, gender, and native language
■ current medical diagnosis
■ name and length of surgical procedure
■ name of surgeon
■ patient's preoperative history, including vital signs, medications, potential or actual drug allergies, medical history, and any communication disabilities or psychosocial problems
■ patient's position during the procedure
■ intraoperative vital signs
■ duration of tourniquet use
■ preoperative medication administered
■ anesthetics, muscle relaxants, and reversal agents administered
■ antibiotics administered
■ nature and treatment of other complications occurring during surgery
■ fluid therapy, including estimated blood loss, the amount and type of fluid administered, and urine output
■ lines present (peripheral, arterial, central venous) and their sites and patency
■ type and number of drains and catheters
■ condition of wound (open, closed, packed)
■ condition of patient at end of procedure, including vital signs and any prostheses present.

Commonly used in place of standard sutures for closure of lacerations and operative wounds, skin staples or clips can secure a wound faster than sutures. In many cases, they are substituted for surface sutures—that is, where cosmetic results are not a prime consideration such as in abdominal closure. When properly placed, staples and clips distribute tension evenly along the suture line, with minimal tissue trauma or compression, facilitating healing and minimizing scarring. Because staples and clips are made from surgical stainless steel, tissue reaction to them is minimal.

TRANSFER TO PACU

Following the operation, a member of the surgical team commonly dresses the patient in a clean gown and then assists with the transfer of the patient to a stretcher. The patient is then covered with warm blankets and secured with safety belts. The side rails are raised to ensure the patient's safety. The anesthesiolo-

gist or nurse anesthetist as well as another member of the surgical team accompany the patient to the PACU. In some institutions, patients who are at high risk for complications are transferred directly from the operating room to the intensive care unit (ICU) for continued specialized care and constant nursing supervision.

Postoperative collaborative care

In the postoperative phase, the third and final phase of the surgical experience, nursing plays a critical role in returning the patient to an optimal level of functioning. The postoperative phase can be further divided into two stages. The first stage, the immediate postanesthesia and postoperative period, is the first few hours after surgery when the patient is recovering from the effects of anesthesia. The second stage, or later postoperative period, is a time for healing and preventing complications.

IMMEDIATE POSTOPERATIVE CARE

The immediate postanesthesia period is a critical time for the patient. Vital physiologic functions must be supported until the effects of the anesthesia abate. Until then, the patient is dependent and drowsy and may be unable to call for assistance.

POSTANESTHESIA CARE UNIT

The immediate postoperative period begins when the patient arrives in the PACU, accompanied by the anesthesiologist or nurse-anesthetist. Before the transfer staff depart, be sure to obtain all pertinent surgical information to guide the patient's care. (See *Obtaining background information.*) When providing care, your goal is to meet the patient's physical and emotional needs, thereby minimizing the development of postoperative complications. Factors such as lack of oxygen, pain, and sudden movement may threaten his physiologic equilibrium.

Recovery from general anesthesia takes longer than induction. During maintenance, anesthesia uptake occurs in muscle and fat. Because fat has a sparse blood supply, it surrenders the anesthesia more slowly, providing a reserve of anesthetic that serves to maintain brain and blood levels. A patient's recovery time will also depend on which preoperative medication he received, the specific anesthetic used, the duration of anesthetic administration, the dosage in relation to patient's body size, the patient's percentage of body fat, and his individual response to the anesthetic.

During recovery from general anesthesia, reflexes return in reverse order to the way they disappear. The normal sequence of return is responsiveness to stimuli, drowsiness, awake but disoriented, and alert and oriented. Keep in mind that hearing is the first sense to return; explain your actions to the patient, and be careful not to make careless remarks in his presence.

Thanks to the use of short-acting anesthetics, the average PACU stay lasts less than 2 hours. Expect to assess the patient every 10 to 15 minutes initially, then as his condition warrants. During this time, continue to monitor him for respiratory and cardiovascular complications. Obstruction and hypoventilation may lead to inadequate respiratory function and postoperative hypoxia. Disruptions in cardiovascular function may include arrhythmias and hypotension.

Patient evaluation and monitoring. Perform the following postanesthesia care measures:
- Check the patient's airway. Feel for the amount of air exchange. Start the patient's oxygen at the flow rate ordered. Note rate, depth, and quality of respirations.
- Note the presence or absence of protective throat reflexes.
- Take pulse rate, initiate pulse oximetry and ECG monitoring, if ordered, and then take blood pressure readings. Note rate and quality of pulse. Compare all vital-sign readings with the patient's preoperative and intraoperative values.
- Determine the patient's level of consciousness (LOC).
- Observe the patient's skin color; check the mucous membrane inside the lower lip and also his nail beds.
- For any I.V. infusions, note the type and amount of fluid, infusion rate, catheter position, and site location.
- Observe the presence and condition of any drains and tubes.
- Make sure that tubes aren't kinked or occluded and are properly attached to the suction or drainage bag.
- Assess any dressings. If they're soiled, note the color, type, odor, and amount of drainage.
- If irrigants are being infused, note the amount and type.

Other measures include properly positioning the patient, encouraging respiratory exercises, removing secretions, minimizing hypothermia, and administering reversal agents and I.V. fluids.

The doctor may use anticholinesterase agents, such as neostigmine and pyridostigmine, to reverse nondepolarizing agents. To reverse opioid analgesics, he may use naloxone. Monitor the patient who receives reversal agents closely; the effects of these agents may wear off, leaving the patient vulnerable to respiratory depression.

Fear, pain, hypothermia, anxiety, and confusion can cause emotional distress for the patient. He may fall or become delirious. Interventions to maintain his physical and emotional well-being include raising side rails, making sure that his body is in proper alignment, keeping him warm, administering analgesics, providing reassurance, and taking steps to protect his dignity and privacy. Document your care measures and other patient information.

TRANSFER TO THE PATIENT CARE AREA
Regardless of whether the patient is discharged from the PACU to the medical-surgical unit, the ICU, or the short-procedure unit, safety remains the major consideration. A scoring system will usually quantify the patient's readiness for transfer. Common criteria used to evaluate the patient's readiness include the following:
- recovery from effects of anesthesia
- quiet and unlabored respirations
- vital signs stable at preoperative level
- hemodynamic stability
- ability to summon help when needed
- only moderate or light drainage from any site
- physiologic effects of narcotic stabilized
- satisfactory LOC with patent airway
- essential care completed by PACU staff
- adequate urine output, at least 30 ml/hour
- report given to staff on transfer unit; unit prepared to receive patient
- complete documentation of patient's progress and status.

ONGOING POSTOPERATIVE CARE
When assessing the patient after his return to the patient care unit, be systematic yet sensitive to his needs. Compare your findings with intraoperative and preoperative assessment findings, and report any significant changes immediately.

CHECKING VITAL SIGNS
Begin by verifying that the patient has a patent airway and by checking his respiratory rate, rhythm, and depth. Excessive sedation from analgesics or a general anesthetic can cause respiratory depression. Respiratory depression may also occur if reversal agents begin to wear off.

Observe for tracheal deviation from the midline. As you auscultate the lungs, note any chest asymmetry, unequal lung expansion, or use of accessory muscles. Diminished breath sounds at the lung bases commonly occur in patients who inhaled an anesthetic and in those with COPD or a heavy smoking habit. Encourage deep breathing to promote elimination of the anesthetic and optimal gas exchange and acid-base balance. Encourage coughing if the patient has

●

secretions. Use this opportunity to assess the patient's LOC by testing his ability to follow commands.

Assessing for cyanosis. Circumoral, nail-bed, or sublingual cyanosis denotes an arterial oxygen saturation level of less than 80%. Earlobe cyanosis, which usually accompanies COPD, may be exacerbated by anesthesia. Also assess for other signs and symptoms of respiratory distress, including nasal flaring, inspiratory or expiratory grunts, changes in posture to ease breathing, and progressive disorientation. You may use a pulse oximeter to supplement your assessment. This monitor will help you determine life-threatening levels of oxygen saturation (70% or less).

Taking pulse rate. Take the patient's pulse rate for 1 minute. An irregular rhythm may reflect the effects of anesthesia or may be a preexisting arrhythmia such as atrial fibrillation. Assess the rate and quality of radial and pedal pulses, and note any dependent edema. Compare these data to the preoperative assessment to confirm any significant changes. An overly rapid pulse rate may signal pain, bleeding, dehydration, or shock. Correlate pulse rate with blood pressure, urine output, and overall clinical status to verify any of the above conditions.

Taking blood pressure. Systolic pressure shouldn't vary more than 15% from the preoperative reading (except in patients who experience preoperative hypotension). Administration of I.V. fluids and blood products during surgery can increase both systolic and diastolic pressures. Also, be aware of any drugs given during surgery so you can evaluate their potential vasodilative or vasoconstrictive effects.

Usually, the patient is placed in the lateral decubitis or semiprone position after surgery. Remember that rapid position changes may cause orthostatic hypotension associated with lingering vasodilative effects of the anesthetic. Conversely, postoperative pain may increase systolic pressure by causing sympathetic stimulation.

Measuring temperature. The route varies with the patient's age and the type of surgery he's had. In infants and young children, rectal temperature is preferred over axillary temperature. In an adult cardiac patient, though, rectal temperature can cause vagal stimulation; therefore, take oral or axillary temperature if possible. Don't take oral temperature if the patient is still groggy from the effects of anesthesia. Tympanic membrane thermometer systems are gaining popularity, so you may find yourself using one of these.

Keep in mind that slowing of basal metabolism associated with anesthesia may cause postoperative hy-pothermia. A cold operating room or I.V. solution may also lower the patient's temperature. Provide warm blankets as necessary. Equally likely, the patient may experience a slight fever—the result of the body's response to the trauma of surgery. Fever may also signal infection or dehydration.

EXAMINING THE SURGICAL WOUND
First, note the wound's location and describe its length, width, and type (horizontal, transverse, or puncture). Next, document the type of dressing, if any. If the dressing is stained by drainage, estimate the quantity and note its color and odor. Or, if the patient has a drainage device, record the amount and color of drainage; make sure the device remains secure. If the patient has an ileostomy or colostomy, note any output. Describe the sutures, staples, or Steri-Strips used to close the wound, and assess approximation of wound edges.

ASSESSING THE ABDOMEN
First, observe for changes in abdominal contour. Abdominal dressings and tubes or other devices may distort this contour. To detect abdominal asymmetry, stand at the foot of the patient's bed to view the abdomen. Also, observe for Cullen's sign—a bluish hue around the umbilicus that commonly accompanies intra-abdominal or peritoneal bleeding.

Auscultate for bowel sounds in all four quadrants for at least 1 minute per quadrant. You probably won't be able to detect bowel sounds for at least 6 hours after surgery because general anesthetics slow peristalsis. If the doctor handled the patient's intestines, bowel sounds will be absent for longer than usual.

If the patient has a nasogastric (NG) tube, regularly check its patency. If you suspect tube displacement, try to aspirate gastric contents. Or confirm proper tube placement by instilling air with a bulb syringe while you auscultate over the epigastric area.

PROVIDING COMFORT
Many postsurgical patients are unable to assume a comfortable position because of incisional pain, activity restrictions, immobilization devices, or an array of tubes and monitoring lines. Therefore, assess the patient's level of comfort and offer analgesics, as ordered. Discuss specific measures the patient can take to prevent or reduce incision pain. (See *Relieving acute pain.*) Although most patients will tell you when they experience severe pain, some may suffer silently. Increased pulse rate and blood pressure may provide the only clues to their condition.

Recognize that emotional support can do much to relieve pain but doesn't replace adequate analgesia. Physical measures, such as repositioning, back rubs, and creating a comfortable environment in the patient's room, can also promote comfort and enhance the effectiveness of analgesics.

After administering an analgesic, always document the dose, administration route, and patient's response.

RECORDING INTAKE AND OUTPUT
When recording postoperative intake of food and oral fluids, remember to include ice chips as well as I.V. fluids and blood products. If the patient receives peritoneal dialysis or three-way bladder irrigation after surgery, you'll probably keep a separate flow sheet to identify positive or negative fluid balance.

Expect urine output for an adult to measure a minimum of 0.5 to 1 ml/kg/hour. After surgery, however, the patient may have difficulty voiding; this occurs when medications such as atropine depress parasympathetic stimulation. Monitor the patient's intake and palpate his bladder regularly to assess the need for catheterization. Because some anesthetics slow peristalsis, the patient may not defecate until his bowel sounds return.

Other sources of output include perspiration, NG contents, and wound drainage. A Hemovac or other type of closed wound suction allows you to measure drainage precisely via wound drainage tubes. Wound drainage can be estimated by observing the amount of staining on dressings.

When documenting output, note the source of output; its quantity, color, and consistency; and the duration of output. Notify the doctor of significant changes, such as a change in the color and consistency of NG contents from dark green to "coffee grounds."

PREVENTING POSTOPERATIVE COMPLICATIONS
After surgery, take steps to avoid complications. Be ready to recognize and manage them if they occur. (See *Detecting and managing postoperative complications,* pages 44 to 47.) To avoid extending the patient's hospital stay and to speed his recovery, perform the following measures to prevent complications.

Turning and repositioning. Performed every 2 hours, turning and repositioning the patient promotes circulation, thereby reducing the risk of skin breakdown especially over bony prominences. When the patient is in a lateral recumbent position, tuck pillows under bony prominences to reduce friction and promote comfort. Each time you turn the patient, carefully inspect the skin to detect redness or other signs of breakdown. Keep in mind that turning and repositioning may be contraindicated in some

(Text continues on page 47.)

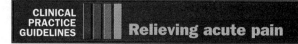

CLINICAL PRACTICE GUIDELINES — **Relieving acute pain**

Following are selected portions of the clinical practice guidelines for pain management developed by the Agency for Health Care Policy and Research of the U.S. Department of Health and Human Services.

Nonpharmacologic management
- Include in patient teaching procedural and sensory information, instructions to decrease treatment- and activity-related pain (such as pain caused by deep breathing or coughing), and relaxation techniques.
- Supplement pharmacologic interventions with cognitive-behavioral interventions (such as distraction and imagery) and physical interventions (such as heat, cold, and massage).
- Encourage the patient to perform simple relaxation strategies. Basic approaches require only a few minutes to teach. Periodically reinforce and coach him in their use as appropriate.
- Consider that transcutaneous electrical nerve stimulation may reduce pain and improving physical function.

Special considerations for elderly patients
Keep the following points in mind:
- Many elderly people suffer multiple chronic, painful illnesses and take multiple medications. They're at greater risk for drug-drug and drug-disease interactions.
- Pain assessment presents unique problems in the elderly because these patients may exhibit physiologic, psychologic, and cultural changes associated with aging.
- Many health care providers and patients alike mistakenly consider pain to be a normal part of aging. Elderly patients sometimes believe that pain can't be relieved and are stoic in reporting their pain. The frail and oldest-old (older than age 85) are at particular risk for undertreatment of pain.
- Aging need not alter pain thresholds or tolerance. The similarities between elderly and younger patients are far more common than the differences.
- Cognitive impairment, delirium, and dementia are serious barriers to assessing pain in the elderly. Sensory problems such as visual changes may also interfere with the use of some pain assessment scales.
- Observe for behavioral cues to pain, such as restlessness and agitation. But remember that their absence doesn't negate the presence of pain.
- Nonsteroidal anti-inflammatory drugs can be used safely in elderly people, but their use requires vigilance for adverse effects, especially gastric and renal toxicity.
- Opioids are safe and effective in elderly patients when used appropriately. Elderly people are more sensitive to analgesic effects of opiate drugs; they experience higher peak effect and longer duration of pain relief.

Detecting and managing postoperative complications

Despite your best efforts, complications sometimes still occur. By knowing how to recognize and manage them, you can limit their effects.

Complication	Description	Assessment	Interventions
ABDOMINAL DISTENTION	■ Sluggish peristalsis and paralytic ileus usually last 24 to 72 hours postoperatively and cause abdominal distention. Nonabsorbable gas accumulates in the intestine and passes to the atonic portion of the bowel, remaining there until tone returns.	■ Increasing adominal girth ■ Complaints of feeling bloated	■ Encourage ambulation. ■ Keep the patient on nothing by mouth until bowel sounds return ■ Insert a rectal tube or a nasogastric (NG) tube, as ordered. ■ Keep the NG tube patent and functioning properly.
PARALYTIC ILEUS	■ A common postsurgical complication, paralytic ileus occurs whenever autonomic innervation of the GI tract becomes disrupted. Causes include intraoperative manipulation of intestinal organs, hypokalemia, wound infection, and medications such as codeine, morphine, and atropine.	■ Diminished bowel sounds in all four quadrants ■ Little or no passage of flatus or stool	■ Encourage ambulation and administer medications such as dexpanthenol, as ordered. ■ If the ileus doesn't resolve within 24 to 48 hours, insert an NG tube, as ordered. ■ Keep the NG tube patent and functioning properly.
CONSTIPATION	■ Postoperative constipation usually results from colonic ileus caused by diminished GI motility and impaired perception of rectal fullness. Although primarily a problem of elderly postoperative patients, assess for constipation in any patient receiving opiates or anticholinergics.	■ Feelings of abdominal fullness or nausea	■ Encourage ambulation. ■ Administer stool softeners, laxatives, and nonnarcotic analgesics, as ordered.
ALTERED BODY IMAGE	■ The mental image a patient holds of himself contributes greatly to his identity and self-esteem. A drastic change in this image following surgery normally arouses anxiety and emotional tension. The patient becomes insecure and will likely grieve for his former self-image. Grieving may last up to 1 year.	■ Comments from the patient that indicate depression or insecurity ■ Constantly inspecting his incision or talking about it	■ Listen to the patient and be attentive to his behavior. ■ Assess what changes in appearance mean to him. ■ Assure him that feelings of anxiety and depression are normal. ■ Discuss the grieving process with him. ■ Provide support to the patient and his family. ■ Ask if they would like to talk with a patient who has successfully adapted to a similar alteration. ■ Encourage the patient to participate as much as possible in his care, and help him anticipate the reactions and comments of others. ■ Identify the patient's coping strategies. ■ If he uses denial as a coping mechanism, accept it but don't reinforce this behavior.

Detecting and managing postoperative complications *(continued)*

Complication	Description	Assessment	Interventions
ATELECTASIS AND PNEUMONIA	■ In atelectasis, incomplete lung expansion causes the distal alveoli to collapse. After surgery, this complication usually results from hypoventilation and excessive retained secretions, which provide an excellent medium for bacterial growth and set the stage for stasis pneumonia. ■ In stasis pneumonia, an acute inflammation, the alveoli and bronchioles become plugged with a fibrous exudate, making them firm and inelastic.	*For atelectasis* ■ Diminished or absent breath sounds over the affected area ■ Flatness on percussion ■ Decreased chest expansion and mediastinal shift toward the side of collapse ■ Fever; restlessness or confusion; worsening dyspnea, and elevated blood pressure, pulse rate, and respiratory rate *For pneumonia* ■ Sudden onset of shaking chills with high fever and headache ■ Diminished breath sounds or telltale crackles over the affected lung area ■ Dyspnea, tachypnea, and sharp chest pain that's exacerbated by inspiration ■ Productive cough with pinkish or rust-colored sputum ■ Cyanosis with hypoxemia, confirmed by arterial blood gas measurement ■ Chest X-rays with patchy infiltrates or areas of consolidation	■ Encourage the patient to deep-breathe and cough every hour while he's awake. (*Note:* Coughing is contraindicated in patients who have undergone neurosurgery or eye surgery.) ■ Show him how to use an incentive spirometer to facilitate deep breathing. ■ Perform chest physiotherapy, if ordered. ■ Administer antibiotics, if ordered. ■ Administer humidified air or oxygen to loosen secretions, as ordered. ■ Elevate the head of the patient's bed to reduce pressure on the diaphragm and to allow lung expansion. ■ Reposition the patient at least every 2 hours to prevent pooling of secretions.
HYPOVOLEMIA	■ Characterized by reduced circulating blood volume, hypovolemia may result from blood loss, severe dehydration, third-space fluid sequestration (as in burns, peritonitis, intestinal obstruction, or acute pancreatitis), or abnormal fluid loss (as in excessive vomiting or diarrhea). This complication develops when the patient loses from 15% to 25% of his total blood volume.	■ Hypotension and a rapid, weak pulse ■ Cool, clammy, and perhaps slightly mottled skin ■ Rapid, shallow respirations ■ Oliguria or anuria ■ Lethargy	■ To increase blood pressure, administer I.V. crystalloids, such as normal saline solution or lactated Ringer's solution. ■ To restore urine output and fluid volume, administer colloids, such as plasma, albumin, or dextran.
POSTOPERATIVE PSYCHOSIS	■ Postoperative mental aberrations may have a physiologic or psychological origin. Physiologic causes include cerebral anoxia, fluid and electrolyte imbalance, malnutrition, and drugs such as tranquilizers, sedatives, and narcotics. Psychological causes include fear, pain, and disorientation.	■ Changes in baseline mental status	■ Reorient the patient frequently to person, place, and time. ■ Place a clock and calendar in his room where he can see them. ■ Keep changes in his environment to a minimum, and make sure that familiar objects are close by. ■ Call the patient by his preferred name, and encourage him to move about. ■ Make sure he wears clean eyeglasses and has a working hearing aid, if appropriate. ■ Protect the patient from harm. ■ Use sedatives and restraints only if necessary.

(continued)

Detecting and managing postoperative complications *(continued)*

Complication	Description	Assessment	Interventions
SEPTICEMIA	■ Septicemia, a severe systemic infection, may result from a break in asepsis during surgery or wound care or from peritonitis (as in ruptured appendix or ectopic pregnancy). The most common cause of postoperative septicemia is	■ Fever, chills, rash, abdominal distention, prostration, pain, headache, nausea, or diarrhea	■ Obtain specimens (blood, wound, and urine) for culture and sensitivity tests to verify cause and guide treatment. ■ Administer antibiotics, as ordered. ■ Monitor vital signs and level of consciousness to detect septic shock.
SEPTIC SHOCK	■ *Escherichia coli.* Septic shock occurs when endotoxins are released into the bloodstream. The endotoxins stimulate the release of chemical mediators that decrease vascular resistance, resulting in dramatic hypotension.	*Early stages* ■ Fever; chills; warm, dry, flushed skin; slightly altered mental status; increased pulse and respiratory rates; decreased or normal blood pressure; and reduced urine output *Late stages* ■ Pale, moist, cold skin ■ Significant decrease in mentation, pulse and respiratory rates, blood pressure, and urine output	■ Administer I.V. antibiotics, as ordered. ■ Monitor serum peak and trough levels to help ensure effective therapy. ■ Give I.V. fluids and blood or blood products to restore circulating blood volume.
THROMBO-PHLEBITIS	■ Postoperative venous stasis associated with immobility predisposes the patient to thrombophlebitis—an inflammation of a vein, usually in the leg, accompanied by clot formation. ■ High-risk patients include those with a history of varicose veins, hypercoagulation, or cardiovascular disease; elderly or obese patients; and women taking oral contraceptives	■ Complaints of leg pain, functional impairment, or edema (although majority of calf vein thrombi are asymptomatic) ■ Increased calf circumference ■ Engorgement of the cavity behind the medial malleolus (early clue to edema) ■ Increase in temperature in the affected leg ■ Areas of cordlike venous segments	■ Elevate the affected leg and apply warm compresses. ■ Offer analgesics, as ordered. ■ Administer I.V. heparin, if ordered, to prevent clot formation. ■ During this therapy, monitor prothrombin and partial thromboplastin times daily.
PULMONARY EMBOLISM	■ If a clot breaks away, it may become lodged in the lung, causing a pulmonary embolism. This obstruction of a pulmonary artery interrupts blood flow, thereby decreasing gas exchange in the lungs.	■ Sudden anginal or pleuritic chest pain ■ Dyspnea ■ Rapid, shallow respirations ■ Cyanosis ■ Restlessness ■ Thready pulse ■ Fine to coarse crackles over the affected lung area	■ Administer oxygen by face mask or nasal cannula, as ordered, to improve tissue perfusion. ■ Administer an analgesic and I.V. heparin, as ordered. ■ Elevate the head of the patient's bed to relieve dyspnea. ■ Provide emotional support to decrease anxiety.
URINE RETENTION	■ Despite normal kidney function, absence of obstruction, and a full bladder, the patient may not be able to void spontaneously within 12 hours after surgery. ■ Retention is usually transient and reversible.	■ Absence of voided urine (major indication) ■ Distended bladder above the level of the symphysis pubis ■ Complaints of discomfort or pain ■ Restlessness, anxiety ■ Diaphoresis ■ Hypertension ■ Overflow (overdistended bladder dispels enough urine to relieve the pressure within it)	■ Avoid making the patient anxious. ■ Help him ambulate as soon as possible after surgery, unless contraindicated. ■ Assist the patient to a normal voiding position and, if possible, leave him alone. ■ Turn the water on so the patient can hear it, and pour warm water over his perineum. ■ Lightly stroke the inner aspect of his thigh.

Detecting and managing postoperative complications *(continued)*

Complication	Description	Assessment	Interventions
WOUND INFECTION	■ Wound infection is the most common wound complication as well as the second most common nosocomial infection. ■ It's also a major factor in wound dehiscence (the partial or total disruption of a surgical wound).	■ Increased tenderness at wound site ■ Deep pain at the wound site ■ Edema, especially from the third to fifth day after the operation ■ Increased pulse rate and temperature and an elevated white blood cell count ■ Temperature pattern of spikes in the afternoon or evening; returns to normal by morning (aerobic organisms)	■ Obtain a wound culture and sensitivity test, as ordered. ■ Administer antibiotics, as ordered. ■ Irrigate the wound with an appropriate solution, as ordered. ■ Monitor wound drainage.
DEHISCENCE AND EVISCERATION	■ Complete dehiscence leads to evisceration (the abrupt protrusion of wound contents). ■ Abdominal wounds are more likely to dehisce and eviscerate than thoracic incisions.	*To detect wound dehiscence* ■ Gushes of serosanguineous fluid from the wound ■ Report of a "popping sensation" after retching or coughing. *To detect evisceration:* ■ Protruding wound contents ■ Coils of intestine possibly extruding from the abdomen	■ Stay with the patient; have a colleague notify the doctor. ■ If an abdominal wound dehisces, help the patient to low Fowler's position, with knees bent. This will decrease abdominal tension. ■ Cover the extruding wound contents with warm normal saline soaks. ■ Monitor the patient's vital signs.

patients, such as those who have undergone neurologic or musculoskeletal surgery that demands immobilization postoperatively.

Deep breathing and coughing. Deep breathing promotes lung expansion, which helps clear anesthetics from the body. (Note that it doesn't increase intracranial pressure.) Along with coughing, it also lowers the risk of pulmonary and fat emboli and hypostatic pneumonia associated with secretion buildup in the airways. Encourage the patient to cough and deep-breathe at least every 2 hours, and show him how to use an incentive spirometer. Encourage him to splint the incision to promote greater comfort.

Monitoring nutrition and fluids. Adequate nutrition and fluid intake is essential to ensure proper hydration, promote healing, and provide energy to match the increased basal metabolism associated with surgery. If the patient has a protein deficiency or compromised immune function preoperatively, expect to deliver supplemental protein via parenteral nutrition to promote healing. If he has renal failure, this treatment would be contraindicated because his inability to break down protein could lead to dangerously high blood nitrogen levels.

Promoting exercise and ambulation. Early postoperative exercise and ambulation can significantly reduce the risk of thromboembolism as well as improve ventilation and brighten the patient's outlook. Perform passive range-of-motion (ROM) exercises or, better yet, encourage active ROM exercises to prevent joint contractures and muscle atrophy and to promote circulation. These exercises can also help you assess the patient's strength and tolerance.

Before encouraging ambulation, have the patient dangle his legs over the side of the bed and perform deep-breathing exercises. His tolerance of this step is usually a key predictor of out-of-bed tolerance. Begin ambulation by helping the patient walk a few feet from his bed to a sturdy chair. Then have him gradually progress each day from ambulating in his room to ambulating in the hallway, with or without assistance, as necessary. Document frequency of ambulation and patient tolerance, including use of analgesics.

DISCHARGE PLANNING
Planning for the patient's discharge should begin during your first contact with him. Include his family or other caregivers to ensure proper home care. Components of a discharge plan include medication, diet, activity, home care procedures, potential complications, return appointments, and referrals.

Recognizing potential problems early will help your discharge plan succeed. Assess the strengths and limitations of the patient and family. Consider physiologic factors, such as general physical and functional abilities, current medications, and general nutritional status; psychological factors, such as self-concept, motivation, and learning abilities; and social factors, such as duration of care needed, types of services available, and family involvement in the patient's care. The initial nursing history and preoperative assessment as well as subsequent assessments can provide useful information for tailoring the contents of your plan to the patient's individual needs.

Consider providing written materials as a reference for the patient at home. Make sure, however, that you reinforce readings with personal teaching.

Medications. Educate the patient about the purpose of drug therapy, proper dosages and routes, special instructions, how long the regimen will last, potential adverse effects, and when to contact the doctor. Working with the patient and pharmacist, try to establish a medication schedule that fits the patient's lifestyle. If the hospital schedule proves inconvenient for the patient at home, he may become lax about taking his medication.

Diet. Discuss dietary restrictions with the patient and, if appropriate, the family member or caregiver who will prepare his meals. Assess the patient's usual dietary intake. How well does the patient understand his prescribed diet? Discuss the cost of the diet and how the patient's restrictions may affect other family members. Recommend a good diet book. Refer the patient to a dietitian if appropriate.

Activity. After surgery, many patients are advised not to lift anything that's heavy such as a basket of laundry. Restrictions usually last 4 to 6 weeks after surgery. Make sure the patient and his family understand the reasons behind these rules. Discuss how limitations will affect the patient's daily routine. Let him know when he can return to work, driving, and sexual activity. If the patient seems unlikely to comply fully with restrictions, discuss possible compromises.

Home care procedures. Use clear, nontechnical language, and include close friends or family members when providing instruction about home care. After he watches you demonstrate a procedure, have him (or his caregiver) perform a return demonstration.

Make it clear to the patient that the equipment he uses at home may differ from the equipment at your health care facility; discuss what's available to him at home. If he needs to rent or purchase special equipment, such as a hospital bed or walker, give him a list of suppliers in the area.

Teach the patient about changing his wound dressing. Tell him to keep the incision clean and dry, and teach proper hand-washing technique. Discuss when the patient can take a shower or bath, and specify which method he should use.

Potential complications. Make sure the patient can recognize signs and symptoms of wound infection and other potential complications. Provide written instructions about reportable signs and symptoms, such as bleeding or discharge from an incision or acute incision pain. Advise the patient to call the doctor with any questions.

Return appointments. If the patient feels well at home, he may neglect his return appointment. Stress the importance of this appointment, and make sure the patient has the doctor's office telephone number. If the patient has no means of transportation, refer him to an appropriate community resource.

Referrals. Reassess whether the patient needs a referral to a home care agency or other community resource. The decision will depend on the patient's physical and psychological well-being, his social status, and the needs of his family. Discuss with the family how they will handle the patient's return home. In some hospitals, the responsibility for making referrals falls to a home care coordinator or discharge planning nurse.

Selected readings

American Hospitals Formulary Service: Drug Information. Bethesda, Md.: American Society of Health System Pharmacists, Inc., 1997.

Holland, C.A. "Conscious Sedation Policy Development and Review," *American Association of Nurse Anesthetists Journal* 63(3):196-97, June 1995.

Kiviniemi, K. "Conscious Awareness and Memory During General Anesthesia," *American Association of Nurse Anesthetists Journal* 62(5):441-49, Obtober 1994.

Maser, R.E., et al. "Glucose Monitoring of Patients with Diabetes Mellitus Receiving General Anesthesia: A Study of the Practices of Anesthesia Providers in a Large Community Hospital," *American Association of Nurse Anesthetists Journal* 64(4):357-61, August 1996.

Miller, R.D., ed. *Anesthesia,* 4th ed. New York: Churchill Livingstone, 1994.

Nelson, M.S., et al. "Competency Verification for Conscious Sedation," *Journal of Emergency Nursing* 22(2):116-19, April 1996.

Vitello, I., et al. "Management of Sedation: The Nursing Perspective," *Critical Care Nurse,* Supplement 1-16, August 1996.

Cardiovascular disorders

Although people are living longer than ever before, they're living increasingly with chronic conditions or the sequelae of acute ones. Of these conditions, cardiovascular disorders head the list. In North America, more than 60 million people suffer from some form of cardiovascular disorder—many from a combination of disorders—and the numbers rise yearly.

Nurses will be dealing with cardiovascular patients more often, regardless of the practice setting. To provide effective care for these patients, nurses need a clear understanding of cardiovascular anatomy and physiology, assessment techniques, diagnostic tests, and management of the disorders that plague this body system. Such knowledge allows nurses to better promote recovery, improve patient compliance, and ensure adequate home care.

Anatomy and physiology review

The heart is a four-chambered muscle about the size of a closed fist. Roughly cone-shaped, it weighs about 10½ to 12½ oz (300 to 350 g) in an adult male and 9 to 10½ oz (250 to 300 g) in an adult female.

The heart lies substernally in the mediastinum, between the second and sixth ribs. About one-third of the organ lies to the right of the midsternal line; the remainder, to the left. In most people, the heart rests obliquely, with the right side almost in front of the left, the broad part at the top, and the pointed end (apex) at the bottom. However, its position varies with body build; in a tall, thin person, the heart lies more vertically; in a short, stocky person, it lies more horizontally.

HEART WALL
This wall consists of three layers. A thick myocardium, composed of interlacing bundles of cardiac muscle fibers, forms most of the heart wall. A thin layer of endothelial tissue forms the inner endocardium. An outer epicardium makes up the outside layer.

The pericardium is a fibroserous sac that surrounds the heart and the roots of the great vessels. It consists of the serous pericardium and the fibrous pericardium. The serous pericardium consists of the parietal layer, which lines the inside of the fibrous pericardium, and the visceral layer, which adheres to the surface of the heart. Between the two layers is the pericardial space, which contains a few drops of pericardial fluid to lubricate the surfaces of the space and allows the heart to move easily during contraction. (See *Inside the heart,* page 50.)

CHAMBERS
The heart contains four hollow chambers: two atria and two ventricles. The right atrium lies in front and to the right of the left atrium. It receives blood from the superior and inferior venae cavae. The left atrium, smaller but with thicker walls than the right atrium, forms the uppermost part of the heart's left border, extending to the left of and behind the right atrium. It receives blood from the pulmonary veins. The interatrial septum separates the right and left atria.

The right and left ventricles make up the two lower chambers. Both are large and thick-walled. The right ventricle lies behind the sternum and forms the largest part of the sternocostal surface and inferior border of the heart. The left ventricle is larger than the right because it must contract against high resistance with enough force to eject blood into the aorta and the rest of the body. Its wall is two to three times thicker (8 to 15 mm) than that of the right ventricle (4 to 5 mm). The left ventricle forms the apex and

Inside the heart

The heart's internal structure includes the pericardium, 3 layers of the heart wall, 4 chambers, 11 openings, and 4 valves.

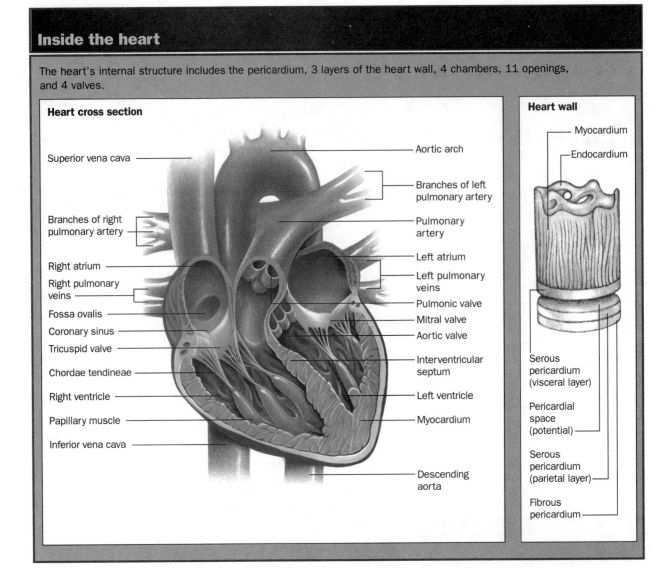

Heart cross section

- Superior vena cava
- Branches of right pulmonary artery
- Right atrium
- Right pulmonary veins
- Fossa ovalis
- Coronary sinus
- Tricuspid valve
- Chordae tendineae
- Right ventricle
- Papillary muscle
- Inferior vena cava

- Aortic arch
- Branches of left pulmonary artery
- Pulmonary artery
- Left atrium
- Left pulmonary veins
- Pulmonic valve
- Mitral valve
- Aortic valve
- Interventricular septum
- Left ventricle
- Myocardium
- Descending aorta

Heart wall

- Myocardium
- Endocardium
- Serous pericardium (visceral layer)
- Pericardial space (potential)
- Serous pericardium (parietal layer)
- Fibrous pericardium

most of the left border of the heart and its diaphragmatic surface.

VALVES

Four valves keep blood flowing in one direction through the heart: two atrioventricular (AV) valves and two semilunar valves.

The AV valves separate the atria from the ventricles. The right AV valve, commonly called the tricuspid valve, has three triangular cusps, or leaflets. It controls the flow of blood through the right atrioventricular orifice. Thin but strong tendinous cords known as chordae tendineae attach the cusps of the tricuspid valve to the papillary muscles in the right ventricle. The left AV valve, called the mitral or bicuspid valve, guards the left atrioventricular opening.

This valve contains two cusps, a large anterior and a smaller posterior. Chordae tendineae attach these two cusps to papillary muscles in the left ventricle.

The pulmonic and aortic valves compose the semilunar valves. Both valves have three cusps shaped like half-moons, and both open and close passively in response to pressure changes caused by ventricular contraction and blood ejection. The pulmonic valve guards the orifice between the right ventricle and the pulmonary artery. The aortic valve guards the orifice between the left ventricle and the aorta.

CARDIAC CONDUCTION SYSTEM

An electrical conduction system regulates myocardial contraction. This system includes the nerve fibers of

Cardiac conduction

In the heart's conduction system, specialized fibers spread an impulse quickly throughout the heart's muscle cell network, causing a generalized contraction. This illustration shows the elements of this conduction system.

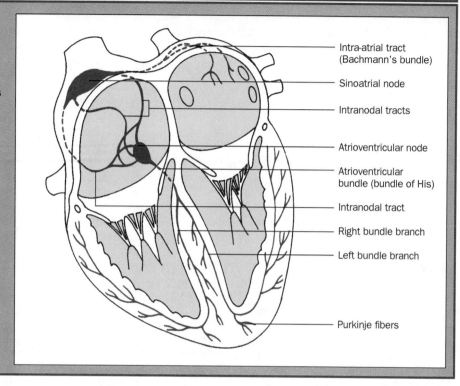

- Intra-atrial tract (Bachmann's bundle)
- Sinoatrial node
- Intranodal tracts
- Atrioventricular node
- Atrioventricular bundle (bundle of His)
- Intranodal tract
- Right bundle branch
- Left bundle branch
- Purkinje fibers

the autonomic nervous system (ANS) and specialized nerves and fibers in the heart. (See *Cardiac conduction.*)

The ANS involuntarily increases or decreases heart action to meet the individual's metabolic needs.

Both sympathetic and parasympathetic nerves participate in the control of cardiac function. With the body at rest, the parasympathetic nervous system controls the heart through branches of the vagus nerve (CN X). Heart rate and electrical impulse propagation are very slow.

In times of activity or stress, the sympathetic nervous system takes control. It stimulates the heart's nerves and fibers to fire and conduct more rapidly and the ventricles to contract more forcefully.

PACEMAKER CELLS

Myocardial cells have specialized pacemaker cells that allow electrical impulse conduction. Pacemaker cells control heart rate and rhythm (a property known as automaticity). Therefore, any myocardial muscle cell can control initiation of contractions under certain circumstances.

Normally, the sinoatrial (SA) node (located on the endocardial surface of the right atrium, near the superior vena cava) paces the heart. SA node firing spreads

an impulse throughout the right and left atria by way of intranodal and intra-atrial pathways, resulting in atrial contraction through a sequence of cardiac activation (depolarization).

The AV node (located low in the septal wall of the right atrium, immediately above the coronary sinus opening) then takes up impulse conduction. Normally, the AV node forms the only electrical connection between the atria and ventricles. It initially slows the impulse, delaying ventricular activity and allowing blood to fill from the atria. Then conduction speeds through the AV node and a network of fibers called the bundle of His.

The bundle of His arises in the AV node and continues along the right intraventricular septum. It divides in the ventricular septum to form the right and left bundle branches. Its fibers rapidly spread the impulse throughout both ventricles.

Purkinje fibers, the distal portions of the left and right bundle branches, fan across the subendocardial surface of the ventricles from the endocardium through the myocardium. As the impulse spreads throughout the distal conduction system, it prompts ventricular contraction through a change in electrical (action) potential in reponse to the stimulus.

Action potential occurs in two steps: depolarization and repolarization. In depolarization, the cell membrane's permeability to sodium increases, causing a rapid influx of sodium into the cells. (Calcium also enters but through slow channels.) Potassium moves out of the cell, creating an electrical current. When sodium reaches a certain level, an electrical impulse is created.

Repolarization returns the cell to its resting state. Cell membrane permeability to sodium decreases. Sodium leaves the cell and potassium returns to the inside.

CARDIAC CYCLE

The cardiac cycle describes the period from the beginning of one heartbeat to the beginning of the next. During this cycle, electrical and mechanical events must occur in the proper order and to the proper degree to provide adequate blood flow to all body parts. The cardiac cycle has two phases: systole and diastole.

Systole. At the beginning of systole, the ventricles contract, increasing pressure and forcing the mitral and tricuspid valves shut. This valvular closing prevents blood backflow into the atria and coincides with the first heart sound, known as S_1 or the *lub* of *lub-dub*. As the ventricles contract, ventricular pressure builds until it exceeds that in the pulmonary artery and the aorta. Then the aortic and pulmonic valves open, and the ventricles eject blood into the aorta and the pulmonary artery.

Diastole. When the ventricles empty and relax, ventricular pressure falls below that in the pulmonary artery and the aorta. At the beginning of diastole, the semilunar valves close to prevent blood backflow into the ventricles. This coincides with the second heart sound, known as S_2 or the *dub* of *lub-dub*.

As the ventricles relax, the mitral and tricuspid valves open and blood begins to flow into the ventricles from the atria. When the ventricles become full near the end of diastole, the atria contract to send the remaining blood to the ventricles. Then a new cardiac cycle begins as the heart enters systole.

CARDIAC OUTPUT AND STROKE VOLUME

Cardiac output refers to the amount of blood that the heart pumps in 1 minute. Stroke volume, the amount of blood ejected with each beat multiplied by the number of beats per minute, determines cardiac output. Stroke volume depends on three major factors:
- preload—the stretch of heart muscle fibers caused by blood volume in the ventricles at the end of diastole

- afterload—the pressure in the aorta and other arteries leading from the ventricles that must be overcome for ejection to occur
- contractility—the myocardium's inherent ability to contract normally.

Understanding the cardiac cycle helps to assess the heart's hemodynamics. Many cardiac dysfunctions cause abnormal findings that correlate with specific events in the cardiac cycle.

BLOOD VESSELS

About 60,000 miles of arteries, arterioles, capillaries, venules, and veins keep blood circulating to and from every functioning cell in the body. (See *Major blood vessels,* opposite, and *Blood vessels: Form follows function,* page 54.) This network has two branches: the systemic circulation and the pulmonary circulation.

SYSTEMIC CIRCULATION

Through the systemic circulation, blood carries oxygen and other nutrients to body cells and transports waste products for excretion. At specific sites, the pumping action of the heart that forces blood through the arteries becomes palpable. This regular expansion and contraction of the arteries is called the pulse.

The major artery—the aorta—branches into vessels that supply specific organs and areas of the body. The left common carotid, the left subclavian, and the innominate arteries arise from the arch of the aorta and supply blood to the brain, arms, and upper chest. As the aorta descends through the thorax and abdomen, its branches supply GI and genitourinary organs, the spinal column, and the lower chest and abdominal muscles. Then the aorta divides into the iliac arteries, which further divide into femoral arteries.

As the arteries divide into smaller units, the number of vessels increases dramatically, thereby increasing the area of perfusion. At the end of the arterioles and the beginning of the capillaries, strong sphincters control blood flow into the tissues. They dilate to permit more flow when needed, close to shunt blood to other areas, or constrict to increase blood pressure.

Although the capillary bed contains the smallest vessels, it supplies blood to the largest area. Capillary pressure is extremely low to allow for the exchange of nutrients, oxygen, and carbon dioxide with body cells. From the capillaries, blood flows into venules and, eventually, into veins.

Valves in the veins prevent blood backflow, and the pumping action of skeletal muscles assists venous return. The veins merge until they form two main branches—the superior and inferior vena cavae—that return blood to the right atrium.

Major blood vessels

This illustration shows the body's major arteries and veins.

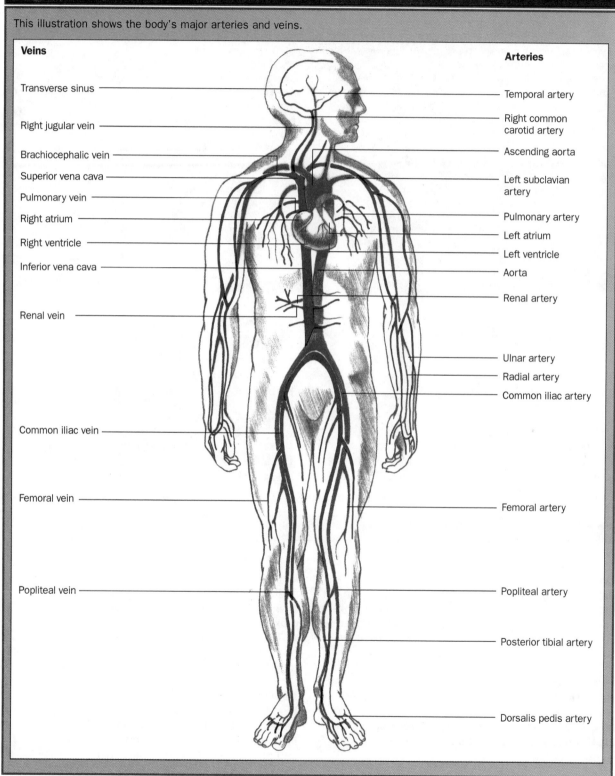

Veins

- Transverse sinus
- Right jugular vein
- Brachiocephalic vein
- Superior vena cava
- Pulmonary vein
- Right atrium
- Right ventricle
- Inferior vena cava
- Renal vein
- Common iliac vein
- Femoral vein
- Popliteal vein

Arteries

- Temporal artery
- Right common carotid artery
- Ascending aorta
- Left subclavian artery
- Pulmonary artery
- Left atrium
- Left ventricle
- Aorta
- Renal artery
- Ulnar artery
- Radial artery
- Common iliac artery
- Femoral artery
- Popliteal artery
- Posterior tibial artery
- Dorsalis pedis artery

Blood vessels: Form follows function

As blood courses through the vascular system, it travels through five distinct types of blood vessels: arteries, arterioles, capillaries, venules, and veins. Vessel diameter and composition depend on specific function.

In the aorta, vascular resistance to blood flow is almost nil, and mean arterial pressure remains almost constant at 100 mm Hg. When blood reaches the arterioles, which have much smaller diameters, vascular resistance has risen enough to reduce mean blood pressure to 85 mm Hg. When blood crosses the arterioles to the capillaries, vascular resistance causes the mean blood pressure to fall to 35 mm Hg.

Blood pressure is only about 15 mm Hg when blood begins its return to the heart. Venous pressure continues to decline to 0 to 6 mm Hg when blood reaches the right atrium. Blood pressure decreases despite a steady increase in venous diameter. Why? Because many veins are collapsed much of the time by pressure from the surrounding tissues.

Vessel structure

Differences in blood pressure are reflected in vessel structure:
- Arteries have thick, muscular walls to accommodate the flow of blood at high speeds and pressures.
- Arterioles have thinner walls than arteries. They can constrict or dilate as needed to control blood flow to the capillaries.
- The capillaries, which are microscopic vessels, have walls composed of only a single layer of endothelial cells.
- Venules gather blood from the capillaries but have thinner walls than arterioles.
- Veins have thinner walls than arteries but have larger diameters because of the low blood pressures required for venous return to the heart. Veins of the extremities and neck have valves that open in the direction of blood flow to prevent venous backflow.

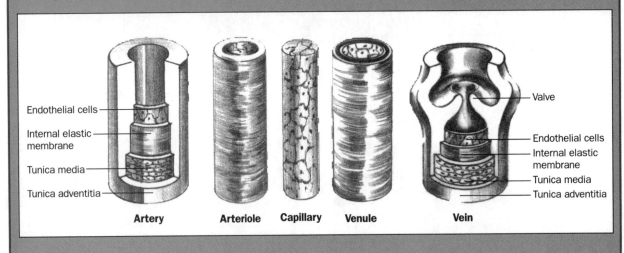

Endothelial cells
Internal elastic membrane
Tunica media
Tunica adventitia

Artery **Arteriole** **Capillary** **Venule** **Vein**

Valve
Endothelial cells
Internal elastic membrane
Tunica media
Tunica adventitia

CORONARY CIRCULATION
Blood flowing through the heart's chambers doesn't exchange oxygen and other nutrients with the myocardial cells. Instead, a specialized part of the systemic circulation, the coronary circulation, supplies blood to the heart. (See *The heart's blood supply*.)

PULMONARY CIRCULATION
Blood travels to the lungs to pick up oxygen and release carbon dioxide as follows:
- Unoxygenated blood travels from the right ventricle through the pulmonic semilunar valve into the pulmonary arteries.

- Blood passes through progressively smaller arteries and arterioles into the capillaries of the lungs.
- Blood reaches the alveoli and exchanges carbon dioxide for oxygen.
- The oxygenated blood then returns via venules and veins to the pulmonary veins, which carry it back to heart's left atrium.

BLOOD PRESSURE
Blood pressure refers to the pressure exerted on the blood vessels by the blood as it flows through them. Pressure regulating mechanisms—neural, hormonal, and physical—interact to ensure that enough blood is

The heart's blood supply

The heart relies on the coronary arteries and their branches to supply itself with oxygenated blood and on the cardiac veins to remove oxygen-depleted blood. During left ventricular systole, blood is ejected into the aorta. During diastole, blood flows into the coronary ostia and then through the coronary arteries to nourish the heart muscle.

The right coronary artery supplies blood to the right atrium (including the sinoatrial and atrioventricular nodes of the conduction system), part of the left atrium, most of the right ventricle, and the inferior part of the left ventricle.

The left coronary artery, which splits into the anterior descending and circumflex arteries, supplies blood to the left atrium, most of the left ventricle, and most of the interventricular septum. Many collateral arteries connect the branches of the right and left coronary arteries.

The cardiac veins lie superficial to the arteries. The largest vein, the coronary sinus, lies in the posterior part of the coronary sulcus and opens into the right atrium. Most of the major cardiac veins empty into the coronary sinus, except for the anterior cardiac veins, which empty into the right atrium.

Anterior view

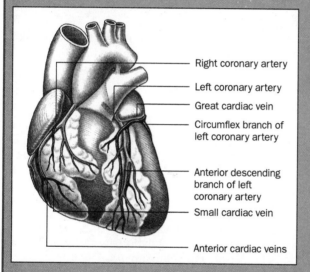

- Right coronary artery
- Left coronary artery
- Great cardiac vein
- Circumflex branch of left coronary artery
- Anterior descending branch of left coronary artery
- Small cardiac vein
- Anterior cardiac veins

Posterior view

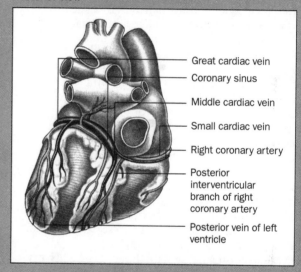

- Great cardiac vein
- Coronary sinus
- Middle cardiac vein
- Small cardiac vein
- Right coronary artery
- Posterior interventricular branch of right coronary artery
- Posterior vein of left ventricle

channeled to or diverted from the right part of the body at the right time.

Neural regulators

Neural regulators include baroreceptors and chemoreceptors. Baroreceptors are nerve endings embedded in blood vessels that are sensitive to the stretching of vessel walls. They are found in the walls of the internal carotid arteries, aortic arch, and in most large arteries of the neck and thorax. When vessel walls stretch in response to increasing blood volume, baroreceptors signal the central nervous system to inhibit the vasoconstrictor center in the medulla and to stimulate the vagal center. This causes peripheral vasodilation, decreased heart rate, and less vigorous contractions, decreasing arterial blood pressure. Conversely, when baroreceptors detect decreased blood pressure, they induce peripheral vasoconstriction, in-

creased heart rate, and more vigorous contractions. However, with continued stimulation, such as with chronic hypertension, baroreceptors lose their ability to control arterial pressure changes.

Chemoreceptors are nerve endings located in the walls of the carotid arteries, aorta, and medullary area of the brain stem. Chemoreceptors respond to abnormally low levels of dissolved oxygen and carbon dioxide in the blood, stimulating sympathetic activity and inhibiting parasympathetic activity. This action causes a reflex increase in arterial pressure.

Hormonal regulators

Four hormonal regulators control arterial pressure: secretion of norepinephrine and epinephrine by the adrenal glands; secretion of renin by the juxtaglomerular cells of the kidneys, with subsequent formation of angiotensin I and II; secretion of antidiuretic hormone by the hypothalamus; and secretion of prostaglandins by various body tissues.

Norepinephrine and epinephrine are released by the adrenal medulla and cause effects similar to direct sympathetic stimulation of the cardiovascular system: increased heart rate, blood pressure, automaticity, and contractility. These hormones achieve their effects by stimulating the sympathetic system's alpha and beta receptors throughout the vasculature. Alpha stimulation causes vasoconstriction; beta stimulation causes vasodilation.

Renin is released by the kidney when blood pressure drops excessively. Persisting in the blood up to an hour, this enzyme acts on the plasma protein angiotensinogen to form the hormone angiotensin I. When blood containing this hormone reaches the lungs, an enzyme in the small vessels of the lungs catalyzes its conversion to angiotensin II. Angiotensin II strongly constricts arterioles, raising arterial pressure, and moderately constrict veins, promoting venous return to the heart and providing additional blood to pump against the increased pressure. Angiotensin II has a direct effect on the kidneys, decreasing excretion of salt and water. It also causes the adrenal cortex to secrete aldosterone, further decreasing salt and water excretion. This reduced fluid loss tends to increase blood volume and raise blood pressure.

Antidiuretic hormone is secreted by the hypothalamus in response to decreased blood pressure. Like angiotensin, it is a vasoconstrictor. It acts on the renal tubules to promote water retention, which in turn increases plasma volume and thus increases peripheral resistance and blood pressure.

Various prostaglandins are thought to be involved in blood pressure regulation. In general, prostaglandins A and E dilate arteries and veins, while prostaglandin F constricts veins.

Physical regulators

Vascular stress relaxation and capillary fluid shift are physical regulators of blood pressure. These mechanisms are slower than the other regulators mentioned.

Stress relaxation allows a blood vessel to compensate for sudden shifts in volume and pressure by adjusting its diameter without prolonging a change in its diameter and tension. A rapid increase in blood volume and pressure distends the blood vessel but causes only a transient increase in tension. The converse is also true.

Capillary fluid shift is a compensatory mechanism that regulates fluid exchange across the capillary membranes in response to arterial pressure. With a sharp increase in arterial pressure, capillary hydrostatic pressure increases, causing more fluid to shift into the interstitial spaces. As a result, less fluid is circulat-

ing and blood pressure decreases. The converse is also true.

Assessment

Assessment aims to identify and evaluate changes in the patient's cardiac function—changes that may disrupt or threaten his life. Baseline information obtained during assessment will help guide your intervention and follow-up care.

Note, however, that if your patient is in a cardiac crisis, you'll have to rethink your assessment priorities. The patient's condition and the clinical situation will dictate what steps to take.

HISTORY

Begin your assessment with a thorough history. Ask open-ended questions and listen carefully to the patient's responses; also, closely observe his nonverbal behavior.

CHIEF COMPLAINT

Ask your patient why he's seeking medical care. Document the answer in the patient's own words. If he can't identify a single chief complaint, ask more specific questions, such as, "What made you seek medical care at this time?"

Ask the patient how long he's had the problem, how it affects his daily routine, and when it began. Find out about any associated signs and symptoms. Ask about the location, radiation, intensity, and duration of any pain and about any precipitating, exacerbating, or relieving factors. Try to obtain as accurate a description as possible of any chest pain.

Let the patient describe his problem in his own words. Avoid leading questions. Use familiar expressions rather than medical terms whenever possible. If the patient is not in distress, ask questions requiring more than a yes-or-no answer. (See *Key questions for assessing cardiac function*.)

MEDICAL HISTORY

Ask about any history of cardiac-related disorders, such as hypertension, diabetes mellitus, hyperlipidemia, congenital heart defects, or syncope. Other questions to ask include:

■ Have you ever had severe fatigue not caused by exertion?

■ Do you use alcohol, tobacco, or caffeine?

■ Do you take any prescription, over-the-counter, or recreational drugs? If so, which ones?

■ Are you allergic to any drugs, foods, or other products? If so, describe the reaction you experienced.

In addition, ask the female patient:

■ Have you begun menopause?

- Do you use oral contraceptives or estrogen?
- Have you ever experienced any medical problems during pregnancy? Have you ever had pregnancy-induced hypertension?

FAMILY HISTORY

Information about the patient's blood relatives may suggest a specific cardiac problem. Ask him if anyone in his family has ever had hypertension, diabetes mellitus, coronary artery disease (CAD), vascular disease, or hyperlipidemia.

SOCIAL HISTORY

Obtain information about your patient's occupation, educational background, living arrangements, daily activities, and family relationships. Explore any potentially stressful circumstances. Be sure to ask about his employment, exercise habits, and diet.

Throughout the history-taking session, note the appropriateness of the patient's responses, his speech clarity, and his mood so that you can better identify changes later on.

PHYSICAL EXAMINATION

Before assessing the patient's cardiovascular system, you must assess the factors that reflect cardiovascular function. These include general appearance, body weight, vital signs, and related body structures.

Prepare for the examination by washing your hands and gathering the necessary equipment. Choose a room that affords privacy. Adjust the thermostat if necessary; cool temperatures may alter the patient's skin temperature and color, heart rate, and blood pressure. Make sure the room is quiet. If possible, close the door and windows, and turn off radios and noisy equipment.

Combine parts of the assessment, as needed, to conserve time and the patient's energy. If the patient experiences cardiovascular difficulties, alter the order of your assessment as needed. For example, if he develops chest pain and dyspnea, quickly check his vital signs and then auscultate the heart.

If a female patient feels embarrassed about exposing her chest, explain each assessment step beforehand and use drapes appropriately, exposing only the area being assessed at the moment.

ASSESSING APPEARANCE

Begin by observing the patient's general appearance, particularly noting weight and muscle composition. Is he well developed, well nourished, alert, and energetic? Document any departures from the norm. Does the patient appear older than his chronological age or seem unusually tired or slow-moving?

Measuring height and weight. Accurately measure and record the patient's height and weight. These

---

Key questions for assessing cardiac function

Ask the following questions to help the patient more accurately describe his symptoms of cardiovascular illness:

- Can you point to the site of your pain?
- Do you get a burning or squeezing sensation in your chest?
- What relieves the pain?
- Do you ever feel short of breath? Does a particular body position seem to bring this on? Which one? How long does shortness of breath last? What relieves it?
- How many pillows do you use for sleeping?
- Has sudden breathing trouble ever awakened you from sleep?
- Do you ever wake up coughing? How often?
- Have you ever coughed up blood?
- Does your heart ever pound or skip a beat? If so, when does this happen?
- Do you ever get dizzy or faint? What seems to bring this on?
- Do your feet or ankles swell? At what time of day? Does anything relieve the swelling?
- Do you urinate more frequently at night?
- Do any activities tire you? Which ones? Have you had to limit your activities or rest more often while doing them?

---

measurements will help guide treatment plans, determine medication dosages, assist with nutritional counseling, and detect fluid overload. Fluctuations in weight may prove significant, especially when extreme. For example, a patient developing heart failure may gain several pounds overnight.

Next, assess for cachexia—weakness and muscle wasting. Observe the amount of muscle bulk in the upper arms, thighs, and chest wall. For a more precise measurement, calculate the percentage of body fat. For men, this should be 12%; for women, 18%. A patient with chronic cardiac disease may develop cachexia, losing body fat and muscle mass, though edema may mask these effects. Loss of the body's energy stores slows healing and impairs immune function.

ASSESSING VITAL SIGNS

This includes measurement of temperature, blood pressure, and pulse and respiratory rates.

Measuring temperature. Fever can indicate cardiovascular inflammation or infection. Mild to moderate fever usually occurs 2 to 5 days after a myocardial infarction (MI), when the healing infarct passes through the inflammatory stage. It can also accompany acute pericarditis. Higher elevations accompany infections such as infective endocarditis, which causes fever spikes.

Increased metabolism will lead to fever and heightened cardiac workload. As a result, you need to assess a febrile patient with heart disease for signs of increased cardiac workload, such as tachycardia.

Taking blood pressure. First palpate and then auscultate the blood pressure in an arm or a leg. Wait 3 to 5 minutes between measurements. Normally, blood pressure measures less than 140/90 mm Hg in a resting adult and 78/46 to 114/78 mm Hg in a young child.

According to the American Heart Association, blood pressure above 140/90 mm Hg on three successive readings indicates hypertension. However, emotional stress caused by the physical examination may elevate blood pressure. If the patient's blood pressure is high, allow him to relax for several minutes and measure again to rule out anxiety.

When assessing a patient's blood pressure for the first time, take measurements in both arms. A difference of 10 mm Hg or more between arms may indicate thoracic outlet syndrome or other forms of arterial obstruction.

If the blood pressure is elevated in both arms, measure the pressure in the thigh. Wrap a large cuff around the patient's upper leg at least 1″ (2.5 cm) above the knee. Place the stethoscope over the popliteal artery, located on the posterior surface slightly above the knee joint. Listen for sounds when the bladder of the cuff is deflated. High pressure in the arms with normal or low pressure in the legs suggests aortic coarctation.

Determining pulse pressure. Subtract diastolic pressure from systolic pressure. The result reflects pulse pressure—arterial pressure during the resting phase of the cardiac cycle—which normally ranges from 30 to 50 mm Hg.

Pulse pressure rises when the stroke volume increases, as in exercise, anxiety, or bradycardia. It also rises when peripheral vascular resistance or aortic distention declines, as in anemia, hyperthyroidism, fever, hypertension, aortic coarctation, or aging.

Pulse pressure diminishes when a mechanical obstruction exists, as in mitral or aortic stenosis; when the peripheral vessels constrict, as in shock; or when stroke volume declines, as in heart failure, hypovolemia, or tachycardia.

Checking radial pulse. If you suspect cardiac disease, palpate for a full minute to detect any arrhythmias. Normally, an adult's pulse ranges from 60 to 100 beats/minute. Its rhythm should feel regular, except for a subtle slowing on expiration caused by changes in intrathoracic pressure and vagal response.

Evaluating respirations. Observe for eupnea—a regular, unlabored, and bilaterally equal breathing pattern. Tachypnea may indicate low cardiac output. Dyspnea, a possible indicator of heart failure, may not be evident at rest. However, the patient may pause after only a few words to take a breath. A Cheyne-Stokes respiratory pattern may accompany severe heart failure, although it's more commonly associated with coma.

ASSESSING THE SKIN

Because normal skin color can vary widely among individuals, ask the patient if his present skin tone is normal. Then inspect the skin color and note any cyanosis. Examine the underside of the tongue, buccal mucosa, and conjunctiva for signs of central cyanosis. Inspect the lips, tip of the nose, earlobes, and nail beds for signs of peripheral cyanosis.

In a dark-skinned patient, inspect the oral mucous membranes, such as the lips and gingivae, which normally appear pink and moist but will be ashen if cyanotic. Because the color range for normal mucous membranes is narrower than that for the skin, they provide a more accurate assessment.

Central cyanosis suggests reduced oxygen intake or transport from the lungs to the bloodstream, conditions that may occur with heart failure. Peripheral cyanosis suggests constriction of peripheral arterioles, a natural response to cold or anxiety or a result of hypovolemia, cardiogenic shock, or a vasoconstrictive disease.

When evaluating the patient's skin color, also observe for flushing and pallor. Flushing can result from medications, excess heat, or anxiety or fear. Pallor can result from anemia or increased peripheral vascular resistance caused by atherosclerosis.

Next, assess the patient's perfusion by evaluating arterial flow adequacy. With the patient lying down, elevate one of his legs 12″ (30 cm) above heart level for 60 seconds. Next, tell him to sit up and dangle both legs. Compare the color of both legs. The leg that was elevated should show mild pallor compared with the other leg. Color should return to the pale leg in about 10 seconds, and the veins should refill in about 15 seconds. Suspect arterial insufficiency if the patient's foot shows marked pallor, delayed color return that ends with a mottled appearance, or delayed venous filling or if the leg shows marked redness.

Touch the patient's skin; it should feel warm and dry. Cool, clammy skin results from vasoconstriction, which occurs when cardiac output is low, as in shock. Warm, moist skin results from vasodilation, which occurs when cardiac output is high—for example, during exercise.

Next, evaluate skin turgor by grasping and raising the skin between two fingers and then letting it go. Normally, the skin returns to its original position immediately. Taut, shiny skin that can't be grasped may result from ascites or the marked edema that accompanies heart failure Skin that doesn't return to the original position immediately exhibits tenting, a sign of decreased skin turgor, which may result from dehydration, especially if the patient takes diuretics. It also may result from age or malnutrition or as an adverse reaction to corticosteroid treatment.

Next, observe the skin for signs of edema. Inspect the patient's arms and legs for symmetrical swelling. Because edema usually affects lower or dependent areas of the body first, be especially alert when assessing the arms, hands, legs, feet, and ankles of an ambulatory patient or the buttocks and sacrum of a bedridden patient. Determine the type of edema present (pitting or nonpitting) as well as its location, extent, and symmetry (unilateral or symmetrical). If the patient has pitting edema, assess the degree of pitting.

Edema can result from heart failure or venous insufficiency caused by varicosities or thrombophlebitis. Chronic right-sided heart failure may even cause ascites, which leads to generalized edema and abdominal distention. Venous compression may result in localized edema along the path of the compressed vessel.

While inspecting the patient's skin, note the location, size, number, and appearance of any lesions. Dry, open lesions on the lower extremities accompanied by pallor, cool skin, and lack of hair growth signify arterial insufficiency, perhaps caused by arterial peripheral vascular disease. Wet, open lesions with red or purplish edges that appear on the legs may result from the venous stasis associated with venous peripheral vascular disease.

ASSESSING THE ARMS AND LEGS
Inspect the hair on the patient's arms and legs. Hair should be distributed symmetrically and should grow thicker on the anterior surface of the arms and legs. If not, it may indicate diminished arterial blood flow to the arms and legs.

Note whether the length of the arms and legs is proportionate to the length of the trunk. Long, thin arms and legs may indicate Marfan syndrome, a congenital disorder that causes cardiovascular problems, such as aortic dissection, aortic valve incompetence, and cardiomyopathy.

ASSESSING THE FINGERNAILS
Fingernails normally appear pinkish with no markings. A bluish color in the nail beds indicates peripheral cyanosis.

To estimate the rate of peripheral blood flow, assess capillary refill in the fingernails. Apply pressure to the patient's fingernail for 5 seconds. Then remove the pressure and observe how rapidly the normal color returns to the fingernail. Note how many seconds it takes for the color to return to the nail. In a patient with a good arterial supply, color should return in less than 3 seconds. Delayed capillary refill suggests reduced circulation to that area, a sign of low cardiac output, which may lead to arterial insufficiency.

Assess the angle between the nail and the cuticle. An angle of 180 degrees or greater indicates finger clubbing. Check for enlarged fingertips with spongey, slightly swollen nail bases. Finger clubbing commonly indicates chronic tissue hypoxia.

The shape of the nails should be smooth and rounded. A concave depression in the middle of a thin nail indicates koilonychia (spoon nail), a sign of iron deficiency anemia.

Finally, check for splinter hemorrhages—small, thin, red or brown lines that run from the base to the tip of the nail. Splinter hemorrhages develop in patients with bacterial endocarditis.

ASSESSING THE EYES
Inspect the eyelids for xanthelasmas—small, slightly raised, yellowish plaques that usually appear around the inner canthus. These plaques result from lipid deposits and may signal severe hyperlipidemia, a risk factor of cardiac disease.

Observe the color of the sclerae. Yellowish sclerae may be the first sign of jaundice, which occasionally results from liver congestion caused by right-sided heart failure.

Next, check for arcus senilis—a thin grayish ring around the edge of the cornea. A normal occurrence in old age, arcus senilis can indicate hyperlipidemia in patients under age 65.

Using an ophthalmoscope, examine the retinal structures, including the retinal vessels and background. The retina is normally light yellow to orange, and the background should be free from hemorrhages and exudates. Structural changes, such as narrowing or blocking of a vein where an arteriole crosses over, indicate hypertension. Soft exudates may suggest hypertension or subacute bacterial endocarditis.

ASSESSING FOR HEAD MOVEMENT
A slight, rhythmic bobbing of the head in time with the heartbeat (Musset's sign) may accompany the high back pressure caused by aortic insufficiency or aneurysm.

Estimating CVP

To estimate a patient's central venous pressure (CVP), determine the height from the right atrium to the highest level of visible pulsation in the jugular vein. Follow the steps listed below.

■ Place the patient at a 45-degree angle and use tangential lighting to observe the internal jugular vein. Note the highest level of visible pulsation.
■ Locate the angle of Louis, or sternal notch, by palpating the clavicles where they join the sternum (the suprasternal notch). Place two of your fingers on the suprasternal notch and slide them down the sternum until they reach a bony

protuberance. This is the angle of Louis. The right atrium lies about 2″ (5 cm) below this point.
■ Measure the vertical distance between the highest level of visible pulsation and the angle of Louis. Normally, this distance is less than 1⅛″ (3 cm). Add 2″ to this figure to estimate the distance between the highest level of pulsation and the right atrium. A distance greater than 4″ (10 cm) may indicate elevated CVP and right-sided heart failure.

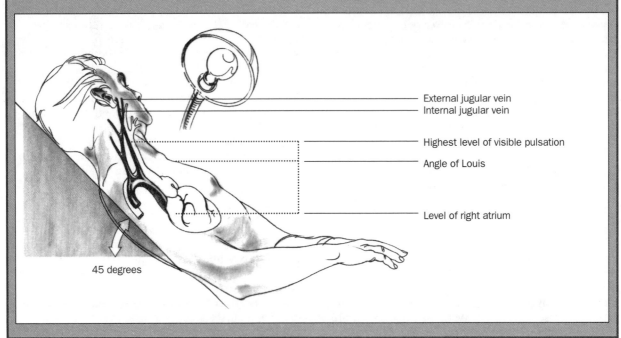

External jugular vein
Internal jugular vein

Highest level of visible pulsation

Angle of Louis

Level of right atrium

45 degrees

INSPECTION
Inspect the patient's chest and thorax. Expose the anterior chest and observe its general appearance. Normally, the lateral diameter is twice the anteroposterior diameter. Note any deviations from typical chest shape.

Checking for jugular vein distention. When the patient is supine, the neck veins normally protrude; when the patient stands, they normally lie flat. To check for jugular vein distention, place the patient in semi-Fowler's position with the head turned slightly away from the side being examined. Use tangential lighting (lighting from the side) to cast small shadows along the neck. This will allow you to see pulse wave movement better. Distended jugular veins indicate

high right atrial pressure and an increase in fluid volume caused by right-sided heart dysfunction.

Characterize distention as mild, moderate, or severe. Determine the degree of distention in fingerbreadths above the clavicle or in relation to the jaw or clavicle. Also note the amount of distention in relation to head elevation.

You can use jugular vein distention to obtain a rough estimate of central venous pressure (CVP). (See *Estimating CVP*.) In addition, observing pulsations of the right internal jugular vein will help to assess right-sided heart dynamics.

Inspecting the precordium. Before inspecting the area over the heart, place the patient in the supine position, with the head flat or elevated for respiratory comfort. Stand to the right of the patient. Then identify the necessary anatomic landmarks. (See *Inspecting and palpating the precordium.*)

Using tangential lighting to cast shadows across the chest, watch for chest wall movement, visible pulsations, and exaggerated lifts or heaves (strong outward thrusts palpated over the chest during systole) in all areas of the precordium. Ask an obese patient or a patient with large breasts to sit during inspection. This brings the heart closer to the anterior chest wall and makes pulsations more noticeable.

Normally, you'll see pulsations at the point of maximal impulse (PMI) of the apical impulse. The apical impulse (pulsations at the apex of the heart) normally appears in the fifth intercostal space at or just medial to the midclavicular line. This impulse reflects the location and size of the heart, especially of the left ventricle. In thin adults and in children, you may see a slight sternal movement and pulsations over the pulmonary arteries or the aorta as well as visible pulsations in the epigastric area.

Abnormal findings. Inspection may reveal barrel chest (rounded thoracic cage caused by chronic obstructive pulmonary disease), pectus excavatum (depressed sternum), scoliosis (lateral curvature of the spine), or kyphosis (convex curvature of the thoracic spine). If severe enough, these conditions can impair cardiac output by preventing chest expansion and inhibiting heart muscle movement.

Retractions (visible indentations of the soft tissue covering the chest wall) or the use of accessory muscles to breathe typically results from a respiratory disorder but may also indicate respiratory effects of cardiovascular disorders, such as a congenital heart defect or heart failure.

Other abnormal findings include:
■ any visible pulsation to the right of the sternum, a possible indication of aortic aneurysm
■ a pulsation in the sternoclavicular or epigastric area, a possible indication of aortic aneurysm
■ a sustained, forceful apical impulse, a possible indication of left ventricular hypertrophy, which increases blood pressure and may cause cardiomyopathy and mitral regurgitation
■ a laterally displaced apical impulse, a possible sign of left ventricular hypertrophy.

PALPATION

Palpate the peripheral pulses and precordium. Make sure that the patient is positioned comfortably, draped appropriately, and kept warm. Also, warm your hands and remember to use gentle to moderate pressure.

Palpating pulses. During assessment of vital signs, you palpated the radial pulse. Now palpate the other

Inspecting and palpating the precordium

Use the guidelines below when inspecting and palpating the precordium.

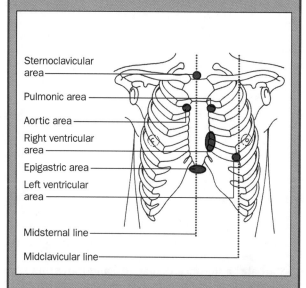

- Sternoclavicular area
- Pulmonic area
- Aortic area
- Right ventricular area
- Epigastric area
- Left ventricular area
- Midsternal line
- Midclavicular line

■ Locate the six precordial areas by using the anatomic landmarks named for the underlying structures.
■ Palpate (or inspect) the *sternoclavicular area*, which lies at the top of the sternum at the junction of the clavicles.
■ Move to the *aortic area*, located in the second intercostal space on the right sternal border.
■ Assess the *pulmonic area*, found in the second intercostal space on the left sternal border.
■ Palpate the *right ventricular area*, the point where the fifth rib joins the left sternal border.
■ Then assess the *left ventricular area (apical area)*, which falls at the fifth intercostal space at the midclavicular line (see illustration).
■ Finally, palpate the *epigastric area*, located at the base of the sternum between the cartilage of the left and right seventh ribs.

major pulse points to assess blood flow to the tissues. The larger central arteries (the carotids) lie closer to the heart, have slightly higher pressures, and demonstrate pulsations earlier than the peripheral arteries. This makes the carotids easier to palpate.

Palpate the carotid, brachial, radial, femoral, popliteal, dorsalis pedis, and posterior tibial pulses. These arteries are close to the body surface and lie over bones, making palpation easier. Press gently over the pulse sites; excess pressure can obliterate the pulsation, making the pulse appear absent. Also, palpate only one carotid artery at a time; simultaneous palpation can slow the pulse or decrease blood pressure, causing the patient to faint.

Look for the following:
- pulse rate—varies with age and other factors; in adults, usually ranges from 60 to 100 beats/minute
- pulse rhythm—should be regular
- symmetry—pulses should be equally strong bilaterally
- contour—the wavelike flow of the pulse, the upstroke and downstroke, should be smooth
- strength—pulses should be easily palpable; obliterating the pulse should require strong finger pressure.

Grade the pulse amplitude bilaterally at each site. Use a pulse rating scale such as a 3+ scale, in which 0 = absent, 1 = weak, 2 = normal, and 3 = bounding. Document any variations in rate, rhythm, contour, symmetry, and strength.

Palpating the precordium. Follow a systematic palpation sequence covering the sternoclavicular, aortic, pulmonic, right ventricular, left ventricular (apical), and epigastric areas. Use the pads of the fingers to effectively assess large pulse sites; finger pads are especially sensitive to vibrations.

Start at the sternoclavicular area and move methodically through the palpation sequence down to the epigastric area. At the sternoclavicular area, you may feel pulsation of the aortic arch, especially in a thin or average-build patient. In a thin patient, you may palpate a pulsation in the abdominal aorta over the epigastric area.

To locate the apical impulse, place your fingers in the fifth intercostal space at or just medial to the midclavicular line. Usually, you palpate the apical pulse best at the PMI; light palpation should reveal a tap with each heartbeat over a space roughly ¾″ (2 cm) in diameter.

Moderately strong, the apical impulse demonstrates a swift upstroke and downstroke early in systole, caused by left ventricular movement. It normally lasts for about one-third of the cardiac cycle if the heart rate is under 100 beats/minute. It should correlate with the first heart sound and carotid pulsation.

You should not be able to palpate pulsations over the aortic, pulmonic, or right ventricular area.

Abnormal findings. Palpation may reveal:
- a weak pulse—indicating low cardiac output or increased peripheral vascular resistance, as in arterial atherosclerotic disease. Elderly patients commonly have weak pedal pulses. Absence of a pulse in a warm foot with normal color carries little significance.
- a strong bounding pulse—occurs in hypertension and in high cardiac output states such as exercise, pregnancy, anemia, and thyrotoxicosis

- an apical impulse that exerts unusual force and lasts longer than one-third of the cardiac cycle—a possible indication of increased cardiac output
- a displaced or diffuse impulse—a possible indication of left ventricular hypertrophy
- a pulsation in the aortic, pulmonic, or right ventricular area—a sign of chamber enlargement or valvular disease
- a pulsation in the sternoclavicular or epigastric area—a sign of an aortic aneurysm
- a palpable thrill (fine vibration)—the main indication of blood flow turbulence, usually related to valvular dysfunction; determine how far the thrill radiates and make a mental note to listen for a murmur at this site during auscultation
- a heave (a strong outward thrust during systole) along the left sternal border—an indication of right ventricular hypertrophy
- a heave over the left ventricular area—a sign of a ventricular aneurysm. Note that a thin patient may experience a heave with exercise, fever, or anxiety because of increased cardiac output and more forceful contraction.
- a displaced PMI—a possible indication of left ventricular hypertrophy caused by volume overload from mitral or aortic stenosis, septal defect, acute MI, or other disorder.

PERCUSSION
Mediate percussion of the heart's borders enables you to estimate the organ's size. Beginning at the anterior left axillary line, percuss toward the sternum in the fifth intercostal space. The percussion note changes from resonance to dullness at the left border of the heart, usually near the PMI. Locate the left border of the heart at the midclavicular line in the fifth intercostal space. If the border extends to the left of the midclavicular line, the heart—and especially the left ventricle—may be enlarged. The right border of the heart lies under the sternum and cannot be percussed.

Note, however, that chest X-rays provide more accurate information and usually eliminate the need for percussion. Also, lung problems that commonly accompany cardiovascular disorders reduce the accuracy of percussion.

AUSCULTATION
The cardiovascular system requires more auscultation than any other body system.

Auscultating the precordium. Practice auscultating and identifying heart sounds in the precordium. First gain experience identifying normal heart sounds, rates, and rhythms. Then auscultate patients with known abnormal sounds, seeking help from experts to identify findings.

Expect some difficulty. Even with a stethoscope, the amount of tissue between the source of the sound and the outer chest wall can affect what you hear. Fat, muscle, and air tend to reduce sound transmission. When auscultating an obese patient or one with a muscular chest wall or hyperinflated lungs, sounds may seem distant and difficult to hear.

Make sure that the room remains as quiet as possible. If the patient has special equipment, such as an oxygen nebulizer or a suction device, perform auscultation with the equipment turned off, if possible.

Select a stethoscope with a chestpiece that's an appropriate size for the patient's chest. Consider choosing a pediatric chestpiece for a thin adult. Use the diaphragm of the stethoscope to detect the normal higher-pitched heart sounds (S_1 and S_2). Use the bell to identify low-pitched sounds, such as mitral murmurs and gallops.

Help the patient into a supine position, either flat or at a comfortable elevation. If you're right-handed, stand at the patient's right side. This allows you to manipulate the stethoscope with your dominant hand.

If the heart sounds seem faint or undetectable, reposition the patient. Alternative positioning may enhance the sounds or make them seem louder by bringing the heart closer to the chest's surface. Common alternative positions include a seated, forward-leaning position and the left-lateral decubitus position.

Because clothing and surgical dressings will muffle heart sounds or render them inaudible, open the front of the patient's gown and drape the patient appropriately.

Explain the procedure to the patient, and instruct him to breathe normally, inhaling through the nose and exhaling through the mouth. Finally, warm the stethoscope chestpiece by rubbing it between your hands.

Identify cardiac auscultation sites. Most normal heart sounds result from vibrations created by the opening and closing of the heart valves. When valves close, they suddenly terminate the motion of blood; when valves open, they accelerate the motion of blood. This sudden acceleration or deceleration is responsible for producing heart sounds. Auscultation sites lie not directly over the valves, but over the pathways the blood takes as it flows through chambers and valves. (See *Auscultation sites and abnormal heart sounds,* pages 64 and 65.)

Now auscultate, listening selectively for each cardiac cycle component. Move the stethoscope slowly and methodically over the four main auscultation sites.

You'll need to concentrate to hear these relatively quiet sounds. Closing your eyes while you listen may help. Noise from stethoscope movement (especially over chest hair) or patient movement or shivering will prevent you from hearing sounds clearly. So keep your hand steady, and ask the patient to remain as still as possible.

Begin by listening for a few cycles to become accustomed to the rate and rhythm of the sounds. Two sounds normally occur: the first heart sound (S_1) and the second heart sound (S_2). They sound relatively high pitched and are separated by a silent period.

You'll characterize heart sounds by their pitch (frequency), intensity (loudness), duration, quality (such as musical or harsh), location, and radiation. The timing of heart sounds in relation to the cardiac cycle is particularly important. Normal heart sounds last only a fraction of a second and are followed by slightly longer periods of silence.

The first heart sound—the *lub* of *lub-dub*—marks the beginning of systole. It occurs as the mitral and tricuspid valves close. The closing of these valves immediately precedes elevation of ventricular pressure, aortic and pulmonic valve opening, and ejection of blood into the circulation. All this occurs within one-third of a second.

The mitral valve actually closes slightly before the tricuspid valve. An experienced examiner may be able to discriminate the corresponding sound (split S_1), which sounds somewhat like *li-lub*. However, an inexperienced examiner may confuse a split S_1 with an abnormal extra sound occurring just before S_1.

The first heart sound is louder in the mitral and tricuspid listening areas (*LUB-dub*) and softer in the aortic and pulmonic areas (*lub-DUB*). Comparing the loudness of the normal heart sounds at each site will help you differentiate systole from diastole. Learning to identify phases of the cardiac cycle will enable you to time abnormal sounds.

The second heart sound—the *dub* of *lub-dub*—occurs at the beginning of diastole. The S_2 sound coincides with the closing of the aortic and pulmonic valves; it's louder in the aortic and pulmonic areas of the chest. At these sites, the sequence sounds like *lub-DUB*. The second heart sound coincides with the pulse downstroke. At normal rates, the diastolic pause between S_2 and the next S_1 exceeds the systolic pause between S_1 and S_2.

During auscultation, S_2 may have a split sound like that of a broken syllable. This may occur normally when the aortic and pulmonic valves don't close at exactly the same time. A split S_2 commonly occurs in healthy children and young adults.

At each auscultatory site, use the diaphragm to listen closely to S_1 and S_2 and compare them. Next, listen to the systolic period and the diastolic period. Then, auscultate again, using the bell of the stethoscope. If you hear any sounds during the diastolic or

Auscultation sites and abnormal heart sounds

When auscultating for heart sounds, place the stethoscope over four different sites. Follow the same auscultation sequence during every cardiovascular assessment.

■ Place the stethoscope in the second intercostal space along the right sternal border. In the aortic area, blood moves from the left ventricle during systole, crossing the aortic valve and flowing through the aortic arch.
■ Move to the pulmonic area, located in the second intercostal space at the left sternal border. In the pulmonic area, blood ejected from the right ventricle during systole crosses the pulmonic valve and flows through the main pulmonary artery.

■ Assess in the third auscultation site, the tricuspid area, which lies in the fifth intercostal space along the left sternal border. In the tricuspid area, sounds reflect blood movement from the right atrium across the tricuspid valve, filling the right ventricle during diastole.
■ Finally, listen in the mitral area, located in the fifth intercostal space near the midclavicular line. (If the patient's heart is enlarged, the mitral area may be closer to the anterior axillary line.) In the mitral, or apical, area, sounds represent blood flow across the mitral valve and left ventricular filling during diastole.

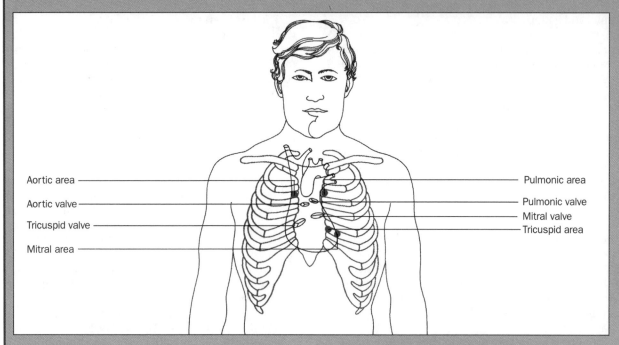

Aortic area
Aortic valve
Tricuspid valve
Mitral area

Pulmonic area
Pulmonic valve
Mitral valve
Tricuspid area

systolic period or any variations in S_1 and S_2, document the characteristics of the sound. Note the auscultatory site and the part of the cardiac cycle during which it occurred.

Abnormal heart sounds. Auscultation may detect first and second heart sounds that are accentuated, diminished, or inaudible. These abnormalities may result from pressure changes, valvular dysfunctions, or conduction defects. A prolonged, persistent, or reversed split sound may result from a mechanical or electrical problem. Auscultation may reveal a third heart sound, a fourth heart sound, or both.

Third heart sound. Also known as S_3 or a ventricular gallop, this low-pitched sound is heard best with the bell of the stethoscope. Its rhythm resembles a horse galloping, and its cadence resembles the word "Kentuc-KY" (*lub-dub-by*). Listen for S_3 with the patient supine or in the left-lateral decubitus position.

S_3 usually occurs during early to mid-diastole, at the end of the passive filling phase of either ventricle. It may signify that the ventricle is not compliant enough to accept the filling volume without additional force. If the right ventricle is noncompliant, the sound will occur in the tricuspid area; if the left ventricle is noncompliant, in the mitral area. A heave may be palpable when the sound occurs.

Implications of abnormal heart sounds

Upon detecting an abnormal heart sound, you must accurately identify the sound as well as its location and timing in the cardiac cycle. This information will help you identify the possible cause of the sound. The chart below lists abnormal heart sounds with their possible causes.

Abnormal heart sound	Timing	Possible causes
ACCENTUATED S₁	Beginning of systole	Mitral stenosis, fever
DIMINISHED S₁	Beginning of systole	Mitral regurgitation, severe mitral regurgitation with calcified immobile valve, heart block
ACCENTUATED S₂	End of systole	Pulmonary or systemic hypertension
DIMINISHED OR INAUDIBLE S₂	End of systole	Aortic or pulmonic stenosis
PERSISTENT S₂ SPLIT	End of systole	Delayed closure of the pulmonic valve, usually from overfilling of the right ventricle, causing prolonged systolic ejection time
REVERSED OR PARADOXICAL S₂ SPLIT (appears on expiration and disappears on inspiration)	End of systole	Delayed ventricular stimulation, left bundle-branch block or prolonged left ventricular ejection time
S₃ (ventricular gallop)	Early diastole	Normal in children and young adults, overdistention of ventricles in rapid-filling segment of diastole, mitral insufficiency or ventricular failure
S₄ (atrial gallop or presystolic extra sound)	Late diastole	Forceful atrial contraction from resistance to ventricular filling late in diastole, left ventricular hypertrophy, pulmonic stenosis, hypertension, coronary artery disease, and aortic stenosis
PERICARDIAL FRICTION RUB (grating or leathery sound at left sternal border; usually muffled, high pitched, and transient)	Throughout systole and diastole	Pericardial inflammation

S_3 may occur normally in a child or young adult. In a patient over age 30, it usually indicates a disorder such as right- or left-sided heart failure, pulmonary congestion, intracardiac shunting of blood, MI, anemia, or thyrotoxicosis.

Fourth heart sound. This abnormal heart sound, known as S_4, occurs late in diastole, just before the pulse upstroke. It immediately precedes the S_1 of the next cycle and is associated with acceleration and deceleration of blood entering a chamber that resists additional filling. Also known as an atrial or presystolic gallop, it occurs during atrial contraction.

The fourth heart sound shares the same cadence as the word "TEN-nes-see" (*le-lub-dub*). Heard best with the bell of the stethoscope and with the patient supine, S_4 may occur in the tricuspid or mitral area, depending on which ventricle is dysfunctional.

Although rare, S_4 may occur normally in a young patient with a thin chest wall. In most cases, however, it indicates cardiovascular disease, such as acute MI, hypertension, CAD, cardiomyopathy, angina, anemia, elevated left ventricular pressure, or aortic stenosis. If the sound persists, it may indicate impaired ventricular compliance or volume overload. S_4 commonly appears in elderly patients with age-related systolic hypertension and aortic stenosis.

Summation gallop. Occasionally a patient may have both a third and a fourth heart sound. Auscultation may reveal two separate abnormal heart sounds and two normal sounds. Usually, the patient has tachycardia and a shortened diastole. S_3 and S_4 occur so close together that they appear to be one sound—a summation gallop.

Murmurs. Longer than a heart sound, a murmur occurs as a vibrating, blowing, or rumbling noise. Just as turbulent water in a stream babbles as it passes through a narrow point, turbulent blood flow produces a murmur.

If you detect a murmur, identify where it's loudest, pinpoint when in the cardiac cycle it occurs, and describe its pitch, pattern, quality, and intensity.

Location and timing. Murmurs may occur in any cardiac auscultatory site and may radiate from one site to another. To identify the radiation area, auscultate from the site where the murmur seems loudest to the farthest site where it's still heard. Note the anatomic landmark of this farthest site.

Determine if the murmur occurs during systole (between S_1 and S_2) or diastole (between S_2 and the next S_1). Pinpoint when in the cardiac cycle the murmur occurs—for example, mid-diastole or late systole. Occasionally, murmurs occur during both portions of the cycle (continuous murmur).

Pitch. Depending on the rate and pressure of blood flow, a murmur's pitch may be high, medium, or low. You can hear a *low-pitched murmur* with the bell of the stethoscope, but not with the diaphragm; a *high-pitched murmur* with the diaphragm, but not with the bell; a *medium-pitched murmur* with both.

Pattern. Crescendo occurs when the velocity of blood flow increases and the murmur becomes louder. *Decrescendo* occurs when velocity decreases and the murmur becomes quieter. A *crescendo-decrescendo pattern* describes a murmur with increasing loudness followed by increasing softness.

Quality. The volume of blood flow, the force of the contraction, and the degree of valve compromise all contribute to murmur quality. Terms used to describe quality include musical, blowing, harsh, rasping, rumbling, or machinelike.

Intensity. Use the following standard, six-level grading scale to describe the intensity of a murmur:
- grade 1—extremely faint; barely audible even to the trained ear
- grade 2—soft and low; easily audible to the trained ear
- grade 3—moderately loud; about equal to the intensity of normal heart sounds
- grade 4—loud with a palpable thrill at the murmur site
- grade 5—very loud with a palpable thrill; audible with the stethoscope in partial contact with the chest
- grade 6—extremely loud with a palpable thrill; audible with the stethoscope over (but not in contact with) the chest.

Causes. An *innocent* or *functional murmur* may appear in a patient without heart disease. Heard best in the pulmonic area, it occurs early in systole and seldom exceeds grade 2 in intensity. When the patient changes from a supine to a sitting position, the murmur may disappear. If fever, exercise, anemia, anxiety, pregnancy, or other factors increase cardiac output, the murmur may increase in intensity. Innocent murmurs affect up to 25% of all children but usually disappear by adolescence.

Elderly patients who experience changes in the aortic valve structures and the aorta also experience a nonpathologic murmur. This murmur occurs as a short systolic murmur heard best at the left sternal border.

Pathologic murmurs may occur during systole or diastole and may affect any heart valve. They may result from valvular stenosis (inability of the valves to open properly), valvular insufficiency (inability of the valves to close properly, allowing regurgitation of blood), or a septal defect (a defect in the septal wall separating two heart chambers).

Other abnormal heart sounds. During auscultation, three other abnormal sounds may occur: clicks, snaps, and rubs.

Clicks. These high-pitched abnormal heart sounds result from tensing of the chordae tendineae structures and mitral valve cusps. Initially, the mitral valve closes securely, but a large cusp prolapses into the left atrium. The click usually precedes a late systolic murmur caused by regurgitation of a little blood from the left ventricle into the left atrium. Clicks occur in 5% to 10% of young adults and affect more women than men.

To detect the high-pitched click of mitral valve prolapse, place the stethoscope diaphragm at the apex and listen during mid- to late systole. To enhance the sound, have the patient sit or stand, and listen along the lower left sternal border.

Snaps. Upon placing the stethoscope diaphragm medial to the apex along the lower left sternal border, you may detect an opening snap immediately after S_2. The snap resembles the normal S_1 and S_2 in quality; its high pitch helps differentiate it from an S_3. Because the opening snap may accompany mitral or tricuspid stenosis, it usually precedes a mid- to late diastolic murmur—a classic sign of stenosis. It results from the stenotic valve attempting to open.

Rubs. To detect a pericardial friction rub, use the diaphragm of the stethoscope to auscultate in the third left intercostal space along the lower left sternal border. Listen for a harsh, scratchy, scraping, or squeaking sound that occurs throughout systole, diastole, or both. To enhance the sound, have the patient sit upright and lean forward or exhale. A rub usually indicates pericarditis.

AUSCULTATION OF ARTERIES

Auscultate the carotid, femoral, and popliteal arteries as well as the abdominal aorta. (See *Performing arterial auscultation*.) Over the carotid, femoral, and popliteal arteries, auscultation should reveal no sounds; over the abdominal aorta, it may detect bowel sounds, but no vascular sounds.

During auscultation of the central and peripheral arteries, you may notice a bruit—a continuous sound caused by turbulent blood flow. A bruit over the carotid artery usually indicates atherosclerosis; over the femoral or popliteal arteries, narrowed vessels; and over the abdominal aorta, an aneurysm (weakness in the arterial wall that allows a sac to form) or a dissection (a tear in the layers of the arterial wall).

DIAGNOSTIC TESTING

Today, safe and effective nursing care means, in part, becoming fully familiar with commonly performed diagnostic tests and keeping up with rapid advances in testing. These advances have allowed earlier diagnosis and treatment of cardiovascular disorders. For instance, in certain patients, echocardiography—a noninvasive, risk-free test—can provide as much diagnostic information on valvular heart disease as cardiac catheterization—an invasive, high-risk test.

Technological advances have also improved the precision of diagnostic tests. Previously, diagnosis of acute MI depended solely on serial 12-lead electrocardiogram (ECG) and cardiac enzyme studies. Today, electrophysiologic and nuclear imaging tests can pinpoint the exact location and extent of cardiac damage within hours of an acute MI, allowing more effective treatment.

Commonly used diagnostic tests include the following:
- chest X-ray—to detect cardiac enlargement, pulmonary congestion, pleural effusion, and calcium deposits in or on the heart; to show placement of a pacemaker, hemodynamic monitoring lines, or tracheal tubes
- cardiac enzyme levels—to aid in diagnosis of MI and monitor progress of healing
- ECG tracings (including exercise ECG, continuous ambulatory ECG, and pulse wave tracings)—to graphically record electrical current generated by the heart and thus detect conduction abnormalities, arrhythmias, hypertrophy, pericarditis, electrolyte imbalances, MI (including site and extent), and the heart's response to exercise and daily physical and psychological stress
- imaging studies (such as echocardiography and magnetic resonance imaging)—to allow visualization of the heart and its structures in order to evaluate functioning and possible complications
- radionucleide imaging (such as positron emission tomography, thallium scanning, technetium [Tc 99m]

Performing arterial auscultation

Use these steps when auscultating the carotid, femoral, and popliteal arteries and the abdominal aorta.

- Ask the patient to hold his breath while you auscultate.
- Assess the carotid arteries by auscultating with the bell of the stethoscope on both sides of the trachea, as shown.
- To evaluate the femoral and popliteal arteries, place the bell of the stethoscope over the pulse sites that you palpated earlier in the assessment.
- Auscultate the abdominal aorta by listening to the epigastric area.

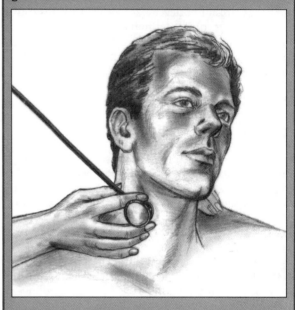

pyrophosphate scanning, and multiple-gated acquisition scanning)—to detect healthy tissue from damaged or diseased tissue and to identify heart regions that don't contract normally
- cardiac catheterization and coronary angiography (see discussion later in this chapter)
- hemodynamic monitoring—to assess cardiac function and determine the effectiveness of therapy by measuring cardiac output, mixed venous oxygen saturation, intracardiac pressures, and blood pressure.

Abdominal aneurysm

An abnormal dilation in the arterial wall, an abdominal aneurysm typically occurs in the aorta between the renal arteries and the iliac branches. These aneurysms, which develop slowly, can be fusiform (spindle-shaped) or saccular (pouchlike).

Abdominal aneurysms begin most commonly in hypertensive white men ages 50 to 80. More than 50% of patients with untreated abdominal aneurysms die of hemorrhage and shock from aneurysmal rupture within 2 years of diagnosis. More than 85% die within 5 years.

CAUSES

About 95% of abdominal aortic aneurysms result from arteriosclerosis or atherosclerosis; the rest, from cystic medial necrosis, trauma, syphilis, and other infections.

Abdominal aneurysms begin when a focal weakness occurs in the muscular layer of the aorta (tunica media) as a result of degenerative changes. This causes the inner layer (tunica intima) and outer layer (tunica adventitia) to stretch outward. Blood pressure within the aorta progressively weakens the vessel walls and enlarges the aneurysm.

DIAGNOSIS AND TREATMENT

Because an abdominal aneurysm seldom produces symptoms, it's typically detected inadvertently on a routine X-ray or during a physical examination.

Several tests can confirm a suspected abdominal aneurysm. Abdominal ultrasonography or echocardiography can determine the size, shape, and location of the aneurysm. Anteroposterior and bilateral X-rays of the abdomen can detect aortic calcification. Computed tomography scanning can note the aneurysm's effect on nearby organs.

An abdominal aneurysm usually requires resection of the aneurysm and Dacron graft replacement of the aortic section. If the aneurysm is small and produces no symptoms, surgery may be delayed, with regular physical examination and ultrasonography performed to monitor its progression. Large or symptomatic aneurysms risk rupture and need immediate repair.

In acute dissection, emergency treatment before surgery includes resuscitation with fluid and blood replacement, I.V. propranolol to reduce myocardial contractility, I.V. nitroprusside to reduce and maintain systolic blood pressure at 100 to 120 mm Hg, and analgesics to relieve pain. An arterial line and indwelling urinary catheter will monitor the patient's condition.

COLLABORATIVE MANAGEMENT

Care of the patient with an abdominal aneurysm focuses on preoperative preparation for surgery and postoperative care to promote optimal body function.

ASSESSMENT

Most patients with abdominal aneurysms are asymptomatic until the aneurysm enlarges and compresses surrounding tissue. A large aneurysm may produce signs and symptoms that mimic renal calculi, lumbar disk disease, and duodenal compression.

The patient may complain of gnawing, generalized, steady abdominal pain or of low back pain that's unaffected by movement. He may have a sensation of gastric or abdominal fullness caused by pressure on the GI structures.

Sudden onset of severe abdominal pain or lumbar pain that radiates to the flank and groin from pressure on lumbar nerves may signify enlargement and imminent rupture. If the aneurysm ruptures into the peritoneal cavity, severe and persistent abdominal and back pain, mimicking renal or ureteral colic, occurs. If it ruptures into the duodenum, GI bleeding occurs with massive hematemesis and melena.

Inspection of the patient with an intact abdominal aneurysm usually reveals no significant findings. However, if the person is not obese, you may note a pulsating mass in the periumbilical area. Auscultation of the abdomen may reveal a systolic bruit over the aorta caused by turbulent blood flow in the widened arterial segment. Hypotension occurs with aneurysm rupture.

Palpation of the abdomen may disclose some tenderness over the affected area and a pulsatile mass; however, avoid deep palpation to locate the mass because this may cause the aneurysm to rupture.

NURSING DIAGNOSES AND COLLABORATIVE PROBLEMS

Based on these nursing diagnoses, you'll establish patient outcomes.

Anxiety related to possible aneurysm rupture. The patient will:
- state feelings of anxiety
- use support systems and perform stress-reduction techniques to assist with coping
- show fewer physical signs of anxiety.

Risk for injury related to possible aneurysm rupture. The patient will:
- avoid activities that increase risk of rupture
- identify the signs of aneurysm rupture and what emergency measures to take
- understand the prescribed medical regimen and importance of follow-up care.

Fluid volume deficit related to hemorrhage caused by aneurysm rupture. The patient will:
- regain normal fluid and blood volume that will remain normal, as evidenced by stable vital signs
- produce adequate urine volume.

Knowledge deficit related to aneurysm, its treatment, and follow-up. The patient will:

- verbalize information about the disease and its treatment
- demonstrate preoperative and postoperative instructions
- state the need for medical follow-up.
Altered renal tissue perfusion related to aneurysm rupture. The patient will:
- maintain hemodynamic status within acceptable parameters
- maintain fluid balance.

PLANNING AND IMPLEMENTATION
The following measures help the patient with an abdominal aneurysm.
- If the patient's condition is acute or becomes acute, expect him to be admitted to the intensive care unit (ICU).
- Administer ordered medications to control the aneurysm's progression. Provide analgesics to relieve pain, if present.
- Prepare the patient for elective surgery, as indicated, or emergency surgery if a rupture occurs. In an emergency, a pneumatic antishock garment may be used while transporting him to the operating room.
- Observe the patient for signs of rupture, which may be immediately fatal. Watch closely for any signs of acute blood loss: decreasing blood pressure; increasing pulse and respiratory rates; cool, clammy skin; restlessness; and decreased sensorium.
- Assess the patient's vital signs, especially blood pressure, every 4 hours or more frequently, depending on the severity of his condition.
- Evaluate kidney function by obtaining blood samples for blood urea nitrogen, creatinine, and electrolyte levels. Measure his intake and output.
- Monitor complete blood count for evidence of blood loss, reflected in decreased hemoglobin, hematocrit, and red blood cell count.
- If the patient's condition is acute, obtain an arterial sample for arterial blood gas analysis as ordered, and monitor cardiac rhythm. Insert an arterial line to allow for continuous blood pressure monitoring. Assist with insertion of a pulmonary artery line to assess hemodynamic balance.
- Allow the patient to express his fears and concerns about the diagnosis. Offer him and his family psychological support. Anticipate additional emotional needs should the aneurysm rupture.
- If the patient is being admitted to the ICU, help ease the family's fears about this type of care, the threat of impending rupture, and any planned surgery.
- If the patient developed complications or requires assistance with his postoperative care and adjustment, provide a referral for home care.

Patient teaching
- Take time to provide appropriate explanations and answer all questions.
- If the patient hasn't had surgery, give him instructions about any limitations or activity restrictions and the signs and symptoms of possible rupture.
- Explain the surgical procedure and the expected postoperative care in the ICU for patients undergoing complex abdominal surgery (I.V. lines, endotracheal and nasogastric intubation, mechanical ventilation).
- Teach the patient and family about any restrictions required after surgery.
- Review the signs and symptom of possible complications, including infection.
- Instruct the patient to take all medications as prescribed and to carry a list of them at all times in case of an emergency.
- Tell the patient not to push, pull, or lift heavy objects until the doctor gives him permission.
- Instruct the patient and family in any measures related to wound care, if appropriate.
- Encourage the patient to make appointments for follow-up care as required.

EVALUATION
Achievement of patient outcomes determines whether collaborative management has succeeded. For a patient with an abdominal aneurysm, evaluation focuses on improved coping skills, adequate safety, fluid balance, and hemodynamic status.

Angina pectoris

Angina pectoris is a term used to describe chest pain that results from an imbalance between myocardial oxygen supply and demand. Angina is common, although its exact incidence is unknown.

Three types of angina have been identified: stable angina, unstable angina, and Prinzmetal's (variant) angina. Stable angina is the most common and predictable form, occurring with a known amount of activity or stress. In this type of angina, the duration and intensity of the pain remain stable.

Unstable angina occurs with increasing frequency, severity, and duration. The pain is unpredictable and may occur with decreasing levels of activity or stress and at rest. Patients with unstable angina are at high risk for myocardial infarction (MI).

Prinzmetal's angina is an atypical form that occurs without an identified precipitating cause. It usually occurs at the same time each day, often waking the patient from sleep. It is caused by coronary artery spasms. An atherosclerotic lesion may or may not be present.

CAUSES

Angina pectoris results from coronary artery disease or any cardiac disease that impedes blood flow. Hypermetabolic conditions, such as anemia, exercise, thyrotoxicosis, stimulants such as caffeine, hyperthyroidism, and emotional stress, can increase myocardial oxygen demand, thereby precipitating angina. Heart failure, congenital heart defects, pulmonary hypertension, left ventricular hypertrophy, and cardiomyopathy can cause a decrease in blood and oxygen supply to the myocardium, leading to anginal attacks.

The coronary arteries normally supply the myocardium with blood to meet its metabolic needs during varying workloads. When the heart needs more blood, the vessels dilate. As the vessels become occluded, they cannot dilate sufficiently to supply the myocardium with blood for normal workloads. A growing mass of plaque in the vessel collects platelets, fibrin, and cellular debris. Platelet aggregations are known to release prostaglandins, which can cause vessel spasm. This in turn promotes platelet aggregation, causing a vicious cycle of events.

Myocardial ischemia develops if the blood supply through the coronary vessels or the oxygen content of the blood is inadequate to meet metabolic demands. Either the supply or the demand is altered. In some patients, the coronary arteries can supply adequate blood when the patient is at rest, but when he attempts activity or becomes stressed in some other manner, angina develops. Myocardial cells become ischemic within 10 seconds of coronary artery occlusion. After several minutes of ischemia, the heart's pumping function is reduced. This reduction deprives the ischemic cells of much-needed oxygen and glucose. The cells convert to an anaerobic metabolism that leaves lactic acid as a waste product. As the lactic acid accumulates, pain develops.

Angina pectoris is usually transient, lasting only 3 to 5 minutes. If blood flow is quickly restored, the patient experiences no permanent myocardial damage. However, reduced blood flow lasting more than 30 minutes causes irreversible damage to myocardial cells.

DIAGNOSIS AND TREATMENT

Diagnostic tests are commonly used to determine the extent and location of the angina and coronary artery disease. These may include electrocardiography (ECG), stress testing, radioisotope imaging, and coronary angiography.

In approximately 25% to 30% of patients with angina, the ECG remains normal. An ECG taken during pain may show transient ischemic attacks with ST-segment elevation. It also may suggest the coronary artery involved and the amount of cardiac muscle affected by the ischemic event. With a stress ECG, ECG or vital sign changes may indicate ischemia.

Radioisotope imaging techniques may show "cold spots," regions of poor perfusion or ischemia that appear as areas of diminished or absent activity. Coronary angiography reveals any partial or complete blockage of the artery.

The goal of treatment is to minimize the discrepancy between the heart's demand for oxygen and the ability of the coronary arteries to meet this demand. Treatment is aimed at maintaining the patient's physical activity at a level below that which causes his pain. Additional measures include adopting a diet designed to achieve the patient's ideal weight, eliminating any possible risk factors associated with heart disease, and treating hypertension if it's present.

Pharmacologic measures are used to prevent angina or to provide relief from it if it occurs, thereby reducing the risk of MI. Three main classes of drugs are used in the treatment of angina: nitrates, beta-adrenergic blockers, and calcium channel blockers.

Nitrates, including nitroglycerin and longer-acting nitrate preparations, are used in both the acute and long-term management of angina. Sublingual nitroglycerin is the drug of choice to treat acute anginal attacks. It acts within 1 to 2 minutes, causing a decrease in the myocardial workload and oxygen demand through venous dilation. This, in turn, reduces preload. It also may improve myocardial oxygen supply by dilating collateral blood vessels and increasing blood flow to the ischemic myocardium. When given in higher doses, arterial dilation occurs. Longer-acting nitroglycerin preparations are used to prevent attacks of angina. The primary problem with long-term nitrate use is the development of tolerance.

Beta-adrenergic blockers, including propranolol, metoprolol, nadolol, and atenolol, are the first line of treatment for patients with chronic angina. They block the stimulating effects of norepinephrine and epinephrine, preventing anginal attacks by reducing heart rate, myocardial contractility, and blood pressure. This, in turn, reduces myocardial oxygen demand. These agents may be used alone or in conjunction with other medications.

Calcium channel blockers, including verapamil, diltiazem, and nifedipine, reduce myocardial oxygen demand and increase myocardial blood and oxygen supply. They're also potent coronary vasodilators, increasing oxygen supply. These drugs are used for long-term prevention of angina.

In addition to these agents, heparin and thrombolytic drugs may be used for patients with unstable angina. Patients with angina, particularly unstable angina, are at risk for MI because of significant narrowing of the coronary arteries. Low-dose aspirin therapy may be prescribed to reduce the risk of platelet aggregation and thrombus formation, which could cause an MI. Angioplasty and coronary artery bypass grafting may be used to relieve symptoms and prolong life in selected subgroups of patients.

COLLABORATIVE MANAGEMENT

Care of the patient with angina focuses on relieving the pain and preventing the progression of ischemia to infarction.

ASSESSMENT

Diagnosis is based on the patient's medical history, a comprehensive description of the characteristics of the chest pain, and physical assessment findings. Laboratory tests may confirm the presence of risk factors. Diagnostic tests reveal information about the overall functioning of the heart.

The cardinal manifestation of angina is chest pain that's typically precipitated by an identifiable event, such as physical activity, strong emotion, stress, eating a heavy meal, or exposure to cold. The pain characteristically begins beneath the sternum and may radiate to the jaw, neck, or arm. It usually lasts less than 15 minutes and is relieved by rest; the classic sequence is activity, pain, rest, relief.

Typically, the pain is described as squeezing, burning, pressing, choking, aching, or bursting, The patient often says the pain feels like "gas," "heartburn," "indigestion," or "a heavy weight on the chest." It usually isn't described as sharp or knifelike. Additional manifestations include dyspnea, diaphoresis, pallor, tachycardia, and great anxiety and fear.

NURSING DIAGNOSES AND COLLABORATIVE PROBLEMS

Based on the following nursing diagnoses, you'll establish patient outcomes.

Altered cardiopulmonary tissue perfusion related to reduced blood flow to the myocardium caused by coronary artery spasm or occlusion. The patient will:
■ maintain adequate myocardial tissue perfusion, as exhibited by a normal heart rate and rhythm and the absence of ischemic ECG changes
■ verbalize an understanding of the prescribed medical regimen and relate the importance of seeking follow-up care for the rest of his life.

Pain related to inadequate oxygen flow to the myocardium as a result of reduced myocardial blood flow. The patient will:
■ experience a reduction in the severity and frequency of anginal attacks by complying with medical or surgical therapy
■ identify the factors that trigger anginal pain
■ verbalize an understanding of what he needs to do when anginal pain occurs.

Activity intolerance related to an imbalance between myocardial oxygen supply and demand. The patient will:
■ identify the activities he needs to avoid and the activities for which he must obtain assistance
■ conserve energy while performing his daily activities
■ participate in a medically supervised exercise program that will help him develop collateral myocardial circulation and increase his activity tolerance level.

Anxiety related to uncertainty of condition. The patient will:
■ verbalize his feelings about the diagnosis
■ demonstrate positive coping mechanisms when dealing with his condition.

Knowledge deficit related to unfamiliarity with diagnostic or therapeutic procedures and the disease. The patient will:
■ verbalize an understanding of the diagnosis and all tests and treatments
■ demonstrate compliance with treatment
■ state the signs and symptoms to report to staff.

PLANNING AND IMPLEMENTATION

The following measures help the patient with angina. (See *Drug therapy for unstable angina,* page 72.)
■ Assess the location, severity, and quality of the patient's pain. Ask him to rate the pain on a scale of 0 to 10.
■ Monitor vital signs and hemodynamic parameters according to the policy of your health care facility.
■ During anginal episodes, monitor blood pressure and heart rate, and take a 12-lead ECG before administering nitroglycerin or other nitrates. Record the duration of pain, the amount of medication required to relieve it, and any accompanying symptoms.
■ Administer nitroglycerin as ordered and note the patient's response. Keep nitroglycerin available for immediate use. Instruct the patient to call immediately whenever he feels chest, arm, or neck pain and before taking nitroglycerin.
■ Place the patient in semi- or high-Fowler's position.
■ Administer oxygen at 4 to 6 L/minute, as ordered, unless contraindicated by chronic pulmonary disease.
■ Ask the patient about any activities that may have precipitated the attack.
■ Monitor the patient for signs of complications, including arrhythmias and progression of ischemia, leading to MI.
■ Maintain bed rest until the patient's condition stabilizes.
■ Space activities to allow the patient to rest between them.
■ Assist with passive range-of-motion (ROM) exercises while the patient is on bed rest; begin a progres-

CLINICAL PRACTICE GUIDELINES

Drug therapy for unstable angina

The following have been adapted from the clinical practice guidelines for angina developed by the Agency for Health Care Policy and Research of the U.S. Department of Health and Human Services. Keep in mind that all medications require a properly written doctor's order.

■ Barring complications, consider I.V. nitroglycerin (NTG) for patients whose symptoms aren't fully relieved with three sublingual NTG tablets and initiation of beta-blocker therapy (when possible) as well as all nonhypotensive high-risk unstable angina patients.

■ Start I.V. NTG at a dose of 5 to 10 µg/minute by continuous infusion, and titrate up by 10 µg/minute every 5 to 10 minutes until relief of symptoms or limiting adverse effects (headache or hypotension with systolic blood pressure [SBP] less than 90 mm Hg or more than 30% below starting mean arterial pressure levels if significant hypertension is present).

■ Switch patients from I.V. NTG to oral or topical nitrate therapy once they've been symptom-free for 24 hours. (Tolerance to nitrates is dose- and duration-dependent and typically becomes significant only after 24 hours of continuous therapy.)

■ Give morphine sulfate at a dose of 2 to 5 mg I.V. to any patient whose symptoms are not relieved after three sublingual NTG tablets or whose symptoms recur with adequate anti-ischemic therapy, unless contraindicated by hypotension or intolerance. Morphine may be repeated every 5 to 30 minutes as needed to relieve symptoms and maintain patient comfort.

■ Start beta blockers (I.V. for high-risk patients; oral for intermediate- and low-risk patients), barring contraindications. Choice of the specific agent is less important than ensuring that appropriate candidates receive this therapy. Don't use beta blockers for patients with heart failure, bronchospasm or a history of asthma, bradycardia (less than 50 beats per minute), or hypotension.

■ During I.V. beta-blocker therapy, monitor heart rate and blood pressure frequently, monitor electrocardiogram readings continuously, and auscultate for crackles or bron-

chospasm. After the initial I.V. load, convert patients without limiting adverse effects to an oral regimen. The target heart rate for beta blockade is 50 to 60 beats/minute.

■ Administer one or a combination of the following drugs to the patient :
– Give I.V. metoprolol in 5-mg increments by slow I.V. infusion (over 1 to 2 minutes) and repeat every 5 minutes for a total initial dose of 15 mg, followed in 1 to 2 hours by 25 to 50 mg by mouth every 6 hours.
– Give I.V. propranolol as an initial dose of 0.5 to 1 mg, followed in 1 to 2 hours by 40 to 80 mg by mouth every 6 to 8 hours.
– Give I.V. esmolol as a starting maintenance dose of 0.1 mg/kg/minute with titration in increments of 0.05 mg/kg/minute every 10 to 15 minutes as tolerated by blood pressure. Continue until the desired therapeutic response has been obtained, limiting symptoms develop, or a dose of 0.2 mg/kg/minute is reached.

■ Use calcium channel blockers to control recurring symptoms in patients already on adequate doses of nitrates and beta blockers, in patients unable to tolerate adequate doses of one or both of these agents, and in patients with Prinzmetal's angina.

■ Choose the individual calcium channel blocker based primarily on the patient's hemodynamic state and risk of adverse effects on contractility and atrioventricular conduction.

■ Continue aspirin once a day at a dose of 80 to 324 mg indefinitely.

■ For patients unable to take aspirin because of a history of hypersensitivity or major GI intolerance, substitute ticlopidine 250 mg twice a day.

■ Give heparin infusion for 2 to 5 days or until revascularization is performed.

sive exercise program, as ordered, once the patient's condition stabilizes.

■ Provide physical and emotional support to the patient and family.

■ Explain all events, tests, and procedures to minimize anxiety.

■ Allow the patient to verbalize his feelings and ask questions; answer questions honestly.

■ Help the patient use coping strategies such as relaxation techniques.

Patient teaching

■ Explain any treatments and procedures. Make sure the patient understands the reasons, the risks, and the

possible need for other interventions (such as angioplasty, bypass surgery, or atherectomy).

■ Help the patient determine which activities precipitate episodes of pain. Help him identify more effective coping mechanisms to deal with stress.

■ Explain all prescribed medications, and stress the need to follow the prescribed drug regimen. Emphasize that drugs used for long-term prevention will not be useful in an acute attack.

■ Advise the patient to carry nitroglycerin at all times. Explain proper storage and the need for a new supply every 6 months.

■ Instruct the patient to take sublingual nitroglycerin before engaging in activities that precipitate angina. Also tell him to take it at the first sign of an attack, re-

peating one tablet every 5 to 10 minutes for a total of three doses. If this brings no relief, tell him to call the doctor or go to the nearest emergency department.
- Advise the patient to sit down or change positions slowly because many of the prescribed drugs can cause dizziness.
- Instruct him in risk-factor reduction, such as losing weight, making dietary changes, reducing stress, and stopping smoking.
- Discuss issues involving sexual activity and the possible need for modification. Review the patient's medications ahead of time for any cardiac drugs that can cause impotence.
- Discuss signs and symptoms that require follow-up care or a call to the doctor.

EVALUATION
Achievement of patient outcomes determines whether collaborative management has succeeded. For a patient with angina, evaluation focuses on pain relief, improved tissue perfusion, activity tolerance, anxiety relief, and adequate knowledge of the disorder and its treatment.

Aortic insufficiency

In this disorder (also called aortic regurgitation), blood flows back into the left ventricle during diastole. The ventricle becomes overloaded and dilated and eventually hypertrophies. The excess fluid volume also overloads the left atrium and eventually the pulmonary system.

Aortic insufficiency by itself occurs most commonly among males. When associated with mitral valve disease, however, it's more common among females. This disorder also may be associated with Marfan syndrome, ankylosing spondylitis, syphilis, essential hypertension, and a ventricular septal defect, even after surgical closure.

CAUSES
Aortic insufficiency may result from rheumatic fever, syphilis, hypertension, endocarditis, or trauma. In some patients, it may be idiopathic.

In this disorder, blood that is propelled forward into the aorta is allowed to flow backward into the left ventricle through an incompetent valve. This causes abnormal filling and a volume overload of the left ventricle. The severity of the valve's incompetence determines the magnitude of the overload.

To compensate for the decrease in systemic circulation, left ventricular stroke volume increases to produce an adequate blood volume for the aorta. A compensatory dilation occurs in the left ventricle, but only a minimal increase in left ventricular end-dias-

tolic pressure develops. These compensatory mechanisms help maintain adequate cardiac output. However, as the condition progresses and the contractile state of the heart declines, cardiac output diminishes.

Left ventricular failure usually occurs. The patient may develop fatal pulmonary edema if a fever, infection, or cardiac arrhythmia develops. The patient also risks myocardial ischemia because left ventricular dilation and elevated left ventricular systolic pressure alter myocardial oxygen requirements.

DIAGNOSIS AND TREATMENT
Cardiac catheterization shows reduced arterial diastolic pressures, aortic insufficiency, other valvular abnormalities, and increased left ventricular end-diastolic pressure.

Chest X-rays display left ventricular enlargement and pulmonary vein congestion. Echocardiography reveals left ventricular enlargement, dilation of the aortic annulus and left atrium, and thickening of the aortic valve. It also shows a rapid, high-frequency fluttering of the anterior mitral leaflet that results from the impact of aortic insufficiency.

Electrocardiography (ECG) shows sinus tachycardia, left ventricular hypertrophy, and left atrial hypertrophy in severe disease. ST-segment depressions and T-wave inversions appear in leads I, aV_L, V_5, and V_6 and indicate left ventricular strain.

Valve replacement is the treatment of choice and should be performed before significant ventricular dysfunction occurs. This may not be possible, however, because signs and symptoms seldom occur until after myocardial dysfunction develops.

Digitalis glycosides, a low-sodium diet, diuretics, vasodilators, and angiotensin-converting enzyme inhibitors are used to treat left-sided heart failure. In acute episodes, supplemental oxygen may be necessary.

COLLABORATIVE MANAGEMENT
Care of the patient with aortic insufficiency requires prompt detection and treatment as well as close monitoring.

ASSESSMENT
In chronic severe aortic insufficiency, the patient may complain that he has an uncomfortable awareness of his heartbeat, especially when lying down. He may report palpitations along with a pounding head.

The patient may experience dyspnea with exertion and paroxysmal nocturnal dyspnea with diaphoresis, orthopnea, and a cough. He may experience fatigue and syncope with exertion or emotion. He may also have a history of anginal chest pain unrelieved by sublingual nitroglycerin.

On inspection, you may note that each heartbeat seems to jar the patient's entire body and that his

Identifying the murmur of aortic insufficiency

A high-pitched, blowing decrescendo murmur that radiates from the aortic valve area to the left sternal border characterizes aortic insufficiency.

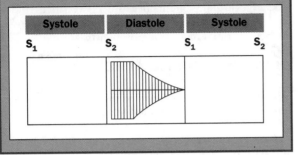

head bobs with each systole. Inspection of arterial pulsations shows a rapidly rising pulse that collapses suddenly as arterial pressure falls late in systole (water-hammer pulse).

The patient's nail beds may appear to be pulsating. If you apply pressure at the nail tip, the root will alternately flush and pale (Quincke's sign). Inspection of the chest may reveal a visible apical impulse. In left-sided heart failure, the patient may have ankle edema and ascites.

In palpating the peripheral pulses, you may note rapidly rising and collapsing pulses (pulsus biferiens). If the patient has cardiac arrhythmias, pulses may be irregular. You'll be able to feel the apical impulse. (The apex will be displaced laterally and inferiorly.) A diastolic thrill probably will be palpable along the left sternal border, and you may be able to feel a prominent systolic thrill in the jugular notch and along the carotid arteries.

Auscultation may reveal an S_3, occasionally an S_4, and a loud systolic ejection sound. A high-pitched, blowing, decrescendo diastolic murmur is heard best at the left sternal border, third intercostal space. Use the diaphragm of the stethoscope to hear it, and have the patient sit up, lean forward, and hold his breath in forced expiration. (See *Identifying the murmur of aortic insufficiency.*)

You also may hear a midsystolic ejection murmur at the base of the heart. It may be a grade 5 or 6 and typically is higher pitched, shorter, and less rasping than the murmur heard in aortic stenosis. Another murmur that may occur is a soft, low-pitched, rumbling, middiastolic or presystolic bruit (Austin Flint murmur). This murmur is heard best at the base of the heart.

Place the stethoscope lightly over the femoral artery, and you'll notice a booming, pistol-shot sound

and a to-and-fro murmur (Duroziez's sign). Arterial pulse pressure is widened. Taking blood pressure may be difficult because you can auscultate the patient's pulse without inflating the cuff. To determine systolic pressure, note when Korotkoff sounds start to muffle.

NURSING DIAGNOSES AND COLLABORATIVE PROBLEMS

Based on these nursing diagnoses, you'll establish patient outcomes.

Altered cardiopulmonary tissue perfusion related to left ventricular dilation and elevated left ventricular systolic pressure. The patient will:
- state relief of symptoms
- identify activities that cause chest pain and avoid or seek assistance with these activities
- show no ischemic changes on his ECG.

Decreased cardiac output related to aortic insufficiency caused by damage to the aortic valve. The patient will:
- exhibit a pulse rate and blood pressure that remain within set limits and be free of arrhythmias
- describe signs and symptoms of decreased cardiac output, such as dizziness, syncope, clammy skin, fatigue, and dyspnea
- communicate the importance of seeking medical attention if signs and symptoms occur
- express the importance of complying with his ordered diet, medication schedule, and activity level.

Activity intolerance related to decreased tissue oxygenation with exertion caused by aortic insufficiency. The patient will:
- be able to explain how the disease process affects his activity level
- identify measures to prevent or modify fatigue
- incorporate measures to modify fatigue into his daily routine.

Knowledge deficit related to disease, treatment, and care. The patient will:
- verbalize information related to the disease and its treatments
- demonstrate measures for appropriate care.

PLANNING AND IMPLEMENTATION

The following measures help the patient with aortic insufficiency.
- Observe the patient for signs of cardiac arrhythmias, which can increase the risk of pulmonary edema as well as fever and infection.
- Assess the patient's vital signs, weight, and intake and output for changes that suggest fluid overload.
- Monitor the patient for chest pain, which may indicate cardiac ischemia.
- Evaluate the patient's cardiopulmonary function. Notify the doctor if sudden or significant changes occur.
- Watch closely for complications and adverse reactions to drug therapy.

- To improve venous return, keep the patient's legs elevated while he sits in a chair; advise him not to cross his legs.
- Place the patient in an upright position to relieve dyspnea if necessary, and administer oxygen to prevent tissue hypoxia.
- Keep the patient on a low-sodium diet; consult a dietitian to ensure that the patient receives foods that he likes while adhering to the diet restrictions.
- If the patient needs bed rest, stress its importance.
- Assist with bathing if necessary.
- Provide a bedside commode because using a commode puts less stress on the heart than using a bedpan.
- Offer diversional activities that are physically undemanding. Alternate periods of activity and rest to prevent extreme fatigue and dyspnea.
- Regularly evaluate the patient's activity tolerance and degree of fatigue.
- Allow the patient to express his concerns about the effects of activity restrictions on his responsibilities and routines.
- Reassure him that the restrictions are temporary.

Patient teaching
- If the patient is scheduled for valve replacement surgery, explain the procedure and prepare him as necessary.
- Advise the patient to plan for periodic rest in his daily routine to prevent undue fatigue.
- Teach the patient about diet restrictions, medications, symptoms that should be reported, and the importance of consistent follow-up care.
- Tell the patient to elevate his legs whenever he sits.

EVALUATION
Achievement of patient outcomes determines whether collaborative management has succeeded. For a patient with aortic insufficiency, evaluation focuses on improved tissue perfusion and cardiac output, relief of fatigue, and adequate knowledge of the disorder and its treatment.

Arrhythmias

Arrhythmias are changes in heart rate and rhythm that result from abnormal electrical conduction or automaticity. They vary in severity from those that are mild, asymptomatic, and require no treatment (such as sinus arrhythmia, in which the heart rate increases and decreases with respiration) to lethal ventricular fibrillation, which requires immediate intervention.

Arrhythmias are classified according to site of origin as ventricular, atrial, or junctional. (If they're both atrial and junctional, they may be noted as supraventricular.) Their effect on cardiac output and blood pressure, partially influenced by the site of origin, determines their clinical significance.

CAUSES
Arrhythmias may be congenital or may result from myocardial ischemia or infarction, organic heart disease, drug toxicity, or degeneration of conductive tissue necessary to maintain normal heart rhythm (sick sinus syndrome). They may be caused by an abnormal rhythmicity of the sinus node, a shift of the pacemaker function from the sinus node to another part of the atrium, a block in transmission of the impulse through the heart, abnormal conduction pathways through the heart, or the spontaneous generation of impulses from any place along the conduction system.

Normally, when the cardiac impulse has traveled throughout the heart, it has no place to go so it simply dissipates. The heart remains quiet until a new impulse begins in the sinus node. In some circumstances, this mechanism does not occur. Instead, the impulse travels around and around in the cardiac muscle without stopping. This is called re-entry.

Normal automaticity occurs in specialized cells in the atrioventricular (AV) node and Purkinje fibers. Once the action potential is reached, the muscle fiber contracts and the wave of depolarization spreads over the myocardium. Abnormal automaticity develops when the resting potential of the cell membrane is reduced, making the membrane unstable and subject to abnormal conduction patterns and ectopic beats.

Delays in impulse transmission also can occur in the AV node or within the bundle of His and Purkinje fibers.

In a patient with a normal heart, arrhythmias typically produce few symptoms. But even in a normal heart, persistently rapid or highly irregular rhythms can strain the myocardium and impair cardiac output.

DIAGNOSIS AND TREATMENT
The primary diagnostic test is electrocardiography (ECG), which allows detection and identification of arrhythmias. (See *Types of cardiac arrhythmias*, pages 76 to 81.)

Effective treatment aims to return pacer function to the sinus node, increase or decrease the ventricular rate to normal, regain atrioventricular synchrony, and maintain normal sinus rhythm. Such treatment corrects abnormal rhythms through therapy with antiarrhythmic drugs; electrical conversion with precordial shock (defibrillation and cardioversion); physical maneuvers, such as carotid massage and Valsalva's maneuver; temporary or permanent placement of a pacemaker to maintain heart rate; and surgical removal or

(Text continues on page 82.)

Types of cardiac arrhythmias

This chart reviews the features, causes, and treatments of common cardiac arrhythmias. You can compare the features and rhythm strips of the arrhythmias with those of the normal cardiac rhythm strip shown here:

- Ventricular and atrial rates 60 to 100 beats/minute
- Regular and uniform QRS complexes and P waves
- PR interval of 0.12 to 0.2 second
- QRS duration <0.12 second
- Identical atrial and ventricular rates, with constant PR interval.

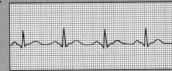

Arrhythmia and features	Causes	Treatment
SINUS ARRHYTHMIA 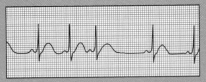 ■ Irregular atrial and ventricular rhythms ■ Normal P wave before QRS complex	■ A normal variation of normal sinus rhythm in athletes, children, and elderly people ■ Also seen in digitalis toxicity and inferior wall myocardial infarction (MI)	■ Atropine, if rate decreases below 40 beats/minute
SINUS TACHYCARDIA 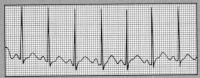 ■ Atrial and ventricular rates regular ■ Rate >100 beats/minute; rarely >160 beats/minute ■ Normal P wave before QRS complex	■ Normal physiologic response to fever, exercise, anxiety, pain, dehydration; may also accompany shock, left-sided heart failure, cardiac tamponade, hyperthyroidism, anemia, hypovolemia, pulmonary embolism, anterior wall MI ■ May also occur with atropine, epinephrine, isoproterenol, quinidine, caffeine, alcohol, and nicotine use	■ Correction of underlying cause
SINUS BRADYCARDIA 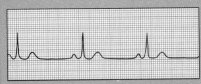 ■ Regular atrial and ventricular rhythms ■ Rate <60 beats/minute ■ Normal P wave before QRS complex	■ Normal in well-conditioned heart, such as in an athlete ■ Increased intracranial pressure; increased vagal tone due to bowel straining, vomiting, intubation, mechanical ventilation; sick sinus syndrome; hypothyroidism; inferior wall MI ■ May also occur with anticholinesterase, beta blockers, digitalis glycosides, and morphine use	■ For low cardiac output, dizziness, weakness, altered level of consciousness, or low blood pressure: 0.5 mg atropine every 5 minutes to total of 2 mg ■ Temporary pacemaker or isoproterenol, if atropine fails; may need permanent pacemaker
SINOATRIAL ARREST OR BLOCK (SINUS ARREST) 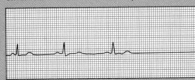 ■ Atrial and ventricular rhythms normal except for missing complex ■ Normal P wave before QRS complex ■ Pause not equal to a multiple of the previous sinus rhythm	■ Acute infection ■ Coronary artery disease, degenerative heart disease, acute inferior wall MI ■ Vagal stimulation, Valsalva's maneuver, carotid sinus massage ■ Digitalis, quinidine, or salicylate toxicity ■ Pesticide poisoning ■ Pharyngeal irritation caused by endotracheal intubation ■ Sick sinus syndrome	■ Atropine 0.5 mg I.V. to treat symptoms ■ Temporary or permanent pacemaker for repeated episodes

Types of cardiac arrhythmias *(continued)*

Arrhythmia and features	Causes	Treatment

WANDERING ATRIAL PACEMAKER

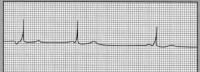

- Atrial and ventricular rates vary slightly
- Irregular PR interval
- P waves irregular with changing configuration, indicating they're not all from sinoatrial (SA) node or single atrial focus; may appear after the QRS complex
- QRS complexes uniform in shape but irregular in rhythm

Causes
- Rheumatic carditis as a result of inflammation involving the SA node
- Digitalis toxicity
- Sick sinus syndrome

Treatment
- No treatment if asymptomatic
- Treatment of underlying cause if symptomatic

PREMATURE ATRIAL CONTRACTION (PAC)

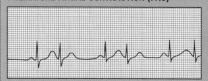

- Premature, abnormal-looking P waves, differing in configuration from normal P waves
- QRS complexes after P waves, except in very early or blocked PACs
- P wave often buried in the preceding T wave or identified in the preceding T wave

Causes
- Coronary or valvular heart disease, atrial ischemia, coronary atherosclerosis, heart failure, acute respiratory failure, chronic obstructive pulmonary disease (COPD), electrolyte imbalance, and hypoxia
- Digitalis toxicity; aminophylline, adrenergic, or caffeine use
- Anxiety

Treatment
- If occurring more than six times per minute or increasing in frequency, digitalis glycosides, quinidine, verapamil, or propranolol; after revascularization surgery, propranolol
- Treatment of underlying cause

PAROXYSMAL ATRIAL TACHYCARDIA (PAROXYSMAL SUPRAVENTRICULAR TACHYCARDIA)

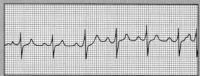

- Atrial and ventricular rates regular
- Heart rate >160 beats/minute; rarely exceeds 250 beats/minute
- P waves regular but aberrant; difficult to differentiate from preceding T wave; precede QRS complexes
- Sudden onset and termination of arrhythmia

Causes
- Intrinsic abnormality of atrioventricular (AV) conduction system
- Physical or psychological stress, hypoxia, hypokalemia, cardiomyopathy, congenital heart disease, MI, valvular disease, Wolff-Parkinson-White syndrome, cor pulmonale, hyperthyroidism, systemic hypertension
- Digitalis toxicity; caffeine, marijuana, central nervous system stimulant use

Treatment
- Vagal stimulation, Valsalva's maneuver, carotid sinus massage
- Adenosine by rapid I.V. bolus injection to rapidly convert arrhythmia
- Propranolol, quinidine, verapamil, or edrophonium to alter AV node conduction and maintain normal rhythm
- Elective cardioversion if patient is symptomatic and unresponsive to drugs

(continued)

Types of cardiac arrhythmias *(continued)*

Arrhythmia and features	Causes	Treatment
ATRIAL FLUTTER 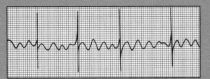 ■ Atrial rhythm regular; 250 to 400 beats/minute ■ Ventricular rate variable, depending on degree of AV block, usually 60 to 100 beats/minute ■ Sawtooth P-wave configuration possible (F waves) ■ QRS complexes uniform in shape but often irregular in rate	■ Heart failure, tricuspid or mitral valve disease, pulmonary embolism, cor pulmonale, inferior wall MI, carditis ■ Digitalis toxicity	■ Digitalis glycosides (unless arrhythmia is due to digitalis toxicity), verapamil, propranolol, or quinidine ■ May require synchronized cardioversion or atrial pacemaker
ATRIAL FIBRILLATION 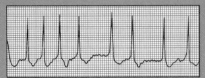 ■ Atrial rhythm grossly irregular; rate >400 beats/minute ■ Ventricular rate grossly irregular ■ QRS complexes of uniform configuration and duration ■ PR interval indiscernible ■ No P waves, or erratic, irregular, baseline fibrillatory P waves	■ Heart failure, COPD, thyrotoxicosis, constrictive pericarditis, ischemic heart disease, sepsis, pulmonary embolus, rheumatic heart disease, hypertension, mitral stenosis, digitalis toxicity (rarely), atrial irritation, complication of coronary bypass or valve replacement surgery ■ Nifedipine and digitalis glycoside use	■ Digitalis glycosides (unless the cause) and quinidine to slow ventricular rate and to convert rhythm to normal sinus rhythm ■ May require elective cardioversion for rapid ventricular rate ■ Treatment of underlying cause
JUNCTIONAL RHYTHM 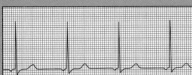 ■ Atrial and ventricular rates regular ■ Atrial rate 40 to 60 beats/minute ■ Ventricular rate 40 to 60 beats/minute (60 to 100 beats/minute is accelerated junctional rhythm) ■ P waves before, hidden in, or after QRS complex; inverted, if visible ■ PR interval (when present) <0.12 second ■ QRS complex configuration and duration normal, except in aberrant conduction	■ Inferior wall MI or ischemia, hypoxia, vagal stimulation, sick sinus syndrome ■ Acute rheumatic fever ■ Valve surgery ■ Digitalis toxicity	■ Atropine for symptomatic slow rate ■ Pacemaker insertion if refractory to drugs ■ Discontinuation of digitalis glycosides if appropriate

Types of cardiac arrhythmias *(continued)*

Arrhythmia and features	Causes	Treatment

PREMATURE JUNCTIONAL CONTRACTIONS (JUNCTIONAL PREMATURE BEATS)

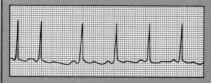

- Atrial and ventricular rhythms irregular
- P waves inverted; may precede, be hidden within, or follow QRS complex
- PR interval <0.12 second, if P wave precedes QRS complex
- QRS complex configuration and duration normal

■ MI or ischemia
■ Digitalis toxicity; excessive caffeine or amphetamine use

■ Correction of underlying cause
■ Quinidine, atropine, or disopyramide, as ordered
■ Discontinuation of digitalis glycosides if appropriate
■ May require pacemaker

FIRST-DEGREE AV BLOCK

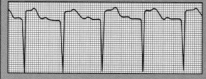

- Atrial and ventricular rhythms regular
- PR interval >0.20 second
- P wave preceding each QRS complex; QRS complex normal

■ May be seen in a healthy person
■ Inferior wall myocardial ischemia or infarction, hypothyroidism, hypokalemia, hyperkalemia
■ Digitalis toxicity; quinidine, procainamide, or propranolol use

■ Cautious use of digitalis glycosides
■ Correction of underlying cause
■ Atropine may be used if PR interval exceeds 0.26 second or bradycardia develops

SECOND-DEGREE AV BLOCK MOBITZ I (WENCKEBACH)

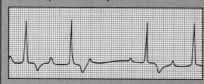

- Atrial rhythm regular
- Ventricular rhythm irregular
- Atrial rate exceeds ventricular rate
- PR interval progressively, but only slightly, longer with each cycle until QRS complex disappears (dropped beat); PR interval shorter after dropped beat

■ Inferior wall MI, cardiac surgery, acute rheumatic fever, and vagal stimulation
■ Digitalis toxicity; propranolol, quinidine, or procainamide use

■ Treatment of underlying cause
■ Atropine or temporary pacemaker for symptomatic bradycardia
■ Discontinuation of digitalis glycosides if appropriate

(continued)

Types of cardiac arrhythmias *(continued)*

Arrhythmia and features	Causes	Treatment
SECOND-DEGREE AV BLOCK **MOBITZ II** 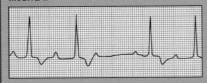 ■ Atrial rate regular ■ Ventricular rhythm regular or irregular, with varying degree of block ■ P-P interval constant ■ QRS complexes periodically absent	■ Severe coronary artery disease, anterior MI, acute myocarditis ■ Digitalis toxicity	■ Isoproterenol for symptomatic bradycardia ■ Temporary or permanent pacemaker ■ Discontinuation of digitalis glycosides if appropriate
THIRD-DEGREE AV BLOCK **(COMPLETE HEART BLOCK)** 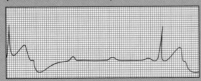 ■ Atrial rate regular ■ Ventricular rate slow and regular ■ No relation between P waves and QRS complexes ■ No constant PR interval ■ QRS interval normal (nodal pacemaker) or wide and bizarre (ventricular pacemaker)	■ Inferior or anterior wall MI, congenital abnormality, rheumatic fever, hypoxia, postoperative complications of mitral valve replacement, Lev's disease (fibrosis and calcification that spreads from cardiac structures to the conductive tissue), and Lenègre's disease (conductive tissue fibrosis) ■ Digitalis toxicity	■ Atropine or isoproterenol for symptomatic bradycardia ■ Temporary or permanent pacemaker
JUNCTIONAL TACHYCARDIA 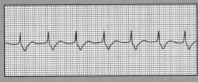 ■ Atrial rate >100 beats/minute; however, P wave may be absent, be hidden in QRS complex, or precede T wave ■ Ventricular rate >100 beats/minute ■ P wave inverted ■ QRS complex configuration and duration normal ■ Onset of rhythm often sudden, occurring in bursts	■ Myocarditis, cardiomyopathy, inferior wall MI or ischemia, acute rheumatic fever, valve replacement surgery ■ Digitalis toxicity	■ Temporary atrial pacemaker to override the rhythm ■ Carotid sinus massage, elective cardioversion ■ Propranolol, verapamil, or edrophonium ■ Discontinuation of digitalis glycosides if appropriate

Types of cardiac arrhythmias *(continued)*

Arrhythmia and features	Causes	Treatment
PREMATURE VENTRICULAR CONTRACTION (PVC) 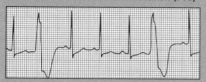 ■ Atrial rate regular ■ Ventricular rate irregular ■ QRS complex premature, usually followed by a complete compensatory pause ■ QRS complex wide and distorted, usually >0.14 second ■ Premature QRS complexes occurring singly, in pairs, or in threes; alternating with normal beats; focus from one or more sites ■ Most ominous when clustered, multifocal, with R wave on T pattern	■ Heart failure; old or acute myocardial ischemia, infarction, or contusion; myocardial irritation by ventricular catheter, such as a pacemaker; hypercapnia; hypokalemia; hypocalcemia ■ Drug toxicity (digitalis glycosides, aminophylline, tricyclic antidepressants, beta-adrenergics [isoproterenol or dopamine]) ■ Caffeine, tobacco, or alcohol use ■ Psychological stress, anxiety, pain, exercise	■ Lidocaine I.V. bolus and drip infusion or procainamide or quinidine ■ Treatment of underlying cause ■ Discontinuation of drug causing toxicity ■ Potassium chloride I.V. if induced by hypokalemia
VENTRICULAR TACHYCARDIA 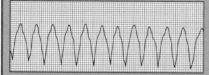 ■ Ventricular rate 140 to 220 beats/minute, regular or irregular ■ QRS complexes wide, bizarre, and independent of P waves ■ P waves not discernible ■ May start and stop suddenly	■ Myocardial ischemia, infarction, or aneurysm; coronary artery disease; rheumatic heart disease; mitral valve prolapse; heart failure; cardiomyopathy; ventricular catheters; hypokalemia; hypercalcemia; pulmonary embolism ■ Digitalis, procainamide, epinephrine, or quinidine toxicity ■ Anxiety	■ Lidocaine, procainamide, or bretylium I.V. ■ Cardiopulmonary resuscitation (CPR) if pulses are absent, following advanced cardiac life support (ACLS) protocol ■ Synchronous cardioversion
VENTRICULAR FIBRILLATION 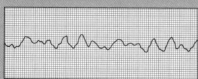 ■ Ventricular rhythm rapid and chaotic ■ QRS complexes wide and irregular; no visible P waves	■ Myocardial ischemia or infarction, untreated ventricular tachycardia, R-on-T phenomenon, hypokalemia, alkalosis, hyperkalemia, hypercalcemia, electric shock, hypothermia ■ Digitalis, epinephrine, or quinidine toxicity	■ Defibrillation ■ Epinephrine and lidocaine, procainamide, or bretylium I.V. ■ CPR ■ Treatment of underlying cause
VENTRICULAR STANDSTILL (ASYSTOLE) 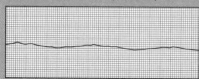 ■ No atrial or ventricular rate or rhythm ■ No discernible P waves, QRS complexes, or T waves	■ Myocardial ischemia or infarction, aortic valve disease, heart failure, hypoxemia, hypokalemia, severe acidosis, electric shock, ventricular arrhythmias, AV block, pulmonary embolism, heart rupture, cardiac tamponade, hyperkalemia, electromechanical dissociation ■ Cocaine overdose	■ CPR, following ACLS protocol ■ Endotracheal intubation ■ Pacemaker ■ Treatment of underlying cause

cryotherapy of an irritable ectopic focus to prevent recurring arrhythmias.

Arrhythmias may respond to treatment of the underlying disorder, such as correction of hypoxia, pain, or fever. However, those associated with heart disease may require continuing and complex treatment.

COLLABORATIVE MANAGEMENT

Care of the patient with an arrhythmia focuses on prompt detection and early treatment so that the heart can return to its normal rhythm.

ASSESSMENT

Depending on the type of arrhythmia, the patient may exhibit symptoms ranging from pallor, cold and clammy extremities, reduced urine output, palpitations, and weakness to chest pain, dizziness and syncope.

NURSING DIAGNOSES AND COLLABORATIVE PROBLEMS

Based on the following nursing diagnoses, you'll establish these patient outcomes.

Altered cerebral tissue perfusion related to decreased cardiac output from an arrhythmia. The patient will:
- develop no complications, such as stroke or seizures, from altered cerebral tissue perfusion
- maintain adequate cerebral perfusion, as evidenced by proper orientation to time, person, and place
- maintain hemodynamic stability.

Anxiety related to potential for an arrhythmia to become life-threatening. The patient will:
- express feelings of anxiety
- use support systems to assist with coping
- experience diminished physical symptoms of anxiety.

Decreased cardiac output related to decreased left ventricular filling time caused by the arrhythmia. The patient will:
- exhibit no signs of decreased cardiac output, such as hypotension and altered tissue perfusion
- recover a normal cardiac rhythm that will remain normal
- communicate understanding of medical therapy to treat and prevent arrhythmias.

Knowledge deficit related to newly diagnosed arrhythmia. The patient will:
- verbalize an understanding of the potential causes of the arrhythmia
- verbalize an understanding of the medical regimen (such as medications or pacemaker)
- verbalize an understanding of possible procedures, such as cardioversion and electrophysiologic studies.

PLANNING AND IMPLEMENTATION

The following measures help the patient with an arrhythmia.

- Assess the patient's level of consciousness (LOC), including orientation to time, person, and place; if you note any changes in mental status, notify the doctor.
- Monitor the patient for signs of irritability, dizziness, and light-headedness.
- Evaluate the monitored patient's ECG regularly for arrhythmias, and document any arrhythmias that you detect.
- Notify the doctor if a monitored patient exhibits an arrhythmia or if a change in pulse pattern or rate occurs in an unmonitored patient.
- As ordered, obtain an ECG tracing in an unmonitored patient to confirm and identify the type of arrhythmia present.
- Be prepared to initiate cardiopulmonary resuscitation, if indicated, when a life-threatening arrhythmia occurs.
- Assess an unmonitored patient for rhythm disturbances. If the patient's pulse rate is abnormally rapid, slow, or irregular, watch for signs of hypoperfusion, such as hypotension and diminished urine output.
- Monitor for predisposing factors, such as fluid and electrolyte imbalance, and signs of drug toxicity, especially in a patient taking digitalis glycosides.
- If an arrhythmia occurs, carefully monitor the patient's cardiac, electrolyte, and overall clinical status to determine the effect on cardiac output.
- When life-threatening arrhythmias develop, rapidly assess the patient's LOC, blood pressure, and pulse and respiratory rates. Monitor his ECG continuously.
- After pacemaker insertion, monitor the patient's pulse rate regularly and watch for signs of pacemaker failure and decreased cardiac output. Watch closely for premature ventricular contractions, a sign of myocardial irritation, and check threshold daily.
- Administer medications as ordered, and prepare to assist with medical procedures (such as cardioversion) if indicated.
- To prevent arrhythmias postoperatively, provide adequate oxygen and reduce cardiac workload while carefully maintaining metabolic, neurologic, respiratory, and hemodynamic status.
- To avoid temporary pacemaker malfunction, install a fresh battery before each insertion. Carefully secure the external catheter wires and the pacemaker box.
- Encourage the patient to verbalize his feelings and concerns.
- Explain all tests and procedures in terms the patient and family can understand. Answer their questions honestly.

Patient teaching

- Explain to the patient the importance of taking all ordered medications at the proper time intervals.

■ Teach him how to take his pulse and recognize an irregular rhythm, and instruct him to report any changes to the doctor.

■ If the patient has a permanent pacemaker, warn him about environmental and electrical hazards, as indicated by the pacemaker manufacturer. Although hazards may not present a problem, in doubtful situations a 24-hour ambulatory ECG (Holter monitor) may be helpful.

■ Tell the patient to report any light-headedness or syncope.

■ Stress the importance of scheduling and keeping appointments for regular checkups.

EVALUATION

Achievement of patient outcomes determines whether collaborative management has been successful. For a patient with an arrhythmia, evaluation focuses on maintenance of LOC, adequate cardiac function, relief of anxiety, and adequate knowledge of the disease and required therapy.

Cardiogenic shock

Sometimes called pump failure, cardiogenic shock is a condition of diminished cardiac output that severely impairs tissue perfusion. It occurs as a serious complication in nearly 15% of all patients who are hospitalized with an acute myocardial infarction (MI). Cardiogenic shock typically affects patients whose area of infarction involves 40% or more of left ventricular muscle mass; in such patients, mortality may exceed 85%. Most patients in cardiogenic shock die within 24 hours of onset; the prognosis for those who survive is poor.

CAUSES

Cardiogenic shock can result from any condition that causes significant left ventricular dysfunction with reduced cardiac output, such as MI (most common), myocardial ischemia, papillary muscle dysfunction, and end-stage cardiomyopathy.

Other causes include myocarditis and decreased myocardial contractility after cardiac arrest and prolonged cardiac surgery. Mechanical abnormalities of the ventricle, such as acute mitral or aortic insufficiency or an acutely acquired ventricular septal defect or ventricular aneurysm, may also result in cardiogenic shock.

Regardless of the cause, left ventricular dysfunction initiates a series of compensatory mechanisms that attempt to increase cardiac output and, in turn, maintain vital organ function. As cardiac output falls, aortic and carotid baroreceptors activate sympathetic

nervous responses. These compensatory responses increase heart rate, left ventricular filling pressure, and peripheral resistance to flow in order to enhance venous return to the heart. This action initially stabilizes the patient but later causes deterioration with rising oxygen demands on the already compromised myocardium. These events constitute a vicious circle of low cardiac output, sympathetic compensation, myocardial ischemia, and even lower cardiac output.

Death usually ensues because the vital organs can't overcome the deleterious effects of extended hypoperfusion.

DIAGNOSIS AND TREATMENT

Pulmonary artery pressure monitoring reveals increased pulmonary artery pressure (PAP) and pulmonary artery wedge pressure (PAWP), reflecting a rise in left ventricular end-diastolic pressure (preload) and heightened resistance to left ventricular emptying (afterload) caused by ineffective pumping and increased peripheral vascular resistance. Thermodilution catheterization reveals a reduced cardiac index.

Invasive arterial pressure monitoring shows systolic arterial pressure less than 80 mm Hg caused by impaired ventricular ejection. Arterial blood gas (ABG) analysis may show metabolic and respiratory acidosis and hypoxia.

Electrocardiography (ECG) may demonstrate evidence of acute MI, ischemia, or ventricular aneurysm. Serum enzyme measurements reveal elevated levels of creatine kinase (CK), lactate dehydrogenase (LD), aspartate aminotransferase, and alanine aminotransferase, which indicate MI or ischemia and suggest heart failure or shock. CK-MB (an isoenzyme of CK that occurs in cardiac tissue) and LD isoenzyme levels may confirm acute MI.

Cardiac catheterization and echocardiography reveal other conditions that can lead to pump dysfunction and failure, such as cardiac tamponade, papillary muscle infarct or rupture, ventricular septal rupture, pulmonary emboli, venous pooling (associated with venodilators and continuous or intermittent positive-pressure breathing), and hypovolemia.

Treatment aims to enhance cardiovascular status by increasing cardiac output, improving myocardial perfusion, and decreasing cardiac workload with combinations of cardiovascular drugs and mechanical-assist techniques.

I.V. drugs may include dopamine, a vasopressor that increases cardiac output, blood pressure, and renal blood flow; amrinone or dobutamine, inotropic agents that increase myocardial contractility; and norepinephrine, when a more potent vasoconstrictor is necessary. Nitroprusside, a vasodilator, may be used with a vasopressor to further improve cardiac output by decreasing peripheral vascular resistance (after-

How the intra-aortic balloon pump works

Made of polyurethane, the intra-aortic balloon is attached to an external pump console by means of a large-lumen catheter. The balloon is inserted through the femoral artery into the descending thoracic aorta. The illustrations below show the direction of blood flow when the pump inflates and deflates the balloon.

Balloon inflation

The balloon inflates as the aortic valve closes and diastole begins. The increased pressure increases perfusion to the coronary arteries.

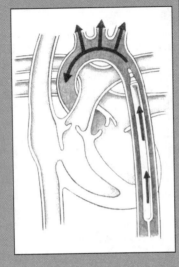

Balloon deflation

The balloon deflates before systole (before the aortic valve opens). Deflation reduces resistance to ejection of blood from the left ventricle (afterload), lessening cardiac workload. Improved ventricular ejection, which significantly improves cardiac output, and a subsequent vasodilation in the peripheral vessels lead to lower preload volume.

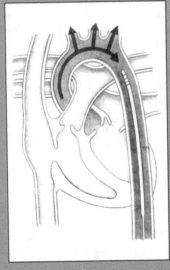

load) and reducing left ventricular end-diastolic pressure (preload). However, the patient's blood pressure must be adequate to support nitroprusside therapy and must be monitored closely.

Treatment may also include the intra-aortic balloon pump (IABP), a mechanical-assist device that at-tempts to improve coronary artery perfusion and decrease cardiac workload. (See *How the intra-aortic balloon pump works.*)

When drug therapy and IABP insertion fail, a ventricular-assist device may be used.

COLLABORATIVE MANAGEMENT

Care of the patient in cardiogenic shock focuses on quick assessment, diagnosis, and interventions. The patient will be treated aggressively to increase cardiac output and maintain adequate tissue perfusion. Interventions may include vasoactive medications, intra-aortic balloon pump, pulmonary artery catheterization, and frequent ongoing assessments.

ASSESSMENT

Typically, the patient's history includes a disorder that severely decreases left ventricular function (such as MI or cardiomyopathy). Patients with underlying cardiac disease may complain of anginal pain because of decreased myocardial perfusion and oxygenation. Urine output is usually less than 20 ml/hour.

Inspection usually reveals pale skin, decreased sensorium, and rapid, shallow respirations. Palpation of peripheral pulses may detect a rapid, thready pulse. The skin feels cold and clammy.

Blood pressure measurement usually discloses a mean arterial pressure of less than 60 mm Hg and a narrowing pulse pressure. In a patient with chronic hypotension, the mean pressure may fall below 50 mm Hg before he exhibits any signs of shock. Auscultation of the heart detects gallop rhythm, faint heart sounds and, possibly (if shock results from rupture of the ventricular septum or papillary muscles), a holosystolic murmur.

Although many of these clinical features also occur in heart failure and other shock syndromes, they are usually more profound in cardiogenic shock. Patients with pericardial tamponade may have distant heart sounds.

NURSING DIAGNOSES AND COLLABORATIVE PROBLEMS

Based on these nursing diagnoses, you'll establish patient outcomes.

Altered cardiopulmonary tissue perfusion related to decreased cardiac output caused by left ventricular dysfunction. The patient will:
- exhibit no cardiac arrhythmias
- remain free from chest pain
- exhibit ABG values within the normal range.

Decreased cardiac output related to left ventricular dysfunction caused by myocardial injury. The patient will:
- have a heart rate and blood pressure within the normal range
- regain and maintain normal cardiac output.

Fear related to threat of death caused by cardiogenic shock. The patient will:

- identify and verbalize his fears
- use support systems to diminish his fears
- exhibit fewer physical symptoms of fear.

Knowledge deficit related to disease process, treatments and procedures, and long-term implications of the disease. The patient will:

- relate information about immediate needs and on-going care
- ask appropriate questions
- verbalize an understanding of the disease, treatments, and possible complications.

PLANNING AND IMPLEMENTATION
The following measures help the patient in cardiogenic shock.

- In the intensive care unit (ICU), start an I.V. infusion of normal saline or lactated Ringer's solution using a large-bore (14G to 18G) catheter, which allows easier administration of later blood transfusions.
- Administer oxygen by face mask or artificial airway to ensure adequate oxygenation of tissues.
- Adjust the oxygen flow rate to a higher or lower level, as ABG measurements indicate. Many patients will need 100% oxygen, and some will require 5 to 15 cm H_2O of positive end-expiratory or continuous positive airway pressure ventilation.
- Administer an osmotic diuretic such as mannitol, if ordered, to increase renal blood flow and urine output.
- When a patient is on the IABP, move him as little as possible. Never flex his "ballooned" leg at the hip because this may displace or fracture the catheter. Never place the patient in a sitting position for any reason (including chest X-rays) while the balloon is inflated; the balloon will tear through the aorta and result in immediate death.
- During use of the IABP, assess pedal pulses and skin temperature and color to ensure adequate peripheral circulation.
- Check the dressing over the IABP insertion site frequently for bleeding, and change it according to your facility's protocol. Also check the site for hematoma or signs of infection, and culture any drainage.
- If the patient becomes hemodynamically stable, gradually reduce the frequency of balloon inflation to wean him from the IABP.
- When weaning the patient from the IABP, watch for ECG changes, chest pain, and other signs of recurring cardiac ischemia as well as shock.
- Monitor and record blood pressure, pulse, respiratory rate, and peripheral pulses every 1 to 5 minutes until the patient stabilizes.
- Record hemodynamic pressure readings every 15 minutes. Monitor cardiac rhythm continuously. Systolic blood pressure less than 80 mm Hg usually results in inadequate coronary artery blood flow, cardiac ischemia, arrhythmias, and further complications of low cardiac output.
- If blood pressure drops below 80 mm Hg, increase the oxygen flow rate and notify the doctor immediately.
- Keep in mind that a progressive drop in blood pressure accompanied by a thready pulse generally signals inadequate cardiac output from reduced intravascular volume. Notify the doctor, and increase the I.V. infusion rate.
- Using a pulmonary artery catheter, closely monitor PAP, PAWP and, if equipment is available, cardiac output. A high PAWP indicates heart failure, increased systemic vascular resistance, decreased cardiac output, and decreased cardiac index and should be reported immediately.
- Insert an indwelling urinary catheter if necessary to measure hourly urine output. If output is less than 30 ml/hour in adults, increase the fluid infusion rate but watch for signs of fluid overload, such as an increase in PAWP. Notify the doctor if urine output doesn't improve.
- Determine how much fluid to give by checking blood pressure, urine output, central venous pressure (CVP), or PAWP. (To increase accuracy, measure CVP at the level of the right atrium, using the same reference point on the chest each time.)
- Monitor ABG values, complete blood count, and electrolyte levels.
- During therapy, assess skin color and temperature and note any changes. Cold, clammy skin may be a sign of continuing peripheral vascular constriction, indicating progressive shock.
- Plan your care to allow frequent rest periods, and provide as much privacy as possible.
- Allow family members to visit and comfort the patient as much as possible. Allow them to express their anger, anxiety, and fear.

Patient teaching
- Because the patient and his family may be anxious about the ICU and about the IABP and other devices, offer explanations and reassurance.
- Prepare the patient and his family for a probable fatal outcome, and help them find effective coping strategies

EVALUATION
Achievement of patient outcomes determines whether collaborative management has succeeded. For a patient in cardiogenic shock, evaluation focuses on improved tissue perfusion and cardiac output.

Cardiomyopathy

This disorder of the heart muscle occurs in three major forms: dilated, restrictive, and hypertrophic cardiomyopathy. Dilated cardiomyopathy occurs when myocardial muscle fibers become extensively damaged. Disturbances in myocardial metabolism and gross dilation of the ventricles without proportional compensatory hypertrophy cause the heart to take on a globular shape and to contract poorly during systole. Dilated cardiomyopathy leads to intractable heart failure, arrhythmias, and emboli. Usually not diagnosed until its advanced stages, this form of cardiomyopathy carries a poor prognosis.

Restrictive cardiomyopathy is characterized by restricted ventricular filling and failure to contract completely during systole. This disorder of the myocardial musculature results in low cardiac output and, eventually, endocardial fibrosis and thickening. If severe, it's irreversible.

Hypertrophic cardiomyopathy (also called idiopathic hypertrophic subaortic stenosis) is a primary disease of the cardiac muscle characterized by disproportionate, asymmetrical thickening of the interventricular septum, particularly in the anterior-superior part. Depending on whether stenosis is obstructive or nonobstructive, cardiac output may be low, normal, or high. If cardiac output is normal or high, the disorder may go undetected for years. Low cardiac output may lead to potentially fatal heart failure. The course of the illness varies; some patients demonstrate progressive deterioration. Others remain stable for several years.

CAUSES

The primary cause of all three forms of cardiomyopathy is unknown. Occasionally, also for unknown reasons, the dilated form occurs secondary to one of the following conditions:
- viral infections
- muscle disorders, such as myasthenia gravis and progressive muscular dystrophy
- infiltrative disorders, such as hemochromatosis and amyloidosis
- sarcoidosis
- endocrine disorders, such as hyperthyroidism and pheochromocytoma
- nutritional disorders, such as thiamine deficiency and kwashiorkor (protein deficiency)
- alcoholism
- pregnancy, especially in multiparous women over age 30 with preeclampsia or malnutrition.

In amyloidosis, infiltration of amyloid into the intracellular spaces in the myocardium, endocardium, and subendocardium may lead to restrictive cardiomyopathy syndrome.

About half of all cases of hypertrophic cardiomyopathy are transmitted as an autosomal dominant trait.

Dilated cardiomyopathy produces a diffuse degeneration of myocardial fibers. All four chambers enlarge and dilate. Initially, the ventricles enlarge, which results in impaired contractility and eventually leads to heart failure.

In restrictive cardiomyopathy, the ventricular walls are excessively rigid, impeding ventricular filling. Myocardial contractility with systole is usually unaffected. The ventricles lose their elasticity from the fibrotic infiltrations into the myocardium, endocardium, and subendocardium. The tightening heart muscle interferes with ventricular diastolic filling. As filling pressures increase, cardiac output decreases. Eventually, cardiac failure and mild ventricular hypertrophy occur.

In hypertrophic cardiomyopathy, the left ventricle walls (particularly the interventricular septum) thicken and encroach on the left ventricular chamber, impeding flow. Septal hypertrophy may obstruct the left ventricular outflow during systole. Diastolic dysfunction commonly occurs in the form of stiffness of the left ventricle during diastolic filling. This stiffness raises left ventricular end-diastolic pressure, which eventually results in elevation of left atrial, pulmonary venous, and pulmonary capillary pressure. These patients are at risk for endocarditis.

DIAGNOSIS AND TREATMENT

Diagnosis is based on a complete history and physical examination to rule out other known causes of heart failure.

Although no single test confirms dilated cardiomyopathy, the patient may undergo an electrocardiogram (ECG) and angiography to rule out ischemic heart disease. The ECG may also show biventricular hypertrophy, sinus tachycardia, atrial enlargement and, in 20% of patients, atrial fibrillation. In addition, a chest X-ray demonstrates cardiomegaly (usually affecting all heart chambers), pulmonary congestion, or pleural effusion. Multiple-gated acquisition scanning and echocardiography show decreased left ventricular function and decreased wall motion.

In restrictive cardiomyopathy, the ECG may show low-voltage complexes, hypertrophy, or atrioventricular conduction defects. Arterial pulsation reveals blunt carotid upstroke with small volume. In advanced stages of the disease, a chest X-ray shows massive cardiomegaly affecting all four chambers of the heart.

Echocardiography rules out constrictive pericarditis as the cause of restricted filling by detecting increased left ventricular muscle mass and differences in end-diastolic pressures between the ventricles. Cardiac catheterization demonstrates increased left ventricular end-diastolic pressure and rules out constrictive pericarditis as the cause of restricted filling.

Most useful in diagnosing hypertrophic cardiomyopathy, echocardiography shows increased thickness of the interventricular septum and abnormal motion of the anterior mitral leaflet during systole (in obstructive hypertrophic cardiomyopathy, this leads to occluded left ventricular outflow). Cardiac catheterization reveals elevated left ventricular end-diastolic pressure and possibly mitral insufficiency. The ECG usually demonstrates left ventricular hypertrophy, ST-segment and T-wave abnormalities, deep waves (from hypertrophy, not infarction), left anterior hemiblock, ventricular arrhythmias, and possibly atrial fibrillation. Phonocardiography confirms an early systolic murmur.

Treatment for dilated cardiomyopathy seeks to correct the underlying causes and to improve the heart's pumping ability with digitalis glycosides, diuretics, oxygen, and a sodium-restricted diet. It may also include prolonged bed rest, selective use of steroids and, possibly, pericardiotomy, which is still investigational. Vasodilators reduce preload and afterload, thereby decreasing congestion and increasing cardiac output. Acute heart failure requires vasodilation with I.V. nitroprusside or nitroglycerin. Long-term treatment may include prazosin, hydralazine, isosorbide dinitrate and, for the patient on prolonged bed rest, anticoagulants. When these treatments fail, carefully selected patients may undergo a heart transplant.

Although no therapy currently exists for restricted ventricular filling, digitalis glycosides, diuretics, and a sodium-restricted diet ease symptoms of heart failure. Oral vasodilators—such as isosorbide dinitrate, prazosin, and hydralazine—may control intractable heart failure. Anticoagulant therapy may prevent thrombophlebitis in the patient on prolonged bed rest.

In hypertrophic cardiomyopathy, treatment seeks to relax the ventricle and to relieve outflow tract obstruction. Propranolol, a beta-adrenergic blocking agent, slows heart rate and increases ventricular filling by relaxing the obstructing muscle, thereby reducing angina, syncope, dyspnea, and arrhythmias. However, propranolol may aggravate symptoms of cardiac decompensation. Atrial fibrillation necessitates cardioversion to treat the arrhythmia and, because of the high risk of systemic embolism, anticoagulant therapy until fibrillation subsides.

If drug therapy fails, the patient may undergo surgery. Ventricular myotomy (resection of the hypertrophied septum) alone or combined with mitral valve replacement may ease outflow tract obstruction and relieve symptoms. This procedure may cause complications, such as complete heart block and ventricular septal defect.

COLLABORATIVE MANAGEMENT

Care of the patient with cardiomyopathy focuses on minimizing the signs and symptoms of heart failure and treating any arrhythmias that develop.

ASSESSMENT

The patient with dilated cardiomyopathy may develop shortness of breath (orthopnea, exertional dyspnea, paroxysmal nocturnal dyspnea), fatigue, and an irritating dry cough at night. Other manifestations include edema, liver engorgement, jugular vein distention, peripheral cyanosis, sinus tachycardia, atrial fibrillation, and diffuse apical impulses. Auscultation may reveal a pansystolic murmur (mitral and tricuspid regurgitation secondary to cardiomegaly and weak papillary muscles) or S_3 and S_4 gallop rhythms.

Restrictive cardiomyopathy produces fatigue, dyspnea, orthopnea, chest pain, generalized edema, liver engorgement, peripheral cyanosis, pallor, and S_3 or S_4 gallop rhythms.

In hypertrophic cardiomyopathy, clinical features include angina pectoris, arrhythmias, dyspnea, syncope, heart failure, systolic ejection murmur (of medium pitch, heard along the left sternal border and at the apex), pulsus biferiens, and irregular pulse (with atrial fibrillation.

NURSING DIAGNOSES AND COLLABORATIVE PROBLEMS

Based on the following nursing diagnoses, you'll establish patient outcomes.

Decreased cardiac output related to alteration in cardiac structure and ventricular dysfunction. The patient will:
■ exhibit hemodynamic stability, including vital signs within acceptable parameters
■ remain free of complications.

Fluid volume excess related to mechanical dysfunction of the heart. The patient will:
■ tolerate restrictions without problems
■ remain free of signs and symptoms of fluid excess.

Activity intolerance related to imbalance between oxygen supply and demand. The patient will:
■ exhibit vital signs within acceptable parameters during activity
■ demonstrate skill in conserving energy.

Ineffective individual coping related to disease process and fear of death. The patient will:
■ verbalize feelings freely
■ demonstrate positive coping mechanisms.

Knowledge deficit related to all aspects of disease and its treatment. The patient will:
■ verbalize correct information about the disease and its treatment
■ identify signs and symptoms of possible complications and need to seek medical treatment.

PLANNING AND IMPLEMENTATION
The following measures help the patient with cardiomyopathy.

■ In the patient with acute heart failure, monitor for signs of progressive failure (decreased arterial pulses, increased neck vein distention) and compromised renal perfusion (oliguria, increased blood urea nitrogen and serum creatinine levels, and electrolyte imbalances).

■ If the patient takes vasodilators, check blood pressure and heart rate frequently. If he becomes hypotensive, stop the infusion and place him in the supine position, with his legs elevated to increase venous return and to ensure cerebral blood flow. Keep the patient on bed rest until blood pressure returns to normal.

■ In the acute phase, monitor heart rate and rhythm, blood pressure, urine output, and pulmonary artery pressure readings to help guide treatment.

■ Administer medications as ordered. Before dental work or surgery, administer prophylaxis for subacute bacterial endocarditis.

■ Weigh the patient daily.

■ Monitor the patient receiving diuretics for signs of resolving congestion (decreased crackles and dyspnea) or too-vigorous diuresis. Check serum potassium level for hypokalemia, especially if therapy includes digitalis glycosides.

■ Assess the patient's tolerance of activities before ambulation.

■ Monitor vital signs and ECG during any periods of activity.

■ Provide appropriate diversionary activities for the patient on prolonged bed rest.

■ Balance activity and rest periods; assist with energy conservation measures.

■ Warn the patient against strenuous physical activities such as running. Syncope or sudden death may follow well-tolerated exercise.

■ Be aware that therapeutic restrictions and an uncertain prognosis usually cause profound anxiety and depression. Offer support and encourage the patient to express his feelings.

■ Be flexible with visiting hours. If the patient faces a prolonged hospitalization, try to obtain permission for him to spend occasional weekends at home.

■ If the patient needs additional help in coping with his restricted lifestyle, refer him for psychosocial counseling.

Patient teaching
■ Emphasize the need to take digitalis glycosides as prescribed; advise him to watch for adverse effects, such as as anorexia, nausea, vomiting, and yellow vision.

■ If propranolol is prescribed, warn the patient not to stop taking it abruptly; doing so could cause rebound effects, resulting in MI or sudden death.

■ Instruct the patient to record and report weight gain.

■ If the patient must restrict sodium intake, tell him to read food labels, avoid canned foods, pickles, smoked meats, and excessive use of table salt.

■ Because the patient faces an increased risk of sudden cardiac arrest, encourage family members to learn cardiopulmonary resuscitation and how to access the emergency medical system.

EVALUATION
Achievement of patient outcomes determines whether collaborative management has succeeded. For a patient with cardiomyopathy, evaluation focuses on improved cardiac output as evidenced by good color; warm, dry skin; clear lungs; improved fluid balance; activity tolerance; improved coping; and adequate knowledge.

Coronary artery disease

The primary effect of coronary artery disease (CAD), also called atherosclerotic heart disease, is loss of oxygen and nutrients to myocardial tissue because of diminished coronary blood flow. Fatty fibrous plaques, possibly including calcium deposits, narrow the lumens of coronary arteries, reducing the volume of blood that can flow through them.

Nearly epidemic in the Western world, CAD is more prevalent in men, whites, and middle-aged and elderly people than in women or in people of other races and ages. More than 50% of men age 60 or older show signs of CAD on autopsy.

CAUSES
Atherosclerosis, the most common cause of CAD, has been linked to many risk factors. Age, sex, a family history of CAD, and race are nonmodifiable factors. However, with good medical care and appropriate lifestyle changes, the patient can modify other risk factors, such as the following:

■ *Blood pressure.* Systolic blood pressure greater than 160 mm Hg or diastolic blood pressure greater than 95 mm Hg increases the risk.

■ *Serum cholesterol levels.* Increased low-density lipoprotein levels and decreased high-density lipoprotein levels substantially increase the risk.

■ *Smoking.* Cigarette smokers are twice as likely to have a myocardial infarction (MI) and four times as likely to experience sudden death. The risk dramatically drops within 1 year after smoking ceases.

Understanding coronary artery spasm

In coronary artery spasm, a spontaneous, sustained contraction of one or more coronary arteries causes ischemia and dysfunction of the heart muscle. This disorder may also cause Prinzmetal's angina and even myocardial infarction (MI) in patients with unoccluded coronary arteries.

Causes

The direct cause of coronary artery spasm is unknown, but possible contributing factors include:
- altered influx of calcium across the cell membrane
- intimal hemorrhage into the medial layer of the blood vessel
- hyperventilation
- elevated catecholamine levels
- fatty buildup in the lumen.

Signs and symptoms

The major symptom of coronary artery spasm is angina. But unlike classic angina, this pain commonly occurs spontaneously and may be unrelated to physical exertion or emotional stress; it may, however, follow cocaine use. The pain is usually more severe than classic angina, lasts longer, and may be cyclic—recurring every day at the same time.

Ischemic episodes may cause arrhythmias, altered heart rate, lower blood pressure and, occasionally, fainting due to decreased cardiac output. Spasm in the left coronary artery may result in mitral valve prolapse, producing a loud systolic murmur and, possibly, pulmonary edema, with dyspnea, crackles, and hemoptysis. MI and sudden death may occur.

Treatment

After diagnosis by coronary angiography and 12-lead electrocardiography, the patient may receive calcium channel blockers (verapamil, nifedipine, or diltiazem) to reduce coronary artery spasm and to decrease vascular resistance, and nitrates (nitroglycerin or isosorbide dinitrate) to relieve chest pain. During cardiac catheterization, the patient with clean arteries may receive ergotamine to induce the spasm and aid in the diagnosis.

Nursing interventions

When caring for a patient with coronary artery spasm, explain all necessary procedures and teach him how to take his medications safely. For calcium antagonist therapy, monitor the patient's blood pressure, pulse rate, and cardiac rhythm strips to detect arrhythmias.

For nifedipine and verapamil therapy, monitor digoxin levels and check for signs of digitalis toxicity. Because nifedipine may cause peripheral and periorbital edema, watch for fluid retention.

Because coronary artery spasm is sometimes associated with atherosclerotic disease, advise the patient to stop smoking, avoid overeating, drink alcoholic beverages sparingly, and maintain a balance between exercise and rest.

- *Obesity.* Excessive weight raises the risk of diabetes mellitus, hypertension, and elevated serum cholesterol levels.
- *Physical activity.* Regular exercise reduces the risk.
- *Stress.* Added stress or type A personality increases the risk.
- *Diabetes mellitus.* This disorder raises the risk, especially in women.
- *Other modifiable factors.* Increased levels of serum fibrinogen and uric acid, elevated hematocrit, reduced vital capacity, high resting heart rate, thyrotoxicosis, and use of oral contraceptives heighten the risk.

Uncommon causes of reduced coronary artery blood flow include dissecting aneurysms, infectious vasculitis, syphilis, and congenital defects in the coronary vascular system. Coronary artery spasms may also impede blood flow. (See *Understanding coronary artery spasm*.)

CAD is a progressive disease characterized by the formation of atheromas or plaques in the intimal and medial layers of large and medium-sized arteries. An unknown factor—believed to be injury, inflammation

of the endothelial cells lining the artery, or a mural thrombus (a clot in the arterial wall from injury)—initiates atherosclerotic plaque development. Lipoproteins and fibrous tissue accumulate in the arterial wall. As part of the normal inflammatory process, the damaged endothelium promotes adhesion and aggregation of platelets and attracts leukocytes to the area.

Macrophage contact with platelets, cholesterol, and other blood components stimulates the smooth muscle cells and connective tissue within the vessel wall to proliferate abnormally. Blood flow at this stage may not be affected; however, a yellowish fatty streak may be apparent on the inner lining of the artery.

As the smooth-muscle cells enlarge, collagen fibers accumulate, cholesterol builds up, and fibrous plaques appear as white, elevated areas protruding into the arterial lumen and fixed to the intimal layer. The developing plaque gradually narrows the vessel lumen and impairs its ability to dilate in response to increased oxygen demands. As the plaque expands, it can produce severe stenosis or total arterial occlusion.

The final stage is the development of complex lesions consisting of lipids, fibrous tissue, collagen, calcium, cellular debris, and capillaries. These calcified lesions can ulcerate or rupture, stimulating thrombosis. The thrombus may rapidly occlude the vessel lumen or it may embolize to occlude distant vessels.

When a coronary artery goes into spasm or is occluded by plaque, blood flow to the myocardium supplied by that vessel decreases, causing angina pectoris, the classic symptom of CAD. Failure to remedy the occlusion causes ischemia and, eventually, myocardial tissue infarction.

DIAGNOSIS AND TREATMENT

Until the patient experiences signs and symptoms of arterial narrowing, the diagnosis is typically presumed, based on the history and physical examination findings and on the existence of risk factors.

Possible diagnostic tests include the following:
- *Electrocardiography (ECG)* during angina shows ischemia, as demonstrated by T-wave inversion or ST-segment depression and, possibly, arrhythmias, such as premature ventricular contractions. ECG results may be normal during pain-free periods. Arrhythmias may occur without infarction, secondary to ischemia.
- *Exercise ECG* may provoke chest pain and ECG signs of myocardial ischemia in response to physical exertion. Monitoring of electrical rhythm may demonstrate T-wave inversion or ST-segment depression in the ischemic areas.
- *Coronary angiography* reveals coronary artery stenosis or obstruction, collateral circulation, and the arteries' condition beyond the narrowing.
- *Myocardial perfusion imaging* with thallium-201 during treadmill exercise detects ischemic areas of the myocardium, visualized as "cold spots."

The goal of treatment in patients with CAD is to reduce myocardial oxygen demand or increase the oxygen supply and reduce pain. Activity restrictions may be required to prevent pain. Rather than eliminating activities, performing them more slowly often averts pain. Stress-reduction techniques are also essential, especially if known stressors precipitate pain.

Drug therapy consists primarily of nitrates, such as nitroglycerin, isosorbide dinitrate, or beta-adrenergic blockers.

Obstructive lesions may need atherectomy or coronary artery bypass graft (CABG) surgery using vein or arterial grafts. Percutaneous transluminal coronary angioplasty (PTCA) may be performed during cardiac catheterization to compress fatty deposits and relieve occlusion. Intracoronary stents also may be used.

Laser angioplasty corrects occlusion by vaporizing fatty deposits with the excimer or hot-tip laser device. Rotational ablation (or rotational atherectomy) removes plaque with a high-speed, rotating burr covered with diamond crystals.

Because CAD is so widespread, prevention is important. Dietary restrictions aimed at reducing the intake of calories (in obesity), salt, fats, and cholesterol minimize the risk, especially when supplemented with regular exercise. Abstention from smoking and stress reduction are also essential.

Other preventive actions include controlling hypertension (with diuretics or beta blockers), controlling elevated serum cholesterol or triglyceride levels (with antilipemics such as clofibrate), and minimizing platelet aggregation and the danger of blood clots (with aspirin, for example).

COLLABORATIVE MANAGEMENT

Care of the patient with CAD focuses on aggressive management of risk factors to slow the atherosclerotic process and reduce the risk of complications.

ASSESSMENT

The classic symptom of CAD is angina, the direct result of inadequate flow of oxygen to the myocardium. The patient usually describes the pain as a burning, squeezing, or crushing tightness in the substernal or precordial chest that may radiate to the left arm, neck, jaw, or shoulder blade. He typically clenches his fist over his chest or rubs his left arm when describing the pain. Nausea, vomiting, fainting, sweating, and cool extremities may accompany the tightness.

Angina commonly occurs after physical exertion but may also follow emotional excitement, exposure to cold, or a large meal. Angina can also develop during sleep and may awaken the patient.

The patient's history will suggest any pattern to the type and onset of pain. If the pain is predictable and relieved by rest or nitrates, it's called stable angina. If it increases in frequency and duration and is more easily induced, it's referred to as unstable or unpredictable angina. Unstable angina generally indicates extensive or worsening disease and, untreated, may progress to MI. An effort-induced pain that occurs with increasing frequency and with decreasing provocation is referred to as crescendo angina. If severe pain occurs at rest without provocation, it's called Prinzmetal's or variant angina.

Inspection may reveal evidence of atherosclerotic disease, such as xanthelasma and xanthoma. Ophthalmoscopic inspection may show increased light reflexes and arteriovenous nicking, suggesting hypertension, an important risk factor for CAD.

Palpation can uncover thickened or absent peripheral arteries, signs of cardiac enlargement, and abnormal contraction of the cardiac impulse, such as left ventricular akinesia or dyskinesia.

Auscultation may detect bruits, an S_3, an S_4, or a late systolic murmur (in mitral insufficiency).

NURSING DIAGNOSES AND COLLABORATIVE PROBLEMS

Based on the following nursing diagnoses, you'll establish patient outcomes.

Altered cardiopulmonary tissue perfusion related to reduced blood flow to the myocardium caused by coronary artery spasm, narrowing, or occlusion. The patient will:
- maintain adequate myocardial tissue perfusion, as exhibited by a normal heart rate and rhythm and the absence of ischemic ECG changes
- verbalize an understanding of the prescribed medical regimen and relate the importance of seeking continued follow-up care.

Pain related to inadequate oxygen flow to the myocardium as a result of reduced myocardial blood flow. The patient will:
- identify the factors that trigger anginal pain
- verbalize an understanding of what he needs to do when anginal pain occurs
- experience a reduction in the severity and frequency of anginal attacks by complying with medical or surgical therapy.

Activity intolerance related to an imbalance between myocardial oxygen supply and demand. The patient will:
- identify the factors and activities he needs to avoid and the activities for which he must obtain assistance
- recognize modifications to conserve energy while performing his daily activities
- participate in a medically supervised exercise program that will help him develop collateral myocardial circulation and increase his activity tolerance level.

Knowledge deficit related to all aspects of the disease process and treatment. The patient will:
- verbalize measures to decrease modifiable risk factors
- state signs and symptoms to report to the doctor
- recognize events that may precipitate symptoms
- demonstrate an understanding of all procedures and treatments necessary.

Ineffective management of therapeutic regimen related to required lifestyle changes. The patient will:
- verbalize the importance of lifestyle changes related to diet, exercise, stress, and smoking
- adhere to lifestyle changes associated with therapeutic regimen
- demonstrate compliance with the treatment plan.

PLANNING AND IMPLEMENTATION

The following measures help the patient with CAD.
- Assess the location, severity, and quality of the patient's pain. Ask him to rate the pain on a scale of 0 to 10.
- Monitor vital signs and hemodynamic parameters according to the policy of your health care facility.
- Assess cardiopulmonary status, including heart sounds.
- Assess skin color and mucous membranes for signs of oxygenation; monitor pulse oximetry and arterial blood gas (ABG) levels, as ordered.
- Administer oxygen as ordered and as reflected by pulse oximetry or ABG levels.
- Monitor bowel sounds and urine output, both of which may decrease with poor perfusion.
- Administer vasodilators, such as nitroglycerin, to increase perfusion.
- Monitor the ECG for changes indicating ischemia; watch for possible arrhythmias.
- Prepare the patient for PTCA or CABG surgery, as indicated.
- After cardiac catheterization, monitor the patient's catheter site for bleeding and hematoma formation, evaluate his distal pulses, and periodically check his serum potassium level. To counter the diuretic effect of the dye, increase the I.V. flow rate and make sure the patient drinks plenty of fluids. Add potassium to the I.V. fluid, as ordered.
- After rotational ablation, monitor the patient for chest pain, hypotension, coronary artery spasm, and bleeding from the catheter site. Provide heparin and antibiotics for 24 to 48 hours, as ordered.
- During anginal episodes, monitor blood pressure and heart rate, and take a 12-lead ECG before administering nitroglycerin or other nitrates. Record the duration of pain, the amount of medication required to relieve it, and any accompanying symptoms.
- Administer nitroglycerin as ordered, and note the patient's response. Keep nitroglycerin available for immediate use. Instruct the patient to call immediately whenever he feels chest, arm, or neck pain and before taking nitroglycerin.
- Place the patient in semi- or high-Fowler's position.
- Administer oxygen at 4 to 6 L/minute, as ordered, unless contraindicated by chronic pulmonary disease.
- Question the patient about any factors or activities that may have precipitated the attack.
- Monitor the patient for signs of complications, including arrhythmias and progression of ischemia, leading to MI.
- Assess the patient's activity level, and note any incidences of chest pain with activity.
- Space activities to allow the patient to rest between them.
- Assist with passive range-of-motion exercises during bed rest; begin a progressive exercise program as ordered.

HEALTHY LIVING — Reducing the risk of CAD

Teach your patient how to reduce the risk of coronary artery disease (CAD) by adopting the following healthy behaviors:

- stress reduction techniques
- diet low in fat and cholesterol (with saturated fat intake of less than 10%, nonsaturated fat intake less the 30% of daily food intake, and cholesterol intake reduced to 250 to 300 mg/day)
- exercise and weight reduction
- smoking cessation
- caffeine intake reduction
- alcohol intake in moderation or not at all
- medical follow-up for such disorders as diabetes and hypertension.

Patient teaching

- Explain any treatments, procedures, and surgeries to the patient. Before cardiac catheterization, make sure he knows why it's necessary, understands the risks, and realizes that it may indicate a need for other interventional therapies. After catheterization, review the expected course of treatment with the patient and his family.
- Explain that recurrent angina after PTCA or rotational ablation may signal recurring obstruction.
- Help the patient determine which activities precipitate episodes of pain. Help him identify and select more effective coping mechanisms to deal with stress.
- Explain all aspects of medication therapy. Stress the need to follow the prescribed drug regimen.
- Encourage the patient to maintain the prescribed low-sodium diet and, if indicated for obesity, a low-calorie diet.
- Encourage regular, moderate exercise. Refer the patient to a cardiac rehabilitation center or cardiovascular fitness program near his home or workplace.
- Discuss issues involving sexual activity and possible modifications. Ahead of time, review the patient's medications for any drugs that can cause impotence.
- Explain the signs and symptoms that require follow-up care or doctor notification.
- If necessary, refer the patient to a program to stop smoking. (See *Reducing the risk of CAD*.) Make any other necessary referrals for home care (to ensure compliance), rehabilitation, support groups, or other organized activities.

EVALUATION

Achievement of patient outcomes determines whether collaborative management has succeeded. For a patient with CAD, evaluation focuses on improved tissue perfusion, pain relief, improved activity tolerance, and adequate knowledge of the disease and its treatment.

Heart failure

When the myocardium can't pump effectively enough to meet the body's metabolic needs, heart failure occurs. Pump failure usually occurs in a damaged left ventricle (left-sided heart failure). However, it may occur in the right venticle, either as primary failure or as secondary failure due to left ventricular dysfunction. Left- and right-sided heart failure may also develop simultaneously.

Heart failure is classified as high-output or low-output, acute or chronic, left-sided (systolic), or right-sided (diastolic), and forward or backward. (See *Categorizing heart failure*.)

For many patients, the symptoms of heart failure restrict their ability to perform activities of daily living, severely affecting their quality of life. Advances in diagnostic and therapeutic techniques have greatly improved the outlook for these patients, but the prognosis still depends on the underlying cause and its response to treatment.

CAUSES

Heart failure commonly results from a primary abnormality of the heart muscle (such as an infarction) that impairs ventricular function to the point that the heart can no longer pump sufficient blood. It can also result from causes not related to myocardial function. These include:

- mechanical disturbances in ventricular filling during diastole, which result from blood volume that's insufficient for the ventricle to pump (occur in mitral stenosis secondary to rheumatic heart disease or constrictive pericarditis and atrial fibrillation)
- systolic hemodynamic disturbances—such as excessive cardiac workload caused by volume overload or pressure overload—that limit the heart's pumping ability (can result from mitral or aortic insufficiency, which causes volume overload, and aortic stenosis or systemic hypertension, which results in increased resistance to ventricular emptying)

In addition, certain conditions can predispose the patient to heart failure, particularly if he has some form of underlying heart disease. These include:

- arrhythmias—such as tachyarrhythmias, which can reduce ventricular filling time; bradycardia, which can reduce cardiac output; and arrhythmias that disrupt the normal atrial and ventricular filling synchrony
- pregnancy and thyrotoxicosis—which increase demand for cardiac output

Categorizing heart failure

Although heart failure is usually classified by the site of failure (left-sided, right-sided, or both), it may also be classified by level of cardiac output (high-output or low-output), stage (acute or chronic), and direction (forward or backward). These classifications represent different clinical aspects of heart failure, not distinct diseases.

Left-sided (or systolic) failure

Failure of the left ventricle to pump blood to the vital organs and periphery is usually caused by myocardial infarction (MI). Decreased left ventricular output causes fluid to accumulate in the lungs, precipitating dyspnea, orthopnea, and paroxysmal nocturnal dyspnea.

Right-sided (or diastolic) failure

Resulting from failure of the right ventricle to pump sufficient blood to the lungs, this type usually is caused by disorders that increase pulmonary vascular resistance, such as pulmonary embolism, pulmonic stenosis, and pulmonary hypertension. Right ventricular failure produces congestive hepatomegaly, ascites, and edema.

High-output failure

Failure with an elevated cardiac output occurs when tissue demands for oxygenated blood exceed the heart's ability to supply it. High-output failure occurs in arteriovenous fistula, hyperthyroidism, anemia, sickle cell anemia, beriberi, Paget's disease of the bone, and thyrotoxicosis.

Low-output failure

Failure with decreased cardiac output is caused by decreased pumping ability of the myocardium. Low-output failure occurs in coronary artery disease, hypertension, primary myocardial disease, and valvular disease.

Acute failure

This failure occurs suddenly, as in MI or ruptured cardiac valve. The sudden reduction in cardiac output results in systemic hypotension without peripheral edema. Acute failure may occur in a chronic condition—for example, when a patient with chronic heart failure experiences acute heart failure with MI. It may also occur in any condition that stresses an already diseased heart.

Chronic failure

This type of heart failure occurs gradually and is sustained for long periods. The arterial blood pressure doesn't drop, but peripheral edema is present. Chronic failure may occur in cardiomyopathy or multivalvular disease or in a healed, extensive MI.

Forward failure

In this type of heart failure, the heart fails to expel enough blood into the arterial system. Sodium and water retention result from decreased renal perfusion and excessive proximal tubular sodium reabsorption or excessive distal tubular reabsorption, through activation of the renin-angiotensin-aldosterone system.

Backward failure

When backward failure occurs, one ventricle fails to empty its contents normally, and end-diastolic ventricular pressures rise. The pressures and volume in the atrium and venous system behind the failing ventricle also rise, and sodium and water retention occur because of the elevated systemic venous and capillary pressures and the resulting transudation of fluid into the interstitial space.

■ pulmonary embolism—which elevates pulmonary artery pressures that can cause right-sided heart failure
■ infections—which increase metabolic demands, further burdening the heart
■ anemia—which requires increased cardiac output to meet the oxygen needs of the tissues
■ increased physical activity, emotional stress, increased sodium or water intake, or failure to comply with the prescribed treatment regimen—which are all underlying risk factors for heart disease.

Heart rate and stroke volume determine cardiac output. When stroke volume decreases, the heart normally compensates by increasing the rate. In heart failure, the heart may not be able to contract efficiently enough to maintain adequate stroke volume or beat fast enough to compensate. Stroke volume and cardiac output may continue to decrease as the heart weakens from increased workload or decreased oxygenation.

Left-sided heart failure involves impairment of the left side of the heart's function. A decrease in cardiac output occurs with pulmonary congestion and an increase in left atrial and left ventricular end-diastolic pressures. Pulmonary artery wedge pressure (PAWP) increases, resulting in fluid accumulation in the interstitial spaces of the lungs; this, in turn, causes pulmonary edema, a life-threatening condition. If the pulmonary edema is severe, capillary fluid moves into the alveoli, impairing gas exchange in the lungs.

In right-sided heart failure, an accumulation of blood backing up into the systemic venous system causes an increase in right atrial, right ventricular end-diastolic, and systemic venous pressures. Later effects include edema in the peripheral tissues and congestion of the abdominal organs. Because of the effects of gravity, edema is most pronounced in dependent parts of the body, such as the lower legs when the person is upright. The accumulation of fluid is evidenced as weight gain. As venous distention pro gresses, blood backs up into the hepatic veins and the liver becomes engorged. If engorgement is severe, hepatic function becomes impaired.

Pulmonary congestion can lead to pulmonary edema. Decreased perfusion to major organs, especially the brain and kidneys, can cause these organs to fail. MI can occur because the oxygen demands of the overworked heart can't be sufficiently met.

DIAGNOSIS AND TREATMENT

Electrocardiography reflects heart strain, enlargement, or ischemia. It may also reveal atrial enlargement, tachycardia, and extrasystole.

Chest X-rays show increased pulmonary vascular markings, interstitial edema, or pleural effusion and cardiomegaly.

Pulmonary artery pressure monitoring typically demonstrates elevated pulmonary artery pressure and PAWP, elevated left ventricular end-diastolic pressure in left-sided heart failure, and elevated right atrial or central venous pressure in right-sided heart failure.

The aim of therapy is to improve pump function by reversing the compensatory mechanisms that produce the clinical effects. Heart failure can usually be controlled quickly by the following treatments:
- diuresis (with diuretics, such as furosemide, hydrochlorothiazide, spironolactone, ethacrynic acid, bumetanide, or triamterene) to reduce total blood volume and circulatory congestion
- prolonged bed rest
- oxygen administration to increase oxygen delivery to the myocardium and other vital organ tissues
- inotropic drugs, such as digoxin, to strengthen myocardial contractility; sympathomimetics, such as dopamine and dobutamine, in acute situations; or amrinone, to increase contractility and produce arterial vasodilation
- vasodilators to increase cardiac output or angiotensin-converting enzyme inhibitors to decrease afterload
- antiembolism stockings to prevent venostasis and thromboembolism formation.

After recovery, the patient usually must continue taking digitalis glycosides, diuretics, and potassium supplements and must remain under medical supervision. If the patient with valve dysfunction has recurrent acute heart failure, surgical replacement may be necessary.

COLLABORATIVE MANAGEMENT

Care of the patient with heart failure focuses on reducing the heart's oxygen demand. This involves ensuring physical and psychological rest, administering and monitoring multiple-drug therapy, improving the contractility of the heart, and managing symptoms. (See *Managing uncomplicated heart failure,* pages 96 and 97.)

ASSESSMENT

The patient's history reveals a disorder or condition that can precipitate heart failure. The patient commonly complains of shortness of breath, which occurs in early stages during activity and, in late stages, also at rest. He may report that dyspnea worsens at night when he lies down. He may use two or three pillows to elevate his head to sleep or may have to sleep sitting up in a chair. He may relate that his shortness of breath wakes him up soon after he falls asleep, causing him to sit bolt upright to catch his breath. In many cases, he may remain dyspneic, coughing and wheezing even when he sits up (paroxysmal nocturnal dyspnea).

The patient may report that his shoes or rings have become too tight, a result of peripheral edema. He may also report increasing fatigue, weakness, insomnia, anorexia, nausea, and a sense of abdominal fullness (particularly in right-sided heart failure).

Inspection may reveal a dyspneic, anxious patient in respiratory distress. In mild cases, dyspnea may occur while the patient is lying down or active; in severe cases, it's not related to position. The patient may have a cough that produces pink, frothy sputum. You may note cyanosis of the lips and nail beds, pale skin, diaphoresis, dependent peripheral and sacral edema, and jugular vein distention. Ascites may also be present, especially in patients with right-sided heart failure. If heart failure is chronic, the patient may appear cachectic.

When palpating the pulse, you may note that the skin feels cool and clammy. The pulse rate will be rapid, and pulsus alternans may be present. You may also detect hepatomegaly and, possibly, splenomegaly.

Percussion reveals dullness over fluid-filled lung bases.

Auscultation of the blood pressure may detect decreased pulse pressure, reflecting reduced stroke volume. Heart auscultation may disclose third and four heart sounds. Lung auscultation reveals moist, bibasilar crackles. If pulmonary edema is present, you'll hear crackles throughout the lung, accompanied by rhonchi and expiratory wheezing.

NURSING DIAGNOSES AND COLLABORATIVE PROBLEMS

Based on these nursing diagnoses, you'll establish patient outcomes.

Decreased cardiac output related to reduced stroke volume caused by mechanical, structural, or electrophysiologic heart problems. The patient will:
- maintain a normal pulse rate and blood pressure
- be free of dizziness, syncope, arrhythmias, and chest pain
- express an understanding of why he must comply with the prescribed diet, take medications as ordered, and maintain an appropriate activity level.

Fluid volume excess related to blood pooling in the pulmonary system or the systemic circulation caused by myocardial damage. The patient will:
- restrict fluid intake, as ordered, so that it doesn't exceed fluid output
- regain and maintain baseline weight
- regain and maintain central venous and pulmonary artery pressures within normal limits (if available).

Ineffective breathing pattern related to fatigue caused by pulmonary congestion. The patient will:
- regain his baseline respiratory rate and maintain stable respirations
- regain and maintain arterial blood gas values within normal limits
- exhibit an ability to conserve energy while performing activities of daily living.

Knowledge deficit related to disease process, treatments and procedures, and long-term implications of the disease. The patient will:
- relate information about immediate needs and ongoing care
- ask appropriate questions
- verbalize accurate information about the disease and treatment.

Altered nutrition: Less than body requirements, related to fatigue. The patient will:
- consume enough calories to maintain ideal body weight
- consume six to eight small meals a day
- conserve energy before mealtimes.

Impaired skin integrity related to decreased tissue perfusion. The patient will:
- verbalize an understanding of basic skin care
- maintain strong peripheral pulses
- experience no skin breakdown.

PLANNING AND IMPLEMENTATION

The following measures help the patient with heart failure. (See *Treating heart failure,* page 98.)
- Assess the patient's vital signs for increased respiratory and heart rates and for narrowing pulse pressure; also assess his mental status.

- Provide continuous cardiac monitoring during acute and advanced disease stages to identify and manage arrhythmias promptly.
- Administer medications such as digitalis glycosides as ordered.
- Watch for calf pain and tenderness. To prevent deep vein thrombosis due to vascular congestion, assist the patient with range-of-motion exercises. Enforce bed rest, and apply antiembolism stockings.
- Place the patient in Fowler's position. Administer supplemental oxygen, as ordered, to ease his breathing.
- Auscultate the heart for abnormal sounds and the lungs for crackles or rhonchi.
- Report changes in the patient's condition immediately.
- Weigh the patient daily to help detect fluid retention, and observe for peripheral edema. Record abdominal girth at least every shift.
- Watch for jugular vein distention and peripheral edema; measure the circumference of lower extremities and note any changes.
- Administer diuretics as ordered.
- Assess intake and output frequently. Monitor I.V. intake and urine output (especially if the patient is receiving diuretics).
- Frequently monitor blood urea nitrogen and serum creatinine, potassium, sodium, chloride, and magnesium levels.
- Anticipate fluid and sodium restrictions.
- Organize all activities to provide maximum rest periods.
- Maintain a quiet environment to promote rest.
- Complete referrals for any necessary home care for follow-up assessment and instructions.

Patient teaching
- Advise the patient to avoid foods high in sodium content, such as canned and commercially prepared foods and dairy products, to curb fluid overload.
- Teach the patient that he must replace the potassium lost through diuretic therapy by taking a prescribed potassium supplement and eating potassium-rich foods, such as bananas, apricots, and orange juice.
- Stress the need for regular medical checkups and periodic blood tests to monitor drug levels.
- Stress the importance of taking digitalis glycosides exactly as prescribed. Tell the patient to watch for and immediately report signs of toxicity, such as anorexia, vomiting, confusion, slow or irregular pulse rate and, in elderly patients, flulike symptoms.
- Tell the patient to notify the doctor if his pulse rate is unusually irregular or less than 60 beats/minute; if

(Text continues on page 98.)

Managing uncomplicated heart failure

DRG
Average length of stay: 6.1 days
Date:

	Day 1	Days 2 to 3

MEDICAL INTERVENTIONS	■ History and physical; rule out myocardial infarction
	■ Standing orders (medications):
	  –Diuretics
	  –Angiotensin-converting enzyme (ACE) inhibitor
	  –Digoxin
	■ +/– Potassium/magnesium
	■ +/– Oxygen (O_2)
		■ If not already started:
		  – +/– ACE inhibitor (isosorbide if contraindicated)
		  – +/– Medication titration
		  – +/– Digoxin

NURSING INTERVENTIONS	■ Admission data base ■ +/– Cardiac monitoring ■ Vital signs (VS) and respiratory assessment every 2 to 4 hr (ICU), every 4 to 8 hr (on floor) ■ Arterial oxygen saturation (SpO_2) every 4 to 8 hr ■ Intake and output (I & O) every 8 hr ■ Daily weight ■ Head of bed raised to 45 degrees	■ Cardiac, respiratory assessment every 4 to 8 hr ■ SpO_2 every 4 to 8 hr ■ I & O ■ Daily weight
SOCIAL WORK	■ Respond to identified high-risk patient.	■ Evaluate patient compliance with medication regimen. ■ Evaluate family support at home.
NUTRITION	■ +/– Nothing by mouth or low-sodium diet ■ Fluid restriction ____ml/day	■ Low-sodium diet ■ Fluid restriction_____ml/day
TESTS	■ Complete blood count (CBC), blood chemistries, coagulation study, cardiac enzymes: #1 ___, #2_____, #3_____ ■ Chest X-ray (CXR), arterial blood gas (ABG) analysis, electrocardiogram (ECG)	■ Blood chemistry, CXR, ECG, (+/–) cardiac enzymes #3 ____ ■ Evaluation of left ventricular function: multiple-gated acquisition scan, echocardiogram
CONSULTS	■ Cardiology	
ACTIVITY	■ Bed rest	■ Out of bed to chair
PATIENT EDUCATION	■ Explain routine of cardiac intensive care unit/floor. ■ Teach the importance of complying with the current medication regimen.	■ Educate patient and family about scheduled tests. ■ Educate patient about medications.
DISCHARGE PLANNING	■ Evaluate support system at home.	■ Discuss advanced directives with patient and family.
KEY PATIENT OUTCOMES	■ Patient demonstrates improved cardiac output, breath sounds, and respiratory effort and rate. Date met_____Not met _____ Initials _____ ■ Patient verbalizes and exhibits understanding of plan of care. Date met _____Not met _____Initials _____	■ Patient can state purpose of scheduled tests. Date met_____Not met _____ Initials_____ ■ Patient can list the medications he is taking and differences among them. Date met_____Not met _____ Initials_____
	Signature _____	Signature _____

Key: +/– indicates may or may not be appropriate for the patient.

Adapted with permission from Veterans Affairs Maryland Health Care System at Baltimore.

Days 4 to 5	Day 6

■ Differentiate between systolic and diastolic dysfunction.
■ Rule out coronary artery disease and hypertension.
■ Medications:
  –Beta blockers
  –Calcium channel blockers
  –Diuretics (judiciously)
	■ Rule out chronic obstructive pulmonary disease.

■ Continue:
  –Assessments
  –VS, SpO$_2$, I & O every 8 hr
  –Daily weight
	■ Continue to monitor respiratory and cardiac status.
	■ VS, SpO$_2$, I & O every 8 hr
	■ Daily weight

■ Evaluate high-risk patients in need of placement services.	
■ Fluid restriction ____ml/day	■ Fluid restriction ____ml/day
■ +/– Evaluation of ischemic process: pharmacologic and exercise stress tests	■ +/– Evaluation for revascularization, cardiac catheterization ■ +/– Pulmonary function tests
■ Nutrition	
■ Up in room and hallway	■ Up to bathroom and hallway (or at baseline) ■ Able to perform activities of daily living independently
■ Teach patient types of food to avoid. ■ Teach importance of constant, daily activity and exercise.	■ Teach patient and family about signs and symptoms of worsening heart failure. ■ Give patient educational material.
■ Evaluate need for home health nurse on discharge to check medical and dietary compliance, daily weight, signs and symptoms to report.	■ Emphasize importance of keeping follow-up appointments.
■ Patient can state dietary restrictions. *Date met* _____*Not met* _____*Initials* _____ ■ Patient demonstrates increased activity tolerance. *Date met* _____*Not met* _____*Initials* _____	■ Patient can state signs and symptoms of worsening heart failure (including increased shortness of breath, dyspnea on exercise, weight gain) and when to return to emergency care. *Date met* _____*Not met* _____*Initials* _____ ■ Patient can list lifestyle modifications (if any). *Date met* _____*Not met* _____*Initials* _____ ■ Patient can state "normal" weight to maintain. *Date met* _____*Not met* _____*Initials* _____ ■ SpO$_2$ on room air will be >90%. *Date met* _____*Not met* _____*Initials* _____
Signature _____	*Signature* _____

Key: +/– indicates may or may not be appropriate for the patient.

CLINICAL PRACTICE GUIDELINES ▌▌▌ **Treating heart failure**

The following important points are adapted from clinical practice guidelines for heart failure developed by the Agency for Health Care Policy and Research of the U.S. Department of Health and Human Services.

Patient teaching
Include these points in your teaching:
■ Encourage regular exercise, such as walking or cycling, for all patients with stable heart failure. Recent studies show that exercise is safe and may improve functional status and decrease symptoms.
■ Set dietary sodium restrictions as close to 2 g/day as possible; tell patients never to exceed 3 g daily.
■ Caution against excessive fluid intake. However, fluid restrictions are unnecessary unless a patient develops hyponatremia.
■ Instruct patients to keep a daily record of body weight and to call the doctor if they gain 3 to 5 lb (1.4 to 2.3 kg) or more within 1 week or since the previous doctor visit.
■ Make sure that patients receive accurate information about their prognosis in order to make decisions and plans for the future (such as advance directives and durable power of attorney).
■ Because noncompliance is a problem, discuss the importance of compliance at follow-up visits, and assist patients in removing barriers to compliance, such as cost, adverse effects, or complexity of the treatment regimen.

Drug therapy
Medications are prescribed for patients with heart failure for two basic reasons: to reduce mortality and to reduce

symptoms and improve functional status. Drug therapy may include the following (keep in mind that all medications require a properly written doctor's order):
■ Give diuretics—such as thiazide, loop, thiazide-related, and potassium-sparing diuretics—to help reduce symptoms of volume overload, such as orthopnea, paroxysmal nocturnal dyspnea, dyspnea on exertion, pulmonary rales, third heart sound, jugular venous distention, hepatic engorgement, ascites, peripheral edema, pulmonary vascular congestion, or pulmonary edema that appears on chest X-ray.
■ Consider using angiotensin-converting enzyme (ACE) inhibitors—such as enalapril maleate, captopril, lisinopril, and quinapril—as sole therapy for symptoms of left-ventricular systolic dysfunction (such as fatigue or mild dyspnea on exertion) if the patient has no signs or symptoms of volume overload.
■ Digoxin increases the force of ventricular contraction in the patient with left-ventricular systolic dysfunction. Add digoxin to the therapeutic regimen if symptoms persist despite optimal doses of ACE inhibitors and diuretics.
■ Don't use anticoagulants routinely unless the patient has a history of systemic or pulmonary embolism or recent atrial fibrillation.

he experiences dizziness, blurred vision, shortness of breath, persistent dry cough, palpitations, increased fatigue, paroxysmal nocturnal dyspnea, swollen ankles, or decreased urine output; or if he gains 3 to 5 lb (1.4 to 2.3 kg) in 1 week.

EVALUATION
Achievement of patient outcomes determines whether collaborative management has succeeded. For a patient with heart failure, evaluation focuses on adequate cardiac function, fluid balance, oxygenation, and knowledge of the disease and treatment regimen.

Hypertension

This disorder is marked by persistent elevation of diastolic or systolic blood pressure. Generally, a sustained systolic pressure of 140 mm Hg or more or a diastolic

pressure of 90 mm Hg or more qualifies as hypertension.

Hypertension is classified according to its cause, severity, and type. The two major types are *essential* (also called primary or idiopathic) *hypertension,* the most common (90% to 95% of cases), and *secondary hypertension,* which results from renal disease or another identifiable cause. *Malignant hypertension* is a severe, fulminant form of hypertension that commonly arises from both types. (See *Understanding malignant hypertension.*)

Hypertension affects more than 60 million adults in North America. Blacks are twice as likely as whites to be affected and four times as likely to die of the disorder.

Essential hypertension usually begins insidiously as a benign disease and slowly progresses to an accelerated or malignant state. If untreated, even mild hypertension can cause significant complications and a high mortality rate. However, treatment with stepped care offers patients an improved prognosis.

Understanding malignant hypertension

Malignant hypertension is a medical emergency characterized by marked blood pressure elevation; papilledema; retinal hemorrhages and exudates; and manifestations of hypertensive encephalopathy, such as severe headache, vomiting, visual disturbances, transient paralysis, seizures, stupor, and coma. Cardiac decompensation and acute renal failure may also develop.

The average age at diagnosis is 40, and the disorder affects more men than women. Before the availability of effective antihypertensives, most patients died within 2 years. Even with effective treatment, however, at least half of the patients die within 5 years.

Causes
The cause of malignant hypertension isn't known. However, studies do show that dilation of cerebral arteries and generalized arteriolar fibrinoid necrosis contribute to this disorder. The cerebral arteries dilate because markedly high arterial pressure overrides normal regulation of cerebral blood flow. The resulting excess in cerebral blood flow produces encephalopathy.

Treatment
Emergency treatment aims to quickly reduce blood pressure and identify the underlying cause.
■ Diazoxide given rapidly I.V. can begin to reduce blood pressure in 1 to 3 minutes. Nitroprusside and trimethaphan, given by continuous infusion, may be tried. Other drugs for maintaining long-term control of blood pressure include hydralazine and methyldopa.
■ With suspected pheochromocytoma, drugs that release additional catecholamines—such as methyldopa, reserpine, and guanethidine—are contraindicated.
■ Furosemide and digitalis glycosides may be used to treat associated heart failure.

Hypertension is a major risk factor for cerebral coronary, renal and peripheral vascular diseases, cerebrovascular accident (CVA), cardiac disease, and renal failure. Complications occur late in the disease and can attack any organ system. Cardiac complications may include angina, myocardial infarction (MI), heart failure, arrhythmias, and sudden death. Neurologic complications include cerebral infarction and hypertensive encephalopathy. Hypertensive retinopathy can cause blindness. Renovascular hypertension can lead to renal failure.

CAUSES
The cause of essential hypertension is unknown. Family history, race, stress, obesity, a diet high in sodium or saturated fat, use of tobacco or oral contraceptives, sedentary lifestyle, and aging have all been studied to determine their role in the development of hypertension.

Secondary hypertension may result from renovascular disease; renal parenchymal disease; pheochromocytoma; primary hyperaldosteronism; Cushing's syndrome; diabetes mellitus; dysfunction of the thyroid, pituitary, or parathyroid gland; coarctation of the aorta; pregnancy; and neurologic disorders. Use of oral contraceptives may be the most common cause of secondary hypertension, probably because these drugs activate the renin-angiotensin-aldosterone system. (See *How hypertension develops,* page 100.)

DIAGNOSIS AND TREATMENT
Diagnostic tests may be used to identify predisposing factors and help identify the cause of hypertension.

Urinalysis may show protein, red blood cells, or white blood cells (suggesting renal disease) or glucose (suggesting diabetes mellitus). Excretory urography may reveal renal atrophy, indicating chronic renal disease; one kidney that is more than $5/8''$ (1.6 cm) shorter than the other suggests unilateral renal disease.

Serum potassium levels less than 3.5 mEq/L may indicate adrenal dysfunction (primary hyperaldosteronism). Blood urea nitrogen (BUN) levels that are normal or elevated to more than 20 mg/dl and serum creatinine levels that are normal or elevated to more than 1.5 mg/dl suggest renal disease.

Other tests that help detect cardiovascular damage and other complications include electrocardiography, which may show left ventricular hypertrophy or ischemia, and chest X-rays, which may demonstrate cardiomegaly.

Although essential hypertension has no cure, drugs and modifications in diet and lifestyle can control it. Lifestyle changes are usually tried first, especially in early, mild cases. If these are ineffective, treatment progresses in a stepwise manner to include various types of antihypertensives. This stepped-care approach may need modification. For instance, most blacks respond poorly to beta-adrenergic blockers but for unknown reasons respond well to a combination

How hypertension develops

Increased blood volume, cardiac rate, and stroke volume, or arteriolar vasoconstriction that increases peripheral resistance causes blood pressure to rise. Hypertension may also result from the breakdown or inappropriate response of the following intrinsic regulatory mechanisms.

Renin-angiotensin system

Renal hypoperfusion causes the release of renin. Angiotensinogen, a liver enzyme, converts the renin to angiotensin I, which increases preload and afterload. Angiotensin I then converts to angiotensin II in the lungs. A powerful vasoconstrictor, angiotensin II also helps increase preload and afterload by stimulating the adrenal cortex to secrete aldosterone. This serves to increase sodium reabsorption. Next comes hypertonic-stimulated release of antidiuretic hormone from the pituitary gland. This, in turn, increases water absorption, plasma volume, cardiac output, and blood pressure.

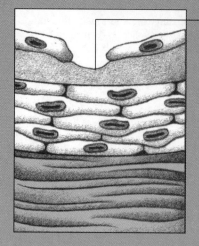

Damage from increased blood pressure

Autoregulation

Several intrinsic mechanisms work to change an artery's diameter to maintain tissue and organ perfusion despite fluctuations in systemic blood pressure. These mechanisms include stress relaxation and capillary fluid shift. In stress relaxation, blood vessels gradually dilate when blood pressure rises to reduce peripheral resistance. In capillary fluid shift, plasma moves between vessels and extravascular spaces to maintain intravascular volume.

When blood pressure drops, baroreceptors in the aortic arch and carotid sinuses decrease their inhibition of the medulla's vasomotor center. This action increases sympathetic stimulation of the heart by norepinephrine. And this increases cardiac output by strengthening the contractile force, raising the heart rate, and augmenting peripheral resistance by vasoconstriction. Stress also can stimulate the sympathetic nervous system to increase cardiac output and peripheral vascular resistance.

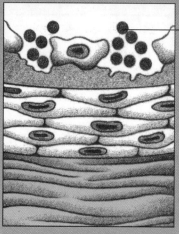

Angiotensin

Blood vessel damage

Sustained hypertension damages blood vessels. Vascular injury begins with alternating areas of dilation and constriction in the arterioles. Increased intra-arterial pressure damages the endothelium (top illustration). Independently, angiotensin induces endothelial wall contraction, allowing plasma to leak through interendothelial spaces (middle illustration). Eventually, plasma constituents deposited in the vessel wall cause medial necrosis (bottom illustration).

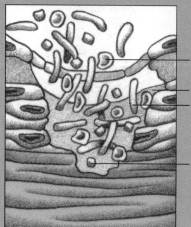

Protein with fibrin deposits

Medial necrosis

Fibrinogen

Platelet

of diuretics and angiotensin-converting enzyme inhibitors. Many elderly patients can be treated with diuretics alone. (See *Stepped care for hypertension.*)

Treatment of secondary hypertension includes correcting the underlying cause and controlling hypertensive effects. Severely elevated blood pressure (hypertensive crisis) may be refractory to medications and may be fatal.

COLLABORATIVE MANAGEMENT

Care of the patient with hypertension focuses on early identification and prompt treatment to reduce the blood pressure to more normal levels. Emphasis is also placed on the patient's adherence with the plan of care to prevent the serious consequences of noncompliance.

ASSESSMENT

Many people with hypertension have no symptoms; in them, the disorder is revealed incidentally during evaluation for another disorder or during a routine blood pressure screening program. When symptoms do occur, they reflect the effect of hypertension on the organ systems.

The patient may report awakening with a headache in the occipital region, which subsides spontaneously after a few hours. This symptom usually is associated with severe hypertension. He may also complain of dizziness, palpitations, fatigue, and impotence.

With vascular involvement, the patient may complain of nosebleeds, bloody urine, weakness, and blurred vision. Complaints of chest pain and dyspnea may indicate cardiac involvement.

Inspection may reveal peripheral edema in late stages when heart failure is present. Ophthalmoscopic evaluation may reveal hemorrhages, exudates, and papilledema in late stages if hypertensive retinopathy is present.

Palpation of the carotid artery may disclose stenosis or occlusion. Palpation of the abdomen may reveal a pulsating mass, suggesting an abdominal aneurysm. Enlarged kidneys may point to polycystic disease, a cause of secondary hypertension.

Systolic or diastolic pressure, or both, may be elevated. A rise in diastolic blood pressure from a sitting to a standing position suggests essential hypertension, whereas a fall in blood pressure from the sitting to the standing position indicates secondary hypertension.

An abdominal bruit may be heard just to the right or left of the umbilicus midline or in the flanks if renal artery stenosis is present. Bruits may also be heard over the abdominal aorta and carotid and femoral arteries.

Stepped care for hypertension

Recently, the National Institutes of Health revised its stepped-care approach to hypertension. The latest guidelines follow.

Step 1
Initial therapy to reduce high blood pressure includes lifestyle modifications, such as weight reduction, increased physical activity, and moderation of sodium and alcohol intake as well as smoking cessation.

Step 2
If lifestyle changes don't adequately reduce blood pressure, therapy with a single drug should be started. Diuretics and beta blockers are preferred because they've been shown to reduce cardiovascular illness and mortality in long-term controlled clinical trials.

If the patient has other underlying medical problems, alternative drugs (such as angiotensin-converting enzyme inhibitors, calcium channel blockers, $alpha_1$-receptor blockers, and labetalol) may be substituted.

Step 3
If initial therapy fails to control blood pressure sufficiently in 1 to 3 months and the patient is compliant and not experiencing significant adverse reactions, three options for subsequent therapy should be considered: increased drug dose, substitution of another drug, or addition of a second agent from a different class.

Step 4
Although some patients may respond adequately to therapy with a single drug, frequently a second or third agent and, if not already prescribed, a diuretic must be added if the desired blood pressure reduction hasn't been achieved.

NURSING DIAGNOSES AND COLLABORATIVE PROBLEMS

Based on these nursing diagnoses, you'll establish patient outcomes.

Decreased cardiac output related to problems with plasma volume, peripheral resistance, and stroke volume. The patient will:
■ exhibit reduction in blood pressure
■ remain free from signs and symptoms of decreased cardiac output
■ demonstrate vital signs and hemodynamic parameters within normal limits.

HEALTHY LIVING

Living with hypertension

Many patients with hypertension are required to follow a sodium-restricted diet as part of their treatment plan. To ensure compliance, help reduce the risk of complications, and promote healthy living with hypertension, give the following specific instructions:

- Read labels to determine sodium content.
- Know that sodium is present in large amounts in commercial preparations such as baking powder, meat tenderizer, and soy sauce.
- Be aware that sodium often is added to canned, boxed, and some frozen foods and that not all dietetic foods are sodium-free.
- Avoid canned, smoked, pickled, or cured meat and fish products, pickled or preserved vegetables, and fast foods.
- Choose foods that are baked, broiled, boiled, or roasted without salted gravies or juices.
- Be aware that sodium substitutes may be used, but that they may contain potassium.
- Contact the local chapter of the American Heart Association for information about low-sodium diets.

To help the patient prepare low-sodium meals, be sure to include the following instructions:

- Don't add salt at the table.
- Use no salt preparation (if you're on a 2 g sodium diet); use only half the salt called for in the recipe (if you're on a 4 g sodium diet)
- Rinse any canned products to be used and heat them in tap water.
- Use natural spices, herbs, and condiments, such as pepper, parsley, chili, horseradish, lemon, cloves, and onion and garlic powder, liberally.
- Avoid using herb salts and such items as steak sauce, catsup, and marinade.

Fluid volume excess related to increased sodium intake, decreased cardiac output, and compromised renin-angiotensin-aldosterone mechanism. The patient will:
- demonstrate stable weight
- exhibit decreasing signs of fluid overload.

Risk for injury related to complications of hypertension. The patient will:
- keep regular appointments for blood pressure evaluation to detect persistent or serious elevations
- seek medical attention immediately for any abnormal signs or symptoms
- avoid dysfunction of any organ system, especially the cardiovascular and renal systems.

Knowledge deficit related to hypertension and its treatment. The patient will:
- acknowledge the need to learn about hypertension and its control and express a desire to do so

- participate in a learning situation to gain knowledge about hypertension and its treatment
- express an understanding of hypertension and the methods used to control it.

Noncompliance related to the lifelong need for antihypertensive therapy and the misconception that such therapy is needed only during symptomatic periods. The patient will:
- express an understanding of the need for lifelong therapy even when he lacks overt signs and symptoms
- comply with prescribed treatments, as shown by normal blood pressure and absence of organ dysfunction.

PLANNING AND IMPLEMENTATION
The following measures help the patient with hypertension.
- Monitor and record level of consciousness for changes indicating decreased cerebral perfusion; watch for dizziness, headache, blurred vision, and confusion.
- Monitor heart rate and rhythm, respirations, and blood pressure frequently. Note any signs of irregular pulses, complaints of palpitations, or dramatic increases in blood pressure.
- Administer antihypertensive therapy as ordered; monitor for signs of adverse reactions.
- Monitor intake and output frequently; obtain daily weights.
- Assess for signs of fluid retention. such as dependent or sacral edema and ascites.
- Monitor laboratory studies, such as urine specific gravity, blood urea nitrogen, creatinine, electrolyte and hemoglobin levels; and hematocrit.
- Assess the patient's intake of sodium; consult the dietitian for assistance with reducing sodium intake.
- Monitor the patient closely for complications associated with hypertension. Assess for signs of malignant hypertension, including severe headache, vomiting, seizures, stupor and coma.
- If malignant hypertension develops, anticipate administering emergency medications, such as diazoxide, nitroprusside, trimethaphan, hydralazine, or methyldopa.
- Monitor the patient for signs of orthostatic hypotension related to medication therapy. If this symptom occurs, have the patient change positions gradually and sit at the edge of the bed for a few minutes before rising.

Patient teaching
- Teach the patient to use a self-monitoring blood pressure cuff and to record the reading at least twice weekly in a journal for review by the doctor at every office appointment.

- Tell him to take his blood pressure at the same time each day and after the same type of activity.
- Tell the patient and family to keep a record of antihypertensive drugs used in the past, including which ones were or weren't effective. Suggest recording this information on a card so the patient can show it to his doctor.
- To encourage compliance with antihypertensive therapy, suggest establishing a daily routine for taking medication. Warn him that uncontrolled hypertension may cause CVA and MI. Tell him to report adverse effects to the doctor.
- Help the patient examine and modify his lifestyle. Suggest stress-reduction techniques, dietary changes, and an exercise program, particularly aerobic walking, to improve cardiac status and reduce obesity and serum cholesterol levels.
- Help the obese patient plan a weight-loss diet.
- Advise the patient to avoid high-sodium foods (pickles, potato chips, canned soups, cold cuts), table salt, and foods high in cholesterol and saturated fat. Also advise him to avoid high-sodium antacids and over-the-counter cold and sinus medications containing harmful vasoconstrictors. (See *Living with hypertension*.)

EVALUATION

Achievement of patient outcomes determines whether the collaborative management has been successful. For a patient with hypertension, evaluation focuses on improved cardiac function, restoration of fluid balance, maintenance of safety, and adequate knowledge of the disorder and its treatment.

Mitral insufficiency

Also known as mitral regurgitation, mitral insufficiency occurs when a damaged mitral valve allows blood from the left ventricle to flow back into the left atrium during systole. As a result, the atrium enlarges to accommodate the backflow. The left ventricle also dilates to accommodate the increased volume of blood from the atrium and to compensate for diminishing cardiac output.

Mitral insufficiency tends to be progressive. As left ventricular dilation continues to lead to left atrial and ventricular enlargement, the insufficiency increases further.

CAUSES

Damage to the mitral valve can result from rheumatic fever, hypertrophic cardiomyopathy, mitral valve prolapse, myocardial infarction (MI), severe left-sided heart failure, or ruptured chordae tendineae.

In older patients, mitral insufficiency may result from calcification of the mitral annulus. The cause is unknown, but it may be linked to a degenerative process. Mitral insufficiency is sometimes associated with congenital anomalies, such as transposition of the great arteries.

Mitral insufficiency occurs during systole, when much pressure is generated within the left ventricle. Blood is ejected forward into the aorta and also backward into the left atrium through the mitral valve, which is not completely closed. The backward flow of blood causes left atrial and left ventricular enlargement. The left atrium responds to the large volume of blood it is receiving during systole by becoming dilated and hypertrophic. The left ventricle responds to the large amount of blood lost to the left atrium by trying to pump harder to preserve cardiac output. This causes hypertrophy of the left ventricle and increased left ventricular and end-diastolic pressure, eventually resulting in left-sided heart failure.

Over time, the increased blood flow to the left atrium causes a rise in left atrial pressure. This pressure is reflected backward into both the pulmonary venous and arterial system with an increase in pulmonary artery pressure. With continued high pressures, right-sided heart failure can develop.

DIAGNOSIS AND TREATMENT

Cardiac catheterization detects mitral insufficiency with increased left ventricular end-diastolic volume and pressure, increased atrial and pulmonary artery wedge pressures, and decreased cardiac output.

Chest X-rays demonstrate left atrial and ventricular enlargement, pulmonary venous congestion, and calcification of the mitral leaflets in long-standing mitral insufficiency and stenosis.

Echocardiography reveals abnormal motion of the valve leaflets, left atrial enlargement, and a hyperdynamic left ventricle. Electrocardiography (ECG) may show left atrial and ventricular hypertrophy, sinus tachycardia, and atrial fibrillation.

The nature and severity of associated symptoms determine treatment in valvular heart disease. The patient may need to restrict activities to avoid extreme fatigue and dyspnea.

Heart failure requires digoxin, diuretics, a sodium-restricted diet and, in acute cases, oxygen. Other appropriate measures include anticoagulant therapy to prevent thrombus formation around diseased or replaced valves and prophylactic antibiotics before and after surgery or dental care.

If the patient has severe signs and symptoms that can't be managed medically, he may need open-heart surgery with cardiopulmonary bypass for valve replacement. Valvuloplasty may be used in elderly patients with end-stage disease who can't tolerate general anesthesia.

Identifying the murmur of mitral insufficiency

A high-pitched, rumbling pansystolic murmur that radiates from the mitral area to the left axillary line characterizes mitral insufficienciy.

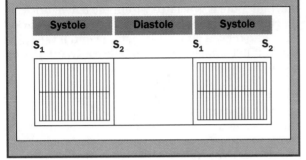

Systole	Diastole	Systole
S_1	S_2	S_1	S_2

COLLABORATIVE MANAGEMENT

Care of the patient with mitral insufficiency requires prompt detection and treatment as well as close monitoring.

ASSESSMENT

Depending on the disorder's severity, the patient may either be asymptomatic or may complain of orthopnea, exertional dyspnea, fatigue, weakness, weight loss, chest pain, and palpitations.

Inspection may reveal jugular vein distention with an abnormally prominent *a* wave. You may also note peripheral edema.

Auscultation may detect a soft first heart sound (S_1) that may be buried in the systolic murmur. A grade 3 to 6 holosystolic murmur, most characteristic in mitral insufficiency, is heard best at the apex. (See *Identifying the murmur of mitral insufficiency*.) You'll also hear a split S_2 and a low-pitched S_3. The S_3 may be followed by a short, rumbling diastolic murmur. An S_4 may be evident in patients with recent onset of severe mitral insufficiency who are in normal sinus rhythm.

Auscultation of the lungs may reveal crackles if the patient has pulmonary edema.

Palpation of the chest may disclose a regular pulse rate with a sharp upstroke. You can probably palpate a systolic thrill at the left sternal border. In patients with marked pulmonary hypertension, you may be able to palpate a right ventricular tap and the shock of the pulmonic valve closing. When the left atrium is markedly enlarged, it may be palpable along the sternal border late during ventricular systole. (It resembles a right ventricular lift.) Abdominal palpation may reveal hepatomegaly if the patient has right-sided heart failure.

NURSING DIAGNOSES AND COLLABORATIVE PROBLEMS

Based on these nursing diagnoses, you'll establish patient outcomes.

Activity intolerance related to fatigue and dyspnea. The patient will:
■ state the activities that increase fatigue or dyspnea, then avoid them or request assistance to perform them
■ perform self-care activities as tolerated.

Decreased cardiac output related to the disease process. The patient will:
■ comply with the prescribed treatment regimen to enhance cardiac output
■ avoid manifestations of profoundly decreased cardiac output, such as shock and tissue ischemia
■ remain hemodynamically stable.

Fluid volume excess related to pulmonary edema. The patient will:
■ respond to treatment measures to alleviate excess fluid, as evidenced by a normal respiratory rate and pattern and fluid output that exceeds intake
■ take measures to prevent or minimize pulmonary edema, such as adhering to dietary and activity restrictions
■ regain and maintain normal pulmonary function.

Knowledge deficit related to the disease and its treatment. The patient will:
■ verbalize information about the disease and its treatment
■ demonstrate measures to adequately manage the disease and comply with therapy.

PLANNING AND IMPLEMENTATION

The following measures help the patient with mitral insufficiency.
■ Provide periods of rest alternating with activity to prevent excessive fatigue. Organize all activities to provide maximum rest periods.
■ Allow the patient to express his concerns about the effects of activity restrictions on his responsibilities and routines. Assure him that the restrictions are temporary.
■ Maintain a quiet environment to promote rest.
■ Provide oxygen to prevent tissue hypoxia, as needed and ordered; place the patient in Fowler's position to ease breathing.
■ Monitor vital signs, arterial blood gas values, intake and output, daily weights, blood chemistry studies, chest X-rays, and ECG. Notify the doctor of any abnormal findings. Also assess mental status.
■ Provide continuous cardiac monitoring during acute and advanced disease stages to identify and manage arrhythmias promptly.
■ Administer medications such as digitalis glycosides, as ordered.

- Watch for calf pain and tenderness.
- To prevent deep vein thrombosis due to vascular congestion, assist the patient with range-of-motion exercises.
- Enforce bed rest and apply antiembolism stockings.
- Report changes in the patient's condition immediately.
- Observe the patient for signs and symptoms of left-sided heart failure, pulmonary edema, and adverse reactions to drug therapy.
- Before giving penicillin (the antibiotic of choice), ask the patient if he's ever had a hypersensitivity reaction to it. Even if he hasn't, warn him that such a reaction is possible. Administer antibiotics on time to maintain consistent drug levels in the blood.
- Weigh the patient daily to help detect fluid retention, and observe for peripheral edema.
- Administer diuretics as ordered.
- Assess intake and output frequently. Monitor I.V. intake and urine output (especially if the patient is receiving diuretics).
- Auscultate the heart for abnormal sounds and the lungs for crackles or rhonchi.
- Frequently monitor blood urea nitrogen and serum creatinine, potassium, sodium, chloride, and magnesium levels.
- Record abdominal girth at least every shift.
- Watch for jugular vein distention and peripheral edema; measure the circumference of the lower extremities and note any changes.
- Anticipate fluid and sodium restrictions; if sodium is restricted, consult with the dietitian to ensure that the patient receives as many favorite foods as possible while he's on the restricted diet.

Patient teaching

- Prepare the patient for valve replacement or valvuloplasty, as indicated.
- Teach the patient about diet restrictions, medications, signs and symptoms that should be reported, and the importance of consistent follow-up care.
- Explain all tests and treatments.
- If valve replacement or valvuloplasty is scheduled, teach the patient and family about the surgery or procedure and what care to expect afterward.
- Make sure the patient and his family understand the need to comply with prolonged antibiotic therapy and follow-up care and the need for additional antibiotics during dental surgery.
- Instruct the patient and his family to watch for and report early signs of heart failure, such as dyspnea and a hacking, nonproductive cough.

EVALUATION
Achievement of patient outcomes determines whether the collaborative management has been suc-cessful. For a patient with mitral insufficiency, evaluation focuses on activity tolerance, improved cardiac function, adequate fluid balance, and adequate knowledge of the disease process and treatment regimen.

Myocardial infarction

Myocardial infarction (MI) results from reduced blood flow through one of the coronary arteries, which causes myocardial ischemia and necrosis. The infarction site depends on the vessels involved. For instance, occlusion of the circumflex coronary artery causes a lateral wall infarction; occlusion of the left anterior coronary artery causes an anterior wall infarction. True posterior and inferior wall infarctions result from occlusion of the right coronary artery or one of its branches. Right ventricular infarctions can also result from right coronary artery occlusion, can accompany inferior infarctions, and may cause right-sided heart failure. In transmural (Q wave) MI, tissue damage extends through all myocardial layers; in subendocardial (non–Q wave) MI, only the innermost layer is usually damaged.

Men are more susceptible to MI than premenopausal women, although the incidence is rising among women who smoke or take oral contraceptives. The incidence in postmenopausal women is similar to that in men.

In North America and western Europe, MI is one of the most common causes of death, which usually results from cardiac damage or complications. Mortality is about 25%. However, more than 50% of sudden deaths occur within 1 hour after onset of signs and symptoms, before the patient reaches the hospital. Of those who recover, up to 27% of men and 44% of women die within 1 year of having an MI.

Complications associated with acute MI include arrhythmias, cardiogenic shock, heart failure causing pulmonary edema, and pericarditis. Other complications include rupture of the atrial or ventricular septum, ventricular wall, or valves; ventricular aneurysms; mural thrombi causing cerebral or pulmonary emboli; and extensions of the original infarction. Dressler's syndrome (post-MI pericarditis) can occur days to weeks after an MI and cause residual pain, malaise, and fever.

Typically, elderly patients are more prone to complications and death. Psychological problems can also occur, either from the patient's fear of another MI or from an organic brain disorder caused by tissue hypoxia. Occasionally, a patient may undergo a personality change.

What happens in MI

When blood supply to the myocardium is interrupted, the following events occur:

Injury to the endothelial lining of the coronary arteries causes platelets, white blood cells, fibrin, and lipids to converge at the injured site. Foam cells, or resident macrophages, congregate under the damaged lining and absorb oxidized cholesterol, forming a fatty streak that narrows the arterial lumen. Signs and symptoms are undetectable at this stage.

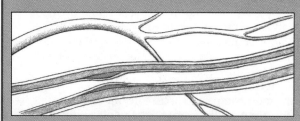

Because the arterial lumen narrows gradually, collateral circulation develops, which helps to maintain myocardial perfusion distal to the obstructed vessel. The patient may experience chest pain when myocardial demand for oxygen increases.

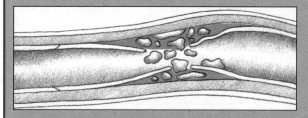

When myocardial oxygen demand exceeds what the collateral circulation can supply, myocardial metabolism shifts from aerobic to anaerobic, producing lactic acid, which stimulates pain nerve endings. The patient experiences worsening angina that requires rest and medication for relief.

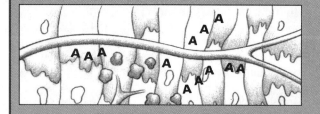

Lacking oxygen, the myocardial cells die. This decreases contractility, stroke volume, and blood pressure. At this stage, the patient develops tachycardia, hypotension, diminished heart sounds, cyanosis, tachypnea, and poor perfusion to vital organs.

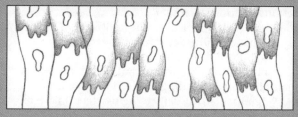

Hypotension stimulates baroreceptors, which in turn stimulate adrenal glands to release epinephrine and norepinephrine. These catecholamines increase heart rate and cause peripheral vasoconstriction, further increasing myocardial oxygen demand. The patient develops tachyarrhythmias, changes in pulses, decreased level of consciousness, and cold, clammy skin.

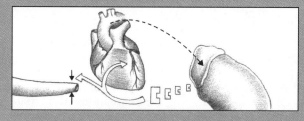

Damaged cell membranes in the infarcted area leak their intracellular contents into the systemic vascular circulation. Levels of serum enzyme (creatine kinase [CK], CK-MB, aspartate aminotransferase, and lactate dehydrogenase) and potassium rise, and the patient experiences ventricular arrhythmias.

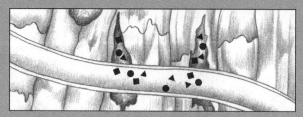

CAUSES

MI results from occlusion of one of the coronary arteries. Such occlusion can stem from atherosclerosis, thrombosis, platelet aggregation, or coronary artery stenosis or spasm. Predisposing factors include:

- aging
- diabetes mellitus
- elevated serum triglyceride, low-density lipoprotein, and cholesterol levels and decreased serum high-density lipoprotein levels
- excessive intake of saturated fats, carbohydrates,

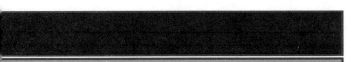

All myocardial cells are capable of spontaneous depolarization and repolarization, so the electrical conduction system may be affected by infarct, injury, and ischemia. The patient may have a fever, leukocytosis, tachycardia, and ECG signs of tissue ischemia (altered T waves), injured tissue (altered ST segment), and infarcted tissue (deep Q waves).

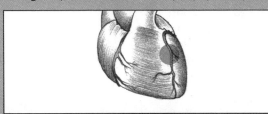

Extensive damage to the left ventricle may impair the ventricle's pumping ability, allowing blood to back up into the left atrium and, eventually, into the pulmonary veins and capillaries. In the patient, this may produce dyspnea, orthopnea, tachypnea, and cyanosis, along with crackles in the lungs on auscultation. Pulmonary artery pressure and pulmonary artery wedge pressure are increased.

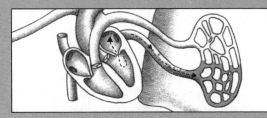

As back pressure rises, fluid crosses the alveolar-capillary membrane, impeding diffusion of oxygen (O_2) and carbon dioxide (CO_2). The patient experiences increasing respiratory distress. Laboratory studies may show decreased partial pressure of arterial oxygen and arterial pH and increased partial pressure of arterial carbon dioxide.

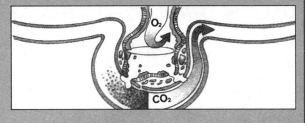

or salt
■ hypertension
■ obesity
■ family history of coronary artery disease (CAD)
■ sedentary lifestyle
■ smoking

stress or a type A personality (aggressive, competitive attitude, addiction to work, chronic impatience).

In addition, use of such drugs as amphetamines or cocaine can cause an MI. (See *What happens in MI*.)

DIAGNOSIS AND TREATMENT

For critical diagnostic test results, see *MI: Key abnormal diagnostic findings,* page 108. Echocardiography shows ventricular wall dyskinesia with a transmural MI and helps evaluate the ejection fraction.

Scans using I.V. technetium (Tc 99m) can identify acutely damaged muscle by picking up accumulations of radioactive nucleotide, which appears as a "hot spot" on the film. Myocardial perfusion imaging with thallium-201 reveals a "cold spot" in most patients during the first few hours after a transmural MI.

The goals of treatment are to relieve chest pain, to stabilize heart rhythm, and to reduce cardiac workload. Treatment includes revascularization to preserve myocardial tissue. Arrhythmias, the most common problem during the first 48 hours after MI, may require antiarrhythmics, possibly a pacemaker and, rarely, cardioversion.

Drug therapy usually includes:
■ lidocaine for ventricular arrhythmias; if lidocaine is ineffective, procainamide, quinidine sulfate, bretylium, or disopyramide
■ atropine I.V. or a temporary pacemaker for heart block or bradycardia
■ nitroglycerin (sublingual, topical, transdermal, or I.V.); calcium channel blockers, such as nifedipine, verapamil, or diltiazem (sublingual, oral, or I.V.); or isosorbide dinitrate (sublingual, oral, or I.V.) to relieve pain by redistributing blood to ischemic areas of the myocardium, increasing cardiac output, and reducing myocardial workload
■ morphine I.V., the drug of choice for pain, sedation, and preload reduction; and possibly meperidine or hydromorphone
■ drugs that increase contractility or blood pressure
■ inotropic drugs, such as dobutamine or amrinone, to enhance myocardial contractility
■ beta-adrenergic blockers, such as propranolol or timolol, after acute MI to help prevent reinfarction
■ aspirin for its antiplatelet effect.

The following other therapies may also be used:
■ Oxygen is usually administered (by face mask or nasal cannula) at a modest flow rate for 24 to 48 hours; a lower concentration is necessary if the patient has chronic obstructive pulmonary disease.
■ Bed rest with a bedside commode is enforced to decrease cardiac workload.
■ Pulmonary artery catheterization may be performed to detect left- or right-sided heart failure and to monitor response to treatment, but it's not a routine procedure.

MI: Key abnormal diagnostic findings

To help diagnose a myocardial infarction (MI), the patient will undergo a 12-lead electrocardiogram (ECG) as well as serum laboratory analysis. Expect the following results:

■ serial 12-lead ECG revealing serial ST-segment depression in subendocardial MI and ST-segment elevation and Q waves (representing scarring and necrosis) in transmural MI; however, be aware that during the first few hours after an MI, the ECG may be normal or inconclusive
■ total serum creatine kinase (CK) level above 175 U/L for men and above 140 U/L for women (*Note:* Different measurement methods give different ranges. Check the normal range used by the laboratory at your health care facility.)
■ CK-MB isoenzyme level that starts to rise within 4 hours of an acute MI, peaks in 12 to 48 hours, and usually returns to normal in 24 to 48 hours (Persistent elevations or increasing levels indicate ongoing myocardial damage.)
■ lactate dehydrogenase (LD) isoenzyme ratio (LD1-LD2) above 1.

■ An intra-aortic balloon pump may be used for cardiogenic shock.
■ Revascularization therapy can be used if the patient is less than age 70 and doesn't have a history of cerebrovascular accident, bleeding, GI ulcers, marked hypertension, recent surgery, or chest pain lasting longer than 6 hours. Thrombolytic therapy with intracoronary or systemic streptokinase (I.V) or tissue plasminogen activator must be started within 6 hours after the MI. The best response occurs when treatment begins within the first hour after onset of symptoms. (See *Treating acute MI with streptokinase.*)
■ Cardiac catheterization, percutaneous transluminal coronary angioplasty (PTCA), and coronary artery bypass grafting may also be performed.

COLLABORATIVE MANAGEMENT

Care of the patient with an MI focuses on relieving chest pain, maintaining cardiovascular stability, decreasing cardiac workload, and preventing complications. Risk factor control is a major focus in long-term management. Rapid assessment and early diagnosis are crucial.

ASSESSMENT

Typically, the patient reports the cardinal symptom of MI—persistent, crushing substernal pain that may ra-
diate to the left arm, jaw, neck, and shoulder blades. The pain—commonly described as heavy, squeezing, or crushing—may persist for 12 or more hours. However, in some patients—particularly elderly patients or those with diabetes—pain may not occur; in others, it may be mild and may be confused with indigestion. Research indicates that the pain experience differs in men and women.

Patients with CAD may report increasing anginal frequency, severity, or duration (especially when not precipitated by exertion, a heavy meal, or cold and wind). The patient may also report a feeling of impending doom, fatigue, nausea, vomiting, and shortness of breath. Sudden death, however, may be the first and only indication of MI.

Inspection may reveal an extremely anxious and restless patient with dyspnea and diaphoresis. If right-sided failure is present, you may note jugular vein distention. Within the first hour after an anterior MI, about 25% of patients exhibit signs of sympathetic nervous system hyperactivity, such as tachycardia and hypertension. Up to 50% of patients with an inferior MI exhibit signs of parasympathetic nervous system hyperactivity, such as bradycardia and hypotension.

In patients who develop ventricular dysfunction, auscultation may disclose a fourth heart sound (S_4), an S_3, paradoxical splitting of S_2, and decreased heart sounds. A systolic murmur of mitral insufficiency may be heard with papillary muscle dysfunction secondary to infarction. A pericardial friction rub may also be heard, especially in patients who have a transmural MI or have developed pericarditis.

Fever is unusual at the onset of MI. However, a low-grade fever may develop during the next few days.

NURSING DIAGNOSES AND COLLABORATIVE PROBLEMS

Based on the following nursing diagnoses, you'll establish patient outcomes.

Altered cardiopulmonary tissue perfusion related to narrowing or closure of one or more coronary arteries. The patient will:
■ seek emergency intervention immediately to minimize myocardial damage
■ exhibit no arrhythmias on the electrocardiogram (ECG)
■ regain adequate cardiac tissue perfusion.
Risk for injury related to complications of MI. The patient will:
■ seek immediate medical treatment if complications arise
■ avoid permanent deficits caused by complications of MI.

Treating acute MI with streptokinase

In the early stages of acute myocardial infarction (MI), therapy with the thrombolytic drug streptokinase can dissolve the clot in an occluded artery. This action restores perfusion and limits the size of an infarction.

How streptokinase works

Streptokinase is a first-generation thrombolytic that hastens fibrinolysis. It joins plasminogen to form a complex that then reacts with additional plasminogen to form plasmin. This proteolytic enzyme dissolves the clot and relieves the occlusion.

Because streptokinase causes antibodies to it to form, an allergic response may occur with subsequent administration. The antibodies usually last up to 6 months but can remain even longer. So a patient can't receive repeat streptokinase therapy for at least 6 months.

Procedure

Streptokinase may be given I.V. through central venous or intracoronary access immediately following cardiac catheterization. However, during treatment of acute MI, the I.V. route is most commonly used.

To prevent potential allergic reactions, steroids and antihistamines may be given to the patient. In some cases, the streptokinase is then administered over 30 to 60 minutes. Other protocols and regimens are continuously being investigated to achieve the highest rate of reperfusion.

Nursing considerations

During the infusion:
- Monitor the patient's blood pressure for hypotension, an adverse effect of streptokinase. If hypotension occurs,

stop the drug until blood pressure returns to a safe level, and then restart the infusion.

After streptokinase therapy:
- Be alert for signs of bleeding. Because streptokinase alters the natural clotting mechanisms, it can produce hemorrhaging, especially at the site of recent surgery, needle puncture, or trauma.
- Avoid giving the patient I.M. or I.V. injections for 24 hours.
- Check the infusion site for bleeding every 15 minutes for 1 hour, every 30 minutes for the next 2 hours, and then once every hour until the catheter is removed.
- Watch for signs and symptoms of GI bleeding.

If a peripheral intracoronary catheter is used:
- Maintain alignment and immobility of the affected extremity. Don't raise the head of the bed more than 15 degrees.
- When checking the site for bleeding, document the patient's pulse rate, color, temperature, and sensitivity of both extremities.
- Apply direct pressure to the infusion site for at least 30 minutes after catheter removal. Assess the affected extremity distal to the pressure point, and keep the patient on bed rest for at least 6 hours with his leg straight and the head of the bed elevated no more than 15 degrees.

Risk for fluid volume deficit related to anticoagulant and thrombolytic therapy. The patient will:
- exhibit hemodynamic status within acceptable parameters
- remain free of signs and symptoms of bleeding.

Pain related to myocardial tissue ischemia. The patient will:
- express relief of chest discomfort after treatment
- avoid new episodes of chest pain and exhibit no ischemic changes on the ECG
- comply with the prescribed treatment regimen to prevent further tissue ischemia.

Ineffective individual coping related to fear of death, anxiety, denial, or depression. The patient will:
- display feelings appropriate to stage of disease
- exhibit adequate positive coping strategies.

Activity intolerance related to imbalance between oxygen demand and supply. The patient will:
- participate in desired activities

- perform activities of daily living
- display vital signs within acceptable parameters during activity
- be free of signs and symptoms indicating intolerance.

Knowledge deficit related to disease process, treatments and procedures, and long-term implications of the disease. The patient will:
- relate information about his immediate needs and ongoing care
- ask appropriate questions
- verbalize accurate information about the disease, treatment, procedures, and long-term implications.

PLANNING AND IMPLEMENTATION

The following measures help the patient with MI.
- On admission to the intensive care unit (ICU), monitor and record the patient's ECG, blood pressure, temperature, and heart and breath sounds.

- Continuously monitor ECG rhythm strips to detect heart rate and rhythm changes. Analyze rhythm strips and place a representative strip in the patient's chart if you assess any new arrhythmias, if chest pain occurs, or at least once each shift or according to health care facility policy.
- Watch for crackles, cough, tachypnea, and edema, which may indicate impending left-sided heart failure.
- Administer vasoactive medications as ordered, and observe for adverse effects and benefits.
- Carefully monitor daily weight, intake and output, respiratory rate, serum enzyme levels, ECG waveforms, and blood pressure.
- Auscultate for adventitious breath sounds periodically. (A patient on bed rest commonly has atelectatic crackles, which may disappear after coughing). Also auscultate for S_3 or S_4 gallops.
- Monitor arterial blood gas levels as ordered, assess hemodynamic status according to your health care facility's protocol, and watch for increasing pulmonary artery wedge pressure and decreasing cardiac output.
- Prepare the patient for diagnostic procedures and for PTCA and thrombolytic therapy, as indicated.
- Provide a stool softener to prevent straining during defecation, which causes vagal stimulation and may slow the heart rate. Allow the patient to use a bedside commode, and provide as much privacy as possible.
- Check the patient's blood pressure after administering nitroglycerin, especially after the first dose.
- During episodes of chest pain, monitor ECG tracings, blood pressure, and pulmonary artery catheter measurements (if applicable) to determine changes.
- Apply antiembolism stockings or compression boots to help prevent venostasis and thrombophlebitis.
- Assess the patient's degree of pain. Record the severity, location, type, and duration of pain.
- Administer analgesics as ordered. Avoid giving I.M. injections because absorption from muscles is unpredictable and I.V. administration provides more rapid symptomatic relief.
- Organize patient care and activities to allow periods of uninterrupted rest.
- Ask the dietary department to provide a clear-liquid diet until nausea subsides. A low-cholesterol, low-sodium diet without caffeine-containing beverages may be ordered.
- Provide opportunities for the patient to express his feelings about himself and the illness.
- Allow choices when appropriate. Help the patient identify strengths and areas of control.
- Administer antianxiety medications as ordered.
- Assist with range-of-motion exercises.
- If the patient is immobilized by a severe MI, turn him often.

- Monitor vital signs for changes before, during, and immediately after activity.
- Provide assistance with self-care activities.
- Provide for rest periods, especially after meals.
- Assist with the cardiac rehabilitation program, and provide positive reinforcement for achievements.
- Arrange referrals for any needed in-home rehabilitation, support groups, and other organized activities.

Patient teaching

- Explain procedures to the patient and his family and answer their questions honestly.
- Explain the ICU environment and routine. Remember, you may need to repeat explanations once the emergency situation has resolved
- Promote compliance with the prescribed medication regimen and other treatments. Thoroughly explain dosages and therapy. Inform the patient of adverse drug effects, and advise him to watch for and report signs of toxicity (for example, anorexia, nausea, vomiting, mental depression, vertigo, blurred vision, and yellow vision if he's receiving a digitalis glycoside).
- Review dietary restrictions with the patient. If he must follow a low-sodium or low-fat and low-cholesterol diet, provide a list of foods to avoid. Ask the dietitian to speak to the patient and his family.
- Encourage the patient to participate in a cardiac rehabilitation program. The doctor and the exercise physiologist should determine the level of exercise, discuss it with the patient, and secure his agreement to a stepped-care program.
- Counsel the patient to resume sexual activity progressively. He may need to take nitroglycerin before sexual intercourse to prevent chest pain from the increased activity.
- Explain the signs and symptoms that require follow-up care or doctor notification.
- Advise the patient to report typical or atypical chest pain. Post-MI syndrome produces chest pain that must be differentiated from recurrent MI, pulmonary infarction, and heart failure.
- Stress the need to stop smoking. If necessary, refer the patient to a support group.

EVALUATION
Achievement of patient outcomes determines whether collaborative management has succeeded. For a patient with MI, evaluation focuses on improved tissue perfusion, decreased risk of injury, improved comfort, adequate coping, improved activity tolerance, and adequate knowledge of the disease process and treatment regimen.

Thrombophlebitis

An acute condition characterized by inflammation and thrombus formation, thrombophlebitis may occur in deep or superficial veins. It typically occurs at the valve cusps because venous stasis encourages the accumulation and adherence of platelets and fibrin. (See *Major venous pathways of the leg.*) Thrombophlebitis usually begins with localized inflammation alone (phlebitis), but such inflammation rapidly provokes thrombus formation. Rarely, venous thrombosis develops without associated inflammation of the vein (phlebothrombosis).

Deep vein thrombophlebitis affects small veins, such as the lesser saphenous vein, or large veins, such as the iliac, femoral, and popliteal veins and the vena cava. It is more serious than superficial vein thrombophlebitis because it affects the veins deep in the leg musculature that carry 90% of the venous outflow from the leg. The incidence of deep vein thrombophlebitis involving the subclavian vein is rising with the increased use of subclavian vein catheters.

Some studies indicate that up to 35% of hospitalized patients develop deep vein thrombophlebitis. Some hospitalized patients are more at risk than others; however, the risk of developing deep vein thrombophlebitis increases dramatically after age 40 and triples with each additional 20 years.

The major complications of thrombophlebitis are pulmonary embolism and chronic venous insufficiency. (See *Dealing with chronic venous insufficiency,* page 112.)

Superficial vein thrombophlebitis is usually self-limiting and, because these veins have fewer valves than the deep veins, is less likely to cause complications.

CAUSES

Virchow, in 1846, identified three major factors that promote development of venous thrombosis. Known as Virchow's triad, they include hypercoagulability, venous stasis, and intimal damage.

Deep vein thrombophlebitis may be idiopathic, but it is more likely to occur in conjunction with certain diseases, treatments, injuries, or other factors, such as the following:
■ hypercoagulability states—cigarette smoking; circulating lupus anticoagulant; deficiencies of antithrombin III, protein C, or protein S; disseminated intravascular coagulation; estrogen use; dysfibrinogenemia; myeloproliferative diseases; systemic infection
■ intimal damage—infection, infusion of irritating I.V. solutions, trauma, venipuncture

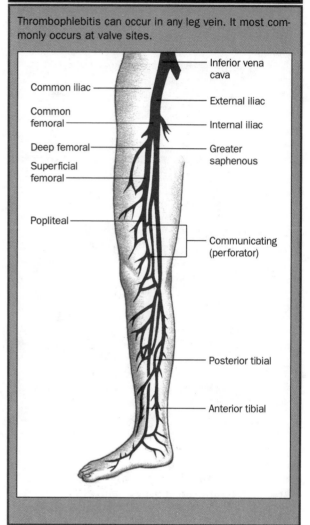

Major venous pathways of the leg

Thrombophlebitis can occur in any leg vein. It most commonly occurs at valve sites.

Common iliac
Common femoral
Deep femoral
Superficial femoral
Popliteal

Inferior vena cava
External iliac
Internal iliac
Greater saphenous
Communicating (perforator)
Posterior tibial
Anterior tibial

■ neoplasms—lung, ovary, pancreas, stomach, testicles, urinary tract
■ surgery—abdominal, genitourinary, orthopedic, thoracic
■ fracture—spine, pelvis, femur, tibia
■ venous stasis—acute myocardial infarction, heart failure, dehydration, immobility, incompetent vein valves, postoperative convalescence, cerebrovascular accident
■ venulitis—Behçet's disease, homocystinuria, thromboangiitis obliterans
■ other—pregnancy, previous deep vein thrombosis.

A thrombus develops when platelets adhere to the endothelium. Where the platelets adhere to collagen, adenosine diphosphate is released. This is also re-

Chronic venous insufficiency results from the valvular destruction of deep vein thrombosis, usually in the iliac and femoral veins and occasionally in the saphenous veins. It's often accompanied by incompetence of the communicating veins of the ankle, causing increased venous pressure and fluid migration into the interstitial tissue.

Signs and symptoms
Chronic venous insufficiency causes chronic edema and swelling in the affected leg, which leads to tissue fibrosis and induration; skin discoloration from extravasation of blood in subcutaneous tissue; and stasis ulcers around the ankle.

Treatment
Appropriate treatment for small stasis ulcers consists of bed rest, elevation of the legs, warm soaks, and antimicrobial therapy for infection.

Treatment to counteract increased venous pressure, the result of reflux from the deep venous system to superficial veins, may include compression dressings, such as a sponge rubber pressure dressing or a zinc gelatin boot (Unna's boot). This therapy begins after massive swelling subsides.

Large stasis ulcers unresponsive to conservative treatment may require excision and skin grafting. Care includes daily inspection to assess healing and measures similar to those for varicose veins.

leased from the damaged tissues and disrupted platelets. Adenosine diphosphate produces platelet aggregation resulting in a platelet plug.

As the thrombus increases in diameter and length, venous obstruction occurs. The resulting inflammatory process can destroy the valves of the veins, thus initiating venous insufficiency.

DIAGNOSIS AND TREATMENT
Diagnosis must rule out arterial occlusive disease, lymphangitis, cellulitis, and myositis. Diagnosis of superficial vein thrombophlebitis is based on physical findings, whereas diagnosis of deep vein thrombophlebitis is based on characteristic test findings.

Venous duplex ultrasonography identifies reduced blood flow to a specific area and any obstruction to venous flow. Plethysmography measures electrical resistance as a result of changes in blood volume due to deep vein thrombosis distal to the affected area; it's less accurate than ultrasonography in detecting calf vein thrombi. Venography identifies the thrombi or obstruction in lower extremity veins.

In deep vein thrombophlebitis, treatment includes bed rest, with elevation of the affected arm or leg; application of warm, moist compresses to the affected area; and analgesics. After the acute episode subsides, the patient may begin to ambulate while wearing antiembolism stockings (applied before he gets out of bed).

Treatment may also include anticoagulants (initially, heparin; later, warfarin) to prolong clotting time. However, the full anticoagulant dose must be discontinued during any surgical procedure to avoid the risk of hemorrhage. After some types of surgery, especially major abdominal or pelvic operations, prophylactic doses of anticoagulants may reduce the risk of deep vein thrombophlebitis.

For lysis of acute, extensive deep vein thrombophlebitis, treatment should include streptokinase or urokinase if the risk of bleeding doesn't outweigh the potential benefits of thrombolytic treatment.

Rarely, deep vein thrombophlebitis may cause complete venous occlusion, which necessitates venous interruption through simple ligation to vein plication, or clipping. Embolectomy may be done if clots are being shed to the pulmonary and systemic vasculature and other treatment is unsuccessful. Caval interruption with transvenous placement of an umbrella filter can trap emboli, preventing them from traveling to the pulmonary vasculature.

Therapy for severe superficial vein thrombophlebitis may include an anti-inflammatory drug such as indomethacin, along with antiembolism stockings, warm compresses, and elevation of the affected leg.

COLLABORATIVE MANAGEMENT
Care of the patient with thrombophlebitis focuses on treatment of the inflammatory process, prevention of further clotting or extension of the disease, and restoration of venous blood flow.

ASSESSMENT
In both deep vein and superficial vein thrombophlebitis, clinical features vary with the site of inflammation and the length of the affected vein. Up to 50% of patients with deep vein thrombophlebitis may be asymptomatic, but others may complain of some tenderness, aching, or severe pain in the affected leg or arm as well as fever, chills, and malaise. Perform your physical examination carefully because much of the patient's subsequent care will depend on your findings.

Inspection may reveal redness, swelling, and cyanosis of the affected leg or arm. Some patients with deep vein thrombophlebitis of a leg vein may have a positive Homans' sign (pain on dorsiflexion of the foot), but this is considered an unreliable sign. A positive cuff sign (elicited by inflating a blood pressure cuff until pain occurs) may be present in deep vein thrombophlebitis of either the arm or leg. When palpated, the affected leg or arm may feel warm.

Patients with superficial vein thrombophlebitis may also be asymptomatic, or they may complain of pain localized to the thrombus site. Inspection may disclose redness and swelling at the site and surrounding area. When palpated, the area feels warm, and a tender, hard cord extends over the affected vein's length.

Extensive vein involvement may cause lymphadenitis.

NURSING DIAGNOSES AND COLLABORATIVE PROBLEMS

Based on these nursing diagnoses, you'll establish patient outcomes.

Altered peripheral tissue perfusion related to obstruction in venous flow. The patient will:
■ report a decrease in edema and inflammation
■ exhibit palpable peripheral pulses with pink, dry warm skin
■ exhibit quick capillary refill.

Altered protection related to increased risk of bleeding caused by anticoagulant therapy. The patient will:
■ communicate an understanding of bleeding precautions
■ incorporate bleeding precautions into daily life
■ show no signs or symptoms of bleeding.

Risk for injury related to potential for pulmonary emboli. The patient will:
■ identify the signs and symptoms of pulmonary emboli and report any occurrence immediately
■ maintain adequate ventilation
■ develop no pulmonary emboli.

Pain related to inflammation of a vessel wall. The patient will:
■ express feelings of comfort following analgesic administration
■ use bed rest and warm compresses to reduce inflammation and, thus, pain
■ report the alleviation of pain when thrombophlebitis is eradicated.

Knowledge deficit related to thrombophlebitis, contributing factors, and treatment. The patient will:
■ verbalize signs and symptoms of thrombophlebitis and possible contributing factors
■ verbalize an understanding of the medication regimen
■ report signs and symptoms of changes indicating possible complications.

PLANNING AND IMPLEMENTATION

The following measures help the patient with thrombophlebitis.
■ Apply warm compresses or a covered aquathermia pad to increase circulation to the affected area and to relieve pain and inflammation.

■ Administer heparin I.V., as ordered, with an infusion monitor or pump to control the flow rate, if necessary.
■ Mark, measure, and record the circumference of the affected arm or leg daily, and compare this measurement with that of the other arm or leg.
■ To ensure the accuracy and consistency of serial measurements, mark the skin over the area and measure at the same spot daily.
■ Perform neurovascular checks on the affected extremity, and compare your findings to other side; assess pulses distal to the area; monitor the temperature, color, and condition of the affected extremity; and ask the patient if he feels any numbness or tingling. Report any significant changes.
■ Enforce bed rest as ordered, and elevate the patient's affected arm or leg. If you plan to use pillows to elevate the leg, position them so that they support its entire length to avoid compressing the popliteal space.
■ To prevent thrombophlebitis in high-risk patients, perform range-of-motion exercises while the patient is on bed rest, use intermittent pneumatic calf massage during lengthy surgical or diagnostic procedures, apply antiembolism stockings postoperatively, and encourage early ambulation.
■ Measure partial thromboplastin time regularly for the patient on heparin therapy. Measure prothrombin time for the patient on warfarin (therapeutic anticoagulation values for both are one and one-half to two times control values).
■ Assess the affected extremity for pain, pallor, pulselessness, and paresthesia, and notify the doctor if any of these occur.
■ Watch for signs and symptoms of bleeding, such as tarry stools, coffee-ground vomitus, and ecchymoses. Watch for oozing of blood at I.V. sites, and assess gums for excessive bleeding.
■ Be alert for signs of pulmonary emboli (crackles, dyspnea, hemoptysis, sudden changes in mental status, restlessness, and hypotension).
■ Give analgesics to relieve pain, as ordered.
■ Change the patient's position frequently to minimize the risks of prolonged bed rest.

Patient teaching
■ Before discharge, emphasize the importance of follow-up blood studies to monitor the effects of anticoagulant therapy.
■ If the patient is being discharged on heparin therapy, teach him or a family member how to give subcutaneous injections. If he requires further assistance, arrange for a home health care nurse.
■ Tell the patient to avoid crossing legs and prolonged sitting or standing to help prevent a recurrence.

- Teach the patient how to properly apply and use antiembolism stockings.
- Tell him to report any complications, such as cold, blue toes.
- To prevent bleeding, encourage the patient to use an electric razor and avoid medications that contain aspirin.

EVALUATION

Achievement of patient outcomes determines whether or not the collaborative management has been successful. For a patient with thrombophlebitis, evaluation focuses on improved peripheral tissue perfusion, maintenance of safety, promotion of comfort, and adequate knowledge of the disorder and its treatment.

Treatments and procedures

Various treatments and procedures are available for patients with cardiovascular disease. Advances in therapy have helped save hundreds of lives and allowed many cardiac patients to lead normal lives.

CARDIAC CATHETERIZATION

In cardiac catheterization, a catheter is inserted into the heart and surrounding vessels to relay detailed information about the structure and performance of the heart, valves, and circulatory system. The procedure typically takes place in a cardiac catheterization laboratory.

The procedure is used to locate and measure coronary lesions, evaluate ventricular function, and measure heart pressure and oxygen saturation levels. During the procedure, the electrocardiogram (ECG) is continuously monitored, often with angiography. Usually only one side of the heart is catheterized, although both sides may be.

Right-sided catheterization is used to:
- assess right ventricular function
- determine tricuspid and pulmonic valve patency
- detect intracardiac shunts
- diagnose pulmonary hypertension
- measure cardiac output.

Left-sided catheterization is used to:
- assess left ventricular function
- determine mitral and aortic valve patency.

PROCEDURE

The catheter is inserted through either the brachial artery (Sones procedure) or the femoral artery (Judkins procedure). It's then passed to the aortic root (coronary artery openings). During this procedure,

the patient's heart rate and rhythm are continually monitored.

Right-sided catheterization. In this procedure, a multilumen catheter is passed through the superior or inferior vena cava into the right atrium, to the right ventricle, and into the pulmonary artery. A fluoroscope is used to monitor the catheter's passage. Pressures in each chamber are measured and recorded, blood samples are withdrawn for oxygen analysis, pulmonary artery and capillary pressures are measured, and cardiac output is calculated.

Left-sided catheterization. In this procedure, a single-lumen catheter is advanced into the aorta, through the aortic valve, and into the left ventricle. Heart activity is recorded by cineangiography (filming) to identify ventricular areas that don't pump properly.

The single-lumen catheter is then removed, and two specially shaped catheters are inserted to study the left and right coronary arteries. Cineangiography is used to identify such problems as a narrowed or blocked coronary artery.

During left-sided catheterization, angioplasty may be performed, anticoagulants may be injected, and left ventricular function may be evaluated before bypass surgery. A biopsy may be performed to diagnose myocarditis or rejection of a transplanted heart.

COLLABORATIVE MANAGEMENT

Care of the patient undergoing cardiac catheterization involves thorough preparation, close monitoring during and after the procedure, and providing follow-up instructions and medical care.

Preparation
- Obtain baseline vital signs.
- Document the presence and intensity of peripheral pulses; mark the sites with an indelible marker to help locate them later.
- Note the patient's anxiety and activity levels, and the presence and pattern of any chest pain.
- Identify any known allergies, particularly to iodine or shellfish, which suggest sensitivity to the radiopaque dye used in angiography. Alert the doctor to allergies.
- Be aware that the patient may receive nitroglycerin during the test to dilate coronary vessels and aid visualization.
- Check with the doctor before withholding any medications. If your patient is scheduled for early morning catheterization, withhold foods and fluids after midnight of the preceding day.
- Alert the doctor to changes in the patient's condition.

- Make sure the patient understands why he's scheduled for catheterization.
- Tell him that the insertion site will be cleaned and prepped. Explain that he won't receive general anesthesia but may be given a mild I.V. or oral sedative before or during the procedure.
- Warn him that he may feel a warm sensation, light-headedness, or nausea for a few moments after the dye injection.
- Explain that he'll have to cough or breathe deeply as instructed during the test.
- Tell the patient he'll need to remain on strict bed rest (lying down) for several hours after the procedure.
- Advise him to notify you immediately if he has any chest pain during or after the procedure.

Monitoring and aftercare

- Following the Judkins procedure, tell the patient to keep his leg straight for at least 6 to 8 hours. Elevate the head of the bed no more than 30 degrees. Following the Sones procedure, tell the patient to keep his arm straight for at least 3 hours. To immobilize the leg or arm, place a sandbag over it.
- Monitor for bleeding, the most serious risk. If bleeding occurs, remove the pressure dressing and apply firm manual pressure; notify the doctor.
- For the first hour after catheterization, monitor vital signs every 15 minutes and inspect the dressing frequently for signs of bleeding and hematoma formation.
- Check skin color, temperature, and pulses distal to the insertion site. An absent or weak pulse may signify an embolus or another problem that needs immediate attention.
- Notify the doctor of any changes in peripheral pulses.
- Monitor heart rhythm and be alert for complaints of chest pain. If heart rhythm or vital signs change, or if the patient has chest pain (possible indications of arrhythmias, angina, or myocardial infarction [MI]), monitor the ECG closely and notify the doctor.
- Encourage the patient to drink fluids to flush out the radiopaque dye. Monitor urine output, especially in cases of impaired renal function.
- Check with the doctor about resuming medications that were withheld before catheterization.
- Before discharge, make sure vital signs, hemodynamic parameters, and ECG recordings are within acceptable parameters. The patient should be alert and oriented, without signs of any mental confusion, and able to tolerate fluids and food without problems. The catheter dressing site should be clean and dry with no evidence of bleeding or infection.
- Make appointments for office visits or additional testing and procedures. Provide emotional support to

help the patient deal with the diagnosis and make possibly life-changing decisions.

Patient teaching

- Make sure the patient receives and understands instructions regarding aftercare, activities, and follow-up measures.
- Describe the signs and symptoms of complications.
- Tell the patient to check the catheter insertion site for signs of bleeding and infection. Demonstrate measures to keep the site clean.
- Encourage the patient to resume his previous level of activity as tolerated.
- Advise him to keep all appointments for follow-up care.

COMPLICATIONS
Some possible complications of cardiac catheterization can be life threatening. (See *Complications of cardiac catheterization*, page 116.)

CORONARY ARTERY BYPASS GRAFTING
Coronary artery bypass grafting (CABG) is used to circumvent one or more occluded coronary arteries with an autologous graft (usually a segment of the internal mammarian artery or the saphenous vein from the leg) to restore blood flow to the myocardium. This may prevent myocardial infarction in a patient with acute or chronic myocardial ischemia. CABG also can relieve anginal pain, improve cardiac function, and enhance the patient's quality of life.

PROCEDURE
Surgery, performed under general anesthesia, begins with graft harvesting of a segment from the internal mammarian artery (preferred) or the saphenous vein. The heart is then exposed and cardiopulmonary bypass is initiated. The heart is stopped to reduce oxygen demands and protect the heart during surgery.

For each artery bypassed, one end of the graft is sutured to the ascending aorta and the other end to a patent coronary artery distal to the occlusion. Cardiopulmonary bypass is then discontinued, epicardial pacing electrodes are implanted, and a chest tube is inserted.

COLLABORATIVE MANAGEMENT
Care of the patient undergoing CABG surgery involves providing instructions and caring for the patient's changing cardiovascular needs.

Preparation
- Make sure the patient understands the reason for the procedure and is familiar with the equipment and procedures used in the intensive care unit (ICU) or

Complications of cardiac catheterization

Cardiac catheterization imposes more patient risk than most other diagnostic tests. Although infrequent, complications can become life-threatening. Observe the patient closely during the procedure and afterward until he's stable. Keep in mind that some complications arise in both left-sided and right-sided catheterization; others result only from catheterization of one side. In either case, notify the doctor promptly, and carefully document complications and their treatments.

Complications and causes	Signs and symptoms
LEFT- OR RIGHT-SIDED CATHETERIZATION	
CARDIAC TAMPONADE ■ Perforation of heart wall by catheter	Arrhythmias, tachycardia, hypotension, chest pain, diaphoresis, cyanosis, distant heart sounds
ARRHYTHMIAS ■ Cardiac tissue irritated by catheter	Irregular heartbeat, palpitations, ventricular tachycardia, ventricular fibrillation
HEMATOMA OR BLOOD LOSS AT INSERTION SITE ■ Bleeding at insertion site from vein or artery damage	Bloody dressing, limb swelling or increased girth, hypotension, tachycardia, color changes in affected extremity
HYPOVOLEMIA ■ Diuresis from angiography contrast medium	Hypotension, tachycardia, pallor, diaphoresis
INFECTION (SYSTEMIC) ■ Poor aseptic technique ■ Catheter contamination	Fever, tachycardia, chills and tremors, unstable blood pressure
INFECTION AT INSERTION SITE ■ Poor aseptic technique	Swelling, warmth, redness, and soreness at insertion site; purulent discharge at insertion site
MYOCARDIAL INFARCTION ■ Emotional stress induced by procedure ■ Plaque dislodged by catheter tip that travels to a coronary artery (left-sided catheterization only) ■ Occlusion of diseased artery by contrast media or catheter during procedure	Chest pain, possibly radiating to left arm, back, or jaw; cardiac arrhythmias; diaphoresis, restlessness, or anxiety; thready pulse; nausea and vomiting
PULMONARY EDEMA ■ Excessive fluid administration	Early stage: tachycardia, tachypnea, dependent crackles, diastolic (S_3) gallop. Acute stage: dyspnea; rapid, noisy respirations; cough with frothy, blood-tinged sputum; cyanosis with cold, clammy skin; tachycardia; hypertension
REACTION TO CONTRAST MEDIUM ■ Allergy to iodine	Fever, agitation, hives, itching, difficulty breathing
LEFT-SIDED CATHETERIZATION	
ARTERIAL EMBOLUS OR THROMBUS IN LIMB ■ Injury to artery during catheter insertion ■ Plaque dislodged from artery wall by catheter	Slow or faint pulse distal to insertion site; loss of warmth, sensation, and color in arm or leg distal to insertion site; sudden pain in extremity
CEREBROVASCULAR ACCIDENT OR TRANSIENT ISCHEMIC ATTACK ■ Blood clot or plaque dislodged by catheter tip that travels to brain	Hemiplegia or paresis, aphasia, lethargy, confusion or decreased level of consciousness
RIGHT-SIDED CATHETERIZATION	
PULMONARY EMBOLISM ■ Dislodged blood clot	Shortness of breath, tachypnea, tachycardia, chest pain, pink-tinged sputum
THROMBOPHLEBITIS ■ Vein damaged during catheter insertion	Vein that is hard, sore, cordlike, and warm (vein may look like a red line above catheter insertion site); swelling at site
VAGAL RESPONSE ■ Vagus nerve endings irritated in sinoatrial node, atrial muscle tissue, or atrioventricular junction	Hypotension, bradycardia, nausea

procedures used in the intensive care unit (ICU) or postanesthesia care unit (PACU).

■ Describe early postoperative events. Tell the patient that he'll awaken from surgery with an endotracheal tube in place and be connected to a mechanical ventilator and a cardiac monitor. He may have in place a nasogastric tube, mediastinal tubes, an indwelling urinary catheter, arterial lines, epicardial pacing wires and, possibly, a pulmonary artery catheter. Reassure him that this equipment should cause him little discomfort and will be removed as soon as possible. Tell him that medication will be available if needed.

■ The evening before surgery, have the patient shower with antiseptic soap. Restrict food and fluids after midnight, and provide a sedative if ordered.

■ On the morning of surgery, also provide a sedative as ordered.

■ Immediately before surgery, assist with pulmonary artery catheterization and insertion of arterial lines. Begin cardiac monitoring.

Monitoring and aftercare

■ Assess the patient for signs of hemodynamic compromise, such as severe hypotension, decreased cardiac output, and shock. Check and record vital signs every 5 to 15 minutes until the patient's condition stabilizes. Monitor the ECG for heart rate and rhythm.

■ Tell the doctor if you detect serious abnormalities. Be prepared to assist with epicardial pacing or, if necessary, cardioversion or defibrillation.

■ Maintain arterial pressure within established guidelines to prevent inadequate tissue perfusion or hemorrhage and graft rupture. Monitor pulmonary artery, central venous, and left atrial pressures, as ordered.

■ Frequently evaluate peripheral pulses, capillary refill time, and skin temperature and color. Auscultate for heart sounds. Notify the doctor of any abnormalities.

■ Assess breath sounds, chest excursion, and symmetry of chest expansion to check tissue oxygenation.

■ Check arterial blood gas (ABG) results every 2 to 4 hours. Adjust ventilator settings as needed to maintain established ABG values.

■ Monitor intake and output. Assess for electrolyte imbalances, especially hypokalemia.

■ Maintain chest tube drainage pressure (usually −10 to −40 cm H_2O).

■ Check regularly for hemorrhage, excessive drainage (more than 200 ml/hour), and suddenly decreased drainage from mediastinal tubes (or no drainage at all).

■ Give analgesics and other drugs as ordered.

■ Assess for symptoms of cerebrovascular accident (altered level of consciousness, pupillary changes, weakness and loss of movement in extremities, ataxia, aphasia, dysphagia, sensory disturbances), pulmonary

embolism (chest pain, dyspnea, hemoptysis, pleural friction rub, cyanosis, hypoxemia), and impaired renal perfusion (decreased urine output, elevated blood urea nitrogen and serum creatinine levels).

■ After the ventilator and endotracheal tube are removed, promote chest physiotherapy and begin incentive spirometry. Encourage the patient to cough, turn frequently, and breathe deeply.

■ Assist with range-of-motion (ROM) exercises as ordered.

■ Establish a discharge plan. (See *After CABG.*)

Patient teaching

■ Instruct the patient to tell the doctor if he has signs of infection (fever; sore throat; or redness, swelling, or drainage from the leg or chest incisions) or possible arterial reocclusion (angina, dizziness, dyspnea, rapid or irregular pulse, or prolonged recovery time from exercise).

■ Explain postpericardiotomy syndrome. Tell the patient to report fever, muscle and joint pain, weakness, or chest discomfort.

■ Warn the patient about possible postoperative depression, which may develop weeks after discharge. Reassure him that this symptom is normal and should pass quickly.

■ Make sure the patient understands the dosage, administration route, and possible adverse effects of all prescribed medications.

■ Encourage the patient to make recommended dietary changes, especially sodium and cholesterol restrictions, to help prevent recurrent arterial occlusion.

■ Explain the need for at least 8 hours of sleep a night, afternoon rest periods, and frequent rest during

---

DISCHARGE READY **After CABG**

After undergoing coronary artery bypass graft (CABG) surgery and before discharge, the patient should exhibit the following criteria:

■ adequate cardiac output, as evidenced by normal blood pressure and pulse rate

■ adequate tissue perfusion, as evidenced by urine output of at least 30 ml/hour

■ vital signs and hemodynamic parameters within acceptable limits

■ alertness and proper orientation to time, place, and person

■ absence of complications, such as arrhythmias, fluid and electrolyte imbalances, or pericardial tamponade, which could alter his cardiac output

■ adequate fluid and electrolyte balance.

activities. Tell the patient that he can climb stairs, engage in sexual activity, take baths and showers, and do light chores, as appropriate. Tell him to follow exercise guidelines and avoid lifting objects heavier than 10 lb (4.5 kg), driving a car, or doing strenuous work (such as lawn mowing or vacuuming), as the doctor recommends.

■ Provide referrals for sources of information and support and for home care, if necessary.

COMPLICATIONS

Postoperative complications include arrhythmias, hypertension or hypotension, cardiac tamponade, thromboembolism, hemorrhage, postpericardiotomy syndrome, and MI. Noncardiac complications include cerebrovascular accident, postoperative depression or emotional instability, pulmonary embolism, decreased renal function, and infection. Problems such as graft rupture or closure or the development of atherosclerosis in other coronary arteries sometimes necessitate repeat surgery.

HEART TRANSPLANTATION

In heart transplantation for end-stage cardiac disease, a diseased heart is replaced with a healthy one from a brain-dead donor. Most patients can expect to experience infection or tissue rejection after transplantation.

PROCEDURE

Heart transplantation can be performed using either of two techniques. In an *orthotopic transplant,* a large portion of the recipient's right and left atria is retained and the donor heart is implanted to the atria. Cardiopulmonary bypass is used during the surgery. Temporary pacemaker wires and chest drainage catheters are inserted.

In a *heterotopic transplant,* the donor heart is placed parallel to the recipient's heart. The right side of the patient's heart can continue to function and the dysfunctional left side is bypassed.

An artificial heart can be implanted in similar procedures until a donor heart is available.

COLLABORATIVE MANAGEMENT

Care of the patient receiving a heart transplant involves thorough preparation, close monitoring of all body systems, and thorough patient teaching and discharge planning.

Preparation

■ Provide strong emotional support for the patient and family members. Discuss the procedure, possible complications, and the impact of transplantation and a prolonged recovery period. Encourage all family members to express their concerns and to ask questions; if necessary, refer them for psychological counseling.

■ Explain what to expect before surgery, including food and fluid restrictions and the need for intubation and mechanical ventilation.

■ If possible, arrange a tour of the PACU and the ICU. Describe postoperative isolation measures and the tests used to detect tissue rejection and other complications.

■ Explain the immunosuppressant drug regimen to combat rejection.

Monitoring and aftercare

■ Maintain isolation precautions according to your facility's protocol.

■ Administer immunosuppressant drugs as ordered.

■ Immunosuppressants typically mask obvious signs of infection; watch for more subtle signs, such as fever above 100° F (37.8° C).

■ Administer prophylactic antibiotics and maintain strict asepsis when caring for incision and drainage sites.

■ Assess the patient for signs of hemodynamic compromise, such as severe hypotension, decreased cardiac output, and shock.

■ Check and record vital signs every 15 minutes until the patient's condition stabilizes.

■ Monitor the ECG for disturbances in heart rate and rhythm from myocardial irritability or ischemia, fluid and electrolyte imbalances, hypoxemia, or hypothermia. If you detect abnormalities, notify the doctor and assist with epicardial pacing.

■ To ensure adequate myocardial perfusion, maintain arterial pressure within established parameters. Also monitor pulmonary artery, central venous, and left atrial pressures.

■ Frequently auscultate for heart sounds and evaluate peripheral pulses, capillary refill time, and skin temperature and color. Notify the doctor of any abnormalities.

■ Evaluate tissue oxygenation by assessing breath sounds, chest excursion, and symmetry of chest expansion. Check ABG levels every 2 to 4 hours, and adjust ventilator settings as needed.

■ Maintain chest tube drainage at the prescribed negative pressure (usually –10 to –40 cm H_2O). Check chest tubes every hour for patency, and regularly assess for hemorrhage, excessive drainage (more than 200 ml/hour), or sudden decrease or cessation of drainage.

■ Continually assess the patient for signs of tissue rejection. Be alert for decreased electrical activity on the ECG, right axis shift, atrial arrhythmias, conduction defects, ventricular gallop, ventricular failure, jugular vein distention, malaise, lethargy, weight gain, and increased T-cell count. Report any of these signs immediately.

■ As ordered, administer antiarrhythmic, inotropic, pressor, and analgesic medications as well as I.V. fluids and blood products.

- Monitor intake and output, and assess for hypokalemia and other electrolyte imbalances.
- Evaluate for the effects of denervation. Look for an elevated resting heart rate or a sinus rhythm that's unaffected by respirations. A lack of heart rate variation in response to changes in position, Valsalva's maneuver, or carotid massage indicates complete denervation.
- Remember that atropine, anticholinergics, and edrophonium may have no effect on a denervated heart and that the effects of quinidine, digoxin, and verapamil may vary.
- Throughout the patient's recovery period, assess him carefully for complications. Watch especially for signs of CVA (altered level of consciousness, pupillary changes, weakness and loss of movement in the extremities, ataxia, aphasia, dysphagia, sensory disturbances), pulmonary embolism (dyspnea, cough, hemoptysis, chest pain, pleural friction rub, cyanosis, hypoxemia), and impaired renal perfusion (decreased urine output, elevated blood urea nitrogen and serum creatinine levels).
- After weaning the patient from the ventilator and removing the endotracheal tube, promote chest physiotherapy.
- Begin incentive spirometry and encourage the patient to cough, turn frequently, and breathe deeply.
- Assist with ROM exercises as ordered.
- Provide referrals for home care.

Patient teaching
- Explain that the doctor will schedule frequent (weekly to monthly) myocardial biopsies to check for signs of tissue rejection. Stress the importance of keeping these appointments, and reassure the patient that biopsies don't require hospitalization.
- Instruct the patient to immediately report any signs and symptoms of rejection (fever, weight gain, dyspnea, lethargy, weakness) or infection (chest pain, fever, sore throat, or redness, swelling, or drainage from the incision site).
- Explain that postpericardiotomy syndrome often develops after open-heart surgery. Tell him to call his doctor if he experiences fever, muscle and joint pain, weakness, and chest discomfort.
- During the initial recovery period, advise him to try to sleep at least 8 hours a night, to rest briefly each afternoon, and to take breaks during physical activity.
- Tell him he can climb stairs, engage in sexual activity, take baths and showers, and do light housework and other chores as allowed by the doctor.
- Warn against lifting objects heavier than 10 lb (4.5 kg), driving, or doing heavy work (such as mowing the lawn or vacuuming), as the doctor recommends.
- Provide instructions for a home exercise program.

- If the patient shows signs of denervation, advise him to rise slowly from a sitting or lying position to minimize orthostatic hypotension.
- Make sure he knows the dosage, schedule, and adverse effects of prescribed drugs.
- Encourage him to follow his prescribed diet, especially sodium and fat restrictions.
- Before discharge, make sure the patient and family members understand all instructions on activity, diet, wound care, and medications and that they can identify the signs and symptoms of rejection.

COMPLICATIONS
The major complication of heart transplantation is rejection. The patient is also at risk for complications of open-heart surgery, such as hypothermia, coagulation problems, fluid and electrolyte imbalances, hemorrhage, thrombosis or embolism, and respiratory, renal, GI, and central nervous system complications.

IMPLANTABLE CARDIAC DEFIBRILLATOR
The primary mechanism of sudden cardiac death is ventricular fibrillation. A patient who's had one episode of ventricular fibrillation (which carries a high risk of further episodes of ventricular tachyarrhythmia) is a good candidate for an implantable cardiac defibrillator (ICD).

The ICD consists of a pulse generator and a lead system. It continuously analyzes the patient's cardiac rhythm and delivers an internal electrical discharge when ventricular fibrillation or tachycardia occurs.

PROCEDURE
The ICD is implanted through a medial sternotomy or lateral thoracotomy. Separate leads (the defibrillating electrodes) are sutured to the ventricular wall and attached to the epicardium. The pulse generator is placed in a pocket under the patient's skin. The latest generators incorporate antitachycardia pacing, low-energy cardioversion, high-energy defibrillation, and bradycardia backup pacing.

When the ICD senses a ventricular tachyarrhythmia, it discharges a small shock (25 to 30 joules) to defibrillate the heart automatically. If the initial discharge doesn't end the arrhythmia, the device can discharge up to four more times, increasing the voltage each time. The unit usually lasts 3 years or for up to 100 discharges. In an emergency, defibrillation or cardioversion can be performed without damage to the ICD.

COLLABORATIVE MANAGEMENT
Care of the patient undergoing ICD insertion requires thorough preparation, preoperative and postoperative monitoring, and patient teaching.

Preparation
■ Tell the patient that small incisions will be made on the left side of his chest, right shoulder, and abdomen.
■ Advise him that he'll be able to feel the unit discharge once it's implanted. (Some patients describe the sensation as a sudden blow to the chest.)

Monitoring and aftercare
■ Assess and document continuous ECG rhythm, vital signs, mental status, heart and breath sounds, and urine output as well as any changes in these parameters.
■ If arrhythmias occur, document the ICD response. Institute advanced cardiac life support if the ICD does not successfully convert the arrhythmia.
■ If necessary, provide a referral for follow-up home care.

Patient teaching
■ Warn the patient that if ventricular arrhythmias occur, he'll probably experience sudden faintness or shortness of breath (or both), followed by the discharge and a return to a feeling of well-being. The episode usually lasts less than 30 seconds.
■ Make sure that the patient and family understand what to expect if arrhythmias occur. If the ICD fires, the patient should be transported by ambulance to the hospital and the number of ICD discharges should be reported.
■ Teach the patient and family the signs and symptoms of infection.
■ Explain activity limitations.
■ Suggest that the family obtain a home defibrillator in case the ICD fails to convert the arrhythmia at home; instruct family members how to use the equipment before the patient is discharged.
■ Recommend that family members learn to perform cardiopulmonary resuscitation (CPR) in case the ICD doesn't convert the rhythm after firing a specified number of times. Refer them to appropriate sources for training.
■ Instruct the family to initiate CPR if the patient experiences cardiac arrest and not to wait for the ICD to fire.

COMPLICATIONS
Possible complications include infection, cardiac tamponade, and thromboembolism.

PACEMAKER INSERTION
Temporary or permanent, pacemakers are battery-operated generators that emit timed electrical signals, triggering contraction of the heart muscle and controlling the heart rate when the heart's natural pacemaker is irreversibly disrupted. Temporary pacemakers may be used in emergency situations or before a permanent pacemaker is implanted.

Pacemakers are categorized according to their capabilities. (See *Understanding pacemaker codes.*)

PROCEDURE
A temporary pacemaker may be used after transcutaneous pacing by a pulse generator. A transvenous pacemaker is inserted via the subclavian or jugular vein into the right ventricle. Transthoracic pacing—used only in emergencies—involves needle insertion of leads into the heart. An epicardial pacemaker is inserted during open-heart surgery to permit rapid treatment of postoperative complications.

A permanent pacemaker can be implanted under general anesthesia through a thoracotomy, but most are implanted under local anesthesia. The electrode catheter is inserted through a vein and guided into the heart chamber that's appropriate for the type of pacemaker. The pulse generator is set and attached to the leads, then implanted into a pocket of muscle in the patient's chest or abdominal wall.

COLLABORATIVE MANAGEMENT
Care of the patient undergoing pacemaker insertion requires thorough preparation, close monitoring during and after the procedure, and follow-up with instructions and medical care.

Preparation
■ In an emergency, briefly explain the procedure to the patient if possible. For permanent implantation, ensure that the patient understands the procedure and the need for an artificial pacemaker, the potential complications, and the alternatives. Review pacemaker terminology.
■ Before permanent implantation, obtain baseline vital signs and record a 12-lead ECG or rhythm strip. Evaluate radial and dorsalis pedis pulses and assess the patient's mental status.
■ Restrict food and fluids for 12 hours before the procedure.
■ Explain that a sedative may be given before the procedure and that the upper chest or abdomen will be shaved and scrubbed with an antiseptic solution.
■ Inform the patient that his hands may be restrained in the operating room so that they don't touch the sterile area and that his chest or abdomen will be draped with sterile towels.
■ Unless he's scheduled to undergo a thoracotomy, explain that he'll receive a local anesthetic and that he'll be in the operating room for about an hour.
■ Make sure that the patient or a responsible family member has signed a consent form.

Understanding pacemaker codes

Chamber paced	Chamber sensed	Response to sensing	Programmable functions and rate modulation	Antitachyarrhythmia functions
V (ventricle)	V	T (triggers pacing)	P (programmable rate, output, or both)	P (pacing)
A (atrium)	A	I (inhibits pacing)	M (multiprogrammable rate, output, sensitivity)	S (shock)
D (dual A + V)	D	D (dual, T + I)	C (communicating functions, such as telemetry)	D (dual, P + S)
O (none)	O	O (none)	R (rate modulation) O (none)	O (none)

Monitoring and aftercare

- Provide continuous ECG monitoring.
- Document the type of insertion, lead system, pacemaker mode, and pacing guidelines.
- Take vital signs every 30 minutes until the patient stabilizes, and monitor the ECG for signs of pacemaker problems.
- Be on guard for signs of a perforated ventricle and cardiac tamponade. Ominous signs include persistent hiccups, distant heart sounds, pulsus paradoxus, hypotension accompanied by narrow pulse pressure, increased venous pressure, bulging neck veins, cyanosis, decreased urine output, restlessness, and complaints of fullness in the chest. Report any of these signs immediately, and prepare the patient for emergency surgery.
- If the patient's condition worsens dramatically and he requires defibrillation, follow these guidelines to avoid damaging the pacemaker: Place the paddles at least 4″ (10 cm) from the pulse generator, and avoid anterior-posterior paddle placement. Have a backup temporary pacemaker available. If your patient has an external pacemaker, turn it off. Keep the current under 200 joules if possible.

Assess the area around the incision for swelling, tenderness, and hematoma, but don't remove the occlusive dressing for the first 24 hours without a doctor's order. When you remove it, check the wound for drainage, redness, and unusual warmth or tenderness.
- After 24 hours, begin passive ROM exercises for the affected arm if ordered. Progress to active ROM in 2 weeks.
- Before discharge, ensure that the patient has met certain criteria. (See *After pacemaker insertion,* page 122.)

Patient teaching

- Tell the patient to take his pulse every day before getting out of bed and to record his heart rate, the date, and the time. Stress the importance of calling the doctor immediately if his pulse rate drops below the minimal pacemaker setting or if it exceeds 100 beats/minute.
- Advise him to report difficulty breathing, dizziness, fainting, or swollen hands or feet. Also have him report redness, warmth, pain, drainage, or swelling at the insertion site.
- Warn him against placing excessive pressure over the insertion site, moving suddenly or jerkily, or extending his arms over his head for 8 weeks after discharge.
- Tell the patient that he may bathe and shower normally, engage in sexual activity, and follow his other normal routines.
- Urge him to follow dietary and exercise instructions.
- Remind the patient to carry his pacemaker identification at all times and to show his card to airline clerks when he travels; the pacemaker will set off metal detectors but won't be harmed.
- Explain precautions involving electrical or electronic devices that could disrupt the pacemaker. Advise the patient to inform any doctor that he has an implanted pacemaker before undergoing certain diagnostic tests, such as magnetic resonance imaging.
- The doctor may provide instructions for testing the pacemaker by using a transistor radio or telephone.
- Stress the importance of keeping scheduled follow-up appointments.

COMPLICATIONS

Early complications include serous or bloody drainage from the insertion site, swelling, ecchymosis, incisional pain, and impaired mobility; less common complications include venous thrombosis, embolism, infection, pneumothorax, pectoral or diaphragmatic muscle stimulation from the pacemaker, arrhythmias, cardiac tamponade, heart failure, and abnormal pacemaker operation with lead dislodgment. Late complications (up to several years) include failure to capture, failure to sense, firing loss, and pacemaker rejection.

PERCUTANEOUS TRANSLUMINAL CORONARY ANGIOPLASTY

Percutaneous transluminal coronary angioplasty (PTCA) is a nonsurgical and less costly alternative to CABG surgery for treating coronary artery disease. Patients undergoing PTCA must also be acceptable candidates for emergency CABG surgery in case PTCA is not successful.

PROCEDURE

Coronary arteriography confirms the size and location of the lesion in the coronary artery. Temporary pacemaker wires are inserted in case transient heart block occurs during the procedure.

A guide wire is inserted percutaneously into the femoral artery (or other site), and a catheter is inserted into the coronary artery. Angiography is used to locate the lesion.

A small double-lumen balloon-tipped catheter is introduced through the guide wire and repeatedly inflated with a solution of normal saline and contrast medium for 15 to 30 seconds to compress the athero-sclerotic plaque against the artery wall. Pressure gradients are measured to confirm success.

The catheter is left in place for 18 hours after the procedure to provide access in case coronary artery occlusion develops. Afterward, the patient is returned to the ICU or PACU for monitoring.

COLLABORATIVE MANAGEMENT

Care of the patient undergoing PTCA requires preparing him for the procedure, monitoring his condition afterward, and providing instructions for follow-up visits and home care.

Preparation

- Make sure the patient understands the procedure, its risks, and alternatives.
- Tell him that a catheter will be inserted into an artery in the groin area and that he may feel pressure as the catheter moves along the vessel.
- Advise him that the procedure lasts from 1 to 4 hours and that he'll lie flat on a hard table during that time.
- Explain that he'll be awake during the procedure and may be asked to take deep breaths to allow visualization of the radiopaque balloon catheter. He may also have to answer questions about how he's feeling and alert the doctor if he's experiencing angina.
- Warn him that he may feel a hot, flushing sensation or transient nausea as the contrast medium is injected.
- Check the patient's history for allergies, especially to shellfish, iodine, or contrast medium. Report such allergies to the doctor.
- Tell the patient that an I.V. line will be inserted. Explain that the groin area of both legs will be shaved and cleaned with an antiseptic and that he'll experience a brief stinging sensation when a local anesthetic is injected.
- Restrict the patient's food and fluid intake for at least 6 hours before the procedure or as ordered.
- Ensure that coagulation studies, complete blood count, serum electrolyte studies, and blood typing and crossmatching have been performed.
- Palpate the bilateral distal pulses (usually the dorsalis pedis or posterior tibial pulses), and mark them with an indelible marker so that you can locate them later.
- Take the patient's baseline vital signs, and assess the color, temperature, and sensation in his extremities.
- Before the patient goes to the catheterization laboratory, sedate him as ordered and put a 5-lb (2.2-kg) sandbag on the bed to be used later for applying direct pressure on the arterial puncture site.

Monitoring and aftercare

■ After the procedure, the patient will receive I.V. heparin and nitroglycerin and require continuous arterial and ECG monitoring.

■ Keep the patient's leg straight and elevate the head of the bed no more than 15 degrees (15 to 30 degrees at mealtimes).

■ Monitor vital signs every 15 minutes for the first hour, then every 30 minutes for 2 hours, and then hourly for the next 5 hours. If vital signs are unstable, tell the doctor and check them every 5 minutes.

■ Assess the peripheral pulses distal to the catheter insertion site as well as the color, temperature, and capillary refill time of the extremity. If pulses are difficult to palpate because of the arterial catheter, use a Doppler stethoscope to hear them. Tell the doctor if pulses are absent.

■ Assess the catheter insertion site for hematoma, ecchymosis, or hemorrhage. If you detect an expanding ecchymotic area, mark the area to determine the rapidity of expansion, and obtain a blood sample for hemoglobin and hematocrit analysis, as ordered.

■ If bleeding occurs, apply direct pressure and notify the doctor.

■ Monitor cardiac rate and rhythm continuously. Report any changes or chest pain to the doctor.

■ Administer I.V. fluids as ordered to promote excretion of the contrast medium; assess for signs of fluid overload (distended neck veins, atrial and ventricular gallops, dyspnea, pulmonary congestion, tachycardia, hypertension, and hypoxemia).

■ After the arterial catheter is removed, apply direct pressure for at least 30 minutes and then apply a pressure dressing. Assess vital signs frequently, as above.

■ Before discharge, make sure the patient's condition is stable: that cardiac and hemodynamic parameters are within acceptable values, vital signs are within normal limits, and sudden angina-like pain is absent. The ECG should show no signs of ischemia. Signs and symptoms of abrupt reclosure, such as diaphoresis, tachycardia, chest pain, and anxiety, should be absent. The catheter site should be free of bleeding or infection. In addition, the patient should be using support systems to assist with coping. If necessary, provide referrals for follow-up home care.

Patient teaching

■ Make sure the patient understands activity limitations and the time frame for resuming activities.

■ Confirm the medication regimen and explain the purpose of all prescriptions.

■ Tell him to report bleeding or bruising at the arterial puncture site to the doctor.

■ Schedule a follow-up stress thallium imaging test and angiography, as recommended by the doctor.

COMPLICATIONS

PTCA precludes many surgical risks but can cause serious complications. Coronary artery rupture, cardiac tamponade, myocardial ischemia or infarction, or death can occur with arterial dissection during dilatation; abrupt reclosure of the coronary artery is usually manifested by chest pain.

Other possible complications include closure of a side branch of a coronary artery, coronary artery spasm, decreased coronary artery blood flow, allergic reactions to the contrast medium, and arrhythmias during catheter manipulation. In rare cases, thrombi may embolize, causing a cerebrovascular headache.

VENTRICULAR ASSIST DEVICE

A temporary life-sustaining treatment for a failing heart (such as for a patient awaiting a heart transplant), a ventricular assist device (VAD) provides total mechanical support to the heart and circulation by diverting systemic blood flow from a diseased ventricle into a centrifugal pump. It's usually used to assist the left ventricle but may also assist the right ventricle or both ventricles.

PROCEDURE

The VAD is inserted into the left or right ventricle. Insertion is easier when the patient's chest is open, as for surgery. Up to 10 L/minute of blood is diverted from the heart, routed to the pump, and returned to the pulmonary artery or the aorta. As the patient's condition improves, the patient is gradually weaned from the VAD.

COLLABORATIVE MANAGEMENT

Care of the patient undergoing VAD insertion requires thorough preparation, close monitoring during and after the procedure, and follow-up with instructions and medical care.

Preparation

■ Make sure the patient understands the procedure. Answer all his questions.

■ Tell the patient about food and fluid restrictions before surgery.

■ Explain that his cardiac function will be continuously monitored, using an electrocardiogram, a pulmonary artery catheter, and an arterial line.

■ Prepare the patient's chest as instructed.

■ Provide emotional support to the patient and members of the family.

Monitoring and aftercare

■ Use a kinetic therapy bed. Place an air mattress or sheepskin on the patient's bed to help position him and avoid skin breakdown.

- As the anesthetic wears off, administer analgesics as ordered.
- Keep the patient immobilized to prevent accidental extubation, contamination, or disconnection of the device. Use soft restraints on both of his hands.
- Be aware that most VAD patients are chemically paralyzed, so neurologic assessment findings may be inappropriate indicators of perfusion.
- If appropriate, adjust the VAD pump, maintain cardiac output at 5 to 8 L/minute, pulmonary artery wedge pressure at 10 to 20 mm Hg, central venous pressure at 8 to 16 mm Hg, mean blood pressure above 60 mm Hg, and left atrial pressure at 4 to 12 mm Hg.
- Monitor the patient for signs and symptoms of poor perfusion and ineffective pumping: arrhythmias, hypotension, cool skin, slow capillary refill, oliguria or anuria, confusion, restlessness, and anxiety.
- Administer heparin, as ordered, to prevent clotting in the pump head and thrombus formation.
- Provide enteral or parenteral feedings to maintain adequate nutrition.
- Check mediastinal chest drainage (more than 75 ml/hour may require blood replacement.)
- Check for bleeding, especially at the operative sites.
- Monitor prothrombin time, partial thromboplastin time, and hemoglobin and hematocrit levels every 4 hours. Notify the doctor of abnormal findings.
- Be alert for signs and symptoms of infection. Assess incisions and the cannula insertion site for signs of infection, and culture any suspicious exudate.
- Monitor the patient's white blood cell count and differential daily, and take rectal or core temperatures every 4 hours.
- Using aseptic technique, change the dressing over the cannula insertion sites daily.
- Provide supportive care such as lubricating the skin every 4 hours. Perform passive ROM exercises every 2 hours.
- Before discharge, teach the patient how to care for the VAD insertion site and to be alert for complications.

Patient teaching

- Reinforce all aspects of disease process management.
- Make sure the patient understands why he needs a VAD and the procedure for inserting it.
- Explain the reason for using restraints after the procedure.
- Advise the patient about possible complications.

COMPLICATIONS

VADs carry a high risk of complications, such as blood cell damage and thrombi formation, leading to pulmonary embolism, cerebrovascular accident, and other complications.

Selected references

Cerrato, P. "New Acute MI Guidelines," *RN* 60(1):25-26, January 1997.

Chase, S. "Pharmacology in Practice: Antiarrhythmics," *RN* 60(5):41-48, May 1997.

Diseases, 2nd ed. Springhouse Pa.: Springhouse Corp., 1997.

Heart and Stroke Facts: 1996 Statistical Supplement. Dallas: American Heart Association, 1996.

Hudak, C.M., et al. *Critical Care Nursing: A Holistic Approach,* 6th ed. Philadelphia: Lippincott–Raven Pubs., 1994.

Huddleston, S.S., and Ferguson, S.G. *Critical Care and Emergency Nursing,* 3rd ed. Springhouse Notes Series. Springhouse, Pa.: Springhouse Corp., 1997.

Illustrated Manual of Nursing Practice, 2nd ed. Springhouse, Pa.: Springhouse Corp., 1994.

Nursing98 Drug Handbook. Springhouse, Pa.: Springhouse Corp., 1998.

Ondrusek, R.S. "Spotting an MI Before It's an MI," *RN* 59(4):26-30, April 1996.

Phipps, W.J., et al. *Medical-Surgical Nursing: Concepts and Clinical Practice,* 5th ed. St. Louis: Mosby–Year Book, Inc., 1995.

Possanza, C.P. "What You Should Know about Coronary Artery Bypass Graft Surgery," *Nursing96* 26(2):48-50, February 1996.

Ruppert, S.D., et al. *Dolan's Critical Care Nursing: Clinical Management Through the Nursing Process,* 2nd ed. Philadelphia: F.A. Davis Co., 1996.

Stamatis, S.J., and Spadoni, S.M. "Getting to the Heart of IABP Therapy," *RN* 60(1):38-45, January 1997.

Swearingen, P.L., and Keen, J.H. *Manual of Critical Care: Applying Nursing Diagnoses to Adult Critical Illness,* 3rd ed. St. Louis: Mosby–Year Book, Inc., 1995.

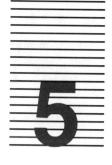

Respiratory disorders

5

The respiratory system functions primarily to exchange oxygen and carbon dioxide in the lungs and tissues and to regulate acid-base balance. Any change in this system affects every other body system. Conversely, changes in other body systems may reduce the lungs' ability to provide oxygen. For instance, any acute disease heightens the body's oxygen demand and increases the work of breathing. Also, a debilitating, acute disease makes a patient more susceptible to secondary infections, which may also affect the lungs. Even a mild illness can predispose the patient to respiratory complications.

Many patients are diagnosed with severe acute and chronic respiratory problems. To help your patients, you need sharp clinical skills and the newest insights into causes and pathophysiology of respiratory disorders.

Anatomy and physiology review

The respiratory system consists of the upper and lower airways, the lungs, and the thoracic cage. (See *Structures of the lower respiratory system*, page 126.)

The upper airways (nose, mouth, nasopharynx, oropharynx, laryngopharynx, and larynx) warm and humidify inspired air and handle taste, smell, and mastication. They protect the respiratory system from infection and foreign body inhalation by involuntary defense mechanisms: sneezing, coughing, gagging, and spasm.

The lower airways (trachea, bronchi, and lungs) also use coughing and spasm as defense mechanisms. Beginning at the bottom of the trachea, the bronchi split into right and left branches. Growing progressively smaller, the right and left mainstem bronchi

further divide into secondary and tertiary bronchi, then into bronchioles, and finally into alveoli.

The lungs hang suspended in the right and left pleural cavities at the hilum, a pleural cavity depression where the bronchi, blood vessels, nerves, and lymphatics enter the lungs. Formed by the pleural membrane, the pleural cavities are lined with thin tissue—the parietal pleural membrane. This membrane doubles back onto itself to form the outer covering of the lungs, called the visceral pleural membrane. A lubricant coats both membranes to reduce irritation from lung expansion and contraction. The membranes are separated by a minute, pleural space that holds a slight negative pressure to help lung expansion and contraction.

The mainstem bronchi enter the pleural cavities at the hilum. The right mainstem bronchus, which is shorter, wider, and more vertical than the left mainstem bronchus, supplies air to the right lung, and the left mainstem bronchus supplies air to the left lung. The right lung is larger, has three lobes and handles 55% of the gas exchange. The smaller left lung, with two lobes, extends slightly lower in the thorax; it's crowded by the heart.

At the hilum, the mainstem bronchi divide into five secondary (lobar) bronchi. The right bronchus divides to supply the upper, middle, and lower lobes of the right lung, and the left bronchus divides to supply the upper and lower lobes of the left lung. The lobar bronchi further divide into tertiary (segmental) bronchi, which carry air to smaller bronchopleural segments. Within these segments, the bronchi continue to branch into progressively smaller bronchi and bronchioles. The larger bronchi consist of cartilage, smooth muscle, and epithelium; however, as the bronchi become smaller, they lose first the cartilage and then the smooth muscle until, finally, the smallest (respiratory) bronchioles consist of only a single

Structures of the lower respiratory system

The upper and lower airways and the thoracic cage work together to exchange carbon dioxide and oxygen in the lungs. Shown below are the main structures of the lower respiratory tract.

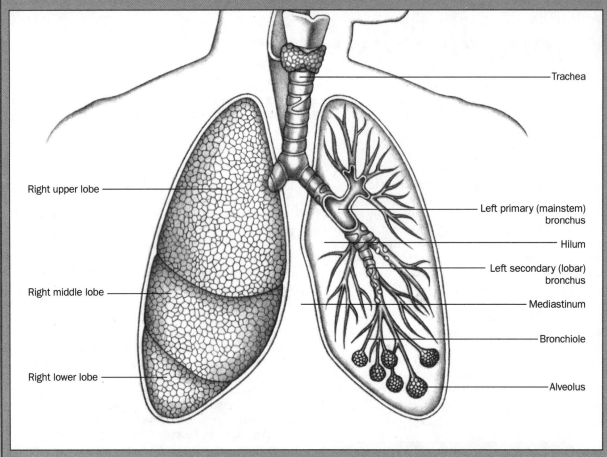

Trachea

Left primary (mainstem) bronchus

Hilum

Left secondary (lobar) bronchus

Mediastinum

Bronchiole

Alveolus

Right upper lobe

Right middle lobe

Right lower lobe

layer of epithelial cells. These bronchioles lead to the alveolar ducts and alveoli. Gas exchange occurs in the respiratory bronchioles, alveolar ducts, and alveoli.

THORACIC CAGE

Composed of bone and cartilage, the thoracic cage supports and protects the lungs. The vertebral column and 12 pairs of ribs form the posterior portion of the cage and permit the lungs to expand and contract. Posteriorly, certain landmarks help identify specific vertebrae. In 90% of the population, the most prominent vertebra on a flexed neck is the seventh cervical vertebra (C7); for the remaining 10%, it's the first thoracic vertebra (T1). You can locate a specific vertebra

by counting down along the vertebrae from T1. The ribs, which form the major portion of the thoracic cage, extend from the thoracic vertebrae toward the anterior thorax. They're numbered from top to bottom, like the vertebrae.

The anterior thoracic cage—the manubrium, sternum, xiphoid process, and ribs—also protects the mediastinal organs (heart, aorta, and great vessels) that lie between the right and left pleural cavities. Ribs 1 through 7 attach directly to the sternum; ribs 8 through 10 attach to the cartilage of the preceding rib. The other two pairs of ribs are free-floating. Rib 11 ends anterolaterally, and rib 12 ends laterally. The lower parts of the rib cage (the costal margins) near the xiphoid process form the borders of the costal angle—an angle of about 90 degrees in a normal person.

Above the anterior thorax is a depression called the suprasternal notch. Because this notch isn't covered by the rib cage like the rest of the thorax, it allows you to palpate the trachea.

INSPIRATION AND EXPIRATION
Breathing involves inspiration, an active process, and expiration, normally a passive one. Inspiration relies on respiratory muscle function; expiration on the effects of pressure differences in the lungs.

PULMONARY CIRCULATION
Oxygen-depleted blood is ejected from the right ventricle into the pulmonary artery, flows into the left and right pulmonary arteries, then into the arterioles. Subsequently it flows through progressively smaller vessels until it reaches the single-celled endothelial capillaries serving the alveoli. Here, oxygen and carbon dioxide diffusion takes place. After passing through the pulmonary capillaries, blood flows through progressively larger vessels, enters the main pulmonary veins, and flows into the left atrium.

EXTERNAL AND INTERNAL RESPIRATION
Effective respiration requires gas exchange in the lungs (external respiration) and in the tissues (internal respiration).

External respiration occurs through ventilation (gas distribution into and out of the pulmonary airways), pulmonary perfusion (blood flow from the right side of the heart, through the pulmonary circulation, and into the left side of the heart), and diffusion (gas movement from an area of greater to lesser concentration through a semipermeable membrane). Internal respiration occurs only through diffusion. These processes are vital to maintain adequate oxygenation and acid-base balance.

VENTILATION
Adequate ventilation depends upon the nervous, musculoskeletal, and pulmonary systems for the requisite lung pressure changes. Any dysfunction in these systems increases breathing effort and diminishes breathing effectiveness.

Nervous system effects. Although ventilation is largely involuntary, a patient can control its rate and depth, such as by performing breathing exercises to reduce stress. Involuntary breathing results from neurogenic stimulation of the respiratory center in the medulla and the pons. The medulla controls the rate and depth of respiration; the pons moderates the

rhythm of the switch from inhale to exhale. Specialized neurovascular tissue alters these phases of the breathing process automatically and instantaneously.

When carbon dioxide in the blood diffuses into the cerebrospinal fluid, specialized tissue in the respiratory center of the brain stem responds. At the same time, peripheral chemoreceptors in the aortic arch and the bifurcation of the carotid arteries respond to reduced oxygen levels in the blood. When the carbon dioxide level rises or the oxygen level falls noticeably, the respiratory center of the medulla responds by initiating respiration.

Musculoskeletal effects. The medulla stimulates contraction of the diaphragm and the external intercostals, the major muscles of breathing. The diaphragm descends to expand the length of the chest cavity while the external intercostals contract to expand the anteroposterior diameter. These actions produce the changes in intrapulmonary pressure that cause inspiration.

Pulmonary effects. During inspiration, air flows through the right and left mainstem bronchi into increasingly smaller bronchi, then into bronchioles, alveolar ducts, alveolar sacs, and alveoli. This normal airflow distribution can be altered by many factors, including the airflow pattern, the volume and location of the functional residual capacity (air retained in the alveoli that prevents their collapse during respiration), the amount of intrapulmonary resistance, and the presence of lung disease. If disrupted, the airflow distribution follows the path of least resistance. For example, an intrapulmonary obstruction or forced inspiration would cause the air to distribute unevenly.

Other musculoskeletal and intrapulmonary factors can affect airflow. Normal breathing requires active inspiration and passive expiration; forced breathing, as in emphysema, demands both active inspiration and expiration and activates accessory muscles of respiration. The muscles require additional oxygen to work, combining less efficient ventilation with an increased workload.

Other alterations in airflow that increase oxygen and energy demand and cause respiratory muscle fatigue include changes in compliance (distensibility of the lungs and thorax) and resistance (interference with airflow in the tracheobronchial tree).

PULMONARY PERFUSION
Perfusion aids external respiration. Optimal pulmonary blood flow allows alveolar gas exchange, but many factors may interfere with gas transport to the alveoli. For example, a cardiac output of less than the average of 5 L/minute reduces blood flow, cutting gas

exchange. Also, elevated pulmonary and systemic resistance reduces blood flow, and abnormal or insufficient hemoglobin picks up less oxygen for exchange. Gravity can affect oxygen and carbon dioxide transport by influencing pulmonary circulation. Gravity pulls more unoxygenated blood to the lower and middle lung lobes relative to the upper lobes, where most of the tidal volume also flows. As a result, neither ventilation nor perfusion is uniform throughout the lung. Areas of the lung where perfusion and ventilation are similar have good ventilation-perfusion matching and the most efficient gas exchange.

DIFFUSION

In diffusion, molecules of oxygen and carbon dioxide move between the alveoli and the capillaries. Partial pressure exerted by one gas in a mixture of gases dictates the direction of movement, which is always from an area of greater to lesser concentration.

Successful diffusion requires an intact alveolocapillary membrane. Both the alveolar epithelium and the capillary endothelium are composed of a single layer of cells. Between these layers are minute interstitial spaces filled with elastin and collagen. Normally, oxygen and carbon dioxide move easily through all of these layers. Oxygen moves from the alveoli into the bloodstream, where it's taken up by hemoglobin in the red blood cells (RBCs). Once there, it displaces carbon dioxide (the by-product of metabolism), which diffuses from the RBCs into the blood and then to the alveoli. Most transported oxygen binds with hemoglobin to form oxyhemoglobin, while a small portion dissolves in the plasma (measurable as the partial pressure of artieral oxygen[PaO_2]).

OXYGEN DELIVERY TO TISSUES

After oxygen binds to hemoglobin, the RBCs travel to the tissues. At this point, the blood cells contain more oxygen and the tissue cells contain more carbon dioxide. Internal respiration occurs when, through cellular diffusion, the RBCs release oxygen and absorb carbon dioxide. The RBCs then transport the carbon dioxide back to the lungs for expiration.

Oxygen delivery to the tissues depends on the lungs to put oxygen in the blood (arterial oxygen saturation and PaO_2), hemoglobin to carry the oxygen (hemoglobin level), and a pump to move the blood to the tissues (cardiac output).

ACID-BASE BALANCE

Because carbon dioxide is more soluble than oxygen, it dissolves in the blood. There, most of it forms bicarbonate (base) and smaller amounts form carbonic acid (acid). In the lungs, bicarbonate is converted to carbon dioxide and water for expiration.

In response to signals from the medulla, the lungs can change the rate and depth of ventilation. This change allows for adjustment of the amount of carbon dioxide lost to help maintain acid-base balance. For example, in metabolic alkalosis (resulting from excess bicarbonate retention or metabolic acid loss), the rate and depth of ventilation decrease so that carbon dioxide can be retained, increasing carbonic acid levels. In metabolic acidosis (resulting from excess acid retention or excess bicarbonate loss), the lungs increase the rate and depth of ventilation to exhale excess carbon dioxide, reducing carbonic acid levels.

When the lungs function inadequately, they can actually produce an acid-base imbalance. For example, they can cause respiratory acidosis through hypoventilation, which causes carbon dioxide retention. The lungs can also cause respiratory alkalosis through hyperventilation, which causes exhalation of increased amounts of carbon dioxide.

Assessment

By performing a thorough respiratory assessment, you can evaluate both obvious and subtle respiratory changes. This section reviews the techniques for obtaining an accurate health history and performing a complete physical examination.

HISTORY

Build your nursing history by asking the patient open-ended questions as systematically as possible to avoid overlooking important information. You may have to conduct the interview in several short sessions, depending on the severity of your patient's condition, his expectations, and time constraints.

Begin to establish a rapport with the patient by explaining who you are and what you'll do. Try to gain his trust by being sensitive to his concerns and feelings. Be alert to nonverbal responses that support or contradict his verbal responses. He may, for example, deny chest pain verbally but reveal it through his facial expression. If the patient's verbal and nonverbal responses contradict each other, explore this with him to clarify your assessment.

CHIEF COMPLAINT

Ask your patient to tell you about his chief complaint. Use such questions as "When did you first notice that you didn't feel well?" "What's happened since then that brings you here today?" Because many respiratory disorders are chronic, be sure to ask him how the latest episode compared with previous episodes and what relief measures were helpful or unhelpful.

Record the patient's age, sex, marital status, occupation, education, religion, and ethnic background. These factors provide clues to potential risks and to the patient's interpretation of his respiratory condition. Advanced age, for example, suggests physiologic changes such as decreased vital capacity. Or the patient's occupation may alert you to problems related to hazardous materials. Also, don't forget to ask him for the name, address, and phone number of a relative who can be contacted in an emergency.

Once you've obtained demographic data, ask the patient to describe his symptoms chronologically. Concentrate on:

■ onset. When did the symptom first occur? Did it appear suddenly or gradually?

■ incidence. How often does the symptom occur?

■ duration. How long does the symptom last?

■ manner. How does the symptom change over time? For example, is the pain described as constant, intermittent, steadily worsening, or crescendo-decrescendo?

Use precise terms to describe the patient's answers, such as "30 minutes after meals," "twice a day," or "for 3 hours."

Next, ask the patient to characterize his symptoms. Have him describe:

■ aggravating factors. What increases the symptom's intensity? For example, if he has dyspnea, how many blocks can he walk before he feels short of breath?

■ alleviating factors. What relieves the symptom? Has he tried any home remedies, such as an over-the-counter medication or a change in sleeping position?

■ associated factors. Do other symptoms occur at the same time as the primary symptom?

■ location. Where does he experience the symptom? Can he pinpoint it? Does it radiate to other areas?

■ quality. What feeling accompanies the symptom? Has he felt anything similar before? Ask him to characterize the symptom in his own words. Document his description, including the words he chooses to describe pain—for example, sharp, stabbing, or throbbing.

■ duration. How long did the symptom last?

■ setting. Where was he when the symptom occurred? What was he doing? Who was with him? Be sure to document your findings.

MEDICAL HISTORY

The information you gain from the patient's medical history helps you understand his present symptoms. It also helps to identify patients at risk for developing respiratory difficulty.

Focus first on identifying previous respiratory problems, such as asthma or emphysema. Such a history provides instant clues to the patient's current condition. Then, ask about childhood illnesses. Infan-

tile eczema, atopic dermatitis, or allergic rhinitis, for example, may precipitate current respiratory problems such as asthma. Obtain an immunization history (especially of influenza and pneumococcal vaccination), which may provide clues about the potential for respiratory disease.

Next, ask what problems caused the patient to see a doctor or required hospitalization in the past. Again, pay particular attention to respiratory problems. For example, chronic sinus infection or postnasal discharge may lead to recurrent bronchitis. And, repeated episodes of pneumonia involving the same lung lobe may accompany bronchogenic carcinoma.

Ask the patient to describe the prescribed treatment, whether he followed the treatment plan, and whether the treatment helped. Determine if he's suffered any traumatic injuries. If he has, note when they occurred and how they were treated.

The history should also include brief personal details. Ask the patient if he smokes; if he does, ask when he started and how many cigarettes he smokes per day. By calculating his smoking in pack-years, you can assess his risk for respiratory disease. To estimate pack-years, use this simple formula: number of packs smoked per day multiplied by the number of years the patient has smoked. For example, a patient who's smoked 2 packs of cigarettes a day for 42 years has accumulated 84 pack-years.

Also ask about his alcohol use and his diet because nutritional status may influence his risk of respiratory infection.

FAMILY HISTORY

Through a family history, you can determine whether your patient is at risk for hereditary or infectious respiratory diseases. First, ask if any of his immediate blood relatives (parents, siblings, or children) have had cancer, sickle cell anemia, heart disease, or a chronic illness, such as asthma or emphysema. Remember that diabetes can lead to cardiac and, possibly, respiratory problems. If an immediate relative has one or more of these disorders, ask for more information about the patient's maternal and paternal grandparents, aunts, and uncles.

Then ask him if he lives with anyone who has an infectious disease, such as influenza or tuberculosis.

SOCIAL HISTORY

Assess your patient's psychosocial history for lifestyle (including sex habits or drug use that may be connected to pulmonary disorders related to acquired immunodeficiency syndrome) as well as home, community, and other environmental factors that may influence how he deals with his respiratory problems. These include interpersonal relationships, occupation, mental status, stress management, and coping style.

EMERGENCY ASSESSMENT

Typically, you'll proceed with the physical examination after taking the patient's history. At times, though, you won't take much of a history because the patient reports or develops an ominous sign or experiences acute respiratory distress.

If the patient develops acute respiratory distress, immediately assess his airway, breathing, and circulation (ABCs). If these are absent, call for help and start cardiopulmonary resuscitation.

If the patient has a patent airway, is breathing, and has a pulse, quickly check for these signs of impending crisis:

- Is the patient having trouble breathing (dyspnea)?
- Is he using accessory muscles to breathe? If chest excursion measures less than the normal 1¹/₄″ to 2¹/₄″ (3 to 6 cm), he'll use accessory muscles when he breathes. Look for shoulder elevation, intercostal muscle retraction, and use of scalene and sternocleidomastoid muscles.
- Has his level of consciousness diminished?
- Is he confused, anxious, or agitated?
- Does he change his body position to ease breathing?
- Does his skin look pale, diaphoretic, or cyanotic?

SETTING PRIORITIES

If your patient is in respiratory distress, establish priorities for your nursing assessment. Don't assume the obvious. Note both positive and negative factors, starting with the most critical (the ABCs) and progressing to less critical factors.

Although you won't have time to go through each step of the nursing process, make sure you gather enough data to clarify the problem. Remember, a single sign or symptom has many possible meanings. Rely on a group of findings for problem solving and appropriate intervention.

Adapt your assessment to the patient's condition, the resources available, and your own knowledge and skill. In an emergency, increase efficiency with close teamwork. For example, you could take a quick history while a second nurse begins appropriate interventions.

EXPLORING SIGNS AND SYMPTOMS

Examine your patient for the following respiratory indicators.

Dyspnea. This symptom occurs when breathing is inappropriately difficult for the activity being performed. It usually occurs with strenuous exertion; if it occurs at rest or during a mild activity, such as dressing or walking, suspect a respiratory problem.

Document the onset and severity of dyspnea carefully, including when the patient first noticed being short of breath. A sudden onset may indicate such disorders as pneumothorax or pulmonary embolus, whereas a gradual onset suggests a slowly progressive disorder such as emphysema.

Evaluate the type and degree of dyspnea. Qualitative and quantitative descriptions of dyspnea vary among patients.

Pay particular attention to orthopnea (increased dyspnea when supine), which may indicate pulmonary or cardiac disorders, such as pulmonary hypertension or left-sided heart failure. Extreme obesity, diaphragmatic paralysis, asthma, or chronic obstructive pulmonary disease (COPD) may also cause orthopnea.

Chest pain. If your patient reports chest pain, ask him to describe its precise location and type. Also, find out if the pain radiates to other parts of the body. Crushing pain that radiates to the arm may indicate myocardial infarction. Substernal pain, a sharp, stabbing pain in the middle of the chest, may indicate spontaneous pneumothorax. Tracheal pain, a burning sensation that intensifies with deep breathing or coughing, suggests oxygen toxicity or aspiration. Esophageal pain, a burning sensation that intensifies with swallowing, may indicate local inflammation.

If your patient complains of a stabbing, knifelike pain that increases with deep breathing or coughing, he may be experiencing pleural pain associated with pulmonary infarction, pneumothorax, or pleurisy. If he describes chest wall pain (localized chest pain and tenderness), he may be suffering from infection or inflammation of the chest wall, intercostal nerves, or intercostal muscles. Another possible cause: blunt chest trauma.

No matter what type of pain he describes, remember to assess associated factors, such as breathing, body position, and ease or difficulty of moving.

Hemoptysis. This sign, coughing up blood, may result from violent coughing or from a serious disorder, such as pneumonia, lung cancer, lung abscess, tuberculosis, pulmonary embolism, bronchiectasis, or left-sided (systolic) heart failure. If hemoptysis is mild (sputum streaked with blood), reassure the patient and report this finding to the doctor. Ask the patient when he first noticed it and how often it occurs. If hemoptysis is severe (frank bleeding), place the patient in a semi-recumbent position, call the doctor immediately, and note the patient's pulse rate, blood pressure, and general condition. When his condition stabilizes, ask if he's ever experienced similar bleeding.

PHYSICAL EXAMINATION

Before assessing your patient's respiratory system, inspect his skin. This will give you an overview of the patient's clinical status as well as an assessment of the degree of peripheral oxygenation. A dusky or bluish skin tint (cyanosis) may indicate decreased oxygen content in the arterial blood.

Distinguishing central from peripheral cyanosis is important. Central cyanosis results from hypoxemia and affects all body organs. It may appear in patients with right-to-left cardiac shunting or a pulmonary disease that causes hypoxemia such as chronic bronchitis. The cyanosis appears on the skin; on the mucous membranes of the mouth, lips, and conjunctivae; or in other highly vascular areas, such as the earlobes, tip of the nose, or nail beds. Dark-skinned patients may be more difficult to assess for central cyanosis. In these patients, inspect the oral mucous membranes and lips. If a dark-skinned patient has central cyanosis, these areas will appear ashen gray rather than bluish. Facial skin may appear pale gray or ashen in a cyanotic black-skinned patient and yellowish brown in a cyanotic brown-skinned patient.

In contrast, peripheral cyanosis results from vasoconstriction, vascular occlusion, or reduced cardiac output. Commonly seen in patients exposed to cold, peripheral cyanosis appears in the nail beds, nose, ears, and fingers. Peripheral cyanosis doesn't affect the mucous membranes.

Next, assess the patient's nail beds and toes for abnormal enlargement. This condition, called clubbing, results from chronic tissue hypoxia. Nail thinning accompanied by an abnormal alteration of the angle of the finger and toe bases distinguishes clubbing.

PREPARING FOR RESPIRATORY ASSESSMENT
After obtaining a general picture of the patient's oxygenation, assess his respiratory system. You'll need a quiet, well-lit environment and specific equipment, such as a stethoscope with a diaphragm (a pediatric-size diaphragm for a child), a felt-tip pen, a ruler, and a tape measure.

To assess the chest and lungs, use inspection, palpation, percussion, and auscultation. Be familiar with all of the equipment and techniques before using them on a patient.

To begin, have the patient sit in a position that allows access to the anterior and posterior thorax. Provide a gown that offers easy access to the chest and back without requiring unnecessary exposure. Make sure the patient isn't cold because shivering may alter breathing patterns.

If the patient can't sit up, use the supine semi-Fowler's position to assess the anterior chest wall and the side-lying position to assess the posterior thorax. Keep in mind that these positions may cause some distortion of findings. If the patient is an infant or a small child, seat the child on the parent's lap.

You may find it easier to inspect, palpate, percuss, and auscultate the patient's anterior chest before the posterior. However, this section covers inspection of the whole chest, then palpation, percussion, and auscultation of the whole chest.

INSPECTION
Basic assessment of respiratory function requires determination of the rate, rhythm, and quality of the patient's respirations as well as inspection of chest configuration, chest symmetry, skin condition, and accessory muscle use. It should also include assessment for nasal flaring. Accomplish these steps by inspecting the patient's breathing and the anterior and posterior thorax, and noting any abnormal findings.

Respiration. Because respiratory rates vary with age, be aware of the normal rate range for your patient. If he's eupneic, the respiratory rate is within the normal range for the patient's age-group.

When assessing respiratory rate, count the number of respirations, each composed of an inspiration and an expiration, for 1 full minute. For an infant or a patient with periodic or irregular breathing, monitor the respirations for more than 1 minute to determine the rate accurately. Assess the duration of any periods lacking spontaneous respiration (apnea), and alert the doctor to any alteration in the breathing pattern. Also note any abnormal respiratory patterns, such as tachypnea (persistent, rapid, shallow breathing) and bradypnea (abnormally decreased respiratory rate).

Assess the quality of respiration by observing the type and depth of breathing. Also assess the method of ventilation by having the patient lie supine to expose the chest and abdominal walls. Adult female patients commonly exhibit thoracic breathing when sitting, which involves an upward and outward motion of the chest; infants, males, and supine females usually exhibit abdominal breathing, which uses the abdominal muscles. Patients with COPD may exhibit pursed-lip breathing, which prevents small airway collapse during exhalation. Forced inspiration or expiration may alter assessment findings; therefore, ask the patient to breathe normally.

Note the depth of breathing, assessing for shallow chest wall expansion (hypopnea) or unusually deep chest wall expansion (hyperpnea). Use your judgment to assess the depth of breathing, but be sure to use the terms hypopnea or hyperpnea, not hypoventilation or hyperventilation. Detecting hypoventilation or hyperventilation requires a measurement of partial pressure of carbon dioxide in arterial blood.

Anterior thorax. After assessing respiration, inspect the thorax for structural deformities, such as a concave or convex curvature of the anterior chest wall over the sternum. Inspect between and around the ribs for visible sinking of soft tissues (retractions). Assess the patient's respiratory pattern for symmetry. Look for any abnormalities in skin color or alterations in muscle tone. For future documentation, note the location of any abnormalities according to regions delineated by imaginary lines on the thorax.

Initially inspect the chest wall to identify the shape of the thoracic cage. In an adult, the thorax should have a greater diameter laterally (side to side) than anteroposteriorly (front to back).

Note the angle between the ribs and the sternum at the point immediately above the xiphoid process. This angle, called the costal angle, should be less than 90 degrees in an adult; it widens if the chest wall is chronically expanded, as in barrel chest.

To inspect the anterior chest for symmetry of movement, have the patient lie supine. Stand at his feet and carefully observe his resting and deep breathing for equal expansion of the chest wall. At the same time, watch for the abnormal collapse of part of the chest wall during inspiration along with an abnormal expansion of the same area during expiration (paradoxical movement); this indicates a loss of normal chest wall function.

Next, check for use of the accessory muscles of respiration by observing the sternocleidomastoid, scalene, and trapezius muscles in the shoulders and neck. During normal inspiration and expiration, the diaphragm and external intercostal muscles alone should easily maintain the breathing process. Hypertrophy of any of the accessory muscles may indicate frequent use, especially if found in an older adult patient, but may be normal in a well-conditioned athlete. Also observe the position the patient assumes to breathe when sitting. A patient who depends on accessory muscles may assume a "tripod position," which involves resting the arms on the knees or on the sides of a chair.

Observe the patient's skin on the anterior chest for any unusual color, lumps, or lesions, and note the location. Unless the patient has been exposed to significant sun or heat, the skin color of his chest should match the rest of his complexion. Further inspect the chest for the location of the underlying ribs and other bones, cartilage, and lung lobes. An abnormality noted on the skin may reflect a problem in the underlying structure. Also check for any chest wall scars from surgery. If the patient hasn't mentioned surgery, ask about it now.

Posterior thorax. To inspect the posterior chest, observe the patient's breathing again and assess for the same characteristics as in the anterior chest wall. If he can't sit in a backless chair or lean forward against a supporting structure, have him lie in a lateral posi-

tion. However, this may distort findings in some situations. For example, if he's obese, he may not be able to expand the lower lung fully from the lateral position, so breath sounds on that side would be diminished.

Abnormal findings. During inspection, note all abnormal findings. For example, a unilateral absence of chest movement may indicate previous surgical removal of that lung, a bronchial obstruction, or a collapsed lung caused by air or fluid in the pleural space. Delayed chest movement may indicate congestion or consolidation of the underlying lung. However, paradoxical movement commonly occurs after trauma or in flail chest (fractures of two or more ribs in two or more places).

Inspection also may reveal structural deformities of the chest wall resulting from defects of the sternum, rib cage, or vertebral column. These deformities have many variations and may be congenital, acute, or progressive. A concave sternal depression, called funnel chest (pectus excavatum), and a convex deformity, called pigeon chest (pectus carinatum), are two thoracic defects that can hinder breathing by preventing full chest expansion. Also, COPD may cause a rounded chest wall (barrel chest).

Other structural deformities of the posterior thorax that may alter ventilation include an anteroposterior curvature of the spine (kyphosis) and a lateral and anteroposterior curvature of the spine (kyphoscoliosis). These deformities can compress one lung while allowing an overexpansion of the opposite lung, eventually leading to respiratory dysfunction. Acute changes in the thoracic wall from trauma, such as fractured ribs or a flail chest, also alter the ventilatory process by allowing uneven chest expansion. These deformities also cause pain, which leads to shallow breathing, worsening respiratory distress.

Nonstructural abnormalities found on inspection include visible vein paths (superficial venous patterns), which could indicate underlying vascular or heart disease. Rib prominence suggests malnutrition, and a layer of fat over the ribs indicates obesity.

PALPATION

By carefully palpating the trachea and the anterior and posterior thorax, you'll be able to detect structural and skin abnormalities, areas of pain, and chest asymmetry. (See *Sequences for chest palpation.*)

Trachea and anterior thorax. First, palpate the trachea for position. Observe whether the patient uses accessory neck muscles to breathe.

Next, palpate the suprasternal notch. In most patients, the arch of the aorta lies close to the surface, just behind the suprasternal notch. Use your fingertips to gently evaluate the strength and regularity of the patient's aortic pulsations there. Then palpate the thorax to assess the skin and underlying structures. Gentle palpation shouldn't be painful, so assess any complaints of pain for localization, radiation, and severity. Be especially careful to palpate any areas that looked abnormal during inspection. If necessary, support the patient during the procedure with one hand while using your other hand to palpate one side at a time, continuing to compare sides. Note any unusual findings, such as masses, crepitus, skin irregularities, or painful areas.

If the patient complains of chest pain, attempt to determine the cause by palpating the anterior chest. Certain disorders—such as musculoskeletal pain, an irritation of the nerves covering the xiphoid process, or an inflammation of the cartilage connecting the bony ribs to the sternum (costochondritis)—cause increased pain during palpation. These disorders may also produce pain during inspiration, causing the patient to breathe shallowly. On the other hand, palpation does not worsen pain caused by cardiac or pulmonary disorders, such as angina or pleurisy.

Next, palpate the costal angle. The area around the xiphoid process contains many nerve endings, so be gentle to avoid causing pain. If a patient frequently uses the internal intercostal muscles to breathe, these muscles will eventually pull the chest cavity upward and outward. If this has occurred, the costal angle will be greater than the normal 90 degrees.

Posterior thorax. Palpate the patient's posterior thorax in a similar manner, using the palmar surface of the fingertips of one or both hands. During the process, identify bony structures, such as the vertebrae and the scapulae.

To determine the location of any abnormalities, identify the first thoracic vertebra (with the patient's head tipped forward) and count the number of spinous processes from this landmark to the abnormal finding. Use this reference point for documentation. Also identify the inferior scapular tips and medial borders of both bones to define the margins of the upper and lower lung lobes posteriorly. Locate and describe all abnormalities in relation to these landmarks. Remember to evaluate abnormalities, such as use of accessory muscles or complaints of pain.

Abnormal findings. Palpation may show that the trachea isn't midline. This could result from a collapse of lung tissue (atelectasis), thyroid enlargement, or fluid accumulation in the pleural space (pleural effusion). A tumor or collapsed lung (pneumothorax) may also displace the trachea to one side. In atelectasis, the trachea shifts to the affected side; in pneumothorax, to the unaffected side.

Sequences for chest palpation

Follow this guide to conduct a thorough chest palpation. The numerical sequence ensures that all areas are examined and that bilateral findings can be easily compared.

Posterior

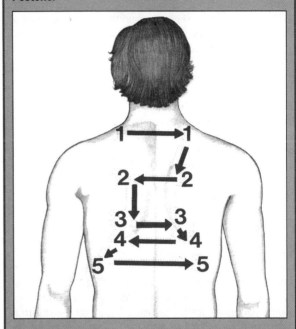

Anterior

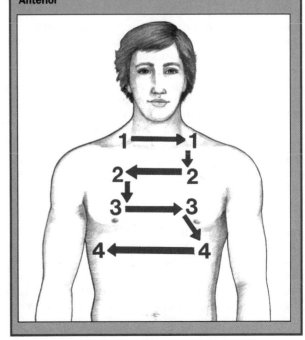

Tenderness on palpation of the anterior chest could indicate musculoskeletal inflammation, especially if the patient complains of chest pain of unknown origin.

Palpation producing a crackly sound similar to the noise of crumpling cellophane paper suggests subcutaneous emphysema. Report this to the doctor immediately because it indicates air leakage into the subcutaneous tissue from a breach somewhere in the respiratory system.

Absent or delayed chest movement during respiratory excursion may indicate previous surgical removal of the lung, complete or partial obstruction of the airway or underlying lung, or diaphragmatic dysfunction on the affected side.

Tactile fremitus. Because sound travels more easily through solid structures than through air, assessing for tactile fremitus (the palpation of vocalizations) helps you learn about the contents of the lungs.

The patient's vocalization should produce vibrations of equal intensity on both sides of the chest. Normally, vibrations should occur in the upper chest, close to the bronchi, and then decrease and finally disappear toward the periphery of the lungs.

Conditions that restrict air movement, such as pleural effusion or COPD with overinflated lungs, cause decreased tactile fremitus. Conditions that consolidate tissue or fluid in a portion of the pleural area, such as a lung tumor, pneumonia, or pulmonary fibrosis, increase tactile fremitus. A grating feeling may signify a pleural friction rub.

PERCUSSION

This assessment technique helps you determine the boundaries of the lungs and how much gas, liquid, or solid exists in them. Percussion can effectively assess structures as deep as 1¾″ to 3″ (4.5 to 7.5 cm). Accurate percussion of the thorax requires that you practice to master the technique as well as become familiar with the characteristic sounds.

The most commonly used technique is mediate percussion, or striking one finger with another. Immediate percussion—direct tapping on the chest to elicit sound—produces vibrations that are somewhat more difficult to identify.

To percuss correctly, follow these guidelines. Choose a quiet environment and proceed systematically, percussing the anterior, lateral, and posterior chest over the intercostal spaces. (See *Sequences for chest percussion and auscultation.*) Avoid percussing over bones because their density produces a dull sound that yields no useful information. Percussion over a healthy lung elicits a resonant sound hollow and loud, with a low pitch and long duration.

To percuss the anterior chest, have the patient sit facing forward, hands resting at the side of the body. Following the anterior percussion sequence (starting at the apices and working downward), percuss and compare sound variations from one side to the other. Anterior chest percussion should produce resonance from below the clavicle to the fifth intercostal space on the right (where dullness occurs close to the liver) and to the third intercostal space on the left (where dullness occurs near the heart).

Next, percuss the lateral chest to obtain information about the left upper and lower lobes and about the right upper, middle, and lower lobes. The patient's left arm should be positioned on his head. Repeat the sequence on the right side, with the patient's right arm on his head. Lateral chest percussion should produce resonance to the sixth or eighth intercostal space.

Finally, percuss the posterior thorax according to the percussion sequence. Posterior percussion should sound resonant to the level of T10.

Abnormal findings. Hyperresonance and dullness are the most common abnormal percussion findings. (See *Characterizing and interpreting percussion sounds,* page 136.) Hyperresonance may result from air in the pleural space, commonly caused by a pneumothorax or overinflation of the lung, as occurs in emphysema. Dullness may result from a consolidation of fluid or tissue, in many cases with pneumonia or atelectasis. Flatness over the lung bases with the patient sitting upright indicates pleural effusion, masses, or hemothorax.

AUSCULTATION

Auscultate the anterior, lateral, and posterior thorax to detect normal and abnormal breath sounds. Auscultate directly on the patient's skin because clothing or linen interferes with accuracy. Before placing the stethoscope's diaphragm on the patient's skin, warm it between your hands.

If the patient has significant hair growth over the areas to be auscultated, wet the hair to decrease sound blurring. Tell the patient to take deep breaths through the mouth (nose breathing may alter the findings), and caution him against breathing too deeply or too rapidly, to prevent light-headedness or dizziness.

During auscultation, first identify normal breath sounds and then assess and identify abnormal sounds. Practice auscultation on a normal chest to gain confidence. Specific breath sounds occur normally only in certain locations; therefore, the same sound heard anywhere else in the lung field constitutes an important abnormality requiring appropriate documentation.

Sequences for chest percussion and auscultation

To conduct a complete examination, percuss and auscultate along the points shown on the posterior shoulders. Then follow the sequence shown. Remember to compare findings from one side of the body with those from the other side.

Posterior   **Anterior**

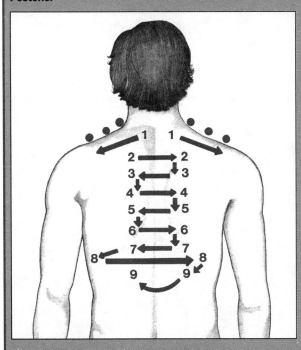

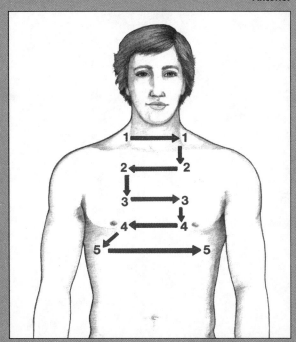

Left lateral   **Right lateral**

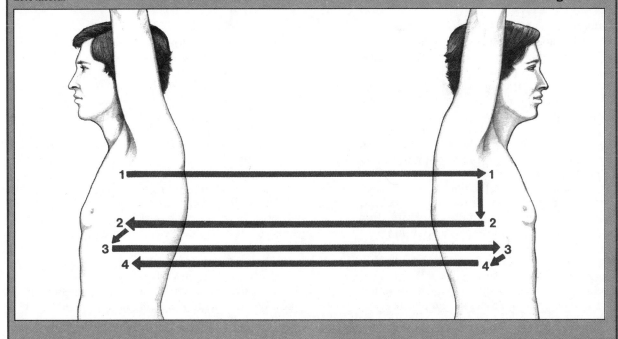

Characterizing and interpreting percussion sounds

Several kinds of sounds may emanate from percussion. Known as flat, dull, resonant, hyperresonant, or tympanic, these sounds determine the location and density of various structures.

During percussion, determining other tonal characteristics, such as pitch, intensity, and quality, will also help you identify respiratory structures. Use this chart as a guide.

CHARACTER				IMPLICATIONS
Sound	Pitch	Intensity	Quality	
FLATNESS	High	Soft	Extremely dull	These sounds are normal over the sternum. Over the lung, they may indicate atelectasis or pleural effusion.
DULLNESS	Medium	Medium	Thudlike	Normal over the liver, heart, and diaphragm, these sounds over the lung may point to pneumonia, tumor, atelectasis, or pleural effusion.
RESONANCE	Low	Moderate to loud	Hollow	Over the lung, these sounds are normal.
HYPERRESONANCE	Lower than resonance	Very loud	Booming	These sounds are normal over a child's lung. Over an adult's lung, they may indicate emphysema, chronic bronchitis, asthma, or pneumothorax.
TYMPANY	High	Loud	Musical, drumlike	Over the stomach, these sounds are normal; over the lung, they suggest tension pneumothorax.

Anterior and lateral thorax. Systematically auscultate the anterior and lateral thorax for normal as well as abnormal breath sounds, following the same sequence used for percussion. Begin at the upper lobes, and move from side to side and down, comparing side-to-side findings. Always assess one full breath (inspiration and expiration) at each point.

To assess the right middle lung lobe, auscultate breath sounds laterally at the level of the fourth to the sixth intercostal spaces, following the lateral auscultation sequence, which is the same as the lateral percussion sequence. Although difficult to assess, especially in a female patient with large breasts, the right middle lobe is a common site of aspiration pneumonia, so it requires special attention.

Normal breath sounds include tracheal, bronchial, bronchovesicular, and vesicular sounds. Tracheal sounds, which are harsh and discontinuous, occur over the trachea and are heard equally during inspiration and expiration. Bronchial sounds are coarse, loud, and high-pitched and occur over the manubrium. They have a prolonged expiratory phase and re-

sult from a high rate of turbulent air flow through the large bronchi. Bronchovesicular sounds are soft breezy sounds that are two notes lower in pitch than bronchial sounds. Anteriorly, they can be heard over the mainstem bronchi in the first and second intercostal areas. Posteriorly, they are heard between the scapulae. Inspiration and expiration rates are equal. Vesicular sounds, low-pitched and continuous, occur in the periphery of the lungs and are prolonged during inspiration.

Classify normal and abnormal breath sounds according to location, intensity (amplitude), characteristic sound, pitch (tone), and duration during the inspiratory and expiratory phases. When assessing duration, time the inspiratory and expiratory phases to determine the ratio. Also, when classifying sounds, keep in mind that higher-pitched breath sounds have a higher tone than lower-pitched ones and that louder breath sounds have more intensity than softer ones. When describing specific sounds, identify the quality using specific terms, such as high-pitched or harsh.

For the last step in auscultation, identify the inspiratory and expiratory phase of normal and abnormal breath sounds. Also determine whether the sound occurs during inspiration, expiration, or both. Do this by placing one hand on the patient's chest wall during auscultation: If the sound occurs as the thorax expands, it's part of inspiration; if the sound occurs as the thorax contracts, it's part of expiration.

Posterior thorax. Auscultate the posterior thorax in the same pattern as the percussion sequence. During auscultation, remain aware of the patient's breathing pattern. Breathing too rapidly or deeply causes an excessive loss of carbon dioxide, which may result in vertigo or syncope.

In a normal adult, adolescent, or older child, bronchovesicular breath sounds (air moving through the bronchial airways) should occur over the interscapular area; vesicular breath sounds (air moving through the alveoli) should occur in the suprascapular and infrascapular areas. Note any absent, decreased, or adventitious breath sounds. For example, bronchovesicular sounds auscultated in the periphery of the lungs are adventitious. Crackles and rhonchi (gurgles) are also adventitious; if you hear them, ask the patient to cough, and then listen again.

Diaphragmatic excursion. This technique allows you to evaluate your patient's diaphragm movement. Normal diaphragmatic excursion is 1¼" to 2¼" (3 to 6 cm). Failure of the diaphragm to contract downward may indicate paralysis or muscle flattening, a condition that results from COPD.

Voice resonance. To assess voice resonance, instruct the patient to say "ninety-nine." As he speaks, auscultate in the usual sequence. The voice normally sounds muffled and indistinct during auscultation. The sound appears loudest medially and softest in the lung periphery. However, conditions producing lung tissue consolidation cause bronchophony—the greater resonance that allows you to hear "ninety-nine" clearly during auscultation.

To test increased resonance further, ask the patient to repeat the letter "e," which should sound muffled and indistinct on auscultation. If the letter sounds like "a" and the voice sounds nasal or bleating, you've heard egophony, another sign of consolidation.

To perform another test for increased resonance, ask the patient to whisper the words "one, two, three." On auscultation, these words should be barely audible. If the words sound distinct and understandable, you have heard whispered pectoriloquy, which suggests lung tissue consolidation resulting from such conditions as a lung tumor, pneumonia, or pulmonary fibrosis.

These abnormal voice sounds occur because sound vibrations travel with greater intensity through a solid structure than through a normal, air-filled lung.

Abnormal findings. Document adventitious breath sounds by labeling the sound or describing its characteristics. Although either method is correct, most nurses use a description of the sound with or without a label. Adventitious breath sounds may indicate fluid within alveoli, opening of compressed alveoli, secretions in small or large airways, narrowed airways, or pleural membrane inflammation.

Certain adventitious breath sounds, including crackles, wheezes, rhonchi, subcutaneous emphysema, and pleural friction rubs, may appear in any lung lobe.

By the end of the assessment, a cluster of abnormal signs and symptoms may point to a particular disorder.

Adult respiratory distress syndrome

A severe form of hypoxemic respiratory failure, adult respiratory distress syndrome (ARDS) can occur in association with a variety of clinical situations that result in direct or indirect lung injury. Previously known as shock, stiff, white, wet, or Da Nang lung, ARDS is now referred to in more descriptive terms, such as noncardiogenic or exudative pulmonary edema and acute respiratory distress syndrome.

CAUSES
Although a variety of clinical situations can lead to ARDS, the most common causes are sepsis, aspiration, and multiple trauma. Regardless of the etiology, the prominent features are the same: damage to the alveolocapillary membrane, abnormal gas exchange with refractory hypoxemia, bilateral diffuse pulmonary infiltrates, and absence of hydrostatic or cardiogenic pulmonary edema.

Other common causes of ARDS include anaphylaxis, diffuse pneumonia (especially viral), drug overdose (for example, heroin, aspirin, or ethchlorvynol), idiosyncratic drug reaction (to ampicillin or hydrochlorothiazide), inhalation of noxious gases (such as nitrous oxide, ammonia, and chlorine), near-drowning, and oxygen toxicity.

Less common causes of ARDS include coronary artery bypass grafting, hemodialysis, leukemia, acute miliary tuberculosis, pancreatitis, thrombotic thrombocytopenic purpura, uremia, and venous air embolism.

In ARDS, damage to the alveolocapillary membrane leads to increased permeability and allows fluid to accumulate in the lung interstitium, alveolar spaces, and small airways, causing the lung to stiffen. This impairs gas exchange, reducing oxygenation of pulmonary capillary blood. Difficult to recognize, the disorder can prove fatal within 48 hours of onset.

Although this four-stage syndrome can progress to intractable and fatal hypoxemia, patients who recover may have little or no permanent lung damage.

In some patients, this syndrome may coexist with disseminated intravascular coagulation (DIC). Whether ARDS stems from DIC or develops independently remains unclear.

DIAGNOSIS AND TREATMENT
Arterial blood gas (ABG) analysis is the primary diagnostic test. (Hypoxemia, despite increased supplemental oxygen, is the hallmark of ARDS.) The initial blood pH usually reflects respiratory alkalosis. As ARDS worsens, ABG values show respiratory acidosis and metabolic acidosis despite oxygen therapy.

Pulmonary artery catheterization helps identify the cause of pulmonary edema by measuring pulmonary artery wedge pressure (PAWP).

Pulmonary artery and mixed venous blood sampling shows decreased oxygen saturation, reflecting tissue hypoxia.

Serial chest X-rays in early stages show bilateral infiltrates. In later stages, findings demonstrate lung fields with a ground-glass appearance and, eventually (with irreversible hypoxemia), "whiteouts" of both lung fields.

Therapy focuses on correcting the cause of the syndrome, preventing progression of life-threatening hypoxemia and respiratory acidosis, and preventing complications of therapy. Supportive care consists of administering humidified oxygen by a tight-fitting mask, which facilitates the use of continuous positive airway pressure (CPAP). However, this therapy alone seldom fulfills the ARDS patient's ventilatory requirements. If the patient's hypoxemia does not subside with this treatment, he may require intubation, mechanical ventilation, and positive end-expiratory pressure (PEEP). Other supportive measures include fluid restriction, diuretic therapy, and correction of electrolyte and acid-base imbalances.

When a patient with ARDS needs mechanical ventilation, sedatives, narcotics, or neuromuscular blocking agents (such as vecuronium) may be prescribed to minimize restlessness (and thereby reduce oxygen consumption and carbon dioxide production) and to facilitate ventilation.

When ARDS results from fatty emboli or a chemical injury, a short course of high-dose corticosteroids may help, if given early. Treatment with sodium bicarbonate may be necessary to reverse severe metabolic acidosis. Fluids and vasopressors may be needed to maintain blood pressure. Nonviral infections require treatment with antimicrobial drugs.

COLLABORATIVE MANAGEMENT
Care of the patient with ARDS focuses on maintaining adequate gas exchange, preventing further lung injury, and preventing failure of nonpulmonary organs.

ASSESSMENT
Be alert for rapid, shallow breathing; dyspnea; tachycardia; hypoxemia; intercostal and suprasternal retractions; crackles and rhonchi; restlessness; apprehension; mental sluggishness; and motor dysfunction. ARDS is staged from I to IV, and each stage has typical signs. (See *Recognizing stages of ARDS*.)

NURSING DIAGNOSES AND COLLABORATIVE PROBLEMS
Based on the following nursing diagnoses, you'll establish patient outcomes.

Anxiety related to potential for ARDS to develop into acute respiratory failure and possible death. The patient will:
- state or write down feelings of anxiety about his condition and possible death
- use support systems to assist with coping
- demonstrate diminished physical symptoms of anxiety.

Impaired gas exchange related to direct or indirect lung injury. The patient will:
- demonstrate adequate gas exchange with therapy, evidenced by ABG values that return to normal and restoration of normal respiratory function
- recover from ARDS with no residual lung damage.

Inability to sustain spontaneous ventilation related to pulmonary edema and fibrosis. The patient will:
- recover from lung tissue damage
- resume spontaneous ventilation with treatment
- regain and maintain normal ABG values

Risk for complications related to invasive procedures, treatments, and severity of disease. The patient will:
- remain free from any complications
- demonstrate hemodynamic and respiratory values within acceptable parameters

PLANNING AND IMPLEMENTATION
These measures help the patient with ARDS:
- Frequently assess the patient's respiratory status. Be alert for inspiratory retractions. Note respiratory rate, rhythm, and depth. Watch for dyspnea and accessory muscle use. Listen for adventitious or diminished breath sounds. Check for clear, frothy sputum, indicating pulmonary edema.

Recognizing stages of ARDS

The following signs and symptoms characterize stage I through IV of adult respiratory distress syndrome (ARDS).

Stage I
The patient may complain of dyspnea, especially on exertion. Respiratory and pulse rates are normal to high. Auscultation may reveal clear but diminished breath sounds.

Stage II
Respiratory distress becomes more apparent. The patient may use accessory muscles to breathe and may appear pallid, anxious, and restless. He may have a dry cough with thick, frothy sputum and bloody, sticky secretions. Palpation may disclose cool, clammy skin. Tachycardia and tachypnea may accompany elevated blood pressure. Auscultation may detect basilar crackles. (Stage II signs and symptoms may be incorrectly attributed to other causes such as multiple trauma.)

Stage III
The patient may struggle to breathe. A check of vital signs reveals tachypnea (more than 30 breaths/minute), tachycardia with arrhythmias (usually premature ventricular contractions), and a labile blood pressure. The patient may have a productive cough and pale, cyanotic skin. Auscultation may disclose crackles and rhonchi. The patient will need intubation and ventilation.

Stage IV
At this late stage, the patient has acute respiratory failure with severe hypoxia. His mental status is deteriorating, and he may become comatose. His skin appears pale and cyanotic. Spontaneous respirations are not evident. Bradycardia with arrhythmias accompanies hypotension. Metabolic and respiratory acidosis develop. When ARDS reaches this stage, the patient is at high risk for fibrosis. Pulmonary damage becomes life-threatening.

■ Maintain a patent airway by suctioning. Use sterile, nontraumatic technique. Ensure adequate humidification to help liquefy tenacious secretions.

■ If the patient is on mechanical ventilation, drain any condensate from the tubing promptly to ensure maximum oxygen delivery.

■ Be prepared to administer CPAP to the patient with severe hypoxemia.

■ To maintain PEEP, suction only as needed. High-frequency jet ventilation may also be required.

■ With pulmonary artery catheterization, know the desired PAWP level; check readings as indicated, and watch for decreasing mixed venous oxygen saturation.

■ Check ventilator settings frequently. Monitor ABG levels; document and report changes in arterial oxygen saturation as well as metabolic and respiratory acidosis and changes in partial pressure of arterial oxygen.

■ Provide emotional support. Answer the patient's and family members' questions as fully as possible to allay their fears and concerns.

■ Provide alternative means of communication for the patient on mechanical ventilation.

■ Give sedatives, as ordered, to reduce restlessness. Administer sedatives or analgesics at regular intervals if patient is receiving neuromuscular blocking agents.

■ If the patient has a pulmonary artery catheter in place, change dressings according to hospital guidelines, using strict aseptic technique.

■ Reposition the patient often.

■ Note and record any changes in respiratory status, temperature, or hypotension that may indicate a deteriorating condition. Notify the doctor.

■ Record caloric intake. Administer tube feedings and parenteral nutrition, as ordered. To promote health and prevent fatigue, arrange for alternate periods of rest and activity.

■ Maintain joint mobility by performing passive range-of-motion exercises. If possible, help the patient perform active exercises.

■ Provide meticulous skin care. To prevent skin breakdown, reposition the endotracheal tube from side to side every 24 hours.

■ Be alert for signs of treatment-induced complications, including arrhythmias, DIC, GI bleeding, infection, malnutrition, paralytic ileus, pneumothorax, pulmonary fibrosis, renal failure, thrombocytopenia, and tracheal stenosis.

■ Because PEEP may lower cardiac output, check for hypotension, tachycardia, and decreased urine output.

■ Evaluate the patient's nutritional intake.

Patient teaching
■ Explain the disorder to the patient and his family. Tell them what signs and symptoms may occur, and review the treatment that may be required.

■ Orient the patient and his family to the unit and hospital surroundings. Provide them with simple explanations and demonstrations of treatments.

■ Tell the recuperating patient that recovery will take some time and that he'll feel weak for a while. Urge him to share his concerns with staff members.

EVALUATION

Evaluation of patient outcomes determines the success of collaborative management. For the patient with ARDS, evaluation focuses on adequate oxygenation and absence of complications.

Asthma

A chronic reactive airway disorder, asthma involves episodic, reversible airway obstruction resulting from bronchospasms, increased mucus secretions, and mucosal edema. The patient's attack may range from mild wheezing and dyspnea to life-threatening respiratory failure. Signs and symptoms of bronchial airway obstruction may or may not persist between acute episodes.

Although this common respiratory condition can strike at any age, about half of all asthma patients are under age 10, with boys in this age-group affected twice as often as girls. About one-third of patients first develop asthma between ages 10 and 30; in this group, incidence is the same in both sexes.

CAUSES

Hereditary factors are important: About one-third of all asthma patients share the disease with at least one immediate family member. Asthma may result from sensitivity to specific external allergens (extrinsic) or from internal, nonallergenic factors (intrinsic). Allergens that cause extrinsic asthma (atopic asthma) include pollen, animal dander, house dust or mold, kapok or feather pillows, food additives containing sulfites, and any other sensitizing substance. Extrinsic asthma begins in childhood and is commonly accompanied by other manifestations of atopy (type I, immunoglobulin E [IgE]–mediated allergy), such as eczema and allergic rhinitis.

In intrinsic asthma (nonatopic asthma), no extrinsic substance can be identified. Most episodes are preceded by a severe respiratory tract infection (especially in adults). Irritants, emotional stress, endocrine changes, fatigue, temperature and humidity variations, and exposure to noxious fumes may aggravate intrinsic asthma attacks. In many asthmatics, especially children, intrinsic and extrinsic asthma coexist.

In asthma, the tracheal and bronchial linings overreact to various stimuli, causing episodic smooth-muscle spasms that severely constrict the airways. Mucosal edema and thickened secretions further block the airways.

IgE antibodies, attached to histamine-containing mast cells and receptors on cell membranes, initiate intrinsic asthma attacks. When exposed to an antigen such as pollen, the IgE antibody combines with the antigen. On subsequent exposure to the antigen, mast cells degranulate and release mediators.

These mediators cause the bronchoconstriction and edema of an asthma attack. As a result, expiration decreases, trapping gas in the airways and causing alveolar hyperinflation. Atelectasis may develop in some lung regions. The increased airway resistance causes labored breathing.

Contributors to bronchoconstriction may include hereditary predisposition; sensitivity to allergens or irritants such as pollutants; viral infections; aspirin, beta blockers, nonsteroidal anti-inflammatory drugs, and other drugs; tartrazine (a yellow food dye); psychological stress; cold air; and exercise.

DIAGNOSIS AND TREATMENT

Diagnosis includes arterial blood gas (ABG) analysis, skin testing to determine allergies, and bronchial challenge testing to evaluate the clinical significance of allergens identified by skin testing.

The best treatment for asthma is prevention by identifying and avoiding precipitating factors, such as environmental allergens or irritants. Usually, such stimuli can't be eliminated. Desensitization to specific antigens may be more helpful in children than in adults with bronchial asthma.

Drug therapy usually includes inhaled corticosteroids and bronchodilators. Inhaled steroid medications reduce airway inflammation and should be taken whether or not the patient has symptoms. Breakthrough medications, usually bronchodilators, are most effective when used soon after an attack begins. Drugs used include rapid-acting epinephrine, terbutaline, aminophylline, theophylline and theophylline-containing oral preparations, oral sympathomimetics, corticosteroids, and aerosolized sympathomimetics, such as metaproterenol and albuterol.

Low-flow oxygen may be required, as may antibiotics if infection is evident. Fluid replacement may also be necessary.

Status asthmaticus must be treated promptly to prevent progression to fatal respiratory failure. The patient with increasingly severe asthma who doesn't respond to drug therapy is usually admitted to the intensive care unit for treatment with corticosteroids, epinephrine, sympathomimetic aerosol sprays, and I.V. aminophylline. He'll need frequent ABG analysis and pulse oximetry, particularly after ventilator therapy or a change in oxygen concentration. The patient may require endotracheal intubation and mechanical ventilation if his partial pressure of arterial carbon dioxide ($PaCO_2$) rises.

Avoiding asthma triggers

Tell your patient that avoiding the following common triggers and taking certain steps can reduce the frequency and severity of asthma attacks.

Triggers to avoid at home
- Foods, such as nuts, chocolate, eggs, shellfish, and peanut butter; flour, cereals, and other grains
- Beverages, such as orange juice, wine, beer, and milk
- Mold spores and pollens from flowers, trees, grasses, hay, and ragweed
- Dander from rabbits, cats, dogs, hamsters, gerbils, and chickens
- Feather or hair-stuffed pillows, down comforters, wool clothing, and stuffed toys
- Insect parts such as those from dead cockroaches
- Medicines such as aspirin, certain antibiotics (which can cause anaphylaxis), and drugs containing dyes or tartrazine
- Vapors from cleaning solvents, paint, paint thinners, and liquid chlorine bleach
- Fluorocarbon spray products, such as furniture polish, starch, cleaners, and room deodorizers
- Scents from spray deodorants, perfumes, hair sprays, talcum powder, and cosmetics
- Cloth-upholstered furniture, carpets, and draperies, which collect dust
- Brooms and dusters that raise dust
- Dirty filters on hot-air furnaces and air conditioners that blow dust into the air
- Dust from vacuum cleaner exhaust

Triggers to avoid at work
- Dust, vapors, or fumes from wood products (western red cedar, some pine and birch woods, mahogany); coffee, tea, or papain; metals (platinum, chromium, and nickel sulfate) and soldering fumes; and cotton, flax, and hemp
- Mold from decaying hay

Triggers to avoid outdoors
- Cold air, hot air, or sudden temperature changes (such as when entering an air-conditioned store in the summer)
- Excessive humidity or dryness
- Changes in seasons
- Smog
- Automobile exhaust

Steps to take at home
- Install a bedroom air-conditioner with a filter, and keep the filter clean.
- Avoid long walks when pollen counts are high.
- Consider finding a new home for a pet.
- Use smooth, not fuzzy, washable blankets.
- Hang lightweight, washable cotton or synthetic-fiber curtains, and use washable cotton throw rugs on bare floors.
- Clean your bedroom daily by damp dusting and damp mopping. Keep the door to your bedroom closed.

General steps to take
- Avoid exposure to people with the common cold, flu, and other viruses.
- Avoid overexertion or extreme emotions, such as fear, anger, frustration, laughing too hard, or crying.
- Avoid smoke from cigarettes, cigars, and pipes. Don't smoke and don't stay in a room with people who do.
- Drink plenty of fluids, at least six to eight glasses a day.
- Avoid sleeping pills and sedatives. They may make your breathing slower and more difficult. Instead, try propping yourself up on extra pillows while waiting for your antianxiety medication to work.

COLLABORATIVE MANAGEMENT

Care of the patient with asthma focuses on maintaining oxygenation during an acute attack and preventing future attacks. (See *Avoid asthma triggers*.)

ASSESSMENT

An asthma attack may begin dramatically, with severe, multiple symptoms, or insidiously, with gradually increasing respiratory distress. Typically, the patient reports exposure to a particular allergen, followed by a sudden onset of dyspnea, wheezing, and tightness in the chest accompanied by a cough that produces thick, clear or yellow sputum. Look for:
- complaints of suffocation
- visibly dyspneic and able to speak only a few words between breaths
- use of accessory respiratory muscles to breathe
- profuse sweat and increased anteroposterior thoracic diameter
- hyperresonance
- vocal fremitus
- tachycardia, tachypnea, mild systolic hypertension, harsh respirations with both inspiratory and expiratory wheezes
- prolonged expiratory phase of respiration
- diminished breath sounds
- cyanosis, confusion, and lethargy, indicating onset of life-threatening status asthmaticus and respiratory failure

- signs of airway obstructive disease (decreased flow rates and forced expiratory volume in 1 second (FEV_1))
- low-normal or decreased vital capacity, and increased total lung and residual capacities
- abnormal findings during asthmatic episodes, but normal pulmonary function between attacks.
- decreased partial pressure of arterial oxygen and $PaCO_2$
- in severe asthma, normal or increased $PaCO_2$, indicating severe bronchial obstruction (FEV_1 will probably be less than 25% of the predicted value)
- improved airflow with treatment; however, even when the asthma attack appears controlled, the spirometric values (FEV_1 and forced expiratory flow) remain abnormal (between 25% and 75% of vital capacity), necessitating frequent ABG analyses or pulse oximetry measurements
- abnormal residual volume for the longest period—up to 3 weeks after the attack
- high serum IgE levels from an allergic reaction
- increased eosinophil count in complete blood count with differential
- possible hyperinflation with areas of focal atelectasis shown in X-rays.

NURSING DIAGNOSES AND COLLABORATIVE PROBLEMS

Based on the following nursing diagnoses, you'll establish patient outcomes.

Impaired gas exchange related to bronchoconstriction and mucosal edema caused by an acute asthma attack. The patient will:
- regain normal gas exchange
- recover from an acute asthma attack with no residual lung damage.

Ineffective airway clearance related to increased thick mucus secretions and fatigue. The patient will:
- cough and deep-breathe adequately to expectorate secretions
- demonstrate skill in conserving energy while attempting to clear airway
- maintain a patent airway.

Ineffective breathing pattern related to labored breathing. The patient will:
- achieve maximum lung expansion with adequate ventilation
- recover and maintain normal respiratory rate and pattern
- experience diminished dyspnea.

Anxiety related to inability to breathe and interference with activities. The patient will:
- verbalize fears related to breathing problems
- demonstrate measures to decrease anxiety during an attack.

PLANNING AND IMPLEMENTATION

These measures help the patient with asthma:
- Control exercise-induced asthma with oxygenation, by having the patient rest and use diaphragmatic and pursed-lip breathing.
- Assess the patient's respiratory status for deterioration.
- In an acute attack, find out if the patient has and used a nebulizer; make sure he has access to an albuterol or metaproterenol inhaler. Instruct him to take only two to three puffs every 4 hours, or check with his doctor. (Excessive nebulizer use can progressively weaken the patient's response and mask underlying inflammation. Extended overuse rarely leads to cardiac arrest.)
- As ordered, administer humidified oxygen by nasal cannula at 2 L/minute to ease breathing and increase arterial oxygen saturation during an acute asthma attack. Later, adjust oxygen to suit the patient's vital functions and ABG measurements.
- Administer drugs and I.V. fluids as prescribed. Continue epinephrine or a sympathomimetic for a patient experiencing an acute attack. Administer aminophylline I.V. as a loading dose. Follow with I.V. drip administration, as ordered. When possible, use an I.V. infusion pump. Simultaneously, give a loading dose of corticosteroidal medication I.V. or I.M., as prescribed.
- Combat dehydration with I.V. fluids until the patient can tolerate oral fluids to help loosen secretions.
- Monitor the patient's compliance with drug therapy regimen.
- Monitor plasma drug levels of theophylline because oral absorption may vary.
- With long-term corticosteroid therapy, watch for cushingoid adverse reactions.
- Encourage the patient to express his fears and concerns about his illness. Answer his questions honestly. Encourage him to identify and comply with care measures and activities that promote relaxation.
- Reassure the patient during an asthma attack and stay with him. Place him in semi-Fowler's position, and encourage diaphragmatic breathing.

Patient teaching

- Teach the patient and family members or friends about diaphragmatic and pursed-lip breathing. Advise him to perform relaxation exercises.
- Teach the patient how to use an oral or turbo-inhaler. Tell him about possible adverse reactions and when to notify the doctor.
- Supervise the patient's drug regimen, checking for proper use of a metered-dose inhaler. The addition of spacer devices may help optimize drug delivery.
- Show the patient how to breathe deeply. Instruct him to cough up secretions accumulated overnight and to allow time for medications to work.

- Emphasize consistency of medications for maximum benefits, even though he is feeling well.
- Urge the patient to drink plenty of fluids (at least six 8-oz glasses daily) to help loosen secretions and maintain hydration.
- Tell the patient to eat a well-balanced diet to prevent respiratory infection and fatigue. Teach him to avoid substances that trigger an attack.

EVALUATION

Evaluation of patient outcomes determines the success of collaborative management. For the patient with asthma, evaluation focuses on adequate oxygenation and knowledge.

Chronic obstructive pulmonary disease

The most common chronic lung disease, chronic obstructive pulmonary disease (COPD) is chronic airway obstruction that results from emphysema, chronic bronchitis, asthma, or any combination of these disorders. Usually, more than one of these underlying conditions coexist; in most cases, bronchitis and emphysema occur together. COPD affects males more than females, probably because until recently men were more likely to smoke heavily.

CAUSES

Predisposing factors include cigarette smoking, recurrent or chronic respiratory infections, air pollution, and allergies. Smoking is by far the most important of these factors; it impairs ciliary action and macrophage function and causes inflammation in airways, increased mucous production, destruction of alveolar septa, and peribronchiolar fibrosis. Early inflammatory changes may reverse if the patient stops smoking before lung destruction is extensive. Familial and hereditary factors (such as deficiency of alpha$_1$-antitrypsin) may also predispose a person to COPD.

In emphysema, recurrent inflammation associated with release of proteolytic enzymes from lung cells causes bronchiolar and alveolar wall damage and, ultimately, destruction. Loss of lung supporting structure results in decreased elastic recoil and airway collapse on expiration. Destruction of alveolar walls decreases surface area for gas exchange.

In chronic bronchitis, hypertrophy and hyperplasia of bronchial mucous glands, increased goblet cells, damage to cilia, squamous metaplasia of columnar epithelium, and chronic leukocytic and lymphocytic infiltration of bronchial walls as well as widespread inflammation, distortion, narrowing of airways and mucus within the airways produce resistance in small airways and cause severe ventilation-perfusion imbalance.

DIAGNOSIS AND TREATMENT

Diagnostic tests include chest X-rays, pulmonary function tests, arterial blood gas (ABG) analysis, electrocardiography, and red blood cell (RBC) count.

Treatment is designed to relieve symptoms and prevent complications. Because most COPD patients receive outpatient treatment, they need comprehensive patient teaching to help them comply with therapy and understand the nature of this chronic, progressive disease. If programs in pulmonary rehabilitation are available, encourage the patient to enroll.

Smoking cessation and avoidance of other respiratory irritants is the most important treatment.

Bronchodilators alleviate bronchospasm and enhance mucociliary clearance of secretions. Antibiotics are used to treat respiratory infections. I.V. steroids (such as Solu-Medrol or Solu-Cortef) may be used to mediate any inflammatory response.

Low concentrations of oxygen may be prescribed. High flow rates are usually avoided as they may hinder the respiratory drive in the COPD patient, whose drive is usually based on hypoxemia.

Pneumococcal vaccination and annual influenza vaccination are helpful preventive measures.

COLLABORATIVE MANAGEMENT

Care of the patient with COPD focuses on maintaining air exchange and teaching self-care and energy conservation.

ASSESSMENT

The patient's history may disclose that he is a long-time smoker with shortness of breath, chronic cough and, possibly, anorexia with resultant weight loss and a general feeling of malaise. Look for:
- barrelchest
- breathing through pursed lips with accessory muscle use
- peripheral cyanosis, clubbed fingers and toes, and tachypnea
- decreased tactile fremitus and decreased chest expansion
- hyperresonance
- decreased breath sounds, crackles, and wheezing during inspiration, a prolonged expiratory phase with grunting respirations, and distant heart sounds.

NURSING DIAGNOSES AND COLLABORATIVE PROBLEMS

Based on the following nursing diagnoses, you'll establish patient outcomes.

Activity intolerance caused by fatigue related to chronic tissue hypoxia. The patient will:

- identify controllable factors that contribute to fatigue
- skillfully conserve energy while performing daily activities at a tolerable level
- seek assistance when necessary to complete an activity.

Impaired gas exchange related to lung tissue changes caused by recurrent inflammation. The patient will:
- demonstrate adequate ventilation
- maintain a respiratory rate at baseline level
- exhibit no signs of acute hypoxia, such as confusion, restlessness, or severe anxiety.

Ineffective airway clearance related to increased bronchial secretions caused by recurrent lung inflammation. The patient will:
- cough effectively
- expectorate sputum to keep the airway open
- skillfully perform bronchial hygiene to clear secretions from the airway.

PLANNING AND IMPLEMENTATION

These measures help the patient with COPD:
- If prescribed, perform chest physiotherapy, including postural drainage and chest percussion and vibration, several times daily.
- Schedule respiratory treatments at least 1 hour before or after meals. Provide mouth care after bronchodilator therapy.
- Make sure the patient receives adequate fluids (at least 3 qt [3 L] a day) to loosen secretions.
- Administer bronchodilators and steroids, as ordered, and record the patient's response.
- Monitor the patient's respiratory function regularly. Perform the activities needed for ABG analyses and pulmonary function studies, as ordered.
- Monitor the patient's RBC count for increases (signs of increasing lung and vascular congestion).
- Watch for complications, such as respiratory tract infections, cor pulmonale, spontaneous pneumothorax, respiratory failure, and peptic ulcer disease.
- Provide a high-calorie, protein-rich diet to promote health and healing. Give small, frequent meals to conserve the patient's energy and prevent fatigue.
- Have the patient alternate rest and activity periods to conserve energy and prevent fatigue.
- Provide supportive care, and help the patient adjust to lifestyle changes imposed by a chronic illness.
- Answer the patient's questions about his illness honestly. Encourage him to express his fears and concerns, and stay with him during periods of extreme stress and anxiety.
- Include the patient and family members or friends in care-related decisions. Refer them to appropriate support services as needed.

Patient teaching

- Tell the patient to avoid crowds and people with known infections and to receive influenza and pneumococcus immunizations.
- If the patient is receiving home oxygen therapy, explain treatment rationales and proper use of equipment. If the patient requires a transtracheal catheter, teach him catheter care, precautions, and follow-up care.
- Teach the patient and family members how to perform postural drainage and chest percussion. The patient should maintain each position for about 10 minutes, while a family member performs percussion and directs the patient to cough. Also teach the patient coughing and deep-breathing techniques to promote good ventilation and mobilize secretions.
- Review the patient's medications and explain the rationale, dosage, and adverse effects related to the prescribed drug. Teach him to report adverse reactions to the doctor immediately. Show him how to use an inhaler correctly, if appropriate.
- Encourage the patient to eat high-calorie, protein-rich foods. Urge him to drink plenty of fluids to prevent dehydration and to help loosen secretions.
- If the patient smokes, urge him to stop. Provide him with smoking cessation resources or counseling, if necessary.
- Urge the patient to avoid respiratory irritants, such as automobile exhaust fumes, aerosol sprays, and industrial pollutants. Suggest that he install an air conditioner with an air filter in his home.
- Warn the patient that exposure to blasts of cold air may precipitate bronchospasm. Tell him to avoid cold, windy weather and to cover his mouth and nose with a scarf or mask if he must go outside.
- If appropriate, describe signs and symptoms of peptic ulcer disease. Instruct the patient to check his stools every day for blood and to notify the doctor if he has persistent nausea, vomiting, heartburn, indigestion, constipation, diarrhea, or bloody stools.
- Tell the patient about signs and symptoms that suggest ruptured alveolar blebs and bullae. Explain the seriousness of possible spontaneous pneumothorax. Urge him to notify the doctor if he feels sudden, sharp pleuritic pain that's exacerbated by chest movement, breathing, or coughing.

EVALUATION

Evaluation of patient outcomes determines the success of collaborative management. For the patient with COPD, evaluation focuses on adequate ventilation and air exchange, maximization of energy level, and adequate knowledge.

Cor pulmonale

Also called right ventricular hypertrophy, cor pulmonale occurs at the end stage of various chronic disorders that affect lung function or structure (except congenital heart disease or diseases that affect the left side of the heart). It invariably follows certain disorders of the lungs, pulmonary vessels, chest wall, or respiratory control center. Because cor pulmonale usually occurs late in chronic obstructive pulmonary disease (COPD) and other irreversible diseases, the prognosis is poor.

The disorder accounts for about 25% of all types of heart failure, and it's most common in patients who smoke and who have COPD.

CAUSES

Cor pulmonale may result from:
- disorders that affect pulmonary parenchyma (such as pulmonary fibrosis, pneumoconiosis, cystic fibrosis, periarteritis nodosa, and tuberculosis)
- pulmonary diseases that affect the airways (such as COPD and bronchial asthma)
- vascular diseases (such as vasculitis, pulmonary emboli, or external vascular obstruction resulting from a tumor or an aneurysm)
- chest wall abnormalities, including thoracic deformities (such as kyphoscoliosis and pectus excavatum)
- other external factors, including obesity, living at high altitude, and neuromuscular disorders (such as muscular dystrophy and poliomyelitis).

In cor pulmonale, pulmonary hypertension increases the heart's workload. To compensate, the right ventricle hypertrophies to force blood through the lungs. However, the compensatory mechanism eventually fails, and larger amounts of blood remain in the right ventricle at the end of diastole. This causes ventricular dilation. Cardiac output drops, resulting in tissue hypoxia. In response to hypoxia, the bone marrow produces more red blood cells, resulting in polycythemia. Then, the blood's viscosity increases, further aggravating pulmonary hypertension, increasing the right ventricle's workload, and causing heart failure.

DIAGNOSIS AND TREATMENT

Diagnostic tests include pulmonary artery catheterization (revealing elevated pressures), echocardiography, chest X-ray, and arterial blood gas (ABG) analysis. Electrocardiography (ECG) discloses arrhythmias, such as premature atrial and ventricular contractions and atrial fibrillation during severe hypoxia. The ECG may also show right bundle-branch block, right axis deviation, prominent P waves and inverted T wave in right precordial leads, and right ventricular hypertrophy.

Other tests include pulmonary function tests and serum hematocrit (typically over 50%). If the patient's liver is affected, serum hepatic enzyme levels will show an elevated serum level of aspartate aminotransferase and serum bilirubin level may be elevated.

Therapy for the patient with cor pulmonale aims to reduce hypoxemia, increase exercise tolerance and, when possible, correct the underlying condition.

Besides bed rest, treatment may include digitalis glycosides such as digoxin and antibiotics for an underlying respiratory tract infection. (Usually, sputum culture and sensitivity tests determine which antibiotic the patient receives.) To treat primary pulmonary hypertension, the patient may receive a potent pulmonary artery vasodilator, such as diazoxide, nitroprusside, or hydralazine.

The patient may need oxygen administered by mask or cannula in concentrations ranging from 24% to 40%, depending on his partial pressure of arterial oxygen. In acute disease, therapy may also include mechanical ventilation.

The patient may benefit from a low-sodium diet, restricted fluid intake and, possibly, a diuretic (furosemide, for example) to reduce edema.

Occasionally, the patient with cor pulmonale may require phlebotomy to decrease red blood cell mass. Anticoagulation with small doses of heparin can decrease the risk of thromboembolism.

COLLABORATIVE MANAGEMENT

Care of the patient with cor pulmonale focuses on maintaining oxygenation and fluid balance.

ASSESSMENT

As long as the heart can compensate for the increased pulmonary vascular resistance, your patient will report signs and symptoms associated with the underlying disorder, occurring mostly in the respiratory system. Look for:
- complaints of a chronic productive cough, exertional dyspnea, wheezing respirations, fatigue, and weakness
- dyspnea (even at rest) that worsens on exertion, tachypnea, orthopnea, edema, weakness, and right upper quadrant discomfort
- dependent edema and distended neck veins. Also drowsiness and alterations in consciousness.
- tachycardia and a weak pulse (from decreased cardiac output)
- enlarged and tender liver
- hepatojugular reflux

- prominent parasternal or epigastric cardiac impulse
- crackles, rhonchi, and diminished breath sounds.

With disease secondary to upper airway obstruction or damage to the respiratory control center, auscultation findings may be normal except for a right ventricular lift, a gallop rhythm, and a loud pulmonic component of the second heart sound (S_2).

With tricuspid insufficiency, you'll hear a pansystolic murmur at the lower left sternal border. The murmur's intensity increases when the patient inhales, distinguishing it from a murmur caused by mitral valve disease, a right ventricular early murmur that increases on inspiration and can be heard at the left sternal border or over the epigastrium, and a systolic pulmonary ejection sound.

NURSING DIAGNOSES AND COLLABORATIVE PROBLEMS

Based on the following nursing diagnoses, you'll establish patient outcomes.

Activity intolerance related to hypoxemia caused by cor pulmonale. The patient will:
- identify controllable factors and activities that cause fatigue and dyspnea
- demonstrate methods of conserving energy while carrying out daily activities
- seek assistance as needed to perform activities of daily living.

Fluid volume excess related to right-sided heart failure caused by cor pulmonale. The patient will:
- tolerate restricted fluid and sodium intake without physical or emotional discomfort
- maintain normal fluid balance, as exhibited by no weight gain, intake and output balance, and the absence of edema.

Risk for injury related to potential for polycythemia-induced thromboembolism. The patient will:
- use measures to prevent emboli formation, such as passive exercise, antiembolism stockings, and regular position changes
- comply with anticoagulation therapy or scheduled phlebotomy, as ordered
- develop no thromboembolism.

PLANNING AND IMPLEMENTATION

These measures help the patient with cor pulmonale:
- Listen to the patient's fears and concerns about his illness. Remain with him when he feels severe stress and anxiety.
- Encourage him to identify actions and care measures that promote comfort and relaxation. Include him in care-related decisions whenever possible.
- Because the patient may tire easily, provide small, frequent feedings rather than three heavy meals. Avoid scheduling respiratory treatments immediately before meals.

- Reposition the bedridden patient often to prevent atelectasis.
- Provide meticulous respiratory care, including oxygen therapy and, for COPD patients, pursed-lip breathing exercises. Encourage the patient to rinse his mouth after respiratory therapies.
- Pace care activities to avoid patient fatigue.
- Periodically measure ABG levels and watch for signs and symptoms of respiratory failure, such as a change in pulse rate; deep, labored respirations; and increased fatigue produced by exertion.
- Prevent fluid retention by limiting the patient's fluid intake to 1 to 2 qt (1 to 2 L) daily and by providing a low-sodium diet.
- Clarify the need for restricting fluids, especially if the patient has underlying COPD. (Most patients with COPD are encouraged to drink up to 10 glasses of water daily.)

Patient teaching

- Make sure the patient understands the importance of maintaining a low-sodium diet, weighing himself daily, and immediately reporting edema. He should promptly report any weight gain of 2 to 3 lb (1 to 1.5 kg) over 1 to 2 days.
- Tell the patient to schedule frequent rest periods and to perform his breathing exercises regularly.
- Because pulmonary infection usually exacerbates cor pulmonale (and COPD), tell the patient to watch for and immediately report early signs and symptoms of infection, such as increased sputum production, change in sputum color, increased coughing or wheezing, chest pain, fever, and tightness in the chest. Tell the patient to avoid crowds and people known to have infections, especially during the flu season.
- Warn the patient to avoid nonprescription medications that may depress ventilatory drive, such as sedatives. Teach him to check his radial pulse before taking digoxin or any digitalis glycoside. Tell him to notify the doctor if he detects a pulse rate change.
- Urge the patient to discuss influenza and pneumonia immunizations with the doctor. Help him obtain the vaccines, if appropriate.
- Tell the patient to add potassium-rich foods to his daily diet if he takes a potassium-wasting diuretic.
- If the patient needs supplemental oxygen therapy at home, refer him to a social service agency that can help him obtain the equipment and care. As needed, arrange for follow-up examinations.

EVALUATION

Evaluation of patient outcomes determines the success of collaborative management. For the patient with cor pulmonale, evaluation focuses on fluid balance, activity tolerance, and adequate knowledge.

Flail chest

A complication of blunt trauma, flail chest occurs when a portion of the chest wall "caves in," causing a loss of chest wall integrity and inadequate lung inflation.

CAUSES
Flail chest can result from motor vehicle accidents, sports, fights, and blast injuries.

Normally, the chest wall expands during inspiration, drawing air into the lungs. But in flail chest, the injured free-floating section retracts as the patient inhales. During expiration, the flail section moves contrary to the rest of the chest wall, bulging outward. As a result, the patient can't expel air effectively. Palpation of the chest may reveal crepitus.

DIAGNOSIS AND TREATMENT
Chest X-ray may show localized atelectasis from decreased ventilation. Arterial blood gas (ABG) values may indicate hypoxemia.

Treatment of flail chest may include endotracheal (ET) intubation and mechanical ventilation along with neuromuscular blocking agents, sedatives, and antianxiety agents. I.V. muscle relaxants may be prescribed to relieve muscular tension. Also, the patient may need surgical repair for an air leak.

COLLABORATIVE MANAGEMENT
Care of the patient with flail chest focuses on maintaining oxygenation and supplying pain relief.

ASSESSMENT
The patient's history usually includes blunt trauma to the chest. Look for:
- complaints of severe pain from the rib fractures and extreme shortness of breath
- restlessness, with shallow, rapid respirations, and cyanosis
- paradoxical movements of the chest wall, with a section of the wall moving in on inspiration and out on expiration
- bony crepitus palpable at the fracture site and subcutaneous crepitus
- diminished breath sounds on auscultation.

NURSING DIAGNOSES AND COLLABORATIVE PROBLEMS
Based on the following nursing diagnoses, you'll establish patient outcomes.

Inability to sustain spontaneous ventilation related to altered chest wall. The patient will:

- maintain a respiratory rate within 5 breaths/minute of baseline
- show normal ABG levels
- breathe spontaneously once ventilatory support is withdrawn.

Pain related to air pressure change in pleural cavity. The patient will:
- report chest comfort following analgesic administration
- sit upright to increase comfort.

PLANNING AND IMPLEMENTATION
These measures help the patient with flail chest:
- Monitor patient's vital signs every 15 to 60 minutes to detect tachypnea and tachycardia, early indications of respiratory distress.
- Monitor ABG levels and report deviations promptly to determine the need for changes to the therapeutic regimen.
- Monitor for spontaneous breathing.
- Position the patient in semi-Fowler's or Fowler's position to increase comfort.
- Administer analgesics as prescribed and monitor the patient's response to the medications.
- Schedule activities and repositioning to follow analgesic administration.
- Monitor for arrhythmias, especially in anterior flail chest.

Patient teaching
- Teach the patient relaxation techniques.
- Explain all procedures, and include the patient and family members in care decisions when possible.
- Explain the workings of the ventilator and reassure the patient that he will be able to breathe on his own once the ET tube is removed.

EVALUATION
Evaluation of patient outcomes determines the success of collaborative management. For the patient with flail chest, evaluation focuses on adequate oxygenation and pain relief.

Laryngeal cancer

Squamous cell carcinoma constitutes about 95% of laryngeal cancers. Rare laryngeal cancer forms — adenocarcinoma and sarcoma — account for the rest. The disease affects approximately five times more men than women, and most victims are between ages 50 and 65.

Laryngeal cancer is classified by its location:
- supraglottis (false vocal cords)
- glottis (true vocal cords)

- subglottis (rare downward extension from vocal cords).

A tumor on the true vocal cord seldom spreads because underlying connective tissues lack lymph nodes. On the other hand, a tumor on another part of the larynx tends to spread early. Metastasis, when it does occur, usually presents as diffuse pulmonary nodules. Other sites include the mediastinal lymph nodes, the liver, and the brain.

CAUSES

The cause of laryngeal cancer is unknown. Major risk factors include smoking and alcoholism. Minor risk factors include chronic inhalation of noxious fumes, familial disposition, and a history of frequent laryngitis and vocal straining.

DIAGNOSIS AND TREATMENT

The usual diagnostic workup includes laryngoscopy, xeroradiography, biopsy, laryngeal tomography and computed tomography scans, and laryngography to visualize and define the tumor and its borders. Chest X-ray findings can help detect metastases.

Early lesions may respond to laser surgery or radiation therapy; advanced lesions to laser surgery, radiation therapy, and chemotherapy. Treatment aims to eliminate cancer and preserve speech. If speech preservation isn't possible, speech rehabilitation may include esophageal speech or prosthetic devices. Surgical techniques to construct a new voice box are experimental.

In early disease, laser surgery destroys precancerous lesions; in advanced disease, it can help clear obstructions. Other surgical procedures vary with tumor size and include cordectomy, partial or total laryngectomy, supraglottic laryngectomy, and total laryngectomy with laryngoplasty.

Radiation therapy alone or combined with surgery can produce complications, including airway obstruction, pain, and loss of taste.

Chemotherapy alone is minimally beneficial in treating laryngeal cancer.

COLLABORATIVE MANAGEMENT

Care of the patient with laryngeal cancer focuses on preventing and managing adverse effects of treatment and maximizing speech.

ASSESSMENT

Varied assessment findings in laryngeal cancer depend on tumor location and stage. Stage 0 is asymptomatic. In stage I, you'll hear complaints of local throat irritation or hoarseness that lasts about 2 weeks. Stages II and III include hoarseness, sore throat, and voice volume reduced to a stage whisper. In stage IV, the patient complains of pain radiating to the ear, dysphagia, and dyspnea. And in advanced stage IV, palpation may detect a neck mass or enlarged cervical lymph nodes.

NURSING DIAGNOSES AND COLLABORATIVE PROBLEMS

Based on the following nursing diagnoses, you'll establish patient outcomes.

Impaired swallowing related to presence of tumor. The patient will:
- consume a nutritionally balanced diet with sufficient calories
- maintain his weight within a normal range
- exhibit no signs or symptoms of aspiration pneumonia.

Impaired verbal communication related to presence of tumor. The patient will:
- communicate his needs and desires without undue frustration
- use an alternate method of communication as necessary
- use available resources to maximize his communication skills.

Ineffective airway clearance related to presence of tumor. The patient will:
- cough effectively and expectorate any sputum
- maintain a patent airway
- maintain arterial blood gas values within a normal range.

PLANNING AND IMPLEMENTATION

These measures help the patient with laryngeal cancer:
- Provide supportive psychological, preoperative, and postoperative care to minimize complications and speed recovery.
- Encourage the patient to describe his concerns before surgery.
- Help the patient choose a temporary, alternative way to communicate, such as writing or using sign language or an alphabet board.
- If appropriate, arrange for a well-adjusted laryngectomee to visit him.
- Postoperatively, after a partial laryngectomy, monitor vital signs. Be especially alert for fever, which indicates infection. Record fluid intake and output, and watch for dehydration. Also, be alert for and report postoperative complications.
- Give I.V. fluids and, usually, tube feedings for the first 2 days after surgery; then, resume oral fluids. Keep the tracheostomy tube (inserted during surgery) in place until tissue edema subsides.
- Make sure the patient doesn't use his voice until the doctor gives permission (usually 2 to 3 days postoperatively). Then, caution the patient to whisper until he heals completely.

■ If the patient has a total laryngectomy, as soon as he returns to his room, position him on his side and elevate his head 30 to 45 degrees. When you move him, remember to support the back of his neck. This will prevent tension on sutures and possible wound dehiscence.

■ If the patient has a laryngectomy tube in place, care for it as you would a tracheostomy tube. Shorter and thicker than a tracheostomy tube, the laryngectomy tube stays in place until the stoma heals (about 7 to 10 days).

■ To prevent crusting of the laryngectomy stoma, provide adequate room humidification. Remove crusts with petroleum jelly, antimicrobial ointment, and moist gauze.

■ Provide frequent mouth care. Clean the patient's tongue and the sides of his mouth with a soft toothbrush or a terry washcloth, and rinse his mouth with a deodorizing mouthwash.

■ Suction gently. Unless ordered otherwise, do not attempt deep suctioning, which could penetrate the suture line. Suction through both the tube and the patient's nose because the patient can no longer blow air through his nose. Suction his mouth gently.

■ Give analgesics, as ordered. Keep in mind that opioid analgesics depress respiration and inhibit coughing.

■ Support the patient through inevitable grieving. If his depression becomes severe, consider referring him for appropriate counseling.

■ If the patient will undergo chemotherapy (typically with methotrexate or bleomycin), assess bone marrow and pulmonary function before treatment begins. Once treatment is under way, reassess these functions. Also, monitor for renal toxicity related to chemotherapy.

Patient teaching

■ Before partial or total laryngectomy, teach the patient good oral hygiene practices. If appropriate, instruct a male patient to shave off his beard to facilitate postoperative care.

■ Explain postoperative procedures, such as suctioning, nasogastric tube feeding, and laryngectomy tube care. Carefully discuss the effects of these procedures (breathing through the neck and speech alteration, for example).

■ Prepare the patient for other functional losses. Forewarn him that he won't be able to smell aromas, blow his nose, whistle, gargle, sip, or suck on a straw.

■ Reassure the patient that speech rehabilitation measures (including laryngeal speech, esophageal speech, an artificial larynx, and various mechanical devices) may help him communicate again.

■ Teach the patient and family member or friend how to care for his stoma. Give him written instruc-

tions for the care as well as signs and symptoms of infection to report to the doctor.

■ Review with the patient the supplies he will need and provide a list of sources.

■ Encourage the patient to take advantage of services and information offered by the American Speech-Learning-Hearing Association, the International Association of Laryngectomees, the American Cancer Society, or the local chapter of the Lost Chord Club.

EVALUATION

Evaluation of patient outcomes determines the success of collaborative management. For the patient with laryngeal cancer, evaluation focuses on airway patency, ability to communicate, and adequate nutrition and knowledge.

Lung cancer

The most common forms of lung cancer are squamous cell (epidermoid) carcinoma, small-cell (oat cell) carcinoma, adenocarcinoma, and large-cell (anaplastic) carcinoma. The most common site is the wall or epithelium of the bronchial tree.

For most patients, the prognosis is poor, depending on the extent of the cancer when diagnosed and the cells' growth rate. Only about 13% of patients with lung cancer survive 5 years after diagnosis. Although the disease is largely preventable, it's the most common cause of cancer death in men. In women, lung cancer ranks with breast cancer as a leading cause of death.

CAUSES

Lung cancer's exact cause remains unclear. Risk factors include tobacco smoking, exposure to carcinogenic and industrial air pollutants (asbestos, arsenic, chromium, coal dust, iron oxides, nickel, radioactive dust, and uranium), and genetic predisposition.

Most malignant lung tumors originate in the cells lining the bronchi. They usually invade adjacent structures, including the pleura, blood vessels, chest wall, and diaphragm. Metastasis occurs early, especially in small-cell carcinoma. The first site of metastasis is usually the lymph nodes. Distant metastatic sites include the brain, bone, bone marrow, other lung, liver, adrenal glands, and skin.

DIAGNOSIS AND TREATMENT

Diagnostic tests include chest X-rays, cytologic sputum analysis, and bronchoscopy. Needle biopsy of the lungs may be performed using biplanar fluoroscopic visual control to locate peripheral tumors. Tissue biopsy of metastatic sites (including supraclavicular and mediastinal nodes and pleura) helps to assess the extent of the disease. Thoracentesis allows chemical and cytologic examination of pleural fluid. Additional studies include chest tomography, bronchography, esophagography, and angiocardiography (contrast studies of bronchial tree, esophagus, and cardiovascular tissues).

Tests to detect metastasis include a bone scan (abnormal findings may lead to a bone marrow biopsy, typically recommended in patients with small-cell carcinoma), a computed tomography scan of the brain, liver function studies, and gallium scans of the liver and spleen.

Various combinations of surgery, radiation therapy, and chemotherapy improve the prognosis and prolong patient survival. Because lung cancer is usually advanced at diagnosis, most treatment is palliative.

Surgery is the primary treatment for stage I, stage II, or selected stage III squamous cell carcinoma, adenocarcinoma, and large-cell carcinoma, unless the tumor is inoperable or other conditions (such as cardiac disease) rule out surgery. Surgery may involve partial lung removal (wedge resection, segmental resection, lobectomy, radical lobectomy) or total removal (pneumonectomy, radical pneumonectomy).

Preoperative radiation therapy may reduce tumor size to allow for surgical resection and may also improve response rates. Radiation therapy is ordinarily recommended for stage I and stage II lesions, for stage III disease confined to the involved hemithorax and the ipsilateral supraclavicular lymph nodes, and if surgery is contraindicated. Radiation therapy usually begins about 1 month after surgery (to allow the wound to heal). It's directed at the chest area most likely to develop metastasis.

Chemotherapy drug combinations of fluorouracil, vincristine, mitomycin, cisplatin, and vindesine induce a response rate of 30% to 50% yet have little effect on long-term survival. Promising combinations of drugs for treating small-cell carcinomas include cyclophosphamide, doxorubicin, and vincristine; cyclophosphamide, doxorubicin, vincristine, and etoposide; and etoposide, cisplatin, cyclophosphamide, and doxorubicin.

Immunotherapy is investigational. Nonspecific regimens using bacille Calmette-Guérin vaccine or, possibly, *Corynebacterium parvum* offer the most promise.

In laser therapy, also largely investigational, a laser beam is directed through a bronchoscope to destroy local tumors.

COLLABORATIVE MANAGEMENT
Care of the patient with lung cancer focuses on promoting air exchange and maximizing activity level.

ASSESSMENT
Because early lung cancer may cause no symptoms, the disease is typically advanced when diagnosed. While taking the patient's history, be sure to assess his exposure to carcinogens. If he's a smoker, determine pack-years. Look for:
- chief complaints of coughing (induced by tumor stimulation of nerve endings), hemoptysis, dyspnea (from the tumor occluding air flow) and, sometimes, hoarseness (from tumor or tumor-bearing lymph nodes pressing on the laryngeal nerve)
- shortness of breath when he walks or exerts himself
- finger clubbing; edema of the face, neck, and upper torso; dilated chest and abdominal veins (superior vena cava syndrome); weight loss; and fatigue
- enlarged lymph nodes and liver
- dullness over the lung fields in a patient with pleural effusion
- decreased breath sounds, wheezing, and pleural friction rub (with pleural effusion).

NURSING DIAGNOSES AND COLLABORATIVE PROBLEMS
Based on the following nursing diagnoses, you'll establish patient outcomes.

Anticipatory grieving related to poor prognosis. The patient will:
- express his feelings about his diagnosis and the potential for death
- maintain control by making decisions about his care
- use appropriate behaviors to cope with the threat of death.

Fatigue related to hypoxia caused by impaired gas exchange. The patient will:
- explain the relationship between fatigue and his activity level
- employ measures to prevent and modify fatigue.

Impaired gas exchange related to pulmonary dysfunction. The patient will:
- express feelings of comfort in maintaining adequate air exchange
- perform his activities of daily living as tolerated
- maintain his respiratory rate within 5 breaths/ minute of his baseline.

PLANNING AND IMPLEMENTATION
These measures help the patient with lung cancer:
- Provide comprehensive supportive care and patient teaching to minimize complications and speed the patient's recovery from surgery, radiation therapy, and chemotherapy.
- Urge the patient to voice his concerns, and schedule time to answer his questions. Be sure to explain

procedures before performing them to help reduce his anxiety.

■ Teach the patient relaxation techniques to lessen his anxiety and lower his body's oxygen demand.

■ Monitor the patient's respiratory status. Obtain arterial blood gas measurements regularly, as ordered.

■ Administer oxygen as ordered.

■ Elevate the head of the bed.

■ Encourage the patient to pace his activities.

■ Ask the dietary department to provide soft, nonirritating, protein-rich foods. Encourage the patient to eat high-calorie, high-protein between-meal snacks.

■ Give antiemetics and antidiarrheals as needed with chemotherapy. Evaluate the effectiveness of any medication administered.

■ Schedule patient care to help him conserve his energy.

■ Impose reverse isolation if bone marrow suppression develops during chemotherapy.

■ Provide meticulous skin care to minimize skin breakdown.

Patient teaching

■ Before surgery, supplement and reinforce what the doctor told the patient about the disease and the operation.

■ If the patient is receiving chemotherapy or radiation therapy, discuss possible adverse effects of these treatments and which reactions to report. Teach him ways to avoid complications such as infection.

■ Teach high-risk patients how to reduce their chances of developing lung cancer or recurrent cancer. (See *Reducing the risk of lung cancer*.)

■ Refer smokers to local branches of the American Cancer Society or Smokenders. Provide information about group therapy, individual counseling, and hypnosis.

■ Urge all heavy smokers over age 40 to have a chest X-ray annually and cytologic sputum analysis every 6 months. Also encourage patients who have recurring or chronic respiratory tract infections, chronic lung disease, or a nagging or changing cough to seek prompt medical evaluation.

EVALUATION

Evaluation of patient outcomes determines the success of collaborative management. For the patient with lung cancer, evaluation focuses on adequate air exchange, relief of anxiety, activity tolerance, and adequate knowledge.

HEALTHY LIVING

Reducing the risk of lung cancer

Although the exact cause of lung cancer isn't known, there are known risk factors. Encourage your patient to take the following steps to minimize his risk.

■ Don't smoke. Cigarette smoking is the leading risk factor for lung cancer; pipe and cigar smoking also pose a danger.

■ Avoid places where people are smoking. Secondary smoke can be as damaging to the lungs as primary smoke.

■ Use protective respiratory equipment on the job or working around the house. Exposure to asbestos, polycyclic hydrocarbons, arsenic, and radon can precipitate lung cancer.

■ Reduce residential radon exposure. Have your home tested, and improve ventilation in closed areas such as basements.

■ Eat less fat and more vegetables. A healthy diet strengthens the immune system and is associated with lower cancer incidence.

■ When possible, avoid urban pollution. Carbon monoxide and other invisible gases can damage the lungs.

Occupational lung disease

Characterized by pulmonary fibrosis, occupational lung diseases are pneumoconioses caused by lung damage in the workplace. Coal worker's pneumoconiosis, silicosis, and asbestosis are examples.

Also known as black lung, coal miner's disease, miner's asthma, anthracosis, and anthracosilicosis, coal worker's pneumoconiosis is a progressive nodular pulmonary disease. The disease occurs in two forms: simple and complicated. With the simple form, the patient has characteristically limited lung capacity. In the complicated form, fibrous tissue masses form in the lungs.

A person's risk for coal worker's pneumoconiosis depends on various factors, including length of exposure to coal dust (usually 15 or more years), intensity of exposure (dust count and size of inhaled particles), his proximity to the mine site, the silica content of the coal (anthracite is highest), and his susceptibility. Anthracite miners in the eastern United States are the most affected.

The most common form of pneumoconiosis, silicosis is a progressive disease characterized by nodular lesions, which commonly progress to fibrosis. It's classified according to the severity of the pulmonary disease and the rapidity of its onset and progression, although it usually occurs as a simple illness without symptoms.

Those who work around silica dust, such as foundry workers, boiler scalers, and stonecutters, have the highest incidence of the disease. Silica in its pure form occurs in the manufacture of ceramics (flint) and building materials (sandstone). It occurs in mixed form in the production of construction materials (cement). It's also found in powder form (silica flour) in paints, porcelain, scouring soaps, and wood fillers, and in the mining of gold, lead, zinc, and iron.

Sandblasters, tunnel workers, and others exposed to high concentrations of respirable silica may develop acute silicosis after 1 to 3 years. Those exposed to lower concentrations of free silica can develop accelerated silicosis, usually after about 10 years of exposure.

Asbestosis is characterized by diffuse interstitial pulmonary fibrosis, resulting from prolonged exposure to airborne asbestos particles. Asbestosis may develop 15 to 20 years after regular exposure to asbestos ceases. Asbestos exposure also causes pleural plaques and mesotheliomas of the pleura and the peritoneum. A potent cocarcinogen, asbestos heightens a cigarette smoker's risk for lung cancer. In fact, an asbestos worker who smokes is 90 times more likely to develop lung cancer than a smoker who never worked with asbestos.

Asbestos-related diseases may also develop in family members of asbestos workers from exposure to stray fibers shaken off the workers' clothing at home. Furthermore, asbestosis may develop in the general public from exposure to fibrous asbestos dust in public buildings, such as schools and factories, or waste piles from a nearby asbestos plant.

CAUSES

Inhalation and prolonged retention of respirable coal dust particles (less than 5 microns wide) cause coal worker's pneumoconiosis. Asbestosis follows prolonged inhalation of respirable asbestos fibers (about 50 microns long and 0.5 micron wide). Silicosis results from the inhalation and pulmonary deposition of respirable crystalline silica dust, mostly from quartz. Although particles up to 10 microns in diameter can be inhaled, the disease-causing particles deposited in the alveolar space usually have a diameter of only 1 to 3 microns.

In the simple type of pneumoconiosis, macules (coal dust–laden macrophages) form around terminal and respiratory bronchioles and are surrounded by a halo of dilated alveoli. At the same time, supporting tissues atrophy and harden, causing permanent small-airway dilation (focal emphysema). Simple coal work-

er's pneumoconiosis may progress to the complicated form—most likely if the disease begins after a relatively short exposure.

Complicated coal worker's pneumoconiosis may involve one or both lungs. Fibrous tissue masses enlarge and coalesce, grossly distorting pulmonary structures as the disease progressively destroys vessels, alveoli, and airways.

In asbestosis, the inhaled fibers travel down the airway and penetrate respiratory bronchioles and alveolar walls. They become encased in a brown, iron-rich, proteinlike sheath (ferruginous bodies or asbestosis bodies) in sputum or lung tissue. Interstitial fibrosis may develop in lower lung zones, causing pathologic changes in lung parenchyma and pleurae. Raised hyaline plaques may form in the parietal pleura and the diaphragm and in pleura adjacent to the pericardium.

Nodules in silicosis occur when alveolar macrophages ingest silica particles, which they can't process. As a result, the macrophages die and release proteolytic enzymes into surrounding tissue. The enzymes inflame the tissue, attracting other macrophages and fibroblasts. These produce fibrous tissue to wall off the reaction, resulting in a nodule that has an onionskin appearance.

These nodules develop adjacent to the terminal and respiratory bronchioles. Although frequently accompanied by bullous changes in both lobes, nodules concentrate in upper lung lobes. If the disease doesn't progress, the patient may experience only minimal physiologic disturbances, with no disability. Occasionally, however, the fibrotic response accelerates, engulfing and destroying a large lung area.

DIAGNOSIS AND TREATMENT

In simple pneumoconiosis, chest X-rays show small opacities (less than 3/8" [10 mm] in diameter) that are widespread but more prominent in the upper lung zones. In complicated pneumoconiosis, X-rays show one or more large opacities, some with cavitation.

Pulmonary function studies indicate a vital capacity that's normal in simple pneumoconiosis but decreased in the complicated form, decreased forced expiratory volume in 1 second (FEV_1) in the complicated form, and a normal ratio of FEV_1 to forced vital capacity.

Treatment aims to relieve respiratory symptoms, manage hypoxia and cor pulmonale, and avoid respiratory tract irritants and infections. Treatment also includes observation for developing tuberculosis.

Respiratory signs and symptoms may be relieved by bronchodilator therapy with theophylline or aminophylline (if bronchospasm is reversible), oral or inhaled beta-adrenergics (such as metaproterenol), corticosteroids (such as oral prednisone or aerosolized beclomethasone), or inhalable cromolyn sodium. Chest physiotherapy may be used to mobilize and remove secretions.

Other measures include increased fluid intake (at least 3 qt [3 L] daily) and respiratory therapy with aerosolized preparations, inhaled mucolytics, and intermittent positive-pressure breathing or incentive spirometry. Diuretic agents, digitalis glycosides, and sodium restriction may be ordered to treat cor pulmonale.

In serious illness, oxygen may be administered by cannula or mask (usually 1 to 2 qt [1 to 2 L] per minute) if the patient has chronic hypoxia or by mechanical ventilation if partial pressure of arterial oxygen falls below 40 mm Hg.

Respiratory tract infections require prompt administration of antibiotics.

COLLABORATIVE MANAGEMENT
Care of the patient with pneumoconiosis focuses on maintaining oxygenation and establishing coping strategies.

ASSESSMENT
Whether the patient has simple or complicated pneumoconiosis, his history will disclose exposure to coal dust, asbestos, or silica. In the simple form, he is typically asymptomatic, especially if he's a nonsmoker.

If the patient has complicated pneumoconiosis, he may report exertional dyspnea and a cough, occasionally producing inky black sputum (from avascular necrosis and cavitation). He may also have milky, gray, clear, or coal-flecked sputum or yellow, green, or thick sputum with recurrent bronchial and pulmonary infections. Look for:
- tachypnea, barrel chest, and clubbing of the fingers
- hyperresonant lungs with areas of dullness
- diminished breath sounds, crackles, rhonchi, and wheezes and an intensified ventricular gallop on inspiration—a hallmark of cor pulmonale.

NURSING DIAGNOSES AND COLLABORATIVE PROBLEMS
Based on the following nursing diagnoses, you'll establish patient outcomes.

Fatigue related to hypoxia caused by impaired gas exchange as a result of pneumoconiosis. The patient will:
- identify activities that cause or increase fatigue
- modify daily routine to allow rest periods
- perform self-care without fatigue.

Impaired gas exchange related to fibrotic lung tissue masses caused by pneumoconiosis. The patient will:
- maintain normal arterial blood gas values
- have no signs of hypoxia, such as irritability, restlessness, change in skin color, change in level of consciousness, or shortness of breath while at rest.

Knowledge deficit related to complex treatment regimen required to manage pneumoconiosis. The patient will:
- express an interest in learning how to manage coal worker's pneumoconiosis
- learn how to perform measures used to manage coal worker's pneumoconiosis
- verbalize an understanding of and demonstrate the skill needed to perform necessary respiratory care measures.

PLANNING AND IMPLEMENTATION
These measures help the patient with occupational lung disease:
- Help the patient adjust to lifestyle changes required by chronic illness.
- Answer his questions, and encourage him to express his concerns.
- Include the patient and family members in care-related decisions.
- Provide high-calorie, high-protein foods, and offer small, frequent meals to conserve the patient's energy and prevent fatigue.
- Encourage daily activity. Provide diversionary activities as appropriate. To conserve the patient's energy and prevent fatigue, alternate periods of rest and activity.
- Make sure the patient receives adequate fluids to loosen secretions.
- Perform chest physiotherapy, including postural drainage and chest percussion and vibration, several times daily.
- Schedule respiratory therapy at least 1 hour before or after meals. Provide mouth care after inhalation therapy.
- If the patient requires incentive spirometry, assist him to a comfortable sitting or semi-Fowler's position to promote optimal lung expansion.
- Administer medications, as prescribed. Record the patient's response to drug therapies.
- Assess for changes in baseline respiratory function. Be alert for changes in sputum quality and quantity. Watch for restlessness, increased tachypnea, and changes in breath sounds. Report these changes immediately.
- Watch for complications such as pulmonary hypertension, cor pulmonale, and tuberculosis.

Patient teaching
- Advise the patient to avoid crowds and people with known infections and to obtain influenza and pneumococcus immunizations.
- If the patient receives home oxygen therapy, explain its purpose. Teach him how to use the equipment.
- Teach the patient and family members how to perform chest physiotherapy with postural drainage and

chest percussion. Tell the patient to maintain each position for about 10 minutes and then to perform percussion and coughing exercises. Also teach him coughing and deep-breathing techniques to promote good ventilation and to remove secretions.

■ Show the patient how to use an incentive spirometer properly, and tell him why he needs it.

■ Explain the medication regimen to the patient and family members. Discuss the dosages, adverse effects, and purposes of prescribed drugs.

■ Encourage the patient to follow a high-calorie, high-protein diet and to drink plenty of fluids to prevent dehydration and help loosen secretions.

■ If the patient smokes, urge him to stop. Provide him with further information, or refer him for counseling.

■ As appropriate, provide information about coal worker's pneumoconiosis, including prevention. Educate workers and employers concerning the importance of wearing effective respirators in the workplace.

EVALUATION
Evaluation of patient outcomes determines the success of patient outcomes. For the patient with occupational lung disease, evaluation focuses on adequate oxygenation, activity tolerance, and adequate knowledge.

Pleural effusion and empyema

Normally, the pleural space contains a small amount of extracellular fluid that lubricates the pleural surfaces. But if fluid builds up from either increased production or inadequate removal, pleural effusion results. An accumulation of pus and necrotic tissue in the pleural space results in empyema, a type of pleural effusion. Blood (hemothorax) and chyle (chylothorax) may also collect in this space.

The incidence of pleural effusion increases with congestive heart failure (the most common cause), parapneumonia, cancer, and pulmonary embolism.

CAUSES
Pleural effusion may be transudative or exudative. Transudative effusions arise from congestive heart failure, hepatic disease with ascites, peritoneal dialysis, hypoalbuminemia, and disorders that increase extravascular volume. They consist of an ultrafiltrate of plasma containing a low concentration of protein. The effusion stems from an imbalance of osmotic and hydrostatic pressures. Normally, the balance of these pressures in parietal pleural capillaries causes fluid to move into the pleural space; balanced pressure in visceral pleural capillaries promotes reabsorption of this fluid. But when excessive hydrostatic pressure causes excessive fluid to pass across intact capillaries, a transudative pleural effusion results.

Exudative effusions can result from tuberculosis, subphrenic abscess, pancreatitis, bacterial or fungal pneumonitis or empyema, cancer, parapneumonia, pulmonary embolism (with or without infarction), collagen disease (lupus erythematosus and rheumatoid arthritis), myxedema, intra-abdominal abscess, esophageal perforation, and chest trauma. They occur when capillary permeability increases, with or without changes in hydrostatic and colloid osmotic pressures, allowing protein-rich fluid to leak into the pleural space.

Empyema usually stems from an infection in the pleural space. The infection may be idiopathic or may be related to pneumonitis, cancer, perforation, penetrating chest trauma, or esophageal rupture.

DIAGNOSIS AND TREATMENT
With thoracentesis, analysis of aspirated fluid can differentiate between a transudate, an exudate, and empyema. Transudative effusion usually has a specific gravity below 1.015 and less than 3 g/dl of protein. Exudative effusion usually has a ratio of protein in the fluid to serum of more than or equal to 0.5, pleural fluid lactate dehydrogenase (LD) of greater than or equal to 200 IU, and a ratio of LD in pleural fluid to LD in serum of more than or equal to 0.6.

Aspirated fluid in empyema reveals acute inflammatory white blood cells and microorganisms, showing leukocytosis. Fluid in empyema and rheumatoid arthritis (sometimes the cause of an exudative pleural effusion) shows an extremely decreased pleural fluid glucose level.

Pleural effusion from esophageal rupture or pancreatitis usually has fluid amylase levels higher than serum levels. Fluid may be tested for lupus erythematosus cells, antinuclear antibodies, and neoplastic cells. Also, it may be analyzed for color and consistency; acid-fast bacillus, fungal, and bacterial cultures; and triglycerides (in chylothorax).

Other diagnostic tests include negative tuberculin skin test or, in exudative pleural effusion, a pleural biopsy to confirm tuberculosis or cancer.

Depending on the amount of fluid present, symptomatic effusion may require thoracentesis to remove fluid or careful monitoring of the patient's own reabsorption of the fluid. Chemical pleurodesis—the instillation of a sclerosing agent through the chest tube to create adhesions between the two pleura—may prevent recurrent effusions.

The patient with empyema needs one or more chest tubes inserted after thoracentesis. These tubes allow purulent material to drain. He may also need surgical removal of the thick coating over the lung or rib resection to allow open drainage and lung expansion. He'll also require parenteral antibiotics and, if he has hypoxia, oxygen administration.

Hemothorax requires drainage to prevent fibrothorax formation.

COLLABORATIVE MANAGEMENT

Care of the patient with pleural effusion focuses on maintaining oxygenation and facilitating chest drainage.

ASSESSMENT

The patient's history characteristically shows underlying pulmonary disease. If he has a large amount of effusion, he'll typically complain of dyspnea. If he has pleurisy, he may report pleuritic chest pain. If he has empyema, he may also complain of a general feeling of malaise. Look for:

- trachea deviated away from the affected side, with empyema and fever
- decreased tactile fremitus with a large amount of effusion; dullness over the effused area that doesn't change with respiration
- diminished or absent breath sounds over the effusion and a pleural friction rub during both inspiration and expiration (disappears as fluid accumulates in the pleural space)
- bronchial breath sounds, sometimes with the patient's pronunciation of the letter *e* sounding like the letter *a*.

NURSING DIAGNOSES AND COLLABORATIVE PROBLEMS

Based on the following nursing diagnoses, you'll establish patient outcomes.

Risk for infection related to introduction of foreign object (thoracentesis needle, chest tube, or both) into chest cavity. The patient will:

- maintain a normal temperature and white blood cell count
- develop no empyema; if empyema is already present, it won't become worse following invasive treatment.

Impaired gas exchange related to ineffective breathing pattern. The patient will:

- maintain adequate ventilation with treatment
- have no signs or symptoms of hypoxia
- regain and maintain normal arterial blood gas (ABG) values.

Ineffective breathing pattern related to compromised lung expansion. The patient will:

- report the ability to breathe comfortably with effective treatment

- perform activities of daily living without dyspnea
- regain his normal breathing pattern when the condition is eradicated.

Anxiety related to diagnosis and lack of knowledge. The patient will:

- verbalize fears and concerns
- demonstrate positive coping skills.

PLANNING AND IMPLEMENTATION

These measures help the patient with pleural effusion:

- Administer oxygen and, in empyema, antibiotics, as ordered. Record the patient's response to these care measures.
- Encourage deep-breathing exercises and use of an incentive spirometer to promote deep breathing and lung expansion.
- After thoracentesis, watch for respiratory distress and signs of pneumothorax (sudden onset of dyspnea and cyanosis).
- Monitor the patient's respiratory status frequently. Obtain ABG analysis if signs and symptoms of hypoxia develop.
- Ensure chest tube patency by watching for fluctuations in the tubing. Record the amount, color, and consistency of any tube drainage.
- Follow your facility's policy for milking the tube. Keep petroleum gauze at the bedside in case of chest tube dislodgment.
- Don't clamp the chest tube; doing so may cause tension pneumothorax.
- Provide meticulous chest tube care, and use aseptic technique for changing dressings around the tube insertion site in the patient with empyema.
- If the patient has open drainage through a rib resection or intercostal tube, use contact precautions. The patient usually needs weeks of such drainage to obliterate the space, so make home health nurse referrals if he'll be discharged with the tube in place.
- Throughout therapy, listen to the patient's fears and concerns and remain with him during periods of extreme stress and anxiety. Encourage him to identify care measures and actions that will make him comfortable and relaxed. Then, try to perform these measures and encourage the patient to do so, too.

Patient teaching

- Explain all tests and procedures to the patient, including thoracentesis, and answer his questions.
- Before thoracentesis, tell the patient to expect a stinging sensation from the local anesthetic and a feeling of pressure when the needle is inserted. Instruct him to tell you immediately if he feels uncomfortable or has trouble breathing during the procedure.

- If the patient developed pleural effusion because of pneumonia or influenza, tell him to seek medical attention promptly whenever he gets a chest cold.
- Teach the patient the signs and symptoms of respiratory distress and when to notify his doctor.
- Fully explain the medication regimen, including adverse effects. Emphasize the importance of completing the prescribed drug regimen.
- If the patient smokes, urge him to stop.

EVALUATION
Evaluation of patient outcomes determines the success of collaborative management. For the patient with pleural effusion, evaluation focuses on adequate oxygenation and absence of infection.

Pneumonia

An acute infection of the lung parenchyma that commonly impairs gas exchange, pneumonia can be classified in several ways: It may be viral, bacterial, fungal, protozoal, mycobacterial, mycoplasmal, or rickettsial in origin.

Based on location, pneumonia may be classified as bronchopneumonia, lobular pneumonia, or lobar pneumonia. Bronchopneumonia involves distal airways and alveoli; lobular pneumonia, part of a lobe; and lobar pneumonia, an entire lobe.

Additionally, the infection can be classified as primary, secondary, or aspiration pneumonia. Primary pneumonia results directly from inhalation or aspiration of a pathogen and includes pneumococcal and viral pneumonia. Secondary pneumonia may follow initial lung damage from a noxious chemical or other insult (superinfection) or a hematogenous spread of bacteria from a distant area. Aspiration pneumonia starts with inhalation of foreign matter, such as vomitus or food particles.

Pneumonia occurs in both sexes and at all ages. More than 3 million cases of pneumonia occur annually in the United States. The infection carries a good prognosis for patients with normal lungs and adequate immune systems. In debilitated patients, however, bacterial pneumonia ranks as the leading cause of death. Pneumonia is also the leading cause of death from infectious disease.

CAUSES
Certain predisposing factors increase the risk of pneumonia. For bacterial and viral pneumonia, these include chronic illness and debilitation, cancer (particularly lung cancer), abdominal and thoracic surgery, atelectasis, common colds or other viral respiratory infections, chronic respiratory disease (chronic obstructive pulmonary disease, asthma, bronchiectasis, cystic fibrosis), influenza, smoking, malnutrition, alcoholism, sickle cell disease, tracheostomy, exposure to noxious gases, aspiration, and immunosuppressant therapy.

Aspiration pneumonia is more likely to occur in older adults or debilitated patients, those receiving nasogastric (NG) tube feedings, and those with an impaired gag reflex, poor oral hygiene, or a decreased level of consciousness.

In bacterial pneumonia, in any part of the lungs, an infection initially triggers alveolar inflammation and edema. Capillaries become engorged with blood, causing stasis. As the alveolocapillary membrane breaks down, alveoli fill with blood and exudate, resulting in atelectasis. In severe bacterial infections, the lungs assume a heavy, liverlike appearance, as in adult respiratory distress syndrome (ARDS).

Viral infection, which typically causes diffuse pneumonia, first attacks bronchiolar epithelial cells, causing interstitial inflammation and desquamation. It then spreads to the alveoli, which fill with blood and fluid. In advanced infection, a hyaline membrane may form. As with bacterial infection, severe viral infection may clinically resemble ARDS.

In aspiration pneumonia, gastric juices or hydrocarbons trigger similar inflammatory changes and inactivate surfactant over a large area, leading to alveolar collapse. Acidic gastric juices may directly damage the airways and alveoli. Particles in the aspirated gastric juices may obstruct the airways and reduce airflow, which in turn leads to secondary bacterial pneumonia.

DIAGNOSIS AND TREATMENT
Confirming tests include chest X-rays to disclose infiltrates. Sputum specimen for Gram stain and culture and sensitivity tests show acute inflammatory cells. Cultures help determine the causative organism. Other tests include white blood cell count, arterial blood gas (ABG) analysis, and pulse oximetry. Bronchoscopy with bronchoalveolar lavage or transtracheal aspiration allows the collection of material for culture.

The patient needs antimicrobial therapy, based on the causative agent. Therapy should be reevaluated early in the course of treatment. (See *Managing uncomplicated pneumonia*, pages 158 and 159.)

Supportive measures include humidified oxygen therapy for hypoxia, bronchodilator therapy, antitussives, mechanical ventilation for respiratory failure, a high-calorie diet and adequate fluid intake, bed rest, and an analgesic to relieve pleuritic chest pain. A patient with severe pneumonia who's on mechanical ventilation may need positive end-expiratory pressure to maintain adequate oxygenation.

COLLABORATIVE MANAGEMENT

Care of the patient with pneumonia focuses on maintaining oxygenation and preventing complications.

ASSESSMENT

In bacterial pneumonia, the patient may report pleuritic chest pain, a cough, excessive sputum production, and chills. Look for:
- fever and shakes
- sputum that is creamy yellow, suggesting staphylococcal pneumonia
- green sputum, denoting *Pseudomonas* organisms
- sputum with currant-jelly appearance, indicating *Klebsiella*
- clear sputum, indicating there's no infective process
- dullness when you percuss, in advanced cases of all types of pneumonia
- crackles, wheezing, or rhonchi over the affected lung area as well as decreased breath sounds and decreased vocal fremitus.

NURSING DIAGNOSES AND COLLABORATIVE PROBLEMS

Based on the following nursing diagnoses, you'll establish patient outcomes.

Risk for infection related to potential for sepsis, lung abscess, and other complications. The patient will:
- develop no signs or symptoms of a second infection, such as neurologic dysfunction (suggestive of meningitis) or cardiac dysfunction (suggestive of endocarditis)
- comply with the prescribed treatment to limit pneumonia's severity and minimize the potential for other infections.

Impaired gas exchange related to acute infection of the lung parenchyma. The patient will:
- maintain his respiratory rate within 5 breaths of baseline
- regain and maintain normal blood gas levels
- express feelings of comfort in maintaining air exchange with treatment.

Ineffective airway clearance related to thick sputum production. The patient will:
- use correct bronchial hygiene to facilitate sputum removal
- consume sufficient fluids to decrease sputum thickness
- cough and expectorate sputum effectively
- maintain a patent airway.

Risk for complications related to progression of disease and treatment. The patient will:

- remain free from any complications
- demonstrate measures to reduce the risk of complications.

PLANNING AND IMPLEMENTATION

These measures help the patient with pneumonia:
- Administer supplemental oxygen if the patient's partial pressure of oxygen in arterial blood falls below 55 to 60 mm Hg. If he has an underlying chronic lung disease, give oxygen cautiously.
- In severe pneumonia that requires endotracheal intubation or a tracheostomy, provide thorough respiratory care and suction often.
- Monitor the patient's ABG levels, especially if he's hypoxic.
- Assess the patient's respiratory status. Auscultate breath sounds at least every 4 hours.
- Obtain sputum specimens as needed, using suction if necessary.
- Administer antibiotics, as prescribed, and pain medication, as needed.
- Administer I.V. fluids and electrolyte replacement, if needed, for fever and dehydration.
- Evaluate the effectiveness of medications, and check the patient for adverse reactions.
- Provide a high-calorie, high-protein diet of soft foods to offset the calories the patient uses to fight the infection. If necessary, supplement oral feedings with NG tube feedings or parenteral nutrition.
- Monitor fluid intake and output and nutritional intake.
- To prevent aspiration during NG tube feedings, elevate the patient's head, and check the tube position. Administer a moderate volume slowly to avoid causing vomiting.
- If the patient has an endotracheal tube, inflate the tube cuff before feeding. Keep his head elevated for at least ½ hour after feeding.
- To control the spread of infection, dispose of secretions properly. Tell the patient to sneeze and cough into a disposable tissue, and tape a waxed bag to the side of the bed for used tissues.
- Provide a quiet, calm environment, with frequent rest periods. Make sure the patient has diversionary activities appropriate to his age.
- Listen to the patient's fears and concerns, and remain with him during periods of severe stress and anxiety. Encourage him to identify actions and care measures that promote comfort and relaxation.
- Whenever possible, include the patient in decisions about his care.
- Include family members in all phases of the patient's care, and encourage them to visit.

(Text continues on page 160.)

CLINICAL PATH

Managing uncomplicated pneumonia

DRG#: 481
Average length of stay (LOS): 8 days
Actual LOS:
Initiation date:
Exclusions: Patients in ICU; blood cultures; severe COPD

	Day 1 (Admission)	Days 2 to 3
MEDICAL INTERVENTIONS	■ History and physical: Evaluation for fever, dyspnea, cough, sputum, I.V. drug abuse, alcohol use, tobacco use, epidemiological history ■ Supplemental oxygen; nebulizer treatments, if wheezing ■ Blood and sputum cultures ■ Antipyretics, expectorants, antibiotics ■ I.V. fluids ■ Possible respiratory isolation to rule out tuberculosis ■ Review of standing medications	■ Daily assessment; evaluation for recovery, effectiveness of antibiotics ■ Lab culture assessment for results, sensitivities ■ Antibiotic adjustment, as needed ■ Continued supplemental oxygen, as needed
NURSING INTERVENTIONS	■ Complete database. ■ Measure pulse oximetry every 4 to 8 hr. ■ Check vital signs every 4 hrs if temperature exceeds 101° F. ■ Assess breath sounds and respiratory symptoms every shift. ■ Ensure that blood and sputum samples are collected for culture before starting antibiotics.	■ Evaluate patient recovery, ability to perform activities of daily living (ADLs). ■ Check vital signs every shift (or every 4 hr if abnormal). ■ Assess breath sounds every shift. ■ Measure pulse oximetry every shift if needed.
SOCIAL WORK	■ Response to assessed need if patient has inadequate support systems or needs assistance with discharge	■ Continued screening for additional support, as necessary
NUTRITION	■ Regular diet as tolerated, or special diet	■ Regular or special diet
TESTS	■ Admission bloodwork: blood chemistries, complete blood count (CBC), liver function tests, chest X-ray (CXR), electrocardiogram (ECG) ■ Acute serology for patient with atypical pneumonia ■ Urinalysis (UA), urine and sputum culture and sensitivity, two blood cultures, Gram stain	■ Bronchoscopy or computed tomography (CT) if postobstructive pneumonia develops
CONSULTS	■ Respiratory therapy (nebulizers, chest physiotherapy, oxygen) ■ Pulmonary consult as needed	■ Ensure that ordered consults are obtained. ■ Arrange for physical therapy as needed.
ACTIVITY	■ Keep patient on bed rest; allow up as tolerated. ■ Assess for fall risk if unsteady.	■ Allow patient up as tolerated. ■ Assess for fall risk, if unsteady.
PATIENT EDUCATION	■ Assist patient to identify pertinent signs and symptoms. ■ Discuss disease process, signs and symptoms, risk factors. ■ Assess prior compliance. ■ Instruct in coughing and deep breathing; assess return demonstration.	■ Continue planned education.
DISCHARGE PLANNING	■ Assess learning needs: risk factors, preventive measures (pneumococcal and influenza vaccines, hand washing, tissue disposal.	■ Discuss influence of environmental factors on illness. ■ Discuss dietary, drug, and activity regimens.
KEY PATIENT OUTCOMES	■ Pulse oximetry >90% *Date met* _____ *Not met* _____ *Initials* _____ ■ Respiratory rate 16 to 20 *Date met* _____ *Not met* _____ *Initials* _____ ■ Decreased anxiety, shortness of breath *Date met* _____ *Not met* _____ *Initials* _____	■ Pulse oximetry >90% *Date met* _____ *Not met* _____ *Initials* _____ ■ Respiratory rate 16 to 20 *Date met* _____ *Not met* _____ *Initials* _____ ■ Decreased anxiety, shortness of breath *Date met* _____ *Not met* _____ *Initials* _____ ■ Temperature <100° F *Date met* _____ *Not met* _____ *Initials* _____
	SIGNATURE _____	**SIGNATURE** _____

Adapted with permission from Veterans Affairs Maryland Health Care System at Baltimore.

Days 4 to 6	**Day 7**	**Day 8**
■ Daily assessment ■ Assessment for home oxygen; order, as needed ■ Possible discontinuation of pulse oximetry ■ Referral to physical therapy (PT) or occupational therapy (OT) if patient needs assistance with ADLs	■ I.V. to oral antibiotics ■ Discharge plan: Send prescriptions to pharmacy, arrange follow-up clinic appointment(s), consider repeat CXR ■ Patient notification of planned discharge so he can arrange transportation	■ Discharge when patient is afebrile for 24 hr on oral antibiotics ■ Discharge-summary dictation ■ Appropriate follow-up arrangements ■ Discharge instructions discussed with patient and caregiver ■ Written order for discharge
■ Assess patient daily. ■ Check vital signs every shift.	■ Verify patient's ability to transfer, ambulate, perform ADLs. ■ Recommend PT or OT if not previously addressed. ■ Arrange for prosthetic equipment if needed.	■ Attach discharge note to discharge/transfer sheet. ■ Complete education.
■ Complete insurance form for home oxygen, if necessary.	■ Assist in travel arrangements for discharge if necessary.	■ Provide transportation as needed.
■ Regular or special diet	■ Regular or special diet	■ Evaluation of patient tolerance for routine diet
■ Draw specimens for CBC, blood chemistry.		
■ Arrange for PT or OT as needed.		
■ Verify patient's baseline performance, ability to perform ADLs.	■ Allow activity as tolerated.	■ Evaluate return to baseline function.
■ Assess knowledge learned. ■ Reinforce knowledge as needed.	■ Assess knowledge learned. ■ Reinforce knowledge as needed. ■ Add new teaching as patient and caregiver are able to absorb previous teaching.	
■ Evaluate need for prosthetic equipment, such as a cane or walker.		■ Patient and caregiver aware of follow-up for repeat CXR, clinic contact name, telephone number, how to refill prescriptions.
■ Patient aware of behaviors needed for home health management: drugs, activity, diet, smoking cessation, removal of environmental factors. *Date met*____*Not met*____*Initials*____	■ Pulse oximetry > 88% or home oxygen arranged *Date met*____*Not met*____*Initials*____ ■ Absence of adventitious breath sounds *Date met*____*Not met*____*Initials*____ ■ Temperature < 100° F *Date met*____*Not met*____*Initials*____ ■ Patient aware of planned discharge on next day *Date met*____*Not met*____*Initials*____	Discharge to home with: ■ Pulse oximetry >88% or home oxygen arranged ■ Patient afebrile off I.V. antibiotics *Date met*____*Not met*____*Initials*____
SIGNATURE _____	**SIGNATURE** _____	**SIGNATURE** _____

Patient teaching

■ Explain all procedures (especially intubation and suctioning) to the patient and family members.
■ Emphasize the importance of adequate rest to promote full recovery and prevent a relapse. Explain that the doctor will advise the patient when he can resume full activity and return to work.
■ Review the patient's medication. Stress the need to take the entire course of medication, even if he feels better, to prevent a relapse.
■ Teach the patient procedures and therapies for clearing lung secretions, such as deep-breathing and coughing exercises as well as home oxygen therapy. Explain deep breathing and pursed-lip breathing.
■ Urge the patient to drink 2 to 3 qt (2 to 3 L) of fluid a day to maintain adequate hydration and keep mucus secretions thin for easier removal.
■ Teach the patient and family members about chest physiotherapy. Explain that postural drainage, percussion, and vibration help to mobilize and remove mucus from the lungs.
■ Urge all bedridden and postoperative patients to perform deep-breathing and coughing exercises frequently. Position such patients properly to promote full aeration and drainage of secretions.
■ Advise patients to avoid using antibiotics indiscriminately for minor infections. Doing so could result in upper airway colonization with antibiotic-resistant bacteria. If pneumonia develops, the organisms that produce the pneumonia may require treatment with more toxic antibiotics.
■ Encourage the high-risk patient to ask his doctor about an annual influenza vaccination and the pneumococcal pneumonia vaccination, which the patient would receive only once.
■ Urge the patient to avoid irritants that stimulate secretions, such as cigarette smoke, dust, and significant environmental pollution. If necessary, refer him to community programs or agencies that can help him stop smoking.
■ Discuss ways to avoid spreading the infection to others. Remind the patient to sneeze and cough into tissues and to dispose of the tissues in a waxed or plastic bag. Advise him to wash his hands thoroughly after handling contaminated tissues.

EVALUATION

Evaluation of patient outcomes determines the success of collaborative management. For the patient with pneumonia, evaluation focuses on adequate oxygenation, prevention of complications, and adequate knowledge.

Pneumothorax

An accumulation of air or gas between the parietal and visceral pleurae characterizes pneumothorax. The amount of air or gas trapped in the intrapleural space determines the degree of lung collapse. The most common types of pneumothorax are open, closed, and tension.

CAUSES

Pneumothorax results from a break in the chest wall, or the lung, allowing air into the pleural space. Open pneumothorax, also called an open or sucking chest wound, occurs with penetrating wounds, insertion of a central venous catheter, chest surgery, transbronchial biopsy, thoracentesis, or closed pleural biopsy.

Blunt chest trauma may cause a closed pneumothorax, when the chest wall is intact, but the trauma ruptures the lung wall and air leaks. Closed pneumothorax can also occur with rupture by high intrathoracic pressures during mechanical ventilation. Spontaneous pneumothorax, another type of closed pneumothorax, is more common in men than in women. It's common in older patients with chronic pulmonary disease, but may affect healthy, tall, young adults. Causes include ruptured congenital blebs, ruptured emphysematous bullae, and erosion of tubercular or cancerous lesions into the pleural space.

Tension pneumothorax, where the air in the pleural space is under higher pressure than in adjacent lung and vascular structures, occurs with penetrating chest wounds treated with an airtight dressing, and occlusion or malfunction of a chest tube. It can also arise during mechanical ventilation, when a fractured rib punctures a lung; following a chest injury; and with high-level positive end-expiratory pressure that ruptures alveolar blebs.

In an open pneumothorax, air flows directly into the pleural cavity. As the air pressure in the pleural cavity becomes positive, the lung collapses on the affected side, resulting in substantially decreased total lung capacity, vital capacity, and lung compliance. The resulting ventilation-perfusion imbalances lead to hypoxia.

With a closed pneumothorax, air enters the pleural space from within the lung, causing increased pleural pressure and preventing lung expansion during normal inspiration. Both types of closed pneumothorax, traumatic and spontaneous, can result in a collapsed lung with hypoxia and decreased total lung capacity, vital capacity, and lung compliance. The total amount of lung collapse can range from 5% to 95%.

In tension pneumothorax, air in the pleural space is under higher pressure than air in adjacent lung and vascular structures. The air cannot escape, and the accumulating pressure causes the lung to collapse. As air continues to accumulate and intrapleural pressures rise, the mediastinum shifts away from the affected side and decreases venous return. This forces the heart, trachea, esophagus, and great vessels to the unaffected side, compressing the heart and the contralateral lung. Without immediate treatment, the patient can rapidly die.

DIAGNOSIS AND TREATMENT

Chest X-rays reveal air in the pleural space and, possibly, a mediastinal shift, confirming the diagnosis. Arterial blood gas (ABG) studies may show hypoxemia, possibly accompanied by respiratory acidosis and hypercapnia. Arterial oxygen saturation levels may fall initially but typically return to normal within 24 hours.

Typically, treatment is conservative for spontaneous pneumothorax with no signs of increased pleural pressure (indicating tension pneumothorax), with lung collapse less than 30%, and with no dyspnea or other indications of physiologic compromise. Such treatment consists of bed rest, careful monitoring (blood pressure and pulse and respiratory rates), oxygen administration and, possibly, aspiration of air with a large-bore needle attached to a syringe.

If more than 30% of the lung collapses, treatment to reexpand the lung includes placing a thoracostomy tube in the second or third intercostal space in the midclavicular line. The thoracostomy tube then connects to an underwater seal or to low-pressure suction.

Recurring spontaneous pneumothorax requires thoracotomy and pleurectomy. These procedures prevent recurrence by causing the lung to adhere to the parietal pleura.

Traumatic and tension pneumothorax require chest tube drainage; traumatic pneumothorax may also require surgical repair. Analgesics may be prescribed.

COLLABORATIVE MANAGEMENT

Care of the patient with a pneumothorax focuses on maintaining oxygenation and relieving pain and anxiety.

ASSESSMENT

The patient history reveals sudden, sharp, pleuritic pain. He may report that chest movement, breathing, and coughing exacerbate the pain. He may also report shortness of breath. Look for:

- asymmetrical chest wall movement with overexpansion and rigidity on the affected side
- cyanotic appearance
- in tension pneumothorax, distended neck veins, pallor, and anxiety. (The presence of these signs confirms increased central venous pressure.)
- crackling beneath the skin, indicating subcutaneous emphysema (air in tissues) and decreased vocal fremitus
- decreased or absent breath sounds over the collapsed lung
- hypotension with tension pneumothorax
- no signs or symptoms with spontaneous pneumothorax, which releases only a small amount of air into the pleural space
- in tension pneumothorax, tracheal deviation away from the affected side and a weak and rapid pulse. Percussion may demonstrate hyperresonance on the affected side.

NURSING DIAGNOSES AND COLLABORATIVE PROBLEMS

Based on the following nursing diagnoses, you'll establish patient outcomes.

Altered tissue perfusion related to decreased oxygen availability in blood. The patient will:
- restrict his activities to reduce tissue oxygen need until pneumothorax is resolved
- exhibit no signs or symptoms of tissue hypoxia.

Impaired gas exchange related to air trapped in pleural space impeding lung expansion. The patient will:
- regain and maintain adequate ventilation with prompt treatment
- regain and maintain normal ABG levels
- show resolution of pneumothorax on chest X-ray with treatment.

Pain related to air pressure change in pleural cavity. The patient will:
- express feelings of chest comfort following analgesic administration
- sit upright to increase comfort
- become pain free with resolution of pneumothorax.

Knowledge deficit related to disease and its treatment. The patient will:
- verbalize information related to pneumothorax and its treatment
- state signs and symptoms to doctor.

PLANNING AND IMPLEMENTATION

These measures help the patient with pneumothorax:
- Keep the patient as comfortable as possible (usually sitting upright), and administer analgesics as necessary. Painful respirations will be shallow and have poor gas exchange.

■ Assess the patient's respiratory status. Monitor ABG levels regularly, as prescribed.

■ Watch for complications, signaled by pallor, gasping respirations, and sudden chest pain. Carefully monitor vital signs at least every hour for indications of shock, increasing respiratory distress, or mediastinal shift. Listen for breath sounds over both lungs.

■ Watch for signs of tension pneumothorax (especially if the patient has chest tubes inserted). These include falling blood pressure and rising pulse and respiratory rates, which could be fatal without prompt treatment.

■ Assess the effectiveness of analgesics, and monitor for adverse reactions.

■ Listen to the patient's fears and concerns. Offer reassurance as appropriate. Include the patient and family members in care decisions whenever possible.

■ Reassure the patient. Explain pneumothorax, its causes, and all diagnostic tests and procedures.

■ If the patient is having surgery or chest tubes inserted, explain why he needs these procedures. Reassure him that the chest tubes will make him more comfortable.

Patient teaching

■ Encourage the patient to perform deep-breathing exercises every waking hour.

■ Discuss the potential for recurrent spontaneous pneumothorax, and review its signs and symptoms. Emphasize the need for immediate medical intervention if these should occur.

EVALUATION

Evaluation of patient outcomes determines the success of collaborative management. For the patient with pneumothorax, evaluation focuses on adequate oxygenation and tissue perfusion, pain relief, and adequate knowledge.

Pulmonary embolism

An obstruction of the pulmonary arterial bed, pulmonary embolism occurs when a mass—such as a dislodged thrombus—lodges in a pulmonary artery branch, partially or completely obstructing it. This causes a ventilation-perfusion mismatch, resulting in hypoxemia as well as intrapulmonary shunting.

Pulmonary embolism strikes approximately 500,000 adults each year in the United States, causing 50,000 deaths. The prognosis varies. Although the pulmonary infarction that results from embolism may be so mild as to be asymptomatic, massive embolism (more than 50% obstruction of pulmonary arterial circulation) and infarction can cause rapid death.

CAUSES

In most patients, pulmonary embolism results from a dislodged thrombus that originates in the leg veins. More than half of such thrombi arise in the deep veins of the legs; usually, multiple thrombi arise. Other, less common sources of thrombi include the pelvic, renal, and hepatic veins, the right side of the heart, and the upper extremities.

In rare cases, pulmonary embolism results from other types of emboli, including bone, air, fat, amniotic fluid, tumor cells, or a foreign object, such as a needle, catheter part, or talc from drugs intended for oral administration that are injected I.V. by addicts. (See *Who's at risk for pulmonary embolism?*)

A thrombus results from vascular wall damage, venous stasis, or hypercoagulability of the blood. Trauma, clot dissolution, sudden muscle spasm, intravascular pressure changes, or a change in peripheral blood flow can cause the thrombus to loosen or fragment. The thrombus—now called an embolus—then floats to the heart's right side and enters the lung through the pulmonary artery. There, the embolus may dissolve, continue to fragment, or grow.

By occluding the pulmonary artery, the embolus prevents alveoli from producing enough surfactant to maintain alveolar integrity. As a result, alveoli collapse and atelectasis develops. If the embolus enlarges, it may clog most or all of the pulmonary vessels and cause death.

DIAGNOSIS AND TREATMENT

Diagnostic tests include a lung perfusion scan and a ventilation scan (usually performed together). Pulmonary angiography, although the most definitive test, is only used if the diagnosis can't be confirmed any other way and anticoagulant therapy would put the patient at significant risk. Electrocardiography helps distinguish pulmonary embolism from myocardial infarction and a chest X-ray helps rule out other pulmonary disease. Other tests include arterial blood gas (ABG) analysis and magnetic resonance imaging.

The goals of treatment are to maintain adequate cardiovascular and pulmonary function until the obstruction resolves and to prevent any recurrence. Most emboli resolve within 10 to 14 days.

Treatment for an embolism caused by a thrombus usually consists of oxygen therapy, as needed, and anticoagulation with heparin to inhibit new thrombus formation. The patient on heparin therapy needs daily coagulation studies (partial thromboplastin time [PTT]). He may also receive warfarin for 3 to 6 months, depending on his risk factors; if so, his prothrombin time (PT) will be monitored daily and then biweekly.

Fibrinolytic therapy with urokinase, streptokinase, or alteplase may be needed if the patient has a massive pulmonary embolism and undergoes shock. Initially, these thrombolytic agents dissolve clots within 12 to 24 hours. Seven days later, they lyse clots to the same degree as heparin therapy alone.

Vasopressors are used if the embolus causes hypotension.

Antibiotics, not anticoagulants, are needed if the patient has a septic embolus, along with evaluation for the infection's source (most likely endocarditis).

An umbrella filter, inserted into the vena cava, may be necessary if the patient can't take anticoagulants or develops recurrent emboli during anticoagulant therapy. The umbrella device filters blood returning to the heart and lungs.

Rotating compression stockings may be applied to the patient's legs to prevent postoperative venous thromboembolism. Or he may be given a combination of heparin and dihydroergotamine, which is more effective than heparin alone.

The patient with a fat embolus needs oxygen therapy. He may also need mechanical ventilation, corticosteroids and, if pulmonary edema arises, diuretics.

COLLABORATIVE MANAGEMENT
Care of the patient with a pulmonary embolus focuses on maintaining adequate anticoagulation and preventing complications.

ASSESSMENT
The patient's history may reveal a predisposing condition. Look for:
■ complaints of shortness of breath for no apparent reason as well as pleuritic or anginal pain
■ tachycardia with low-grade fever
■ with circulatory collapse, a weak, rapid pulse rate and hypotension
■ a cough that produces blood-tinged sputum
■ less commonly, chest splinting, massive hemoptysis, leg edema, and, with a large embolus, cyanosis, syncope, and distended neck veins
■ with circulatory collapse, restlessness—a sign of hypoxia
■ a warm, tender area in the extremities, a possible area of thrombosis
■ transient pleural friction rub and crackles at the embolus site
■ an S_3 and S_4 gallop, with increased intensity of the pulmonic component of S_2

In pleural infarction, the patient's history may include heart disease and left-sided (or systolic) heart failure. He may complain of sudden, sharp pleuritic

Who's at risk for pulmonary embolism?

Many disorders and treatments heighten the risk of pulmonary embolism. At particular risk are surgical patients. For example, the anesthetic used during surgery can injure lung vessels, and surgery itself or prolonged bed rest can promote venous stasis, which compounds the risk.

Predisposing disorders
■ Autoimmune hemolytic anemia
■ Cardiac disorders and procedures, especially heart failure, atrial fibrillation, cardiac arrest, defibrillation, or cardioversion
■ Diabetes mellitus
■ Infection
■ Long-bone fracture
■ Lung disorders, especially chronic types
■ Osteomyelitis
■ Polycythemia vera
■ Sickle cell disease
■ History of thromboembolism, thrombophlebitis, thrombocytosis, or vascular insufficiency
■ Varicose veins

Venous stasis
■ Age over 40
■ Burns
■ Obesity
■ Orthopedic casts
■ Pregnancy or recent childbirth
■ Prolonged bed rest or immobilization

Venous injury
■ I.V. drug abuse
■ I.V. therapy
■ Leg or pelvic fractures or injuries
■ Surgery, particularly of the legs, pelvis, abdomen, or thorax

Increased blood coagulability
■ Cancer
■ High-estrogen oral contraceptives

chest pain accompanied by progressive dyspnea. The patient may have a fever and cough up blood-tinged sputum. Auscultation may reveal a pleural friction rub.

NURSING DIAGNOSES AND COLLABORATIVE PROBLEMS
Based on the following nursing diagnosis, you'll establish patient outcomes.

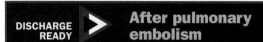

DISCHARGE READY > **After pulmonary embolism**

After treatment for pulmonary embolism, the patient will meet the following criteria before discharge:

- heparin discontinued, and patient receiving maintenance dose of oral warfarin*
- anticoagulation at therapeutic level (International Normalized Ratio between 2 and 3)*
- oxygen saturation >95% on room air
- no signs of bleeding
- medication list and written instructions for administration given to patient
- verbalized understanding of anticoagulation precautions and signs and symptoms to report to the doctor
- appointment made for ongoing labwork to monitor anticoagulation
- follow-up doctor appointment made.

* Some patients may be discharged on home I.V. heparin therapy and oral warfarin. The home infusion agency and the doctor monitor the conversion from I.V. heparin to oral anticoagulant therapy.

Altered cardiopulmonary perfusion related to obstruction of pulmonary artery. The patient will:
- regain and maintain cardiopulmonary tissue perfusion and cellular oxygenation
- show no signs and symptoms of pulmonary infarction or emboli extension
- eliminate risk factors, when possible, to prevent recurrence.
   Anxiety related to situational crisis. The patient will:
- express his feelings of anxiety
- cope with his condition without showing signs of severe anxiety.
   Impaired gas exchange related to collapsed alveoli. The patient will:
- regain and maintain adequate ventilation
- regain and maintain normal ABG levels
- show no signs and symptoms of severe hypoxia.

PLANNING AND IMPLEMENTATION
These measures help the patient with pulmonary embolus:
- Administer the anticoagulant heparin, as ordered, by I.V. push or by continuous drip. Don't administer I.M. injections.
- Monitor coagulation studies daily. Effective heparin therapy raises PTT to about 2½ times normal.

- During heparin therapy, watch closely for epistaxis, petechiae, and other signs of abnormal bleeding. Also check the patient's stools for occult blood.
- Watch for possible anticoagulant treatment complications, including gastric bleeding, cerebrovascular accident, and hemorrhage.
- As ordered, give oxygen by nasal cannula or mask. If breathing is severely compromised, provide endotracheal intubation with assisted ventilation, as ordered.
- If the patient has pleuritic chest pain, administer the prescribed analgesic.
- If needed, provide incentive spirometry to help the patient with deep breathing. Provide tissues and a bag for easy disposal of tissues.
- Monitor the patient's respiratory status closely. If he has worsening dyspnea, check his ABG levels.
- After the patient's condition stabilizes, encourage him to move about and assist him with isometric and range-of-motion exercises. Never vigorously massage his legs; doing so could cause thrombi to dislodge.
- If the patient needs surgery, make sure he ambulates as soon as possible afterward to prevent venous stasis.
- Check the patient's temperature and the color of his feet to detect venous stasis.

Patient teaching
- Explain all procedures and treatments to the patient and his family members.
- Teach the patient and his family members the signs and symptoms of thrombophlebitis and pulmonary embolism.
- Teach the patient on anticoagulant therapy the signs of bleeding (bloody stools, blood in urine, large bruises).
- Tell the patient he can help prevent bleeding by shaving with an electric razor and by brushing his teeth with a soft toothbrush.
- Make sure the patient understands the importance of taking his medication exactly as ordered. Tell him not to take any other medications, especially aspirin, without asking the doctor.
- Teach the patient taking warfarin not to significantly vary the amount of vitamin K he takes in daily. Doing so could interfere with anticoagulation stabilization.
- Stress the importance of follow-up laboratory tests, such as PT, to monitor anticoagulant therapy.
- Tell the patient that he must inform all his health care providers—including dentists—that he's receiving anticoagulant therapy.
- To prevent pulmonary emboli in a high-risk patient, encourage him to walk and exercise his legs,

wear support or antiembolism stockings, and avoid crossing or massaging his legs.

EVALUATION

Evaluation of patient outcomes determines the success of collaborative management. For the patient with a pulmonary embolism, evaluation focuses on adequate circulation, oxygenation, and knowledge. (See *After pulmonary embolism.*)

Respiratory acidosis

This acid-base disturbance is characterized by reduced alveolar ventilation and manifested by hypercapnia (partial pressure of arterial carbon dioxide greater than 45 mm Hg). Respiratory acidosis can be acute (resulting from sudden failure in ventilation) or chronic (resulting from long-term pulmonary disease).

The prognosis depends on the severity of the underlying disturbance and the patient's general clinical condition.

CAUSES

Factors that predispose a patient to respiratory acidosis include:
- drugs, such as narcotics, anesthetics, hypnotics, and sedatives, which depress the respiratory control center's sensitivity
- central nervous system (CNS) trauma, such as medullary injury, which may impair ventilatory drive
- chronic metabolic alkalosis, which may occur when respiratory compensatory mechanisms attempt to normalize pH by decreasing alveolar ventilation
- myasthenia gravis and poliomyelitis, in which respiratory muscles fail to respond properly to respiratory drive, reducing alveolar ventilation.

In addition, respiratory acidosis can result from an airway obstruction or parenchymal lung disease that interferes with alveolar ventilation or from chronic obstructive pulmonary disease (COPD), asthma, severe adult respiratory distress syndrome, chronic bronchitis, large pneumothorax, extensive pneumonia, and pulmonary edema.

Respiratory acidosis progresses through six basic steps, with the patient displaying specific signs and symptoms at each step. (See *What happens in respiratory acidosis,* page 166.)

DIAGNOSIS AND TREATMENT

For typical test results, see *Respiratory acidosis: Key abnormal test values,* page 167.

Treatment aims to correct the source of alveolar hypoventilation. If alveolar ventilation is significantly reduced, the patient may need mechanical ventilation until the underlying condition can be treated. This includes bronchodilators, oxygen, and antibiotics in COPD; drug therapy for conditions such as myasthenia gravis; removal of foreign bodies from the airway in cases of obstruction; antibiotics for pneumonia; dialysis to eliminate toxic drugs; and correction of metabolic alkalosis.

Dangerously low pH levels (less than 7.15) can produce profound CNS and cardiovascular deterioration and may require administration of I.V. sodium bicarbonate. In chronic lung disease, elevated CO_2 levels may persist despite treatment.

COLLABORATIVE MANAGEMENT

Care of the patient with respiratory acidosis focuses on maintaining ventilation and oxygenation and relieving anxiety.

ASSESSMENT

The patient may initially complain of headache and dyspnea. He may also have a predisposing condition for respiratory acidosis. Look for:
- patient who's dyspneic and diaphoretic and may report nausea and vomiting
- bounding pulses
- rapid, shallow respirations, tachycardia and, possibly, hypotension
- ophthalmoscopic evidence of papilledema
- a level of consciousness (LOC) ranging from restlessness, confusion, and apprehension to somnolence, with a fine or flapping tremor (asterixis) and depressed reflexes.

NURSING DIAGNOSES AND COLLABORATIVE PROBLEMS

Based on the following nursing diagnoses, you'll establish patient outcomes.

Fear related to threat of death. The patient will:
- identify and express his fear
- use available support systems to help him cope with fear
- show no physical signs or symptoms of fear.

Impaired gas exchange related to alveolar hypoventilation. The patient will:
- regain and maintain normal arterial blood gas (ABG) values
- exhibit no signs or symptoms of profound CNS or cardiovascular deterioration

What happens in respiratory acidosis

These six steps explain the basic pathophysiology of respiratory acidosis.

1. Pulmonary ventilation diminishes
When pulmonary ventilation decreases, retained carbon dioxide (CO_2) in the red blood cells combines with water to form excess carbonic acid (H_2CO_3). The H_2CO_3 dissociates into free hydrogen (H^+) and bicarbonate ions (HCO_3^-).

At this stage, the patient's arterial blood gas (ABG) studies show increased partial pressure of arterial carbon dioxide ($PaCO_2$; over 45 mm Hg) and reduced blood pH (below 7.35).

2. Oxygen saturation drops
As pH falls and 2,3-diphosphoglycerate (2,3-DPG) increases in red blood cells, 2,3-DPG alters hemoglobin so that it releases oxygen. This reduced hemoglobin, which is strongly basic, picks up H^+ and CO_2, eliminating some free H^+ and excess CO_2.

At this stage, the patient's arterial oxygen saturation levels decrease, and the hemoglobin dissociation curve shifts to the right.

3. Respiratory rate rises
Whenever $PaCO_2$ increases, CO_2 levels increase in all tissues and fluids, including the medulla and cerebrospinal fluid. CO_2 reacts with water to form H_2CO_3, which dissociates into H^+ and HCO_3^-. Elevated $PaCO_2$ and H^+ stimulate the medulla, increasing respirations to blow off CO_2.

This stage produces rapid, shallow respirations and diminishing $PaCO_2$ levels.

4. Blood flow to brain increases
The free H^+ and excess CO_2 dilate cerebral blood vessels and increase blood flow to the brain, causing cerebral edema and depressed central nervous system activity.

At this stage, the patient experiences headache, confusion, lethargy, nausea, and vomiting.

5. Kidneys compensate
As respiratory mechanisms fail, increasing $PaCO_2$ stimulates the kidneys to retain HCO_3^- and sodium ions (Na^+) and to excrete H^+. As a result, more sodium bicarbonate $NaHCO_3^-$) is available to buffer free H^+. Ammonium ions (NH_4^+) are also excreted to remove H^+.

A patient in this condition has increased urine acidity and ammonium levels, elevated serum pH and HCO_3^- levels, and shallow, depressed respirations.

6. Acid-base balance fails
As H^+ concentration overwhelms compensatory mechanisms, H^+ ions move into the cells and potassium ions (K^+) move out. Without sufficient oxygen, anaerobic metabolism produces lactic acid. Electrolyte imbalance and acidosis critically depress brain and cardiac function.

In a patient in this condition, ABG values show elevated $PaCO_2$ and decreased partial pressure of arterial oxygen and pH levels. The patient experiences hyperkalemia, arrhythmias, tremors, decreased level of consciousness and, possibly, coma.

■ demonstrate compliance with the prescribed treatment for the underlying cause of respiratory acidosis.

Ineffective breathing pattern related to rapid shallow respirations. The patient will:
■ reestablish his respiratory rate within normal limits
■ express a feeling of comfort with his breathing pattern
■ have normal breath sounds on auscultation.

PLANNING AND IMPLEMENTATION
These measures help the patient with respiratory acidosis:
■ Be prepared to treat or remove the underlying cause such as an airway obstruction.

■ Maintain adequate hydration by administering I.V. fluids.
■ Give oxygen (only at low concentrations in patients with COPD) if the level of partial pressure of oxygen in arterial blood drops.
■ Give aerosolized or I.V. bronchodilators as prescribed.
■ Start mechanical ventilation if hypoventilation can't be corrected immediately. Maintain a patent airway and provide adequate humidification if acidosis requires mechanical ventilation.
■ Perform tracheal suctioning regularly and chest physiotherapy, if prescribed.
■ Be alert for and immediately report critical changes in the patient's respiratory, CNS, and cardiovascular

functions. Also monitor and report variations in ABG levels and electrolyte status.

■ Reassure the patient as much as possible, depending on his LOC. Allay the fears and concerns of family members by keeping them informed about the patient's status.

Patient teaching

■ Tell the patient who's recovering from a general anesthetic to turn, cough, and perform deep-breathing and coughing exercises frequently to prevent respiratory acidosis.

■ If the patient receives home oxygen therapy for COPD, stress the importance of maintaining the dose at the ordered flow rate.

■ Explain the reasons for ABG analysis. Discuss the blood-drawing technique and tell the patient that he may feel slight discomfort from the needle stick.

■ Alert the patient to possible adverse effects of prescribed medications. Tell him to call the doctor if any occur.

EVALUATION

Evaluation of patient outcomes determines the success of collaborative management. For the patient with respiratory acidosis, evaluation focuses on adequate ventilation and knowledge.

Respiratory alkalosis

Marked by a decrease in the partial pressure of arterial carbon dioxide to less than 35 mm Hg and a rise in blood pH above 7.45, respiratory alkalosis results from alveolar hyperventilation.

CAUSES

Predisposing conditions to respiratory alkalosis include:

■ congestive heart failure
■ central nervous system (CNS) injury to the respiratory control center
■ extreme anxiety
■ fever
■ overventilation during mechanical ventilation
■ pulmonary embolism
■ salicylate intoxication (early).

Uncomplicated respiratory alkalosis leads to a decrease in hydrogen ion concentration, which raises the blood pH. Hypocapnia occurs when the lungs eliminate more carbon dioxide than the body pro-

---

Respiratory acidosis: Key abnormal test values

The following arterial blood gas values confirm respiratory acidosis:

■ partial pressure of arterial carbon dioxide above the normal 45 mm Hg
■ pH typically below the normal range of 7.35 to 7.45
■ bicarbonate (HCO_3^-) levels normal (22 to 26 mEq/L) in acute respiratory acidosis but elevated (above 26 mEq/L) in chronic respiratory acidosis (elevated HCO_3^- levels indicate partial or complete compensation).

---

duces at the cellular level. In the acute stage, respiratory alkalosis is also called hyperventilation syndrome.

In extreme respiratory alkalosis, related cardiac arrhythmias may fail to respond to conventional treatment. Seizures may also occur.

DIAGNOSIS AND TREATMENT

For typical test results, see *Respiratory alkalosis: Key abnormal test values,* page 168. Serum electrolyte studies may also be performed to detect metabolic acid-base disorders.

In respiratory alkalosis, treatment attempts to eradicate the underlying condition—for example, by removing ingested toxins or by treating fever, sepsis, or CNS disease. In severe respiratory alkalosis, the patient may need to breathe into a paper bag, which helps relieve acute anxiety and increase carbon dioxide levels. If respiratory alkalosis results from anxiety, sedatives and tranquilizers may help the patient.

Prevention of hyperventilation in patients receiving mechanical ventilation requires monitoring arterial blood gas (ABG) levels and adjusting dead-space or minute volume.

COLLABORATIVE MANAGEMENT

Care of the patient with respiratory alkalosis will focus on maintaining normal ventilation and relieving anxiety.

ASSESSMENT

The patient's history may reveal a predisposing factor associated with respiratory alkalosis. The patient may complain of light-headedness or paresthesia (numbness and tingling in his arms and legs). Look for:

■ anxiety, with visibly rapid breathing

Respiratory alkalosis: Key abnormal test values

The following arterial blood gas values confirm respiratory alkalosis and rule out compensation for metabolic acidosis:

- partial pressure of arterial carbon dioxide ($PaCO_2$) below 35 mm Hg
- pH rising in proportion to a fall in $PaCO_2$ in the acute stage but dropping toward normal (7.35 to 7.45) in the chronic stage
- bicarbonate level normal (22 to 26 mEq/L) in the acute stage but below normal (less than 22 mEq/L) in the chronic stage.

- in severe cases, tetany may be apparent, with visible twitching and flexion of the wrists and ankles
- tachycardia and deep, rapid breathing

NURSING DIAGNOSES AND COLLABORATIVE PROBLEMS

Based on the following nursing diagnoses, you'll establish patient outcomes.

Anxiety related to cause of respiratory alkalosis. The patient will:
- identify and express feelings of anxiety
- use stress-reduction techniques to prevent or minimize anxiety
- exhibit a decrease in physical anxiety symptoms when respiratory alkalosis resolves.

Impaired gas exchange related to alveolar hyperventilation. The patient will:
- regain and maintain normal ABG values
- show no signs or symptoms of severe respiratory alkalosis, such as cardiac arrhythmias and seizures
- comply with prescribed treatment to correct the cause of respiratory alkalosis.

Ineffective breathing pattern related to deep, rapid breathing. The patient will:
- regain a normal respiratory rate and pattern
- express a feeling of comfort with his breathing pattern
- have normal breath sounds on auscultation.

PLANNING AND IMPLEMENTATION

These measures help the patient with respiratory alkalosis:
- Provide supportive care for the underlying cause of respiratory alkalosis, as ordered.
- Watch for and report changes in neurologic, neuromuscular, and cardiovascular functioning.
- Remember that twitching and cardiac arrhythmias may be associated with alkalemia and electrolyte imbalances. Monitor ABG and serum electrolyte levels closely. Report any variations immediately.
- Stay with the patient during periods of extreme stress and anxiety. Offer reassurance and maintain a calm, quiet environment.
- If the patient is coping with anxiety-induced respiratory alkalosis, help him identify factors that precipitate anxiety. Also help him find coping mechanisms and activities that promote relaxation.

Patient teaching
- Explain all care procedures to the patient. Allow ample time to answer his questions.
- Teach the patient anxiety-reducing techniques, such as guided imagery, meditation, or yoga. Teach him how to counter hyperventilation with a controlled-breathing pattern.

EVALUATION
Evaluation of patient outcomes determines the success of collaborative management. For the patient with respiratory alkalosis, evaluation focuses on adequate ventilation and relief of anxiety.

Respiratory failure

When the lungs can't adequately maintain arterial oxygenation or eliminate carbon dioxide, acute respiratory failure results. Unchecked and untreated, the condition leads to tissue hypoxia. In patients with essentially normal lung tissue, acute respiratory failure usually produces a partial pressure of arterial carbon dioxide ($PaCO_2$) above 50 mm Hg and a partial pressure of arterial oxygen (PaO_2) below 50 mm Hg.

These limits, however, don't apply to patients with chronic obstructive pulmonary disease (COPD). These patients consistently have a high $PaCO_2$ (hypercapnia) and a low PaO_2 (hypoxemia) level. So, for them, only acute deterioration in arterial blood gas (ABG) values (especially a pH <7.35) —and corresponding clinical deterioration—signals acute respiratory failure.

CAUSES
Acute respiratory failure may develop from any condition that increases the work of breathing and decreases the respiratory drive. These conditions may result from respiratory tract infection (such as bronchitis or pneumonia), bronchospasm, or accumulated secretions secondary to cough suppression. Other common causes are related to ventilatory failure, in which the brain fails to direct respiration, and gas exchange failure, in which respiratory structures fail to function properly.

Normal ventilation is impaired, resulting in decreased oxygen passing into the bloodstream, and accumulation of carbon dioxide. ABG levels become abnormal, as described above. Tissue hypoxia, metabolic acidosis, and respiratory and cardiac arrest are among possible complications.

DIAGNOSIS AND TREATMENT

The key diagnostic test, ABG analysis, shows progressively deteriorating values and pH. In patients with essentially normal lung tissue, a pH below 7.35 usually indicates acute respiratory failure. In patients with COPD, the pH deviation from the normal value is even lower.

Chest X-ray may identify underlying pulmonary diseases or conditions, such as emphysema, atelectasis, lesions, pneumothorax, infiltrates, and effusions.

Acute respiratory failure constitutes an emergency. The patient will need cautious oxygen therapy (nasal prongs, a nonrebreather mask, or a Venturi mask) to raise his PaO_2. If significant respiratory acidosis persists, mechanical ventilation with an endotracheal or a tracheostomy tube may be necessary. High-frequency ventilation may be initiated if the patient doesn't respond to conventional mechanical ventilation. Treatment routinely includes antibiotics (for infection), bronchodilators and, possibly, corticosteroids.

If the patient also has cor pulmonale and decreased cardiac output, fluid restriction and administration of positive inotropic agents, vasopressors, and diuretics may be ordered.

COLLABORATIVE MANAGEMENT

Care of the patient with respiratory failure focuses on maintaining oxygenation and relieving anxiety.

ASSESSMENT

Because acute respiratory failure is life-threatening, you probably won't have time to conduct an in-depth patient interview. Instead, you'll rely on family members or the patient's medical records to discover the precipitating incident. Look for:
■ cyanosis of the oral mucosa, lips, and nail beds; nasal flaring; and ashen skin
■ yawning and use of accessory muscles to breathe; restlessness, anxiety, depression, lethargy, agitation, or confusion
■ usually tachypnea, which signals impending respiratory failure
■ cold, clammy skin and asymmetrical chest movement, which suggests pneumothorax. If tactile fremitus is present, it decreases over an obstructed bronchi or pleural effusion but increases over consolidated lung tissue.

■ hyperresonance, especially in patients with COPD; when cause is atelectasis or pneumonia, percussion usually produces a dull or flat sound
■ diminished breath sounds; in pneumothorax, absent breath sounds; in other cases, such adventitious breath sounds as wheezes (in asthma) and rhonchi (in bronchitis). If you hear crackles, suspect pulmonary edema.

NURSING DIAGNOSES AND COLLABORATIVE PROBLEMS

Based on the following nursing diagnoses, you'll establish patient outcomes.

Impaired gas exchange related to altered oxygen supply caused by the underlying pulmonary condition. The patient will:
■ exhibit PaO_2 and breath sounds that return to baseline
■ experience no dyspnea
■ use correct bronchial hygiene to keep airways clear, which enhances oxygenation.

Ineffective airway clearance related to decreased energy, fatigue, or presence of tracheobronchial secretions. The patient will:
■ cough and deep-breathe adequately to expectorate secretions
■ demonstrate skill in conserving energy while attempting to clear airway
■ maintain a patent airway.

Ineffective breathing pattern related to decreased energy or fatigue caused by underlying pulmonary condition or metabolic acidosis. The patient will:
■ achieve maximum lung expansion with adequate ventilation
■ demonstrate skill in conserving energy while carrying out activities of daily living
■ exhibit a respiratory rate and pattern and ABG values that return to baseline and remain within this normal range.

PLANNING AND IMPLEMENTATION

These measures help the patient with respiratory failure:
■ To reverse hypoxemia, administer oxygen at appropriate concentrations to maintain PaO_2 at a minimum pressure range of 50 to 60 mm Hg. The patient with COPD usually requires only small amounts of supplemental oxygen.
■ Maintain a patent airway. If your patient retains carbon dioxide, encourage him to cough and breathe deeply with pursed lips. If he's alert, have him use an incentive spirometer. If he's intubated and lethargic, reposition him every 1 to 2 hours. Use postural drainage and chest physiotherapy to help clear secretions.

- Perform oral hygiene measures frequently.
- Position the patient for comfort and optimal gas exchange.
- Auscultate for chest sounds. Report any changes in ABG values immediately. Notify the doctor of any deterioration in oxygen saturation levels as detected by pulse oximetry
- Check ventilator settings, cuff pressures, oximetry, and capnometry values often and ABG values as clinically indicated to ensure correct fraction of inspired oxygen (FIO_2) settings.
- Suction the trachea as needed after hyperoxygenation. Provide humidification to liquefy secretions.
- Prevent infection by using sterile technique while suctioning and by changing ventilator tubing every 24 hours.
- Prevent tracheal erosion that can result from an overinflated artificial airway cuff compressing the tracheal wall's vasculature. Use the minimal-leak technique and a cuffed tube with high residual volume (low-pressure cuff), a foam cuff, or a pressure-regulating valve on the cuff. Measure cuff pressure every 8 hours.
- Implement measures to prevent nasal tissue necrosis. Position and maintain the nasotracheal tube midline within the nostrils, and provide meticulous care. Periodically, loosen the tape securing the tube to prevent skin breakdown. Avoid excessive movement of any tubes, and make sure that the ventilator tubing has adequate support.
- Monitor changes in oximetry or capnometry values after each change in the FIO_2 setting. Perform ABG analysis as clinically indicated.
- When suctioning the patient, check for any changes in sputum quality, consistency, odor, or color.
- Watch for complications of mechanical ventilation, such as reduced cardiac output, pneumothorax or other barotrauma, increased pulmonary vascular resistance, diminished urine output, increased intracranial pressure, and GI bleeding.
- Routinely assess endotracheal (ET) tube position and patency. Make sure the tube is placed properly and taped securely. Immediately after intubation, auscultate the lung fields to check for accidental intubation of the esophagus or the mainstem bronchus, which may have occurred during ET tube insertion. Also be alert for transtracheal or laryngeal perforation, aspiration, broken teeth, nosebleeds, vagal reflexes such as bradycardia, arrhythmias, and hypertension.
- Monitor for signs of stress ulcers, which are common in intubated patients, especially those in the intensive care unit. Inspect gastric secretions for blood, especially if the patient has a nasogastric tube or reports epigastric tenderness, nausea, or vomiting. Also

monitor hematocrit and hemoglobin levels, and check all stools for blood.
- Orient the patient to the treatment unit. Most patients with acute respiratory failure receive intensive care. Acquainting the patient with procedures, sounds, and sights helps to minimize his anxiety.
- Apply soft wrist restraints for the confused patient as prescribed. This will prevent him from disconnecting the oxygen setup. However, remember that these restraints can increase anxiety, fear, and agitation. Check restraints and release them every 1 to 2 hours.
- If the patient is on mechanical ventilation, help him communicate without words. Offer him a pen and tablet, a word chart, or an alphabet board.
- Maintain the patient in a normothermic state to reduce his body's demand for oxygen.
- Pace patient care activities to maximize his energy level and provide needed rest.

Patient teaching
- Describe all tests and procedures to the patient and family members. Discuss the reasons for suctioning, chest physiotherapy, blood tests and, if used, soft wrist restraints.
- If the patient is intubated or has a tracheostomy, explain why he can't speak. Suggest alternative means of communication.
- Identify reportable signs of respiratory infection.
- If applicable, teach the patient about the effects of smoking. Provide resources to help him stop smoking.

EVALUATION
Evaluation of patient outcomes determines the success of collaborative management. For the patient with respiratory failure, evaluation focuses on adequate oxygenation and relief of anxiety.

Sleep apnea

Absence of respiration during sleep, sleep apnea in the adult is usually the result of upper airway obstruction. Patients whose upper airways are anatomically narrow, as in obesity, tonsillar hypertrophy, micrognathia, and macroglossia, are more likely to develop obstructive sleep apnea. The incidence is highest in obese middle-aged men.

CAUSES
A narrow airway and weak pharyngeal muscles are the primary cause. Alcohol or sedative consumption before sleeping may worsen the condition.

In sleep apnea, loss of normal pharyngeal muscle tone allows the pharynx to collapse passively during inspiration. The collapsed pharynx blocks the airway, causing loud, sonorous breathing and airway occlusion.

DIAGNOSIS AND TREATMENT
Weight loss and strict avoidance of alcohol and sedatives are the first steps in management and are curative for a small number of patients.

Nasal continuous positive airway pressure (CPAP) is used during sleep to keep the airway open.

Supplemental oxygen may be used to lessen the nocturnal oxygen desaturation, but may also lengthen the apnea episode.

Uvulopalatopharyngoplasty, resection of the pharyngeal soft tissue and amputation of ⅝" (15 mm) of the free edge of the soft palate and uvula, is helpful in some cases of retropalatal airway occlusion.

Nasal septoplasty is performed in patients with gross anatomic nasal septal deformity.

Tracheotomy is the definitive surgical procedure for sleep apnea. However, it's rarely used because of its many adverse effects.

COLLABORATIVE MANAGEMENT
Care of the patient with sleep apnea focuses on patient education and emotional support.

ASSESSMENT
The patient's history will reveal complaints of daytime somnolence, morning sluggishness and headaches, daytime fatigue, and cognitive impairment. Look for:
- complaints of recent weight gain and impotence
- family members' reports of loud, cyclical snoring, breath cessation, restlessness, and thrashing extremities during sleep
- narrowed nasopharynx if the patient has macroglossia, septal deviation, tumors, or enlarged adenoids
- in sleep, loud snoring interrupted by episodes of increasingly strong ventilatory effort that fail to produce airflow; a first breath accompanied by a loud snort
- apneic episodes lasting as long as 1 to 2 minutes, revealed by polysomnography
- decreased oxygen saturation during sleep and bradyarrhythmias.

NURSING DIAGNOSES AND COLLABORATIVE PROBLEMS
Based on the following nursing diagnoses, you'll establish patient outcomes.

Sleep pattern disturbance related to internal factors. The patient will:
- sleep 8 hours a night
- report being well rested

> ### Using nasal CPAP
>
> This illustration shows the continuous positive-airway pressure (CPAP) apparatus. In a patient with sleep apnea, CPAP applies positive pressure to the airway to prevent obstruction during inspiration.
>
>
> Inlet valve
> Oxygen tubing
> Positive end-expiratory pressure valve
> Inflation valve

- exhibit no sleep-related behavioral symptoms, such as restlessness, irritability, lethargy, or disorientation

Inability to sustain spontaneous ventilation related to airway obstruction. The patient will:
- have normal arterial blood gas levels
- have a normal breathing pattern while sleeping
- report no feelings of fatigue.

PLANNING AND IMPLEMENTATION
These measures help the patient with sleep apnea:
- Assist the patient with measures to promote sleep.
- Institute CPAP, as ordered.
- Monitor respiratory status, especially at night while sleeping; note and report any periods of apnea.
- Reassure the patient that sleep apnea is correctable with treatment.
- Help the patient deal with the alterations in self-image.
- Refer the patient to a trained sex counselor if impotence is a problem.

Patient teaching
- Encourage the obese patient to follow a low-calorie, low-fat diet.
- Explain that he may be able to reduce the frequency of CPAP treatments if he loses weight.
- Ask the patient to demonstrate use of the system to make sure he can prevent excess leakage and maintain the prescribed pressures. Teach him how to clean the mask and change the air filter. (See *Using nasal CPAP.*)

- Explain to the patient that he must use CPAP every night, even if he feels well after the initial treatments. Apneic episodes will recur if he doesn't use CPAP as directed. Emphasize that he should call his doctor if symptoms recur despite CPAP.

EVALUATION

Evaluation of patient outcomes determines the success of collaborative management. For the patient with sleep apnea, evaluation focuses on a restful sleep pattern and adequate patient knowledge.

Tuberculosis

An acute or chronic infection, tuberculosis is characterized by pulmonary infiltrates and by formation of granulomas with caseation, fibrosis, and cavitation. The American Lung Association estimates that active disease afflicts nearly 14 of every 100,000 persons.

The disease is twice as common in men as in women and four times as common in nonwhites as in whites. But incidence is highest in people who live in crowded, poorly ventilated, unsanitary conditions, such as those in some prisons, tenement houses, and homeless shelters. The typical newly diagnosed tuberculosis patient is a single, homeless, nonwhite man. With proper treatment, the prognosis is usually excellent.

CAUSES

Tuberculosis results from exposure to *Mycobacterium tuberculosis* and sometimes other strains of mycobacteria. Transmission occurs by coughs or sneezes, which spread infected droplets.

When a person without immunity inhales infected droplets, the bacilli lodge in the alveoli, causing irritation. The immune system responds by sending leukocytes, lymphocytes, and macrophages to surround the bacilli, and the local lymph nodes swell and become inflamed. If the encapsulated bacilli (tubercles) and the inflamed nodes rupture, the infection contaminates the surrounding tissue and may spread through the blood and lymphatic circulation to distant sites— a process called hematogenous dissemination.

After exposure to *M. tuberculosis*, roughly 5% of infected people develop active tuberculosis within 1 year; in the remainder, microorganisms cause a latent infection. The host's immunologic defense system usually destroys the bacillus or walls it up in a tubercle. But the live, encapsulated bacilli may lie dormant within the tubercle for years, reactivating later to cause active infection.

DIAGNOSIS AND TREATMENT

Chest X-rays show nodular lesions, patchy infiltrates (mainly in upper lobes), cavity formation, scar tissue, and calcium deposits. X-rays may not help distinguish between active and inactive tuberculosis.

A skin test reveals infection, but doesn't indicate active disease. In this test, intermediate-strength purified protein derivative or 5 tuberculin units (0.1 ml) are injected intradermally on the forearm and read in 48 to 72 hours. A positive reaction (equal to or more than a 3/8" [10-mm] induration) develops within 2 to 10 weeks after infection with the tubercle bacillus, in both active and inactive tuberculosis.

Stains and cultures of sputum, cerebrospinal fluid, urine, drainage from abscess, or pleural fluid show heat-sensitive, nonmotile, aerobic, acid-fast bacilli.

Computed tomography or magnetic resonance imaging scans allow the evaluation of lung damage or confirm a difficult diagnosis.

A sputum specimen can best be obtained using bronchoalveolar lavage with a protected specimen brush.

Bronchoscopy may be performed if the patient can't produce an adequate sputum specimen.

It may take several of these tests to distinguish tuberculosis from other mimicking diseases (such as lung cancer, lung abscess, pneumoconiosis, and bronchiectasis).

Antitubercular therapy with daily oral doses of isoniazid or rifampin (with ethambutol added in some cases) for at least 9 months usually cures tuberculosis. After 2 to 4 weeks, the disease is no longer infectious and the patient can resume his normal activities while continuing to take medication.

The patient with atypical mycobacterial disease or drug-resistant tuberculosis may require second-line drugs, such as capreomycin, streptomycin, para-aminosalicylic acid, pyrazinamide, and cycloserine.

COLLABORATIVE MANAGEMENT

Care of the patient with tuberculosis focuses on preventing the spread of infection and administering antimicrobial medications.

ASSESSMENT

The patient with a primary infection may complain of weakness and fatigue, anorexia and weight loss, and night sweats. The patient with reactivated tuberculosis may report chest pain and a cough that produces blood or mucopurulent or blood-tinged sputum. He may also have a low-grade fever. Look for:
- dullness over the affected area, a symptom of consolidation or the presence of pleural fluid
- crepitant crackles, bronchial breath sounds, wheezes, and whispered pectoriloquy.

NURSING DIAGNOSES AND COLLABORATIVE PROBLEMS

Based on the following nursing diagnoses, you'll establish patient outcomes.

Altered protection related to potential for recurrence and possible transmission of mycobacterial foci to other areas of the body. The patient will:
- show no signs or symptoms of organ dysfunction outside of the lungs
- comply with the prescribed tuberculosis treatment to eradicate the infection and minimize the risk of other organs becoming infected
- identify and promptly report early signs and symptoms of organ dysfunction.

Impaired gas exchange related to changes in pulmonary tissue. The patient will:
- regain and maintain adequate ventilation
- show no signs or symptoms of hypoxia
- regain and maintain normal arterial blood gas values.

Knowledge deficit related to tuberculosis. The patient will:
- identify the need to learn about tuberculosis
- obtain correct information about tuberculosis
- communicate an understanding of how tuberculosis is contracted and managed and how a recurrence can be prevented.

PLANNING AND IMPLEMENTATION

These measures help the patient with tuberculosis:
- Administer ordered antibiotics and antitubercular agents.
- Give isoniazid and ethambutol with food.
- Because isoniazid can cause hepatitis or peripheral neuritis, monitor levels of aspartate aminotransferase and alanine aminotransferase.
- If the patient receives ethambutol, watch for and report signs of optic neuritis (the doctor probably will discontinue the drug). Assess the patient's vision monthly.
- If the patient receives rifampin, watch for signs of hepatitis, purpura, and a flulike syndrome as well as other complications such as hemoptysis. Monitor liver and kidney function tests throughout therapy.
- Monitor the patient's compliance with treatment.
- Isolate the infectious patient in a quiet, well-ventilated room. Provide diversionary activities, and check on him frequently.
- Place a covered trash can nearby or tape a waxed bag to the bedside for used tissues. Tell the patient to wear a mask outside his room. Visitors and staff members should wear HEPA filter masks in his room.
- Make sure the patient gets plenty of rest. Alternate periods of rest and activity to promote health by conserving energy and reducing oxygen demand.
- Provide the patient with well-balanced, high-calorie foods, in small, frequent meals to conserve energy. (Small, frequent meals may also encourage the anorexic patient to eat more.) If the patient needs oral supplements, consult the dietitian.
- Perform chest physiotherapy, including postural drainage and chest percussion, several times a day.
- Monitor the patient's respiratory status. Auscultate breath sounds frequently.

Patient teaching

- Show the patient and family members how to perform postural drainage and chest percussion. Also, teach the patient coughing and deep-breathing techniques. Tell him to maintain each position for 10 minutes, then perform percussion and cough.
- Teach the patient the adverse effects of his medication, and tell him to report reactions immediately. Emphasize the importance of regular follow-up examinations, and tell the patient and family members the signs and symptoms of recurring tuberculosis. Stress strict adherence to long-term treatment.
- Warn the patient taking rifampin that the drug will temporarily make his body secretions appear orange; reassure him that this effect is harmless. If the patient is a woman, warn her that oral contraceptives may be less effective while she's taking rifampin.
- Teach the patient the signs and symptoms that require medical assessment: increased cough, hemoptysis, unexplained weight loss, fever, and night sweats.
- Stress the importance of eating high-calorie, high-protein, balanced meals.
- Explain respiratory and universal precautions to the hospitalized patient. Before discharge, tell him how to prevent spreading the disease—wear a mask around others—until the doctor says he's not contagious. The patient should tell all his health care providers, including his dentist and eye doctor, that he has tuberculosis so that they can institute infection-control precautions. (See *Preventing the spread of tuberculosis,* page 174.)
- Teach the patient other specific anticontagion steps. Tell him to cough and sneeze into tissues and dispose of tissues properly; wash hands thoroughly in hot, soapy water after handling his own secretions; and wash his eating utensils separately in hot, soapy water.
- Advise anyone exposed to an infected patient to receive tuberculin tests and, if prescribed, chest X-rays and prophylactic isoniazid.
- Emphasize the importance of follow-up appointments.
- Refer the patient to such support groups as the American Lung Association.

HEALTHY LIVING · Preventing the spread of tuberculosis

The steps outlined below will help your patient prevent the spread of tuberculosis.

■ Inform all health care personnel, including the dentist and eye doctor, of your diagnosis so that they can take infection-control precautions.
■ Take all medications as directed to eliminate infection.
■ Wear a mask around others until your doctor says you're no longer contagious.

■ Cover your mouth and nose with a tissue when coughing or sneezing.
■ Carefully dispose of all secretions so that other people won't come in contact with them.
■ Wash your hands thoroughly in hot, soapy water whenever you handle your own secretions.
■ Segregate your eating utensils from others, and wash them separately in hot, soapy water.

EVALUATION

Evaluation of patient outcomes determines the success of collaborative management. For the patient with tuberculosis, evaluation focuses on adequate protection, oxygenation, and knowledge.

Upper respiratory infection

Also known as the common cold, an upper respiratory infection is an acute, usually afebrile, viral infection that causes inflammation of the upper respiratory tract. It accounts for more time lost from school or work than any other cause and is the most common infectious disease. Although it's benign and self-limiting, it can lead to secondary bacterial infections.

CAUSES

Over 100 viruses can cause an upper respiratory infection. Major offenders include rhinoviruses, coronaviruses, myxoviruses, adenoviruses, coxsackieviruses and echoviruses. Occasionally they result from mycoplasma.

Transmission occurs through airborne respiratory droplets, contact with contaminated objects, and hand-to-hand transmission. The virus enters the body through the mucous membrane in the oropharynx. Symptoms are related to the body's immune system dealing with the intruder.

DIAGNOSIS AND TREATMENT

Lacking a specific diagnostic test for upper respiratory infection, diagnosis is usually based on patient history. Treatment focuses on relief of symptoms and includes the following measures.

■ aspirin or acetaminophen to ease myalgia and headache (for children, acetaminophen instead of aspirin)
■ oral fluids to help loosen accumulated respiratory secretions and maintain hydration
■ rest to combat fatigue
■ decongestants to relieve congestion
■ steam to encourage expectoration
■ throat lozenges to relieve soreness.

New evidence suggests that lozenges containing zinc may decrease viral replication in the oropharynx, lessening the severity of the infection's course. The role of vitamin C remains controversial.

COLLABORATIVE MANAGEMENT

Care of the patient with upper respiratory infection focuses on promoting rest and relieving symptoms.

ASSESSMENT

The patient's history will reveal complaints of headache and burning, watery eyes. He may complain of nasal "fullness" and irritating, copious nasal discharge. Look for localized skin irritation around the nares and mouth breathing to compensate for congested sinuses.

NURSING DIAGNOSES AND COLLABORATIVE PROBLEMS

Based on the following nursing diagnosis, you'll establish patient outcomes.

Fatigue related to inability to rest. The patient will:
■ describe and employ measures to prevent or modify fatigue
■ report increased energy.

PLANNING AND IMPLEMENTATION

These measures help the patient with upper respiratory infection:

■ Prevent unnecessary patient fatigue. For instance, avoid scheduling two energy-draining procedures on the same day.

■ Alternate activities with periods of rest. Encourage activities that can be completed in a short period or divided into segments.

■ Encourage the patient to eat foods rich in iron and minerals, unless contraindicated, to help avoid demineralization.

■ Encourage increased fluid intake to help loosen secretions.

■ Administer aspirin (for children, acetaminophen), as ordered for myalgia.

■ Supply hard candies to relieve sore throat.

■ Apply a lubricant to the nostrils for soreness.

Patient teaching

■ Tell the patient to stay in bed, if possible, during the first few days and get plenty of rest.

■ Suggest that he take warm baths or use heating pads to relieve aches and pains.

■ Advise prudent use of nose drops or sprays; overuse may cause rebound congestion.

■ Explain that antibiotics don't cure upper respiratory infections.

■ Teach the patient to control the spread of his infection by frequently washing his hands, covering coughs and sneezes, and not sharing towels and drinking glasses. Warn him to avoid future upper respiratory infections by avoiding people who have colds.

EVALUATION

Evaluation of patient outcomes determines the success of collaborative management. For the patient with an upper respiratory infection, evaluation focuses on adequate knowledge and improved activity level.

Treatments and procedures

Various treatments and procedures can improve airway clearance and gas exchange for patients with respiratory disorders. Tracheotomy and laryngectomy can ensure airway patency.

TRACHEOTOMY

The surgical creation of an opening into the trachea through the neck, tracheotomy is usually performed in the operating room. However, it can be performed at a patient's bedside or in the emergency room.

Tracheotomy is most commonly performed to provide an airway for the intubated patient who needs prolonged mechanical ventilation. It may also be performed to prevent an unconscious or paralyzed patient from aspirating food or secretions; to bypass upper airway obstruction caused by trauma, burns, epiglottitis, or a tumor; or to help remove lower tracheobronchial secretions in a patient who can't clear them.

Although endotracheal (ET) intubation is the treatment of choice in an emergency, tracheotomy may be used if intubation is impossible. For the laryngectomy patient, a permanent tracheostomy in which the skin and the trachea are sutured together provides the necessary stoma.

After creation of the surgical opening, a tracheostomy tube is inserted to permit access to the airway. Selection of a specific tube depends on the patient's condition and the doctor's preference. (See *Comparing tracheostomy tubes,* page 176.)

PROCEDURE

If an ET tube isn't already in place, one is inserted. Then the doctor makes a horizontal incision in the skin below the cricoid cartilage and vertical incisions in the trachea. He places a tracheostomy tube between the second and third tracheal rings, and may also place retraction sutures in the stomal margins to stabilize the opening. Finally, he inflates the tube cuff (if present), provides ventilation, suctions the airway, and provides oxygen by mist.

COLLABORATIVE MANAGEMENT

Care of the patient undergoing tracheotomy requires thorough preparation, close monitoring during and after the procedure, and follow-up with instructions and medical care.

Preparation

■ For an emergency tracheotomy, briefly explain the procedure to the patient, if time permits, and quickly obtain supplies or a tracheotomy tray.

■ For a scheduled tracheotomy, explain the procedure and the need for general anesthesia to the patient and family members. If possible, mention whether the tracheostomy will be temporary or permanent.

■ Set up a communication system with the patient (Magic Slate, letter board, or flash cards), and have him practice using it so that he can communicate comfortably while his speech is limited.

■ If the patient is to have a long-term or permanent tracheostomy, introduce him to someone who has adjusted well to tube and stoma care.

■ Ensure that samples for arterial blood gas (ABG) analysis and other diagnostic tests have been collected.

Comparing tracheostomy tubes

Tracheostomy tubes, made of plastic or metal, come in uncuffed, cuffed, or fenestrated varieties. Tube selection depends on the patient's condition and the doctor's preference.

Tube type	Advantages	Disadvantages
UNCUFFED (plastic or metal) 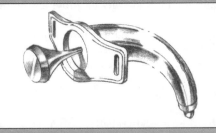	■ Permits free flow of air around tube and through larynx ■ Reduces risk of tracheal damage ■ Allows mechanical ventilation in patient with neuromuscular disease	■ In adults, lack of cuff increases the risk of aspiration. ■ Adapter may be necessary for ventilation.
PLASTIC CUFFED (low pressure and high volume) 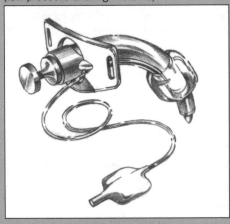	■ Disposable ■ Cuff bonded to tube; won't detach accidentally inside trachea ■ Cuff pressure low and evenly distributed against tracheal wall; no need to deflate periodically to lower pressure ■ Reduces risk of tracheal damage	■ This type may be costlier than other tubes.
FENESTRATED 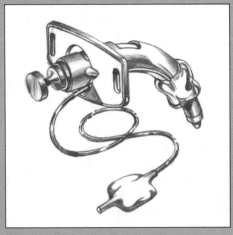	■ Permits speech through upper airway when external opening is capped and cuff is deflated ■ Allos breathing by mechanical ventilation with inner cannula in place and cuff inflated ■ Inner cannula easily removed for cleaning	■ Fenestration may become occluded. ■ Inner cannula can become dislodged.

Monitoring and aftercare

- Auscultate breath sounds every two hours after the procedure. Note crackles, rhonchi, or diminished breath sounds.
- Turn the patient every 2 hours to avoid pooling tracheal secretions.
- As ordered, provide chest physiotherapy to help mobilize secretions and note their quantity, consistency, color, and odor. Provide humidification
- Monitor ABG results and compare them with baseline values.
- Suction the tracheostomy as prescribed to remove excess secretions. Before and after suctioning, oxygenate the patient's lungs to reduce the risk of hypoxemia. Use a gentle twisting motion and apply suction for no longer than 10 seconds. Discontinue suctioning if the patient develops respiratory distress.
- Inflate the cuff with less than 25 cm H_2O (18 mm Hg) of pressure to avoid traumatizing the interior tracheal wall.
- Make sure the tracheal ties are secure but not too tight.
- Using aseptic technique, change the tracheostomy dressing when soiled, or once per shift and check the color, odor, amount, and type of any drainage.
- Have available a sterile tracheostomy tube (with obturator) that's one size smaller than the tube currently being used because the trachea begins to close after the expulsion, making insertion of the same size tube difficult.

Patient teaching

- Tell the patient to notify his doctor of any breathing problems, chest or stoma pain, or change in the amount or color of his secretions.
- Teach the patient to wash the skin around his stoma with a moist cloth. Emphasize the importance of not getting water in his stoma. He should, of course, avoid swimming. When he showers, he should wear a stoma shield or direct the water below his stoma.
- Tell the patient to place a foam filter over his stoma in winter, thereby warming inspired air, and to wear a bib over the filter.
- Teach the patient to bend at his waist during coughing to help expel secretions.

COMPLICATIONS

Tracheotomy can cause serious complications. Within 48 hours after surgery, the patient may develop a hemorrhage at the site, bleeding or edema within the tracheal tissue, aspiration of secretions, pneumothorax, or subcutaneous emphysema. After 48 hours, continued attention to sterile suctioning, careful cuff monitoring, and meticulous stoma care can reduce the risk of complications, such as stoma or pulmonary infection, ischemia and hemorrhage, airway obstruction, hypoxia, and arrhythmias.

LARYNGECTOMY

Laryngectomy removes all or part of the larynx to treat laryngeal cancer. The approach varies with the type and site of the tumor, the extent and location of metastases, and vocal chord mobility.

Total laryngectomy is used to excise a large glottic or supraglottic tumor with vocal cord fixation. A horizontal supraglottic laryngectomy is used for a large tumor when the vocal cords are not involved. For a widespread, unilateral tumor, a vertical hemilaryngectomy is used. For a glottic tumor that is limited to one vocal cord, laryngeal fissure is the procedure of choice.

PROCEDURE

With the patient under general anesthesia, the surgeon makes a midline incision and exposes the trachea. The trachea is incised, and the laryngeal structures are removed. A total laryngectomy removes the true vocal cords, false vocal cords, epiglottis, hyoid bone, cricoid cartilage, and two or three rings of the trachea. When cancer involves the supraglottic portion of the larynx, a horizontal supraglottic laryngectomy is performed. This procedure excises the tip of the larynx (the epiglottis, the hyoid bone, and the false vocal cords), leaving the true vocal cords intact. Speech recovery is excellent in many cases. In a vertical hemilaryngectomy, half of the thyroid gland and subglottis, one false vocal cord, and one true vocal cord are removed. The area is then rebuilt with strap muscles. In a laryngeal fissure, one vocal cord is removed.

COLLABORATIVE MANAGEMENT

Care of the patient undergoing a laryngectomy requires thorough preparation, close monitoring and intense patient teaching.

Preparation

- If the patient is to have a total laryngectomy, explain that he'll breathe through an opening in his neck after surgery. Tell him that he won't be able to smell, blow his nose, whistle, gargle, sip, or suck on a straw after surgery.
- Describe the laryngectomy stoma and show him pictures. Explain that he'll expectorate secretions through his stoma; he'll need periodic suctioning.
- Tell him he'll be taught to perform stoma care and suction for himself.

■ If possible, arrange a meeting with a laryngectomee who has adjusted well to having a stoma.

■ If the patient will be unable to speak after surgery, suggest a communication system, such as flash cards, paper and pencil, or a slate.

■ Coordinate visits by a speech pathologist, who will evaluate the patient, reinforce earlier information, and answer questions about reestablishing speech.

■ Inform the patient that he may have a laryngectomy tube after surgery (shorter and thicker than a tracheostomy tube but requiring the same care) and that it's usually removed after 7 to 10 days.

■ Explain that he'll also have a nasogastric (NG) tube in place for 7 to 10 days; this will provide a route for nourishment until his suture line heals. Mention that he'll begin receiving oral feedings (thick, easy-to-swallow fluids) about 10 days after surgery.

Monitoring and aftercare

■ After surgery, keep emergency resuscitation equipment readily available.

■ Elevate the head of the bed 30 degrees to prevent tension on the incision line, decrease neck edema, and prevent aspiration during feeding.

■ Be sure to support the patient's head, neck, and back for 24 to 48 hours.

■ Periodically auscultate the patient's lungs to detect any pulmonary congestion. Also check the rate and depth of his respirations and observe for accessory muscle use.

■ If the patient has a tracheostomy tube, suction it gently, as ordered, using sterile technique.

■ Provide humidification.

■ If the patient experiences respiratory difficulty, notify the doctor immediately.

■ For 8 hours after surgery, check the incision site hourly for bleeding or signs of hematoma formation (swelling or bulging of the stoma under the skin flap). Report any abnormalities.

■ Perform tracheostomy care every 8 hours or as needed, and check the site for signs of infection. If neck drains are in place, make sure they're patent.

■ As prescribed, give I.V. fluids and NG tube feedings, and monitor intake and output. If the patient experiences discomfort, give analgesics and sedatives, as prescribed, through the NG tube or I.V. line. Keep in mind that narcotics depress respirations and inhibit coughing.

■ To help relieve the patient's anxiety, use the communication system you developed before surgery.

■ If he has had a partial laryngectomy, tell him not to use his voice until the doctor gives permission. Reassure him that speech rehabilitation will enable him to speak again.

Patient teaching

■ Teach the patient how to perform stoma care using clean technique.

■ Tell him to clean the inner cannula of his tube with hydrogen peroxide and water daily.

■ Explain that he must suction the outer cannula to keep his airway patent when he feels congested, when his breathing sounds raspy or wheezy, or when excess mucus forms. Tell him to watch for bloody secretions, which may indicate local trauma.

■ Have him demonstrate correct cleaning and suctioning techniques. Emphasize the importance of daily stoma care, using warm water, to maintain a patent airway, promote healing, and prevent infection.

■ Warn him not to use tissues, loose cotton, or soap during cleaning because these may get in his airway. Warn against swimming.

■ Tell him to wear a bib or dressing over the stoma to act as a filter, to warm incoming air, and to humidify his home, especially during the winter.

■ Tell him to notify the doctor of any signs of respiratory infection (fever, cough, yellow or green drainage from the stoma, or surrounding erythema).

■ Stress the importance of follow-up appointments to monitor for recurrence of cancer.

■ Provide emotional support and help the patient adjust to his new self-image. Suggest that he contact the International Association of Larngectomees.

COMPLICATIONS

Immediate complications following laryngectomy include pneumonia, atelectasis, and wound infection. Others may appear as much as 2 weeks later. Secretions leaking from the wound 10 days after surgery may indicate a pharyngeal fistula. The carotid artery may rupture 8 to 20 days after a wound infection or sooner as a result of surgical injury or weakening from preoperative radiation.

THORACOTOMY

A surgical incision into the thoracic cavity, thoracotomy is done to locate and examine abnormalities such as tumors, bleeding sites, or thoracic injuries; to perform a biopsy; or to remove diseased lung tissue. Lung excision may involve pneumonectomy, lobectomy, segmental resection, or wedge resection.

Pneumonectomy is the excision of an entire lung. After pneumonectomy, chest cavity pressures stabilize and, over time, fluid fills the cavity where lung tissue was removed, preventing significant mediastinal shift. Following lobectomy, the removal of one of the five long lobes, the remaining lobes expand to fill the entire pleural cavity.

Segmental resection is the removal of one or more lung segments and preserves more functional tissue than lobectomy. Remaining lung tissue needs to be reexpanded.

Wedge resection, the removal of a small portion of the lung without regard to segments, preserves the most functional tissue. Remaining lung tissue needs to be reexpanded.

Thoracotomy is usually performed to remove part or all of a lung to spare healthy lung tissue from disease. Pneumonectomy is usually performed to treat bronchogenic cancer but may also be used to treat tuberculosis, bronchiectasis, or lung abscess. It's used only when a less radical approach can't remove all diseased tissue. Lobectomy can treat bronchogenic cancer, tuberculosis, lung abscess, emphysematous blebs or bullae, benign tumors, or localized fungal infections. Segmental resection is commonly used to treat bronchiectasis. Wedge resection preserves the most functional tissue of all the surgeries but can treat only a small, well-circumscribed lesion.

Other types of thoracotomy and their indications include the following:

■ Exploratory thoracotomy is done to examine the chest and pleural space in evaluating chest trauma and tumors.

■ Decortication is used to help reexpand the lung in a patient with empyema. It involves the removal or stripping of the thick, fibrous membrane covering the visceral pleura.

■ Thoracoplasty is performed to remove part or all of one rib and reduce the size of the chest cavity. It decreases the risk of mediastinal shift when tuberculosis has reduced lung volume.

PROCEDURE

After the patient is anesthetized, the surgeon performs a thoracotomy using one of three approaches: posterolateral thoracotomy, anterolateral thoracotomy, or median sternotomy.

Once the incision is made, the surgeon takes a biopsy, locates and ties off sources of bleeding, locates and repairs injuries within the thoracic cavity, or spreads the ribs and exposes the lung area for excision.

After completing the procedure requiring the thoracotomy, the surgeon closes the chest cavity and applies a dressing.

COLLABORATIVE MANAGEMENT

Care of the patient undergoing a thoracotomy requires thorough preparation, close monitoring during and after the procedure, and follow-up with instructions and medical care.

Preparation

■ Explain the thoracotomy procedure to the patient, and inform him that he'll receive a general anesthetic. Prepare him psychologically, according to his condition. A patient having a lung biopsy, for example, faces the fear of cancer as well as the fear of surgery and needs ongoing emotional support. In contrast, a patient with a chronic lung disorder, such as tuberculosis or a fungal infection, may view having a lung excision as a cure for his ailment.

■ Inform the patient that, postoperatively, he may have chest tubes in place and may receive oxygen. Teach him coughing and deep-breathing techniques. Explain that he'll use these after surgery to facilitate lung reexpansion. Also teach him how to use an incentive spirometer; record the volumes he achieves to provide a baseline.

■ If a pneumonectomy is to be performed, arrange for laboratory studies, as ordered. Tests to assess cardiac function may include pulmonary function tests, electrocardiography, chest X-ray, arterial blood gas analysis, bronchoscopy and, possibly, cardiac catheterization.

Monitoring and aftercare

■ If the patient had a pneumonectomy, make sure he lies only on his operative side or his back until he's stabilized. This prevents fluid from draining into the unaffected lung if the sutured bronchus opens.

■ If the patient has a chest tube in place, make sure it's functioning and monitor him for signs and symptoms of tension pneumothorax, such as dyspnea, chest pain, an irritating cough, vertigo, syncope, or anxiety. If the patient develops any of these signs or symptoms, palpate his neck, face, and chest wall for subcutaneous emphysema and palpate his trachea for deviation from midline. Auscultate his lungs for decreased or absent breath sounds on the affected side. Then, percuss them for hyperresonance. If you suspect tension pneumothorax, notify the doctor at once and help him to identify the cause.

■ Provide analgesics, as prescribed.

■ Have the patient begin coughing and deep-breathing exercises as soon as he's stabilized. Auscultate his lungs, place him in semi-Fowler's position, and have him splint his incision to facilitate coughing and deep breathing. Have him cough every 2 to 4 hours until his breath sounds clear.

■ Perform passive range-of-motion (ROM) exercises the evening of surgery and two or three times daily thereafter. Progress to active ROM exercises.

Patient teaching

■ Tell the patient to perform coughing and deep-breathing exercises to prevent complications. Advise him to report any changes in sputum characteristics to his doctor.

■ Teach the patient to perform ROM exercises to maintain mobility of his shoulder and chest wall.

■ Tell the patient to avoid contact with people who have upper respiratory tract infections and to refrain from smoking.

■ As necessary, provide the patient with instructions for wound care and dressing changes.

COMPLICATIONS

Hemorrhage, infection, and tension pneumothorax are possible. Additional complications include bronchopleural fistula and empyema. A lung excision may also cause a persistent air space that the remaining lung tissue doesn't expand to fill. Removal of up to three ribs may be necessary to reduce chest cavity size and allow lung tissue to fit the space.

Selected references

Angelucci, P. "A New Weapon Against ARDS," *RN* 59(11):22-24. November 1996.

Beare, P.G., and Myers, J.L. *Principles and Practice of Adult Health Nursing,* 2nd ed. St Louis: Mosby–Year Book, Inc., 1994.

Carroll, P. "Pulse Oximetry at Your Fingertips," *RN* 60(2):22-26, February 1997.

Handbook of Medical-Surgical Nursing. 2nd ed. Springhouse, Pa.: Springhouse Corp., 1998.

Illustrated Manual of Nursing Practice, 2nd ed.. Springhouse, Pa.: Springhouse Corp., 1994.

Majoros, K.A., and Moccia, J.M. "Pulmonary Embolism: Targeting an Elusive Enemy," *Nursing96* 26(4):26-32, April 1996.

Mathews, P.J. "Ventilator-Associated Infections, Part I: Reducing the Risks," *Nursing97* 27(2):59-61, February 1997.

Nursing98 Drug Handbook. Springhouse, Pa.: Springhouse Corp., 1998.

Phipps, W.J., et al. *Medical-Surgical Nursing: Concepts and Clinical Practice,* 5th ed. St. Louis: Mosby–Year Book, Inc., 1995.

Polaski, A.L., and Tatro, S.E. *Luckmann's Core Principles and Practice of Medical-Surgical Nursing.* Philadelphia: W.B. Saunders Co., 1996.

6

Gastrointestinal disorders

Anatomy and physiology review

The site of the body's digestive processes, the gastrointestinal (GI) system has the critical task of supplying essential nutrients to fuel the brain, heart, and lungs. GI function also profoundly affects the quality of life by its impact on overall health.

The GI system has two major components: the alimentary canal and the accessory GI organs. The alimentary canal, or GI tract, is a hollow muscular tube that begins in the mouth and extends to the anus. It includes the pharynx, esophagus, stomach, small intestine, and large intestine. Accessory organs aiding GI function include the salivary glands, liver, biliary duct system (gallbladder and bile ducts), and pancreas. (See *Reviewing GI structure and innervation,* pages 182 and 183.)

Together, the GI tract and accessory organs serve two major functions: digestion, the breaking down of food and fluid into simple chemicals that can be absorbed into the bloodstream and transported throughout the body, and elimination of waste products from the body through excretion of feces.

DIGESTION AND ELIMINATION
Digestion starts in the mouth, with chewing, salivation (the beginning of starch digestion), and swallowing (deglutition).

When a person swallows a food bolus, the upper esophageal (hypopharyngeal) sphincter relaxes, allowing food to enter the esophagus. In the esophagus, peristaltic waves, activated reflexively by the glossopharyngeal nerve, propel food toward the stomach. As food moves through the esophagus, glands in the esophageal mucosal layer lubricate the bolus and pro-

tect the esophageal mucosal layer from being damaged by poorly chewed foods.

STOMACH
By the time the food bolus is on its way to the stomach, the cephalic phase of digestion has already begun. In this phase, the stomach secretes hydrochloric acid and pepsin in response to stimuli from smelling, tasting, chewing, or thinking of food. When food enters the stomach through the cardiac sphincter, the stomach wall distends, initiating the gastric phase of digestion. In this phase, distention stimulates the antral mucosa of the stomach to release gastrin. Gastrin, in turn, stimulates the stomach's motor functions and gastric juice secretion by the gastric glands. These highly acidic digestive secretions (pH of 0.9 to 1.5) are mainly pepsin, hydrochloric acid, intrinsic factor, and proteolytic enzymes. (See *Sites and mechanisms of gastric secretion,* page 184.)

The stomach has three major motor functions: storing food, mixing food with gastric juices, and slowly parceling food into the small intestine for further digestion and absorption. Except for alcohol, little food absorption normally occurs in the stomach. Peristaltic contractions churn the food into tiny particles and mix it with gastric juices, forming a thick, almost liquid food bolus known as chyme. After mixing, stronger peristaltic waves move the chyme into the antrum, where it's backed up against the pyloric sphincter before being released into the duodenum, triggering the intestinal phase of digestion.

The rate of stomach emptying depends on a complex interplay of factors, including gastrin release and neural signals caused by stomach wall distention and the enterogastric reflex. In this reaction, the duodenum releases secretin and gastric-inhibiting peptide,

(Text continues on page 185.)

◆◆◆ **181**

Reviewing GI structure and innervation

The GI tract is a hollow tube extending from the lips to the anal opening. Along its entire length are glands and accessory organs devoted to breaking down foods into useful components and eliminating unabsorbed residues. The tract walls alternate muscle tissue with nerve tissue and blood vessels to regulate peristalsis, digestion, and absorption. The diagram below shows the system's major anatomic structures.

GI tract

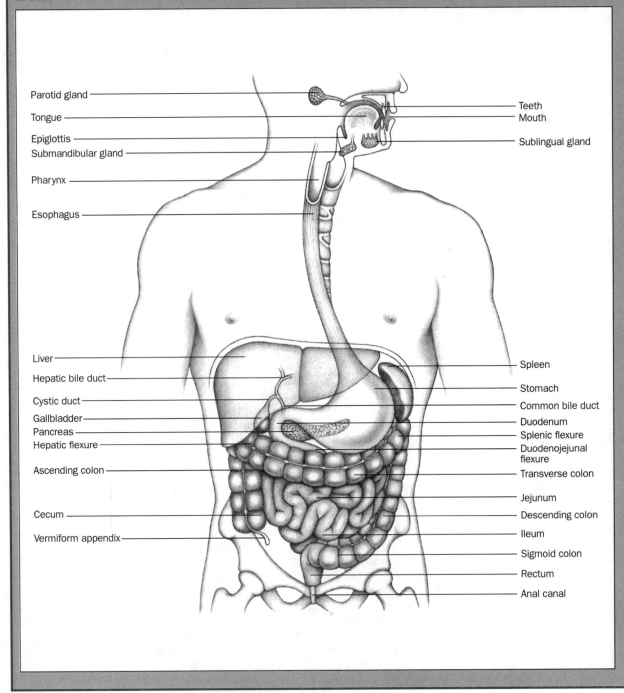

Parotid gland
Tongue
Epiglottis
Submandibular gland
Pharynx
Esophagus
Liver
Hepatic bile duct
Cystic duct
Gallbladder
Pancreas
Hepatic flexure
Ascending colon
Cecum
Vermiform appendix

Teeth
Mouth
Sublingual gland
Spleen
Stomach
Common bile duct
Duodenum
Splenic flexure
Duodenojejunal flexure
Transverse colon
Jejunum
Descending colon
Ileum
Sigmoid colon
Rectum
Anal canal

Cellular anatomy

The GI tract wall's innermost layer (tunica mucosa, or mucosa) consists of epithelial and surface cells and loose connective tissue. In the small intestine, epithelial cells elaborate into millions of fingerlike projections (villi) that vastly increase their absorptive surface area. They also secrete gastric and protective juices and absorb nutrients. Surface cells overlie connective tissue (lamina propria), supported by a thin layer of smooth muscle (muscularis mucosae).

The submucosa (tunica submucosa) encircles the mucosa. It's composed of loose connective tissue, blood and lymphatic vessels, and a nerve network (submucosal, or Meissner's, plexus). Around this layer lies the tunica muscularis, composed of skeletal muscle in the mouth, pharynx, and upper esophagus, and of longitudinal and circular smooth-muscle fibers elsewhere in the tract. During peristalsis, longitudinal fibers shorten the lumen length and circular fibers reduce the lumen diameter. At points along the tract, circular fibers thicken to form sphincters. Between the two muscle layers lies another nerve network—myenteric, or Auerbach's, plexus. The stomach wall contains a third muscle layer.

The GI tract's outer covering—the tunica adventitia in the esophagus and rectum, the tunica serosa elsewhere—consists of connective tissue protected by epithelium. Also called the visceral peritoneum, this layer covers most of the abdominal organs and is contiguous with an identical layer (parietal peritoneum) lining the abdominal cavity. The visceral peritoneum becomes a double-layered fold around the blood vessels, nerves, and lymphatics supplying the small intestine and attaches the jejunum and ileum to the posterior abdominal wall to prevent twisting. A similar mesenteric fold attaches the transverse colon to the posterior abdominal wall.

Innervation

Distention of the submucosal or myenteric plexus stimulates neural transmission to the smooth muscle, initiating peristalsis and mixing contractions. Parasympathetic stimulation—via the vagus nerve for most of the intestines and the sacral spinal nerves for the descending colon and rectum—increases gut and sphincter tone and frequency, strength, and velocity of smooth-muscle contractions. Vagal stimulation also increases motor and secretory activities. Sympathetic stimulation, via spinal nerves from levels T6 to L2, reduces peristalsis and inhibits GI activity.

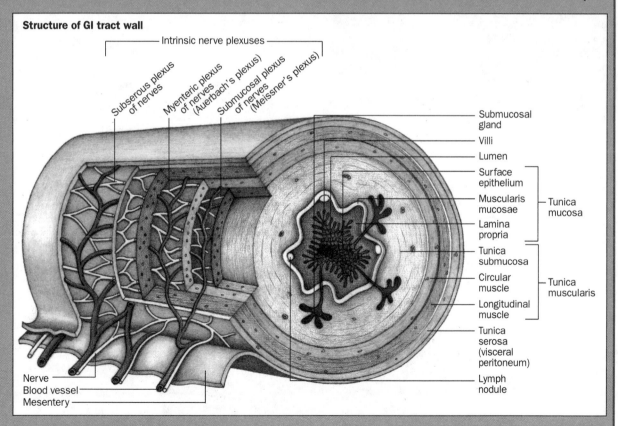

Structure of GI tract wall

Sites and mechanisms of gastric secretion

The body of the stomach lies between the lower esophageal sphincter (LES), or cardiac sphincter, and the pyloric sphincter. Between these sphincters lie the fundus, body, antrum, and pylorus. These areas have a rich variety of mucosal cells that help the stomach carry out its tasks.

Three types of glands secrete 2 to 3 L of gastric juice daily through the stomach's gastric pits. Cardiac glands near the LES and pyloric glands in the pylorus secrete a thin mucus. Gastric glands in the stomach's body and fundus secrete hydrochloric acid (HCl), pepsinogen, intrinsic factor, and mucus.

Specialized cells line the gastric glands, gastric pits, and surface epithelium. Mucous cells in the necks of the gastric glands produce a thin mucus; those in the surface epithelium, a protective alkaline mucus. Both substances lubricate food and protect the stomach from self-digestion by corrosive enzymes and acids.

Argentaffin cells in gastric glands produce the hormone gastrin. Chief cells, primarily in the fundus, produce pepsinogen—the inactive precursor of the proteolytic enzyme pepsin, which breaks down proteins into polypeptides.

Large parietal cells scattered throughout the fundus secrete HCl and intrinsic factor. HCl enzymatically degrades pepsinogen into pepsin and maintains the acid environment favorable for pepsin activity. It also helps disintegrate nucleoproteins and collagens, hydrolyzes sucrose, and inhibits bacterial proliferation. Intrinsic factor promotes vitamin B_{12} absorption in the small intestine.

Stomach structures

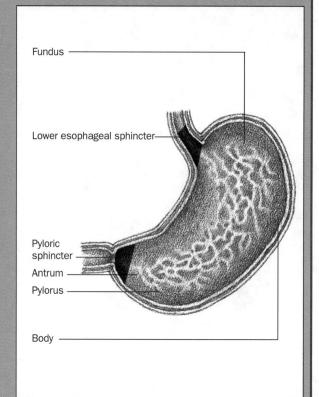

- Fundus
- Lower esophageal sphincter
- Pyloric sphincter
- Antrum
- Pylorus
- Body

Gastric mucosa

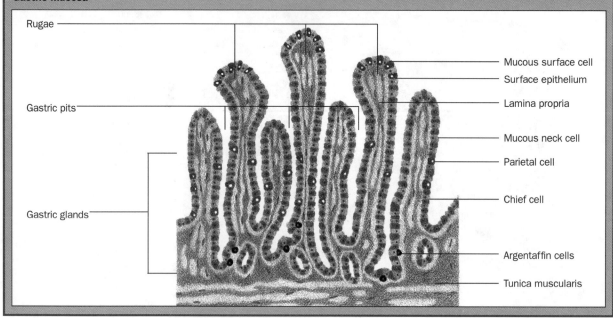

- Rugae
- Gastric pits
- Gastric glands
- Mucous surface cell
- Surface epithelium
- Lamina propria
- Mucous neck cell
- Parietal cell
- Chief cell
- Argentaffin cells
- Tunica muscularis

and the jejunum secretes cholecystokinin (CCK)—all of which act to decrease gastric motility.

SMALL INTESTINE

The small intestine performs most of the work of digestion and absorption. (See *Small intestine: Form affects absorption*, pages 186 and 187.) Here, intestinal contractions and various digestive secretions break down carbohydrates, proteins, and fats and enable the intestinal mucosa to absorb these nutrients, along with water and electrolytes, into the bloodstream for use by the body.

LARGE INTESTINE

By the time chyme passes through the small intestine and enters the ascending colon of the large intestine, it has been reduced to mostly indigestible substances.

The bolus begins its journey through the large intestine at the juncture of the ileum and cecum with the ileocecal pouch. Then the bolus moves up the ascending colon past the right abdominal cavity to the liver's lower border, crosses horizontally below the liver and stomach via the transverse colon, and descends the left abdominal cavity to the iliac fossa through the descending colon.

From there, the bolus travels through the sigmoid colon to the lower midline of the abdominal cavity, then to the rectum, and finally to the anal canal. The anus opens through two sphincters, first a thick, circular smooth muscle under autonomic control then the skeletal muscle under voluntary control.

Circular and longitudinal fibers of the tunica muscularis move and mix intestinal contents, and the longitudinal muscle gives the large intestine its familiar shape. These fibers gather into three narrow bands (taeniae coli) down the middle of the colon and pucker the intestine into characteristic pouches (haustra).

The ascending and descending colons attach directly to the posterior abdominal wall for support. The transverse and sigmoid colons attach indirectly through sheets of connective tissue (mesocolon).

Although the large intestine produces no hormones or digestive enzymes, it continues the absorptive process. Through blood and lymph vessels in the submucosa, the proximal half of the intestine absorbs all but about 100 ml of the remaining water in the colon plus large amounts of sodium and chloride. The large intestine also harbors the bacteria *Escherichia coli, Enterobacter aerogenes, Clostridium perfringens,* and *Lactobacillus bifidus,* which help synthesize vitamin K and break down cellulose into usable carbohydrate. Bacterial action also produces flatus, which helps propel feces toward the rectum. In addition, the mucosa produces alkaline secretions from tubular glands composed of goblet cells. This alkaline mucus lubricates the intestinal walls as food pushes through and protects the mucosa from acidic bacterial action.

In the lower colon, long and relatively sluggish contractions cause propulsive waves known as mass movements. These movements, which normally occur several times a day, propel intestinal contents into the rectum and produce the urge to defecate. Defecation normally results from the defecation reflex, a sensory and parasympathetic nerve-mediated response, along with the person's relaxation of the external anal sphincter.

ACCESSORY ORGANS OF DIGESTION

Allied to the GI tract, the liver, biliary duct system, and pancreas contribute hormones, enzymes, and bile vital to digestion. These organs deliver their secretions to the duodenum through the hepatopancreatic ampulla, also known as the ampulla of Vater and Oddi's sphincter.

LIVER

The body's largest gland (weighing approximately 3 lb [1.4 kg]), the liver is highly vascular and enclosed in a fibrous capsule in the right upper abdominal quadrant. It plays an important role in carbohydrate metabolism, detoxifies various endogenous and exogenous toxins in plasma, and synthesizes plasma proteins, nonessential amino acids, and vitamin A. The liver also stores essential nutrients, such as vitamins K, D, and B_{12}, and iron. What's more, it removes ammonia from body fluids, converting it to urea for excretion in urine, and secretes bile.

Bile is a greenish liquid composed of water, cholesterol, bile salts, electrolytes, and phospholipids. It is important in fat emulsification and intestinal absorption of fatty acids, cholesterol, and other lipids. When bile salts are absent from the intestinal tract, lipids are excreted and fat-soluble vitamins are absorbed poorly. Bile also aids in excretion of conjugated bilirubin (an end product of hemoglobin degradation) from the liver and thereby prevents jaundice. The liver recycles about 80% of bile salts into bile, combining them with bile pigments (biliverdin and bilirubin—the breakdown products of red blood cells) and cholesterol. The liver produces about 500 ml of this alkaline bile in continuous secretion. Enhanced bile production can result from vagal stimulation, release of the hormone secretin, increased liver blood flow, and the presence of fat in the intestine.

The liver metabolizes digestive end products by regulating blood glucose levels. When glucose is being absorbed through the intestine (anabolic state), the liver stores glucose as glycogen. When glucose isn't being absorbed or when blood glucose levels fall (catabolic state), the liver mobilizes glucose to restore blood levels necessary for brain function.

Small intestine: Form affects absorption

Nearly all digestion and absorption takes place in the 20´ (6 m) of small intestine coiled in the abdomen in three major sections: the duodenum, jejunum, and ileum. The duodenum extends from the stomach and contains the hepatopancreatic ampulla (ampulla of Vater, or Oddi's sphincter), an opening that drains bile from the common duct and pancreatic enzymes from the main pancreatic duct.

The jejunum follows the duodenum and leads to the ileum. The small intestine ends in the right lower abdominal quadrant at the ileocecal valve, a sphincter that empties nearly nutrient-free chyme into the large intestine.

A specialized mucosa

Multiple projections of the intestinal mucosa increase the surface area for absorption several hundredfold, as shown in the progressively enlarged views below. Circular projections (Kerckring's folds) are covered by further projections (villi), each containing a lymphatic vessel (lacteal), a venule, capillaries, an arteriole, nerve fibers, and smooth muscle. Each villus is densely fringed with about 2,000 microvilli, resembling a fine brush. The villi are lined with columnar epithelial cells, which dip into the lamina propria between the villi to form intestinal glands (crypts of Lieberkühn).

Small intestine

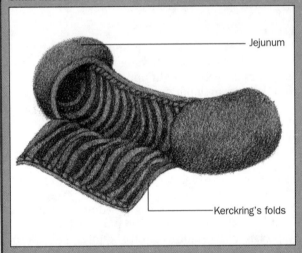

Detail of Kerckring's fold

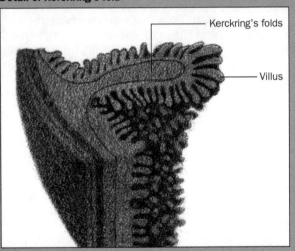

The liver's functional unit, the lobule, consists of a plate of hepatic cells (hepatocytes) that encircle a central vein and radiate outward. The plates of hepatocytes are separated from each other by sinusoids, the liver's capillary system. Lining the sinusoids are reticuloendothelial macrophages (Kupffer's cells), which remove bacteria and toxins that have entered the blood through the intestinal capillaries.

The sinusoids carry oxygenated blood from the hepatic artery and nutrient-rich blood from the portal vein. Unoxygenated blood leaves through the central vein and flows through hepatic veins to the inferior vena cava. Bile, recycled from bile salts in the blood, leaves through bile ducts (canaliculi) that merge into the right and left hepatic ducts to form the common hepatic duct. This common duct joins the cystic duct from the gallbladder to form the common bile duct to the duodenum.

GALLBLADDER

The gallbladder is a 3″ to 4″ (7.5- to 10-cm) long, pear-shaped organ that's joined to the liver's ventral surface by the cystic duct. It stores and concentrates bile produced by the liver. Its 30- to 50-ml storage load increases up to tenfold in potency. Secretion CKK causes gallbladder contraction and relaxation of Oddi's sphincter, releasing bile into the common bile duct for delivery to the duodenum. When the sphincter closes, bile shunts to the gallbladder for storage.

PANCREAS

The pancreas is 6″ to 9″ (15 to 23 cm) long and somewhat flat and lies behind the stomach. Its head and neck extend into the curve of the duodenum and its tail lies against the spleen. The pancreas performs both exocrine and endocrine functions. Its exocrine function involves scattered cells that secrete more than 1 qt (1 L) of digestive enzymes daily. Lobules

The type of epithelial cell dictates its function. Mucus-secreting goblet cells are found on and between the villi on the crypt mucosa. In the proximal duodenum, specialized Brunner's glands also secrete large amounts of mucus to lubricate and protect the duodenum from potentially corrosive acidic chyme and gastric juices.

Other important epithelial cells include Paneth's, argentaffin, undifferentiated, and absorptive cells. Paneth's cells are thought to regulate intestinal flora. Duodenal argentaffin cells produce the hormones secretin and cholecystokinin (CCK). Undifferentiated cells deep within the intestinal glands replace the epithelium. Absorptive cells consist of large numbers of tightly packed microvilli over a plasma membrane containing transport mechanisms for absorption and producing enzymes for the final step in digestion.

The intestinal glands primarily secrete a watery fluid that bathes the villi with chyme particles. Fluid production results from local neural irritation and possibly from hormonal stimulation by secretin and CCK. The microvillous brush border secretes various hormones and digestive enzymes that catalyze final nutrient breakdown.

Detail of villi

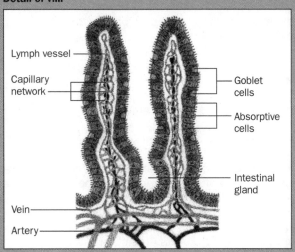

Lymph vessel
Capillary network
Goblet cells
Absorptive cells
Intestinal gland
Vein
Artery

Transverse section of villus

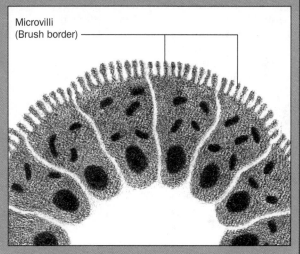

Microvilli (Brush border)

and lobes of the clusters (acini) of enzyme-producing cells release their secretions into ducts that merge into the pancreatic duct. This duct runs the length of the pancreas and joins the bile duct from the gallbladder before entering the duodenum. Vagal stimulation and release of the hormones secretin and CCK control the rate and amount of pancreatic secretion.

The endocrine function of the pancreas involves the islets of Langerhans, which are located between the acinar cells. Over 1 million of these islets house two cell types: beta and alpha. Beta cells secrete insulin to promote carbohydrate metabolism; alpha cells secrete glucagon, which stimulates glycogenolysis in the liver. Both hormones flow directly into the blood, their release stimulated by blood glucose levels.

Assessment

GI signs and symptoms can have many baffling causes. For instance, if your patient is vomiting, what does this sign mean? The patient could be pregnant or could have a viral infection or a severe metabolic disorder such as hyperkalemia. Does your patient merely have indigestion, or is a cardiac crisis building? To help sort out significant symptoms, you'll need to take a thorough patient history. Using inspection, auscultation, palpation, and percussion, you'll probe further by conducting a thorough physical examination.

HISTORY
To help track the development of relevant signs and symptoms over time, remember to develop a detailed

patient history. The history includes the patient's chief complaint, his present illnesses, his previous illnesses, and his family and social history. For best results, establish rapport with the patient by using your best communication skills. Conduct this part of the assessment as privately as possible; many patients feel embarrassed to talk about GI functions. If the patient is in pain, help him into a comfortable position before asking questions.

CHIEF COMPLAINT

Ask the patient why he's seeking care, and record his words verbatim. Ask when he first noticed symptoms, keeping in mind that his answer may indicate only how long the symptoms have been intolerable, not necessarily their true duration.

To establish a baseline for comparison, question the patient about his present state of health. Ask him:
■ How did the problem start? Was it gradual or sudden, with or without previous symptoms? What was he doing when he first noticed it?
■ When did the problem start? Has he had the problem before? If he's in pain, when did that begin? Is the pain continuous, intermittent, or colicky (cramplike)?
■ Ask him to describe the problem. Has he had it before? Was it diagnosed? If he's in pain, does it feel sharp, dull, aching, or burning?
■ Ask him to describe how badly the problem bothers him, on a scale of 1 to 10, for example. Does it keep him from his normal activities? Has it improved or worsened since he first noticed it? Does it wake him at night? If he's in pain, does he double over from it?
■ Where does he feel the problem? Does it spread, radiate, or shift? Where does it hurt most? Does he feel any pain in his shoulder, back, flank, or groin? Some pain may be referred near or far from its origin. (See *Identifying areas of referred pain*.)
■ Does anything seem to bring on the problem? What makes it worse? Does it hurt at the same time each day or with certain positions? Does he notice it after eating or drinking certain foods or after certain activities?
■ Does anything relieve the problem? Does he take any prescribed or over-the-counter (OTC) medications for relief? Has he tried anything else?
■ What else bothers the patient when he has the problem? Has he had nausea, vomiting, dry heaves, diarrhea, or constipation? Has he lost his appetite or lost any weight?
■ When was his last bowel movement? Was it unusual? Has he seen blood in his vomitus or stool? Has his stool changed in size or color or included mucus?
■ Can he eat normally and hold down foods and liquids? Also ask if he's been drinking excessively.

MEDICAL HISTORY

Ask the patient if he's had similar symptoms before. If so, did he see a doctor? What was the medical diagnosis and treatment, if any? Has he had any major acute or chronic illnesses requiring hospitalization? Note the course of the illness, treatment, and any consequences. Record any surgeries in chronologic order, and briefly describe them. Also ask:
■ Has he had peptic ulcer, hiatal hernia, gallbladder disease, diverticulitis, colitis, or inflammatory bowel disease?
■ Are there genetic or environmental causes? Have his family, friends, or coworkers had symptoms similar to his?
■ Has he had cardiac or renal disease, diabetes mellitus, or cancer?
■ Which prescription and OTC medications does he take? (Include dosages and amounts, if known.) Remember that many patients won't mention OTC preparations unless asked. Some of these, such as ibuprofen, aspirin (or drugs containing aspirin), and vitamins, can have GI effects (for example, iron blackens stools).

When asking about recreational drug use and alcohol consumption, remain nonjudgmental to get accurate answers.
■ Does he have any allergies to any drugs, foods, or other agents? If so, have him describe his reaction.
■ Does he exercise? Does he drink caffeinated beverages, such as coffee, tea, and colas? Does he smoke? If so, how much each day? For how many years? Ask what he's had to eat and drink in the last 24 hours, and explore his usual eating habits. Some GI problems can result from certain diets or eating patterns. Ask about any late-night eating or habitually large meals. Because lack of dietary fiber (roughage) may contribute to colorectal cancer and diverticular disease, find out about the patient's fiber intake.

FAMILY HISTORY

Questioning the patient about his family may reveal environmental, genetic, or familial illnesses that influence his current health problems and needs. If his diagnosed or suspected illness has possible familial or genetic tendencies, find out if family members have had similar problems. For example, colon cancer, Crohn's disease, ulcerative colitis, and gallbladder disease tend to run in families; duodenal ulcers occur 35% more commonly in patients with blood group O, suggesting a genetic cause.

SOCIAL HISTORY

Psychological and sociologic factors as well as the physical environment can profoundly affect health. To find out if such factors have contributed to your patient's problem, ask about his occupation, family

Identifying areas of referred pain

Pain may occur relatively near its source or far from it. These illustrations will help you identify the areas and causes of distant, or referred, pain.

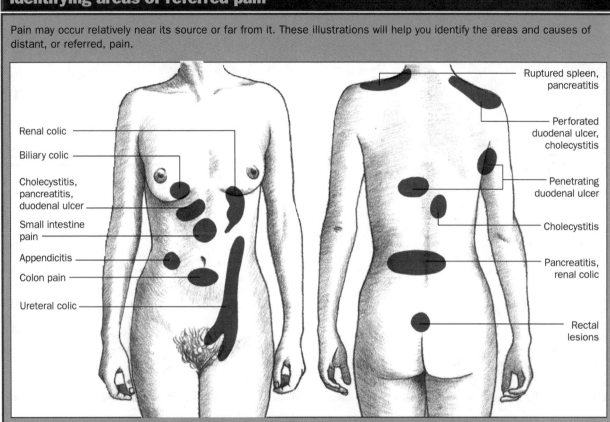

Renal colic
Biliary colic
Cholecystitis, pancreatitis, duodenal ulcer
Small intestine pain
Appendicitis
Colon pain
Ureteral colic

Ruptured spleen, pancreatitis
Perforated duodenal ulcer, cholecystitis
Penetrating duodenal ulcer
Cholecystitis
Pancreatitis, renal colic
Rectal lesions

size, cohabitants, and home environment. Has he been exposed to occupational or environmental hazards? Does he dislike his job? Duodenal ulcers arise more commonly in individuals with marked stress or job responsibility; gastric ulcers, in laborers.

What is his financial status. Inadequate resources can add to the stress of being ill and exacerbate the underlying problem.

Assess his cognition and comprehension levels to help determine his health education needs. Does he understand the importance of appropriate treatment?

PHYSICAL EXAMINATION

Physical assessment of the GI system usually includes evaluation of the mouth, abdomen, liver, and rectum.

To perform a thorough abdominal and rectal assessment, gather the following equipment: gloves, stethoscope, flashlight, measuring tape, felt-tip pen, and a gown and drapes to cover the patient. Make sure that the examination room is private, quiet,

warm, and well lit and that the patient is comfortable and has urinated before you assess the abdomen.

ASSESSING THE ORAL CAVITY

Structural problems or disorders in the oral cavity may affect GI functioning. Here's what to look for:
- Mouth—asymmetry, motility, or malocclusion
- Lips—abnormal color, lesions, nodules, vesicles, or fissures
- Teeth—caries; missing, broken, or displaced teeth; or dental appliances (such as dentures or braces)
- Gums—recession, redness, pallor, hypertrophy, ulcers, or bleeding
- Tongue—deviation to one side, tremors, redness, swelling, ulcers, lesions, or abnormal coatings
- Buccal mucosa—pallor, redness, swelling, ulcers, lesions, or leukoplakia
- Hard and soft palates—redness, lesions, patches, petechiae, or pallor

Identifying abdominal landmarks

To aid accurate abdominal assessment and documentation of findings, envision the patient's abdomen in quadrants. This most commonly used method divides the abdomen into four equal regions by two imaginary lines crossing perpendicularly above the umbilicus.

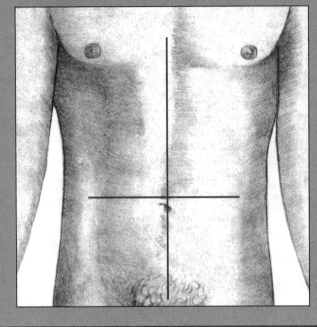

Right upper quadrant (RUQ)
Liver and gallbladder
Pylorus
Duodenum
Head of pancreas
Hepatic flexure of colon
Portions of ascending and
transverse colon

Left upper quadrant (LUQ)
Left liver lobe
Stomach
Body of pancreas
Splenic flexure of colon
Portions of transverse and
descending colon

Right lower quadrant (RLQ)
Cecum and appendix
Portion of ascending colon
Lower portion of right kidney
Bladder (if distended)

Left lower quadrant (LLQ)
Sigmoid colon
Portion of descending colon
Lower portion of left kidney
Bladder (if distended)

■ Pharynx — uvular deviation, tonsil abnormalities, lesions, ulcers, plaques, exudate, or unusual mouth odor (such as sweet and fruity or fetid and musty).

ASSESSING THE ABDOMEN

For consistency, mentally divide the patient's abdomen into four regions, or quadrants. (See *Identifying abdominal landmarks*.) Then, when assessing the abdomen, perform the four basic steps in the following sequence: inspection, auscultation, percussion, and palpation. Remember to auscultate *before* percussing and palpating to avoid altering intestinal activity and bowel sounds.

If the patient has abdominal pain, always auscultate, percuss, and palpate in the painful quadrant last. Otherwise, the patient may tense the abdominal muscles, making further assessment difficult. Watch for signs and symptoms of possible medical emergencies.

When inspecting the patient's entire abdomen, note overall contour and skin integrity, appearance of the umbilicus, and any visible pulsations. Normally, peristalsis isn't visible. In some patients, aortic pulsations may be seen in the epigastric area. Allowing for

various body types, note any localized distention or irregular contours for further assessment.

When inspecting the abdominal skin, look for and document areas of discoloration, striae (lines resulting from rapid or prolonged skin stretching), rashes or other lesions, dilated veins, and scars.

To detect any umbilical or incisional hernias, have the patient raise his head and shoulders while remaining supine. True umbilical or incisional hernias may protrude during this maneuver. Finally, the umbilicus should be midline, concave, and consistent with the color of the rest of the abdomen.

To auscultate for bowel sounds, lightly press the stethoscope diaphragm on the abdominal skin in all four quadrants. Normal peristalsis creates soft, bubbling sounds with no regular pattern, commonly mixed with soft clicks and gurgles, every 5 to 15 seconds. A hungry patient may have a familiar "stomach growl," a condition of hyperperistalsis called borborygmi. Rapid, high-pitched, loud, and gurgling bowel sounds may indicate obstruction.

Sounds at intervals of a minute or longer are hypoactive and normally occur after bowel surgery or when the colon is feces-filled. Remember that bowel sounds can be obscured by a full bladder and that peristalsis and audible bowel sounds may be initiated by gently pressing on the abdominal surface or by having the patient eat or drink something.

Next, use the bell of the stethoscope to auscultate for vascular sounds. Normally, they're absent. Note a bruit, venous hum, or friction rub.

Abdominal percussion helps measure and locate organs and detects excessive accumulation of fluid and air. Percuss in all four quadrants of the abdomen, keeping approximate organ locations in mind as you progress. Percussion sounds depend on the density of underlying structures; dull notes over solids and tympanic notes over air—the predominant abdominal sound. Dull sounds normally occur over the liver and spleen, a lower intestine filled with feces, and a bladder filled with urine. Distinguishing abdominal percussion notes may be difficult in an obese patient.

Keep in mind that abdominal percussion or palpation is contraindicated in patients with suspected abdominal aortic aneurysm or those who have received abdominal organ transplants. It should be performed cautiously in patients with suspected appendicitis.

Abnormal percussion findings usually signal abdominal distention from air accumulation, ascites, or masses. Extremely high-pitched tympanic notes may indicate gaseous bowel distention. Ascites produces shifting dullness, caused by fluid shifting to dependent areas when the patient changes position.

If the patient's abdomen is distended, assess its progression by taking serial measurements of abdominal girth at the level of the umbilicus (marking the point, for reference).

Palpation elicits useful clues about the abdominal wall; the size, condition, and consistency of abdominal organs; the presence and nature of any abdominal masses; and the presence, degree, and location of any abdominal pain. Commonly used techniques include light palpation, deep palpation, and ballottement.

To perform light palpation, gently press your fingertips ½" to ¾" (1.3 to 2 cm) into the abdominal wall. The light touch helps relax the patient. Allow a resistant or jumpy patient to place his hand atop yours and follow along. This usually relaxes him and decreases involuntary muscle contractions.

To begin deep palpation, press the fingertips of both hands about 1½" (4 cm) into the abdominal wall. Move your hands in a slightly circular fashion so that the abdominal wall moves over the underlying structures.

Systematically assess all four quadrants for organ location, masses, and areas of tenderness or increased muscle resistance. If you detect a mass on light or deep palpation, note its location, size, shape, consistency, type of border, degree of tenderness, presence of pulsations, and degree of mobility (fixed or mo-

bile). Deep palpation may evoke rebound tenderness, a possible symptom of peritoneal inflammation.

To accurately assess a patient complaining of generalized tenderness, place your stethoscope on the abdomen and pretend to auscultate, but actually press into the abdomen with the stethoscope as you would with your hands and see if the patient still complains of pain.

Don't palpate a pulsating midline mass; it may be a dissecting aneurysm, with potential to rupture. Report such a mass to the doctor immediately. (See *Eliciting abdominal pain,* page 192.)

Ballottement involves lightly tapping or bouncing your fingertips against the abdominal wall, useful to elicit abdominal muscle resistance or guarding that can be missed with deep palpation. It also may detect the movement or bounce of a freely movable mass. Your fingers should also bounce at the underlying dense liver tissue in the right upper quadrant.

If the patient has ascites, you may need to use deep ballottement. To do so, push your fingertips deeply inward in a rapid motion, then quickly release the pressure, maintaining fingertip contact with the abdominal wall. You should feel the movement of an underlying organ or a movable mass toward your fingertips.

ASSESSING THE LIVER
You can estimate the size and position of the liver through percussion and palpation. (See *Assessing the liver,* page 193.)

Use fist percussion (or blunt percussion) to detect tenderness, a common symptom of gallbladder or liver disease or inflammation. To do this, place one hand flat over the patient's lower right rib cage along the midclavicular line, then strike the back of this hand with your other hand clenched in a fist. Patient discomfort and muscle guarding indicate tenderness.

Use this maneuver only on a patient with unconfirmed inflammation or hepatomegaly, and defer it to the end of the abdominal assessment. Don't perform it if the patient complains of any pain or discomfort during the assessment, particularly over the spleen.

If locating the liver's inferior border through percussion is difficult or impossible, use the scratch test. Lightly place the diaphragm of the stethoscope over the liver's lower border. Auscultate while stroking the patient's abdomen lightly with your right index finger (from well below the level of liver dullness). Start stroking along the midclavicular line at the right iliac crest and move upward, as in percussion. The scratching noise heard through the stethoscope becomes louder over the solid liver.

Usually, palpating the liver in an adult is impossible. If palpable, the liver border usually feels smooth *(Text continues on page 194.)*

Eliciting abdominal pain

Rebound tenderness and the iliopsoas and obturator signs can indicate such conditions as appendicitis and peritonitis. Here's how to elicit these signs.

Rebound tenderness

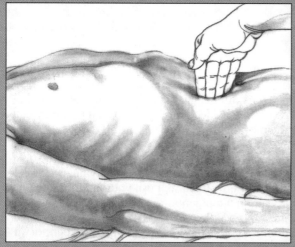

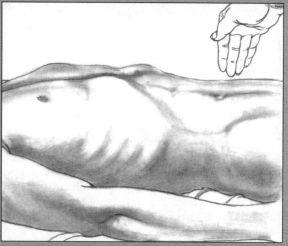

Position the patient supine, with his knees flexed to relax the abdominal muscles. Place your hand gently on the right lower quadrant at McBurney's point—located about midway between the umbilicus and the anterior superior iliac spine.

Slowly and deeply dip your fingers into the area, then release the pressure in a quick, smooth motion. Pain on release—rebound tenderness—is a positive sign. The pain may radiate to the umbilicus.

Caution: To minimize the risk of rupturing an inflamed appendix, don't repeat this maneuver.

Iliopsoas sign

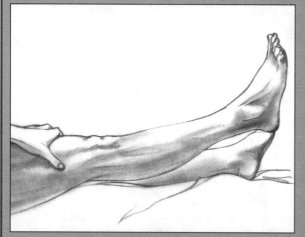

Obturator sign

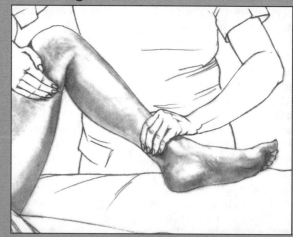

Position the patient supine, with his legs straight. Tell him to raise his right leg upward as you exert slight pressure with your hand.

Repeat the maneuver with the left leg. When testing either leg, increased abdominal pain is a positive result, indicating irritation of the psoas muscle.

Position the patient supine, with his right leg flexed 90 degrees at the hip and knee. Hold the leg just above the knee and at the ankle, then rotate the leg laterally and medially. Pain in the hypogastric region is a positive sign, indicating irritation of the obturator muscle.

Assessing the liver

To assess the liver, you can percuss and attempt to palpate or hook the liver, as shown below.

Liver percussion–anatomic landmarks

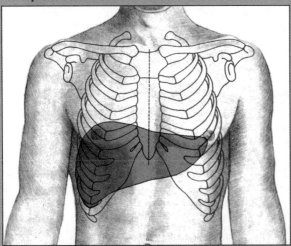

Begin percussing the abdomen along the right midclavicular line, starting below the level of the umbilicus. Move upward until the percussion notes change from tympany to dullness, usually at or slightly below the costal margin. Mark the point of change with a felt-tip pen.

Liver percussion–hand position

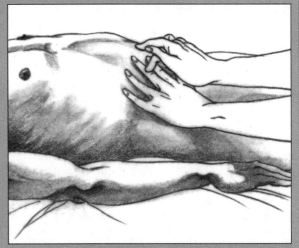

Then percuss downward along the right midclavicular line, starting above the nipple. Move downward until percussion notes change from normal lung resonance to dullness, usually at the fifth to seventh intercostal space. Again, mark the point of change with a felt-tip pen. Estimate liver size by measuring the distance between the two marks.

Liver palpation

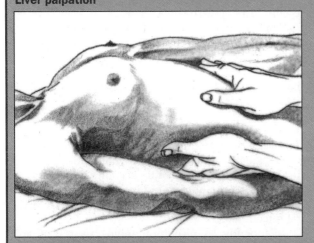

Place one hand on the patient's back at the approximate height of the liver. Place your other hand below your mark of liver dullness on the right lateral abdomen. Point your fingers toward the right costal margin and press gently in and up as the patient inhales deeply. This maneuver may bring the liver edge down to a palpable position.·

Liver hooking

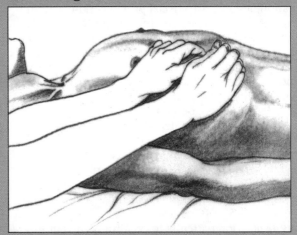

If liver palpation is unsuccessful, try hooking the liver. To do so, stand on the patient's right side at about his shoulder. Place your hands, side by side, below the area of liver dullness. As the patient inhales deeply, press your fingers inward and upward, attempting to feel the liver with the fingertips of both hands.

and firm, with a rounded, regular edge. A palpable liver may indicate hepatomegaly; it also may occur in an extremely thin patient or in the following variations:

- In a child, the liver is proportionately larger, and palpation 1 to 2 fingerbreadths below the ribs is considered normal.
- In a normal variation, Riedel's lobe, the right lobe is elongated toward the right lower quadrant and is palpable below the right costal margin.

ASSESSING THE RECTUM

Usually, you'll perform a routine rectal examination only for patients over age 40, for anyone with a history of bowel elimination changes or anal area discomfort, and for an adult male of any age with a urinary problem.

Because the patient may find it uncomfortable, both physically and psychologically, explain the procedure. Reassure him that the examination, although uncomfortable, should not be painful. Usually, the rectal examination concludes the physical assessment.

To begin, ask an ambulatory patient to stand with his toes pointed inward and bend his body forward over the examination table. The knee-chest position, an excellent alternative for a patient in bed, usually isn't suitable for an ill, elderly, or pregnant patient. Instead, position such a patient in a left lateral Sims' position, with the knees drawn up and the buttocks near the edge of the bed or examination table.

Spread the patient's buttocks to expose the anus and surrounding area. The skin should appear intact and darker than surrounding skin. Inspect the anal area for breaks in the skin, fissures, discharge, inflammation, lesions, scars, rectal prolapse, skin tags, and external hemorrhoids. Ask the patient to strain as though defecating, a way to expose internal hemorrhoids, polyps, rectal prolapse, and fissures.

Next, palpate the external rectum. Put on a glove and apply lubricant to your index finger. As the patient strains again, palpate for any anal outpouchings or bulges, nodules, or tenderness.

Then, palpate the internal rectum. Before beginning, explain that you'll insert your gloved, lubricated finger a short distance into the rectum and he will feel the urge to defecate. Have the patient breathe through the mouth and relax. When the anal sphincter is relaxed, gently insert your finger approximately 2½″ to 4″ (6.5 to 10 cm), angling it toward the umbilicus. (*Note:* Don't attempt force. Wait with your fingertip resting lightly on the sphincter until the sphincter relaxes.)

Rotate your finger systematically to palpate all aspects of the rectal wall for nodules, tenderness, irregularities, and fecal impaction. The rectal wall should feel smooth and soft.

In a female patient, try to feel the posterior side of the uterus through the anterior rectal wall. In a male patient, assess the prostate gland when palpating the anterior rectal wall; the prostate should feel firm and smooth.

With your finger fully inserted, ask the patient to bear down again; this may cause any lesions higher in the rectum to move down to a palpable level. To assess anal sphincter competence, ask the patient to tighten the anal muscles around your finger.

Finally, withdraw your finger and examine it for blood, mucus, or stool. If stool appears, note its color and test a sample for occult blood.

ONGOING ASSESSMENT

Whenever a patient reports a GI complaint, he'll need reassessment. You can't assume, for instance, that a previously assessed dysfunction is causing the patient's present abdominal pain. The pain's nature and location may have changed, indicating more extensive involvement or perhaps a new disorder. To avoid unduly alarming your patient, reassure him that ongoing assessment doesn't necessarily mean he has a significant health problem. Tell him that repeated evaluations aid diagnosis and treatment.

Appendicitis

The most common disease requiring major surgery, appendicitis is an inflammation of the vermiform appendix, a small, fingerlike projection attached to the cecum just below the ileocecal valve.

Appendicitis may occur at any age and affects both sexes equally; however, between puberty and age 25, it's more prevalent in males. Since the advent of antibiotics, the incidence and mortality of appendicitis have declined. If untreated, this disease is invariably fatal.

CAUSES

Although the appendix has no known function, it does regularly fill and empty itself of food. Appendicitis occurs when the appendix becomes inflamed from ulceration of the mucosa or obstruction of the lumen by a fecal mass, a stricture, barium ingestion, or a viral infection.

In appendicitis, ulceration or blockage sets off an inflammatory process that can lead to infection, thrombosis, necrosis, and perforation. The most common and perilous complication occurs when the appendix ruptures or perforates and infected contents spill into the abdominal cavity, causing peritonitis. Other complications include appendiceal abscess and pyelophlebitis.

DIAGNOSIS AND TREATMENT

A moderately elevated white blood cell (WBC) count, with increased numbers of immature cells, supports the diagnosis. Failure of the organ to fill with radiographic contrast agent indicates appendicitis. Diagnosis may also involve ruling out illnesses with similar symptoms, such as bladder infection, diverticulitis, gastritis, ovarian cyst, pancreatitis, renal colic, and uterine disease.

Appendectomy is the only effective treatment. If peritonitis develops, treatment involves GI intubation, parenteral replacement of fluids and electrolytes, and administration of antibiotics.

COLLABORATIVE MANAGEMENT

Care of the patient with appendicitis focuses on preparing him for surgery and promoting recovery.

ASSESSMENT

During the initial phase of appendicitis, the patient typically complains of abdominal pain. Pain may be generalized but, within a few hours, becomes localized in the right lower abdomen (McBurney's point). He may also report anorexia, nausea, and one or two episodes of vomiting. Later signs and symptoms include malaise, constipation or diarrhea (rare), and possibly low-grade fever. Look for:
- a patient who walks bent over to reduce right lower quadrant pain (When sleeping or lying supine, he may keep his right knee bent up to decrease pain.)
- normal bowel sounds
- early on, localized abdominal findings except for diffuse tenderness in the midepigastrium and around the umbilicus
- later, tenderness in the right lower abdominal quadrant that worsens upon coughing or gentle percussion
- rebound tenderness and spasm of the abdominal muscles
- no abdominal tenderness if the appendix is positioned retrocecally or in the pelvis (Instead, rectal or pelvic examination reveals tenderness in the flank.).

Keep in mind that abdominal rigidity and tenderness worsen as the condition progresses. Sudden cessation of abdominal pain signals perforation or infarction.

NURSING DIAGNOSES AND COLLABORATIVE PROBLEMS

Based on the following nursing diagnoses, you'll establish patient outcomes.

Risk for fluid volume deficit related to nausea and vomiting caused by appendicitis. The patient will:
- maintain normal fluid volume as evidenced by normal blood pressure and urine output and absence of dehydration

- experience decreased nausea and vomiting
- recover normal GI function.

Risk for infection related to potential for ruptured or perforated appendix. The patient will:
- exhibit no signs and symptoms of peritonitis, including sudden cessation of abdominal pain followed by pain recurrence that intensifies and becomes constant; other signs and symptoms are fever, tachycardia, hypotension, abdominal distention, increased nausea or vomiting, and inability to pass feces or flatus
- have a WBC count and temperature that will return to normal and remain normal
- state the importance of notifying a health professional immediately if pain suddenly ceases before surgery.

Pain related to inflammation of the vermiform appendix. The patient will:
- express understanding of why pain medication is withheld until diagnosis is confirmed
- obtain pain relief after analgesic administration
- become free from pain.

PLANNING AND IMPLEMENTATION

These measures help the patient with appendicitis:
- Make sure the patient receives nothing by mouth until surgery is performed.
- Administer I.V. fluids to prevent dehydration. Never administer cathartics or enemas because they may rupture the appendix.
- Monitor the patient's vital signs and assess intake and output for signs of dehydration, such as hypotension or fluid imbalance.
- Observe the patient for complications, such as peritonitis, appendiceal abscess, and pyelophlebitis.
- If peritonitis occurs and nasogastric drainage is necessary, record drainage and provide proper mouth and nose care. Expect to administer antibiotic therapy.
- Evaluate the severity and location of abdominal pain. Notify the doctor immediately if pain suddenly ceases.
- Don't administer analgesics until the diagnosis is confirmed because they mask symptoms.
- Place the patient in Fowler's position to reduce pain. Never apply heat to the right lower abdomen; this may cause the appendix to rupture.
- Once the diagnosis is confirmed, prepare the patient for surgery.

Patient teaching
- Teach the patient what happens in appendicitis.
- Explain why analgesic administration may be delayed, and reassure the patient that an analgesic will be administered as soon as possible.

Where calculi collect

Possible locations for calculi to collect include the sites shown at the right.

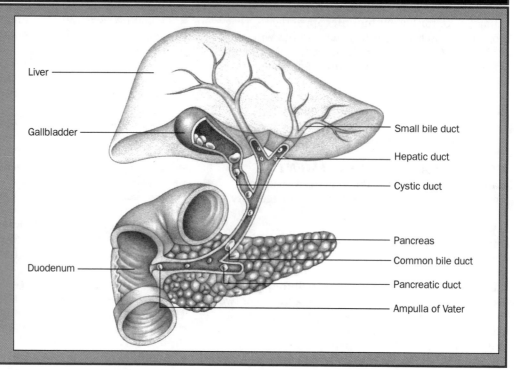

- Liver
- Gallbladder
- Duodenum
- Small bile duct
- Hepatic duct
- Cystic duct
- Pancreas
- Common bile duct
- Pancreatic duct
- Ampulla of Vater

■ Tell the patient that assuming a Fowler's position may help relieve his pain.

■ Emphasize the importance of notifying a health care professional if pain suddenly ends without treatment.

■ Help the patient understand the required surgery and its possible complications.

EVALUATION

Evaluation of patient outcomes determines the success of collaborative management. For the patient with appendicitis, evaluation focuses on fluid balance, reduced risk of infection, improved comfort, and adequate knowledge.

Cholelithiasis and cholecystitis

The leading biliary tract disease, cholelithiasis is the formation of stones or calculi (gallstones) in the gallbladder. Cholecystitis is an inflammation of the gallbladder. The prognosis is usually good with treatment. If infection occurs, the prognosis depends on its severity and response to antibiotics.

CAUSES

These two related disorders stem from a common cause: formation of calculi. Although the exact cause of gallstone formation is unknown, abnormal metabolism of cholesterol and bile salts clearly plays an important role.

Identified risk factors that predispose a person to calculi formation include:

■ high-calorie, high-cholesterol diet, associated with obesity

■ elevated estrogen levels from oral contraceptive use, postmenopausal hormone-replacement therapy, or pregnancy

■ use of clofibrate

■ diabetes mellitus, ileal disease, hemolytic disorders, hepatic disease, or pancreatitis.

The specific disorder that develops depends on where in the gallbladder or biliary tract the calculi collect. (See *Where calculi collect*.) For example, cholelithiasis results when gallstones form and remain in the gallbladder. Cholecystitis, choledocholithiasis, cholangitis, and gallstone ileus usually develop after a gallstone lodges in a duct or in the small bowel, causing an obstruction.

Acute cholecystitis also may result from conditions that alter the gallbladder's ability to fill or empty.

These conditions include trauma, reduced blood supply to the gallbladder, prolonged immobility, chronic dieting, adhesions, prolonged anesthesia, and narcotic abuse.

The formation of gallstones can give rise to a number of related disorders.

In cholecystitis, the gallbladder becomes acutely or chronically inflamed, usually when a stone blocks the cystic duct. The acute form is most common during middle age; the chronic form, among older persons. Prognosis is good with treatment.

In choledocholithiasis, gallstones pass out of the gallbladder and lodge in and obstruct the common bile duct. Prognosis is good unless infection occurs.

In cholangitis, the bile duct becomes infected (associated with choledocholithiasis and cholangiography). Nonsuppurative cholangitis usually responds rapidly to antibiotics. Suppurative cholangitis has a poor prognosis unless surgery to drain the infected bile is performed promptly.

In gallstone ileus, a gallstone obstructs the small bowel by lodging at the ileocecal valve. This condition is most common in elderly persons. The prognosis is good with surgery.

Generally, gallbladder and duct diseases strike during middle age. Between ages 20 and 50, they're six times more common in women, but the odds equalize after age 50. The incidence rises with each succeeding decade.

DIAGNOSIS AND TREATMENT

Ultrasonography and X-rays detect gallstones. Specific procedures include:

■ Plain abdominal X-rays identify gallstones if they contain enough calcium to be radiopaque. X-rays are also helpful in identifying porcelain gallbladder, limy bile, and gallstone ileus.

■ Ultrasonography of the gallbladder confirms cholelithiasis in most patients and distinguishes between obstructive and nonobstructive jaundice; calculi as small as 2 mm can be detected.

■ Oral cholecystography confirms the presence of gallstones (test is being replaced by ultrasonography).

■ Technetium-labeled iminodiacetic acid scan of the gallbladder indicates cystic duct obstruction and acute or chronic cholecystitis if the gallbladder can't be seen.

■ Percutaneous transhepatic cholangiography, imaging performed under fluoroscopic control, supports the diagnosis of obstructive jaundice and visualizes calculi in the ducts.

■ Blood studies may reveal elevated levels of serum alkaline phosphatase, lactate dehydrogenase, aspartate aminotransferase, and total bilirubin. The white blood cell (WBC) count is slightly elevated during a cholecystitis attack.

Surgery, usually elective, remains the most common treatment for gallbladder and duct disease. Surgery is usually recommended if the patient has symptoms frequent enough to interfere with his regular routine; if he has any complications of gallstones; or if he has had a previous attack of cholecystitis.

Procedures may include cholecystectomy; cholecystectomy with operative cholangiography; choledochostomy; exploration of the common bile duct or, possibly, laparoscopic cholecystectomy.

If the patient's gallstones are radiolucent and consist totally or in part of cholesterol, he may be a candidate for gallstone dissolution therapy, using oral chenodeoxycholic acid or ursodiol to partially or completely dissolve gallstones. Limitations are that this prolonged treatment dissolves only small calculi, with a high incidence of adverse reactions and calculi recurrence.

Other, more direct, methods include insertion of a percutaneous transhepatic biliary catheter under fluoroscopic guidance, which permits visualization of the calculi and their removal using a basket-shaped tool called a Dormia basket. Endoscopic retrograde cholangiopancreatography (ERCP) removes calculi with a balloon or basketlike tool passed through an endoscope. Both techniques permit decompression of the biliary tree, allowing bile to flow.

Another technique, lithotripsy, breaks up gallstones with ultrasonic waves. It has been used successfully in some patients with radiolucent calculi.

If the patient is asymptomatic or has recovered from a first attack of biliary colic, noninvasive treatment includes a low-fat diet with replacement of the fat-soluble vitamins A, D, E, and K and administration of bile salts to facilitate digestion and vitamin absorption.

During an acute attack, medications include narcotics for pain relief; antispasmodics and anticholinergics to relax smooth muscles and decrease ductal tone and spasm; and antiemetics to reduce nausea and vomiting. A nasogastric tube may also be inserted and connected to intermittent low-pressure suction to relieve vomiting.

In patients with severe acute cholecystitis, I.V. fluids and I.V. antibiotic therapy often precede surgery. Cholestyramine may be given if the patient has obstructive jaundice with severe itching from accumulation of bile salts in the skin.

The patient with nonsuppurative cholangitis usually responds quickly to antibiotic therapy. Suppurative cholangitis requires antibiotic therapy, prompt surgical correction of the obstruction, and drainage of the infected bile.

COLLABORATIVE MANAGEMENT
Care of the patient with cholelithiasis and cholecystitis focuses on supportive care and close postoperative observation.

ASSESSMENT
Although gallbladder disease may produce no symptoms (even when X-rays reveal gallstones), acute cholelithiasis, acute cholecystitis, and choledocholithiasis produce symptoms of a classic gallbladder attack. Look for:
- complaints of sudden onset of severe steady or aching pain in the midepigastric region or the right upper abdominal quadrant
- pain described as radiating to the back, between the shoulder blades, over the right shoulder blade, or just to the shoulder area (characteristic of biliary colic; commonly requiring treatment in the emergency department).
- reports that the attack followed eating a fatty meal or a large meal after extended fasting
- reports that a sudden night attack caused nausea, vomiting, and chills; possible low-grade fever.
- extended history of milder GI symptoms that preceded the acute attack, including indigestion, vague abdominal discomfort, belching, and flatulence after eating meals or snacks rich in fats
- during an acute attack, severe pain with pallor, diaphoresis, and exhaustion
- in chronic cholecystitis, jaundiced skin, sclerae, and oral mucous membranes may confirm jaundice; specimens may reveal dark-colored urine and clay-colored stools
- tachycardia
- tenderness of abdomen on light palpation (tenderness over the gallbladder increases on inspiration)
- a painless, sausagelike mass when a calculus-filled gallbladder without ductal obstruction is palpated
- hypoactive bowel sounds in acute cholecystitis.

If the patient has cholangitis, he may report a history of choledocholithiasis and classic symptoms of biliary colic. On inspection, jaundice and pain may be evident. He may also have a spiking fever with chills.

In gallstone ileus, the patient may complain of colicky pain that persists for several days, sometimes with nausea and vomiting. You may note abdominal distention on inspection. Auscultation may reveal absent bowel sounds if the patient has a complete bowel obstruction.

NURSING DIAGNOSES AND COLLABORATIVE PROBLEMS
Based on the following nursing diagnoses, you'll establish patient outcomes.

Pain related to inflammation of the gallbladder caused by a gallstone lodged in the cystic duct. The patient will:

- express relief from pain following analgesic administration
- become pain-free following removal of lodged gallstone.

Risk for fluid volume deficit related to nausea and vomiting caused by cholecystitis. The patient will:
- maintain an adequate fluid balance as exhibited by equal intake (I.V. if necessary) and output and normal blood pressure
- exhibit no signs and symptoms of dehydration
- experience a cessation of nausea and vomiting.

Risk for infection related to biliary obstruction caused by one or more gallstones lodging in a duct or the small intestine. The patient will:
- maintain a normal temperature and WBC count
- exhibit no other signs and symptoms of infection, such as chills or acute abdominal pain.

PLANNING AND IMPLEMENTATION
These measures help the patient with cholelithiasis and cholecystitis:
- As ordered, administer narcotic and anticholinergic medications to relieve pain.
- Use relaxation and positioning to help alleviate pain.
- Place the patient in low Fowler's position to minimize pressure on the right upper quadrant.
- If the patient has cholangitis, administer antibiotics, as ordered. Monitor his vital signs closely. Watch for signs of severe toxicity, including confusion, septicemia, and septic shock.
- If the patient is not having surgery, provide a low-fat diet and smaller, more frequent meals to help prevent attacks of biliary colic.
- Replace vitamins A, D, E, and K, and administer bile salts, as ordered.
- If the patient develops nausea or vomits, stay with him and withhold food and fluids. Assess his vital signs and monitor his intake and output for signs of a fluid deficit.
- Give the patient antiemetics to relieve nausea and vomiting.
- After percutaneous transhepatic biliary catheterization or ERCP to remove gallstones, give the patient nothing by mouth until his gag reflex returns. Monitor his intake and output, keeping in mind that urine retention can be a problem. Observe the patient for complications, including cholangitis and pancreatitis.
- Evaluate the effectiveness of medication, and watch for possible adverse reactions.

Patient teaching
- Teach the patient about the disease and the reasons for his symptoms.
- Explain scheduled diagnostic tests, reviewing pretest instructions and necessary aftercare.

- If a low-fat diet is ordered, suggest ways to implement it. If necessary, ask the dietitian to reinforce your instructions. Be sure the patient understands how dietary changes help to prevent biliary colic.
- Review the proper use of prescribed medications, explaining their desired effects and possible adverse reactions, especially those that warrant a call to the doctor.
- Reinforce the doctor's explanation of the ordered treatment, such as surgery, ERCP, or lithotripsy. Be sure the patient fully understands the possible complications, if any, associated with the treatments.

EVALUATION

Evaluation of patient outcomes determines the success of collaborative management. For the patient with gallstones, evaluation focuses on pain relief, adequate nutrition, maintenance of fluid balance, and adequate knowledge.

Cirrhosis

Cirrhosis is the ninth most common cause of death in the United States; among patients ages 35 to 55, it ranks fourth. The disease, which can strike at any age, has four main types: Läennec's, postnecrotic, biliary, and cardiac. Läennec's cirrhosis, the most common, prevails among malnourished alcoholic men and accounts for more than half of all cirrhosis cases. Postnecrotic cirrhosis is more common in women than in men and is the most common type worldwide.

CAUSES

The factors that lead to the development of cirrhosis are not clearly defined. A genetic factor appears important. Some families tend to develop cirrhosis or possess a sensitivity to alcohol. However, many alcoholics don't develop cirrhosis and others develop the disease even though they get adequate nutrition.

Cirrhosis has a diverse etiology, reflecting the varied clinical types:
- Läennec's cirrhosis (alcoholic, nutritional, or portal cirrhosis) follows chronic alcoholism and malnutrition.
- Postnecrotic cirrhosis usually is a complication of viral hepatitis. This type also may follow exposure to liver toxins, such as arsenic, carbon tetrachloride, or phosphorus.
- Biliary cirrhosis links to prolonged biliary tract obstruction or inflammation.
- Cardiac cirrhosis is associated with protracted venous congestion in the liver caused by right-sided heart failure.

- In addition, some patients develop idiopathic cirrhosis.

A chronic hepatic disease, cirrhosis is characterized by diffuse destruction and fibrotic regeneration of hepatic cells. As necrotic tissue yields to fibrosis, this disease alters liver structure and normal vasculature, impairs blood and lymph flow, and ultimately causes hepatic insufficiency.

Depending on the amount of liver damage, cirrhosis can lead to such complications as portal hypertension, bleeding esophageal varices, hepatic encephalopathy, hepatorenal syndrome, and death. Portal hypertension—elevated pressure in the portal vein—occurs when blood flow meets increased resistance from fibrotic tissue that replaces hepatic cells. The disorder may also stem from mechanical obstruction and occlusion of the hepatic veins (Budd-Chiari syndrome).

As pressure in the portal vein rises, blood backs up into the spleen and flows through collateral channels to the venous system, bypassing the liver. Consequently, portal hypertension produces dilated tortuous collateral veins in the submucosa of the lower esophagus known as esophageal varices.

In many patients, the first sign of portal hypertension is bleeding from esophageal varices. Esophageal varices commonly cause massive hematemesis that can quickly result in hemorrhage and hypovolemic shock. If bleeding is not stopped, the patient will die.

DIAGNOSIS AND TREATMENT

Laboratory and other diagnostic tests are required to confirm the diagnosis, establish the type of cirrhosis, and pinpoint complications. Liver biopsy, the definitive test for cirrhosis, detects hepatic tissue destruction and fibrosis.

Abdominal X-rays show liver size and reveal cysts or gas within the biliary tract or liver, liver calcification, and massive ascites. Computed tomography and liver scans determine liver size, identify masses, and visualize hepatic blood flow and obstruction. Esophagogastroduodenoscopy reveals bleeding esophageal varices, stomach irritation or ulceration, or duodenal bleeding and irritation.

Blood studies show liver enzymes (alanine aminotransferase and aspartate aminotransferase), total serum bilirubin, and indirect bilirubin levels are elevated. Total serum albumin and protein levels decrease; prothrombin time is prolonged. Hematocrit and hemoglobin and serum electrolyte levels decrease. Vitamins A, C, and K are deficient. Urine and stool studies show increased urine levels of bilirubin and urobilinogen and lower fecal urobilinogen levels.

Therapy aims to remove or alleviate the underlying cause of cirrhosis, prevent further liver damage, and prevent or treat complications. Vitamins and nutritional supplements promote healing of damaged hepatic cells and improve the patient's nutritional status. Sodium consumption is usually restricted to 500 mg/day and liquid intake is limited to 1½ qt (1.5 L)/day to help manage ascites and edema.

Drug therapy requires special caution because the cirrhotic liver can't detoxify harmful substances efficiently. Antacids may be ordered to reduce gastric distress and decrease the potential for GI bleeding. Potassium-sparing diuretics may be used to reduce ascites and edema. However, diuretics require careful monitoring because fluid and electrolyte imbalance may precipitate hepatic encephalopathy. Vasopressin may be indicated for esophageal varices. Alcohol is prohibited, and sedatives should be avoided.

In patients with ascites, paracentesis may be used to relieve abdominal pressure. However, surgery may be required to divert ascites into venous circulation; if so, a peritoneovenous shunt is used. Shunt insertion results in weight loss, decreased abdominal girth, increased sodium excretion from the kidneys, and improved urine output.

To control bleeding from esophageal varices or other GI hemorrhage, nonsurgical measures are attempted first. These include gastric intubation and esophageal balloon tamponade. In gastric intubation, a tube is inserted and the stomach is lavaged until the contents are clear. If the bleeding is assessed as a gastric ulcer, antacids and histamine-2 receptor antagonists are administered.

In esophageal balloon tamponade, bleeding vessels are compressed to stanch blood loss from esophageal varices. Several forms of balloon tamponade are available, including the Sengstaken-Blakemore tube method, the esophagogastric tube method, and the Minnesota tube method.

Sclerotherapy is performed if the patient continues to hemorrhage despite conservative treatment. A sclerosing agent is injected into the oozing vessels. This agent traumatizes epithelial tissue, which causes thrombosis and leads to sclerosis. If bleeding from the varices doesn't stop within 2 to 5 minutes, a second injection is given below the bleeding site. Sclerotherapy also may be performed prophylactically on nonbleeding varices.

Portal-systemic shunts may be used for patients with bleeding esophageal varices and portal hypertension. Surgical shunting procedures decrease portal hypertension by diverting a portion of the portal vein blood flow away from the liver. These procedures are seldom performed because they can result in bleeding, infection, and shunt thrombosis.

Massive hemorrhage requires blood transfusions. To maintain blood pressure, crystalloid or colloid volume expanders are administered until the blood is available.

COLLABORATIVE MANAGEMENT

Care of the patient with cirrhosis focuses on improving his nutritional status and teaching him about the behavior that causes his condition.

ASSESSMENT

During history taking, you may uncover alcoholism or other diseases or conditions, such as acute viral hepatitis, biliary tract disorders, congestive heart failure, recent blood transfusions, or viral infections. Regardless of the cause, signs and symptoms are similar for all types and vary according to the stage of the disease. Look for:

■ telangiectasis on the cheeks; spider angiomas on the face, neck, arms, and trunk; gynecomastia; umbilical hernia; distended abdominal blood vessels; ascites; testicular atrophy; palmar erythema; clubbed fingers; thigh and leg edema; ecchymosis; and jaundice

■ early, vague signs and symptoms, including abdominal pain, diarrhea, fatigue, nausea, and vomiting

■ as found in early palpation, a large, firm liver with a sharp edge

■ later, complaints of chronic dyspepsia, constipation, pruritus, and weight loss; a tendency for easy bleeding, such as frequent nosebleeds, easy bruising, or bleeding gums

■ later, a decrease in liver size caused by scar tissue and, if palpable, a nodular edge

■ an enlarged spleen.

NURSING DIAGNOSES AND COLLABORATIVE PROBLEMS

Based on the following nursing diagnoses, you'll establish patient outcomes.

Altered nutrition: Less than body requirements, related to adverse GI effects associated with cirrhosis. The patient will:

■ regain lost weight and maintain it

■ consume a balanced diet within his dietary restrictions

■ not become malnourished.

Ineffective breathing pattern related to pressure on diaphragm from ascites and changes in liver function. The patient will:

■ be free from respiratory distress

■ exhibit no dyspnea or hypoxia (cyanosis, restlessness).

Risk for injury related to potential for complications such as bleeding esophageal varices caused by increased portal hypertension. The patient will:

■ develop no bleeding esophageal varices

■ adhere to the treatment regimen to prevent further liver damage and complications such as esophageal varices.

PLANNING AND IMPLEMENTATION
These measures help the patient with cirrhosis:
■ Administer diuretics, potassium, and protein or vitamin supplements, as ordered. Restrict sodium and fluid intake, as ordered.
■ Monitor vital signs, intake and output, and electrolyte levels to determine fluid volume status.
■ To assess fluid retention, measure and record abdominal girth every shift. Weigh the patient daily, and document his weight.
■ Assess respiratory status frequently. Position the patient to ease breathing.
■ Remain with the patient during hemorrhagic episodes.
■ Provide or assist with oral hygiene before and after meals.
■ Determine food preferences, and provide them within the patient's prescribed diet limitations. Offer frequent, small meals.
■ Observe and document the degree of sclerae and skin jaundice.
■ Give the patient frequent skin care, bathe him without soap, and massage him with emollient lotions. Keep his fingernails short. Handle the patient gently; turn and reposition him often to keep the skin intact.
■ Increase the patient's exercise tolerance by decreasing fluid volumes and providing rest periods before exercise.
■ Each time you see the patient, address him by name and say your name. Mention time, place, and date frequently throughout the day. Place a clock and a calendar where he can easily see them.
■ Watch for signs of epigastric fullness and weakness.
■ Observe closely for signs and symptoms of behavioral or personality changes. Report anxiety, restlessness, increasing stupor, lethargy, hallucinations, or neuromuscular dysfunction. Arouse the patient periodically to determine level of consciousness. Watch for asterixis, a sign of developing encephalopathy.
■ Use safety measures to protect the patient from injury. Avoid physical restraints if possible.
■ Allow the patient to express his feelings about having cirrhosis. Offer psychological support and encouragement when appropriate. Offer him and family members a realistic evaluation of his health status, and encouragement for the immediate future.
■ Prepare the patient for necessary medical procedures (such as paracentesis, gastric intubation, esophageal balloon tamponade, sclerotherapy, or por-

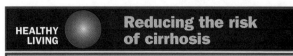

HEALTHY LIVING | **Reducing the risk of cirrhosis**

An alcoholic's odds of developing cirrhosis may be reduced through proper diet and avoidance of alcohol. Although the amount of alcohol consumption needed to produce signs of liver damage remains unknown, people who are alcoholic and malnourished are known to be at greatest risk for cirrhosis. Encourage the patient to maintain an adequate diet. Suggest the use of vitamin supplementation.

tal-systemic shunt insertion), and assist with the procedures as needed.
■ Observe for bleeding gums, ecchymoses, epistaxis, and petechiae.
■ Monitor bowel movements to assess the effectiveness of laxatives and lactulose. Inspect stools for amount, color, and consistency, and test stools and vomitus for occult blood.

Patient teaching
■ To minimize the risk of bleeding, warn the patient against taking nonsteroidal anti-inflammatory drugs. Suggest using an electric razor and a soft toothbrush.
■ Explain the importance of avoiding activities that increase intra-abdominal pressure, such as heavy lifting, vigorous coughing, and straining to have a bowel movement.
■ Advise the patient that rest and good nutrition conserve energy and decrease metabolic demands on the liver. Urge him to eat frequent, small meals. Teach him to alternate periods of rest and activity to reduce oxygen demand and prevent fatigue.
■ Tell the patient how he can conserve energy while performing activities of daily living. For example, suggest that he sit on a bench while bathing or dressing.
■ Stress the need to avoid infections and abstain from alcohol. Refer the patient to Alcoholics Anonymous if appropriate. (See *Reducing the risk of cirrhosis.*)

EVALUATION
Evaluation of patient outcomes determines the success of collaborative management. For the patient with cirrhosis, evaluation focuses on adequate nutrition and supportive care.

Colorectal cancer
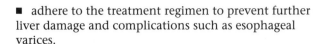

The second most common visceral neoplasm in the United States and Europe, colorectal cancer occurs equally in men and women but is more common in those over age 40.

CAUSES

Although the cause of colorectal cancer is unknown, studies show a greater incidence in areas of higher economic development, suggesting a relation to diet (excess animal fat, particularly beef, and low fiber).

Other risk factors for colorectal cancer include diseases of the digestive tract, a history of ulcerative colitis (cancer typically starts in 11 to 17 years), familial polyposis (cancer almost always develops by age 50), and a family history (first-degree relatives) of the disease.

Malignant tumors of the colon or rectum are almost always adenocarcinomas. About half of these are sessile lesions of the rectosigmoid area; the rest, polypoid lesions.

Colorectal cancer progresses slowly, remaining localized for a long time. Unless the tumor has metastasized, the 5-year survival rate is relatively high: about 80% for rectal cancer and more than 85% for colon cancer. If left untreated, the disease is invariably fatal.

As the tumor grows and encroaches on the abdominal organs, abdominal distention and intestinal obstruction occur. Anemia may develop if rectal bleeding isn't treated.

DIAGNOSIS AND TREATMENT

Digital rectal examination can detect almost 15% of colorectal cancers, revealing suspicious rectal and perianal lesions. Fecal occult blood test can detect blood in stools, a warning sign of rectal cancer.

Proctoscopy or sigmoidoscopy permits visualization of the lower GI tract, detecting up to 66% of colorectal cancers. Colonoscopy permits visual inspection and photography up to the ileocecal valve and provides access for polypectomies and biopsies of suspected lesions. Excretory urography verifies bilateral renal function and allows inspection for displacement of the kidneys, ureters, or bladder by a tumor pressing against these structures.

Barium enema studies, using a dual contrast of barium and air, reveal lesions undetectable manually or visually. Remember that barium examination interferes with colonoscopy or excretory urography. Computed tomography scan allows better visualization if a barium enema is inconclusive or if metastasis to the pelvic lymph nodes is suspected.

Carcinoembryonic antigen, although not specific or sensitive enough for early diagnosis, permits monitoring before and after treatment to detect metastasis or recurrence.

The most effective treatment for colorectal cancer is surgery to remove the malignant tumor and adja-

cent tissues, along with any lymph nodes that may contain cancer cells. After surgery, treatment continues with chemotherapy, radiation therapy, or both.

The type of surgery depends on tumor location:
- *Cecum and ascending colon.* Tumors in these areas call for right hemicolectomy (for advanced disease). Surgery may include resection of the terminal segment of the ileum, cecum, ascending colon, and right half of the transverse colon with corresponding mesentery.
- *Proximal and middle transverse colon.* Surgery consists of right colectomy that includes the transverse colon and mesentery corresponding to midcolic vessels or segmental resection of the transverse colon and associated midcolic vessels.
- *Sigmoid colon.* Surgery usually is limited to the sigmoid colon and mesentery.
- *Upper rectum.* A tumor in this area usually requires anterior or low anterior resection. A newer method, using a stapler, allows much lower resections than previously possible.
- *Lower rectum.* Abdominoperineal resection and permanent sigmoid colostomy are required.

If the patient has metastatic cancer, residual disease, or a recurrent inoperable tumor, he'll need chemotherapy. Chemotherapeutic regimens commonly include fluorouracil combined with levamisole or leucovorin. Researchers are evaluating the effectiveness of fluorouracil with recombinant interferon alfa-2a.

Radiation therapy, used before or after surgery, induces tumor regression.

COLLABORATIVE MANAGEMENT

Care of the patient with colorectal cancer focuses on promoting elimination and providing physical and emotional comfort.

ASSESSMENT

With a tumor on the colon's right side, the patient may have no symptoms in the early stages because the stool is still in liquid form in that part of the colon. However, you may find:
- history of black, tarry stools
- reports of anemia, abdominal aching, pressure, and dull cramps
- in disease progression: reports of weakness, diarrhea, constipation, anorexia, weight loss, and vomiting.

With a tumor on the left side of the colon, expect to find:
- symptoms of obstruction even in the early disease stages because stools are more completely formed when they reach that part of the colon

■ reports of rectal bleeding (commonly ascribed to hemorrhoids)
■ intermittent abdominal fullness or cramping, and rectal pressure
■ in disease progression: constipation, diarrhea, or ribbon- or pencil-shaped stools; reports that passage of flatus or stool relieves pain; reports of bleeding during defecation (dark or bright red blood in the feces), and mucus in or on the stools.

With a rectal tumor, expect:
■ change in bowel habits, in many cases beginning with an urgent need to defecate on arising ("morning diarrhea") or constipation alternating with diarrhea
■ blood or mucus in the stools
■ complaints of a sense of incomplete evacuation
■ in late-stage disease: complaints of pain that begins as a feeling of rectal fullness and progresses to a dull, sometimes constant ache confined to the rectum or sacral region.

During the physical examination, look for:
■ abdominal distention or visible masses
■ enlarged veins, visible from portal obstruction
■ enlarged inguinal and supraclavicular nodes
■ abnormal bowel sounds on abdominal auscultation
■ abdominal masses (right-side tumors usually feel bulky; tumors of the transverse portion are more easily detected).

NURSING DIAGNOSES AND COLLABORATIVE PROBLEMS
Based on the following nursing diagnoses, you'll establish patient outcomes.

Constipation related to presence of a cancerous tumor in the colon or rectal area. The patient will:
■ relieve constipation with changes in lifestyle (such as a high-fiber diet, exercise, and adequate fluid intake) or medication until treatment is complete
■ regain normal bowel pattern with treatment.

Diarrhea related to presence of a cancerous tumor in the colon or rectal area. The patient will:
■ control diarrhea with medication until treatment can be completed
■ exhibit no sign of fluid or electrolyte imbalance
■ develop a normal elimination pattern with treatment, either naturally or through an ostomy.

Fear related to potential for colorectal cancer to recur or metastasize. The patient will:
■ express his fears about the diagnosis
■ use situational support systems to diminish his fears
■ use at least one fear-reducing behavior, such as discussing treatment progress or making decisions about care, each day
■ manifest no physical signs or symptoms of fear.

PLANNING AND IMPLEMENTATION
These measures help the patient with colorectal cancer:
■ Provide comfort measures and reassurance for the patient undergoing radiation therapy. Watch for adverse reactions, such as nausea, vomiting, hair loss, and malaise.
■ Prepare the patient for the adverse effects of chemotherapy, and take steps to minimize these effects. For example, offer a 0.9% sodium chloride mouthwash to help deter mouth ulcers. Watch for complications such as infection.
■ Listen to the patient's fears and concerns, and stay with him during periods of severe stress and anxiety.
■ Encourage the patient to identify and perform actions and care measures that will promote his comfort and relaxation.
■ Whenever possible, include the patient and family members in care decisions.
■ To help prevent infection, use strict aseptic technique when caring for I.V. catheters. Change I.V. tubing and sites as directed by your facility's policy. Have the patient wash his hands before and after meals and after going to the bathroom.
■ Monitor the patient's bowel patterns.
■ Monitor his diet modifications, and assess his nutritional intake.

Patient teaching
■ Throughout therapy, answer the patient's questions and tell him what to expect from surgery and other therapy.
■ Explain to the patient's family members that their positive reactions will foster his adjustment.
■ Tell the patient to follow a high-fiber diet, and teach him about foods to eat or avoid.
■ Tell him to take laxatives or antidiarrheal medications only as prescribed.
■ Emphasize the need for regular checkups because of increased risk of developing another primary cancer. He should have annual screening and follow-up testing.
■ If the patient is to undergo radiation therapy or chemotherapy, explain the treatment.
■ Inform the patient about continued screening for early detection. (See *Reducing the risk of colorectal cancer,* page 204.)
■ Refer the patient to a home health care agency, as necessary.

EVALUATION
Evaluation of patient outcomes determines the success of collaborative management. For the patient with colorectal cancer, evaluation focuses on improved nutrition and elimination, improved comfort, and adequate knowledge.

Crohn's disease

A type of inflammatory bowel disease, Crohn's disease can affect any part of the GI tract but usually involves the terminal ileum and upper colon. The disease extends through all layers of the intestinal wall and may involve regional lymph nodes and the mesentery.

Crohn's disease is most prevalent in adults ages 20 to 40 and in people with a family history of the disease. It is two to three times more common in Jews and less common in blacks. The disease is not considered a predisposing factor for colon or rectal cancer.

Crohn's disease has many names. When it affects only the small bowel, it is also known as regional enteritis. When it also involves the colon or affects only the colon, it is known as Crohn's disease of the colon (also termed granulomatous colitis—inaccurately because not all patients develop granulomas).

CAUSES

Possible causes include allergies and other immune disorders, lymphatic obstruction, and infection (although no infecting organism has been isolated). Genetic factors may matter: Crohn's disease sometimes strikes monozygotic twins, and up to 5% of affected patients have one or more affected relatives.

In Crohn's disease, inflammation spreads slowly and progressively. It begins with lymphadenoma and obstructive lymphedema in the submucosa, where Peyer's patches develop in the intestinal mucosa. Lymphatic obstruction causes edema, with mucosal ulceration and development of fissures, abscesses and, sometimes, granulomas. The mucosa may acquire a characteristic "cobblestone" look.

As the disease progresses, fibrosis occurs, thickening the bowel wall and narrowing the lumen. Serositis (serosal inflammation) also develops, causing inflamed bowel loops to adhere to other diseased or normal loops. This may result in bowel shortening and segmentation, creating a patchwork of healthy and diseased segments. Eventually, the diseased parts of the bowel become thicker, narrower, and shorter.

Anal fistula, resulting from severe diarrhea and enzymatic corrosion of the perineal area, is the most common complication. A perineal abscess may also develop during the active inflammatory state. Fistulas may develop to the bladder or vagina or even to the skin in an old scar area. Other complications include intestinal obstruction, nutritional deficiencies (caused by malabsorption and maldigestion) and, rarely, peritonitis.

DIAGNOSIS AND TREATMENT

Laboratory analysis to detect occult blood in stools is usually positive. Small-bowel X-rays may show irregular mucosa, ulceration, and stiffening. Barium enema that reveals the string sign (segments of stricture separated by normal bowel) supports the diagnosis; this test may also show fissures and narrowing of the lumen.

Sigmoidoscopy and colonoscopy may show patchy areas of inflammation, helping to rule out ulcerative colitis, and characteristic coarse irregularity (cobblestone appearance) of the mucosal surface. When the colon is involved, discrete ulcerations may be evident. Biopsy, performed during sigmoidoscopy or colonoscopy, reveals granulomas in up to half of all specimens.

Laboratory test findings indicate increased white blood cell count and erythrocyte sedimentation rate. Other findings include hypokalemia, hypocalcemia, hypomagnesemia, and decreased hemoglobin levels.

Effective management of Crohn's disease requires drug therapy and significant lifestyle changes, including physical rest and dietary restrictions. In debilitated patients, treatment includes total parenteral nutrition while resting the bowel.

Drug therapy, designed to combat inflammation and relieve symptoms, may include:

- corticosteroids such as prednisone to reduce signs and symptoms of diarrhea, pain, and bleeding by decreasing inflammation
- immunosuppressant agents such as azathioprine to suppress the body's response to antigens
- sulfasalazine to reduce inflammation
- metronidazole to treat perianal complications
- antidiarrheals, such as diphenoxylate and atropine, to combat diarrhea (contraindicated in patients with significant bowel obstruction)
- narcotics to control pain and diarrhea.

Lifestyle changes, such as stress reduction and less physical activity, help to rest the bowel, giving it time to heal. Also essential are dietary changes that decrease bowel activity, including elimination of high-fiber foods (no fruits or vegetables) and foods that irritate the mucosa (such as dairy products, and spicy and fatty foods). Foods that stimulate excessive intestinal activity (such as carbonated or caffeinated beverages) also should be avoided. Vitamins may be prescribed to compensate for the bowel's inability to absorb them.

If complications develop, surgery may be required. Indications for surgery include bowel perforation, massive hemorrhage, fistulas, or acute intestinal obstruction. Colectomy with ileostomy is necessary in many patients with extensive disease of the large intestine and rectum.

COLLABORATIVE MANAGEMENT

Care of the patient with Crohn's disease focuses on providing adequate nutrition and comfort and maintaining bowel elimination.

ASSESSMENT

Generally, the patient reports signs and symptoms of gradual onset, marked by periods of remission and exacerbation. Because signs and symptoms may be intermittent, he may have postponed seeking medical attention for some time.

The patient typically complains of fatigue, fever, abdominal pain, diarrhea (usually without obvious bleeding) and, occasionally, weight loss. Questioning may reveal that his diarrhea worsens after emotional upset or after ingestion of poorly tolerated foods, such as milk, fatty foods, and spices.

The patient with regional enteritis, in many cases a young adult, may report similar signs and symptoms as well as anorexia, nausea, and vomiting. Typically, this patient describes his abdominal pain as steady, colicky, or cramping. It usually occurs in the right lower abdominal quadrant.

Here's what to look for:

- a stool that's soft or semiliquid, without gross blood (distinct from the bloody diarrhea of ulcerative colitis)
- tenderness in the right lower abdominal quadrant; an abdominal mass, indicating adherent loops of bowel.

NURSING DIAGNOSES AND COLLABORATIVE PROBLEMS

Based on the following nursing diagnoses, you'll establish patient outcomes.

Altered nutrition: Less than body requirements, related to malabsorption and diarrhea caused by Crohn's disease. The patient will:

- regain lost weight and maintain it
- eat a well-balanced diet within dietary restrictions and with ordered nutritional supplements
- not become malnourished.

Diarrhea related to bowel changes as a result of Crohn's disease. The patient will:

- develop no fluid or electrolyte disturbance because of diarrhea
- obtain relief from diarrhea by making appropriate changes in his diet and lifestyle and by taking prescribed antidiarrheal agents
- experience a cessation of diarrhea after treatment.

Pain related to inflammation of the bowel caused by Crohn's disease. The patient will:

- avoid stressful situations and foods that contribute to bowel inflammation
- experience a relief of pain after receiving analgesics
- become free from pain with treatment.

PLANNING AND IMPLEMENTATION

These measures help the patient with Crohn's disease:

- Provide a diet that is high in protein, calories, and vitamins in frequent, small meals throughout the day.
- If the patient is receiving parenteral nutrition, provide meticulous site care and monitor his condition closely.
- Give iron supplements and blood transfusions as ordered.
- Administer medications as ordered. Evaluate their effectiveness and watch for adverse reactions.
- If the patient is receiving steroids, watch for adverse reactions such as GI bleeding. Remember that steroids can mask signs of infection.
- Provide good patient hygiene and meticulous oral care if the patient is restricted to nothing by mouth. After each bowel movement, provide careful skin care. Always keep a clean, covered bedpan within the patient's reach. Ventilate the room to eliminate odors.
- Provide emotional support to the patient and family members. Listen to their concerns, and help them cope.

- Schedule care to include rest periods throughout the day.
- Monitor the patient for complications. Watch for fever and pain on urination, which may signal bladder fistula. Abdominal pain, fever, and a hard, distended abdomen may indicate intestinal obstruction.
- Record fluid intake and output (including stools), and weigh the patient daily. Watch for dehydration, and maintain fluid and electrolyte balance. Be alert for signs of intestinal bleeding (bloody stools).
- Monitor hemoglobin levels and hematocrit.

Patient teaching

- Teach the patient about the disease, its symptoms, and its complications. Explain ordered diagnostic tests; make sure he's aware of all pretest dietary restrictions or other pretest guidelines. Answer his questions.
- Emphasize the importance of adequate rest. Explain that limiting physical activity helps to reduce intestinal motility and promote healing.
- Encourage the patient to identify and reduce sources of stress in his life. If stress clearly aggravates his disease, teach him stress-management techniques or refer him for counseling.
- Be sure the patient understands ordered dietary changes. Emphasize the need for a restricted diet, which may be trying, especially for a young patient. Refer him to a dietitian for further instruction, if necessary.
- Give the patient a list of foods to avoid, including milk products, spicy or fried high-residue foods, raw vegetables and fruits, and whole grain cereals. Advise him to avoid carbonated, caffeinated, or alcoholic beverages (because they increase intestinal activity) and extremely hot or cold foods or fluids (because they increase flatus). Remind him to take supplemental vitamins, if prescribed.
- Teach the patient about medications, their desired effects, possible adverse reactions, and when to call his doctor about reactions.
- If the patient smokes, encourage him to quit and help him join a smoking-cessation program. Point out that smoking can aggravate his disease by altering bowel motility.
- Tell the patient to notify his doctor if he experiences signs and symptoms of complications, such as fever, fatigue, weakness, a rapid heart rate, abdominal cramping or pain, vomiting, or acute diarrhea.
- If the patient is scheduled for surgery, provide preoperative teaching. Reinforce the doctor's explanation of the surgery, and mention possible complications.

EVALUATION

Evaluation of patient outcomes determines the success of collaborative management. For the patient with Crohn's disease, evaluation focuses on improved nutrition and elimination, adequate comfort and safety, restored fluid balance, and adequate knowledge.

Diverticular disease

Diverticular disease has two clinical forms. In diverticulosis, diverticula are present but don't cause symptoms. In diverticulitis, a far more serious disorder, diverticula become inflamed and may cause obstruction, infection, or hemorrhage.

CAUSES

A *diverticulum* develops when high intraluminal pressure is exerted on weak areas of the lumen, such as points where blood vessels enter the intestine, causing a break in the muscular continuity of the GI wall. The pressure in the intestinal lumen forces the intestine out, causing a pouch (diverticulum).

Diet, especially highly refined foods, may be a contributing factor. Lack of fiber reduces fecal residue, narrows the bowel lumen, and leads to higher intra-abdominal pressure during defecation.

Diverticulitis occurs when retained undigested food mixed with bacteria accumulates in the diverticulum, forming a hard mass (fecalith). This substance cuts off the blood supply to the diverticulum's thin walls, increasing its susceptibility to attack by colonic bacteria. Inflammation follows bacterial infection.

The most common site for diverticula is the sigmoid colon, but they may develop anywhere, from the proximal end of the pharynx to the anus. Other typical sites are the duodenum, near the pancreatic border or the ampulla of Vater, and the jejunum. Diverticular disease of the stomach is rare and may be a precursor of peptic or neoplastic disease. Diverticular disease of the ileum (Meckel's diverticulum) is the most common congenital anomaly of the GI tract.

DIAGNOSIS AND TREATMENT

Barium studies confirm the diagnosis. In patients with acute diverticulitis, a barium enema may rupture the bowel, so this procedure is withheld until the acute phrase resolves. Radiography may reveal colonic spasm if irritable bowel syndrome accompanies diverticular disease.

Biopsy rules out cancer; however, a colonoscopic biopsy isn't recommended during acute diverticular disease because of the strenuous bowel preparation it requires.

Blood studies may show leukocytosis and an elevated erythrocyte sedimentation rate in diverticulitis, especially if the diverticula are infected. Stool tests detect occult blood in 20% of patients with diverticulitis.

Treatment depends on the type of diverticular disease and the severity of symptoms. Asymptomatic diverticulosis generally requires no treatment. Intestinal diverticulosis that causes pain, mild GI distress, constipation, or difficult defecation may respond to a liquid or bland diet, stool softeners, and occasional doses of mineral oil. These measures relieve symptoms, minimize irritation, and decrease the risk of progression to diverticulitis. After pain subsides, patients also benefit from a high-residue diet and bulk medication such as psyllium.

Treatment of mild diverticulitis without signs of perforation aims to prevent constipation and combat infection. Therapy may include bed rest, a liquid diet, stool softeners, a broad-spectrum antibiotic, meperidine to control pain and relax smooth muscle, and an antispasmodic such as propantheline to control muscle spasms.

For more severe diverticulitis, treatment consists of the above measures and I.V. therapy. A nasogastric (NG) tube to relieve intra-abdominal pressure is usually required.

Patients who hemorrhage need blood replacement and careful monitoring of fluid and electrolyte balance. Such bleeding usually stops spontaneously. If it continues, angiography and infusion of vasopressin into the bleeding vessel are effective. Rarely, surgery may be required.

A colon resection to remove a diseased segment of intestine may be required to treat diverticulitis that fails to respond to medical treatment or that causes severe recurrent attacks in the same area. A temporary colostomy may be created to allow the inflamed bowel to rest.

COLLABORATIVE MANAGEMENT

Care of the patient with diverticulosis focuses on relieving symptoms and reducing the risk of diverticulitis.

ASSESSMENT

Usually, the patient with diverticulosis has no symptoms. Occasionally, he may report intermittent pain in the left lower abdominal quadrant, relieved by defecation or the passage of flatus and alternating bouts of constipation and diarrhea. The assessment usually reveals no clinical findings. Rarely, palpation discloses abdominal tenderness in the left lower quadrant.

In diverticulitis, look for:
■ history of diverticulosis, diagnosed incidentally (possibly during radiographic studies), and low fiber consumption

■ complaints of moderate pain in the left lower abdominal quadrant, described as dull or steady. Straining, lifting, or coughing may aggravate the pain
■ reports of mild nausea, gas, and intermittent bouts of constipation, sometimes accompanied by rectal bleeding and diarrhea
■ appearance of distress
■ palpation that may confirm the patient's reports of left lower quadrant pain
■ low-grade fever
■ recent consumption of foods containing seeds or kernels, such as tomatoes, nuts, popcorn, or strawberries, or indigestible roughage, such as celery or corn. Seeds and undigested roughage can block the neck of a diverticulum, causing diverticulitis.

In acute diverticulitis, look for:
■ reports of muscle spasms and peritoneal irritation
■ guarding and rebound tenderness on palpation
■ upon rectal examination, a tender mass if the inflamed area is close to the rectum.

NURSING DIAGNOSES AND COLLABORATIVE PROBLEMS

Based on the following nursing diagnoses, you'll establish patient outcomes.

Constipation related to changes in the intestinal tract. The patient will:
■ identify factors in his lifestyle that predispose him to constipation
■ change personal habits and thereby encourage a normal elimination pattern
■ regain and maintain a normal elimination pattern.

Risk for infection related to the diverticulum's susceptibility to bacterial activity. The patient will:
■ maintain a normal temperature and white blood cell count
■ have no signs or symptoms of an intestinal infection, such as abdominal distention or pain, diarrhea, or nausea and vomiting
■ remain free from intestinal infection.

Pain related to inflammation. The patient will:
■ express feelings of comfort after analgesic administration
■ have no pain when diverticulitis resolves.

Altered nutrition: Less than body requirements, related to intestinal problems. The patient will:
■ maintain body weight
■ demonstrate intake, advancing to diet as tolerated.

PLANNING AND IMPLEMENTATION

These measures help the patient with diverticulosis:
■ In an acute attack, make sure the patient receives nothing by mouth, and administer ordered I.V. fluids.
■ As symptoms subside, gradually advance the diet, starting with clear liquids.

■ Continue to advance the patient's diet to food. A high-fiber diet is usually ordered.

■ Review elimination patterns with the patient and determine possible causative factors for the disorder.

■ Administer antibiotics, stool softeners, and antispasmodics, as ordered.

■ For severe pain, administer analgesics such as meperidine, as ordered.

■ Maintain bed rest for the patient with acute diverticulitis. Don't let him lift, strain, bend, cough, or perform any other actions that increase intra-abdominal pressure.

■ If the patient expresses anxiety, provide psychological support. Listen to his concerns and offer reassurance, when appropriate.

■ If diverticular bleeding occurs, anticipate angiography and catheter placement for vasopressin infusion. If so, prepare him for the procedure as ordered.

■ If the patient will undergo surgery, provide routine preoperative care. Also perform any special required procedures, such as administering antibiotics or providing a specific diet for several days preoperatively.

■ If symptoms are severe or if he has nausea and vomiting or abdominal distention, insert an NG tube and attach it to intermittent suction, as ordered.

Patient teaching

■ Tell the patient to notify the doctor if he has a temperature above 101° F (38.3° C), abdominal pain that's severe or that lasts for more than 3 days, or blood in his stools. Emphasize that these symptoms indicate complications.

■ In uncomplicated diverticulosis, focus your patient teaching on bowel and dietary habits.

■ Explain what diverticula are and how they form. Teach the patient about necessary diagnostic tests and treatments.

■ Be sure the patient understands the desired actions and possible adverse effects of his prescribed medications.

■ Review recommended dietary changes. Encourage the patient to drink 2 to 3 qt (2 to 3 L) of fluid daily. Emphasize the importance of dietary roughage and the harmful effects of constipation and straining during a bowel movement. Advise him to increase his intake of foods high in undigestible fiber, such as fresh fruits and vegetables, whole grain breads, and wheat or bran cereals. Warn that a fiber-rich diet may temporarily cause flatulence.

■ Advise the patient to relieve constipation with stool softeners or bulk-forming cathartics (with plenty of water; if swallowed dry, they may absorb enough moisture in the mouth and throat to swell and obstruct the esophagus or trachea).

■ Provide preoperative teaching as appropriate. Reinforce the doctor's explanation of the surgery, and discuss possible complications.

■ If a colostomy is constructed during surgery, teach the patient how to care for it. Arrange for a visit with an enterostomal therapist.

EVALUATION

Evaluation of patient outcomes determines the success of collaborative management. For the patient with diverticular disease, evaluation focuses on improved elimination, adequate nutrition, pain relief, and adequate knowledge.

Esophageal cancer

Most common in men over age 60, esophageal cancer is nearly always fatal. The disease occurs worldwide, but it's most common in Japan, Russia, China, the Middle East, and parts of South Africa, where esophageal cancer has reached almost epidemic proportions. In the United States, more than 8,000 cases of esophageal cancer are reported annually.

CAUSES

Although the cause is unknown, several predisposing factors have been identified. These include chronic irritation from heavy smoking or excessive use of alcohol; stasis-induced inflammation, as in achalasia or stricture; previous head and neck tumors; and nutritional deficiency, as in untreated sprue and Plummer-Vinson syndrome.

Esophageal tumors are usually fungating and infiltrating. In most cases, the tumor partially constricts the lumen of the esophagus. Regional metastasis occurs early by way of submucosal lymphatics, in many cases fatally invading adjacent vital intrathoracic organs. If the patient survives primary extension, the liver and lungs are the usual sites of distant metastases. Unusual sites include the bone, kidneys, and adrenal glands.

Most cases (98%) arise in squamous cell epithelium, although a few are adenocarcinomas and, fewer still, melanomas and sarcomas. About half of all squamous cell cancers occur in the lower portion of the esophagus, 40% in the midportion, and the remaining 10% in the upper or cervical esophagus. Regardless of cell type, the prognosis for esophageal cancer is grim: 5-year survival rates are less than 5%, and most patients die within 6 months of diagnosis.

DIAGNOSIS AND TREATMENT

X-rays of the esophagus, with barium swallow and motility studies, delineate structural and filling defects and reduced peristalsis. Chest X-rays or esopha-gography may reveal pneumonitis.

Esophagoscopy, punch and brush biopsies, and ex-foliative cytologic tests confirm esophageal tumors. Bronchoscopy (which is usually performed after an esophagoscopy) may reveal tumor growth in the tra-cheobronchial tree. Endoscopic ultrasonography of the esophagus combines endoscopy and ultrasound technology to measure the depth of penetration of the tumor.

Computed tomography scan may help diagnose and monitor esophageal lesions. Magnetic resonance imaging scan permits evaluation of the esophagus and adjacent structures.

Liver function studies and other laboratory tests may reveal abnormalities. If so, a liver scan and medi-astinal tomography scan can help reveal the extent of the disease.

Esophageal cancer usually is advanced when diag-nosed, so surgery and other treatments can only re-lieve disease effects. Palliative therapy consists of treatment to keep the esophagus open, including esophageal dilatation, laser therapy, and radiation therapy.

Radical surgery can excise the tumor and resect ei-ther the esophagus alone or the stomach and esopha-gus. Either the stomach (gastric pull-up) or a portion of the colon (colon interposition) may be used to re-place the esophagus. Chemotherapy and radiation therapy can slow tumor growth. Gastrostomy or je-junostomy can help provide adequate nutrition. A prosthesis can be used to seal any fistula that devel-ops. Endoscopic laser treatment and bipolar electroco-agulation can help restore swallowing by vaporizing cancerous tissue. If the tumor is in the upper esopha-gus, however, the laser can't be positioned properly. Analgesics are used for pain control.

COLLABORATIVE MANAGEMENT

Care of the patient with esophageal cancer focuses on symptom relief.

ASSESSMENT

Early in the disease, the patient may report a feeling of fullness, pressure, indigestion, or substernal burn-ing. He may also tell of using antacids to relieve GI upset. Later, he may complain of dysphagia and weight loss. The degree of dysphagia varies, depend-ing on the extent of disease. At first, the dysphagia is mild, occurring only after the patient eats solid foods, especially meat. Later, he has difficulty swallowing coarse foods and, in some cases, liquids. Look for:
- complaints of hoarseness (from laryngeal nerve in-volvement) or a chronic cough (possibly from aspira-tion)

- anorexia, vomiting, and regurgitation of food, caused by the tumor size exceeding the limits of the esophagus
- complaints of pain on swallowing or pain that ra-diates to the back
- in the late stages of the disease, thinness, cachex-ia, and dehydration.

NURSING DIAGNOSES AND COLLABORATIVE PROBLEMS

Based on the following nursing diagnoses, you'll es-tablish patient outcomes.

Altered nutrition: Less than body requirements, related to impaired swallowing. The patient will:
- ingest a high-calorie, nutritionally balanced diet naturally or artificially through gastrostomy feedings or parenteral nutrition
- maintain weight
- have no signs or symptoms of malnutrition.

Risk for aspiration related to esophageal blockage. The patient will:
- expectorate secretions without aspiration
- consent to treatments that help prevent aspiration such as a gastrostomy if he has trouble drinking liq-uids
- develop no aspiration pneumonia.

Impaired swallowing related to obstruction. The pa-tient will:
- consent to treatments that improve swallowing, such as periodic dilatation of the esophagus
- develop no malnutrition, aspiration pneumonia, or other complications of impaired swallowing.

Risk for complications related to treatments and proce-dures and invasiveness of the disease. The patient will:
- experience minimal adverse effects of chemothera-py or radiation therapy
- demonstrate measures to cope with adverse effects of treatments.

PLANNING AND IMPLEMENTATION

These measures help the patient with esophageal can-cer:
- Provide high-calorie, high-protein foods. If the pa-tient has trouble swallowing solids, puree or liquefy his food and offer a commercially available nutrition-al supplement. As ordered, provide tube feedings, and prepare him for supplementary parenteral nutrition.
- To prevent food aspiration, place the patient in Fowler's position for meals and allow plenty of time to eat. If he regurgitates food after eating, provide mouth care.
- Prepare the patient for a gastrostomy, as indicated. When using a gastrostomy tube for nutritional sup-port, give food slowly—by gravity—in prescribed amounts (usually 200 to 500 ml). Offer the patient something to chew before each feeding. This pro-

motes gastric secretions and provides some semblance of normal eating.
■ Administer ordered analgesics for pain relief as necessary.
■ Provide comfort measures such as repositioning and distractions to help decrease discomfort.
■ Encourage the patient to identify actions and care measures that will promote his comfort and relaxation. Try to perform these measures, and encourage the patient and family members to do so, too.
■ Protect the patient from infection.
■ After chemotherapy, take steps to decrease adverse effects, such as providing normal saline mouthwash to help prevent mouth ulcers. Allow the patient plenty of rest, and administer medications, as ordered, to reduce adverse effects.
■ Throughout therapy, answer the patient's questions, and tell him what to expect from surgery and other therapies. Listen to his fears and concerns, and stay with him during periods of severe anxiety.
■ Whenever possible, include the patient in care decisions.
■ Anticipate referral to home care to assist with follow-up, teaching, patient care, and support.

Patient teaching

■ Prepare the patient for surgery used to treat esophageal cancer, as indicated.
■ Explain the procedures the patient will undergo after surgery—closed chest drainage, nasogastric suctioning, and placement of gastrostomy tubes.
■ If appropriate, teach family members or friend gastrostomy tube care. This includes checking tube patency before each feeding, providing skin care around the tube, and keeping the patient upright during and after feedings.
■ Stress the importance of adequate nutrition. Ask a dietitian to instruct the patient and family members. If the patient has difficulty swallowing solids, instruct him to puree or liquefy his food and to follow a high-calorie, high-protein diet to minimize weight loss. Also, recommend that he add a commercially available, high-calorie supplement to his diet.
■ Encourage the patient to follow as normal a routine as possible after recovery from surgery and during radiation therapy and chemotherapy. This will help him maintain a sense of control and reduce complications associated with immobility.
■ Advise the patient to rest between activities and to stop any activity that tires him or causes pain.
■ Refer the patient and family members to appropriate organizations such as the American Cancer Society.

EVALUATION

Evaluation of patient outcomes determines the success of collaborative management. For the patient with esophageal cancer, evaluation focuses on improved comfort and adequate knowledge.

Gastritis

Gastritis refers to an inflammation of the gastric mucosa, either acute or chronic.

CAUSES

Acute gastritis has numerous causes, including:
■ chronic ingestion of irritating foods such as hot peppers (or an allergic reaction to them) or alcohol
■ drugs, such as aspirin and other nonsteroidal anti-inflammatory agents (in large doses), cytotoxic agents, caffeine, corticosteroids, antimetabolites, phenylbutazone, and indomethacin
■ ingested poisons, especially ammonia, mercury, carbon tetrachloride, or corrosive substances
■ endotoxins released from infecting bacteria, such as staphylococci, *Escherichia coli*, *Helicobacter pylori*, or salmonella
■ acute illnesses, especially major trauma; burns; severe infection; hepatic, renal, or respiratory failure; or major surgery.

Acute gastritis, the most common stomach disorder, produces mucosal reddening, edema, hemorrhage, and erosion. Chronic gastritis is common among older patients and patients with pernicious anemia. It's often present as chronic atrophic gastritis, in which all stomach mucosal layers are inflamed, with reduced numbers of chief and parietal cells. However, acute or chronic gastritis can occur at any age.

Chronic gastritis usually involves an underlying pathology that results in atrophy of the gastric mucosa. It's associated with pernicious anemia (type A) and infection with *H. pylori* (type B). Individuals with type A chronic gastritis are at risk for developing gastric cancer.

DIAGNOSIS AND TREATMENT

Gastroscopy (commonly with biopsy) confirms gastritis when done before lesions heal (usually within 24 hours), but it's contraindicated after ingestion of a corrosive agent. Laboratory analyses can detect occult blood in vomitus or stool (or both) if the patient has gastric bleeding. If the patient has developed anemia from bleeding, hematocrit and hemoglobin levels are decreased.

Eliminating the cause of gastritis is an immediate therapeutic priority. For example, bacterial gastritis is treated with antibiotics; ingested poisons are neutralized with the appropriate antidote. Once the associated disease is treated or the offending agent is eradicated or neutralized, the gastric mucosa usually will begin to heal.

Treatment of acute gastritis is symptomatic and supportive. Healing usually occurs within a few hours to a few days after the cause has been eliminated. Histamine-2 receptor antagonists, such as cimetidine, ranitidine, or famotidine, may be ordered to block gastric secretion. Antacids may be used as buffering agents.

For critically ill patients, antacids administered hourly, with or without histamine antagonists, may reduce the frequency of acute gastritis episodes. Some patients also require analgesics. Until healing occurs, the patient's oxygen needs, blood volume, and fluid and electrolyte balance must be monitored and maintained.

When gastritis causes massive bleeding, treatment includes blood replacement; iced saline lavage, possibly with norepinephrine; angiography with vasopressin infused in a normal saline solution; and, sometimes, surgery.

A last resort, surgery is performed only if more conservative treatments fail. Vagotomy and pyloroplasty have been used with limited success. Rarely, partial or total gastrectomy may be required.

Because patients with chronic gastritis may be asymptomatic or have only vague complaints, no specific treatment may be necessary, except for avoiding aspirin and spicy foods. If symptoms develop or persist, antacids may be taken. If pernicious anemia is the underlying cause, vitamin B_{12} may be administered parenterally.

COLLABORATIVE MANAGEMENT

Care of the patient with gastritis focuses on immediate elimination of the cause and providing relief of symptoms.

ASSESSMENT

The patient history may reveal one or more causative agents. After exposure to the offending substance, the patient with acute gastritis typically reports rapid onset of symptoms, such as epigastric discomfort, indigestion, cramping, anorexia, nausea, hematemesis, and vomiting. The symptoms may last from a few hours to a few days.

The patient with chronic gastritis may describe similar symptoms or only mild epigastric discomfort. For example, he may report an intolerance for spicy or fatty foods or mild epigastric pain that's relieved by eating. Many patients with chronic atrophic gastritis are asymptomatic.

Heres's what to look for:

- signs of distress, such as fatigue, grimacing, or restlessness, depending on the severity of symptoms
- with gastric bleeding, paleness, tachycardia, and hypotension
- abdominal distention, tenderness, and guarding upon palpation
- increased bowel sounds upon auscultation.

NURSING DIAGNOSES AND COLLABORATIVE PROBLEMS
Based on the following nursing diagnoses, you'll establish patient outcomes.

Altered nutrition: Less than body requirements, related to adverse GI effects. The patient will:
- develop no signs or symptoms of malnutrition
- resume or maintain adequate nutritional intake daily
- regain any weight lost and maintain his weight within a normal range.

Risk for fluid volume deficit related to vomiting. The patient will:
- demonstrate no signs or symptoms of dehydration during acute episodes of gastritis
- maintain normal fluid balance.

Pain related to inflammation of gastric mucosa. The patient will:
- express feelings of comfort after receiving analgesics
- identify factors that increase pain, such as specific foods or stress
- become pain-free with treatment for gastritis and elimination of potential risk factors.

PLANNING AND IMPLEMENTATION
These measures help the patient with gastritis:
- If the patient is vomiting, give antiemetics and replace fluid losses with I.V. fluids, as ordered.
- Monitor his fluid intake and output and electrolyte levels.
- If surgery is necessary, prepare the patient and provide appropriate postoperative care.
- When the patient can tolerate oral feedings, provide a bland diet that takes into account his food preferences. Watch for returning symptoms as you reintroduce food.
- Offer smaller, more frequent servings to reduce the amount of irritating gastric secretions. Help the patient identify specific foods that cause gastric upset, and eliminate them from his diet.
- Administer antacids and other prescribed medications, as ordered. Monitor the patient's response.
- If pain or nausea interferes with the patient's appetite, administer an analgesic or an antiemetic about 1 hour before meals.
- Provide emotional support to help the patient manage his symptoms.

■ Monitor his compliance with the treatment plan and elimination of risk factors in his lifestyle.

Patient teaching
■ Teach the patient about the disorder. Explain the relationship between his symptoms and the causative agents so that he'll understand the need to modify his diet or lifestyle. Answer all of his questions, and explain all necessary diagnostic tests and treatments.
■ If the patient is scheduled for surgery, reinforce the doctor's explanation of the procedure and provide preoperative teaching.
■ Give the patient a list of irritating foods and beverages to avoid, such as spicy and highly seasoned foods, alcohol, and caffeine. Make sure he understands that these changes are lifelong measures to prevent recurrence of gastritis. If necessary, refer him to the dietitian for further instruction.
■ If the patient smokes, encourage him to quit by pointing out that this habit can cause or aggravate symptoms by irritating the gastric mucosa. Refer him to a smoking-cessation program.
■ If appropriate, help the patient identify the need for stress reduction. Teach him stress-reduction techniques, such as meditation, deep breathing, progressive relaxation, and guided imagery.
■ Urge the patient to seek immediate attention for recurring symptoms, such as hematemesis, nausea, or vomiting.
■ To prevent recurrence, stress the importance of taking prophylactic medications as ordered. To reduce gastric irritation, advise the patient to take steroids with milk, food, or antacids. Instruct him to take antacids between meals and at bedtime and to avoid aspirin-containing compounds.
■ Teach family members the importance of supporting the patient as he makes the necessary dietary and lifestyle changes.

EVALUATION
Evaluation of patient outcomes determines the success of collaborative management. For the patient with gastritis, evaluation focuses on adequate nutrition, restored fluid balance, improved comfort, and adequate knowledge.

Gastroesophageal reflux

Popularly known as heartburn, gastroesophageal reflux is the backflow of gastric or duodenal contents, or both, into the esophagus and past the lower esophageal sphincter (LES), without associated belching or vomiting. Reflux may or may not cause symptoms or pathologic changes. Persistent reflux may cause reflux esophagitis, an inflammation of the esophageal mucosa. The prognosis varies with the underlying cause.

CAUSES
Any of the following predisposing factors may lead to reflux:
■ nasogastric intubation for more than 4 days
■ any agent that lowers LES pressure: food; alcohol; cigarettes; anticholinergics, such as atropine, belladonna, and propantheline; and other drugs, such as morphine, diazepam, calcium channel blockers, and meperidine
■ hiatal hernia with incompetent sphincter
■ any condition or position that increases intra-abdominal pressure.

Normally, gastric contents don't back up into the esophagus because the LES creates enough pressure around the lower end of the esophagus to close it. (The sphincter relaxes after each swallow to allow food into the stomach.) Reflux occurs when LES pressure is deficient or pressure within the stomach exceeds LES pressure.

Reflux esophagitis, the primary complication of gastric reflux, can lead to other disorders, including esophageal stricture, esophageal ulcer, and replacement of the normal squamous epithelium with columnar epithelium (Barrett's epithelium). Severe reflux esophagitis can cause anemia from chronic low-grade bleeding of inflamed mucosa.

Chronic pulmonary disease may develop if gastric contents in the patient's throat are aspirated.

DIAGNOSIS AND TREATMENT
Although a careful history and physical examination are essential to the diagnosis, the following tests help to confirm it:
■ esophageal acidity (standard), the most sensitive and accurate measure of reflux
■ gastroesophageal scintillation
■ esophageal manometry, for resting pressure of LES and sphincter competence
■ acid perfusion confirms esophagitis
■ esophagoscopy and biopsy for visualization and tissue sampling of the esophagus (evaluate disease extent and confirm pathologic changes in the mucosa)
■ barium swallow with fluoroscopy to reveal normal findings (except with advanced disease)
■ in children, barium esophagography under fluoroscopic control to show reflux.

Treatment aims to relieve symptoms by reducing reflux through gravity, strengthening the LES with drug therapy, neutralizing gastric contents, and reducing intra-abdominal pressure. (See *Factors affecting LES pressure.*) Treatment should also include a review of lifestyle or dietary habits that affect the patient's LES pressure and reflux symptoms.

In mild cases, diet therapy may reduce symptoms sufficiently. In uncomplicated cases, positional therapy, which relieves symptoms by reducing intra-abdominal pressure, may be useful.

For intermittent reflux, antacids given 1 hour and 3 hours after meals and at bedtime may be effective. Hourly antacid administration may be necessary.

Depending on the patient's bowel status, a nondiarrheal, magnesium-free antacid may be prescribed.

Cholinergic drugs such as bethanechol increase LES pressure. Histamine-2 receptor antagonists, such as cimetidine and ranitidine, reduce gastric acidity. A proton pump inhibitor such as omeprazole (Prilosec) reduces acidity. Metoclopramide has been used with beneficial results. The prokinetic drug cisapride (Propulsid) has been approved for this disorder.

Surgery is usually reserved for patients with refractory symptoms or serious complications. Indications include pulmonary aspiration, hemorrhage, esophageal obstruction or perforation, intractable pain, incompetent LES, or associated hiatal hernia.

Surgical procedures, to create an artificial closure at the gastroesophageal junction, include:
■ Belsey Mark IV operation, Hill posterior gastropexy, and Nissen operation, which all wrap the gastric fundus around the esophagus.
■ Vagotomy or pyloroplasty (which may be combined with an antireflux regimen) modify gastric contents.

COLLABORATIVE MANAGEMENT

Care of the patient with gastroesophageal reflux focuses on promoting dietary changes and symptom management before and after any surgery.

ASSESSMENT

Typically, the patient complains of heartburn, which worsens with vigorous exercise, bending, or lying down. He may report relief from antacids or sitting upright. If asked, he may recall regurgitating without associated nausea or belching. This symptom is commonly described as a feeling of warm fluid traveling up the throat, followed by a sour or bitter taste in the mouth if the fluid reaches the pharynx.

Although heartburn is the most common feature of reflux, the patient may report a variety of signs and symptoms. Look for:
■ reports of a feeling of fluid accumulation in the throat, without a sour or bitter taste (hypersecretion of saliva)
■ odynophagia, possibly followed by a dull substernal ache (possible severe, long-term reflux dysphagia from esophageal spasm, stricture, or esophagitis)
■ bright red or dark brown blood in vomitus

Factors affecting LES pressure

Various dietary and lifestyle factors can increase or decrease lower esophageal sphincter (LES) pressure. Take these factors into account as you plan your patient's care.

Factors that increase LES pressure
■ Protein
■ Carbohydrates
■ Nonfat milk
■ Low-dose ethanol

Factors that decrease LES pressure
■ Fat
■ Whole milk
■ Orange juice
■ Tomatoes
■ Antiflatulents (such as simethicone)
■ Chocolate
■ High-dose ethanol
■ Cigarette smoking
■ Lying on either side
■ Sitting

■ chronic pain that may mimic angina pectoris, radiating to the neck, jaw, and arm (possible esophageal spasm, resulting from reflux esophagitis)
■ nocturnal hypersalivation (rare) that wakes the patient with coughing, choking, and a mouthful of saliva.

NURSING DIAGNOSES AND COLLABORATIVE PROBLEMS

Based on the following nursing diagnoses, you'll establish patient outcomes.

Altered nutrition: Less than body requirements, related to reflux and its interference with eating. The patient will:
■ state foods that contribute to reflux
■ identify appropriate food choices
■ demonstrate a stable weight.

Risk for aspiration related to backflow of stomach or duodenal contents, or both. The patient will:
■ identify measures to prevent aspiration
■ not aspirate
■ have clear, odorless respiratory secretions with clear breath sounds.

Knowledge deficit related to gastroesophageal reflux. The patient will:
■ express an interest in learning about the disorder
■ seek information from a knowledgeable source

■ communicate an understanding of the disorder and its treatment
■ comply with the treatment regimen and avoid or minimize contributing factors.
Pain related to irritation of the esophagus. The patient will:
■ express feelings of pain relief with antacid therapy
■ identify contributing factors that cause or worsen gastroesophageal reflux, such as eating certain foods.

PLANNING AND IMPLEMENTATION
These measures help the patient with gastroesophageal reflux:
■ Develop a diet that takes the patient's food preferences into account while helping to minimize his reflux symptoms. Consult a dietitian, as necessary. Supply a list of foods allowed and foods to avoid.
■ Provide small frequent meals with bland foods while avoiding fatty or acidic foods, chocolate, caffeine, and nicotine.
■ Place the obese patient on a weight reduction diet, as ordered.
■ To reduce intra-abdominal pressure, have the patient sleep in a reverse Trendelenburg position (with the head of the bed elevated 6″ to 12″ (15 to 30.5 cm). He should also avoid lying down immediately after meals and late-night snacks.
■ After surgery, provide care as you would for any patient who has undergone laparotomy. Pay particular attention to the patient's respiratory status because the surgery is performed close to the diaphragm. Administer prescribed analgesics, oxygen, and I.V. fluids. If a thoracic approach was used, give chest physiotherapy, as needed.
■ Administer medications, such as antacids and H$_2$ receptor antagonists, as ordered.
■ Offer the patient emotional and psychological support to help him cope with pain and discomfort. Encourage him to limit activity that would increase intra-abdominal pressure.

Patient teaching
■ Teach the patient about the causes of gastroesophageal reflux, and review his antireflux regimen of medication, diet, and positional therapy.
■ Discuss recommended dietary changes. Advise the patient to sit upright after meals and snacks and to eat small, frequent meals. Explain that he should eat at least 2 to 3 hours before lying down. Tell him to avoid highly seasoned food, acidic juices, bedtime snacks, alcoholic beverages, and foods high in fat or carbohydrates because these reduce LES pressure.
■ Instruct the patient to avoid situations or activities that increase intra-abdominal pressure, such as bending, coughing, vigorous exercise, obesity, constipation, and wearing tight clothing.
■ Caution him to refrain from using any substance that reduces sphincter control, including cigarettes, alcohol, fatty foods, and certain drugs.
■ Encourage compliance with his drug regimen. Review the desired benefits and potential adverse effects.

EVALUATION
Evaluation of patient outcomes determines the success of collaborative management. For the patient with gastroesophageal reflux, evaluation focuses on relief of pain and adequate nutrition, oxygenation, airway, and knowledge.

Hepatitis

Hepatitis is an inflammation of the liver that affects more than 70,000 patients annually in the United States. Five types of viral hepatitis are recognized:
■ *Type A* (infectious or short-incubation hepatitis). The incidence of this type is rising among homosexuals and in persons with immunosuppression related to human immunodeficiency virus infection.
■ *Type B* (serum or long-incubation hepatitis). In moderate prevalence areas, the lifetime risk of infection is 20% to 60% for people of all ages.
■ *Type C.* This type accounts for about 20% of all viral hepatitis and for most posttransfusion hepatitis cases.
■ *Type D* (or delta hepatitis). This type is linked to fulminant hepatitis, which has an extremely high mortality rate. In the United States, type D is associated with transfusion and transplantation from an infectious donor, I.V. drug use, hemodialysis, and needle-stick injuries.
■ *Type E* (formerly grouped with type C under type non-A, non-B). Type E primarily affects patients who have ingested contaminated drinking water, uncooked shellfish, or uncooked fruits and vegetables when visiting developing countries.

CAUSES
The five major forms of viral hepatitis result from infection with the causative viruses: A, B, C, D, or E.
Type A hepatitis is highly contagious and is usually transmitted by the fecal-oral route, commonly within institutions or families. However, it may also be transmitted parenterally. Hepatitis A usually is ingested with contaminated food, milk, or water. Outbreaks of this type are commonly traced to seafood from polluted water.

Type B hepatitis is now known to be spread by contact with contaminated human secretions and feces as well as by direct exchange of contaminated blood. As a result, many nurses, doctors, laboratory technicians, and dentists are commonly exposed to type B hepatitis, often through defective gloves. Transmission also occurs during intimate sexual contact and through perinatal transmission.

Although specific viruses defined as type C hepatitis have been isolated, few patients have tested positive for them—reflecting, perhaps, poor specificity of the test. Usually, this type is transmitted through transfused blood from asymptomatic donors.

Type D hepatitis is found primarily in patients with an acute or a chronic episode of hepatitis B. Type D infection requires the presence of the hepatitis B surface antigen to replicate. For this reason, type D infection can't outlast a type B infection.

Type E hepatitis is a new form that is transmitted enterically, much like type A. No commercially available serologic test for diagnosis is available in the United States.

The most feared complication of all types is life-threatening fulminant hepatitis. Developing in about 1% of patients, it causes unremitting liver failure with encephalopathy. It progresses to coma and commonly leads to death within 2 weeks.

Major complications may be specific to the type of hepatitis:
- Chronic active hepatitis may occur as a late complication of hepatitis B.
- During the prodromal stage of acute hepatitis B, a syndrome resembling serum sickness, characterized by arthralgia or arthritis, rash, and angioedema, may occur. This syndrome may cause misdiagnosis of hepatitis B as rheumatoid arthritis or lupus erythematosus.
- Type D hepatitis can cause a mild or asymptomatic form of type B hepatitis to flare into severe, progressive chronic active hepatitis and cirrhosis.
- Weeks to months after apparent recovery from acute hepatitis A, relapsing hepatitis may develop.

Rarely, hepatitis may lead to pancreatitis, myocarditis, atypical pneumonia, aplastic anemia, transverse myelitis, or peripheral neuropathy.

A fairly common systemic disease, hepatitis is marked by hepatic cell destruction, necrosis, and autolysis, leading to anorexia, jaundice, and hepatomegaly. In most patients, hepatic cells eventually regenerate with little or no residual damage, allowing ready recovery. However, old age and serious underlying disorders make complications more likely. The prognosis is poor if edema and hepatic encephalopathy develop.

DIAGNOSIS AND TREATMENT

In suspected viral hepatitis, a hepatitis profile is routinely performed to establish the type of hepatitis:
- *Type A.* Detection of an antibody to hepatitis A confirms the diagnosis.
- *Type B.* The presence of hepatitis B surface antigens and hepatitis B antibodies confirms the diagnosis.
- *Type C.* Diagnosis depends on serologic testing for the specific antibody 1 or more months after the onset of acute illness. Until then, confirmation is in negative test results for hepatitis A, B, and D.
- *Type D.* Detection of intrahepatic delta antigens or immunoglobulin (Ig) M antidelta antigens in acute disease (or IgM and IgG in chronic disease) establishes the diagnosis.
- *Type E.* Detection of hepatitis E antigens supports the diagnosis; however, so does ruling out hepatitis C.

Additional findings from liver function studies support the diagnosis:
- Serum aspartate aminotransferase and serum alanine aminotransferase levels are increased in the prodromal stage of acute viral hepatitis.
- Serum alkaline phosphatase levels are slightly increased.
- Serum bilirubin levels are elevated, continuing late in the disease, especially if the patient has severe disease.
- Prothrombin time is prolonged (more than 3 seconds longer than normal indicates severe liver damage).
- White blood cell counts commonly reveal transient neutropenia and lymphopenia followed by lymphocytosis.
- Liver biopsy is performed if chronic hepatitis is suspected. (This study is performed for acute hepatitis only if the diagnosis is questionable.)

No specific drug therapy has been developed for hepatitis. However, alpha-interferon is used in selected patients with the chronic form of hepatitis B or C. Though this treatment does not eliminate the virus, it does return liver enzyme levels to normal if the patient's response is good. In other cases, the patient is advised to rest in the early stages of the illness and combat anorexia by eating small, high-calorie, high-protein meals. (Protein intake should be reduced if signs of precoma—lethargy, confusion, mental changes—develop.) Large meals are usually better tolerated in the morning because many patients experience nausea late in the day.

In acute viral hepatitis, hospitalization usually is required only for those patients with severe symptoms or complications. Parenteral nutrition may be required if the patient has persistent vomiting and can't maintain oral intake.

Antiemetics (trimethobenzamide or benzquin-amide) may be given a half hour before meals to relieve nausea and prevent vomiting; phenothiazines have a cholestatic effect and should be avoided. For severe pruritus, the resin cholestyramine, which sequesters bile salts, may be given.

COLLABORATIVE MANAGEMENT

Care of the patient with hepatitis focuses on promoting rest and good nutrition and controlling nausea.

ASSESSMENT

Investigate the patient's history for the source of transmission. Examples are recent exposure to individuals with hepatitis A or B, recent blood transfusions or use of I.V. drugs, and hemodialysis for renal failure. Look for recent body piercing or tattooing (contaminated instruments can transmit hepatitis), travel to a region where hepatitis is endemic, or crowded living conditions.

Be sure to ask about alcohol consumption (highly significant in suspected cirrhosis). Because many alcoholics deliberately underestimate consumption, you may need to interview family members.

The patient's employment history may reveal exposure, such as work in a hospital or laboratory, where the risk of viral exposure from contaminated instruments or waste could be high. Check for possible exposure to toxic chemicals such as carbon tetrachloride, which can cause nonviral hepatitis.

Assessment findings are similar for the different types of hepatitis. Typically, signs and symptoms progress in several stages. In the prodromal (preicteric) stage, here's what you'll see:
- complaints of easy fatigue and anorexia, possibly with mild weight loss
- generalized malaise, depression, headache, weakness, arthralgia, myalgia, photophobia, and nausea with vomiting
- changes in the patient's senses of taste and smell
- fever, with a temperature of 100° to 102° F (37.8° to 38.9° C)
- as the prodromal stage draws to a close, usually within 1 to 5 days before the onset of the clinical jaundice stage, dark-colored urine and clay-colored stools.

In the clinical jaundice stage, here's what to look for:
- pruritus, abdominal pain or tenderness, and indigestion
- early complaints of anorexia, then revived appetite
- jaundice of sclerae, mucous membranes, and skin, which can last for 1 to 2 weeks; indicates damaged liver but doesn't reveal disease severity (hepatitis can occur without jaundice).

During the clinical jaundice stage, look for:
- rashes, erythematous patches, or hives, especially in hepatitis B or C
- abdominal tenderness in the right upper quadrant, an enlarged and tender liver and, in some cases, splenomegaly and cervical adenopathy.

During the recovery or posticteric stage, look for:
- most symptoms decreasing or subsided
- a decrease in liver enlargement. The recovery phase generally lasts from 2 to 12 weeks—sometimes longer in patients with hepatitis B, C, or E.

NURSING DIAGNOSES AND COLLABORATIVE PROBLEMS

Based on the following nursing diagnoses, you'll establish patient outcomes.

Activity intolerance related to fatigue and malaise. The patient will:
- express an understanding of how hepatitis relates to fatigue and why he must comply with activity restrictions
- seek assistance, when needed, to perform self-care activities
- regain energy needed to perform activities of daily living.

Altered nutrition: Less than body requirements, related to adverse GI reactions. The patient will:
- eat a nutritionally balanced, high-protein diet (unless protein is restricted)
- regain any lost weight and maintain weight within a normal range
- avoid signs and symptoms of malnutrition.

Risk for injury related to potential for permanent liver damage. The patient will:
- exhibit normal liver function test results after hepatitis resolves
- avoid signs and symptoms of fulminant hepatitis, cirrhosis, or chronic hepatitis.

PLANNING AND IMPLEMENTATION

These measures help the patient with hepatitis:
- Use standard precautions to prevent disease transmission to anyone, including visitors. (See *Preventing the spread of hepatitis A.*) Watch for signs and symptoms of infection.
- Report all cases of hepatitis to health officials. Ask the patient to name his recent contacts.
- Observe the patient for both desired and adverse effects of medications.
- Watch for signs of complications, such as changes in level of consciousness, ascites, edema, dehydration, respiratory problems, myalgia, and arthralgia.

To prevent transmission of hepatitis, you'll need to observe isolation precautions—and discuss them with your patient to promote his cooperation. According to the most recent recommendations from the Centers for Disease Control and Prevention, standard precautions apply. Specific guidelines include the following:

■ Provide a private room as indicated (necessary for a patient with fecal incontinence or poor hygiene). Wear a gown (when soiling is likely) and gloves (for contact with blood, body fluids, secretions, excretions, or contaminated items).

■ Wash your hands after touching body fluids, blood, secretions, and contaminated items, regardless of whether you were wearing gloves. Wash your hands immediately after removing your gloves and when otherwise indicated to avoid transmission to other patients or environments.

■ Wear a mask or goggles during procedures and patient care activities that are likely to generate splashes or sprays of body fluids, secretions, or excretions.

■ Dispose of needles and syringes in prominently labeled, puncture-resistant containers and don't recap needles and syringes. Dispose of dressings and tissues in the hospital's designated area for contaminated refuse.

■ Dispose of any contaminated bed linens in isolation bags, and label any fecal specimens as "Biohazard."

■ Whenever transporting the patient, use added protection (moisture-resistant pads for a fecally incontinent patient, for example). Notify the staff in the destination area of the patient's arrival so they can take the necessary precautions.

■ At home, tell the patient to use meticulous hygiene after a bowel movement—starting with thorough hand washing. Tell him not to handle food or share food or hand towels.

Patient teaching
After discussing isolation measures, teach the patient who has hepatitis A about how it is transmitted, the incubation period, diagnostic tests, prophylaxis, and who is at high risk for this type of hepatitis. Also, instruct the patient in general hygiene practices to prevent the risk of transmission.

■ Because inactivity may make the patient anxious, include diversionary activities and gradually add activities.

■ Provide rest periods throughout the day, scheduled between treatments and tests.

■ To foster an adequate diet, don't overload the patient's meal tray and include his favorite foods in the meal plan. Too much food may only diminish his appetite. Also take care not to overmedicate him and suppress his appetite.

■ Administer supplemental vitamins and commercial feedings, as ordered. If severe symptoms inhibit oral intake, provide I.V. therapy and parenteral nutrition, as ordered.

■ Administer antiemetics, as ordered.

■ Record the patient's weight daily, and keep accurate intake and output records. Note frequency of defecation and check feces for color, consistency, and amount.

■ Provide adequate fluids (at least 4 qt [4 L] daily) by offering fruit juices, soft drinks, ice chips, and water.

Patient teaching

■ Teach the patient about the disease, its signs and symptoms, and recommended treatments.

■ Explain all necessary diagnostic tests and any special preparations. Point out that the findings from these tests, plus his symptoms, help establish his diagnosis.

■ Stress that complete recovery takes time. The liver takes 3 weeks to regenerate and up to 4 months to return to normal. Advise the patient to avoid contact sports until his liver returns to its normal size, and to check with his doctor before engaging in any strenuous activity.

■ Review measures to prevent spread of the disease, such as washing hands thoroughly and frequently and never sharing food, eating utensils, or toothbrushes. If he has hepatitis A or E, warn him not to contaminate food or water with fecal matter. If he has hepatitis B, C, or D, explain that transmission occurs through exchange of blood or body fluids that contain blood (avoid sexual contact, donating blood, accidental cuts).

■ Emphasize the importance of rest and good nutrition in promoting liver regeneration. Tell the patient to drink adequate fluids and eat a high-calorie, high-protein diet in frequent small meals.

■ Tell the patient who is recuperating at home to weigh himself daily and to report any weight loss greater than 5 lb (2.5 kg) to his doctor.

■ Warn the patient to abstain from alcohol to avoid undue stress on the liver during the illness.

■ Explain to the patient and family members that anyone exposed to the disease through contact with him should receive postexposure prophylaxis as soon as possible. Immune globulin is given for hepatitis C and E, but it has not proved effective.

■ Tell the patient to check with the doctor before taking any medication—even nonprescription drugs—because some medications can precipitate a relapse.

■ Stress the need for continued medical care. Advise the patient to see the doctor again about 2 weeks after the diagnosis. Mention probable monthly follow-up visits for up to 6 months after diagnosis. Also explain that if chronic hepatitis develops, he'll always have to visit the doctor regularly to monitor the disease.

EVALUATION
Evaluation of patient outcomes determines the success of collaborative management. For the patient with hepatitis, evaluation focuses on activity tolerance, injury prevention, and adequate nutrition and knowledge.

Hiatal hernia

Commonly producing no symptoms, hiatal hernia is a defect in the diaphragm that permits a portion of the stomach to pass through the diaphragmatic opening into the chest. Three types of hiatal hernia can occur: a sliding hernia, a paraesophageal (rolling) hernia, or a mixed hernia. (See *Types of hiatal hernia.*)

CAUSES
In a sliding hernia, the muscular collar around the esophageal and diaphragmatic junction loosens, permitting the lower portion of the esophagus and the upper portion of the stomach to rise into the chest. This muscle weakening may be associated with normal aging, or it may be secondary to esophageal carcinoma, kyphoscoliosis, trauma, or surgery. A sliding hernia may also be caused by diaphragmatic malformations.

The cause of a paraesophageal hernia isn't fully understood. One theory says the stomach isn't properly anchored below the diaphragm, permitting the upper portion to slide through the esophageal hiatus.

The intra-abdominal pressure associated with hernias can be caused by such conditions as ascites, preg-

nancy, obesity, constrictive clothing, bending, straining, coughing, Valsalva's maneuver, and extreme physical exertion.

If the hiatal hernia is associated with gastroesophageal reflux, complications include esophagitis, esophageal ulceration, hemorrhage, peritonitis, and mediastinitis. Aspiration of refluxed fluids may lead to respiratory distress, aspiration pneumonia, or cardiac dysfunction from pressure on the heart and lungs. With esophageal stricture and incarceration, a large portion of the stomach is caught above the diaphragm, leading to perforation, gastric ulcer, and strangulation and gangrene of the herniated stomach portion.

In a sliding hernia, both the stomach and the gastroesophageal junction slip up into the chest, placing the gastroesophageal junction above the diaphragmatic hiatus. The patient has symptoms if the lower esophageal reflux (LES) is incompetent and permits gastric reflux and heartburn.

In a paraesophageal or rolling hernia, a part of the greater curvature of the stomach rolls through the diaphragmatic defect. The patient usually doesn't get gastric reflux and heartburn because the closing mechanism of the LES is unaffected.

A mixed hernia has features of both the sliding and rolling hernias.

The incidence of hiatal hernia increases with age. By their sixties, about 60% of people have hiatal hernias. However, most have no symptoms; the hernia is an incidental finding during a barium swallow. Or it may be detected by tests that follow the discovery of occult blood. The prevalence (especially of the paraesophageal type) is higher in women than in men.

DIAGNOSIS AND TREATMENT
Chest X-rays occasionally show an air shadow behind the heart in a large hernia and infiltrates in the lower lung lobes, if the patient has aspirated the refluxed fluids.

Barium swallow with fluoroscopy, the most specific test for hiatal hernia, reveals an outpouching containing barium at the lower end of the esophagus. (Small hernias are difficult to recognize.) This study also shows diaphragmatic abnormalities.

Serum hemoglobin levels and hematocrit may be decreased in patients with paraesophageal hernia. Endoscopy and biopsy differentiate among hiatal hernia, varices, and other small gastroesophageal lesions. These tests also identify the mucosal junction and the edge of the diaphragm indenting the esophagus and can rule out cancer.

Acid perfusion testing indicates that heartburn results from esophageal reflux, and pH studies assess for reflux gastric contents. Esophageal motility studies re-

Types of hiatal hernia

The illustrations below show a normal stomach along with two types of hiatal hernia: sliding and paraesophageal (rolling).

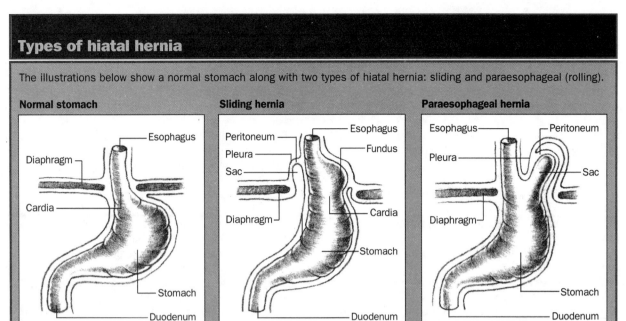

Normal stomach

Esophagus
Diaphragm
Cardia
Stomach
Duodenum

Sliding hernia

Esophagus
Peritoneum
Fundus
Pleura
Sac
Cardia
Diaphragm
Stomach
Duodenum

Paraesophageal hernia

Esophagus
Peritoneum
Pleura
Sac
Diaphragm
Stomach
Duodenum

veal esophageal motor or lower esophageal pressure abnormalities.

Treatment aims to relieve symptoms and to manage and prevent complications. Medical therapy to reduce gastroesophageal reflux consists of medications, activity modifications, and dietary measures.

Antacids help neutralize refluxed fluids (best treatment for intermittent reflux). Histamine-2 receptor antagonists such as cimetidine also modify the acidity of the refluxed fluid. A cholinergic agent, such as bethanechol or metoclopramide, strengthens LES tone.

Restricted activity reduces intermittent reflux, and modified diet may also help.

Rarely, surgery is required when symptoms persist despite medical treatment or if complications develop. Indications for surgery include esophageal stricture, significant bleeding, pulmonary aspiration, or incarceration or strangulation of the herniated stomach portion. Surgical techniques vary greatly, but most create an artificial closing mechanism at the gastroesophageal junction to strengthen the LES. Rare postsurgical complications may include mucosal erosion, ulcers, and bleeding of the gastric pouch; pressure on the left lung due to the size and placement of the pouch; and formation of a volvulus.

Generally, a sliding hernia without an incompetent sphincter produces no reflux or symptoms and therefore requires no treatment. A large rolling hernia, however, should be surgically repaired (even if it pro-duces no symptoms) because of the high risk of complications, especially strangulation.

COLLABORATIVE MANAGEMENT
Care of the patient with hiatal hernia will focus on relieving symptoms and preventing complications.

ASSESSMENT
When a sliding hernia causes symptoms, the patient typically complains of heartburn, indicating an incompetent LES and gastroesophageal reflux. Patient history usually reveals that heartburn occurs from 1 to 4 hours after eating and is aggravated by reclining, belching, or conditions that increase intra-abdominal pressure. Look for:
- heartburn accompanied by regurgitation or vomiting
- complaints of retrosternal or substernal chest pain (typically after meals or at bedtime), reflecting reflux of gastric contents, distention of the stomach, and spasm.

Keep in mind that the patient with a paraesophageal hernia is usually asymptomatic. Symptoms, when present, usually stem from incarceration of a stomach portion above the diaphragmatic opening. Look for:
- report of a feeling of fullness after eating
- if the paraesophageal hernia interferes with breathing, a feeling of breathlessness or suffocation

■ complaints of chest pain resembling angina pectoris

■ dysphagia, especially after very hot or cold foods, alcoholic beverages, or a big meal (may indicate esophagitis, esophageal ulceration, or stricture)

■ bleeding that is mild or massive, frank or occult (may indicate esophagitis or erosion of the gastric pouch)

■ severe pain and shock—symptoms of incarceration (usual in paraesophageal hernia), which requires immediate surgery.

NURSING DIAGNOSES AND COLLABORATIVE PROBLEMS

Based on the following nursing diagnoses, you'll establish patient outcomes.

Risk for aspiration of refluxed stomach fluids. The patient will:

■ comply with the prescribed drug regimen to reduce gastroesophageal reflux

■ modify diet and activity as ordered to reduce gastroesophageal reflux

■ avoid aspiration of refluxed stomach fluids.

Impaired swallowing related to esophagitis, esophageal ulceration, or stricture. The patient will:

■ remain adequately nourished, as shown by a stable weight and absence of signs and symptoms of malnutrition

■ regain ability to swallow normally through medical or surgical therapy.

Pain related to esophageal irritation caused by refluxed stomach fluids. The patient will:

■ express pain relief after taking medications as prescribed

■ take precautions to minimize reflux of stomach contents.

PLANNING AND IMPLEMENTATION

These measures help the patient with a hernia:

■ Develop a diet that takes the patient's food preferences into account and minimizes reflux symptoms. Consult a dietitian as necessary. Supply a list of foods allowed and foods to avoid.

■ Provide small, frequent meals with bland foods while avoiding fatty or acidic foods, chocolate, caffeine, and nicotine.

■ Place the obese patient on a weight reduction diet, as ordered.

■ To reduce intra-abdominal pressure, have the patient sleep in a reverse Trendelenburg position (with the head of the bed elevated 6" to 12" [15 to 30.5 cm]). He should also avoid lying down immediately after meals and late-night snacks.

■ Administer medications, such as antacids and H_2-receptor antagonists, as prescribed.

■ Offer the patient emotional and psychological support to help him cope with pain and discomfort.

■ Encourage limiting activity that would increase intra-abdominal pressure.

Patient teaching

■ To enhance compliance, teach the patient about the disorder.

■ Explain significant symptoms, diagnostic tests, and ordered treatments.

■ Review prescribed medications, explaining their desired actions and possible adverse effects.

■ Tell the patient that he'll need medications for hiatal hernia treatment indefinitely, even after surgical repair.

■ Teach the patient dietary changes to reduce reflux. For example, suggest small, frequent, bland meals to reduce stomach bulk and acid secretion. Advise avoiding beverages and foods that intensify symptoms, such as alcohol and spicy foods.

■ Explain how gravity can help to prevent reflux. Encourage the patient to delay lying down for 2 hours after eating. Suggest elevating the head of the bed on 6" (15-cm) blocks at home.

■ Instruct the patient to avoid activities that increase intra-abdominal pressure, such as coughing, wearing constrictive clothing, and straining.

EVALUATION

Evaluation of patient outcomes determines the success of collaborative management. For the patient with a hiatal hernia, evaluation focuses on relief of pain and adequate nutrition, oxygenation, airway, and knowledge.

Inguinal hernia

When part of an internal organ protrudes through an abnormal opening in the containing wall of its cavity, the patient has a hernia. In an inguinal hernia—the most common type—the large or small intestine, omentum, or bladder protrudes into the inguinal canal.

CAUSES

Inguinal hernias are caused by abdominal muscles weakened by a common congenital malformation, a traumatic injury, or aging. (The malformation may occur in males during the seventh month of gestation, when the testicle descends into the scrotum, preceded by the peritoneal sac. If the sac closes improperly, it leaves an opening through which the intestine can slip, causing a hernia. [See *Inguinal hernia in the male.*]) Another cause is increased intra-abdominal pressure due to heavy lifting, exertion, pregnancy, obesity, excessive coughing, or straining during defecation.

Inguinal hernias can be classified as reducible (if it can be manipulated back into place with relative ease), incarcerated (if it can't be reduced because adhesions have formed in the hernial sac), or strangulated (if part of the herniated intestine becomes twisted or edematous, causing serious complications).

Inguinal hernias can be direct or indirect, depending on the location of the abnormal opening. An indirect hernia causes the abdominal viscera to protrude through the inguinal ring and follow the spermatic cord (in males) or round ligament (in females). A direct hernia is caused by a weakness in the fascial floor of the inguinal canal. The direct form, most common, can develop at any age but is especially prevalent in infants under age 1. This form is three times more common in males.

Inguinal hernia may lead to incarceration or strangulation. Strangulation may seriously interfere with normal blood flow and peristalsis, possibly leading to intestinal obstruction and necrosis.

DIAGNOSIS AND TREATMENT
Although assessment findings are the cornerstone of diagnosis, suspected bowel obstruction requires X-rays and a white blood cell count (may be elevated).

The choice of therapy depends on the hernia type. For a reducible hernia, moving the protruding organ back into place gives temporary relief. A truss may keep the abdominal contents from protruding through the hernial sac. Although a truss can't cure a hernia, it's especially helpful for an older or debilitated patient for whom any surgery is potentially hazardous.

Herniorrhaphy is the preferred surgical treatment for infants, adults, and otherwise healthy older patients. This procedure replaces hernial sac contents into the abdominal cavity and seals the opening. Another effective procedure is hernioplasty, which reinforces the weakened area with steel mesh, fascia, or wire.

A strangulated or necrotic hernia requires bowel resection. Rarely, an extensive resection may require a temporary colostomy.

COLLABORATIVE MANAGEMENT
Care of the patient with an inguinal hernia focuses on providing temporary relief of symptoms and preparing him for surgery and its aftermath.

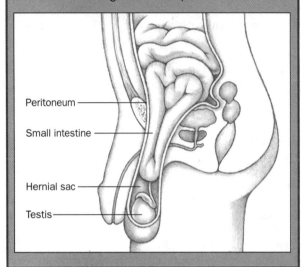

Inguinal hernia in the male

In inguinal hernia, a weakening of the abdominal wall permits a loop of intestine to descend into the scrotum. Constriction by the muscle in the abdominal wall obstructs and strangulates the loop.

Peritoneum

Small intestine

Hernial sac

Testis

ASSESSMENT
The patient history may reveal precipitating factors, such as weight lifting, recent pregnancy, or excessive coughing. Usually, the patient reports the appearance of a lump in the inguinal area when he stands or strains. He may also complain of sharp, steady groin pain, which tends to worsen when tension is placed on the hernia and improve when the hernia is reduced.

Here's what to look for:
■ with a large hernia, obvious swelling in the inguinal area
■ with a small hernia, simply a fullness that disappears as the patient lies down (reducible)
■ characteristic bulging of the inguinal area during Valsalva's maneuver
■ presence of bowel sounds (absence may indicate incarceration or strangulation).

Palpation helps determine size or disclose the presence of a hernia in a male patient.

NURSING DIAGNOSES AND COLLABORATIVE PROBLEMS
Based on the following nursing diagnoses, you'll establish patient outcomes.

Activity intolerance related to presence of an inguinal hernia. The patient will:

- skillfully perform activities to minimize or prevent enlargement of inguinal hernia
- regain his normal activity level, either by wearing a truss or by surgery.

Altered GI tissue perfusion related to hernia incarceration. The patient will:

- express knowledge of signs and symptoms of incarceration and the importance of reporting them immediately
- regain and then maintain normal GI function.

Pain related to the presence of an inguinal hernia. The patient will:

- avoid activities that cause or increase pain
- express relief of pain when wearing a truss
- become free from pain after surgical repair of the hernia.

PLANNING AND IMPLEMENTATION

These measures help the patient with a hernia:

- Apply a truss only after a hernia has been reduced. For best results, apply it in the morning before the patient gets out of bed. Apply powder to protect his skin and inspect it daily.
- Watch for and immediately report signs of incarceration and strangulation.
- Don't try to reduce an incarcerated hernia; doing so may perforate the bowel. If hernial strangulation causes severe intestinal obstruction, tell the doctor immediately. A nasogastric tube may be inserted promptly to empty the stomach and relieve pressure on the hernial sac.
- Monitor the effect of pain medication; try giving medications ½ hour prior to activities.
- Encourage the patient and set realistic goals together. Discuss his feelings and questions about self-care.

Patient teaching

- Explain the inguinal hernia and its treatment. Point out that elective surgery is the treatment of choice. Warn that emergency surgery for a strangulated hernia can require extensive bowel resection, involving a protracted hospital stay and possibly a colostomy.
- Teach the patient who will not undergo surgery to watch for signs and symptoms of incarceration or strangulation. Tell him that severe pain, nausea, vomiting, and diarrhea may indicate complications. Warn him and family members that shock, high fever, and bloody stools are signs of complete obstruction and must be reported at once. Explain that immediate surgery follows such complications.
- If the patient uses a truss, instruct him to bathe daily and apply liberal amounts of cornstarch or baby powder to prevent skin irritation. Warn against applying the truss over clothing because it slips, and point out that a truss doesn't cure a hernia and may be uncomfortable.
- If surgery is scheduled, provide preoperative teaching. Reinforce the doctor's explanation of the surgery and its possible complications.
- Teach the patient how to use abdominal splinting when moving in bed, coughing, or putting any pressure on his abdomen.

EVALUATION

Evaluation of patient outcomes determines the success of collaborative management. For the patient with a hernia, evaluation focuses on improved tissue perfusion, activity tolerance, pain relief, and adequate knowledge.

Intestinal obstruction

Commonly a medical emergency, intestinal obstruction is the partial or complete blockage of the lumen in the small or large bowel. Small-bowel obstruction is far more common (affecting 90% of patients) and usually more serious. Complete obstruction in any part of the bowel, if untreated, can cause death within hours from shock and vascular collapse.

CAUSES

Intestinal obstruction is most likely to occur after abdominal surgery or in persons with congenital bowel deformities. It's caused by either mechanical or neurogenic blockage of the lumen. Mechanical obstruction may result from adhesions or strangulated hernias (usually small-bowel obstruction); carcinomas (large-bowel obstruction); foreign bodies, such as fruit pits, gallstones, or worms; compression of the bowel wall from stenosis; intussusception; volvulus of the sigmoid or cecum; tumors; or atresia. (See *Two types of intestinal obstruction.*)

Nonmechanical obstruction usually results from paralytic ileus (the most common). Paralytic ileus is a physiologic form of intestinal obstruction that usually develops in the small bowel after abdominal surgery. Other nonmechanical causes include electrolyte imbalances; toxicity, as with uremia or generalized infection; neurogenic abnormalities such as spinal cord lesions; and thrombosis or embolism of mesenteric vessels.

Although the obstructions may vary, the underlying pathophysiology is similar. Intestinal obstruction can lead to perforation, peritonitis, septicemia, secondary infection, metabolic alkalosis or acidosis, hypovolemic or septic shock and, if untreated, death.

Two types of intestinal obstruction

Most intestinal obstructions result from intrinsic or extrinsic structures that narrow or close the intestinal lumen. These mechanical obstructions can be congenital or acquired. They include volvulus and intussusception.

In *volvulus*, the intestine twists at least 180 degrees. This produces obstructions both proximal and distal to the loop, blocks intestinal flow, and causes ischemia. Necrosis rapidly occurs. This condition most commonly affects the sigmoid colon, especially in adults. In children, the small bowel is a common site. Other common sites include the stomach and cecum.

In *intussusception*, a portion of the bowel telescopes or invaginates into an adjacent bowel portion. Peristalsis then propels the portion farther into the bowel, pulling more bowel with it. Most common in infants, the condition may be fatal, especially if treatment is delayed more than 24 hours. Strangulation of the intestine usually occurs, with gangrene, shock, and perforation.

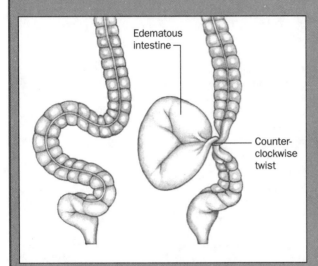

Edematous intestine

Counter-clockwise twist

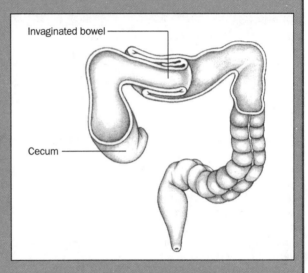

Invaginated bowel

Cecum

DIAGNOSIS AND TREATMENT

Various tests help to establish the diagnosis and pinpoint complications. Abdominal X-rays confirm intestinal obstruction and reveal intestinal gas or fluid. In small-bowel obstruction, a typical "stepladder" pattern emerges, with alternating fluid and gas levels apparent in 3 to 4 hours. In large-bowel obstruction, barium enema reveals a distended, air-filled colon or a closed loop of sigmoid with extreme distention (in sigmoid volvulus).

Serum sodium, chloride, and potassium levels may fall because of vomiting. White blood cell counts may be normal or slightly elevated if necrosis, peritonitis, or strangulation occurs. Serum amylase level may increase, possibly from irritation of the pancreas by a bowel loop. Hemoglobin levels and hematocrit may increase, indicating dehydration.

Sigmoidoscopy, colonoscopy, or barium enema helps find the cause of obstruction; however, these tests are contraindicated if perforation is suspected.

Surgery is usually the treatment of choice. One important exception is paralytic ileus, in which other therapy is usually attempted first. The type of surgery depends on the cause of blockage. For example, if a tumor is obstructing the intestine, a colon resection with anastomosis is performed; if adhesions are obstructing the lumen, these are lysed.

Surgical preparation includes correction of fluid and electrolyte imbalances, decompression of the bowel to relieve vomiting and distention, treatment of shock and peritonitis, and administration of broad-spectrum antibiotics. In many cases, decompression is begun preoperatively with passage of a nasogastric (NG) tube. This tube relieves vomiting, reduces abdominal distention, and prevents aspiration. In strangulating obstruction, preoperative therapy also usually requires blood replacement and I.V. fluids.

Postoperative care involves careful patient monitoring and interventions geared to the type of surgery. Total parenteral nutrition may be ordered if the patient has a protein deficit from chronic obstruction, postoperative or paralytic ileus, or infection.

Nonsurgical treatment may be attempted in some patients with partial obstruction, particularly those who suffer recurrent partial obstruction or who developed it after surgery or a recent episode of diffuse peritonitis.

Nonsurgical treatment usually includes decompression with an NG tube, correction of fluid and electrolyte deficits, administration of broad-spectrum antibiotics, and occasionally total parenteral nutrition. A long nasointestinal tube also may be used for decompression.

Throughout nonsurgical treatment, the patient's condition must be closely monitored. If he fails to improve or his condition deteriorates, surgery is required.

Another indication for nonsurgical treatment is nonmechanical obstruction from adynamic ileus (paralytic ileus). Most of these cases occur postoperatively and disappear spontaneously in 2 to 3 days. However, if the disorder doesn't resolve within 48 hours, treatment consists of decompression with an NG tube. Oral intake is restricted until bowel function resumes; then the diet is gradually advanced.

In the patient with paralytic ileus, decompression occasionally responds to colonoscopy or rectal tube insertion. When paralytic ileus develops secondary to another illness, such as severe infection or electrolyte imbalance, the primary problem must also be treated. Again, if conservative treatment fails, surgery is required.

In both surgical and nonsurgical treatment, drug therapy includes antibiotics and analgesics or sedatives, such as meperidine or phenobarbital (but not opiates because they inhibit GI motility).

COLLABORATIVE MANAGEMENT

Care of the patient with an intestinal obstruction focuses on preparation for surgery and postoperative care that returns the patient to good nutritional status. (See *Managing GI obstruction,* pages 226 and 227.)

ASSESSMENT

The patient's history commonly reveals predisposing factors, such as surgery (especially abdominal), radiation therapy, gallstones, or illnesses that can lead to obstruction, such as Crohn's disease, diverticular disease, or ulcerative colitis. Family history may reveal colorectal cancer.

Hiccups are a common complaint in all types of bowel obstruction. Other specific findings depend on the cause of obstruction—mechanical or nonmechanical—and its location in the bowel.

In mechanical obstruction of the small bowel, you'll find:
- complaints of colicky pain, nausea, vomiting, and constipation; with complete obstruction, vomiting of fecal content
- distended abdomen, the hallmark of all types of mechanical obstruction
- bowel sounds, borborygmi, and rushes (occasionally loud enough to be heard without a stethoscope)
- abdominal tenderness; rebound tenderness in patients with obstruction that results from strangulation with ischemia.

In mechanical obstruction of the large bowel, you'll find:
- commonly, a history of constipation, with a more gradual onset of signs and symptoms than in small-bowel obstruction
- after days of constipation, reports of sudden, colicky abdominal pain, producing spasms that last less than 1 minute and recur every few minutes
- history of constant hypogastric pain, nausea and, in the later stages, vomiting
- orange-brown and foul-smelling vomitus
- abdomen that appears dramatically distended, with visible loops of large bowel
- on auscultation, loud, high-pitched borborygmi
- in partial obstruction, similar but milder signs and symptoms; leakage of liquid stools around the partial obstruction.

Here's what you'll see in nonmechanical obstruction such as paralytic ileus:
- reports of diffuse abdominal discomfort instead of colicky pain; frequent vomiting, which may consist of gastric and bile contents and, rarely, fecal contents; constipation; and hiccups
- with vascular insufficiency or infarction, possible complaints of severe abdominal pain and abdominal distention
- decreased bowel sounds early in the disease, disappearing as the disorder progresses.

NURSING DIAGNOSES AND COLLABORATIVE PROBLEMS

Based on the following nursing diagnoses, you'll establish patient outcomes.

Altered nutrition: Less than body requirements, related to inability to eat. The patient will:
- receive adequate nutrition, either I.V. or total parenteral, until the obstruction is alleviated
- maintain his weight within a normal range
- resume his oral intake after the obstruction is alleviated.

Risk for fluid volume deficit related to inability to ingest oral fluids. The patient will:

- maintain an adequate fluid volume balance, as evidenced by normal vital signs and an I.V. intake that equals his output
- demonstrate no signs or symptoms of dehydration
- ingest fluids orally after the obstruction is alleviated.

Pain related to the pressure and irritation resulting from an intestinal obstruction. The patient will:
- express relief of pain following analgesics
- become free from pain after the obstruction is alleviated.

PLANNING AND IMPLEMENTATION
These measures help the patient with intestinal obstruction:

- Allow the patient nothing by mouth, as ordered, but be sure to provide frequent mouth care to help keep mucous membranes moist. If surgery won't be performed, allow small amounts of ice chips. Avoid lemon-glycerin swabs, which can increase mouth dryness.
- Insert an NG tube to decompress the bowel, as ordered. Attach the tube to low-pressure, intermittent suction. Irrigate the tube with normal saline solution if necessary to maintain patency.
- If ordered, assist with insertion of a weighted nasointestinal tube, such as a Miller-Abbott, Cantor, or Harris tube, to decompress the bowel. Help the patient turn from side to side (or walk around, if he can) to facilitate passage of the tube. Check periodically to make sure the tube is advancing.
- Monitor tube drainage for color, consistency, and amount.
- Listen for bowel sounds, and watch for other signs of resuming peristalsis (passage of flatus and mucus through the rectum).
- Begin and maintain I.V. therapy, as ordered. Provide I.V. fluids to keep levels within normal ranges.
- Look for signs of dehydration (thick, swollen tongue; dry, cracked lips; dry oral mucous membranes).
- Monitor intake and output. Maintain fluid and electrolyte balance by monitoring electrolyte, blood urea nitrogen, and creatinine levels.
- Monitor vital signs frequently. A drop in blood pressure may indicate reduced circulating blood volume due to blood loss from a strangulated hernia. Remember, as much as 10½ qt (10 L) of fluid can collect in the small bowel, drastically reducing plasma volume. Observe closely for signs of shock (pallor, rapid pulse, and hypotension). Provide blood replacement therapy as necessary.
- Monitor urine output carefully to assess renal function, circulating blood volume, and possible urine retention due to bladder compression by the distended intestine. Also measure abdominal girth frequently to detect progressive distention.
- If you suspect bladder compression, catheterize the patient for residual urine immediately after he has voided.
- Administer analgesics, broad-spectrum antibiotics, and other medications, as ordered. Remember that analgesics may be withheld until a diagnosis is confirmed. To ease discomfort, help the patient to change positions frequently.
- After giving medication, monitor the patient for the desired effects and for adverse reactions.
- Continually assess the patient's pain. Remember, colicky pain that suddenly becomes constant could signal perforation.
- Watch for signs and symptoms of metabolic alkalosis (changes in sensorium; slow, shallow respirations; hypertonic muscles; tetany) or acidosis (shortness of breath on exertion; disorientation; and, later, deep, rapid breathing, weakness, and malaise). Watch for signs and symptoms of secondary infection, such as fever and chills.
- Keep the patient in semi-Fowler's or Fowler's position as much as possible to promote pulmonary ventilation and ease respiratory distress from abdominal distention.

Patient teaching
- Teach the patient about his particular disorder, its cause, and signs and symptoms. Listen to his questions and take time to answer them.
- Explain necessary diagnostic tests and treatments and their value.
- Prepare the patient and family members for the possibility of surgery. Provide preoperative teaching, and reinforce the doctor's explanation of the surgery. Demonstrate techniques for coughing and deep breathing, and teach the patient how to use incentive spirometry.
- Tell the patient what to expect postoperatively.
- Review the proper use of prescribed medications, focusing on their correct administration, desired effects, and possible adverse effects.
- Emphasize the importance of following a structured bowel regimen, particularly with mechanical obstruction from fecal impaction. Encourage a high-fiber diet and daily exercise.
- Reassure the patient with paralytic ileus that recurrence is unlikely. However, remind him to report any recurrence of abdominal pain, abdominal distention, nausea, or vomiting.

(Text continues on page 228.)

CLINICAL PATH

Managing GI obstruction

Patient problems:
- Altered elimination patterns
- Alteration in comfort
- Fluid volume deficit
- Anxiety/fear
- Educational needs

Primary diagnosis: GI obstruction
Other:
Tentative DRG #: 180

Expected length of stay (LOS): 4 to 6 days
Actual LOS:
MD:
Discharge planner:
Case manager:
Advance directive: No   Yes

	Day 1	**Day 2**
TESTS	■ Complete blood count (CBC), blood chemistries, magnesium, phosphorus, liver function tests ■ Arterial blood gas analysis* ■ Abdominal X-rays (upright and supine); if volvulus seen, endoscopic intervention or barium enema ■ Chest X-ray ■ Gallbladder sonogram* ■ Urinalysis, electrocardiogram, guaiac stool (occult blood) ■ Computed tomography (CT) scan of abdomen and pelvis with oral or I.V. contrast*	■ CBC, blood chemistries ■ Guaiac stool ■ Paracentesis* ■ Esophagogastroduodenoscopy* ■ Barium enema,* sigmoidoscopy,* or colonoscopy* (depending on site of suspected obstruction) ■ Abdominal obstructive series
MEDICATIONS	■ I.V. hydration ■ Antibiotics* ■ Steroids* ■ Analgesics (meperidine I.M. or I.V.)	■ I.V. hydration ■ Antibiotics* ■ Steroids* ■ Analgesics*
TREATMENTS	■ Nasogastric (NG) tube—low, intermittent ■ Intake and output (I & O) ■ Indwelling urinary catheter*	■ NG tube—low, intermittent ■ I & O ■ Indwelling urinary catheter*
CONSULTS	■ GI ■ Surgical	
ACTIVITIES AND SAFETY	■ Activity as tolerated	■ Activity as tolerated
NUTRITION	■ Nothing by mouth (NPO)	■ NPO
NURSING	■ Perform physical assessment. ■ Assess abdomen for bowel sounds every shift; record results. ■ Take vital signs every shift and as needed. ■ If stool occurs, record number and consistency. ■ Check stool for occult blood. ■ Monitor laboratory values. *Teaching:* ■ Explain reasons for I.V., NG tube, indwelling urinary catheter,* frequent monitoring.	■ Perform physical assessment. ■ Assess abdomen for bowel sounds every shift; record results. ■ Check vital signs twice daily and as needed. ■ If stool occurs, record number and consistency. ■ Check stool for occult blood. ■ Monitor laboratory values. *Teaching:* ■ Review risk factors (previous abdominal or pelvic surgery, chronic constipation, cholelithiasis, ingested foreign body, diverticular disease, inflammatory bowel disease). ■ Explain scheduled tests and preparations.
DISCHARGE PLANNING	■ Initial assessment	
EXPECTED PATIENT OUTCOMES	■ Vital signs stable ■ I.V. site free of infection ■ NG tube patent ■ Abdominal discomfort decreased ■ Patient properly prepared for testing	■ Vital signs stable ■ I.V. site free of infection ■ NG tube patent ■ Abdominal discomfort decreased ■ Patient properly prepared for testing ■ Activity tolerance

*If indicated

Adapted with permission from Staten Island (N.Y.) University Hospital.

Day 3	Day 4	Days 5 to 6
■ Serum electrolytes ■ Upper GI and small bowel series ■ Abdominal CT scan to further evaluate nature of obstruction*		
■ I.V. hydration ■ Antibiotics* ■ Steroids* ■ Analgesics*	■ I.V. heparin lock ■ Antibiotics* ■ Steroids* ■ Analgesics*	■ I.V. heparin lock ■ Antibiotics* ■ Steroids* ■ Analgesics*
■ NG tube: Remove if workup indicates amelioration of process; if workup is questionable, clamp and observe on clear fluids. ■ Indwelling urinary catheter: Remove if no evidence of urinary tract obstruction.* ■ Record I & O.	■ Monitoring of NG tube,* I & O, indwelling urinary catheter*	■ Monitoring of NG tube,* I & O, indwelling urinary catheter*
	■ Nutritional, if patient remains NPO	
■ Activity as tolerated	■ Activity as tolerated	■ Activity as tolerated
■ NPO ■ Clear liquids, if obstruction improves	■ Diet advance	■ Diet advance
■ Physical assessment. ■ Assess abdomen for bowel sounds every shift; record results. ■ Check vital signs twice daily and as needed. ■ Record number and consistency of stool. ■ Check stool for occult blood. ■ Monitor laboratory values. ■ Obtain weight. ■ Assess urine output, if indwelling urinary catheter is removed. ■ Assess I.V. site for change. *Teaching:* ■ Review Day 2 teaching ■ Explain scheduled tests and preparations.	■ Physical assessment *Teaching:* ■ Discharge drugs (dose, adverse effects, indication) ■ Schedule follow-up doctor appointment after discharge. ■ Recurrent symptoms to report: abdominal pain, distention, constipation	■ Physical assessment *Teaching:* ■ Discharge drugs (dose, adverse effects, indication) ■ Schedule follow-up doctor appointment after discharge. ■ Recurrent symptoms to report: abdominal pain, distention, constipation
	■ Discharge when obstruction resolves. ■ Continue hospitalization for further treatment of obstructive cause. ■ Consider surgery if partial small bowel obstruction doesn't improve.	■ Continue hospitalization for further treatment of obstructive cause. *Day 6:* ■ Consider surgery if condition doesn't improve.
■ Vital signs stable ■ Urine output adequate, if indwelling urinary catheter removed ■ I.V. site free of infection ■ Oral intake tolerated* ■ Activity tolerance	■ Vital signs stable ■ Diet tolerated ■ Activities of daily living (ADLs) performed at pre-hospital level of functioning ■ I.V. site free of infection	■ Vital signs stable ■ Diet tolerated ■ ADLs performed at pre-hospital level of functioning ■ I.V. site free of infection

*If indicated

After treatment for intestinal obstruction, the patient will meet the following criteria before discharge:

- vital signs within normal limits for him
- serum glucose, urine glucose, and urine ketone levels returning to normal
- serum electrolyte levels returning to normal
- pain relief
- adequate nutritional intake
- no evidence of pulmonary or other complications
- regular bowel patterns.

EVALUATION

Evaluation of patient outcomes determines the success of collaborative management. For the patient with an intestinal obstruction, evaluation focuses on adequate nutrition, restored fluid balance, pain relief, and adequate knowledge. (See *After intestinal obstruction*.)

Irritable bowel syndrome

A common condition, irritable bowel syndrome is also known as spastic colon, spastic colitis, or mucous colitis. It affects mostly women, with symptoms first emerging before age 40. The prognosis is good.

Irritable bowel syndrome is associated with a higher-than-normal incidence of diverticulitis and colon cancer. Although it usually produces few complications, the disorder may, in rare cases, lead to chronic inflammatory bowel disease.

CAUSES

Although the precise etiology is unclear, irritable bowel syndrome involves a change in bowel motility, reflecting an abnormality in the neuromuscular control of intestinal smooth muscle. Contributing or aggravating factors include anxiety and stress. Initial episodes occur early in life; psychological stress probably causes most exacerbations.

Irritable bowel syndrome may also result from dietary factors, such as fiber, fruits, coffee, alcohol, or foods that are cold, highly seasoned, or laxative. Other possible triggers include hormones, laxative abuse, and allergy to certain foods or drugs.

Irritable bowel syndrome is marked by chronic or periodic diarrhea alternating with constipation. It is accompanied by straining during defecation and abdominal cramps. Because symptoms mimic those of acute abdomen, misdiagnosis occasionally results in unnecessary surgery.

DIAGNOSIS AND TREATMENT

With no definitive test, diagnosis of irritable bowel syndrome typically involves studies to rule out other, more serious, disorders. Barium enema may reveal colonic spasm and a tubular appearance of the descending colon. It also rules out other disorders, such as diverticula, tumors, and polyps. Sigmoidoscopy may disclose spastic contractions. Stool examination for occult blood, parasites, and pathogenic bacteria is negative.

The aim of therapy is to control symptoms through dietary changes, stress management, and lifestyle modifications. Medications are reserved for severe symptoms and are discontinued as the patient learns to control her symptoms through diet and stress reduction.

The type of dietary therapy depends on the patient's symptoms. If she has diarrhea, an elimination diet may help determine whether her symptoms result from food intolerance. In this type of diet, certain foods, such as citrus fruits, coffee, corn, dairy products, tea, and wheat, are sequentially eliminated. Then each food is gradually reintroduced to identify which foods, if any, trigger symptoms.

Other dietary changes may include elimination of sorbitol, an artificial sweetener that can cause diarrhea, abdominal distention, and bloating, and elimination of nonabsorbable carbohydrates (such as beans and cabbage) and lactose-containing foods, all of which can cause flatulence.

To control diarrhea, bran may be added to increase dietary fiber. By increasing the time the stool remains in the bowel, bran helps to promote stool formation.

If the patient has constipation and abdominal pain, her diet should contain at least 15 g daily of high-fiber foods, such as wheat bran, oatmeal, oat bran, rye cereals, prunes, dried apricots, and figs. These foods help to minimize the effect of nonpropulsive colonic contractions that may trap stool or retard its passage, causing abdominal pain. The patient should also increase her water intake to at least eight 8-oz glasses a day.

Counseling to help the patient understand the relationship between stress and her illness is essential, as is instruction in stress-management techniques.

Drug therapy, if required, may include:
- anticholinergic, antispasmodic drugs such as propantheline to reduce intestinal hypermotility
- antidiarrheals such as loperamide to control diarrhea
- laxatives for constipation

- antiemetics such as metoclopramide to relieve heartburn, epigastric discomfort, and fullness after meals
- simethicone to relieve belching and bloating from gas in the stomach and intestines
- mild tranquilizers such as diazepam prescribed for a short time to help reduce psychological stress associated with irritable bowel syndrome
- tricyclic antidepressants if depression accompanies the disorder.

COLLABORATIVE MANAGEMENT

Care of the patient with irritable bowel syndrome focuses on relieving symptoms and promoting dietary changes.

ASSESSMENT

The patient typically reports a history of chronic constipation, diarrhea, or both. She may complain of lower abdominal pain (usually in the left lower quadrant) that is commonly relieved by defecation or passage of gas. She may report bouts of diarrhea, which typically occur during the day, alternating with constipation or normal bowel function. During history taking, investigate possible contributing psychological factors that may have triggered or aggravated symptoms, such as a recent stressful life change. Here's what to look for:

- reports of small stools with visible mucus or small, pasty, and pencil-like stools instead of diarrhea
- complaints of dyspepsia, abdominal bloating, heartburn, faintness, and weakness
- anxiety and fatigue
- normal bowel sounds on auscultation
- a relaxed abdomen
- tympany over a gas-filled bowel.

NURSING DIAGNOSES AND COLLABORATIVE PROBLEMS

Based on the following nursing diagnoses, you'll establish patient outcomes.

Constipation related to change in bowel function. The patient will:

- take steps to prevent constipation
- comply with ordered treatment for irritable bowel syndrome
- regain and maintain normal bowel function.

Diarrhea related to change in bowel function. The patient will:

- avoid foods that cause diarrhea
- adhere to the medication regimen prescribed for irritable bowel syndrome
- regain and maintain normal bowel function.

Pain related to intestinal hypermotility. The patient will:

- express relief from pain following administration of anticholinergic, antispasmodic medication
- experience relief from intestinal hypermotility, as evidenced by normal bowel sounds
- become free from pain.

PLANNING AND IMPLEMENTATION

These measures help the patient with irritable bowel syndrome:

- Assess abdomen for bowel sounds and distention.
- Estimate and document the extent of the nutritional deficit based on body weight; character, color, and texture of hair and skin; presence or absence of corneal plaques; cracked and bleeding gums; and muscle wasting.
- Plan and set goals for normal nutritional maintenance.
- Administer medications, as ordered, to control peristalsis before meals.
- Serve small frequent meals.
- Administer I.V. nutritional supplements.
- Monitor bowel elimination patterns; note frequency and characteristics of stool.
- Monitor fluid and record fluid losses.
- Administer and document electrolyte replacement therapy; watch for signs of electrolyte imbalances, including arrhythmias.
- Monitor and record skin color, turgor, and temperature; level of consciousness; and body temperature.
- Assess and document complaints of pain.
- Be especially alert for vomiting and sudden and severe abdominal pain, guarding, rigidity, or distention; report such symptoms to the doctor immediately.
- Administer appropriate analgesics, as ordered.
- Administer anti-inflammatory medications, as ordered, and document their therapeutic and adverse effects.

Patient teaching

- Explain the disorder to the patient, and reassure her that irritable bowel syndrome can be relieved. Point out, however, that the condition is chronic with no known cure.
- Help the patient understand ordered diagnostic tests. Review all pretest guidelines. Explain that diagnostic tests cannot specifically diagnose irritable bowel syndrome but can rule out other disorders.
- Review the patient's dietary plan; then suggest ways to implement it. Help her schedule meals; the GI tract works best if meals are regular. Show her how to record symptoms and food intake, noting which foods trigger symptoms. Advise her to eat slowly to prevent swallowing air, which causes bloating, and to increase dietary fiber.
- Encourage the patient to drink eight to ten 8-oz glasses of fluids daily to help regulate the consistency

of her stools and promote balanced hydration. Caution her to avoid troublesome beverages, such as carbonated or caffeinated drinks, fruit juices, and alcohol.

■ Discuss the proper use of prescribed drugs, reviewing their desired effects and possible adverse effects.

■ Help the patient implement lifestyle changes to reduce stress. Encourage her to schedule more time for rest and relaxation. Teach her relaxation techniques, such as guided imagery or deep-breathing exercises, and advise her to perform them regularly. If appropriate, suggest professional counseling for stress management.

■ Remind the patient that regular exercise relieves stress and promotes regular bowel function; even a 30-minute walk each day is helpful.

■ Discourage smoking. Warn a smoker that this habit can aggravate her symptoms by altering bowel motility.

■ Explain the need for regular physical examinations. For patients over age 40, emphasize colorectal cancer screening, including annual proctosigmoidoscopy and rectal examinations.

EVALUATION

Evaluation of patient outcomes determines the success of collaborative management. For the patient with irritable bowel syndrome, evaluation focuses on improved elimination and nutrition, pain relief, and adequate knowledge.

Mouth cancer

Cancer of the oral cavity and pharynx is the fourth leading cause of death in African-American men between the ages of 35 and 54. It continues to rise in the nonwhite population.

CAUSES

The combined overuse of tobacco and alcohol is thought to be the primary cause of oral carcinomas, through their destructive effect on the oral mucosa. Other causes include tobacco, alcohol, smokeless tobacco and the use of snuff. Poor nutritional status, family history, poor oral hygiene, low-dose ionizing radiation of the head or neck, occupational exposure to carcinogens, and pollution have also been linked as causes.

Basal cell carcinomas are primarily the result of exposure to sunlight. They occur mainly on the lips and resemble a painless raised scab which evolves into a characteristic ulcer with a pearly border. Generally basal cell carcinomas do not metastasize.

Squamous cell carcinomas account for 90% of oral cancers in the United States. They are slow growing and arise from the lining of the mouth. The patient may complain of a sore or lesion, trouble wearing dentures, mild irritation of the tongue, sore throat, loose teeth, or pain. The tumor may metastasize to the cervical lymph nodes.

Kaposi's sarcoma is a painless red-purple oral plaque that changes to nodular form and is associated with acquired immunodeficiency syndrome.

DIAGNOSIS AND TREATMENT

Evaluating the lesion by biopsy, X-ray of the skull, and computed tomography may help determine if the tumor has spread to other adjacent structures. Other studies include endoscopy by bronchoscopy, esophagoscopy, laryngoscopy, or a combination of the procedures.

Treatment depends on the extent of the cancer and metastasis. Surgery may be required to excise the tumor. If the surgery is extensive, the patient may require tracheostomy due to swelling and increased secretions caused by the procedure. Other treatments may be used alone, in conjunction with the surgery, or together to treat the cancer and include options of radiation and chemotherapy.

COLLABORATIVE MANAGEMENT

Care of the patient with mouth cancer focuses on reducing pain, improving nutritional status, and preparing him for surgery, if necessary.

ASSESSMENT

Assessment includes evaluating oral hygiene of the patient, inspecting the oral cavity, determining oral irritations (such as from dentures) and past medical history. Remember to consider contributing causes and factors. Look for:

■ hemoptysis, which may indicate ulcerative lesion

■ changes in past and current appetite that may affect his nutritional state

■ difficulty chewing or swallowing; speech alterations

■ changes in weight or eating habits

■ lesions, evidence of pain, or restriction of movement in the oral cavity

■ on palpation, altered cervical lymph nodes

■ lesions affecting the patient's psychological and body image.

NURSING DIAGNOSES AND COLLABORATIVE PROBLEMS

Based on the following nursing diagnoses, you'll establish patient outcomes.

Ineffective breathing pattern related to obstruction by tumor, edema, or secretions. The patient will:

- maintain patent airway
- exhibit respiratory rate and character within acceptable parameters.

Altered nutritional status related to altered mucous membrane. The patient will:

- maintain adequate intake of nutrients
- show no weight loss.

Pain related to oral lesions. The patient will:

- report a decrease in pain
- employ measures to alleviate pain.

Anxiety related to diagnosis of cancer. The patient will:

- verbalize feelings and concerns
- demonstrate positive coping mechanisms.

Knowledge deficit related to disease, treatment, and care. The patient will:

- verbalize information about disease
- state measures to cope with disease and treatments.

PLANNING AND IMPLEMENTATION

These measures help the patient with mouth cancer:

- Explain all procedures and treatments to the patient; provide anticipatory teaching and support, especially if he is to receive a tracheostomy.
- Establish alternate communication techniques if the patient is to receive a tracheostomy.
- Suction the patient's airway as needed.
- Suction the tracheostomy and perform adequate pulmonary hygiene as needed.
- Elevate the head of his bed to decrease edema and assist with drainage.
- Assess the effects of medications to decrease oral secretions.
- Monitor the patient's intake and output and weigh him daily.
- Assess bowel sounds and bowel movements.
- Encourage the use of supplements as ordered; consult with the dietitian and assist the patient with food choices.
- Begin nutritional support as ordered, including oral supplements and enteral or parenteral nutrition.
- Review laboratory studies and evaluate supportive methods of nutrition (total parenteral nutrition [TPN], I.V., enteral feedings, oral feedings).
- Give analgesics as ordered and monitor their effects.
- Encourage the patient to express his feelings, and refer him to support groups as indicated.

Patient teaching

- Review medications the patient is taking and ensure that patient and family members are aware of doses, adverse effects, and when to contact the doctor.
- Teach the patient and family member or friend about the disease process.
- Review tracheostomy care, TPN, and enteral feedings as applicable.
- Refer patient to a support group and the American Cancer Society.

EVALUATION

Evaluation of patient outcomes determines the success of collaborative management. For the patient with mouth cancer, evaluation focuses on effective breathing, adequate nutrition, relief of anxiety, and adequate knowledge.

Pancreatic cancer

Pancreatic cancer is the fourth most lethal of all cancers. It occurs most commonly among blacks, particularly in men between ages 35 and 70. Incidence of pancreatic cancer is highest in Israel, the United States, Sweden, and Canada and lowest in Switzerland, Belgium, and Italy. The prognosis is poor: Most patients die within a year of diagnosis.

CAUSES

Evidence suggests that pancreatic cancer is linked to inhalation or absorption of carcinogens that are then excreted by the pancreas. Examples of such carcinogens include:

- cigarette smoke (pancreatic cancer is three to four times more common among smokers)
- excessive fat and protein (a diet high in fat and protein induces chronic hyperplasia of the pancreas, with increased turnover of cells)
- food additives
- industrial chemicals, such as beta-naphthalene, benzidine, and urea.

Other possible predisposing factors include chronic pancreatitis, diabetes mellitus, and chronic alcohol abuse.

Tumors of the pancreas are almost always adenocarcinomas. They usually arise (67% of the time) in the head of the pancreas. Tumors in this location commonly obstruct the ampulla of Vater and common bile duct and metastasize directly to the duodenum. Adhesions anchor the tumor to the spine, stomach, and intestines.

Less commonly, tumors arise in the body and tail of the pancreas. When this happens, large nodular masses become fixed to retropancreatic tissues and the spine. The spleen, left kidney, suprarenal gland, and diaphragm are directly invaded, and the celiac plexus becomes involved, resulting in splenic vein thrombosis and spleen infarction. Among the rarest of pancreatic tumors are islet cell tumors.

In pancreatic cancer, two main tissue types form fibrotic nodes. Cylinder cells arise in ducts and degenerate into cysts, and large, fatty, granular cells arise in parenchyma.

Relatively uncommon, islet cell tumors (insulinomas) may be benign or malignant. They produce symptoms in three stages, and despite treatment, the prognosis is unfavorable.

Stage 1: Slight hypoglycemia produces fatigue, restlessness, malaise, and excessive weight gain.

Stage 2: Compensatory secretion of epinephrine produces characteristic pallor, clamminess, perspiration, palpitations, finger tremors, hunger, decreased temperature, and increased pulse rate and blood pressure.

Stage 3: Severe hypoglycemia results in ataxia, clouded sensorium, diplopia, and episodes of violence and hysteria.

Related to the progression of the disease, complications may include malabsorption of nutrients, insulin-dependent diabetes, liver and GI problems, and mental status changes.

DIAGNOSIS AND TREATMENT

Several tests may be ordered to help diagnose the disease and determine its extent. Percutaneous fine-needle aspiration biopsy of the pancreas may detect tumor cells, and laparotomy with a biopsy is definitive. However, a biopsy may miss relatively small or deep-seated cancerous tissue or create a pancreatic fistula. Retroperitoneal insufflation, cholangiography, scintigraphy and, particularly, barium swallow (to locate the neoplasm and detect changes in the duodenum or stomach relating to cancer of the head of the pancreas) also can be performed to detect the disease.

Ultrasonography helps identify a mass, but not its histology. A computed tomography scan shows greater detail of the mass than ultrasonography. A magnetic resonance imaging scan discloses the tumor's location and size in great detail.

Angiography reveals the tumor's vascular supply. Endoscopic retrograde cholangiopancreatography allows visualization, instillation of contrast medium, and specimen biopsy. A secretin test reveals the absence of pancreatic enzymes and suggests pancreatic duct obstruction and tumors of the body and tail.

Other laboratory tests that support the diagnosis include:
- serum bilirubin (increased)
- serum amylase-lipase (occasionally increased)
- prothrombin time (prolonged)
- aspartate aminotransferase and alanine aminotransferase (elevated enzyme levels when liver cell necrosis is present)
- alkaline phosphatase (markedly elevated, with biliary obstruction)
- plasma insulin immunoassay (shows measurable serum insulin in the presence of islet cell tumors)
- hemoglobin and hematocrit (may show mild anemia)
- fasting blood glucose (may indicate hypoglycemia or hyperglycemia)
- stool studies (may show occult blood if ulceration in the GI tract or ampulla of Vater has occurred)
- specific tumor markers for pancreatic cancer, including carcinoembryonic antigen, pancreatic oncofetal antigen, alpha-fetoprotein, and serum immunoreactive elastase I (all levels elevated in the presence of cancer).

Because pancreatic cancer may metastasize widely before it's diagnosed, treatment seldom cures the disease. Treatment consists of surgery and, possibly, chemotherapy and radiation therapy.

Some surgical procedures raise the survival rate slightly. Total pancreatectomy may increase survival time by resecting a localized tumor or by controlling postoperative gastric ulceration. Cholecystojejunostomy, choledochoduodenostomy, and choledochojejunostomy have partially replaced radical resection. These procedures bypass the obstructing common bile duct extensions, easing jaundice and pruritus. If radical resection isn't indicated and duodenal obstruction is expected to develop later, a gastrojejunostomy is performed.

Whipple's operation, or radical pancreaticoduodenectomy (seldom used), has a high mortality but can obtain wide lymphatic clearance except with tumors located near the portal vein, superior mesenteric vein and artery, and celiac axis.

Although pancreatic cancer usually responds poorly to chemotherapy, recent studies using combinations of fluorouracil, streptomycin, mitomycin, and doxorubicin show a trend toward longer survival time.

Radiation therapy usually doesn't increase long-term survival, although it may prolong life by 6 to 11 months when used as an adjunct to fluorouracil chemotherapy. It also can ease the pain associated with nonresectable tumors.

Medications used in pancreatic cancer include:
- antibiotics to prevent infection and relieve symptoms
- anticholinergics, particularly propantheline, to decrease GI tract spasm and motility and reduce pain and secretions
- antacids to decrease secretion of pancreatic enzymes and suppress peptic activity, thus reducing stress-induced damage to gastric mucosa
- diuretics to mobilize extracellular fluid from ascites
- insulin to provide an adequate exogenous insulin supply after pancreatic resection

■ opioid analgesics to relieve pain (used only after other analgesics fail because morphine, meperidine, and codeine can lead to biliary tract spasm and increase common bile duct pressure)

■ pancreatic enzymes to assist with digestion of proteins, carbohydrates, and fats when pancreatic juices are insufficient because of surgery or obstruction.

Treatment of islet cell tumors consists of enucleation of tumor (if benign) and chemotherapy with streptozocin and fluorouracil and resection to include pancreatic tissue (if malignant). Most islet cell tumors metastasize to the liver only. Some metastasize to the bone, brain, and lungs. Death results from hypoglycemic reactions and widespread metastasis.

COLLABORATIVE MANAGEMENT

Care of the patient with pancreatic cancer focuses on providing adequate nutrition and promoting physical and emotional comfort.

ASSESSMENT

A patient who seeks treatment early in the disease usually reports a dull, intermittent epigastric pain. Later, he may report continuous pain that radiates to the right upper quadrant or dorsolumbar area. He may describe it as colicky, dull, or vague and unrelated to posture or activity, or he may state that meals seem to aggravate the epigastric pain. He also may report anorexia, nausea, vomiting, and a rapid, profound weight loss.

Also look for:

■ jaundice and a palpable, well-defined, large mass in the subumbilical or left hypochondrial region, indicating that the tail of the pancreas is involved

■ a mass that may adhere to the large vessels or the vertebral column and produce a pulsation

■ abdominal bruit on auscultation of the left hypochondrium, if the tumor has involved or compressed the splenic artery.

NURSING DIAGNOSES AND COLLABORATIVE PROBLEMS

Based on the following nursing diagnoses, you'll establish patient outcomes.

Altered nutrition: Less than body requirements, related to adverse GI signs and symptoms. The patient will:

■ obtain relief from GI signs and symptoms with therapy

■ be able to ingest a nutritionally balanced diet daily

■ regain and maintain weight within normal limits.

Anticipatory grieving related to poor prognosis. The patient will:

■ acknowledge feelings about his diagnosis and prognosis

■ seek support from family, friends, and support groups

■ use healthy coping mechanisms to deal with the threat of death.

Risk for complications related to extensive effects of the disease. The patient will:

■ remain safe

■ experience no complications.

Pain related to pancreatic dysfunction. The patient will:

■ express feelings of comfort following analgesic administration

■ use diversionary activities to help minimize pain.

PLANNING AND IMPLEMENTATION

These measures help the patient with pancreatic cancer:

■ If your patient loses weight, replace nutrients by mouth or through an I.V. line or nasogastric (NG) tube. If he gains weight from ascites, impose dietary restrictions such as a low-sodium diet, as ordered.

■ Maintain a 2,500-calorie diet by serving small, frequent meals. Consult the dietitian to ensure proper nutrition, and make mealtimes as pleasant as possible. Administer an oral pancreatic enzyme at mealtimes, if needed. As ordered, give an antacid to prevent stress ulcers.

■ To prevent constipation, administer laxatives, stool softeners, and cathartics, as ordered. Also, modify the patient's diet and increase his fluid intake. To increase GI motility, position him properly during and after meals and assist him with walking.

■ Before surgery, make sure the patient is medically stable, particularly regarding nutrition. This may take 4 to 5 days. If he can't tolerate oral feedings, provide total parenteral nutrition and I.V. fat emulsions to correct deficiencies and maintain a positive nitrogen balance.

■ Give the patient glucose or an antidiabetic agent (such as tolbutamide), as ordered.

■ Ease discomfort from pyloric obstruction with an NG tube.

■ Watch for signs of hypoglycemia or hyperglycemia. Monitor the patient's blood glucose, urine glucose, and acetone levels and his response to treatment.

■ Administer blood transfusions (to combat anemia), vitamin K (to overcome prothrombin deficiency), antibiotics (to prevent postoperative complications), and gastric lavage (to maintain gastric decompression), as ordered.

■ If the patient is receiving chemotherapy, monitor his response and symptomatically treat toxic drug effects.

■ To prevent thrombosis, apply antiembolism stockings and assist with range of motion (ROM) exercises. If thrombosis occurs, elevate the patient's legs and apply moist heat to the thrombus site. Give an anticoagulant, as ordered, to prevent further clot formation and pulmonary embolus.

■ Provide scrupulous skin care to prevent pruritus and necrosis, and keep the patient's skin clean and dry. If he develops overwhelming pruritus, you can prevent excoriation by clipping his nails and having him wear light cotton gloves.

■ To control active bleeding, promote gastric vasoconstriction with medication and with iced saline lavage through an NG tube or a duodenal tube. Replace any lost fluids.

■ Administer analgesics for pain and antibiotics and antipyretics for fever, as ordered. Monitor the patient's pain level and response to administered analgesics.

■ Assess the patient's fluid balance, abdominal girth, metabolic state, and weight daily.

■ Watch for signs of upper GI bleeding. Test stools and emesis for blood, and maintain a flow sheet of frequent hemoglobin and hematocrit determinations.

■ Monitor and document the patient's degree of jaundice daily.

■ Ensure adequate rest and sleep (with a sedative, if necessary). Assist with ROM and isometric exercises, as appropriate.

■ Throughout therapy, answer the patient's questions and tell him what to expect from surgery and other therapies. Listen to his fears and concerns, and stay with him during periods of severe stress and anxiety.

■ Encourage the patient to identify and perform actions and care measures that will promote his comfort and relaxation.

■ Whenever possible, include the patient and family members in care decisions.

Patient teaching

■ Describe expected postoperative procedures and the adverse effects of radiation therapy and chemotherapy.

■ If appropriate, provide information on diabetes.

■ Help the patient and family members cope with the impending reality of death.

■ Refer the patient to resource and support services, such as the social service department, local home health care agencies, hospices, and the American Cancer Society.

■ Encourage as normal a routine as possible, explaining that it will help foster feelings of independence and control.

EVALUATION

Evaluation of patient outcomes determines the success of collaborative management. For the patient with pancreatic cancer, evaluation focuses on ade-

quate nutrition, reduced risk of complications, emotional adjustment, and adequate knowledge.

Pancreatitis

Inflammation of the pancreas, or pancreatitis, occurs in acute and chronic forms and may be caused by edema, necrosis, or hemorrhage. In men, the disorder is commonly associated with alcoholism, trauma, or peptic ulcer; in women, with biliary tract disease. The prognosis is good when pancreatitis follows biliary tract disease but poor when it follows alcoholism. Mortality reaches 60% when pancreatitis is associated with necrosis or hemorrhage.

CAUSES

The most common causes of pancreatitis are biliary tract disease and alcoholism, but the disorder can also result from abnormal organ structure, metabolic or endocrine disorders (such as hyperlipidemia or hyperparathyroidism), pancreatic cysts or tumors, penetrating peptic ulcers, or trauma (blunt or iatrogenic). This disorder also can develop after the use of certain drugs, such as glucocorticoids, sulfonamides, thiazides, and oral contraceptives.

Pancreatitis may be a complication of renal failure, kidney transplantation, open-heart surgery, and endoscopic retrograde cholangiopancreatography (ERCP). Heredity may be a predisposing factor and, in some patients, emotional or neurogenic factors are involved.

Regardless of the cause, pancreatitis involves autodigestion: The enzymes normally excreted by the pancreas digest pancreatic tissue. If pancreatitis damages the islets of Langerhans, diabetes mellitus may follow. Fulminant pancreatitis causes massive hemorrhage and total destruction of the pancreas, resulting in diabetic acidosis, shock, or coma. Respiratory complications include adult respiratory distress syndrome, atelectasis, pleural effusion, and pneumonia. Proximity of the inflamed pancreas to the bowel may cause paralytic ileus. Other complications include GI bleeding, pancreatic abscess, pseudocysts and, rarely, cancer.

DIAGNOSIS AND TREATMENT

The following findings confirm acute pancreatitis:

■ Serum amylase levels above 180 Somogyi U/dl (130 U/L). This is the diagnostic hallmark that confirms acute pancreatitis. Characteristically, serum amylase reaches peak levels in 24 hours after onset of pancreatitis, then returns to normal within 48 to 72 hours despite continued symptoms.

- Urinary amylase level above 80 amylase U/hour (17 U/hour). Because urine amylase is reported in various units of measurement, values differ among laboratories. Check your hospital's normal range for urine amylase. Urine amylase levels remain elevated longer than serum amylase levels.
- Serum lipase levels above 80 U/L. Serum lipase levels along with urine amylase levels remain elevated longer than serum amylase levels.

Supportive laboratory studies include elevated white blood cell count and serum bilirubin level. In many patients, hypocalcemia occurs and appears to be associated with the severity of the disease. Blood and urine glucose tests may reveal transient glycosuria and hyperglycemia. In chronic pancreatitis, significant laboratory findings include elevations in serum alkaline phosphatase, amylase, and bilirubin levels. Serum glucose levels may be transiently elevated. Stools contain elevated lipid and trypsin levels.

Abdominal and chest X-rays differentiate pancreatitis from other diseases that cause similar symptoms and detect pleural effusions. Computed tomography scan and ultrasonography reveal an increased pancreatic diameter; these tests also identify pancreatic cysts and pseudocysts. ERCP shows the anatomy of the pancreas, identifies ductal system abnormalities (such as calcification or strictures), and differentiates pancreatitis from other disorders such as pancreatic cancer.

Treatment goals are to maintain circulation and fluid volume, relieve pain, and decrease pancreatic secretions. Emergency treatment for shock (the most common cause of death in early stage pancreatitis) consists of vigorous I.V. replacement of electrolytes and proteins. Metabolic acidosis, secondary to hypovolemia, and impaired cellular perfusion require vigorous fluid volume replacement. Blood transfusions may be needed if shock occurs. Food and fluids are withheld to allow the pancreas to rest and to reduce pancreatic enzyme secretion.

In acute pancreatitis, nasogastric (NG) tube suctioning is usually required to decrease gastric distention and suppress pancreatic secretions. Prescribed medications may include:

- meperidine to relieve abdominal pain (this drug causes less spasm at the ampulla of Vater than opiates such as morphine)
- antacids to neutralize gastric secretions
- histamine-2 receptor antagonists, such as cimetidine or ranitidine, to decrease hydrochloric acid production
- antibiotics, such as clindamycin or gentamicin, to treat bacterial infections
- anticholinergics to reduce vagal stimulation, decrease GI motility, and inhibit pancreatic enzyme secretion

- insulin to correct hyperglycemia, if present.

Once the crisis begins to resolve, oral low-fat, low-protein foods are gradually introduced. Alcohol and caffeine are eliminated from the diet. If the crisis occurred during treatment with glucocorticoids, oral contraceptives, or thiazide diuretics, these drugs are discontinued.

Surgery usually isn't indicated. However, with such complications as pancreatic abscess or pseudocyst, surgical drainage may be necessary. If biliary tract obstruction causes acute pancreatitis, a laparotomy may be required.

For chronic pancreatitis, treatment depends on the cause. Nonsurgical measures are appropriate if the patient is an unsuitable candidate or refuses surgery. Measures to prevent and relieve abdominal pain are similar to those used in acute pancreatitis. Meperidine usually is the drug of choice; however, pentazocine is also effective. Treatment for diabetes mellitus may include dietary modification, insulin replacement, or antidiabetic agents. Malabsorption and steatorrhea are treated with pancreatic enzyme replacement.

Surgery relieves abdominal pain, restores pancreatic drainage, and reduces the frequency of acute pancreatic attacks. Surgical drainage is required for an abscess or pseudocyst. If biliary tract disease is the underlying cause, cholecystectomy or choledochotomy is performed. A sphincterotomy is indicated to enlarge a pancreatic sphincter that has become fibrotic. To relieve obstruction and allow drainage of pancreatic secretions, pancreaticojejunostomy (anastomosis of the jejunum with the opened pancreatic duct) may be required.

COLLABORATIVE MANAGEMENT

Care of the patient with pancreatitis focuses on providing fluids, relieving pain, and monitoring for shock.

ASSESSMENT

The patient commonly describes intense epigastric pain centered close to the umbilicus and radiating to the back, between the 10th thoracic and 6th lumbar vertebrae. He typically reports that this pain is aggravated by eating fatty foods, consuming alcohol, or lying in a recumbent position. He may also complain of weight loss, with nausea and vomiting.

Investigation may uncover predisposing factors, such as alcoholism, biliary tract disease, or pancreatic disease. Other medical problems, such as peptic ulcer disease or hyperlipidemia, may be discovered. Look for:

- decreased blood pressure, tachycardia, and fever (all indicating respiratory complications), along with dyspnea or orthopnea

> **DISCHARGE READY** > **After pancreatitis**

After treatment for pancreatitis, the patient will meet the following criteria before discharge:

- vital signs within normal limits for him
- serum glucose, urine glucose, and ketone levels returning to normal
- serum electrolyte levels returning to normal
- pain relief
- adequate nutritional intake
- verbalized understanding of disease process and need for lifestyle modifications
- no evidence of pulmonary or other complications.

- changes in behavior and sensorium; possibly related to alcohol withdrawal or indicating hypoxia or impending shock
- abdominal region showing generalized jaundice, Cullen's sign (bluish periumbilical discoloration), and Turner's sign (bluish flank discoloration)
- evidence of steatorrhea in stools, a sign of chronic pancreatitis
- tenderness, rigidity, and guarding during abdominal palpation
- a dull sound while percussing, possibly indicating pancreatic ascites
- absent or decreased bowel sounds on abdominal auscultation, suggesting paralytic ileus.

NURSING DIAGNOSES AND COLLABORATIVE PROBLEMS

Based on the following nursing diagnoses, you'll establish patient outcomes.

Altered nutrition: Less than body requirements, related to malabsorption caused by pancreatic enzyme deficiency. The patient will:
- comply with pancreatic enzyme replacement therapy
- exhibit no signs or symptoms of malnutrition
- regain and maintain normal weight.

Altered protection related to loss of ability to control blood glucose levels naturally, caused by alpha- and beta-cell damage. The patient will:
- communicate his understanding of early signs and symptoms of hypoglycemia and hyperglycemia
- comply with the ordered treatment to control blood glucose levels
- regain and maintain normal serum blood glucose and not have ketones in urine.

Pain related to inflammatory process. The patient will:

- express feelings of comfort following analgesic administration
- avoid eating foods or engaging in activities that precipitate or increase pain
- develop no chronic pain.

PLANNING AND IMPLEMENTATION

These measures help the patient with pancreatitis:
- Assess the patient's level of pain. Evaluate his response to administered analgesics, and monitor for adverse reactions.
- Administer meperidine or other analgesics, as ordered, and document drug effectiveness.
- Restrict the patient to bed rest, and provide a quiet and restful environment.
- Assess pulmonary status at least every 4 hours to detect early signs of respiratory complications.
- Evaluate the patient's present nutritional status and metabolic requirements.
- Keep water and other beverages at the bedside, and encourage the patient to drink plenty of fluids.
- Maintain the NG tube for drainage or suctioning if ordered.
- Provide I.V. fluids and parenteral nutrition, as ordered. As soon as the patient can tolerate it, provide a diet high in carbohydrates, low in proteins, and low in fat.
- Monitor fluid and electrolyte balance, and report any abnormalities. Maintain an accurate record of intake and output.
- Weigh the patient daily and record his weight.
- Monitor serum glucose levels, and administer insulin as ordered.
- Don't confuse thirst due to hyperglycemia (indicated by serum glucose levels up to 350 mg/dl and glucose and acetone in the urine) with dry mouth due to NG intubation and anticholinergics.
- In case of hypocalcemia, keep airway and suction apparatus handy and pad the side rails of the bed.
- Watch for signs and symptoms of calcium deficiency: tetany, cramps, carpopedal spasm, and seizures.
- Place the patient in a comfortable position that also allows maximal chest expansion, such as Fowler's position.
- Allow the patient to express feelings of anger, depression, and sadness related to his condition, and help him cope with these feelings. Encourage use of appropriate physical outlets, such as pounding a punching bag or throwing pillows.
- Counsel the patient to contact a self-help group such as Alcoholics Anonymous, if needed.

Patient teaching

- Emphasize the importance of avoiding factors that precipitate acute pancreatitis, especially alcohol.

- Refer the patient and family members to the dietitian. Stress the need for a diet high in carbohydrates and low in protein and fats. Caution the patient to avoid caffeinated beverages and irritating foods.
- Point out the need to comply with pancreatic enzyme replacement therapy. Tell the patient to take the enzymes with meals or snacks to help digest food and to promote fat and protein absorption. Advise him to watch for and report any of the following signs and symptoms: fatty, frothy, foul-smelling stools; abdominal distention; cramping; and skin excoriation.
- If the patient has chronic pain, teach a family member how to give I.M. injections as ordered.

EVALUATION

Evaluation of patient outcomes determines the success of collaborative management. For the patient with pancreatitis, evaluation focuses on pain relief, adequate nutrition, improved protection (abstinence), and adequate knowledge. (See *After pancreatitis.*)

Peptic ulcer

Occurring as circumscribed lesions in the mucosal membrane, peptic ulcers can develop in the lower esophagus, stomach, duodenum, or jejunum. The major forms are duodenal ulcer and gastric ulcer; both are chronic conditions resulting from contact of the mucosa with gastric juice (especially hydrochloric acid and pepsin).

Duodenal ulcers, which account for about 80% of peptic ulcers, affect the proximal part of the small intestine, with a pattern of remissions and exacerbations; 5% to 10% of patients need surgery. Duodenal ulcers occur most commonly in men between ages 20 and 50.

Gastric ulcers, which affect the stomach mucosa, are most common in middle-aged and older men, especially among the poor and malnourished, and in chronic users of aspirin or alcohol.

CAUSES

Recent findings indicate that bacterial infection with *Helicobacter pylori* is a leading cause of peptic ulcer disease. Two other leading causes include the use of nonsteroidal anti-inflammatory drugs (NSAIDs) and pathologic hypersecretory states such as Zollinger-Ellison syndrome. (See *Causes of peptic ulcer.*)

Peptic ulcers arise from the erosion of the upper GI tract and mucosa by gastric acid and pepsin. Autodigestion of mucosal tissue and ulceration are associated with an increase in acidity of stomach juices or an increased sensitivity of the mucosal surface to erosion.

Causes of peptic ulcer

Although more research is needed to unveil the mechanisms of ulcer formation, several causative factors are known.

- Helicobacter pylori. How the bacterium *H. pylori* produces an ulcer isn't clear. Acid seems to be mainly a contributor to the consequences of the bacterial infection rather than the dominant cause.
- *Drug therapy.* Salicylates and other nonsteroidal anti-inflammatory drugs (NSAIDs), reserpine, or caffeine may erode the mucosal lining. NSAIDs may cause a gastric ulcer by inhibiting prostaglandins (the fatty acids)—particularly the E-series prostaglandins. These substances, present in large quantities in the gastric mucosa, inhibit injury by stimulating secretion of gastric mucus and gastric and duodenal mucosal bicarbonate (a neutralizing agent). They also promote gastric mucosal blood flow, maintain the integrity of the gastric mucosal barrier, and help renew the epithelium after a mucosal injury.
- *Certain illnesses.* Pancreatitis, hepatic disease, Crohn's disease, preexisting gastritis, and Zollinger-Ellison syndrome are associated with ulcer development. In Zollinger-Ellison syndrome, for example, gastrinomas (commonly found in the pancreas) stimulate gastric acid secretion. This large volume of acid eventually erodes the gastric mucosa and contributes to ulcer formation.
- *Blood type.* For unknown reasons, gastric ulcers commonly strike people with type A blood. Duodenal ulcers tend to afflict people with type O blood, perhaps because they don't secrete blood group antigens (mucopolysaccharides, which may serve to protect the mucosa) in their saliva and other body fluids.
- *Genetic factors.* Duodenal ulcers are about three times more common in first-degree relatives of duodenal ulcer patients than in the general population.
- *Exposure to irritants.* Like certain other drugs, alcohol inhibits prostaglandin secretion, triggering a mechanism much like the one produced by NSAIDs. Cigarette smoking also appears to encourage ulcer formation by inhibiting pancreatic secretion of bicarbonate. It also may accelerate the emptying of gastric acid into the duodenum and promote mucosal breakdown.
- *Trauma.* Critical illness, shock, or severe tissue injury from extensive burns or intracranial surgery may lead to a stress ulcer.
- *Psychogenic factors.* Emotional stress may stimulate long-term overproduction of gastric secretions that aid in ulcer production by eroding stomach, duodenal, and esophageal tissue.
- *Normal aging.* The pyloric sphincter may wear down in the course of aging, which permits the reflux of bile into the stomach. This appears to be a common contributor to the development of gastric ulcers in older people.

DIAGNOSIS AND TREATMENT

Barium swallow or upper GI and small-bowel series is the initial test for a patient whose symptoms are not severe. Upper GI endoscopy, or esophagogastroduodenoscopy, confirms the presence of an ulcer and permits biopsy and cytologic studies to rule out *H. pylori* or cancer. Endoscopy is the major diagnostic test for peptic ulcers.

Upper GI tract X-rays reveal abnormalities in the mucosa. Laboratory analysis may detect occult blood in stools. Serologic testing may disclose clinical signs of infection, such as an elevated white blood cell count. Gastric secretory studies show hyperchlorhydria.

Carbon 13 (^{13}C) urea breath test results reflect activity of *H. pylori*. (*H. pylori* contains the enzyme urease, which breaks down orally administered urea containing the radioisotope ^{13}C before it's absorbed systemically. Low levels of ^{13}C in exhaled breath therefore point to *H. pylori* infection.)

Medical management is essentially symptomatic, emphasizing drug therapy, physical rest, dietary changes, and stress reduction. For patients with severe symptoms or complications, surgery may be required.

Drug therapy aims to eradicate *H. pylori*, reduce gastric secretions, protect the mucosa from further damage, and relieve pain. Medications may include:
- bismuth and two other antimicrobial agents, usually tetracycline or amoxicillin and metronidazole
- antacids to reduce gastric acidity
- histamine-2 receptor antagonists, such as cimetidine or ranitidine, to reduce gastric secretion for a short period (up to 8 weeks)
- coating agents, such as sucralfate, for duodenal ulcers; sucralfate forms complexes with proteins at the base of an ulcer, making a protective coat that prevents further digestive action of acid and pepsin
- sedatives and tranquilizers, such as chlordiazepoxide and phenobarbital, for patients with gastric ulcers
- anticholinergics, such as propantheline, to inhibit the vagus nerve effect on the parietal cells and to reduce gastrin production and excessive gastric activity in duodenal ulcers. (These drugs are usually contraindicated in gastric ulcers because they prolong gastric emptying and can aggravate the ulcer.)

Standard therapy also includes rest and decreased activity to help reduce gastric secretions. Diet therapy may consist of eating six small meals daily (or small hourly meals). Some doctors prescribe milk and cream or a bland diet, but the value of such treatments is controversial.

If GI bleeding occurs, emergency treatment begins with passage of a nasogastric tube to allow for iced saline lavage, possibly containing norepinephrine. Gastroscopy allows visualization of the bleeding site and coagulation by laser or cautery to control bleeding. This therapy allows surgery to be postponed until the patient's condition stabilizes.

Surgery is indicated for perforation, unresponsiveness to conservative treatment, suspected cancer, and other complications. The type of surgery chosen for peptic ulcers depends on the location and the extent of the disorder. Choices include bilateral vagotomy, pyloroplasty, and gastrectomy.

COLLABORATIVE MANAGEMENT

Care of the patient with a peptic ulcer focuses on promoting dietary changes and managing symptoms before and after surgery.

ASSESSMENT

The patient typically describes exacerbation and remission of his symptoms, with remissions lasting longer than exacerbations. The patient's history may reveal possible causes or predisposing factors, such as smoking, use of aspirin or other medications, or associated disorders. Look for:
- reports of recent loss of weight or appetite (with peptic ulcer)
- pain in the left epigastrium, described as heartburn or indigestion (often signaling the start of an attack), and a feeling of fullness or distention; in a gastric ulcer, eating worsens the pain; in a duodenal ulcer, food often relieves the pain
- in a gastric ulcer, pain that seldom wakes the patient; in a duodenal ulcer, night pain that often wakes the patient
- in a duodenal ulcer, pain that occurs 90 minutes to 3 hours after eating (whenever the stomach is empty); recent weight gain; vomiting and other digestive disturbances (rare)
- pallor if the patient is anemic from blood loss
- epigastric tenderness in the midline and midway between the umbilicus and the xiphoid process
- hyperactive bowel sounds.

NURSING DIAGNOSES AND COLLABORATIVE PROBLEMS

Based on the following nursing diagnoses, you'll establish patient outcomes.

Altered nutrition: Less than body requirements, related to adverse GI effects. The patient will:
- regain and maintain weight
- consume and tolerate a well-balanced daily diet
- exhibit no signs or symptoms of nutritional deficiencies.

Knowledge deficit related to peptic ulcer. The patient will:
- express a desire to learn about peptic ulcer disease and his treatment regimen
- obtain information about peptic ulcer disease and treatment from appropriate sources

- communicate an understanding of peptic ulcer disease and his ordered treatment.

Risk for fluid volume deficit related to bleeding. The patient will:
- maintain hemodynamic stability, as evidenced by normal vital signs, equal intake and output, and orientation to time, place, and person
- show no evidence of GI bleeding (stools negative for occult blood)
- maintain normal fluid volume balance.

PLANNING AND IMPLEMENTATION
These measures help the patient with peptic ulcer disease:
- Assess the patient's nutritional status and the effectiveness of measures used to maintain it.
- Provide six small meals a day or small hourly meals, as ordered. Tell the patient to eat slowly, chew thoroughly, and have small snacks between meals. Aim for a relaxed and comfortable atmosphere during meals.
- Schedule care so that the patient gets plenty of rest.
- Support the patient emotionally and offer reassurance.
- Administer prescribed medications. Monitor their effectiveness, and watch for adverse reactions.
- Monitor vital signs and hemodynamic status as ordered; note any changes.
- Weigh the patient daily; monitor intake and output.
- Assess skin turgor and mucous membranes for signs of dehydration.
- Check stools for occult blood.
- Continuously monitor the patient for complications: hemorrhage (sudden onset of weakness, fainting, chills, dizziness, thirst, the desire to defecate, and passage of loose, tarry, or even red stools); perforation (acute onset of epigastric pain, followed by lessening of the pain and the onset of a rigid abdomen, tachycardia, fever, or rebound tenderness); obstruction (feeling of fullness or heaviness, copious vomiting of undigested food after meals); and penetration (pain radiating to the back, night distress). If any of the above occurs, notify the doctor immediately.

Patient teaching
- Teach the patient about peptic ulcer disease, and help him recognize its signs and symptoms. Explain scheduled diagnostic tests and ordered therapies. Review symptoms associated with complications, and urge him to notify the doctor if any of these occur. Emphasize the importance of complying with treatment, even after his symptoms disappear.

- Review the proper use of prescribed medications, discussing the desired actions and possible adverse effects of each drug.
- Tell the patient to take antacids 1 hour after meals. If he has cardiac disease or follows a sodium-restricted diet, tell him to take low-sodium antacids. Mention that antacids may affect his bowels (diarrhea with magnesium-containing antacids, constipation with aluminum-containing antacids).
- Warn the patient to avoid aspirin-containing drugs, reserpine, ibuprofen, indomethacin, and phenylbutazone because they irritate the gastric mucosa. For the same reason, advise against too much coffee and alcoholic beverages during exacerbations (moderate alcohol is acceptable during remission).
- Tell the patient to avoid nonprescription medications that contain corticosteroids, aspirin, or other NSAIDs, such as ibuprofen. Explain that these drugs inhibit mucus secretion and leave the GI tract vulnerable to injury from gastric acid. Suggest alternative analgesics such as acetaminophen. Warn against systemic antacids such as sodium bicarbonate because they can cause an acid-base imbalance.
- Encourage the patient to make lifestyle changes. Explain that emotional tension can precipitate an ulcer attack and prolong healing. Help the patient identify anxiety-producing situations, and teach him to perform relaxation techniques such as distraction and meditation.
- If the patient smokes, urge him to stop because smoking stimulates gastric acid secretion. Refer him to a smoking-cessation program.

EVALUATION
Evaluation of patient outcomes determines the success of collaborative management. For the patient with a peptic ulcer, evaluation focuses on adequate nutrition, maintenance of fluid balance and hemodynamic status, and adequate knowledge.

Peritonitis

Although the GI tract normally contains bacteria, the peritoneum is sterile. In peritonitis, however, bacteria invade the peritoneum.

CAUSES
Generally, an infection in the peritoneum results from inflammation and perforation of the GI tract, allowing bacterial invasion. Usually, this is a result of appendicitis, diverticulitis, peptic ulcer, ulcerative colitis, volvulus, strangulated obstruction, abdominal neoplasm, or a stab wound. Peritonitis may also be caused by chemical inflammation after rupture of a

fallopian tube, ovarian cyst, or the bladder; perforation of a gastric ulcer; or released pancreatic enzymes.

In both bacterial and chemical inflammation, fluid containing protein and electrolytes accumulates in the peritoneal cavity and makes the transparent peritoneum opaque, red, inflamed, and edematous. Because the peritoneal cavity is so resistant to contamination, such infection is commonly localized as an abscess instead of disseminated as a generalized infection.

An acute or chronic disorder, peritonitis is an inflammation of the peritoneum, the membrane that lines the abdominal cavity and covers the visceral organs. The inflammation may be generalized or localized as an abscess. Peritonitis commonly decreases intestinal motility and causes intestinal distention with gas. Mortality is about 10%, with bowel obstruction the usual cause of death.

Peritonitis can lead to abscess formation, septicemia, respiratory compromise, bowel obstruction, and shock.

DIAGNOSIS AND TREATMENT
White blood cell count shows leukocytosis (commonly more than 20,000/µl). Abdominal X-rays reveal edematous and gaseous distention of the small and large bowel. With perforation of a visceral organ, the X-ray shows air in the abdominal cavity. Chest X-ray may reveal elevation of the diaphragm. Paracentesis discloses the nature of the exudate and permits bacterial culture so appropriate antibiotic therapy can be instituted.

Peritonitis requires emergency treatment to combat infection, restore intestinal motility, and replace fluids and electrolytes. Antibiotic therapy must match the infecting organism but usually includes cefoxitin with an aminoglycoside or penicillin G and clindamycin with an aminoglycoside. To decrease peristalsis and prevent perforation, the patient should receive nothing by mouth; instead, he requires supportive fluids and electrolytes parenterally.

Supplementary treatment includes an analgesic such as meperidine, nasogastric (NG) intubation to decompress the bowel, and possible use of a rectal tube to ease the passage of flatus.

Surgery, which is necessary as soon as the patient's condition is stable enough to tolerate it, aims to eliminate the source of infection by evacuating the spilled contents and inserting drains.

The surgical procedure varies with the cause of peritonitis. For example, if appendicitis is the cause, an appendectomy is performed; if the colon is perforated, a colon resection may be performed. Occasionally, abdominocentesis may be necessary to remove accumulated fluid. Irrigation of the abdominal cavity with antibiotic solutions during surgery may be appropriate.

COLLABORATIVE MANAGEMENT
Care of the patient with peritonitis focuses on emergency treatment to stop the infection and stabilize the patient for surgery.

ASSESSMENT
The patient's symptoms depend on the stage of the disorder. In the early phase, look for:
- reports of vague, generalized abdominal pain
- with localized peritonitis, pain over a specific area (usually the site of inflammation)
- with generalized peritonitis, diffuse pain over the abdomen
- during auscultation, bowel sounds that disappear as the inflammation progresses
- abdominal rigidity, and then, if peritonitis spreads throughout the abdomen, general tenderness on palpation; local tenderness, if peritonitis remains in a specific area
- rebound tenderness.
    In the later phase, look for:
- reports of increasingly severe and unremitting abdominal pain that increases with movement and respirations
- pain, occasionally, referred to the shoulder or the thoracic area
- abdominal distention, anorexia, nausea, vomiting, and an inability to pass feces and flatus
- fever, tachycardia (a response to the fever), and hypotension
- shallow breathing and little movement, to minimize pain
- with excessive fluid loss, profuse sweating, cold skin, pallor, abdominal distention, and such signs of dehydration as dry mucous membranes
- acute distress (patient may lie very still in bed, commonly with his knees flexed to try to alleviate abdominal pain).

NURSING DIAGNOSES AND COLLABORATIVE PROBLEMS
Based on the following nursing diagnoses, you'll establish patient outcomes.
    Altered GI tissue perfusion related to inflammatory process. The patient will:
- develop increased GI tissue perfusion as inflammation subsides with treatment
- regain and maintain normal GI function with treatment.
    Risk for fluid volume deficit related to excessive fluid loss into abdomen. The patient will:
- maintain hemodynamic stability, as exhibited by normal vital signs

- have no signs and symptoms of ascites, dehydration, and hypovolemic shock
- maintain normal vascular fluid volume balance.
  Pain related to inflammatory process. The patient will:
- express feelings of comfort after analgesic administration
- comply with antibiotic therapy to alleviate inflammation and pain.

PLANNING AND IMPLEMENTATION

These measures help the patient with peritonitis:
- Provide psychological support, and offer encouragement when appropriate.
- Administer medications, such as analgesics and antibiotics, as ordered, and monitor the patient's reaction.
- Assess fluid volume by checking skin turgor, mucous membranes, urine output, weight, vital signs, amount of NG tube drainage, and amount of I.V. infusion. Record intake and output, including NG tube drainage.
- Maintain parenteral fluid and electrolyte administration, as ordered.
- Counteract mouth and nose dryness due to fever, dehydration, and NG intubation with regular hygiene and lubrication.
- Prepare the patient for surgery, as indicated.
- Monitor him for surgical complications if appropriate.
- Maintain bed rest. Place the patient in semi-Fowler's position to help him breathe deeply with less pain and thus prevent pulmonary complications. Encourage coughing and deep breathing.
- If necessary, refer the patient to the hospital's social service department or a home health care agency for services during convalescence.

Patient teaching

- Teach the patient about peritonitis, what caused his problem, and necessary treatments.
- Provide preoperative teaching. Review postoperative care procedures.
- Discuss the proper use of prescribed medications, reviewing their correct administration, desired effects, and possible adverse effects.

EVALUATION

Evaluation of patient outcomes determines the success of collaborative management. For the patient with peritonitis, evaluation focuses on improved comfort, restoration of fluid balance, improved tissue perfusion, and adequate knowledge.

Stomach cancer

Although it's common throughout the world, stomach cancer exhibits unexplained geographic, cultural, and gender differences. For example, incidence is higher in men over age 40 and mortality is high in Japan, Iceland, Chile, and Austria. In the United States, for the past 25 years. the incidence of stomach cancer has fallen 50%, and the death rate is now one-third what it was 30 years ago. This decrease has been attributed, without proof, to the improved, well-balanced diets most Americans enjoy.

CAUSES

Stomach cancer occurs more commonly in some parts of the stomach, with 50% of cases affecting the pyloric area. Although the cause is unknown, predisposing factors, such as gastritis with gastric atrophy, increase the risk. Genetic factors have also been implicated. People with type A blood have a 10% higher risk, and the disease strikes more people who have a family history of such cancer.

Dietary factors may also have an effect. For instance, food type, preparation, and preservation (especially smoked foods, pickled vegetables, and salted fish and meat) increase the risk of stomach cancer. High alcohol consumption and smoking also increase the risk.

This adenocarcinoma rapidly infiltrates the regional lymph nodes, omentum, liver, and lungs by way of the walls of the stomach, duodenum, and esophagus; the lymphatic system; adjacent organs; the bloodstream; and the peritoneal cavity.

The patient's prognosis depends on the stage at diagnosis. Overall, the 5-year survival rate is about 15%.

DIAGNOSIS AND TREATMENT

Barium X-rays of the GI tract with fluoroscopy show changes that suggest stomach cancer: a tumor or filling defect in the outline of the stomach, loss of flexibility and distensibility, and abnormal gastric mucosa with or without ulceration.

Gastroscopy with fiber-optic endoscope helps rule out other diffuse gastric mucosal abnormalities by allowing direct visualization. Gastroscopic biopsy permits evaluation of gastric mucosal lesions. Photography records gastric lesions, used later to judge progression and the effect of treatment.

Gastric acid stimulation test determines whether the stomach secretes acid properly. Blood studies monitor the course of the disease, complications, and treatment, including complete blood count (CBC), chemistry profiles, arterial blood gas, liver function, and a carcinoembryonic antigen radioimmunoassay.

Other tests rule out specific organ metastases: computed tomography scans, chest X-rays, liver and bone scans, and liver biopsy.

Surgery to remove the tumor often is the treatment of choice. Excision of the lesion with appropriate margins is possible in more than one-third of patients. Even in a patient whose disease isn't considered surgically curable, resection eases symptoms and improves the potential benefits of chemotherapy and radiation therapy, which usually follow surgery.

Depending on the nature and extent of the lesion, surgery may consist of gastroduodenostomy, gastrojejunostomy, partial gastric resection, or total gastrectomy. If metastasis has occurred, the omentum and spleen may have to be removed.

Chemotherapy for GI tumors may help control signs and symptoms and prolong survival. Gastric adenocarcinomas respond to several agents, including fluorouracil, carmustine, doxorubicin, and mitomycin. Antiemetics can control nausea, which intensifies as the tumor grows. In the more advanced stages, the patient may need sedatives and tranquilizers to control overwhelming anxiety. Opioid analgesics can relieve severe and unremitting pain.

If the patient has a nonresectable or partially resectable tumor, radiation therapy is effective if combined with chemotherapy. The patient should receive this therapy on an empty stomach but not preoperatively because it may damage viscera and impede healing.

Treatment with antispasmodics and antacids may help relieve GI distress.

COLLABORATIVE MANAGEMENT

Care of the patient with stomach cancer will focus on relief of symptoms.

ASSESSMENT

In the early stages, the patient may complain of pain in his back or in the epigastric or retrosternal areas that's relieved by nonprescription medications. (He may not report this symptom because he doesn't realize its significance.) He typically reports a vague feeling of fullness, heaviness, and moderate abdominal distention after meals. Depending on the cancer's progression, here's what to look for:
- reports of weight loss, appetite disturbance, nausea, and vomiting
- reported coffee-ground vomitus if the tumor is located in the cardia; dysphagia, if the tumor is located in the proximal area of the stomach
- complaints of weakness and fatigue
- a mass in the abdomen and enlarged lymph nodes, especially the supraclavicular and axillary nodes.

NURSING DIAGNOSES AND COLLABORATIVE PROBLEMS

Based on the following nursing diagnoses, you'll establish patient outcomes.

Altered nutrition: Less than body requirements, related to adverse GI effects. The patient will:
- eat a high-protein, high-calorie diet daily
- regain any weight lost and keep his weight within the normal range
- develop no malnutrition.

Fatigue related to anemia. The patient will:
- express an understanding of the relationship between fatigue, activity tolerance, and stomach cancer
- employ measures to prevent and decrease fatigue
- regain his normal energy level when treatment is complete.

Anxiety related to potential threat of death from cancer diagnosis. The patient will:
- express his feelings about his diagnosis and prognosis
- use support systems to assist with coping
- cope with stomach cancer without showing signs of severe anxiety.

PLANNING AND IMPLEMENTATION

These measures help the patient with stomach cancer:
- Provide a high-protein, high-calorie diet to help the patient avoid or recover from the weight loss, malnutrition, and anemia associated with stomach cancer. This diet also helps him tolerate surgery, radiation therapy, and chemotherapy; helps prevent wound dehiscence; and promotes wound healing. Plus, it provides enough protein, fluid, and potassium to aid glycogen and protein synthesis.
- Give the patient dietary supplements, such as vitamins and iron, and provide small, frequent meals. If the patient has an iron deficiency, give him iron-rich foods, such as spinach and dried fruit.
- To stimulate a poor appetite, administer steroids or antidepressants, as ordered. Wine or brandy also may help stimulate the appetite.
- If the patient can't tolerate oral foods, provide parenteral nutrition.
- Monitor the patient's nutritional intake. Weigh him regularly and report excessive weight loss to the doctor. Watch for signs and symptoms of malnutrition.
- Watch for signs of anemia and vitamin B_{12} malabsorption. Monitor CBC and serum vitamin B_{12} levels.
- Administer an antacid to relieve heartburn and acid stomach and a histamine-$_2$ receptor antagonist, such as cimetidine or famotidine, to decrease gastric secretions. Give opioid analgesics, as ordered.
- During radiation therapy, watch for adverse reactions, such as nausea, vomiting, alopecia, malaise, and diarrhea.

■ During chemotherapy, watch for complications, such as infection, and for expected adverse reactions, such as nausea, vomiting, mouth ulcers, and alopecia.

■ During radiation or chemotherapy treatment, offer orange juice, grapefruit juice, ginger ale, or other fluids to minimize nausea and vomiting. Provide comfort measures and reassurance as needed.

■ Watch for surgical complications such as infection.

■ Take measures to prevent fatigue; for example, avoid scheduling two energy-draining activities on the same day or in sequence.

■ Encourage the patient to alternate activities with periods of rest.

■ Structure the patient's environment, taking into account his needs and preferences.

■ Throughout treatment, listen to the patient's fears and concerns, and offer reassurance when appropriate. Stay with him during periods of severe anxiety.

■ Encourage the patient to identify actions and care measures that promote comfort and relaxation. Try to perform these measures, and encourage the patient and family members or a friend to do the same.

■ Whenever possible, include the patient and family members in decisions related to the patient's care.

■ If all treatments fail, keep the patient comfortable and free from unnecessary pain, and provide psychological support. Encourage him to express his feelings and fears and to ask questions about his illness. Answer patient's and family members' questions honestly; evasive answers will make the patient retreat and feel isolated.

■ Advise family members to let the patient talk about his future; encourage them to maintain a realistic outlook.

Patient teaching

■ Provide preoperative teaching for the patient scheduled for surgery.

■ Stress the importance of sound nutrition. Explain that the patient may need vitamins to prevent B_{12} deficiency and iron to prevent or treat anemia.

■ Explain the ordered treatments to the patient and his family members or friends. Describe the adverse effects the treatment may cause, and explain when to notify the doctor.

■ Prepare the patient for chemotherapy's adverse effects, such as nausea and vomiting, and suggest measures that may help relieve these problems, such as drinking plenty of fluids.

■ Encourage the patient to follow his normal routine as much as possible after recovering from surgery and during radiation therapy and chemotherapy. Leading a near-normal life will help foster feelings of independence and control and will reduce complications of immobility.

■ Caution the patient to avoid crowds and people with known infections because chemotherapy and radiation therapy diminish the body's natural resistance to infection.

■ Encourage the patient to learn and practice relaxation and pain management techniques to help control anxiety and discomfort.

■ If appropriate, direct the patient and family members to hospital and community support personnel and services. These include social workers, psychologists, cancer support groups, home health care agencies, and hospices.

EVALUATION

Evaluation of patient outcomes determines the success of collaborative management. For the patient with stomach cancer, evaluation focuses on adequate nutrition, relief of fatigue and anxiety, and adequate knowledge.

Ulcerative colitis

An inflammatory, commonly chronic disease, ulcerative colitis affects the mucosa of the colon. It occurs primarily in young adults, especially women; it is more prevalent among Jews, higher socioeconomic groups, and people with a family history of the disease. The incidence of the disease is unknown; however, some studies indicate that as many as 1 out of 1,000 people are affected. Onset of symptoms seems to peak between ages 15 and 20 and again between ages 55 and 60.

CAUSES

The etiology of ulcerative colitis is unknown, but it may be related to an abnormal immune response in the GI tract, possibly associated with food or bacteria. Although stress is no longer thought to be a cause of ulcerative colitis, studies show that it can increase the severity of an attack.

Ulcerative colitis usually begins in the rectum and sigmoid colon and may extend upward into the entire colon; it rarely affects the small intestine, except for the terminal ileum. It produces congestion, edema (leading to mucosal friability), and ulcerations. Severity ranges from a mild, localized disorder to a fulminant disease that can cause many complications.

Complications depend on the severity and site of inflammation. Nutritional deficiencies are the most common complication, but the disease can also lead to perineal sepsis with anal fissure, anal fistula, perirectal abscess, hemorrhage, and toxic megacolon. A patient with ulcerative colitis has an increased risk of various arthritis types (40 times more than the general population) and cancer (if the disease has persisted more than 10 years since onset).

Other complications include coagulation defects resulting from vitamin K deficiency, erythema nodosum on the face and arms, pyoderma gangrenosum on the legs and ankles, uveitis, pericholangitis, sclerosing cholangitis, cirrhosis, possible cholangiocarcinoma, ankylosing spondylitis, loss of muscle mass, strictures, pseudopolyps, stenosis, and perforated colon, leading to peritonitis and toxemia.

DIAGNOSIS AND TREATMENT

Sigmoidoscopy confirms rectal involvement in most cases by showing increased mucosal friability, decreased mucosal detail, and thick inflammatory exudate. Colonoscopy may determine the extent of the disease and evaluate the strictured areas and pseudopolyps (not performed with active signs and symptoms). Biopsy, performed during colonoscopy, can help confirm the diagnosis.

Barium enema evaluates the extent of the disease and detects complications, such as strictures and carcinoma (not performed with active signs and symptoms). Stool specimen analysis reveals blood, pus, and mucus, but no pathogenic organisms.

Other supportive laboratory tests show decreased serum levels of potassium, magnesium, hemoglobin, and albumin as well as leukocytosis and increased prothrombin time. Erythrocyte sedimentation rate elevation correlates with the severity of the attack.

The goals of treatment are to control inflammation, replace nutritional losses and blood volume, and prevent complications. Supportive treatment includes dietary therapy, bed rest, I.V. fluid replacement, and medications. Blood transfusions or iron supplements may be needed to correct anemia.

Dietary measures depend on disease severity. Patients with severe disease usually receive total parenteral nutrition and are allowed nothing by mouth. Parenteral nutrition also is used for patients awaiting surgery or showing signs of dehydration and debilitation from excessive diarrhea. The goals of parenteral nutrition are to rest the intestinal tract, decrease stool volume, and restore positive nitrogen balance.

The patient with moderate signs and symptoms may receive an elemental feeding source such as Ensure to provide adequate nutrition with minimal bowel stimulation. A low-residue diet may be ordered for the patient with mild signs and symptoms. As signs and symptoms subside, the diet may gradually advance to include a greater variety of foods.

Drug therapy to control inflammation includes corticotropin and adrenal corticosteroids, such as prednisone, prednisolone, and hydrocortisone; sulfasalazine, which has anti-inflammatory and antimicrobial properties, may also be used. Antispasmodics such as tincture of belladonna and antidiarrheals, such as diphenoxylate and atropine, are used only for the patient with frequent, troublesome diarrhea whose ulcerative colitis is otherwise under control. These drugs may precipitate massive dilation of the colon (toxic megacolon) and are generally contraindicated.

Surgery, the treatment of last resort, is performed if the patient has toxic megacolon, if she fails to respond to drugs and supportive measures, or if she finds signs and symptoms unbearable.

The most common surgical technique is proctocolectomy with ileostomy. Total colectomy with ileorectal anastomosis is done in fewer cases because of its mortality rate (2% to 5%). This procedure removes the entire colon and anastomoses the rectum and the terminal ileum. It requires observation of the remaining rectal stump for any signs of cancer or colitis.

Pouch ileostomy, in which a pouch is created from a small loop of the terminal ileum and a nipple valve is formed from the distal ileum, is gaining popularity. The resulting stoma opens just above the pubic hairline; the pouch empties through a catheter inserted in the stoma several times a day. In ulcerative colitis, colectomy to prevent colon cancer is controversial.

Ileoanal reservoir is a newer surgical technique that preserves the anal sphincter and provides the patient with a reservoir made from the ileum and attached to the anal opening. First, the rectal mucosa is excised; then an abdominal colectomy is performed, and a reservoir is constructed and attached. Next, a temporary loop ileostomy is made to allow the new rectal reservoir to heal. Finally, the loop ileostomy is closed after a 3- or 4-month waiting period. Stools from the reservoir are similar to the stools from an ileostomy.

COLLABORATIVE MANAGEMENT

Care of the patient with ulcerative colitis focuses on preventing complications and promoting dietary changes.

ASSESSMENT

Usually, the patient's history will reveal periods of remission of symptoms and exacerbation when she reports mild cramping, lower abdominal pain, and recurrent bloody diarrhea as often as 10 to 25 times daily. She may also experience nocturnal diarrhea. During these periods, she may complain of fatigue, weakness, anorexia, weight loss, nausea, and vomiting. Here's what to look for:
■ stools that may appear liquid, with visible pus and mucus
■ blood in the stools—a cardinal sign of ulcerative colitis
■ abdominal distention, in fulminant disease

- abdominal tenderness; perianal irritation, hemorrhoids, and fissures; and, rarely, rectal fistulas and abscesses.

NURSING DIAGNOSES AND COLLABORATIVE PROBLEMS

Based on the following nursing diagnoses, you'll establish patient outcomes.

Altered nutrition: Less than body requirements, related to inflammation of lower GI tract. The patient will:
- show no further evidence of weight loss
- tolerate oral, tube, or I.V. feedings without adverse effects
- regain and maintain a normal nutritional state.

Diarrhea related to inflammation of lower GI tract. The patient will:
- be able to control diarrhea with medication
- show no signs of skin breakdown in the anal area
- report that her elimination pattern has returned to normal.

Risk for fluid volume deficit related to loss of fluid and electrolytes from diarrhea. The patient will:
- maintain electrolyte values within normal limits
- show no evidence of fluid volume deficit
- maintain stable vital signs and a normal urine output.

PLANNING AND IMPLEMENTATION

These measures help the patient with ulcerative colitis:
- Provide diet therapy as ordered.
- Provide frequent mouth care for the patient who is allowed nothing by mouth.
- After each bowel movement, thoroughly clean the skin around the rectum and apply a soothing and protective agent to the irritated area. Use an air mattress to help prevent skin breakdown.
- Regardless of the ordered diet, monitor and record intake, calorie count, and output, noting the frequency and volume of stools.
- Schedule care to allow frequent rest periods. The patient is usually very tired and weak.
- Administer medications as ordered. Assess regularly for desired effects. Note any adverse reactions such as those from prolonged corticosteroid therapy (moon face, edema, gastric irritation). Be aware that such therapy may mask infection.
- Monitor the fluid and electrolyte status of the patient on total parenteral nutrition. Assess the insertion site for inflammation. Check blood glucose and urine acetone levels every 6 hours.
- Give blood transfusions as ordered.
- Monitor hemoglobin levels and hematocrit.
- Watch for signs of dehydration (poor skin turgor, furrowed tongue) and electrolyte imbalances, especially signs and symptoms of hypokalemia (muscle weakness, paresthesia) and hypernatremia (tachycardia, fever, dry tongue).
- Watch closely for signs and symptoms of complications, such as a perforated colon and peritonitis (fever, severe abdominal pain, abdominal rigidity and tenderness, cool clammy skin) and toxic megacolon (abdominal distention, decreased bowel sounds).
- Support the patient emotionally. Stay with her when she's acutely distressed; check her several times a day and listen to her concerns. Offer reassurance when appropriate.

Patient teaching

- Teach the patient about the disorder and review its signs and symptoms. Explain diagnostic tests and ordered treatments.
- Discuss all ordered dietary changes and help the patient understand how these measures will decrease her symptoms. If she's placed on parenteral nutrition or a restricted diet, reassure her that she will be able to progress to a more advanced diet as her symptoms resolve. In general, caution the patient to avoid GI stimulants, such as caffeine, alcohol, and tobacco products.
- Review the patient's medications with her. Explain the desired actions, dosage, and adverse effects.
- If the patient is scheduled for surgery, reinforce the doctor's explanation of the procedure and its possible complications.
- As part of preoperative teaching, describe the stoma and explain how it differs from normal anatomy. Provide additional patient information as needed (available from the United Ostomy Association).
- Arrange for a visit by an enterostomal therapist and, ideally, a recovered ileostomate.
- After a proctocolectomy and ileostomy, teach stoma care. After a pouch ileostomy, demonstrate procedures to insert the catheter and care for the stoma.
- Emphasize the need for regular physical examinations because of the increased risk of colorectal cancer.

EVALUATION

Evaluation of patient outcomes determines the success of collaborative management. For the patient with ulcerative colitis, evaluation focuses on improved nutrition and elimination, adequate comfort and safety, restored fluid balance, and adequate knowledge.

Treatments and procedures

Various treatments and procedures can be used for patients with GI disorders.

CHOLECYSTECTOMY

When drug therapy, dietary changes, and supportive treatments fail to control gallbladder or biliary duct disease, the patient's gallbladder may need to be removed. Called cholecystectomy, the procedure helps restore biliary flow from the liver to the small intestine.

After gallbladder resection, choledochoduodenostomy (anastomosis of the common bile duct to the duodenum) or choledochojejunostomy (anastomosis of the common bile duct to the jejunum) may be necessary to restore biliary flow.

PROCEDURE

Both abdominal and laparoscopic cholecystectomies are performed under general anesthesia. (See *Understanding cholecystectomy*.)

COLLABORATIVE MANAGEMENT

Care of the patient undergoing cholecystectomy involves relief of preoperative symptoms and postoperative complications related to postcholecystectomy syndrome and obstuction of biliary drainage.

Preparation

■ Explain the planned surgery to the patient, reassuring him that the surgery will relieve his symptoms, and that his recovery should be rapid (4 to 6 weeks) and uneventful.

■ If the patient is scheduled for abdominal surgery, warn him that he'll have a nasogastric (NG) tube for 1 to 2 days and an abdominal drain at the incision site for 3 to 5 days. If appropriate, tell him that a T tube will be inserted in the common bile duct during surgery and may remain for 2 weeks to drain excess bile and allow removal of retained stones.

■ If the patient is scheduled for a laparoscopic approach, tell him of the indwelling urinary catheter in his bladder and the NG tube into his stomach. Reassure him that these tubes will be removed in the postanesthesia room following the procedure. Explain that he will have four small incisions, each covered with a small sterile dressing. Also inform him that he may be discharged the day of surgery or the day after.

■ Teach the patient how to perform coughing and deep-breathing exercises to prevent postoperative atelectasis, which can lead to pneumonia. Tell him that he can take an analgesic before these exercises, to relieve discomfort.

Monitoring and aftercare

■ Monitor and, if necessary, help stabilize the patient's nutritional status and fluid balance. Such measures may include administering vitamin K, blood transfusions, or glucose and protein supplements. Twenty-four hours before surgery, administer only clear liquids. Then, after midnight the night before surgery or as ordered, withhold all food and fluid.

■ Administer preoperative medications and assist with insertion of an NG tube.

■ Ensure that the patient or a responsible family member has signed a consent form.

■ There is no special monitoring required, other than vital signs and monitoring drainage until patient is fully awake. When the patient returns from surgery, place him in low Fowler's position. As ordered, attach the NG tube to low intermittent suction. Monitor the amount and characteristics of drainage from the NG tube as well as from any abdominal drains. Check dressings frequently and change as necessary.

■ If the patient has a T tube in place, frequently assess the position and patency of the tube and drainage bag. The drainage bag should be level with his abdomen to prevent excessive drainage. Also note the amount and characteristics of drainage; bloody or blood-tinged bile normally appears for only the first few hours after surgery. Provide meticulous skin care around the tube insertion site to prevent irritation.

■ After a few days, expect to remove the NG tube, if present, and begin to introduce foods: first liquids, then gradually soft solids. As ordered, clamp the T tube for an hour before and an hour after each meal to allow bile to travel to the intestine to aid digestion. If the patient has had a laparoscopic cholecystectomy, expect him to begin clear liquids when fully recovered from general anesthesia and to resume his normal diet the day of or the day after surgery.

■ Be alert for signs and symptoms of postcholecystectomy syndrome (such as fever, abdominal pain, and jaundice) and other complications involving obstructed bile drainage. For several days after surgery, monitor vital signs and record intake and output every 8 hours. If any complications occur, report them to the doctor and collect urine and stool samples for laboratory analysis of bile content.

■ Assist the patient with ambulation on the first postoperative day, unless contraindicated. Have him cough, deep-breathe, and perform incentive spirometry every 4 hours; as ordered, provide analgesics to ease discomfort during these exercises. Assess his respiratory status every 2 hours to detect hypoventilation and signs of atelectasis.

Patient teaching

■ If the patient is being discharged with a T tube in place, show him how to care for it, stressing the need for meticulous tube care.

■ Tell the patient to immediately report any signs of biliary obstruction: fever, jaundice, pruritus, pain, dark urine, and clay-colored stools.

Understanding cholecystectomy

Gallbladder surgeries include abdominal cholecystectomy and laparoscopic laser cholecystectomy.

Abdominal cholecystectomy

Performed under general anesthesia, this surgery begins with a right subcostal or paramedial incision. The surgeon then surveys the abdomen and uses laparotomy packs to isolate the gallbladder from the surrounding organs. After identifying biliary tract structures, he may use cholangiography or ultrasonography to help identify gallstones. Using a choledoscope, he directly visualizes the bile ducts and inserts a Fogarty balloon-tipped catheter to clear the ducts of stones.

The surgeon ligates and divides the cystic duct and artery and removes the entire gallbladder. Typically, he performs a choledochotomy—the insertion of a T tube into the common bile duct to decompress the biliary tree and prevent bile peritonitis during healing. He may also insert a Penrose drain into the ducts.

Laparoscopic laser cholecystectomy

This surgery begins with several small incisions (1 to 3 cm) on the abdomen—at the umbilicus (for the laparoscope and attached camera) and at the upper midline, right lateral, and right midclavicular (for various grasping and dissecting forceps). Insufflating the abdomen with carbon dioxide allows viewing of the structures. The attached camera transmits to a television monitor, allowing the surgical team to view the procedure. The cystic duct and artery are clipped and divided. Laser or cautery is used to cut and coagulate during removal of the gallbladder from its liver bed. Needle aspiration of bile facilitates gallbladder removal through the incision at the umbilicus.

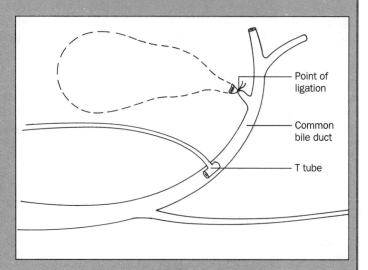

Point of ligation

Common bile duct

T tube

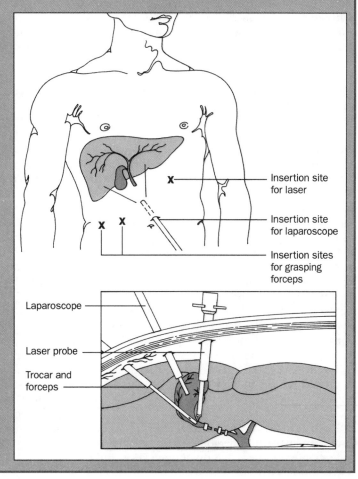

Insertion site for laser

Insertion site for laparoscope

Insertion sites for grasping forceps

Laparoscope

Laser probe

Trocar and forceps

■ Tell the patient that, although there are typically no dietary restrictions, he may wish to avoid excessive fat intake for 4 to 6 weeks.

COMPLICATIONS

Although relatively rare, complications from chole-cystectomy can be grave. Peritonitis, for instance, may occur from obstructed biliary drainage and resultant leakage of bile into the peritoneum. Postchole-cystectomy syndrome, marked by fever, jaundice, and pain, may occur. As in all abdominal surgeries, postoperative atelectasis may result from hampered respiratory excursion if an abdominal surgical approach was used. If a laparoscopic approach was used, bile duct or small-bowel injury may occur during introduction of the trocar.

Other complications include superficial wound infection, prolonged ileus, urine retention, and retained gallstones.

COLON RESECTION

Surgical resection of diseased intestinal tissue and anastomosis of the remaining segments help treat localized obstructive disorders, including diverticulosis (with an area of acute diverticulitis or abscess formation), intestinal polyps, adhesions that cause bowel dysfunction, and malignant or benign intestinal lesions. It's the preferred surgical technique for localized bowel cancer but not for widespread carcinoma, which usually requires massive resection with creation of a temporary or permanent colostomy or an ileostomy.

PROCEDURE

After the patient has received a general anesthetic, the surgeon makes the abdominal incision. The incision site varies, depending on the pathologic site. The surgeon limits the resection to the diseased area and a wide margin of surrounding normal tissue. After excising the diseased colonic tissue, the surgeon then anastomoses the remaining bowel segments to restore patency. End-to-end anastomosis provides the most physiologically sound junction and is the quickest to perform, but it requires that the approximated bowel segments be large enough to prevent postoperative obstruction at the anastomosis site. Side-to-side anastomosis minimizes the danger of obstruction, but this lengthy procedure may be contraindicated in an emergency. After the anastomosis is complete, the surgeon closes the incision and applies a sterile dressing.

COLLABORATIVE MANAGEMENT

Care of the patient undergoing colon resection involves maintaining hydration and nutrition and managing postoperative pain.

Preparation

■ Explain that the surgery will remove a diseased portion of the patient's bowel and will connect the remaining healthy segments. Keep in mind that the patient and his family will probably have many questions about the surgery and its effect on the patient's lifestyle. Take the time to listen to their concerns and to answer their questions.
■ Discuss anticipated postoperative care measures. Tell the patient that he'll awaken from surgery with a nasogastric (NG) tube in place to drain air and fluid from the intestinal tract and prevent distention. Explain that when peristalsis returns, usually within 2 to 3 days, the tube will be removed. Tell him to anticipate ambulation on the first day after surgery to promote return of peristalsis. Also prepare him for the presence of an I.V. line, which will provide fluid replacement, and abdominal drains.
■ To reduce the risk of postoperative atelectasis and pneumonia, teach the patient how to cough and deep-breathe properly and emphasize the need to do so regularly throughout the recovery period. Demonstrate incisional splinting to protect the sutures and reduce discomfort.
■ Before surgery, as ordered, administer antibiotics to reduce intestinal flora and laxatives or enemas to remove fecal contents.

Monitoring and aftercare

■ For the first few days after surgery, carefully monitor intake and output and weigh the patient daily. Maintain fluid and electrolyte balance through I.V. replacement therapy, and check the patient regularly for signs of dehydration, such as decreased urine output and poor skin turgor.
■ Keep the NG tube patent. Warn the patient that, if the tube becomes dislodged, he should never attempt to reposition it himself; doing so could damage the anastomosis.
■ To detect possible complications, carefully monitor the patient's vital signs and closely assess his overall condition. Remember that anastomotic leakage may produce only vague signs and symptoms at first; watch for low-grade fever, malaise, slight leukocytosis, and abdominal distention and tenderness. Also be alert for more extensive hemorrhage from acute leakage; watch for signs and symptoms of hypovolemic shock (precipitous drop in blood pressure and pulse rate, respiratory difficulty, decreased level of consciousness) and bloody stool or wound drainage.
■ Observe the patient for signs of peritonitis or sepsis, caused by leakage of bowel contents into the abdominal cavity. Remember that a patient receiving antibiotics or total parenteral nutrition is at increased

risk for sepsis. Sepsis also may result from "wicking" of colonic bacteria up the NG tube to the oral cavity; to prevent this problem, provide frequent mouth and tube care.

■ Provide meticulous wound care, changing dressings often. Check dressings and drainage sites frequently for signs of infection (purulent drainage, foul odor) or fecal drainage. Also watch for sudden fever, especially when accompanied by abdominal pain and tenderness.

■ Regularly assess the patient for signs of postresection obstruction. Examine the abdomen for distention and rigidity, auscultate for bowel sounds, and note passage of any flatus or feces.

■ Once the patient regains peristalsis and bowel function, take steps to prevent constipation and straining during defecation, both of which can damage the anastomosis. Encourage him to drink plenty of fluids, and administer a stool softener or other laxatives, as ordered. Note and record the frequency and amount of all bowel movements as well as characteristics of the stool.

■ Encourage regular coughing and deep breathing to prevent atelectasis; remind him to splint the incision site as necessary.

■ Refer the patient to a dietitian as needed.

■ Anticipate referral for home care for follow-up and teaching.

Patient teaching

■ Tell the patient to record the frequency and character of bowel movements and to notify the doctor of any changes in his normal pattern. Warn against using laxatives without consulting his doctor.

■ Caution the patient to avoid abdominal straining and heavy lifting until the sutures are completely healed and the doctor grants permission to do so.

■ Tell the patient to maintain the ordered semibland diet until his bowel has healed completely (usually 4 to 8 weeks). In particular, urge him to avoid carbonated beverages and gas-producing foods.

■ Because extensive bowel resection may interfere with the patient's ability to absorb nutrients from food, emphasize the importance of vitamin supplements.

COMPLICATIONS

Several complications can occur in a patient who has had a bowel resection with anastomosis. These include bleeding or leakage from the anastomosis site, peritonitis and resultant sepsis, postresection obstruction, and problems common to all patients undergoing abdominal surgery, such as wound infection and atelectasis.

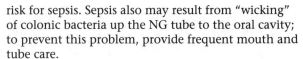

GASTRECTOMY

If chronic ulcer disease doesn't respond to medication, dietary therapy, and rest, gastric surgery may be required to remove diseased tissue and prevent recurrence of ulcers. The surgeon may also excise a malignant tumor, relieve an obstruction or, in an emergency, control severe GI hemorrhage resulting from a perforated ulcer.

Gastric surgery adapts to the location and extent of the disorder. For example, a partial gastrectomy reduces the amount of acid-secreting mucosa. A bilateral vagotomy may relieve ulcer symptoms and eliminate vagal nerve stimulation of gastric secretions. Most commonly, though, two gastric surgeries are combined, such as vagotomy with gastroenterostomy or vagotomy with antrectomy.

PROCEDURE

Surgery begins with an upper abdominal incision, to expose the stomach and part of the intestine. Total gastrectomy, the removal of the entire stomach, requires a more extensive incision.

The rest of the procedure varies, depending on the type of surgery. (See *Understanding common gastric surgeries,* page 250.)

COLLABORATIVE MANAGEMENT

Care of the patient undergoing gastrectomy involves promoting nutrition and fluid replacement and managing pain before and after surgery.

Preparation

■ Before planned surgery, stabilize the patient's fluid and electrolyte balance and nutritional status—all of which may be severely compromised by chronic ulcer disease or other GI disorders. Monitor intake and output, and draw serum samples for hematologic studies. As ordered, begin I.V. fluid replacement and total parenteral nutrition (TPN). As ordered, prepare the patient for abdominal X-rays. On the night before surgery, administer cleansing laxatives and enemas, as necessary. On the morning of surgery, insert a nasogastric (NG) tube.

■ As time permits, discuss postoperative care measures with the patient. Explain that the NG tube will remain in place for 2 to 3 days to remove fluid, blood, and air from the abdominal cavity and to prevent distention; he'll also have abdominal drains inserted at the surgical site and an I.V. line in place for several days.

■ Discuss how surgery will affect his diet, as he gradually resumes oral feeding, progressing from clear liquids to solid foods. If gastric surgery is extensive, he may receive TPN for 1 week or longer.

■ Explain the need for postoperative deep-breathing exercises and coughing to prevent pulmonary compli-

Understanding common gastric surgeries

Besides treating complications of ulcer disease, such as perforation and scarring, the gastric surgeries depicted below help remove obstructions and neoplasms.

Vagotomy with gastroenterostomy

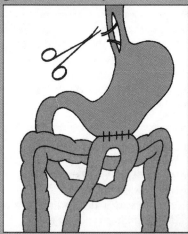

The surgeon resects the vagus nerves and creates a stoma for gastric drainage. Resection may involve selective, truncal, or parietal cell vagotomy, depending on the degree of gastric acid reduction required.

Vagotomy with antrectomy

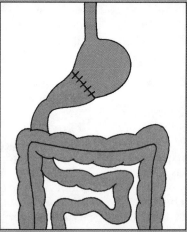

After resecting the vagus nerves, the surgeon removes the antrum, anastomoses the remaining stomach segment to the jejunum, and closes the duodenal stump.

Vagotomy with pyloroplasty

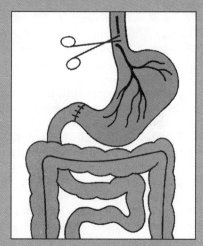

In this procedure, the surgeon resects the vagus nerves and refashions the pylorus to widen the lumen and aid gastric emptying.

Billroth I

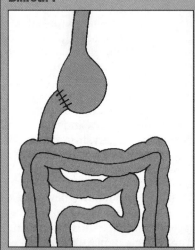

In this partial gastrectomy with a gastroduodenoscopy, the surgeon excises the distal third to half of the stomach and anastomoses the remaining stomach to the duodenum.

Billroth II

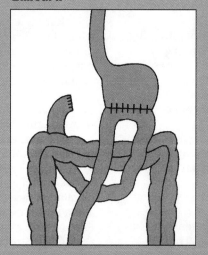

In this partial gastrectomy with a gastrojejunostomy, the surgeon removes the distal segment of the stomach and antrum, anastomoses the remaining stomach and the jejunum, and closes the duodenal stump.

Total gastrectomy

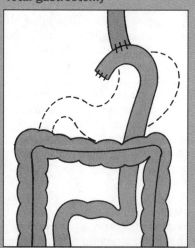

The surgeon removes the entire stomach and attaches the lower end of the esophagus to the jejunum (esophagojejunostomy) at the entrance to the small intestine.

cations. Stress the importance of these activities, even though pain from the incision may inhibit the patient.

■ Remember that he may have unexpressed fears about the surgery and its effect on his lifestyle. Take time to reassure him. Point out that other, more conservative treatments haven't worked and that surgery is now necessary to relieve symptoms and prevent possibly life-threatening complications. Explain that, with successful surgery, he should have a near-normal life with few activity restrictions.

Monitoring and aftercare

■ When the patient awakens after surgery, place him in low Fowler's or semi-Fowler's position—either eases breathing and prevents aspiration if he vomits.

■ Monitor the patient's vital signs frequently until stable, according to your facility's guidelines. Watch especially for hypotension, bradycardia, and respiratory changes, which may signal hemorrhage and shock. Periodically check the wound site, NG tube, and abdominal drainage tubes for bleeding.

■ Maintain tube feedings or TPN and I.V. fluid and electrolyte replacement therapy, as ordered. Monitor blood studies daily. Watch for signs of dehydration, hyponatremia, and metabolic alkalosis, which may result from gastric suctioning. Monitor and record intake and output, including NG tube drainage. Watch for complications associated with TPN or I.V. therapy.

■ Auscultate the patient's abdomen daily for the return of bowel sounds. When they return, notify the doctor, who will order clamping or removal of the NG tube and gradual resumption of oral feeding. During NG tube clamping, watch for nausea and vomiting; if they occur, unclamp the tube immediately and reattach it to suction.

■ Throughout recovery, have the patient cough, deep-breathe, and change position frequently. Provide incentive spirometry, as necessary. Teach him to splint his incision while coughing to help reduce pain. Assess his breath sounds frequently to detect atelectasis.

■ Assess for other complications, including vitamin B_{12} deficiency, anemia (especially common in patients who have undergone total gastrectomy), and dumping syndrome, a potentially serious digestive complication marked by weakness, nausea, flatulence, and palpitations within 30 minutes after a meal.

Patient teaching

■ Tell the patient to notify the doctor immediately if he develops any signs of life-threatening complications, such as hemorrhage, obstruction, or perforation.

■ Explain dumping syndrome and ways to avoid it. Advise the patient to eat small, frequent meals evenly spaced throughout the day. He should chew his food thoroughly and drink fluids between meals rather than with them. He should decrease intake of carbohydrates and salt while increasing fat and protein. After a meal, he should lie down for 20 to 30 minutes.

■ Advise the patient to avoid or limit foods high in fiber, such as fresh fruits and vegetables and whole grain breads.

■ If the doctor has prescribed a GI anticholinergic to decrease motility and acid secretion, instruct the patient to take the drug 30 minutes to 1 hour before meals.

■ If the patient is being discharged on tube feedings, make sure that he and his family understand how to give the feedings.

■ Encourage the patient and family members to help speed healing by identifying and eliminating sources of emotional stress at home and in the workplace, to balance activity and rest, and to schedule a realistic pattern of work and sleep. Suggest that he learn stress management techniques, such as progressive relaxation and meditation. If the patient finds self-management difficult, encourage him to seek professional counseling.

■ Advise the patient to avoid smoking because it alters pancreatic secretions that neutralize gastric acid in the duodenum.

COMPLICATIONS

Gastric surgery carries the risk of serious complications, including hemorrhage, obstruction, dumping syndrome, paralytic ileus, perforation, vitamin B_{12} deficiency, anemia, and atelectasis.

LIVER TRANSPLANTATION

For the patient with a persistent, life-threatening liver disorder, a liver transplant may seem the last best hope. But transplant surgery is performed infrequently because of its risks, its high cost, and the difficulty procuring organs. Typically, it's done only in large teaching centers and is reserved for terminally ill patients who stand a realistic chance of survival. Candidates include patients with congenital biliary abnormalities, inborn errors of metabolism, or end-stage liver disease.

Many qualified transplant candidates are awaiting suitable donor organs, but only some survive the wait. When transplantation *is* performed, the patient faces many challenges to recovery. Besides the complications accompanying extensive abdominal and vascular surgeries, liver transplantation carries a high risk of tissue rejection. However, advances in immunosuppressant therapy and improved surgical techniques and postoperative care have resulted in improved outcomes.

COLLABORATIVE MANAGEMENT

Care of the patient undergoing liver transplantation involes initiation of immunosuppression therapy and pre- and postoperative emotional support of patient and family.

Preparation

■ As ordered, begin immunosuppressant therapy to decrease the risk of tissue rejection, using such drugs as cyclosporine, tacrolimus, and corticosteroids. Explain the need for lifelong therapy to prevent rejection.
■ Before transplant surgery, address the patient's (and family members') emotional needs. Discuss the typical stages of adjustment: overwhelming relief and elation at surviving the operation, followed by anxiety, frustration, and depression as complications set in.

Monitoring and aftercare

■ Focus your aftercare on four areas: maintaining immunosuppressant therapy; monitoring for early signs of rejection and other complications; preventing opportunistic infections, which can lead to rejection; and providing reassurance and emotional support throughout the prolonged recovery period.
■ Monitor vital signs every 15 minutes until stable; monitor for evidence of hemorrhage and rejection.
■ Perform hourly assessments of fluid volume and vital signs required to detect hemorrhage and hypovolemic shock, along with pulses, urine output, level of consciousness, peripheral circulation.
■ Monitor hemoglobin levels and hematocrit daily. Keep 2 units of blood available. Maintain the patency of I.V. lines.
■ If the patient complains of acute pain in the right upper quadrant, cramping pain or tenderness, nausea and vomiting, he may be experiencing vascular obstruction and need emergency thrombectomy.
■ Assess incision site for signs and symptoms of wound infection or abscess.
■ Follow your facility's pulmonary hygiene protocol, to prevent complications.
■ Maintain reverse isolation, note any signs or symptoms of opportunistic infections (fever, chills, leukocytosis or leukopenia, and diaphoresis).
■ Monitor daily weight.
■ Assess for hepatic failure, upper GI bleeding, and renal failure; for early detection, monitor serum amylase daily and electrolytes, blood urea nitrogen, serum creatinine, and potassium levels.

Patient teaching

■ Teach the patient and family members to recognize the early indicators of tissue rejection (pain and tenderness in the right upper quadrant, right flank, or center of the back; fever; tachycardia; jaundice; and changes in the color of urine or stool). Stress the need to call the doctor immediately if any of these signs or symptoms develop.
■ Instruct them to watch for and report any indication of liver failure, such as abdominal distention, bloody stool or vomitus, decreased urine output, abdominal pain and tenderness, anorexia, or altered level of consciousness.
■ To reduce the risk of tissue rejection, advise the patient to avoid contact with anyone who may have a contagious illness. Emphasize the importance of reporting any early signs or symptoms of infection, including fever, weakness, lethargy, and tachycardia.
■ Urge the patient to strictly comply with the prescribed immunosuppressive drug regimen. Explain that noncompliance can trigger rejection, even of a liver that has been functioning well for years. Also warn about potential adverse effects of immunosuppressive therapy, such as infection, fluid retention, acne, glaucoma, diabetes, and cancer.
■ Emphasize the importance of regular follow-up examinations to evaluate the integrity of the surgical site and continued tissue compatibility. If appropriate, suggest that the patient and his family seek psychological counseling to help them cope with the effects of the long and difficult recovery.

COMPLICATIONS

Possible complications include hemorrhage and hypovolemic shock, vascular obstruction, wound infection or abscess, pulmonary insufficiency or failure, opportunistic infections, and rejection and hepatic failure.

PANCREATECTOMY

In pancreatectomy, various resections, drainage procedures, and anastomoses may be used to treat pancreatic diseases that resisted more conservative techniques. It's indicated for palliative treatment of pancreatic cancer as well as chronic pancreatitis, which often stems from prolonged alcohol abuse. It's also used to treat islet cell tumors (insulinomas).

The procedure type depends on the patient's condition, the extent of the disease and its metastasis, and the amount of endocrine and exocrine function the pancreas retains. In many cases, the procedure is determined only after surgical exploration of the abdomen.

PROCEDURE

The surgeon selects the abdominal procedure based on evaluation of the pancreas, liver, gallbladder, and common bile duct. If the disease is localized, he may resect a portion of the pancreas and the surrounding organs. If the surgeon detects either metastatic disease in the liver or lymph nodes or tumor invasion of the aorta or superior mesenteric artery, he may decide to bypass the obstruction to lessen the patient's pain.

COLLABORATIVE MANAGEMENT

Care of the patient undergoing pancreatectomy involves promoting dietary and lifestyle changes and managing symptoms before and after surgery.

Preparation

■ Explain to the patient that the specific procedure will be selected by the surgeon during abdominal exploration. Provide emotional support, and encourage the patient to express his feelings.
■ Give analgesics, as ordered.
■ Arrange for necessary diagnostic studies, as ordered, to help the surgeon determine the existing endocrine and exocrine structure of the pancreas and any anatomic anomalies.
■ For the patient with chronic pancreatitis or cancer, provide enteral or parenteral nutrition before surgery. As ordered, give low-fat, high-calorie feedings to combat the malnutrition and steatorrhea that result from malabsorption.
■ Give meticulous skin care to prevent tissue breakdown that could complicate postoperative healing.
■ If the patient is hyperglycemic, give oral hypoglycemic agents or insulin, as ordered, and monitor blood and urine glucose levels.
■ Monitor the patient with recent history of alcohol abuse for withdrawal signs and symptoms: agitation, tachycardia, tremors, anorexia, and hypertension. Remember that delirium tremens may occur 72 to 96 hours after his last drink and that surgery should be delayed until after this period.
■ If the patient smokes (many patients with pancreatic cancer are heavy smokers), advise him to stop smoking before surgery. Evaluate his pulmonary status to provide baseline information.
■ Instruct the patient in deep-breathing and coughing techniques. Tell him to turn in bed, perform deep-breathing exercises, and cough every 2 hours for 24 to 72 hours after surgery. If incentive spirometry is indicated, instruct him as appropriate.
■ Assess the patient for jaundice and increased hematoma formation—signs of liver dysfunction, which commonly accompanies pancreatic disease. As ordered, arrange for liver function and coagulation studies before surgery. If the patient has a prolonged prothrombin time, expect to give vitamin K to prevent postoperative hemorrhage.
■ Because resection of the transverse colon may be necessary, the doctor may order mechanical and antibiotic bowel preparation as well as prophylactic systemic antibiotics (started 6 hours before surgery and continuing for 72 hours after surgery). Carry out these measures as directed, and expect to assist with insertion of a nasogastric (NG) tube and an indwelling urinary catheter.

Monitoring and aftercare

■ The patient usually spends 48 hours in the intensive care unit after surgery. Monitor his vital signs closely, and administer plasma expanders as ordered. Use central, arterial, or pulmonary catheter readings to evaluate hemodynamic status; correlate these readings with urine output and wound drainage. If central venous pressure and urine output drop, give fluids to avoid hypovolemic shock.
■ Evaluate NG tube drainage, which should be green tinged as bile drains from the stomach.
■ If the patient has a T tube in his common bile duct, evaluate this drainage, too. Normal bile drainage is 600 to 800 ml daily, decreasing as more bile goes to the intestine. Notify the doctor if bile drainage doesn't decrease, as this may indicate a biliary obstruction leading to possibly fatal peritonitis.
■ Assess Penrose or sump drainage from the abdomen, and inspect the dressing and drainage sites for frank bleeding, which may signal hemorrhage. If a pancreatic drain is in place, prevent skin breakdown from highly excoriating pancreatic enzymes by changing dressings frequently or by using a wound pouching system to contain the drainage.
■ Monitor the patient's fluid and electrolyte balance closely, evaluate arterial blood gases, and provide I.V. fluid replacements, as ordered. Keep in mind that constant gastric drainage can cause metabolic alkalosis, signaled by apathy, irritability, dehydration, and slow, shallow breathing. Report these signs and symptoms to the doctor, and expect to administer isotonic fluids. Alternatively, loss of bile and pancreatic secretions can lead to metabolic acidosis, signaled by elevated blood pressure, rapid pulse and respirations, and arrhythmias. Report these signs to the doctor, and give I.V. bicarbonate as ordered.
■ Have I.V. calcium ready because serum amylase levels commonly rise after pancreatic surgery and amylase can bind to calcium. Evaluate serum calcium levels periodically.
■ Check blood glucose levels periodically for possible fluctuations. Give insulin, if ordered.

■ Monitor the patient's respiratory status, being alert for shallow breathing, decreased respiratory rate, and respiratory distress. Administer oxygen, if necessary and ordered. Reinforce deep-breathing techniques, and encourage the patient to cough.

■ Be alert for absent bowel sounds, severe abdominal pain, vomiting, or fever—evidence of fistula development and paralytic ileus. Also, check the patient's wound for redness, pain, edema, unusual odor, or suture line separation. Report any of these findings to the doctor.

■ If no complications develop, expect the patient's GI function to return in 24 to 48 hours. Remove his NG tube as ordered, and start him on fluids.

Patient teaching

■ Teach the patient how to care for his wound, including careful cleaning and dressing each day. Tell him to report any signs of wound infection promptly.

■ As appropriate, teach him to test his urine for ketones or monitor his blood glucose levels. If he had a total pancreatectomy, provide routine diabetic teaching and show him or a responsible family member how to give insulin.

■ If the patient has chronic pancreatitis, stress that he requires continued follow-up and must avoid alcohol. As needed, refer him to an outpatient or chemical dependency clinic.

■ Because pancreatic exocrine insufficiency leads to malabsorption, provide dietary instructions and inform the patient that he may eventually need pancreatic enzyme replacement.

COMPLICATIONS

Major potential complications of pancreatectomy include hemorrhage (during and after surgery), fistulas, abscesses (common with distal pancreatectomy), common bile duct obstruction, and pseudocysts. Subtotal resection sometimes causes insulin dependence, whereas total pancreatectomy always causes permanent and complete insulin dependence.

Selected references

Black, J.M., and Matassarin-Jacobs, E. *Medical-Surgical Nursing: Clinical Management for Continuity of Care,* 5th ed. Philadelphia: W.B. Saunders Co., 1997.

Centers for Disease Control and Prevention. *Prevention of Hepatitis A Through Active or Passive Immunization: Advisory Committee on Immunization Practices.* MMWR Recommendations and Reports, CDC Publication, December 27, 1996.

Illustrated Guide to Diagnostic Tests, 2nd ed. Springhouse, Pa: Springhouse Corp., 1998.

National Digestive Disease Information Clearinghouse. *Stomach and Duodenal Ulcers.* NIH Publication No. 95-38, January 1995.

Nursing98 Drug Handbook. Springhouse, Pa.: Springhouse Corp., 1998.

Tacrolimus Approved for Liver Transplants. Reprinted from Medical Services Bulletin, Pharmaceutical Information Associates, Ltd., May 1994. http:\\pharminfo.com\pubs\msb.

Neurologic disorders

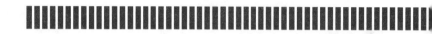

Caring for a patient with a neurologic disorder can be very challenging. Neurologic assessment takes longer than most examinations and requires complex skills. Changes in the patient's condition are often elusive. Some are quite subtle, and some are characteristically latent, uncovered only by systematic testing. Technology has made neurologic tests increasingly accurate but more complex to perform, requiring careful patient preparation and teaching. With a thorough review of the subject and sound clinical skills, you'll successfully administer today's most challenging treatments and procedures.

Anatomy and physiology review

The nervous system coordinates all body functions and enables an individual to adapt to changes in the internal and external environment. The system consists of the central nervous system (CNS)—the brain and spinal cord—plus the peripheral nervous system—the cranial nerves, spinal nerves, and autonomic system. (See *Understanding the central nervous system*, pages 256 and 257, and *Understanding the peripheral nervous system*, pages 258 and 259.)

Bone, meninges, and cerebrospinal fluid (CSF) protect the brain and the spinal cord from shock and infection. Formed of cranial bones, the skull surrounds the brain and opens at the base (the foramen magnum), where the spinal cord exits. The vertebral column protects the spinal cord with 30 vertebrae, each separated by an intervertebral disk for flexibility.

The meninges cover and protect the cerebral cortex and spinal column with three layers of connective tissue: the dura mater, the arachnoid membrane, and the pia mater. Three layers of space between those tis-

sues further cushion the brain and spinal cord against injury.

CSF nourishes cells, transports metabolic waste, and cushions the brain. This colorless fluid circulates through the ventricular system, into the subarachnoid space of the brain and spinal cord, and back to the venous sinuses on top of the brain where it is reabsorbed. The ependymal cells that cover the surface of the choroid plexus (a tangled mass of tiny blood vessels lining the ventricles) constantly produce CSF at a rate of about 150 ml per day.

Two major cell types, neurons and neuroglia, make up the nervous system. The conducting cells of the CNS, neurons (nerve cells) detect and transmit stimuli by electromechanical messages. These specialized cells do not reproduce themselves.

Neuroglia, or glial cells (derived from the Greek word for glue because they hold the neurons together), serve as the supportive cells of the CNS, forming roughly 40% of the brain's bulk. There are four types of neuroglia:

■ Astroglia, or astrocytes, exist throughout the nervous system and form part of the blood-brain barrier. They supply nutrients to the neurons and help maintain their electrical potential.

■ Ependymal cells line the brain's four ventricles and the choroid plexus, and help produce CSF.

■ Microglia phagocytose waste products from injured neurons and are deployed throughout the nervous system.

■ Oligodendroglia support and electrically insulate CNS axons by forming protective myelin sheaths.

NEUROTRANSMISSION
Neurotransmission, the conduction of impulses in the nervous system, occurs through the actions of neurons. Neuron activity may be provoked by touch or

(Text continues on page 260.)

Understanding the central nervous system

The central nervous system includes the brain and spinal cord. The brain consists of the cerebrum, cerebellum, brain stem, and primitive structures that lie below the cerebrum: the diencephalon, limbic system, and reticular activating system (RAS). The spinal cord serves as the primary pathway for messages traveling between peripheral areas of the body and the brain. It also mediates the reflex arc—the natural pathway used in a reflex action.

Cerebrum

The cerebrum consists of hemispheres joined by the corpus callosum, a mass of nerve fibers that allows communication between corresponding centers in the right and left hemispheres. Each hemisphere is divided into four lobes, based on anatomic landmarks and functional differences. The lobes are named for the cranial bones that lie over them (frontal, temporal, parietal, and occipital). The cerebral cortex, the thin surface layer of the cerebrum, is composed of gray matter (unmyelinated cell bodies). The cerebrum has a rolling surface made up of convolutions (gyri) and creases or fissures (sulci).

The frontal lobe influences personality, judgment, abstract reasoning, social behavior, language expression, and movement (in the motor portion). The temporal lobe controls hearing, language comprehension, and storage and recall of memories (although memories are stored throughout the brain). The parietal lobe interprets and integrates sensations, including pain, temperature, and touch. It also interprets size, shape, distance, and texture. The parietal lobe of the nondominant hemisphere, usually the right, is especially important for awareness of body schema (shape). The occipital lobe functions primarily in interpreting visual stimuli.

Brain

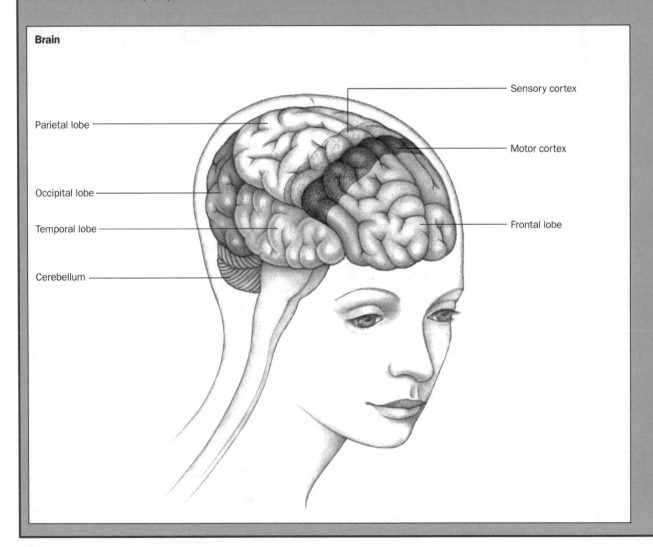

Cerebellum

The cerebellum, which consists of two hemispheres, maintains muscle tone, coordinates muscle movement, and controls balance.

Brain stem

Composed of the midbrain, pons, and medulla oblongata, the brain stem relays messages between upper and lower levels of the nervous system. The cranial nerves originate from the midbrain, pons, and medulla.

The pons connects the cerebellum with the cerebrum and connects the midbrain to the medulla oblongata. It contains one of the respiratory centers. The midbrain mediates the auditory and visual reflexes. The medulla oblongata regulates respiratory, vasomotor, and cardiac function.

Primitive structures

The diencephalon contains the thalamus and hypothalamus, which lie beneath the surface of the cerebral hemispheres. The thalamus relays all sensory stimuli (except olfactory) as they ascend to the cerebral cortex. Thalamic functions include primitive awareness of pain, screening of incoming stimuli, and focusing of attention. The hypothalamus controls or affects body temperature, appetite, water balance, pituitary secretions, emotions, and autonomic functions, including sleep and wake cycles.

The limbic system is a primitive brain area deep within the temporal lobe. Besides initiating primitive drives (hunger, aggression, and sexual and emotional arousal), the limbic system screens all sensory messages traveling to the cerebral cortex.

Reticular activating system

The reticular activating system (RAS), a diffuse network of hyperexcitable neurons fanning out from the brain stem through the cerebral cortex, screens all incoming sensory information and channels it to appropriate areas of the brain for interpretation. RAS activity also stimulates wakefulness; when RAS activity declines, the individual falls asleep.

Spinal cord

The spinal cord joins the brain stem at the level of the foramen magnum and terminates near the second lumbar vertebra.

A cross section of the spinal cord reveals a central H-shaped mass of gray matter divided into dorsal (posterior) and ventral (anterior) horns. Gray matter in the dorsal horns relays sensory (afferent) impulses; in the ventral horns, motor (efferent) impulses. White matter (myelinated axons of sensory and motor nerves) surrounds these horns and forms the ascending and descending tracts.

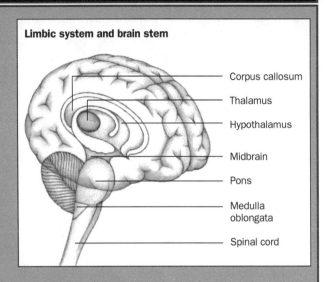

Limbic system and brain stem

- Corpus callosum
- Thalamus
- Hypothalamus
- Midbrain
- Pons
- Medulla oblongata
- Spinal cord

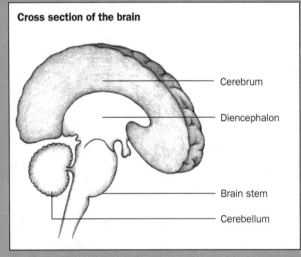

Cross section of the brain

- Cerebrum
- Diencephalon
- Brain stem
- Cerebellum

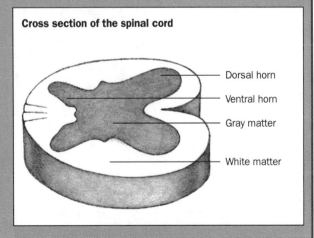

Cross section of the spinal cord

- Dorsal horn
- Ventral horn
- Gray matter
- White matter

Understanding the peripheral nervous system

The peripheral nervous system consists of the cranial nerves, the spinal nerves, and the autonomic nervous system.

Cranial nerves

The 12 pairs of cranial nerves (CNs) transmit motor or sensory messages, or both, primarily between the brain or brain stem and the head and neck. All cranial nerves, except for the olfactory and optic nerves, exit from the midbrain, pons, or medulla oblongata of the brain stem.

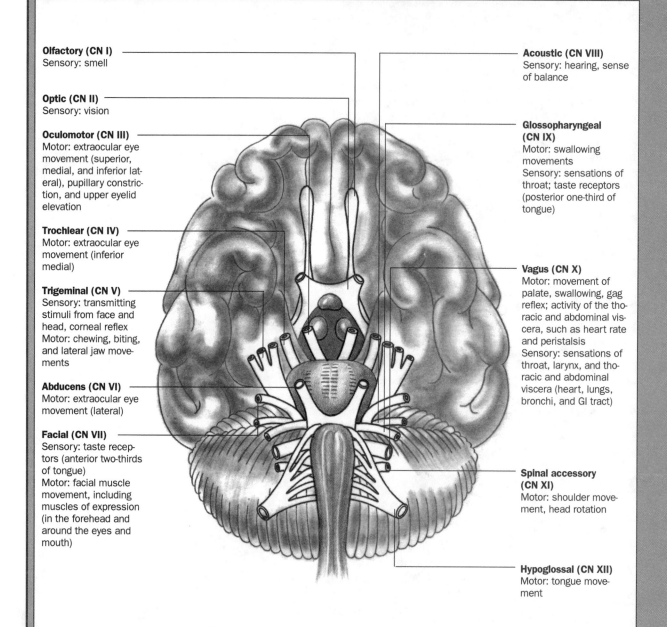

Olfactory (CN I)
Sensory: smell

Optic (CN II)
Sensory: vision

Oculomotor (CN III)
Motor: extraocular eye movement (superior, medial, and inferior lateral), pupillary constriction, and upper eyelid elevation

Trochlear (CN IV)
Motor: extraocular eye movement (inferior medial)

Trigeminal (CN V)
Sensory: transmitting stimuli from face and head, corneal reflex
Motor: chewing, biting, and lateral jaw movements

Abducens (CN VI)
Motor: extraocular eye movement (lateral)

Facial (CN VII)
Sensory: taste receptors (anterior two-thirds of tongue)
Motor: facial muscle movement, including muscles of expression (in the forehead and around the eyes and mouth)

Acoustic (CN VIII)
Sensory: hearing, sense of balance

Glossopharyngeal (CN IX)
Motor: swallowing movements
Sensory: sensations of throat; taste receptors (posterior one-third of tongue)

Vagus (CN X)
Motor: movement of palate, swallowing, gag reflex; activity of the thoracic and abdominal viscera, such as heart rate and peristalsis
Sensory: sensations of throat, larynx, and thoracic and abdominal viscera (heart, lungs, bronchi, and GI tract)

Spinal accessory (CN XI)
Motor: shoulder movement, head rotation

Hypoglossal (CN XII)
Motor: tongue movement

Spinal nerves

The 31 pairs of spinal nerves are named according to the vertebra immediately below the exit point from the spinal cord. Each spinal nerve consists of afferent (sensory) and efferent (motor) neurons, which carry messages to and from particular body regions, called dermatomes.

Autonomic nervous system

The vast autonomic nervous system (ANS) enervates all internal organs. Sometimes known as the visceral efferent nerves, the nerves of the ANS carry messages to the viscera from the brain stem and neuroendocrine system. The ANS has two major divisions: the sympathetic (thoracolumbar) nervous system and the parasympathetic (craniosacral) nervous system.

Sympathetic nervous system. Sympathetic nerves exit the spinal cord between the levels of the first thoracic and second lumbar vertebrae; hence the name thoracolumbar. Once these nerves, called preganglionic neurons, leave the spinal cord, they enter small relay stations (ganglia) near the cord. The ganglia form a chain that disseminates the impulse to postganglionic neurons. The postganglionic neurons reach many organs and glands and can produce widespread, generalized responses.

The physiologic effects of sympathetic activity include vasoconstriction; elevated blood pressure; enhanced blood flow to skeletal muscles; increased heart rate and contractility; heightened respiratory rate; smooth-muscle relaxation of the bronchioles, GI tract, and urinary tract; sphincter contraction; pupillary dilation and ciliary muscle relaxation; increased sweat gland secretion; and reduced pancreatic secretion.

Parasympathetic nervous system. The fibers of the parasympathetic nervous system (also called the craniosacral system) leave the central nervous system (CNS) by way of the cranial nerves from the midbrain and medulla, and also from the spinal nerves between the second and fourth sacral vertebrae (S2 to S4).

After leaving the CNS, the long preganglionic fiber of each parasympathetic nerve travels to a ganglion near a particular organ or gland; the short postganglionic fiber enters the organ or gland. This creates a more specific response involving only one organ or gland.

The physiologic effects of parasympathetic system activity include reduced heart rate, contractility, and conduction velocity; bronchial smooth-muscle constriction; increased GI tract tone and peristalsis with sphincter relaxation; urinary system sphincter relaxation and increased bladder tone; vasodilation of external genitalia, causing erection; pupillary constriction; and increased pancreatic, salivary, and lacrimal secretions. The parasympathetic system has little effect on mental or metabolic activity.

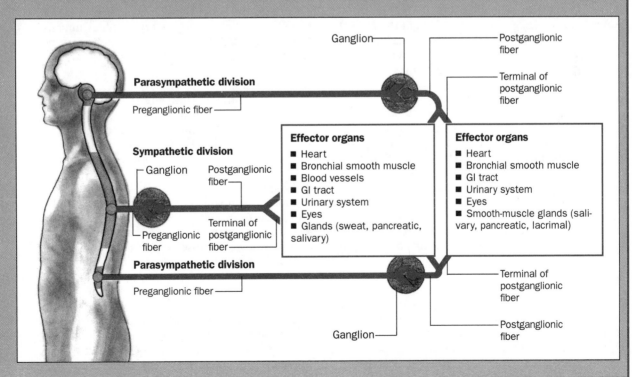

Parasympathetic division

Ganglion

Postganglionic fiber

Terminal of postganglionic fiber

Preganglionic fiber

Sympathetic division

Ganglion

Postganglionic fiber

Terminal of postganglionic fiber

Preganglionic fiber

Effector organs
- Heart
- Bronchial smooth muscle
- Blood vessels
- GI tract
- Urinary system
- Eyes
- Glands (sweat, pancreatic, salivary)

Effector organs
- Heart
- Bronchial smooth muscle
- GI tract
- Urinary system
- Eyes
- Smooth-muscle glands (salivary, pancreatic, lacrimal)

Parasympathetic division

Preganglionic fiber

Terminal of postganglionic fiber

Ganglion

Postganglionic fiber

pressure, heat or cold, external chemicals, or a chemical released by the body, such as histamine. On each neuron, treelike branches called dendrites reach out, detect stimuli, and carry the impulse to the cell body of the neuron. Then a long projection, called an axon, conducts the impulse away from the cell. Some axons are covered by a myelin sheath that allows more rapid impulse transmission.

When the impulse reaches the end of the axon, it stimulates synaptic vesicles in the presynaptic axon terminal to release a neurotransmitter substance into the synaptic cleft (the tiny space that separates one neuron from another). The neurotransmitter substance diffuses across the cleft and binds to special receptors on the cell membrane of the postsynaptic neuron. This stimulates or inhibits stimulation of the postsynaptic neuron.

MAJOR NEURAL PATHWAYS

Sensory impulses are carried to the brain for interpretation via the sensory (afferent or ascending) pathways. Motor impulses are transmitted from the brain to the muscles via the motor (efferent or descending) pathways.

Sensory impulses travel by two major pathways to the sensory cortex in the brain's parietal lobe. Pain and temperature sensations enter the spinal cord through the dorsal horn, then immediately cross over to the opposite side of the cord. These stimuli then travel to the thalamus via the spinothalamic tract. Tactile, pressure, and vibration sensations enter the cord via dorsal root ganglia. These stimuli then travel up the cord in the dorsal column to the medulla, where they cross to the opposite side and enter the thalamus. The thalamus relays all incoming sensory impulses, except olfactory ones, to the sensory cortex in the parietal lobe for interpretation.

Motor impulses that originate in the motor cortex of the frontal lobe reach the lower motor neurons of the peripheral nervous system via upper motor neurons of the pyramidal or extrapyramidal tract. In the pyramidal tract, impulses travel from the motor cortex through the internal capsule to the medulla, where they cross to the opposite side and continue down the spinal cord. In the anterior horn of the spinal cord, impulses are relayed to the lower motor neurons, which carry them via the spinal and peripheral nerves to the muscles, producing a motor response.

Motor impulses that regulate involuntary muscle tone and muscle control travel along the extrapyramidal tract from the promotor area of the frontal lobe to the pons of the brain stem, where they cross to the opposite side. The impulses then travel down the spinal cord to the anterior horn, where they are relayed to the lower motor neurons, which carry the impulses to the muscles.

REFLEX RESPONSES

These responses occur automatically, without any brain involvement, to protect the body. For example, if the brain can't send a message to a patient's leg after a severe spinal cord injury, a stimulus can still cause a knee jerk (patellar) reflex as long as the spinal cord remains intact at the level of the reflex. (See *How the reflex arc functions.*)

Assessment

A complete neurologic assessment helps confirm a suspected neurologic disorder. It establishes a clinical baseline and can offer lifesaving clues to rapid deterioration. Neurologic assessment includes a thorough patient history, a complete physical examination, and a neurologic examination that includes assessment of cerebral function, motor and sensory function, cranial nerves, and reflexes.

HISTORY

Begin by asking about the patient's chief complaint. Then gather details about his medical history, family history, and social history. Also perform a systems review.

Include the patient's family members or close friends when taking the history. Don't assume that the patient remembers details accurately; corroborate them with others to get a better picture.

CHIEF COMPLAINT

To determine the patient's chief complaint, ask why he has come to the health care facility or what's been bothering him. Document the chief complaint in the patient's own words. For the patient with a neurologic disorder, expect any of the following common complaints:
- headaches
- motor disturbances (including weakness, paresis, and paralysis) or seizures
- sensory deviations
- altered level of consciousness (LOC).

Ask the following questions to help the patient elaborate on his signs and symptoms:
- Do you have headaches? How often and when?
- Do you experience episodes of dizziness?
- Do you ever feel a tingling or prickling sensation or numbness anywhere in your body?
- Have you ever had seizures or tremors? Weakness or paralysis in your arms or legs?
- Do you have any difficulty urinating?

How the reflex arc functions

Spinal nerves, which have sensory and motor portions, mediate deep tendon and superficial reflexes. A simple reflex arc requires a sensory (afferent) neuron and a motor (efferent) neuron. The knee-jerk (patellar) reflex illustrates the sequence of events in a normal reflex arc.

First, a sensory receptor detects the mechanical stimulus produced by the reflex hammer striking the patellar tendon. Then, the sensory neuron carries the impulse along its axon via a spinal nerve to the dorsal root, where it enters the spinal cord.

Next, in the anterior horn of the spinal cord, the sensory neuron synapses with a motor neuron, which carries the impulse along its axon via a spinal nerve to the muscle. The motor neuron transmits the impulse to the muscle fibers via stimulation of the motor end plate. This triggers the muscle to contract and the leg to extend.

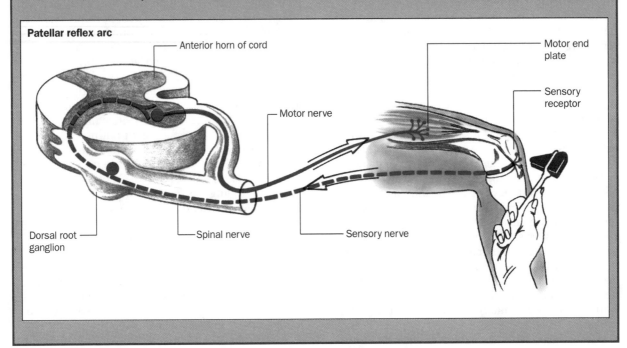

Patellar reflex arc

- Do you have trouble walking?
- How are your memory and ability to concentrate?
- Do you ever have trouble speaking or understanding something someone says to you?
- Do you have trouble reading or writing?

MEDICAL HISTORY

Explore all of the patient's previous major illnesses, recurrent minor illnesses, accidents or injuries, surgical procedures, and allergies. Also explore his health and dietary habits. Does he exercise daily? Does he smoke, drink alcohol, or use illicit drugs?

Ask the patient if he's taking any prescription or over-the-counter drugs. If so, document the name and dosage of each drug, the duration of therapy, and the reason for it. If the patient can't remember which medications he's taking, check those that he's carrying, examining the label and contents yourself.

FAMILY HISTORY

Information about the patient's family members may help uncover hereditary disorders. Ask about diabetes, cardiac or renal disease, high blood pressure, cancer, bleeding disorders, mental disorders, and stroke.

SOCIAL HISTORY

Always consider the patient's cultural and social background when planning his care. For example, what's his religion? Does he actively practice his beliefs? Also note the patient's education level and occupation: Does he have a stable or erratic employment history? Does he live alone or with someone? Does he have any hobbies? How does he view his illness? Assess the patient's self-image as you gather this information.

PHYSICAL EXAMINATION

A complete neurologic assessment provides information about five categories of neurologic function: cerebral function (including LOC, mental status, and language), cranial nerves, motor system and cerebellar function, sensory system, and reflexes. Complex and time-consuming, this assessment can take several hours to complete. Unless you work as a nurse practitioner, you probably won't perform a complete neurologic assessment.

In most cases, you'll perform a neurologic screening assessment. This type of assessment evaluates some of the key indicators of neurologic function and helps identify areas of dysfunction. A neurologic screening assessment usually includes:

- evaluation of LOC (including a brief mental status examination and evaluation of verbal responsiveness)
- selected cranial nerve (CN) assessment (usually CN II, III, IV, VI, X, and XI)
- motor screening (strength, movement, and gait)
- sensory screening (tactile and pain sensations in extremities).

If a screening assessment reveals areas of neurologic dysfunction, you must evaluate those areas in more detail. Finally, you may have to perform a brief neurologic assessment called a *neuro check*. It involves rapid, repeated evaluations of several key indicators of nervous system status: LOC, pupil size and response, verbal responsiveness, extremity strength and movement, and vital signs. After establishing baseline values, you'll be able to detect trends in the patient's neurologic function and transient changes that can be warning signs by regularly evaluating these key indicators.

Always begin with an assessment of cerebral function, including LOC. Because the brain's neurons are extremely sensitive to changes in their internal environment, cerebral dysfunction usually serves as the earliest sign of a developing CNS disorder.

CEREBRAL FUNCTION

Basic assessment of cerebral function includes LOC, communication and, briefly, mental status. Further assessment includes formal evaluation of language skills and a complete mental status evaluation.

Level of consciousness. Assess the patient's level of arousal and orientation. A fully awake patient is alert, with eyes open, and watching his environment. A less-awake patient appears drowsy, has reduced motor activity, and seems less attentive to environmental stimuli. Decreased arousal often precedes disorientation.

Begin by quietly observing the patient's behavior. Is he awake, dozing, or asleep? Moving about or motionless? If awake, what is he doing: resting quietly, watching TV, talking with a visitor, or fidgeting? If the patient is dozing or sleeping, attempt to arouse him by providing an appropriate auditory, tactile, or painful stimulus, in that sequence. Always start with a minimal stimulus.

Speak the patient's name in a normal tone. If he doesn't respond, touch him gently, squeeze his hand, or shake his shoulder.

Use painful stimuli only to assess an unconscious patient or one with a markedly decreased LOC who doesn't respond to other stimuli. To test response to pain, you can apply firm pressure over a nail bed with a blunt hard object, such as a pen, or firmly pinch the Achilles tendon between your thumb and index finger. Never use a pin stick (which can spread infection), pinch a nipple, or rub the sternum, all of which can cause bruising or another injury.

Next, note the type and intensity of stimulus required to get a response. Is the patient's response an appropriate verbal one, unintelligible mumbling, body movement, eye opening, or nothing at all? After you remove the stimulus, how alert is the patient? Wide awake? Drowsy? Drifting to sleep?

After assessing the patient's level of arousal, compare your findings with results of previous assessments. Note any trends; for example, is the patient lethargic more often than usual? Consider any factors that could affect his responsiveness; for example, a normally alert patient may become drowsy after receiving a CNS depressant.

Many clinicians use subjective terms to describe level of arousal, but objective terms are best—for example, to describe lethargy: "awakened when called loudly, then immediately fell asleep."

Assess the patient's orientation—ability of the cerebral cortex to receive and accurately interpret sensory stimuli—which includes three aspects: orientation to time, place, and person. Always ask questions that require information, rather than a yes or no answer.

- *Time.* If oriented to time, most people can state the correct year, month and, usually, date. Most can also differentiate day from night if there's a window. Disorientation to time is one of the first indicators of decreasing LOC.
- *Place.* When he looks around the room, can he conclude that he's in a health care facility? Or does he think he's at home?
- *Person.* Ask him his name and note the response. Self-identity usually remains intact until late in decreasing LOC, making disorientation to person an ominous sign.

To minimize the subjectivity and increase the reliability of LOC assessment, you may use the Glasgow Coma Scale of three objective behaviors: eye opening, verbal responsiveness (which includes orientation), and motor response. (See *Using the Glasgow Coma Scale*.)

Communication. Assess the patient's ability to comprehend speech, writing, numbers, and gestures. Language skills include learning and recalling words, using proper grammar, and structuring message content logically. Speech involves neuromuscular actions of the mouth, tongue, and oropharynx. During the interview and physical assessment, observe the patient's responses.

■ If you suspect a decreased LOC, call the patient's name or gently shake his shoulder to elicit a verbal response.

■ Note how much he says. Does he speak in complete sentences? In phrases? In single words? Does he communicate spontaneously? Or does he rarely speak?

■ Note the quality of his speech. Is it unusually loud or soft? Does he speak clearly, or are his words garbled? What is the rate and rhythm of his speech? If you don't speak his language, seek help from an interpreter or a family member.

■ Are the patient's verbal responses appropriate? Does he have problems finding or articulating words? Does he use made-up words (neologisms)?

■ Can the patient understand and follow commands? Multistep commands?

■ If communication problems arise, is he aware of them? Does he appear frustrated or angry? Does he continue, unaware that you don't comprehend?

■ If you suspect a language difficulty, show the patient a common object, such as a cup or a book, and ask him to name it. Or ask him to repeat a word, such as "dog" or "breakfast."

If the patient appears to have difficulty understanding spoken language, ask him to follow a simple instruction, such as "Touch your nose." If the patient succeeds, try a two-step command, such as "Touch your right knee; then touch your nose."

Keep in mind that language performance tends to fluctuate with the time of day and with changes in physical condition. A healthy individual may experience language difficulty when fatigued. However, increasing language difficulties may indicate deteriorating neurologic status, warranting further evaluation and notification of the doctor.

Impaired language function occurs in dysphasia (impaired ability to use or understand language) or aphasia (inability to use or understand language, or both). Speech problems include articulation difficulties and slurred speech, which may result from facial muscle paralysis. Neuromuscular speech impairment is called dysarthria; voice impairment is called dysphonia.

Using the Glasgow Coma Scale

Originally designed to help predict a patient's survival and recovery after a head injury, the Glasgow Coma Scale assesses level of consciousness (LOC). It minimizes the use of subjective impressions to evaluate LOC by testing and scoring three observations: eye response, motor response, and response to verbal stimuli.

Each response receives a point value. If the patient is alert, can follow simple commands, and is completely oriented to time, person, and place, his score will total 15 points. If the patient is comatose, his score will total 7 or less. A score of 3, the lowest possible score, indicates deep coma and a poor prognosis.

Many health care facilities display the Glasgow Coma Scale on neurologic flowsheets to show changes in the patient's LOC over time.

Observation	Response elicited	Score
EYE RESPONSE	Opens spontaneously	4
	Opens to verbal command	3
	Opens to pain	2
	No response	1
MOTOR RESPONSE	Reacts to verbal command	6
	Reacts to painful stimuli:	
	– Identifies localized pain	5
	– Flexes and withdraws	4
	– Assumes flexor posture	3
	– Assumes extensor posture	2
	No response	1
VERBAL RESPONSE	Is oriented and converses	5
	Is disoriented but converses	4
	Uses inappropriate words	3
	Makes incomprehensible sounds	2
	No response	1

To evaluate the patient's formal language skills, identify the extent and characteristics of his language deficits. Usually performed by a speech pathologist, evaluation may help pinpoint the site of a CNS lesion. For example, identifying expressive aphasia (the patient knows what he wants to say but can't speak the words) may help diagnose a frontal lobe lesion.

If you evaluate the patient's language skills, include:

■ *Spontaneous speech.* After showing the patient a picture, ask him to describe what's going on.

■ *Comprehension.* Ask a series of simple yes-or-no questions and evaluate his answers. Use questions

Mental status screening questions

As part of a neurologic screening assessment, ask the following questions to help identify patients with disordered thought processes. An incorrect answer to any question may indicate a need for a complete mental status examination.

Question	Function screened
What is your name?	Orientation to person
What is today's date?	Orientation to time
What year is it?	Orientation to time
Where are you now?	Orientation to place
How old are you?	Memory
Where were you born?	Remote memory
What did you have for breakfast?	Recent memory
Who is the U.S. president?	General knowledge
Can you count backwards from 20 to 1?	Attention and calculation skills
Why are you here?	Judgment

with obvious answers, for example: "Does it snow in July?" or "Are your pants on fire?"

■ *Naming.* Show the patient various common objects, one at a time, and then ask him to name each one. Typical objects include a comb, a ball, a cup, and a pencil.

■ *Repetition.* Ask him to repeat words or phrases, such as "no ifs, ands, or buts."

■ *Vocabulary.* Have the patient explain the meaning of each of a series of words.

■ *Reading.* Ask him to read printed words on cards and perform the action described, for example: "Raise your hand."

■ *Writing.* Ask the patient to write something, perhaps a story describing a scene or a picture.

■ *Copying figures.* Show the patient several figures, one at a time, and then ask him to copy them. The figures usually become increasingly complex, starting with a circle, an X, and a square and proceeding to a triangle and a star.

Mental status. Performed by a doctor or specially trained nurse, a complete mental status examination provides information about the patient's cognitive, psychological, and intellectual skills. Usually, only a chronically disoriented patient or one with suspected mental status deficits will undergo the complete test.

To identify the need for more in-depth evaluation, you may perform an abbreviated version of the complete mental status examination. This brief screening proves useful if a patient's responses to interview questions seem unreliable or indicate a possible disturbance of memory or cognitive processes. (See *Mental status screening questions.*)

CRANIAL NERVES

CN assessment provides valuable information about the condition of the CNS, particularly the brain stem. Because of their anatomic locations, some cranial nerves are more vulnerable to the effects of increasing intracranial pressure (ICP). Therefore, a neurologic screening assessment of the cranial nerves focuses on these key nerves: the optic (II), oculomotor (III), trochlear (IV), and abducens (VI). Evaluate the other nerves only if the patient's history or symptoms indicate a potential CN disorder or when performing a complete nervous system assessment. (See *Assessing cranial nerves,* pages 265 to 267.)

MOTOR FUNCTION

This portion of the assessment evaluates the ability of the cerebral cortex to plan and initiate motor activity of the pyramidal and extrapyramidal pathways. It also evaluates the ability of the corticospinal tracts to carry motor messages down the spinal cord, of the lower motor neurons to carry efferent impulses to the muscles, and of the muscles to carry out motor commands. Finally, it helps to assess the ability of the cerebellum and basal ganglia to coordinate and fine-tune movement.

A screening assessment always includes examination of the patient's muscle strength (including muscle size and symmetry), arm and leg movement, and gait. Gait reflects the integrated activity of muscle strength and tone, extremity movement and coordination, balance, proprioception (sense of position), and the ability of the cerebral cortex to plan and sequence movements.

Patients who need a complete neurologic examination or who display a motor deficit during the screening assessment may undergo a complete motor system assessment. When performing a complete assessment, proceed from head to toe (for example, moving from the neck to the shoulders, arms, trunk, hips, and finally to the legs), assessing all muscles of the major joints. Then assess the patient's gait and cerebellar functions (balance and coordination).

(Text continues on page 269.)

Assessing cranial nerves

Assessment techniques	Normal findings	Abnormal findings
OLFACTORY (CN I) After checking the patency of both nostrils, have the patient close both eyes. Then occlude one nostril, and hold a familiar, pungent-smelling substance, such as vanilla, tobacco, soap, or peppermint, under his nose and ask its identity. Repeat this technique with the other nostril. If the patient reports detecting the smell but cannot name it, offer a choice, such as, "Do you smell lemon, coffee, or peppermint?"	The patient should be able to detect and identify the smell correctly.	The location of the olfactory nerve makes it especially vulnerable to damage from facial fractures and head injuries. Disorders of the base of the frontal lobe, such as tumors or arteriosclerotic changes, also can damage the nerve. The sense of smell remains intact as long as one of the two olfactory nerves exists; it's permanently lost (anosmia) if both nerves are affected. Anosmia also may result from nonneurologic causes, such as nasal congestion, sinus infection, smoking, or cocaine use. Anosmia also impairs the sense of taste. A complaint about food taste may signal olfactory nerve damage.

OPTIC (CN II) AND OCULOMOTOR (CN III)
To assess the optic nerve, check visual acuity, visual fields, and the retinal structures. To assess the oculomotor nerve, check pupil size, pupil shape, and pupillary response to light. When assessing pupil size, be especially alert for any trends. For example, watch for a gradual increase in the size of one pupil or the appearance of unequal pupils in a patient whose pupils were previously equal.
	The pupils should be equal, round, and reactive to light.	A visual field defect may signal cerebrovascular accident (CVA), head injury, or brain tumor. The area and extent of the loss depend on the location of the lesion. In a blind patient with a nonfunctional optic nerve, light stimulation will fail to produce either a direct or a consensual pupillary response. However, a legally blind patient may have some optic nerve function, which causes the blind eye to respond to direct light. In a patient who is totally blind in only one eye, the pupil of the eye with the intact optic nerve will react to direct light stimulation, whereas the blind eye, because it receives sensory messages from the functional optic nerve, will respond consensually.
		    Increased intracranial pressure (ICP) can put pressure on the oculomotor nerve, causing a change in responsiveness or pupil size on the affected side. If pressure continues to rise, the other oculomotor nerve becomes affected, causing both pupils to change in size and responsiveness. Rising ICP can cause the pupils to become oval or react sluggishly to light shortly before dilating.
		    The hippus phenomenon—brisk pupil constriction in response to light followed by a pulsating dilation and constriction—may be normal in some individuals but may also reflect early oculomotor nerve compression.

OCULOMOTOR (CN III), TROCHLEAR (CN IV), AND ABDUCENS (CN VI) To test the coordinated function of these three nerves, assess them simultaneously by evaluating the patient's extraocular eye movement. Observe each eye for rapid oscillation (nystagmus), movement not in unison with that of the other eye (dysconjugate movement), or inability to move in certain directions (ophthalmoplegia). Also note any complaint of double vision (diplopia).	The eyes should move smoothly and in a coordinated manner through all six directions of eye movement.	Nystagmus may indicate a disorder of the brain stem, the cerebellum, or the vestibular portion of the acoustic nerve (CN VIII). It can also imply drug toxicity, as from the anticonvulsant phenytoin. Increased ICP can put pressure on the trochlear nerve (CN IV), causing impaired extraocular eye movement inferiorly and medially. Increased ICP also can put pressure on the abducens nerve (CN VI), causing impaired extraocular eye movement laterally.

(continued)

Assessing cranial nerves *(continued)*

Assessment techniques	Normal findings	Abnormal findings
TRIGEMINAL (CN V) To assess the sensory portion of this nerve, gently touch the right, then the left side of the patient's forehead with a cotton ball while his eyes are closed. Instruct him to tell you the moment the cotton touches the area. Compare his response on both sides. Repeat the technique on the right and left cheek and on the right and left jaw. Next, repeat the entire procedure using a sharp object. The cap of a disposable ballpoint pen can be used to test light touch (dull end) and sharp stimuli (sharp end). If an abnormality appears, also test for temperature sensation by touching the patient's skin with test tubes filled with hot and cold water and asking him to differentiate between them.)	The patient should report feeling both light touch and sharp stimuli in all three areas (forehead, cheek, and jaw) on both sides of the face.	Peripheral nerve damage can create a loss of sensation in any or all of the three regions supplied by the trigeminal nerve (forehead, cheek, jaw). A lesion in the cervical spinal cord or brain stem can produce impaired sensory function in all three areas.
To assess the motor portion of the trigeminal nerve, ask the patient to clench his jaws. Palpate the temporal and masseter muscles bilaterally, checking for symmetry. Try to open his clenched jaws. Next, watch him opening and closing his mouth for asymmetry.	The jaws should clench symmetrically and remain closed against resistance.	A lesion in the cervical spinal cord or brain stem can produce impaired motor function in regions supplied by the trigeminal nerve, weakening the jaw muscles, causing the jaw to deviate toward the affected side when chewing, and allowing residual food to collect in the affected cheek.
To assess the corneal reflex, stroke a wisp of cotton lightly across a cornea.	The lids of both eyes should close.	An absent corneal reflex may result from peripheral nerve or brain stem damage. However, a diminished corneal reflex commonly occurs in patients who wear contact lenses.
FACIAL (CN VII) To test the motor portion of this nerve, ask the patient to wrinkle his forehead, raise and lower his eyebrows, smile to show teeth, and puff out his cheeks. Also, with the patient's eyes tightly closed, attempt to open the eyelids. With each of these movements, observe closely for symmetry.	Facial movements should be symmetrical.	Unilateral facial weakness can reflect an upper motor neuron problem, such as a CVA or a tumor that has damaged neurons in the facial control area of the motor strip in the cerebral cortex. If the weakness originates in the cerebral cortex, the patient will retain the ability to wrinkle his forehead because the forehead receives motor messages from both hemispheres of the brain—which explains why when one side is damaged, as in a CVA, the other side takes over. However, if the facial nerve itself is damaged, the weakness will extend to the forehead, and the eye on the affected side will not close.
To test the sensory portion of the facial nerve, which supplies taste sensation to the anterior two-thirds of the tongue, first prepare four marked, closed containers, with one containing salt, another sugar, a third, vinegar (or lemon), and a fourth, quinine (or bitters). Then, with the patient's eyes closed, place salt on the anterior two-thirds of his tongue using a cotton swab or dropper. Ask him to identify the taste as sweet, salty, sour, or bitter. Rinse his mouth with water. Repeat this procedure, alternating flavors and sides of the tongue until all four flavors have been tested on both sides. Taste sensations to the posterior third of the tongue are supplied by the glossopharyngeal nerve (CN IX) and are usually tested at the same time.	The patient should have symmetrical taste sensations.	An impaired sense of taste can signify damage to the facial or glossopharyngeal nerve, or it may simply reflect a part of the normal aging process. Chemotherapy or head and neck radiation can also alter taste by damaging taste bud receptors.

Assessing cranial nerves *(continued)*

Assessment techniques	Normal findings	Abnormal findings
ACOUSTIC (CN VIII) To assess the acoustic portion of this nerve, test the patient's hearing acuity. To assess the vestibular portion of this nerve, observe for nystagmus and disturbed balance and note reports of dizziness or room spinning	The patient should be able to hear a whispered voice or a watch ticking. He should have normal eye movement and balance and no dizziness or vertigo.	Hearing loss, nystagmus, disturbance of balance, and dizziness all can indicate acoustic nerve damage.
GLOSSOPHARYNGEAL (CN IX) AND VAGUS (CN X) To assess these nerves, which have overlapping functions, first listen to the patient's voice for indications of a hoarse or nasal quality. Then watch his soft palate when he says "ah." Next, test the gag reflex after warning him. To evoke this reflex, touch the posterior wall of the pharynx with a cotton swab or tongue blade.	The patient's voice should be strong and clear. The soft palate and uvula should rise when he says "ah" and the uvula should remain midline. The palatine arches should remain symmetrical during movement and at rest. The gag reflex should be intact. If it diminishes or the pharynx moves asymmetrically, evaluate the posterior pharyngeal wall to confirm integrity of both cranial nerves.	Glossopharyngeal neuralgia produces paroxysmal pain, which radiates from the throat to the ear. Damage to the glossopharyngeal or vagus nerves impairs swallowing. Furthermore, during swallowing, the palate fails to rise and close off the nasal passageways, allowing nasal regurgitation of fluids. A damaged vagus nerve also can cause loss of the gag reflex and a hoarse or nasal-sounding voice. Finally, because the vagus nerve innervates most viscera through the parasympathetic nervous system, vagal damage can affect involuntary vital functions, producing various disturbances, such as tachycardia, other cardiac arrhythmias, and dyspnea.
SPINAL ACCESSORY (CN XI) Press down on the patient's shoulders while he attempts to shrug against this resistance. Note shoulder strength and symmetry while inspecting and palpating the trapezius muscle. Then apply resistance to his turned head while he attempts to return to a midline position. Note neck strength while inspecting and palpating the sternocleidomastoid muscle. Repeat for the opposite side.	Both shoulders should be able to overcome the resistance equally well. The neck should overcome resistance in both directions.	Unilateral weakness, atrophy, or paralysis of the muscles innervated by the spinal accessory nerve suggests a peripheral nerve lesion. Signs include a drooping shoulder or a scapula that appears displaced toward the affected side.

HYPOGLOSSAL (CN XII)
To assess this nerve, observe the patient's protruded tongue for deviation from midline, atrophy, or fasciculation (fine muscle flickerings indicating lower motor neuron disease).
    Next, instruct the patient to move his tongue rapidly from side to side with the mouth open, to curl his tongue up toward the nose, and to curl his tongue down toward the chin. Then apply resistance to his protruded tongue, using a tongue blade or folded gauze, and ask him to try to push the blade to one side. Repeat on the other side and note the patient's tongue strength.
    Listen to the patient's speech for the sounds *d, l, n,* and *t,* which require use of the tongue to articulate. If his general speech suggests a problem, have him repeat a phrase or a series of words containing these sounds.
	The tongue should be midline, and the patient should be able to move it right and left equally. He also should be able to move the tongue up and down. Pressure exerted by the tongue on the tongue blade should be equal on either side. Speech should be clear.	A peripheral nerve lesion creates a unilateral flaccid paralysis of the tongue, atrophy of the affected side, and deviation of the tongue. A unilateral spastic paralysis of the tongue produces poorly articulated, difficult speech (dysarthria) characterized by an explosive production of words. The tongue deviates toward the unaffected side.

Assessing cerebellar function

Evaluate cerebellar function by assessing balance and coordination.

Balance

To perform this part of the assessment, have the patient perform tandem-gait heel-to-toe walking, the Romberg test, and heel-and-toe walking.

Tandem-gait heel-to-toe walking. Ask the patient to walk heel-to-toe in a straight line, as shown. If she is weak or elderly, stand close by to prevent her from falling. Observe for normal coordination and balance. If she leans or falls to one side, note the direction. When performing heel-to-toe walking, she will tend to lean or fall toward the side of the lesion. If the lesion is midline, she won't be able to perform heel-to-toe walking and will display a wide-based, ataxic gait.

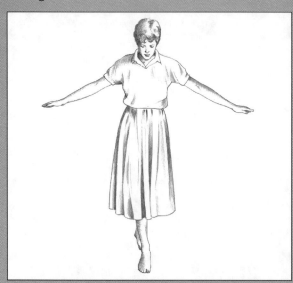

Romberg test. Have the patient stand with her feet together, arms at her sides, and without support. Observe her ability to maintain balance with both eyes open and then with them closed. (Stand nearby in case she loses her balance.) Normally, a small amount of swaying occurs when the eyes are closed.

Note any abnormal problems with balance. When asked to perform the Romberg test, the patient experiencing cerebellar ataxia will have trouble maintaining a steady position with eyes opened or closed. In a positive Romberg test, she'll be able to stand with eyes open but will lose her balance with eyes closed. This indicates damage to the dorsal columns of the spinal cord, which interferes with sense of position in space. If the patient has difficulty with the Romberg test, don't perform further balance testing.

Heel-and-toe walking. First ask the patient to walk on her heels. Then have her walk on her toes. Observe balance, coordination, and ankle strength during both procedures. Note any deviation from the normal ability to walk steadily on the heels and toes.

Coordination

Evaluate the patient's ability to perform rapid alternating movements, the leg coordination test, and point-to-point localization.

Rapid alternating movements. Begin with the arms. Have the seated patient pat one thigh with one hand as rapidly as possible. Then test the other arm, noting speed and rhythm.

Next, have the patient place an open palm on one thigh and then turn her hand over, touching her thigh with the top of her hand, as shown below. Have her repeat this pronation and supination of the hand as rapidly as possible. Note the speed and the degree of effort in performing the maneuver.

Have the patient use the thumb of one hand to touch each finger of the same hand in rapid sequence. Repeat with the other hand. The nondominant hand will perform rapid alternating movement tasks more slowly than the dominant hand.

To assess the legs, have the patient rapidly tap the floor with the ball of one foot. Test each leg separately. Note any slowness or awkwardness in performing rapid alternating movements. Such abnormalities can reflect cerebellar disease or motor weakness associated with extrapyramidal disease.

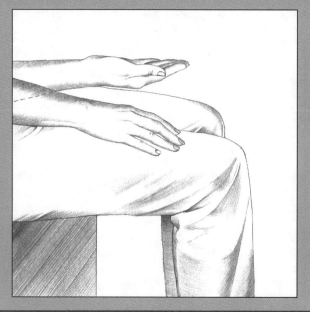

Leg coordination. Have the patient lie supine and place one heel on the shin of her opposite leg just below the knee. Then have her slowly slide her heel along her shin toward her ankle. Repeat with the other leg. Note her ability to position each heel on her shin accurately as well as the ease, speed, and accuracy with which she can move her heel down the shin.

Point-to-point localization. Have the patient stand or sit with her arms extended and then touch her nose. Have her perform the test with both eyes open, and then with them closed.

Next, hold one index finger in front of the patient and ask her to touch it with her index finger. Repeat the maneuver at various positions, as shown. Evaluate her ability to adjust.

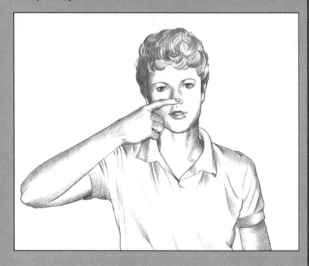

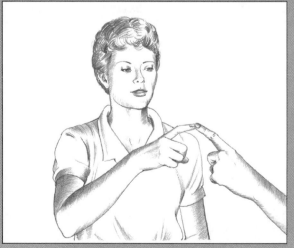

When assessing arm strength, never use hand grasps. The primitive grasp reflex may return with brain dysfunction (especially with frontal lobe involvement), making hand grasps an unreliable indicator. Instead, assess arm strength by asking the patient to push you away as you apply resistance. If this test suggests mild weakness in one arm, confirm your suspicions by evaluating for downward drift and pronation of the arm. To do this, ask the patient to extend both arms, palms up. Then ask him to close his eyes and maintain this position for 20 to 30 seconds. Observe for downward drifting and pronation (palm-down movement) of the arm, which may occur if the patient can't rely on visual clues to keep the weak arm raised.

Assess the patient's movement in response to a command. Instruct the weak patient to open and close each fist or to move each arm without raising it off the bed or examination table. If he fails to respond, observe for spontaneous movements of the arm. For example, note whether the patient uses it for grooming, eating, personal hygiene, or positioning.

If the patient makes no spontaneous movements, use tactile stimuli. Begin with a gentle touch or tickle on the arm. If the patient does not move the arm, use a stronger stimulus. Does he attempt to withdraw the arm or try to push the stimulus away (a purposeful response)? Or does he extend or flex the arm in an abnormal or unusual position (a nonpurposeful response)?

Assess leg movement by first asking the patient to move each leg and foot. If he fails, observe for spontaneous movement. If all else fails and he requires a stimulus stronger than a light touch, press the Achilles tendon firmly between your thumb and index finger. Again, observe for purposeful or nonpurposeful movement.

Remain alert for any involuntary movement of the limbs, trunk, or face. Determine whether the movement is proximal or distal and whether it occurs during sleep. Further assess any involuntary movements for rhythm or repetition, noting the number of repetitions per minute or second. Also note whether the involuntary movement increases, decreases, or stays the same in relation to normal movements and whether other factors appear to exacerbate or alleviate the abnormal movement.

Muscle tone and cerebellar function. For a description of how to assess muscle tone (the underlying tension in the muscle at all times), see Chapter 13, Musculoskeletal disorders. To evaluate cerebellar function, test the patient's balance and coordination. (See *Assessing cerebellar function.*)

SENSORY SYSTEM

This portion of the assessment evaluates how well the sensory receptors detect a stimulus, how well the afferent nerves carry sensory nerve impulses to the spinal cord, and the ability of the sensory tracts in the spinal cord to carry sensory messages to the brain. You'll also assess the sensory, interpretive, and integrative functions of the cerebral cortex.

Basic screening usually evaluates light-touch sensation in all extremities and compares arms and legs for symmetry of sensation. Some experts also recommend assessing the patient's sense of pain and vibration in the hands and feet as well as his ability to recognize objects by touch (stereognosis).

Because the sensory system becomes fatigued with repeated stimulation, complete sensory system testing in all dermatomes tends to give unreliable results. A few screening procedures usually can reveal any dysfunctions.

■ Before beginning, ask about numbness or unusual sensations. Such areas require special attention.

■ With the patient's eyes closed, ask him to say "yes" or "now" when he feels you lightly touch his forearm with a cotton wisp. Allow time for his response, and then lightly touch the same area on his other arm.

■ Compare sensations bilaterally, on his upper arm, back of the hand, thigh, lower leg, and top of the foot. Occasionally skip an area to test the reliability of his responses; be sure to complete the sequence.

■ Be alert for complaints of numbness, tingling, or unusual sensations that accompany the tactile stimulus. Also note the degree of stimulation required. A light, brief touch should evoke a response.

■ If the patient experiences a localized deficit, numbness, or an unpleasant sensation (dysesthesia), perform a complete sensory assessment including two-point discrimination, temperature sensation, position sense, point localization, number identification, superficial pain response to vibration, extinction, and stereognosis.

■ Perform a complete neurologic assessment for a patient with motor or reflex abnormalities or trophic skin changes, such as ulceration, atrophy, or absent sweating.

REFLEXES

Assessment of deep tendon and superficial reflexes reveals the integrity of the sensory receptor organ and evaluates how well afferent nerves relay sensory messages to the spinal cord. It also evaluates how well the spinal cord or brain stem segment mediates the reflex, how well the lower motor neurons transmit messages to the muscles, and how well the muscles respond to the motor message. It's usually reserved for a complete neurologic assessment. (See *Assessing reflexes*, pages 271 and 272.)

You'll also indirectly glean information about the presence or absence of inhibiting brain messages. These messages travel along the corticospinal tract to modify reflex strength.

Reflexes fall into one of three groups: deep tendon, superficial, and pathologic superficial reflexes.

Deep tendon reflexes. These reflexes, also called muscle-stretch reflexes, occur when a sudden stimulus causes the muscle to stretch. Before eliciting this reflex, make sure the patient is relaxed and comfortable because tension or anxiety may diminish the reflex.

Superficial reflexes. You may elicit superficial (also called cutaneous) reflexes, with light, rapid, tactile stimulation, such as stroking or scratching the skin.

Pathologic superficial reflexes. Sometimes called primitive reflexes, these reflexes usually occur in early infancy and disappear with maturity. In adults, pathologic superficial reflexes—such as Babinski's reflex—usually indicate an underlying nervous system disease.

Use a grading scale to rate each reflex. Then document the rating for each reflex at the appropriate site on a stick-figure drawing.

VITAL SIGNS

The CNS, primarily by way of the brain stem and autonomic nervous system, controls the body's vital functions: heart rate and rhythm; respiratory rate, depth, and pattern; blood pressure; and body temperature. However, because these vital control centers lie deep within the cerebral hemispheres and in the brain stem, changes in vital signs (temperature, pulse rate, respiration, and blood pressure) aren't usually early indicators of CNS deterioration. When evaluating the significance of vital sign changes, consider each sign individually as well as in relation to the others.

Temperature. Damage to the hypothalamus or upper brain stem can impair the body's ability to maintain a constant temperature, resulting in profound hypothermia (temperature below 94° F [34.4° C]) or hyperthermia (temperature above 106° F [41.1° C]). Such damage can result from petechial hemorrhages in the hypothalamus or brain stem, trauma (causing pressure, twisting, or traction), or destructive lesions.

Pulse rate. Because the autonomic nervous system controls heart rate and rhythm, pressure on the brain stem and cranial nerves slows the pulse rate by stimulating the vagus nerve.

Bradycardia occurs in the later stages of increasing ICP and usually accompanies a rising systolic blood

Assessing reflexes

You'll use distinct procedures to test each deep tendon, superficial, and pathologic superficial reflex. Reflex assessment helps evaluate the intactness of specific cervical (C), thoracic (T), lumbar (L), and sacral (S) spinal segments. These segments are listed in parentheses after the appropriate reflex.

Deep tendon reflexes

These include the biceps, triceps, brachioradialis, quadriceps, and Achilles reflexes.

Biceps reflex (C5, C6). Have the patient partially flex one arm at the elbow, with the palm facing down. Place your thumb or finger over the biceps tendon. Then tap lightly over your finger with the reflex hammer. An impulse from the tapping should travel to the biceps tendon and cause brisk elbow flexion that's visible and palpable.

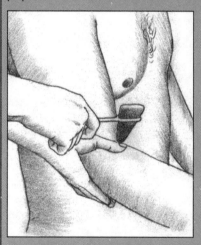

Triceps reflex (C7, C8). Have the patient partially flex one arm at the elbow with the palm facing the body. Support the arm and pull it slightly across the patient's chest. Using a direct blow with the reflex hammer, tap the triceps tendon at its insertion (about 1″ to 2″ [2.5 to 5 cm] above the elbow on the olecranon process of the ulnar bone). Normally, this action causes brisk extension of the elbow with visible and palpable contraction of the triceps muscle.

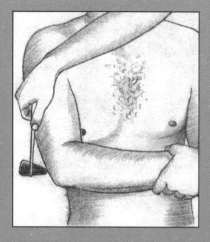

Brachioradialis (supinator) reflex (C5, C6). Position the patient with one arm flexed at the elbow, palm down, and resting in the lap or, if he's lying down, against the abdomen. Then tap the styloid process of the radius with the reflex hammer, about 1″ to 2″ above the wrist. Normally, this action causes elbow flexion, forearm supination, and finger and hand flexion.

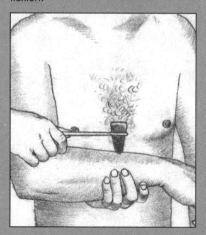

Quadriceps (knee-jerk or patellar) reflex (L2, L3, L4). Seat the patient with his lower legs dangling over the side of the examination table, or place him in the supine position. (For the supine patient, place your hand under his knee, slightly raising and flexing it.) Then tap the patellar tendon with the reflex hammer. The patient's knee should extend and the quadriceps should contract.

Achilles (ankle-jerk) reflex (S1, S2). First, position the patient with his knee bent and his ankle dorsiflexed. For best results, have him sit with his legs dangling from the examination table. Then tap the Achilles tendon, which should cause plantar flexion followed by muscle relaxation.

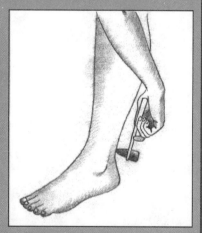

Superficial reflexes

These include the pharyngeal, abdominal, and cremasteric reflexes as well as the anal and bulbocavernous reflexes. Assess the last two, known as perineal reflexes, only in patients with suspected sacral spinal cord or sacral spinal nerve disorders.

(continued)

Assessing reflexes *(continued)*

Pharyngeal reflex (CN IX, CN X). Have the patient open his mouth wide. Then touch the posterior wall of the pharynx with a tongue blade. Normally, this will cause the patient to gag.

Abdominal reflex (T8, T9, T10). Use a fingernail or the tip of the handle of the reflex hammer to stroke one side, and then the opposite side, of the patient's abdomen above the umbilicus. Repeat on the lower abdomen. Normally, the abdominal muscles contract and the umbilicus deviates toward the stimulated side.

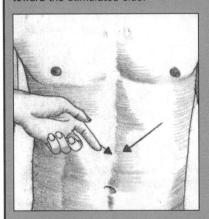

Cremasteric reflex (L1, L2). In a male patient, use a tongue blade to scratch the inner aspect of each thigh gently. This should cause elevation of the testicles.

Anal reflex (S3, S4, S5). Gently scratch the skin at the side of the anus with a blunt instrument, such as a tongue blade or gloved finger. Look for puckering of the anus, a normal response.

Bulbocavernous reflex (S3, S4). In a male patient, apply direct pressure over the bulbocavernous muscle behind the scrotum and gently pinch the foreskin or glans. This action should cause the bulbocavernous muscle to contract.

Pathologic superficial reflexes
These reflexes include the grasp, sucking, snout, and Babinski reflexes. They indicate central nervous system damage.

Grasp reflex. Stimulate the palm of the patient's hand with your fingers. (Because a lack of inhibition by the brain can cause the patient to squeeze very tightly, avoid finger injury or pain by crossing your middle and index fingers before placing them in his palm.) In a positive grasp reflex, the patient's hand will grasp yours upon stimulation, indicating frontal lobe damage, bilateral thalamic degeneration, or cerebral degeneration or atrophy.

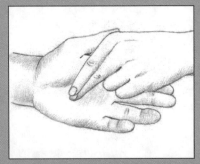

Sucking reflex. Stimulate the patient's lips with a mouth swab. A sucking movement on stimulation can indicate cerebral degeneration.

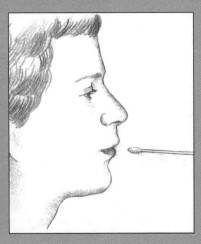

Snout reflex. Gently percuss the oral area with your fingers. This action may make the patient's lips pucker, indicating cerebral degeneration or late-stage dementia.

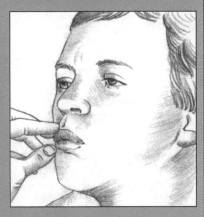

Babinski reflex. Stroke the lateral aspect of the sole of the patient's foot. A positive Babinski reflex occurs when the toes dorsiflex and fan out, indicating upper motor neuron disease.

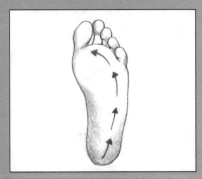

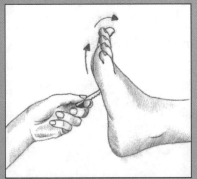

pressure and widening pulse pressure. The patient commonly has a bounding pulse. Cervical spinal cord injuries can also cause bradycardia.

In a patient with acutely increased ICP or a brain injury, tachycardia signals decompensation (a condition in which the body has exhausted its compensatory measures for managing ICP), which rapidly leads to death.

Respiration. Respiratory centers in the medulla and pons control the rate, depth, and pattern of respiration. Neurologic dysfunction, particularly when it involves the brain stem or both cerebral hemispheres, commonly alters respirations. Assessment of respiration provides valuable information about a CNS lesion's site and severity.

One of the first signs of a cerebral or upper brain stem disorder is Cheyne-Stokes respiration. However, this breathing pattern may occur normally in an older patient during sleep, probably the result of generalized brain atrophy from aging.

Spinal cord damage above C7 weakens or paralyzes the respiratory muscles, causing varying degrees of respiratory impairment.

Blood pressure. Pressor receptors in the medulla oblongata of the brain stem constantly monitor blood pressure. In a patient with no history of hypertension, rising systolic blood pressure may signal rising ICP. If ICP continues to rise, pulse pressure widens as systolic pressure climbs and diastolic pressure remains stable or falls. In the late stages of acutely elevated ICP, blood pressure plummets as cerebral perfusion fails, and the patient dies.

Although rare, hypotension accompanying a brain injury is an ominous sign. In addition, cervical spinal cord injuries may interrupt sympathetic nervous system pathways, causing peripheral vasodilation and hypotension.

Altered level of consciousness

Normal cerebral function depends on the continuous activity of the reticular activating system (RAS). Because RAS cells are normally hyperexcitable, disorders that depress central nervous system function usually affect them first. As a result, a change in level of consciousness (LOC) commonly serves as the earliest indication of a neurologic problem. This symptom can take the form of disorientation to time, place, or person.

CAUSES
Decreased LOC—from lethargy to stupor to coma—usually results from neurologic disorders and often signals life-threatening complications of hemorrhage, trauma, or cerebral edema. However, this sign can also result from metabolic, GI, musculoskeletal, urologic, and cardiopulmonary disorders; severe nutritional deficiency; the use of certain drugs; and the effects of toxins.

DIAGNOSIS AND TREATMENT
Diagnostic testing may include X-rays, a computed tomography scan, and magnetic resonance imaging to help differentiate diagnoses. Treatment of the patient with altered LOC will depend on the cause.

COLLABORATIVE MANAGEMENT
Care of the patient with altered LOC focuses on ensuring a safe environment and teaching him about the disorder.

ASSESSMENT
LOC can vary from alertness (response to verbal stimuli) to coma (failure to respond even to painful stimuli). When assessing LOC, it's best to document the patient's exact response to the stimulus—for example, "patient pulled away in response to nail bed pressure"—rather than to just write "stuporous."

The Glasgow Coma Scale, which assesses eye opening as well as verbal and motor responses, provides a quick, standardized assessment of neurologic status. In this test, each response receives a numerical value. A score of 15 for for all three parts is normal; 7 or less indicates coma; 3—the lowest score possible—usually points to brain death.

Patients with altered LOC are likely to display certain characteristics, depending on whether they're disoriented to time, place, or person. A patient who is disoriented to time will often incorrectly identify the year as one past. For example, he may think this is 1972. Bizarre answers, such as 1756 or 2054, suggest a psychiatric disturbance but could indicate lack of cooperation.

A hospitalized patient disoriented to place typically confuses the hospital room with home; a nonhospitalized patient, such as an Alzheimer's patient, may fail to recognize familiar home surroundings and wander off in search of something familiar.

Keep in mind that the patient who *is* oriented to place may not be able to name the hospital, especially if he's been admitted through the emergency department. However, if a patient states the full name of the hospital and later can't recall its name, he may be becoming disoriented to place. A patient who's disoriented to person may not be able to say his name. When asked, he may look baffled or may stammer and finally produce an unintelligible or inaccurate answer.

Rapid deterioration of LOC (minutes to hours) usually indicates an acute neurologic problem requiring immediate intervention. A gradually decreasing LOC (weeks to months) may reflect a progressive or degenerative neurologic disorder.

If the patient's disorientation arises from an organic problem, he's likely to mistake unfamiliar surroundings or people for familiar ones. For example, he may confuse the hospital room with his bedroom or mistake you for a relative. When disorientation originates from psychiatric disturbances such as schizophrenia, the patient's confusion pattern is usually bizarre.

NURSING DIAGNOSES AND COLLABORATIVE PROBLEMS

Based on the following nursing diagnoses, you'll establish patient outcomes.

Risk for injury related to alteration in consciousness. The patient will:
- remain free from injury
- show no further signs of deterioration
- use measures to remain safe.

Ineffective airway clearance related to alteration in consciousness. The patient will:
- maintain a patent airway
- maintain adequate tissue perfusion and oxygenation.

PLANNING AND IMPLEMENTATION

These measures help the patient with altered LOC.
- Reorient the patient to time, place, and person.
- Place familiar objects within reach.
- Monitor the patient closely for signs and symptoms of deterioration; assess his mental status frequently.
- If neurologic status deteriorates, anticipate the need for intubation; hyperoxygenate the patient if head injury is the cause of altered LOC.
- Monitor intracranial pressure (ICP) as indicated, and drain cerebrospinal fluid as necessary.
- Position the patient with his head up, unless contraindicated, to decrease ICP.
- Maintain a quiet environment; don't overly stimulate the patient.
- Assess respirations and breath sounds frequently for changes, and suction the airway as necessary.
- Monitor results of blood studies, including arterial blood gas levels, for changes.
- Institute measures to prevent aspiration, including positioning.

Patient teaching
- Teach family members the signs and symptoms of deterioration and when to notify the doctor immediately.
- Advise the patient and family members about safety measures.
- Explain the disorder and any necessary treatment and follow-up.
- Encourage the patient and family members to comply with his medical regimen.

EVALUATION

Evaluation of patient outcomes determines the success of collaborative management. For the patient with altered LOC, evaluation focuses on the presence of vital signs, neurologic status, and respiratory status within normal parameters; maintenance of safety; and absence of signs or symptoms indicating complications or deterioration in the patient's condition.

Alzheimer's disease

This progressive degenerative disorder of the cerebral cortex (especially the frontal lobe) accounts for more than half of all cases of dementia. An estimated 5% of people over age 65 have a severe form of this disease, and 12% suffer from mild to moderate dementia.

Because this is a primary progressive dementia, the prognosis is poor. Patients typically die of debilitating brain disease 2 to 15 years after the onset of symptoms. The average duration of the illness before death is 8 years.

Complications include injury from the patient's own violent behavior or from wandering or unsupervised activity; pneumonia and other infections, especially if the patient gets insufficient exercise; malnutrition and dehydration; and aspiration.

CAUSES

The cause of Alzheimer's disease is unknown. Pathologic changes involve neuron cell death and a disruption in the neurotransmitter circuits. Factors believed to be connected to the disease include neurochemical factors, such as deficiencies of the neurotransmitters acetylcholine, somatostatin, substance P, and norepinephrine; environmental factors, such as intake of aluminum and manganese; viral factors, such as slow-growing central nervous system viruses; trauma; and genetic factors.

Researchers believe that up to 70% of cases are linked to a genetic abnormality on chromosome 21. They've also isolated a genetic substance (amyloid) that causes brain damage typical of Alzheimer's disease. The brain tissue of Alzheimer's patients has three distinguishing features: neurofibrillary tangles, neuritic plaques, and granulovascular degeneration.

DIAGNOSIS AND TREATMENT

Alzheimer's disease is diagnosed by exclusion. Various tests are performed to rule out other disorders. However, the diagnosis can't be confirmed until death, when pathologic findings come to light at autopsy.

No cure or definitive treatment exists for Alzheimer's disease. Therapy consists of cerebral vasodilators, such as ergoloid mesylates, isoxsuprine, and cyclandelate, to enhance the brain's circulation; hyperbaric oxygen to increase oxygenation to the brain; psychostimulators, such as methylphenidate, to enhance the patient's mood; and antidepressants.

Most other drug therapies are experimental. These include choline salts, lecithin, physostigmine, tacrine, enkephalins, and naloxone, which may slow the disease process.

Another approach to treatment includes avoiding use of antacids, aluminum cooking utensils, and aluminum-containing deodorants to help decrease aluminum intake, one of the suspected environmental factors.

COLLABORATIVE MANAGEMENT

Care of the patient with Alzheimer's disease focuses on maintaining safety and providing support.

ASSESSMENT

As you assess this patient, keep in mind that the onset of Alzheimer's is insidious; changes are almost imperceptible initially but gradually progress to serious problems. The patient history is almost always obtained from a family member or caregiver. Look for:
- initially, reports of very small changes, such as forgetfulness and subtle memory loss, without loss of social skills
- over time, loss of recent memory and difficulty learning and remembering new information
- general deterioration in personal hygiene and appearance and an inability to concentrate
- difficulty with abstract thinking and activities that require judgment
- progressive difficulty in communicating
- severe deterioration of memory, language, and motor function, which in more severe cases eventually results in loss of coordination and an inability to speak or write
- repetitive actions; restlessness; negative personality changes, such as irritability, depression, paranoia, hostility, and combativeness; nocturnal awakenings; and disorientation
- suspicion and fear of imaginary people and situations, misperceptions about his environment,

misidentification of objects and people, and complaints of stolen or misplaced objects
- impaired sense of smell (usually an early symptom), impaired stereognosis (inability to recognize and understand the form and nature of objects by touching them), gait disorders, and tremors
- positive snout reflex (a stroke or tap on his lips or the area just under his nose makes him grimace or pucker his lips)
- in the final stages, urinary or fecal incontinence, twitching, and seizures.

NURSING DIAGNOSES AND COLLABORATIVE PROBLEMS

Based on the following nursing diagnoses, you'll establish patient outcomes.

Altered nutrition: Less than body requirements, related to patient's forgetfulness. The patient will:
- eat meals with supervision to ensure adequate intake
- consume a well-balanced diet provided by the caregiver
- maintain his weight.

Altered thought processes related to progressive deterioration of the cerebral cortex. The family or caregiver will:
- provide a simple daily routine for the patient to perform activities of daily living
- avoid or minimize change in the patient's environment
- demonstrate appropriate interventions, reorientation techniques, and coping skills.

Risk for injury related to negative personality changes and confusion. The patient will:
- remain safe and protected from injury
- perform activities of daily living under supervision.
The family or caregiver will:
- seek assistance with care and consult appropriate resources, as needed, including arrangements for care in a health care facility.

PLANNING AND IMPLEMENTATION

These measures help the patient with Alzheimer's disease.
- Establish an effective communication system with the patient and family members to help them adjust to the patient's altered cognitive abilities. Encourage them to talk about their concerns, and answer their questions honestly. Provide emotional support.
- Because the patient may misperceive his environment, use a soft tone and a slow, calm manner when speaking to him. Allow him sufficient time to answer because his thought processes are slow.
- Monitor the patient's neurologic function, including his emotional and mental states and motor capabilities, for changes indicating further deterioration.

Teaching caregivers about Alzheimer's disease

Counsel family members to expect progressive deterioration in the patient with Alzheimer's disease. To help them plan future patient care, discuss the stages of this relentless and inevitably progressive disease.

Bear in mind that family members may refuse to believe that the disease is advancing. So be sensitive to their concerns and, if necessary, review the information again when they're more receptive.

Forgetfulness
The patient becomes forgetful, especially of recent events. He frequently loses everyday objects such as keys. Aware of his loss of function, he may compensate by relinquishing tasks that might reveal his forgetfulness. Because his behavior isn't disruptive and may be attributed to stress, fatigue, or normal aging, he usually doesn't consult a doctor at this stage.

Confusion
The patient has increasing difficulty at activities that require planning, decision making, and judgment, such as managing personal finances, driving a car, and performing his job. However, he does retain everyday skills, such as personal grooming. Social withdrawal occurs when the patient feels overwhelmed by a changing environment and his inability to cope with multiple stimuli. Travel is difficult and tiring. As he becomes aware of his progressive loss of function, he may become severely depressed.

Safety becomes a concern when the patient forgets to turn off appliances or to recognize unsafe situations such as boiling water. At this point, the family may need to consider day care or a supervised residential facility.

Decline in activities of daily living
The patient at this stage loses his ability to perform daily activities, such as eating or washing, without direct supervision. Weight loss may occur. He withdraws from the family and increasingly depends on the primary caregiver. Communication becomes difficult as his understanding of written and spoken language declines.

Agitation, wandering, pacing, and nighttime awakening are linked to the patient's inability to cope with a multisensory environment. He may mistake his mirror image for a real person (pseudohallucination). Caregivers must be constantly vigilant, which may lead to physical and emotional exhaustion. They may also be angry and feel a sense of loss.

Total deterioration
In the final stage of Alzheimer's disease, the patient no longer recognizes himself, his body parts, or other family members. He becomes bedridden, and his activity consists of small, purposeless movements. Verbal communication stops, although he may scream spontaneously. Complications of immobility may include pressure ulcers, urinary tract infections, pneumonia, and contractures.

■ Administer ordered medications, and note their effects. If the patient has trouble swallowing, ask the pharmacist if you can crush the tablets or open the capsules and mix them with a semisoft food.
■ Provide a safe, structured environment. Allow rest periods between activities because patients with Alzheimer's disease tire easily.
■ Inspect the patient's skin for evidence of trauma, such as bruises or skin breakdown.
■ Encourage the patient to exercise as ordered to help maintain mobility.
■ Foster the patient's independence, and allow ample time to perform tasks.
■ Because the patient may be disoriented or neuromuscular functioning may be impaired, take him to the bathroom at least every 2 hours and make sure he knows the location of the bathroom.
■ Assist the patient with hygiene and dressing as necessary.
■ Encourage sufficient fluid intake and adequate nutrition.

■ Insert and care for a nasogastric tube or a gastrostomy tube for feeding, as ordered.
■ Monitor the patient's fluid and food intake to detect imbalances.
■ Frequently check the patient's vital signs; remember to watch for pneumonia and other infections.
■ Evaluate the family's or caregiver's ability to manage the patient at home.

Patient teaching
■ Teach family members or friends about the disease, the lack of a known cause, and the signs and symptoms. Be sure to explain that Alzheimer's disease progresses at an unpredictable rate to eventual complete memory loss and total physical deterioration. (See *Teaching caregivers about Alzheimer's disease.*)
■ Review the diagnostic tests that will be performed and the treatment the patient will require.
■ Emphasize the patient's need for exercise. Suggest physical activities, such as walking or light housework.

- Stress the importance of diet. Tell the caregiver to limit the number of foods offered so the patient won't have to make decisions. If the patient has coordination problems, suggest aids such as plates with rim guards and cups with lids and spouts.
- Encourage family members to allow the patient as much independence as is possible and safe. Tell them to create a routine to spare him confusion. If the patient becomes belligerent, advise them to remain calm and to try distracting him.
- Refer family members to the social services department and to support groups such as the Alzheimer's Association.

EVALUATION
Evaluation of patient outcomes determines the success of collaborative management. For the patient with Alzheimer's disease, evaluation focuses on physiologic status within acceptable parameters, freedom from injury, and adequate home care or referral to a nursing home.

Amyotrophic lateral sclerosis

Also known as Lou Gehrig's disease (after a well-known baseball player who died of it in 1941), this disease is the most common motor neuron disease of muscular atrophy. Amyotrophic lateral sclerosis (ALS) is a chronic, progressive, and debilitating disease that is invariably fatal.

ALS usually affects people ages 40 to 70. Most patients with ALS die within 3 to 5 years, but some may live as long as 15 years. Death usually results from a complication, such as aspiration pneumonia or respiratory failure.

Reportedly, more than 30,000 Americans have ALS; about 5,000 more are newly diagnosed each year. ALS is about three times more common in men than in women.

Common complications of ALS include respiratory tract infections such as pneumonia, respiratory failure, and aspiration; complications of physical immobility include pressure ulcers and contractures.

CAUSES
The exact cause of ALS is unknown, but about 10% of ALS patients inherit the disease as an autosomal dominant trait. ALS may also be caused by a virus that creates metabolic disturbances in motor neurons or by immune complexes, such as those formed in autoimmune disorders.

Precipitating factors that can cause acute deterioration include severe stress, as from myocardial infarction, traumatic injury, viral infections, and physical exhaustion.

ALS is characterized by progressive degeneration of the anterior horn cells of the spinal cord and cranial nerves and of the motor nuclei in the cerebral cortex and corticospinal tracts.

DIAGNOSIS AND TREATMENT
Although no diagnostic tests are specific to this disease, electromyography, muscle biopsy, nerve conduction studies, and cerebrospinal fluid analysis may aid in its diagnosis. A computed tomography scan and EEG can rule out other disorders, including multiple sclerosis, spinal cord neoplasms, myasthenia gravis, and progressive muscular dystrophy.

There is no cure for ALS. Treatment is supportive, based on the patient's symptoms. Drug therapy may include diazepam for spasticity; quinine for relief of painful muscle cramps that occur in some patients; and I.V. or intrathecal administration of thyrotropin-releasing hormone to improve motor function temporarily in some patients. Riluzole has recently been approved for use in ALS because it can increase the time the patient is able to remain ventilator-free.

Rehabilitative measures can help patients function effectively for a longer period, and mechanical ventilation can help them survive longer.

COLLABORATIVE MANAGEMENT
Care of the patient with ALS focuses on support, protection, and preparation for extended care.

ASSESSMENT
Signs and symptoms of ALS depend on the location of the affected motor neurons and the severity of the disease. Muscle weakness, atrophy, and fasciculation are the principal symptoms. The disease may begin in any muscle group; however, eventually, all muscle groups are involved. Unlike other degenerative disorders, such as Alzheimer's disease, ALS doesn't affect mental function. Look for:
- a family history of ALS if the disease was inherited
- in early stages, reports of fatigue, asymmetrical weakness first noticed in one limb, cramping in affected muscles, fasciculation, and muscle atrophy (most obvious in feet and hands)
- in later stages, progressive weakness in muscles of the arms, legs, and trunk (confirmed by muscle strength tests); brisk and overactive stretch reflexes; fasciculation and atrophy
- with brain stem and cranial nerve involvement, difficulty talking, chewing, swallowing and, ultimately, breathing; decreased breath sounds.

In about 25% of patients, muscle weakness begins in the musculature supplied by the cranial nerves.

When this occurs, the initial patient history reveals difficulty talking, swallowing, and breathing. Occasionally, the patient may report choking. Inspection may reveal some shortness of breath and, occasionally, drooling.

NURSING DIAGNOSES AND COLLABORATIVE PROBLEMS

Based on the following nursing diagnoses, you'll establish patient outcomes.

Ineffective airway clearance related to disease progression. The patient will:
- maintain a patent airway
- demonstrate adequate tissue perfusion and oxygenation.

Anticipatory grieving related to the progression and ultimately fatal outcome of ALS. The patient will:
- express his feelings about the changes in his life and anticipated losses due to ALS
- accept feelings and behavior caused by these changes
- use appropriate coping mechanisms to deal with his grief.

Impaired home maintenance management related to fatigue and loss of muscle strength to perform activities of daily living. The patient will:
- express his need to make home adjustments to perform activities of daily living
- identify and contact individuals or organizations to provide home assistance.

Impaired physical mobility related to progressive deterioration of the nervous system. The patient will:
- attain the highest degree of mobility possible, such as ambulating with assistive devices
- show no evidence of complications related to impaired physical mobility, such as contractures or skin breakdown.

The patient or caregiver will:
- carry out the mobility regimen consistently.

PLANNING AND INTERVENTION

These measures help the patient with ALS.
- Provide emotional and psychological support to the patient and family members. Stay with the patient during periods of severe stress and anxiety. Keep in mind that because his mental status remains intact despite progressive physical degeneration, the patient acutely perceives every change in his condition.
- Implement a rehabilitation program to help the patient maintain his independence as long as possible.
- Have the patient perform active range-of-motion exercises on unaffected muscles to help strengthen them. Stretching exercises are also helpful.

- Help him obtain assistive devices, such as a walker or a wheelchair, when this becomes necessary.
- Depending on the patient's muscular capacity, assist with bathing, personal hygiene, and transfers from wheelchair to bed. Help establish a regular bowel and bladder elimination routine.
- Evaluate his neuromuscular function regularly to assess progression of deterioration.
- To prevent skin breakdown, provide good skin care when the patient's mobility decreases. Turn him often, keep his skin clean and dry, and use pressure-reducing devices, such as an alternating air mattress.
- Inspect his skin regularly for evidence of breakdown.
- If the patient can't talk, provide an alternate means of communication, such as message boards, eye blinking to indicate yes or no, or a computer.
- Administer ordered medications as necessary to relieve the patient's symptoms. Crush tablets and mix them with semisolid food for the patient who has dysphagia.
- Have the patient who has breathing difficulty perform deep-breathing and coughing exercises. Suctioning, chest physiotherapy, and incentive spirometry can help.
- If the patient chooses to use mechanical ventilation to assist his breathing, provide necessary care.
- Monitor the patient's nutritional intake for evidence of malnourishment.
- If the patient has trouble swallowing, give him soft, semisolid foods and position him upright during meals. Gastrostomy and nasogastric tube feedings may be necessary if he can no longer swallow.
- Have suctioning equipment available to prevent aspiration.
- Use a soft cervical collar to help the patient hold his head upright, if needed.
- Frequently assess the patient's respiratory status to detect breathing difficulty. Carefully assess the patient with respiratory involvement for infection, because respiratory complications can be fatal.

Patient teaching

- Teach the patient and family members about ALS and expected signs and symptoms. Make sure they understand that this is a progressive, incurable disease, but that treatments can prolong comfort and independence.
- Teach the patient who has difficulty chewing to cut his food into smaller pieces or to use a blender or food processor to mince food. Suggest thickening minced foods with baby cereal. Teach family members how to administer gastrostomy feedings if these become necessary.
- Caution the patient against eating sticky foods,

such as peanut butter and chocolate. If the patient has drooling problems, suggest that he avoid foods and beverages that increase salivation, such as grapefruit and milk.

■ To help the patient handle increased accumulation of secretions and dysphagia, teach him to suction himself. He should have a suction machine handy at home to reduce the fear of choking.

■ As the patient's condition deteriorates, teach family members how to perform comfort measures and help the patient through this difficult period.

■ Refer them to the social services department and, if appropriate, to a home health care agency, a hospice program, or an ALS support group, such as the Amyotrophic Lateral Sclerosis Association.

EVALUATION
Evaluation of patient outcomes determines the success of collaborative management. For the patient with ALS, evaluation focuses on adequate nutrition; vital signs, neurologic signs, and respiratory status within acceptable parameters; absence of complications; ability to manage bowel or bladder dysfunction, to ambulate with minimal assistance, and to perform activities of daily living; and completion of referrals for additional services as needed.

Bell's palsy

In this disorder, conduction of impulses from the seventh cranial nerve—the nerve responsible for motor innervation of the facial muscles—is blocked, resulting in unilateral facial weakness or paralysis.

Bell's palsy affects all age-groups but most often strikes patients under age 60. Onset is rapid. In 80% to 90% of cases, the disorder subsides spontaneously, with complete recovery in 1 to 8 weeks; however, recovery may take longer in older adults. If the patient experiences only partial recovery, contractures may develop on the paralyzed side of the face. Bell's palsy may recur on the same or opposite side of the face.

CAUSES
Blocked conduction of nerve impulses is caused by an inflammatory reaction around the nerve (usually at the internal auditory meatus). This may result from infection, hemorrhage, tumor, meningitis, or local traumatic injury.

DIAGNOSIS AND TREATMENT
Electromyography helps predict recovery by distinguishing temporary conduction defects from a pathologic interruption of nerve fibers.

Prednisone, an oral corticosteroid, reduces facial nerve edema and improves nerve conduction and blood flow. After the 14th day of prednisone therapy, electrotherapy may help prevent atrophy of facial muscles.

COLLABORATIVE MANAGEMENT
Care of the patient with Bell's palsy focuses on pain control and adequate nutrition.

ASSESSMENT
Perform a neurologic examination, obtain a history, and perform a physical examination. Look for:
■ unilateral facial weakness
■ occasionally, aching pain around the angle of the jaw or behind the ear
■ drooping mouth, causing drooling on the affected side
■ distorted taste perception over the affected anterior portion of the tongue
■ smooth forehead
■ markedly impaired ability to close eye on weak side, Bell's phenomenon (eye rolling upward as eye is closed), and excessive tearing when the patient attempts to close affected eye
■ inability to raise the eyebrow, smile, show the teeth, or puff out the cheek.

NURSING DIAGNOSES AND COLLABORATIVE PROBLEMS
Based on the following nursing diagnoses, you'll establish patient outcomes.
Pain related to nerve stimulation. The patient will:
■ demonstrate measures to minimize pain
■ exhibit positive coping strategies
■ state that his pain is relieved.
Altered nutrition: Less than body requirements, related to pain interfering with ability to eat. The patient will:
■ maintain adequate nutritional intake
■ exhibit weight within acceptable parameters.

PLANNING AND IMPLEMENTATION
These measures help the patient with Bell's palsy.
■ To reduce pain, apply moist heat to the affected side of the face, taking care not to burn the skin.
■ To help maintain muscle tone, massage the patient's face with a gentle upward motion two to three times daily for 5 to 10 minutes, or have him massage his face himself.
■ Apply a facial sling to improve lip alignment.
■ Provide frequent and complete mouth care, being particularly careful to remove residual food that collects between the cheeks and gums.
■ Offer emotional support. Reassure the patient that recovery is likely within 1 to 8 weeks.

Patient teaching

■ Advise the patient to protect his eye by covering it with an eye patch, especially when outdoors. Tell him to keep warm and avoid exposure to dust and wind. When exposure is unavoidable, instruct him to cover his face.

■ To prevent excessive weight loss, help the patient cope with difficulty in eating and drinking. Instruct him to chew on the unaffected side of his mouth. Provide a soft, nutritionally balanced diet, eliminating hot foods and fluids. Arrange for privacy at mealtimes to reduce embarrassment.

■ When the patient is ready, teach him to exercise by grimacing in front of a mirror.

EVALUATION

Evaluation of patient outcomes determines the success of collaborative management. For the patient with Bell's palsy, evaluation focuses on pain control and adequate nutrition.

Brain injury

Injuries to the head may result in a concussion (the most common head injury), a cerebral contusion, or a skull fracture. A concussion results from a blow to the head that jostles the brain and makes it strike the skull, causing temporary neural dysfunction. It usually causes no significant anatomic brain injury but may cause seizures, persistent vomiting, or both. Most concussion patients recover completely within 48 hours; however, repeated concussions have a cumulative effect.

More serious than a concussion, a cerebral contusion is an ecchymosis of brain tissue resulting from a severe blow to the head. This injury disrupts normal nerve functions in the bruised area and may cause loss of consciousness, hemorrhage, edema, and even death. A contusion can cause intracranial hemorrhage or hematoma if the injury causes the brain to strike against bony prominences inside the skull (especially the sphenoidal ridges). Residual headaches and vertigo may complicate recovery. Secondary effects, such as brain swelling, may accompany serious contusions, resulting in increased intracranial pressure (ICP) and herniation. (See the "Skull fracture" entry for information about this type of head injury.)

CAUSES

The blow that causes a concussion is usually sudden and forceful, such as a fall, a motor vehicle accident, or a punch to the head. A cerebral contusion can result from coup-contrecoup or acceleration-decelera-

tion injuries. Such injuries can occur directly beneath the site of impact (coup) when the brain rebounds against the skull from the force of a blow (such as one from a blunt instrument) that drives the brain against the opposite side of the skull (contrecoup), or when the head is hurled forward and stopped abruptly (as in striking a windshield). The brain continues moving and slaps against the skull (acceleration) and then rebounds (deceleration).

DIAGNOSIS AND TREATMENT

Diagnostic tests include a computed tomography scan initially and then possibly magnetic resonance imaging and a radioisotope scan.

Treatment depends on the type of injury. Most patients with a concussion require only bed rest, observation, and acetaminophen for headache.

However, a patient with a cerebral contusion may require immediate emergency treatment, including establishment of a patent airway and a tracheotomy or endotracheal intubation. The patient may need I.V. fluids (dextrose 5% in 0.45% sodium chloride solution), I.V. mannitol to reduce ICP, and restricted fluid intake to decrease intracerebral edema. The patient's ICP may be reduced by maintaining his partial pressure of arterial carbon dioxide ($Paco_2$) between 25 and 30 mm Hg, which will constrict cerebral blood vessels and cause an infarct. Additionally, the patient may require a blood transfusion and a craniotomy.

For seizures resulting from a head injury, the patient may receive an anticonvulsant, usually 10 to 15 mg/kg of I.V. phenytoin sodium given at a rate of no more than 50 mg/minute or according to your health care facility's policy.

COLLABORATIVE MANAGEMENT

Care of the patient with a brain injury focuses on providing pain relief and monitoring his neurologic status.

ASSESSMENT

The patient's history (possibly obtained from others) reveals a traumatic injury to the head followed by a period of unconsciousness. An unconscious patient may appear pale and motionless. If conscious, he may appear drowsy or easily disturbed by any stimulation, such as noise or light.

If he has a concussion, others may report the patient's behavior changes. The patient usually complains of dizziness, nausea, and severe headache. He may also exhibit anterograde or retrograde amnesia. In retrograde amnesia, the patient not only can't recall what happened immediately after the injury, but can't recall what led up to it. Typically, he repeats his questions about the event. The presence of anterograde amnesia and the duration of retrograde amnesia reliably correlate with the injury's severity. Look for:

- in a cerebral contusion, agitation, even violence
- scalp wounds with abrasions, contusions, lacerations, or avulsions
- profuse bleeding, although not usually enough to induce hypovolemic shock
- in severe head injury, a state of shock from other injuries or from medullary failure
- skull tenderness or hematomas
- normal neurologic findings in a patient with a concussion; abnormal findings in a patient with a cerebral contusion or skull fracture
- in a cerebral contusion, hemiparesis, decorticate or decerebrate posturing, and unequal pupillary response.

NURSING DIAGNOSES AND COLLABORATIVE PROBLEMS

Based on the following nursing diagnoses, you'll establish patient outcomes.

Anxiety related to the threat of permanent neurologic injury or death. The patient will:

- express his feelings of anxiety
- use available support systems to help cope with anxiety
- demonstrate fewer physical symptoms caused by anxiety.

Risk for injury related to complications of head injury. The patient will:

- avoid permanent neurologic deficit
- exhibit normal neurologic findings after the head injury heals.

Pain related to altered brain or skull tissue. The patient will:

- maintain normal ICP
- express pain relief with treatment
- obtain complete pain relief after the injury heals.

PLANNING AND IMPLEMENTATION

These measures help the patient with a brain injury.

- Maintain a patent airway.
- Assist with endotracheal intubation or tracheotomy, as necessary.
- Administer medications as ordered. However, don't administer narcotics or sedatives because they may depress respirations, raise $PaCO_2$ levels, and lead to increased ICP. They also can mask changes in neurologic status. Give acetaminophen for pain, as ordered.
- Initially, monitor vital signs continuously and check for additional injuries. Abnormal respirations could indicate a breakdown in the brain's respiratory center and possibly an impending tentorial herniation (a neurologic emergency).

- Monitor the patient's oxygenation status through serial arterial blood gas studies, as ordered, especially if he's intubated.
- Protect the patient from injury by using side rails, assisting him with walking, and staying with him while he uses the bathroom. If he's confused, place him where you can easily observe him.
- If the patient is unconscious, insert a nasogastric (NG) tube to prevent aspiration, but only after a basilar skull fracture has been ruled out. Otherwise, the tube might be inserted into the cranial vault. If the patient has a basilar fracture, insert a soft nasal airway first and then insert the NG tube.
- Monitor the patient's intake and output. The goal is to maintain a normovolumic state.
- Inserted an indwelling urinary catheter if ordered.
- After the patient is stabilized, clean and dress any superficial scalp wounds. Be sure to wear sterile gloves. (If the skin has been broken, the patient may need tetanus prophylaxis.) Assist with suturing if needed. Carefully cover scalp wounds with a sterile dressing, and control any bleeding as necessary.
- Monitor fluid and electrolyte levels and replace them as necessary.
- Assess neurologic status frequently; note any changes in level of consciousness (LOC), alertness, and ability to respond.
- Carefully observe the patient for cerebrospinal fluid (CSF) leakage. Check the bed sheets for a blood-tinged spot surrounded by a lighter ring (halo sign).
- If the patient has CSF leakage, keep the head of the bed flat. Otherwise, elevate it 15 to 30 degrees. Remember that such a patient is at risk for jugular compression, leading to increased ICP, when he's not positioned on his back. Enforce bed rest.
- Position the patient to drain secretions. If you detect CSF leakage from the nose, place a gauze pad under the nostrils. If CSF leaks from the ear, position the patient so his ear drains naturally; don't pack the ear or nose. If required, suction the patient through the mouth, not the nose, to avoid introducing bacteria into CSF.
- Institute seizure precautions, but don't restrain the patient.
- Prepare the patient for a craniotomy, as indicated.
- Continue to check vital signs and neurologic status, including LOC and pupil size, every 15 minutes. If the patient's condition worsens or fluctuates, arrange for a neurosurgical consultation.
- Observe the patient for headache, dizziness, irritability, and anxiety. If his condition worsens, perform a complete neurologic evaluation and notify the doctor.
- Watch for agitated behavior, which may stem from hypoxia or increased ICP.

- Monitor the older patient especially closely. He may have brain atrophy and therefore more space for cerebral edema; ICP may increase, yet cause no signs.
- If the patient remains stable after 4 or more hours of observation, he can be discharged in the care of a family member or friend.
- To decrease the patient's anxiety, speak calmly and explain your actions, even if he's unconscious. Don't make any sudden, unexpected moves. Touch the patient gently.
- If he develops temporary aphasia, provide an alternative means of communication.

Patient teaching
- If the patient is discharged from the emergency department, tell a family member or friend to observe his condition at home for the next 24 to 48 hours. An unaccompanied patient may be hospitalized briefly. Be sure to provide a head injury instruction sheet.
- Tell the caregiver to awaken the patient every 2 hours throughout the night and to ask him his name, location, and the caregiver's identity. Tell the caregiver to return the patient to the hospital if he is difficult to arouse, is disoriented, or has seizures.
- Advise the caregiver to keep the sleep area quiet so the patient can sleep in the 2-hour intervals.
- Tell the patient to return to the health care facility immediately if he experiences a persistent or worsening headache, forceful or constant vomiting, blurred vision, any change in personality, abnormal eye movements, a staggering gait, or twitching.
- Instruct the patient to take nothing stronger than acetaminophen for a headache. Warn him that aspirin may increase the risk of bleeding.
- Instruct the patient who vomits to eat lightly until vomiting stops. (Occasional vomiting is normal after a concussion.)
- Teach the patient to recognize symptoms of postconcussion syndrome: headache, dizziness, vertigo, anxiety, and fatigue. Tell him the syndrome may persist for several weeks.
- Teach the patient and a family member or friend how to care for his scalp wound, if applicable. Emphasize the need to return for suture removal and follow-up evaluation.

EVALUATION
Evaluation of patient outcomes determines the success of collaborative management. For the patient with a brain injury, evaluation focuses on vital signs, neurologic status, and ICP within acceptable parameters; a clean and dry wound; headache relieved by analgesics; and absence of any complications.

Brain tumor

Slightly more common in men than in women, malignant brain tumors affect about 5 out of 100,000 people. Brain tumors can occur at any age. In adults, incidence is highest between ages 40 and 60, and the most common tumor types are gliomas and meningiomas. They usually occur above the covering of the cerebellum (supratentorial tumors).

Most tumors in children occur before age 1 or between ages 2 and 12. The most common are astrocytomas, medulloblastomas, ependymomas, and brain stem gliomas. Brain tumors are one of the most common causes of cancer-related death in children.

In malignant brain tumors, life-threatening complications from increasing intracranial pressure (ICP) include coma, respiratory or cardiac arrest, and brain herniation.

CAUSES
The etiology of brain tumors is unknown. Brain tumors cause central nervous system (CNS) changes by invading and destroying tissues and by secondary effects—primarily compression of the brain, cranial nerves, and cerebral vessels; cerebral edema; and increased ICP.

DIAGNOSIS AND TREATMENT
Diagnostic tests may include the following:
- Skull X-rays, brain scans, computed tomography scans, magnetic resonance imaging, and cerebral angiography help locate the tumor.
- Biopsy of the lesion allows identification of the type and grade. Grade 1 tumors are well differentiated; grade 2, moderately well differentiated; grade 3, poorly differentiated; and grade 4 extremely poorly differentiated. The higher the grade, the poorer the prognosis.

Specific treatments vary with the tumor's histologic type, radiosensitivity, and location. They include surgery, radiation therapy, chemotherapy, and decompression of increased ICP with diuretics, corticosteroids or, possibly, ventriculoatrial or ventriculoperitoneal shunting of the cerebrospinal fluid (CSF).

Treatment of a glioma usually consists of resection by craniotomy, followed by radiation therapy and chemotherapy. The combination of carmustine, lomustine, or procarbazine with radiation therapy is more effective than radiation treatment alone.

For low-grade cystic cerebellar astrocytomas, surgical resection permits long-term survival. For other astrocytomas, treatment consists of repeated surgery, radiation therapy, and shunting of fluid from obstructed CSF pathways. Radiation therapy works best in radiosensitive astrocytomas; some astrocytomas are radioresistant.

Treatment for oligodendrogliomas and ependymomas includes surgical resection and radiation therapy. Medulloblastomas call for surgical resection and possibly intrathecal infusion of methotrexate or another antineoplastic drug. Meningiomas require surgical resection, including dura mater and sometimes, bone.

For schwannomas, microsurgical technique allows complete resection of the tumor and preservation of facial nerves. Although schwannomas are moderately radioresistant, treatment still calls for postoperative radiation therapy.

Treatment for malignant brain tumors also includes chemotherapy with nitrosoureas, which cross the blood-brain barrier and allow other chemotherapeutic agents to cross through as well. Intrathecal and intra-arterial administration maximizes drug action.

Palliative measures for gliomas, astrocytomas, oligodendrogliomas, and ependymomas include dexamethasone for cerebral edema and antacids and histamine-receptor antagonists for stress ulcers. These tumors and schwannomas may also require anticonvulsants.

New treatments under investigation include bone marrow transplantation and hyperthermia.

Treatment of brain tumors can cause several complications. Although rare, surgery can lead to immediate or delayed CNS infections, with symptoms that mimic tumor progression or recurrence. If fever or rapidly progressive neurologic symptoms develop, bacterial and fungal cultures will confirm the infection.

Early delayed radiation encephalopathy may stem from temporary demyelination. Anorexia, somnolence, lethargy, and headache occur 2 to 6 weeks after the therapy but resolve spontaneously in approximately 6 weeks.

Late delayed radiation encephalopathy stems from brain necrosis and small-vessel occlusion. Symptoms can mimic disease advancement and may include intracranial hypertension and focal neurologic dysfunction. Both are irreversible and potentially fatal complications.

Corticosteroid therapy predisposes the patient to cushingoid symptoms, GI ulceration, and steroid psychosis (if used long-term).

COLLABORATIVE MANAGEMENT

Care of the patient with a brain tumor focuses on his treatment regimen and altered lifestyle.

ASSESSMENT

The patient's history usually reveals an insidious onset of signs and symptoms. If the brain tumor has al-

ready been diagnosed, his history may also show an early misdiagnosis—a common occurrence.

Signs and symptoms result from increased ICP. Specific assessment findings vary with the type of tumor, its location, and the degree of invasion. Neurologic assessment findings often help to pinpoint the location of the tumor. (See *Brain tumors: Site-specific signs and symptoms*, page 284, and *Assessing malignant brain tumors*, pages 285 and 286.)

NURSING DIAGNOSES AND COLLABORATIVE PROBLEMS

Based on the following nursing diagnoses, you'll establish patient outcomes.

Impaired gas exchange related to pressure exerted by brain tumor. The patient will:
- maintain a patent airway
- exhibit tissue perfusion and oxygenation within normal limits for patient.

Risk for injury related to neurologic deficits caused by brain tumor. The patient will:
- exhibit neurologic status and ICP within normal parameters
- remain free from injury.

Altered role performance related to neurologic deficits caused by brain tumor. The patient will:
- identify limitations imposed by changes in neurologic function
- seek assistance in performing activities related to role performance, as dictated by tumor growth or adverse reactions
- continue to function in his usual role as much as possible.

Sensory/perceptual alterations (potential for all areas to be affected) related to neurologic deficits caused by brain tumor. The patient will:
- use adaptive equipment (glasses, hearing aid) as needed
- remain safe in his environment.

The patient or caregiver will:
- take an active role in preventing sensory deprivation and isolation.

Powerlessness related to potential inability to control cancer growth or adverse effects of brain tumor. The patient will:
- express feelings of powerlessness over tumor growth and adverse reactions
- participate in planning care and managing adverse reactions
- express feeling of having regained a sense of control.

PLANNING AND IMPLEMENTATION

These measures help the patient with a brain tumor.
- Maintain a patent airway.

(Text continues on page 286.)

Brain tumors: Site-specific signs and symptoms

A brain tumor usually produces signs and symptoms specific to its location. Recognizing these typical effects helps identify the tumor site and guide treatment before and after surgery. It can also help you spot life-threatening complications, such as increasing intracranial pressure and imminent brain herniation. A brain tumor may cause all, some, or none of the effects listed below.

Hypothalamus
- Possible pituitary area tumor extending upward
- Diabetes insipidus
- Loss of temperature control

Frontal lobe
- Expressive or Broca's aphasia (dominant hemisphere)
- Contralateral seizures
- Contralateral motor weakness
- Personality and behavioral changes

Subfrontal lobe
Cranial nerve I (olfactory)
- Loss of smell

Midbrain
Cranial nerve II (optic) and cranial nerve III (oculomotor)
- Ptosis
- Diplopia
- Dilated pupil
- Inability to gaze up, down, or inward (all ipsilateral)
Cranial nerve IV (trochlear)
- Impaired extraocular eye movement inferiorly and medially

Cerebellum
- Disturbed gait
- Impaired balance
- Incoordination

Pituitary (sella turcica)
- Amenorrhea
- Cushingoid signs and symptoms
- Galactorrhea
- Impotence
- Visual field deficits

Cerebellopontile angle
Cranial nerve VII (facial)
- Ipsilateral facial muscle drooping
Cranial nerve VIII (acoustic)
- Tinnitus
- Hearing loss

Occipital lobe
- Visual agnosia (inability to name objects)
- Visual field deficits

Medulla
Cranial nerve IX (glossopharyngeal)
- Difficulty swallowing
Cranial nerve X (vagus)
- Gag and cough reflex loss
- Difficulty swallowing
- Hoarseness
- Projectile vomiting
Cranial nerve XI (spinal accessory)
- Inability to shrug shoulders or turn head toward tumor side
Cranial nerve XII (hypoglossal)
- Tongue protrusion (deviating toward tumor side)
- Respiratory pattern changes

Parietal lobe
- Dyslexia (left side)
- Position sense loss
- Perceptual problems
- Contralateral sensory disturbances
- Visual field deficits

Pons
Cranial nerve V (trigeminal)
- Ipsilateral facial or forehead sensation loss
- Corneal reflex loss
Cranial nerve VI (abducens)
- Ipsilateral inability to gaze outward
Cranial nerve VII (facial)
- Ipsilateral facial muscle drooping

Temporal lobe
- Auditory hallucinations
- Impaired memory (with bilateral tumor)
- Personality changes
- Psychomotor seizures
- Visual field deficits
- Receptive or Wernicke's aphasia (dominant hemisphere)
- Dysarthrias

Assessing malignant brain tumors

Tumor and characteristics	Assessment findings
ASTROCYTOMA ■ Second most common malignant glioma, accounting for 10% of all gliomas ■ Occurs at any age; incidence higher in males than in females ■ Occurs most often in central and subcortical white matter; may originate in any part of the central nervous system ■ Cerebellar astrocytomas usually confined to one hemisphere	**GENERAL** ■ Headache and mental activity changes ■ Decreased motor strength and coordination ■ Seizures and scanning speech ■ Altered vital signs **LOCALIZING** ■ Third ventricle: changes in mental activity and level of consciousness, nausea, and pupillary dilation and sluggish light reflex; paresis or ataxia in later stages ■ Brain stem and pons: ipsilateral trigeminal, abducens, and facial nerve palsies in early stages; cerebellar ataxia, tremors, and other cranial nerve deficits later ■ Third or fourth ventricle or aqueduct of Sylvius: secondary hydrocephalus ■ Thalamus or hypothalamus: various endocrine, metabolic, autonomic, and behavioral changes
EPENDYMOMA ■ Rare glioma; most common in children and young adults ■ Located most often in fourth and lateral ventricles	**GENERAL** ■ Increased intracranial pressure (ICP) and obstructive hydrocephalus ■ Other assessment findings similar to those of oligodendroglioma
GLIOBLASTOMA MULTIFORME ■ Most common glioma, accounting for 60% of all gliomas ■ Peak incidence between ages 50 and 60; more common in men ■ Unencapsulated, highly malignant; grows rapidly and infiltrates the brain; may be enormous before diagnosed ■ Occurs most often in cerebral hemispheres (frontal and temporal lobes) ■ Occupies more than one lobe of affected hemisphere; may spread to opposite hemisphere by corpus callosum; may metastasize into cerebrospinal fluid (CSF), producing tumors in distant parts of the nervous system	**GENERAL** ■ Increased ICP (nausea, vomiting, headache, papilledema) ■ Mental and behavioral changes ■ Altered vital signs (increased systolic pressure, widened pulse pressure, respiratory changes) ■ Speech and sensory disturbances ■ In children, irritability and projectile vomiting **LOCALIZING** ■ Midline: headache (bifrontal or bioccipital) that's worse in morning; intensified by coughing, straining, or sudden head movements ■ Temporal lobe: psychomotor seizures ■ Central region: focal seizures ■ Optic and oculomotor nerves: visual defects ■ Frontal lobe: abnormal reflexes and motor responses
MEDULLOBLASTOMA ■ Rare glioma ■ Incidence highest in children ages 4 to 6 ■ Affects males more than females ■ Frequently metastasizes by way of CSF	**GENERAL** ■ Increased ICP **LOCALIZING** ■ Brain stem and cerebrum: papilledema, nystagmus, hearing loss, perception of flashing lights, dizziness, ataxia, paresthesia of the face, cranial nerve palsies, hemiparesis, suboccipital tenderness; compression of supratentorial area produces other symptoms
MENINGIOMA ■ Most common nonmalignant brain tumor, constituting 20% of primary brain tumors ■ Occurs most frequently among people in their 50s; rare in children; more common in females (ratio 3:2) ■ Arises from the meninges ■ Common locations include parasagittal area, sphenoidal ridge, anterior part of the base of the skull, cerebellopontile angle, and spinal canal ■ Benign, well-circumscribed, highly vascular tumor that compresses underlying brain tissue by invading overlying skull	**GENERAL** ■ Headache, seizures, vomiting, and changes in mental activity. Other assessment findings similar to those of schwannomas **LOCALIZING** ■ Skull changes (bony bulge) over tumor ■ Sphenoidal ridge, indenting optic nerve: unilateral visual changes and papilledema ■ Prefrontal parasagittal: personality and behavioral changes ■ Motor cortex: contralateral motor changes ■ Anterior fossa compressing both optic nerves and frontal lobes: headaches and bilateral vision loss ■ Pressure on cranial nerves, causing varying symptoms

(continued)

Assessing malignant brain tumors *(continued)*

Tumor and characteristics	Assessment findings
OLIGODENDROGLIOMA ■ Third most common glioma, accounting for less than 5% of all gliomas ■ Occurs in middle adult years; more common in women than in men ■ Slow-growing	**GENERAL** ■ Mental and behavioral changes ■ Decreased visual acuity and other visual disturbances ■ Increased ICP **LOCALIZING** ■ Temporal lobe: hallucinations and psychomotor seizures ■ Central region: seizures (one muscle group or unilateral) ■ Midbrain or third ventricle: pyramidal tract symptoms (dizziness, ataxia, paresthesia of the face) ■ Brain stem and cerebrum: nystagmus, hearing loss, dizziness, ataxia, paresthesia of the face, cranial nerve palsies, hemiparesis, suboccipital tenderness, loss of balance
SCHWANNOMA (acoustic neurinoma, neurilemoma, cerebellopontile angle tumor) ■ Accounts for about 10% of all intracranial tumors ■ Onset of symptoms between ages 30 and 60; higher incidence in women ■ Affects the craniospinal nerve sheath, usually cranial nerve VIII; also, V and VII, and to a lesser extent, VI and X on the same side as the tumor ■ Benign, but often classified as malignant because of its growth patterns; slow growing—may be present for years before symptoms occur	**GENERAL** ■ Unilateral hearing loss with or without tinnitus ■ Stiff neck and suboccipital discomfort ■ Secondary hydrocephalus ■ Ataxia and uncoordinated movements of one or both arms due to pressure on brain stem and cerebellum **LOCALIZING** ■ V: early signs including facial hypoesthesia and paresthesia on the side of hearing loss; unilateral loss of corneal reflex ■ VI: diplopia ■ VII: paresis progressing to paralysis (Bell's palsy) ■ X: weakness of palate, tongue, and nerve muscles on same side as tumor

■ Evaluate respiratory changes carefully. Abnormal rate and depth may indicate rising ICP or herniation of the cerebellar tonsils from expanding infratentorial mass.

■ Closely observe the patient for seizure activity. Administer anticonvulsants, as ordered.

■ Carefully document the occurrence, nature, and duration of any seizure activity.

■ Protect the patient's safety.

■ As ordered, administer corticosteroids and osmotic diuretics, such as mannitol, and restrict fluid intake to reduce cerebral edema.

■ Prepare the patient for surgery, as indicated.

■ Because a brain tumor may handicap the patient physically or mentally, begin rehabilitation early. Consult with occupational, physical, or speech therapists, as needed, and provide aids, such as bathroom rails for wheelchair patients.

■ Watch for changes in the patient's neurologic status, and be alert for increased ICP.

■ Monitor his temperature carefully. Fever commonly follows hypothalamic anoxia but may indicate meningitis.

■ Use hypothermia blankets before and after surgery to keep the patient's temperature down and minimize cerebral metabolic demands.

■ Before chemotherapy, give prochlorperazine or another antiemetic, as ordered, to minimize nausea and vomiting.

■ Monitor the patient receiving radiation therapy postoperatively for signs of infection and sinus formation. Because radiation may cause brain inflammation, also watch for signs of rising ICP.

■ Throughout therapy, provide emotional support to help the patient and his family cope with the treatment, potential disabilities, and changes in lifestyle.

■ Regularly evaluate the patient's fluid and electrolyte balance to prevent dehydration.

■ Observe and report signs of stress ulcers: abdominal distention, pain, vomiting, and tarry stools; administer antacids as ordered.

Patient teaching
■ Because some of the antineoplastic agents (carmustine, lomustine, semustine, and procarbazine, for example) used with radiation therapy and surgery can

cause delayed bone marrow depression, tell the patient to watch for and immediately report any signs of infection or bleeding that appear within 4 weeks after the start of chemotherapy.

■ As appropriate, explain the adverse effects of chemotherapy and other treatments. Explain which actions the patient can take to alleviate them.

■ Teach the patient and family members the early signs of tumor recurrence, and encourage their compliance with the treatment regimen.

■ Refer the patient to resource and support services, such as the social service department, home health care agencies, American Brain Tumor Foundation, and the American Cancer Society.

EVALUATION

Evaluation of patient outcomes determines the success of collaborative management. For the patient with a brain tumor, evaluation focuses on vital signs, hemodynamic status, fluid balance, neurologic function, and ICP within normal limits; headaches relieved by oral analgesics; absence of any complications; and understanding of the disease, treatment, and prognosis.

Cerebral aneurysm

This localized dilation of a cerebral artery results from a weakness in the arterial wall. Its most common form is the saccular (berry) aneurysm, a saclike outpouching in a cerebral artery. Cerebral aneurysms commonly rupture, causing subarachnoid hemorrhage. Sometimes bleeding also spills into the brain tissue and forms a clot, causing a potentially fatal increase in intracranial pressure (ICP) and brain tissue damage.

Most cerebral aneurysms occur at bifurcations of major arteries in the circle of Willis and its branches. An aneurysm can produce neurologic symptoms by exerting pressure on the surrounding structures, such as the cranial nerves.

Cerebral aneurysms are much more common in adults than in children. Incidence is slightly higher in women than in men, especially women in their late 40s to middle 50s, but a cerebral aneurysm can occur at any age. About 20% of patients have multiple aneurysms.

The prognosis is usually guarded but depends on the patient's age and neurologic condition, the presence of other diseases, and the extent and location of the aneurysm. About half of all patients with a subarachnoid hemorrhage die immediately. However, with new and better treatment, the prognosis is improving.

Potentially fatal complications after rupture of an aneurysm include subarachnoid hemorrhage and brain tissue infarction. Cerebral vasospasm, probably the most common cause of death after rupture, occurs in about 40% of all patients who suffer a subarachnoid hemorrhage.

Other possible complications include rebleeding, which can occur anytime within the first 6 months but usually occurs in the first 24 to 48 hours after the rupture or 7 to 10 days afterward; meningeal irritation from blood in the subarachnoid space; and hydrocephalus, which can occur weeks or even months after rupture if blood obstructs the fourth ventricle.

CAUSES

Cerebral aneurysm results from a congenital defect of the vessel wall, head trauma, hypertensive vascular disease, advanced age, infection, or atherosclerosis, which can weaken the vessel wall.

DIAGNOSIS AND TREATMENT

The following tests help establish a diagnosis, which usually follows aneurysmal rupture: angiography, lumbar puncture, EEG, computed tomography scan, and magnetic resonance imaging.

Initial emergency treatment includes oxygenation and ventilation. To reduce the risk of rebleeding, the doctor may then attempt to repair the aneurysm, usually by clipping, ligating, or wrapping the aneurysm neck with muscle.

After surgical repair, the patient's condition depends on the extent of damage from the initial bleed and on how successfully resulting complications are treated. Surgery can't improve the patient's neurologic condition unless it removes a hematoma or reduces the compression effect.

When surgical correction is too risky (in the very elderly and in patients with heart, lung, or other serious diseases), when the aneurysm is in a particularly dangerous location, or when vasospasm necessitates a delay in surgery, the patient may receive conservative treatment. This includes:

■ bed rest in a quiet, darkened room, with the head of the bed flat or raised less than 30 degrees (may continue for 4 to 6 weeks if immediate surgery isn't possible)

■ avoidance of coffee, other stimulants, and aspirin

■ codeine or another analgesic, as needed

■ hydralazine or another antihypertensive agent, if the patient is hypertensive

■ a vasoconstrictor to maintain blood pressure at the optimum level (20 to 40 mm Hg above normal), if necessary

■ corticosteroids to reduce cerebral edema and meningeal irritation

- phenobarbital or another sedative to keep the patient relaxed.

COLLABORATIVE MANAGEMENT

Care of the patient with a cerebral aneurysm focuses on preparing him for surgery and lifestyle changes.

ASSESSMENT

Most cerebral aneurysms produce no symptoms until rupture occurs. A history may have to be obtained from a family member if the patient is unconscious or severely neurologically impaired. Look for:
- onset of a very severe headache, accompanied by nausea, vomiting and, commonly, loss of consciousness
- a report that the rupture was preceded by a period of activity, such as exercise, labor and delivery, or sexual intercourse
- patient history of hypertension, infection, or head injury
- occasionally, when the rupture occurs as a slow leak, premonitory symptoms that last for several days, such as headache, stiff back and legs, and intermittent nausea
- with bleeding, meningeal irritation, which can result in nuchal rigidity, back and leg pain, fever, restlessness, irritability, occasional seizures, and blurred vision
- with proximity to the oculomotor nerve, ptosis and vision disturbances (diplopia and vision loss)
- with bleeding into the brain tissue, hemiparesis, unilateral sensory deficits, dysphagia, visual deficits, and altered level of consciousness (LOC).

The following grading system has been developed for ruptured cerebral aneurysm:
- grade I (minimal bleeding): Patient is alert with no neurologic deficit; he may have a slight headache and nuchal rigidity.
- grade II (mild bleeding): Patient is alert with a mild to severe headache, nuchal rigidity and, possibly, third nerve palsy.
- grade III (moderate bleeding): Patient is confused or drowsy with nuchal rigidity and, possibly, a mild focal deficit.
- grade IV (severe bleeding): Patient is stuporous with nuchal rigidity and, possibly, mild to severe hemiparesis.
- grade V (moribund [often fatal]): If nonfatal, patient is in deep coma or decerebrate. Age greater than 70 or the presence of other systemic diseases increases the grade by one.

NURSING DIAGNOSES AND COLLABORATIVE PROBLEMS

Based on the following nursing diagnoses, you'll establish patient outcomes.

Impaired gas exchange related to neurologic deficits. The patient will:
- maintain a patent airway
- demonstrate adequate tissue perfusion and oxygenation as evidenced by laboratory studies within normal parameters for patient.

Altered thought processes related to neurologic impairment caused by a ruptured cerebral aneurysm. The patient will:
- exhibit normal thought processes
- be oriented to time, place, and person
- remain free from injury.

Altered cerebral tissue perfusion related to inadequate oxygenation of cerebral tissue caused by bleeding from a ruptured cerebral aneurysm. The patient will:
- regain adequate cerebral tissue perfusion as exhibited by being oriented to time, place, and person
- demonstrate normal neurologic function.

Risk for injury related to increased ICP caused by a ruptured cerebral aneurysm. The patient will:
- have normal ICP
- experience no signs of permanent neurologic injury, such as paralysis, speech impairment, or memory loss
- remain free from injury.

PLANNING AND INTERVENTION

These measures help the patient with a cerebral aneurysm.
- Establish and maintain a patent airway as needed.
- Administer supplemental oxygen.
- Position the patient to promote pulmonary drainage and prevent upper airway obstruction.
- Following your facility's policy, suction secretions from the airway as necessary to prevent hypoxia and vasodilation from carbon dioxide accumulation. Suction for less than 20 seconds to avoid increased ICP.
- Monitor pulse oximetry levels and arterial blood gas levels frequently, as ordered. Use these values as a guide to determine appropriate needs for supplemental oxygen.
- Frequently check the patient's intake and output, and vital signs.
- Avoid taking the patient's temperature rectally because this could stimulate the vagus nerve and lead to cardiac arrest.
- Give fluids as ordered, and monitor I.V. infusions to avoid overhydration, which may increase ICP.
- Prepare the patient for an emergency craniotomy, if indicated.

■ If surgery can't be performed immediately, institute aneurysm precautions to minimize the risk of rebleeding and increased ICP. Limit visitors, restrict fluids, and warn against performing Valsalva's maneuver.

■ Administer hydralazine or another antihypertensive agent, as ordered.

■ If the patient has third or facial nerve palsy, administer artificial tears to the affected eye, and tape the eye shut at night to prevent corneal damage.

■ Monitor the patient for signs of increasing ICP, such as restlessness, weakness, or a changed speech pattern.

■ Watch for decreased LOC, unilaterally enlarged pupil, onset or worsening of hemiparesis or motor deficit, increased blood pressure, decreased heart rate, worsening or sudden headache, renewed or persistent vomiting, and renewed or worsening nuchal rigidity. These signs and symptoms indicate an enlarging aneurysm, rebleeding, an intracranial clot, vasospasm, or another complication; report them immediately.

■ Carefully monitor the patient's blood pressure. Report any significant changes, particularly a rise in systolic pressure.

■ Turn the patient often and encourage deep breathing and leg movement.

■ Assist with active range-of-motion (ROM) exercises; if the patient is paralyzed, perform passive ROM exercises.

■ Apply elastic stockings or compression boots to the patient's legs to reduce the risk of deep vein thrombosis.

■ Provide frequent nose and mouth care.

■ If the patient can eat, provide a high-fiber diet (bran, salads, and fruit) or provide stool softener or a mild laxative to avoid straining at stool and increased ICP.

■ If the patient has facial weakness, assist him during meals; assess his gag reflex, and place the food in the unaffected side of his mouth. If the patient can't swallow, insert a nasogastric (NG) tube, as ordered, and give all tube feedings slowly.

■ Institute measures to prevent skin breakdown; secure an NG tube by taping the tube so it doesn't press against the nostril.

■ Implement a bowel elimination program based on previous habits. If the patient is receiving steroids, check the stool for blood.

■ Raise the bed's side rails to protect the patient from injury. If possible, avoid using restraints because these can cause agitation and raise ICP.

■ Provide emotional support to the patient and his family members or friends. To minimize stress, encourage use of relaxation techniques. Encourage him to express his concerns if he's able.

Patient teaching

■ Teach the patient, if possible, and his family members about his condition. Encourage a realistic attitude, but don't discourage hope. Answer questions honestly.

■ Explain all tests, neurologic examinations, treatments, and procedures to the patient, even if he's unconscious.

■ Warn the patient who will be treated conservatively to avoid all unnecessary physical activity.

■ If surgery will be performed, provide preoperative teaching, assuring that the patient, if possible, and family members understand the surgery and its possible complications.

■ Before discharge, make a referral to a home health care nurse or a rehabilitation center, when necessary.

■ Teach family members to recognize and immediately report signs of rebleeding, such as headache, nausea, vomiting, and changes in LOC.

EVALUATION

Evaluation of patient outcomes determines the success of collaborative management. For the patient with a cerebral aneurysm, evaluation focuses on vital signs, neurologic status, and laboratory values within normal limits; absence of complications or signs and symptoms of progressing neurologic deficit; absence of skin breakdown or contractures; ability to perform activities within expected parameters; ability to compensate for neurologic deficits, control bowel and bladder function, and maintain adequate nutrition; and participation in rehabilitation programs.

Cerebrovascular accident and transient ischemic attack

Also known as stroke, cerebrovascular accident (CVA) is a sudden impairment of cerebral circulation in one or more of the blood vessels supplying the brain. CVA interrupts or diminishes oxygen supply and commonly causes serious damage or necrosis in brain tissues. The sooner circulation returns to normal after a CVA, the better the chances for complete recovery. However, about half of those who survive a CVA remain permanently disabled and experience a recurrence within weeks, months, or years.

CVA is the third most common cause of death in the United States and the most common cause of neurologic disability. It strikes 500,000 people each year, half of whom die as a result. Although a CVA can strike people of any age, race and sex, it usually affects older adults and is most common in black males.

CVAs are classified according to their progression. The least severe type is a transient ischemic attack (TIA)—a temporary interruption of blood flow, most often in the carotid and vertebrobasilar arteries. A progressive stroke, or stroke-in-evolution (thrombus-in-evolution), begins with a slight neurologic deficit and worsens in a day or two. In a completed stroke, neurologic deficits are maximal at onset.

TIAs can last for seconds or hours and clear within 12 to 24 hours. They usually warn of an impending thrombotic CVA. In fact, TIAs have been reported in 50% to 80% of patients who've had a cerebral infarction from such thrombosis. The age of onset varies. Incidence rises dramatically after age 50 and is highest among blacks and men.

Among the many possible complications of CVA are unstable blood pressure from loss of vasomotor control; fluid imbalances; malnutrition; sensory impairment, including vision problems; and infections, such as encephalitis, brain abscess, and pneumonia. Altered level of consciousness (LOC), aspiration, contractures, and pulmonary emboli also may occur.

CAUSES

Major causes of CVA include cerebral thrombosis, embolism, and hemorrhage. Thrombosis is the most common cause of CVA in middle-aged and older people. CVA results from obstruction of a blood vessel, typically in extracerebral vessels, but sometimes it's in the brain.

Embolism, the second most common cause of CVA, can strike at any age, especially among patients with a history of rheumatic heart disease, endocarditis, posttraumatic valvular disease, or myocardial fibrillation or other cardiac arrhythmias, or after open-heart surgery. It usually develops rapidly—in 10 to 20 seconds—and without warning, most often in the left middle cerebral artery.

Hemorrhage, the third most common cause of CVA, may also occur suddenly at any age. It may result from chronic hypertension or an aneurysm, which causes sudden rupture of a cerebral artery.

Factors that increase the risk of CVA include a history of TIAs, atherosclerosis, hypertension, arrhythmias, electrocardiogram changes, rheumatic heart disease, diabetes mellitus, gout, postural hypotension, heart enlargement, high serum triglyceride levels, lack of exercise, use of oral contraceptives, smoking, and a family history of cerebrovascular disease.

In a TIA, microemboli released from a thrombus probably temporarily interrupt blood flow, especially in the small distal branches of the arterial tree in the brain. Small spasms in those arterioles may impair blood flow and precede the TIA. If the blood vessel is obstructed or ruptures, a CVA occurs. Predisposing factors for TIAs are the same as for thrombotic CVAs.

The symptoms of a TIA correlate with the location of the affected artery and include double vision, unilateral blindness, speech deficits, staggering or uncoordinated gait, unilateral weakness or numbness, falling due to leg weakness, and dizziness.

DIAGNOSIS AND TREATMENT

Diagnostic tests may include cerebral angiography (not routinely done if the CVA results from a subarachnoid hemorrhage or if a carotid study suggests dissection), digital subtraction angiography, computed tomography scan (to rule out hemorrhage), positron emission tomography, single-photon emission tomography, magnetic resonance imaging, transcranial or carotid Doppler studies, cerebral blood flow studies, ophthalmoscopy, EEG, and neuropsychological tests.

Appropriate baseline laboratory studies include urinalysis, coagulation studies, complete blood count, serum osmolality, and tests for electrolyte, glucose, triglyceride, creatinine, and blood urea nitrogen levels.

During an active TIA, treatment seeks to prevent a complete CVA and consists of aspirin or anticoagulants to minimize the risk of thrombosis. After or between attacks, preventive treatment includes carotid endarterectomy or cerebral microvascular bypass.

Medical management of a CVA commonly includes physical rehabilitation, dietary and drug regimens to help decrease risk factors, possible surgery, and care measures to help the patient adapt to specific deficits, such as speech impairment and paralysis.

If the CVA is hemorrhagic, the patient may undergo a craniotomy to remove a hematoma or repair an aneurysm. After a thrombotic CVA, the patient may undergo endarterectomy to remove atherosclerotic plaques from the inner arterial wall, or extracranial-intracranial bypass to circumvent an artery that's blocked by occlusion or stenosis.

Medications useful in CVA include:
- anticonvulsants, such as phenytoin or phenobarbital, to treat or prevent seizures
- stool softeners, such as dioctyl sodium sulfosuccinate, to avoid straining
- corticosteroids, such as dexamethasone, to minimize associated cerebral edema
- anticoagulants, such as heparin, coumadin, or aspirin, if the CVA is related to a thrombus or embolus
- analgesics, such as codeine, to relieve headache that may follow a hemorrhagic CVA; aspirin is usually contraindicated in a hemorrhagic CVA because it increases bleeding tendencies, but it may be useful in preventing TIAs.

COLLABORATIVE MANAGEMENT

Care of the patient with a CVA or TIA focuses on respiratory problems, communication ability, and necessary lifestyle changes.

ASSESSMENT

The patient's history, obtained from a family member or friend if necessary, may uncover one or more risk factors for a CVA. Clinical features of a CVA vary with the artery affected (and, consequently, the portion of the brain it supplies), the severity of the damage, and the extent of collateral circulation that develops to help the brain compensate for decreased blood supply.

When assessing a patient who may have experienced a CVA, remember this: If the CVA occurs in the left hemisphere, it produces signs and symptoms on the right side; if it occurs in the right hemisphere, it produces signs and symptoms on the left side. However, a CVA that causes cranial nerve damage produces signs of cranial nerve dysfunction on the same side as the hemorrhage or infarct. (See *Reviewing neurologic deficits in CVA.*) Look for:

■ a report of either sudden onset of hemiparesis or hemiplegia or gradual onset of dizziness, mental disturbances, or seizures

■ reports of loss of consciousness or changes in LOC, such as a decreased attention span, difficulties with comprehension, forgetfulness, and a lack of motivation

■ in a conscious patient, anxiety, mobility difficulties, and demonstrable communication problems, such as dysarthria, dysphasia or aphasia, and apraxia

■ urinary incontinence

■ loss of voluntary muscle control and hemiparesis or hemiplegia on one side of the body; initially, flaccid paralysis with decreased deep tendon reflexes; later, returned reflexes, increased muscle tone, possible muscle spasticity on the affected side

■ vision changes, such as hemianopia on the affected side and problems with visual-spatial relations

■ sensory losses, ranging from slight impairment of touch to the inability to perceive the position and motion of body parts

■ difficulty interpreting visual, tactile, and auditory stimuli.

NURSING DIAGNOSES AND COLLABORATIVE PROBLEMS

Based on the following nursing diagnoses, you'll establish patient outcomes.

Ineffective airway clearance related to deficits caused by CVA. The patient will:

■ maintain a patent airway

Reviewing neurologic deficits in CVA

A cerebrovascular accident (CVA) can leave one patient with only mild hand weakness and another with complete unilateral paralysis. In both patients, the functional loss reflects damage to the brain area normally perfused by the occluded or ruptured artery. But the damage doesn't stop there. The resulting hypoxia and ischemia produce edema that affects distal parts of the brain, causing further neurologic deficits.

Most CVAs occur in the anterior cerebral circulation and cause symptoms related to damage in the middle cerebral artery, internal carotid artery, or anterior cerebral artery. CVAs can also occur in the posterior circulation. These originate in the vertebral arteries and result in signs and symptoms caused by damage to the vertebral or basilar artery and posterior cerebral artery, resulting in higher mortality. Described below are the signs and symptoms that accompany CVA at the following sites.

Middle cerebral artery
The patient may experience aphasia, dysphasia, reading difficulty (dyslexia), writing inability (dysgraphia), visual field cuts, and hemiparesis on the affected side (more severe in the face and arm than in the leg).

Internal carotid artery
The patient may complain of headaches. Look for weakness, paralysis, numbness, sensory changes, and visual disturbances such as blurring on the affected side. You may also detect altered level of consciousness, bruits over the carotid artery, aphasia, dysphasia, and ptosis.

Anterior cerebral artery
Look for confusion, weakness, and numbness (especially of the arm) on the affected side; paralysis of the contralateral foot and leg with accompanying footdrop; incontinence; loss of coordination; impaired motor and sensory functions; and personality changes (flat affect, distractibility).

Vertebral or basilar artery
The patient may complain of numbness around the lips and mouth and dizziness. Look for weakness on the affected side; visual deficits, such as color blindness, lack of depth perception, and diplopia; poor coordination; dysphagia; slurred speech; amnesia; and ataxia.

Posterior cerebral artery
The patient may experience visual field cuts, sensory impairment, dyslexia, coma, and cortical blindness from ischemia in the occipital area. Usually, paralysis is absent.

- demonstrate tissue perfusion and oxygenation within normal limits for him.

Impaired home maintenance management related to permanent neurologic deficits caused by CVA. The patient will:
- identify changes needed to promote maximum health and safety at home
- seek help from resources and support systems to achieve adequate home maintenance
- continue living successfully at home.

Impaired verbal communication related to neurologic damage to speech center in brain caused by CVA. The patient will:
- use adaptive equipment or speech therapy to improve his ability to communicate
- communicate his needs, thoughts, and feelings without frustration.

Self-esteem disturbance related to sudden devastating change in body function caused by CVA. The patient will:
- verbalize his feelings about his self-esteem
- engage in activities that help him achieve higher physical and emotional wellness
- express a positive self-image.

PLANNING AND IMPLEMENTATION
These measures help the patient with a CVA.
- During the acute phase, maintain a patent airway and oxygenation; loosen constricting clothes; and watch for ballooning of the cheek on the affected side during respiration.
- Insert an artificial airway, and start mechanical ventilation or supplemental oxygen if necessary.
- If the patient is unconscious, position him on his side to allow secretions to drain and to prevent aspiration; if necessary, suction the secretions.
- Also during the acute phase, monitor blood pressure, LOC, pupillary changes, motor function (voluntary and involuntary movements), sensory function, speech, skin color, temperature, signs of increased intracranial pressure (ICP), and nuchal rigidity or flaccidity. Remember, if a CVA is impending, blood pressure rises suddenly, pulse rate is rapid and bounding, and the patient may complain of a headache. Record your observations, and report any significant changes to the doctor.
- If the CVA is ischemic, administer an anticoagulant, such as aspirin, heparin, warfarin, or ticlopidine. Anticipate the use of tissue plasminogen activator for thrombolysis in an acute ischemic CVA within 3 hours of the onset of symptoms.
- Monitor the patient's respiratory status closely for evidence of respiratory depression, aspiration, or infection. Watch for signs of pulmonary emboli, such as chest pains, shortness of breath, dusky color, tachycardia, fever, and changed sensorium.

- If the patient is unresponsive, monitor his arterial blood gas levels often and alert the doctor to increased partial pressure of carbon dioxide or decreased partial pressure of oxygen.
- Maintain fluid and electrolyte balance. If the patient can take liquids orally, offer them as often as fluid limitations permit. Administer I.V. fluids if ordered; never give too much too fast because this can increase ICP.
- Offer the urinal or bedpan every 2 hours. Though an incontinent patient may need one, avoid an indwelling urinary catheter, if possible, because of the risk of infection.
- Ensure adequate nutrition. Check for the gag reflex before offering small oral feedings of semisolid foods. Place the food tray within the patient's view. Have the patient sit upright and tilt his head slightly forward when eating. If the patient has dysphagia or one-sided facial weakness, give him semisoft foods and tell him to chew on the unaffected side of his mouth. If oral feedings aren't possible, insert a nasogastric tube for tube feedings, as ordered.
- Provide careful mouth care.
- Provide meticulous eye care. Remove secretions with a cotton ball and normal saline solution. Instill eye drops as ordered, and patch the affected eye if the patient can't close his eyelid.
- Manage GI problems. Prevent straining at stool to avoid increased ICP; modify the patient's diet or provide stool softeners or laxatives as needed. If the patient vomits (usually during the first few days), keep him positioned on his side to prevent aspiration.
- Position the patient and align his extremities to deal with mobility problems. Use such aids as high-topped sneakers to prevent footdrop and contracture and a convoluted foam, flotation, or pulsating mattress to prevent pressure ulcers.
- To decrease the possibility of pneumonia, turn the patient at least every 2 hours.
- Elevate the affected hand to control dependent edema, and place it in a functional position.
- Perform range-of-motion (ROM) exercises for both the affected and unaffected sides. Teach and encourage the patient to use his unaffected side to exercise his affected side.
- Assess the patient regularly for evidence of complications, such as skin breakdown, contractures, and infection.
- Monitor the patient's progress in his rehabilitation program, if appropriate.
- Maintain communication with the patient. If he's aphasic, set up a simple method to express basic needs; then phrase your questions to match his system. Repeat yourself quietly and calmly, and use gestures if necessary to help him understand. Remember

that even an unresponsive patient can hear; say nothing you wouldn't want him to hear and remember.
■ Give medications as ordered, and watch for and report adverse reactions.
■ Protect the patient from injury. For example, keep the bed's side rails up at all times, and pad the rails if the patient tends to bang them with his feet or arms.
■ Provide psychological support, and establish rapport with the patient. Set realistic short-term goals.
■ Involve his family members in his care when possible, and explain his deficits and strengths.

Patient teaching

■ Teach the patient and his family members about the disorder. Explain the diagnostic tests, treatments, and rehabilitation program.
■ If surgery is scheduled, provide preoperative teaching, explaining the surgery and its possible effects.
■ If necessary, teach the patient to comb his hair, dress, and wash. Involve physical, speech, and occupational therapists as needed, and obtain appliances, such as hand bars by the toilet and ramps.
■ Involve the family in all aspects of the rehabilitation plan, and let them help decide when the patient can return home.
■ Explain the need to follow the ordered exercise program. Then teach the patient how to perform ROM exercises for the affected arm or leg, or teach a family member how to perform passive ROM exercises. Reinforce the importance of wearing slings, splints, or other ordered devices to prevent complications.
■ Have the dietitian teach the patient about any special diet, such as a weight-loss diet for an obese patient, that has been prescribed. Reinforce the dietitian's explanation as necessary.
■ Explain the need to report any signs of an impending CVA, such as a severe headache, drowsiness, confusion, extremity weakness, and dizziness. Emphasize the importance of regular follow-up checkups.
■ Teach the patient and, if necessary, a family member about the schedule, dosage, and adverse effects of prescribed medications, including antiplatelet drugs (such as aspirin and dipyridamole), anticoagulants (such as warfarin), and vasodilators (such as isoxsuprine). Make sure a patient taking aspirin understands that he can't substitute acetaminophen for aspirin. Also, emphasize the importance of follow-up care.
■ Teach the patient and family about the need for safety measures. For example, recommend installing grab bars near the toilet and bathtub, removing throw rugs, and securing carpets to the floor.
■ To reduce the possibility of another CVA, teach them about risk factors, such as smoking and diet. Emphasize the need to maintain an ideal weight and to control such diseases as diabetes or hypertension. Advise all patients (especially those at high risk) about the importance of following a low-cholesterol, low-salt diet; increasing activity; avoiding prolonged bed rest; and minimizing stress.
■ Encourage the patient and family members to contact a local support group and the National Institute of Neurological and Communicative Disorders and Stroke. Refer them to local home health care agencies as necessary.

EVALUATION

Evaluation of patient outcomes determines the success of collaborative management. For the patient with a CVA, evaluation focuses on vital signs and neurologic status within acceptable limits; absence of complications, further neurologic deficits, and skin breakdown and contractures; ability to compensate for neurologic deficit and perform activities within expected parameters; ability to control bowel and bladder function; and participation in rehabilitation programs.

Encephalitis

A severe inflammation of the brain, encephalitis usually results from a mosquito-borne or tick-borne virus. Eastern equine encephalitis can do permanent neurologic damage and is often fatal. It's found in the eastern regions of North, Central, and South America. Western equine encephalitis occurs throughout the western hemisphere; California encephalitis, throughout the United States; St. Louis encephalitis, in Florida and in the western and southern United States; and Venezuelan encephalitis, in South America.

Potential complications associated with viral encephalitis include bronchial pneumonia, urine retention, urinary tract infection, pressure ulcers, seizure disorder, parkinsonism, mental deterioration, and coma.

CAUSES

Encephalitis usually results from infection with arboviruses specific to rural areas. In urban areas, it's usually caused by enteroviruses (coxsackievirus, poliovirus, and echovirus). Other causes include herpesvirus, mumps virus, adenoviruses, and demyelinating diseases after measles, varicella, rubella, or vaccination. The disease may also be transmitted by drinking infected goat's milk and by accidentally injecting or inhaling the virus.

Encephalitis is characterized by intense lymphocytic infiltration of brain tissues and the leptomeninges. This causes cerebral edema, degeneration of the brain's ganglion cells, and diffuse nerve cell destruction.

DIAGNOSIS AND TREATMENT

During an encephalitis epidemic, diagnosis is readily made from clinical findings and patient history. However, sporadic cases are difficult to distinguish from other febrile illnesses, such as gastroenteritis or meningitis. The following tests help establish a diagnosis:

■ Blood analysis or, rarely, cerebrospinal fluid (CSF) analysis identifies the virus and confirms the diagnosis. The common viruses that also cause herpes, measles, and mumps are easier to identify than arboviruses. Arboviruses and herpesviruses can be isolated by inoculating young mice with a specimen taken from the patient.

■ Serologic studies in herpes encephalitis may show rising titers of complement-fixing antibodies.

■ Lumbar puncture reveals elevated CSF pressure in all forms of encephalitis. Despite inflammation, CSF analysis often reveals clear fluid. White blood cell count and protein levels in CSF are slightly elevated, but the glucose level remains normal.

■ EEG reveals such abnormalities as generalized slowing of waveforms.

■ Computed tomography scan may be ordered to check for temporal lobe lesions that indicate herpesvirus and to rule out cerebral hematoma.

The antiviral agent vidarabine monohydrate is effective only against herpes encephalitis and only if it's administered before the onset of coma. Treatment of all other forms of encephalitis is supportive. Drug therapy includes I.V. mannitol to reduce intracranial pressure (ICP) and corticosteroids to reduce cerebral inflammation and resulting edema; phenytoin or another anticonvulsant, usually given I.V.; sedatives for restlessness; and aspirin or acetaminophen to relieve headache and reduce fever.

Other supportive measures include adequate fluid and electrolyte intake to prevent dehydration; appropriate antibiotics for associated infections, such as pneumonia or sinusitis; maintenance of the patient's airway; administration of oxygen to maintain arterial blood gas levels; and maintenance of adequate nutrition, especially during coma. Isolation is unnecessary.

COLLABORATIVE MANAGEMENT

Care of the patient with encephalitis focuses on drug therapy to reduce pain and fever.

ASSESSMENT

Depending on the severity of the disease, all forms of viral encephalitis have similar clinical features. The severity of arbovirus encephalitis may range from subclinical to rapidly fatal, necrotizing disease. Herpes encephalitis also produces signs and symptoms that vary from subclinical to acute and usually fatal fulminating disease. If encephalitis is the primary illness, the patient may be acutely ill when he seeks treatment because the nonspecific symptoms that occurred before acute neurologic symptoms weren't recognized as encephalitis. Look for:

■ patient history including systemic symptoms, such as headache, muscle stiffness, malaise, sore throat, and upper respiratory tract symptoms, that existed for several days before the onset of neurologic symptoms

■ sudden onset of altered level of consciousness (LOC), from lethargy or drowsiness to stupor, or seizures, which may be the only presenting sign of encephalitis

■ confusion, disorientation, or hallucinations

■ demonstrable tremor, cranial nerve palsies, exaggerated deep tendon reflexes, absent superficial reflexes, and paresis or paralysis of the extremities

■ complaints of a stiff neck when the head is bent forward

■ fever, nausea, and vomiting

■ in cerebral hemisphere involvement, possible aphasia; involuntary movements identified on inspection; ataxia; sensory defects, such as disturbances of taste and smell; and poor memory retention.

NURSING DIAGNOSES AND COLLABORATIVE PROBLEMS

Based on the following nursing diagnoses, you'll establish patient outcomes.

Altered thought processes related to brain cell dysfunction. The patient will:

■ remain safe from injury

■ regain orientation to time, place, and person.

Hyperthermia related to infection. The patient will:

■ achieve and remain at a normal temperature

■ sustain no brain damage because of hyperthermia.

Impaired physical mobility related to neurologic dysfunction. The patient will:

■ skillfully perform the prescribed mobility regimen to prevent complications

■ develop no complications

■ regain normal physical mobility.

PLANNING AND IMPLEMENTATION

These measures help the patient with encephalitis.

■ Maintain a quiet environment. Darkening the room may decrease headache. If the patient naps during the day and is restless at night, plan daytime activities to promote nighttime sleep.

■ If the patient has seizures, take precautions to protect him from injury. If he becomes delirious or confused, try often to reorient him; a nearby calendar or a clock may help.

- During the acute phase of the illness, frequently assess neurologic function. Observe for altered LOC and signs of increased ICP (increasing restlessness, plucking at the bedcovers, vomiting, seizures, and changes in pupil size, motor function, and vital signs). Also watch for cranial nerve involvement (ptosis, strabismus, diplopia), abnormal sleep patterns, and behavioral changes.
- Measure and record intake and output; monitor for fluid and electrolyte imbalance. Maintain adequate fluid intake to prevent dehydration, but avoid fluid overload.
- To prevent constipation and minimize the risk of increased ICP resulting from straining, provide a mild laxative or stool softener.
- As ordered, give vidarabine by slow I.V. infusion only. When administering vidarabine, watch for tremor, dizziness, hallucinations, anorexia, nausea, vomiting, diarrhea, pruritus, rash, and anemia. Also watch for adverse effects from other drugs. Check infusion sites often to prevent problems such as infiltration and phlebitis.
- Maintain adequate nutrition by giving small, frequent meals, or supplementary nasogastric tube or parenteral feedings.
- Provide thorough mouth care.
- Carefully position the patient to prevent joint stiffness and neck pain, and turn him often; assist with range-of-motion exercises.
- Watch for complications associated with bed rest, such as skin breakdown, constipation, and muscle weakness.
- Because the illness and frequent diagnostic tests can be frightening, reassure the patient and family.

Patient teaching
- Teach the patient and a family member about the disease and its effects. Explain diagnostic tests and treatments. Be sure to explain procedures to the patient even if he's comatose.
- Explain that behavior changes caused by encephalitis are usually transitory. If a neurologic deficit is severe and appears permanent, refer the patient to a rehabilitation program as soon as the acute phase has passed.

EVALUATION
Evaluation of patient outcomes determines the success of collaborative management. For the patient with encephalitis, evaluation focuses on vital signs, neurologic status, and ICP within normal limits; headache controlled by oral analgesics; absence of any complications; and adequate nutrition and optimal mobility.

Guillain-Barré syndrome

An acute, rapidly progressive, and potentially fatal form of polyneuritis, Guillain-Barré syndrome causes segmented demyelination of peripheral nerves. It affects both sexes equally, usually between ages 30 and 50, striking about 2 out of every 100,000 people.

The clinical course of Guillain-Barré syndrome has three phases. The acute phase begins with the first definitive symptom and ends 1 to 3 weeks later, when no further deterioration is noted. The plateau phase lasts for several days to 2 weeks. The recovery phase, believed to coincide with remyelination and axonal process regrowth, lasts 4 to 6 months. In severe disease, recovery may take 2 to 3 years and may be incomplete. This syndrome is also known as infectious polyneuritis, Landry-Guillain-Barré syndrome, or acute idiopathic polyneuritis.

Because the patient can't use his muscles, complications can occur. These include thrombophlebitis, pressure ulcers, contractures, muscle wasting, aspiration, respiratory tract infections, and life-threatening respiratory and cardiac compromise.

CAUSES
The precise cause of Guillain-Barré syndrome is unknown, but it's thought to be a cell-mediated immune system attack on peripheral nerves in response to a virus. Risk factors include surgery, rabies or swine influenza vaccination, viral illness, Hodgkin's or some other malignant disease, and lupus erythematosus.

The major pathologic effect is segmental demyelination of the peripheral nerves, which prevents normal transmission of electrical impulses along the sensorimotor nerve roots.

DIAGNOSIS AND TREATMENT
Diagnostic tests may include cerebrospinal fluid analysis, electromyography, and electrophysiologic testing.

Treatment is primarily supportive and may consist of endotracheal intubation or tracheotomy if the patient has difficulty clearing secretions and mechanical ventilation if he has respiratory difficulties.

Continuous electrocardiogram monitoring is necessary to identify cardiac arrhythmias. Propranolol may be administered to treat tachycardia and hypotension. Atropine may be administered to treat bradycardia. Marked hypotension may require volume replacement.

Plasmapheresis, which produces a temporary reduction in circulating antibodies, is usually reserved for the most severely affected patients or those whose illness is progressing very rapidly. It's most effective if performed during the first few days of the illness. This procedure does not reverse the symptoms, but it commonly slows or stops their progression.

COLLABORATIVE MANAGEMENT

Care of the patient with Guillain-Barré syndrome focuses on maintaining respiration and regaining strength and mobility.

ASSESSMENT

Most patients seek treatment when the syndrome is in the acute stage. The history typically reveals a minor febrile illness (usually an upper respiratory tract infection or, less often, GI infection) 1 to 4 weeks before the current symptoms. Look for:

■ reports of tingling and numbness (paresthesia) that began in the legs and progressed to the arms, the trunk and, finally, the face (tends to vanish quickly); stiffness and pain in the calves, such as a severe charley horse, and in the back

■ muscle weakness (the major neurologic sign) and sensory loss, usually in the legs (in later stages, in the arms); rapid progression of symptoms beyond the legs in 24 to 72 hours

■ a loss of position sense and diminished or absent deep tendon reflexes

■ with cranial nerve involvement, difficulty talking, chewing, and swallowing (paralysis of the ocular, facial, and oropharyngeal muscles revealed in tests).

Remember that muscle weakness sometimes develops in the arms first (descending type), rather than in the legs (ascending type), or in the arms and legs simultaneously. In mild cases, muscle weakness may affect only the cranial nerves or may not occur at all.

NURSING DIAGNOSES AND COLLABORATIVE PROBLEMS

Based on the following nursing diagnoses, you'll establish patient outcomes.

Risk for impaired skin integrity related to immobility. The patient will:

■ communicate an understanding of preventive skin care measures

■ experience no skin breakdown.

Impaired physical mobility related to an inability to move muscles. The patient will:

■ develop no complications from immobility, such as contractures, venous stasis, thrombus formation, or skin breakdown

■ regain mobility with no permanent deficits.

The caregiver will:

■ carry out the patient's physical regimen.

Ineffective breathing pattern related to weakness or paralysis of respiratory muscles. The patient will:

■ maintain adequate ventilation naturally or with mechanical support

■ regain and maintain normal arterial blood gas (ABG) measurements when the syndrome resolves

■ recover normal breathing patterns when the syndrome resolves.

PLANNING AND IMPLEMENTATION

These measures help the patient with Guillain-Barré syndrome.

■ Turn and reposition the patient, and encourage coughing and deep breathing.

■ Begin respiratory support at the first sign of dyspnea (in adults, a vital capacity less than 800 ml or decreasing partial pressure of arterial oxygen [PaO_2]).

■ Continually assess the patient's respiratory function. Auscultate for breath sounds regularly. If respiratory muscles are weak, take serial vital capacity recordings. Use a respirometer with a mouthpiece or a face mask for bedside testing.

■ If respiratory failure becomes imminent, establish an emergency airway with an endotracheal tube. Be prepared to begin and maintain mechanical ventilation.

■ To prevent aspiration, test the gag reflex, and elevate the head of the bed before giving the patient anything to eat. If the gag reflex is absent, give nasogastric feedings until this reflex returns.

■ Monitor the patient's vital signs and level of consciousness.

■ Obtain ABG measurements as baseline and as ordered. Monitor pulse oximetry readings because neuromuscular disease results in primary hypoventilation with hypoxemia and hypercapnia; watch for PaO_2 below 70 mm Hg, which signals respiratory failure. Be alert for confusion and tachypnea—signs of rising partial pressure of arterial carbon dioxide ($PaCO_2$).

■ Provide meticulous skin care to prevent skin breakdown and contractures. Establish a strict turning schedule and reposition the patient every 2 hours. Use alternating pressure pads at points of contact.

■ Inspect his skin regularly for evidence of skin breakdown.

■ Perform passive range-of-motion exercises within the patient's pain limits, possibly using a Hubbard tank. Remember that the proximal muscle group of the thighs, shoulders, and trunk will be the most tender and will cause the most pain on passive movement and turning. When the patient's condition stabilizes, change to gentle stretching and active assistance exercises.

■ As the patient regains strength and can tolerate a vertical position, apply toe-to-groin elastic bandages or an abdominal binder to prevent postural hypotension, if necessary. Monitor blood pressure and pulse rate during tilting periods.

- Inspect the patient's legs regularly for signs of thrombophlebitis (localized pain, tenderness, erythema, edema, positive Homans' sign). To prevent thrombophlebitis, apply antiembolism stockings or compression boots and give prophylactic anticoagulants, as ordered.
- Administer medications as ordered. Analgesics may be prescribed to relieve muscle stiffness and spasm.
- If the patient has facial paralysis, provide eye and mouth care every 4 hours. Protect the corneas with isotonic eyedrops and conical eye shields.
- Offer the bedpan every 3 to 4 hours. Encourage adequate fluid intake (2 qt [2 L/day]) unless contraindicated. If urine retention develops, begin intermittent catheterization, as ordered. Record intake and output every 8 hours.
- To prevent or relieve constipation, offer prune juice and a high-fiber diet. If necessary, give daily or alternate-day suppositories (glycerin or bisacodyl) or enemas, as ordered.
- Monitor the patient's muscle function daily to assess pattern and degree of function.
- Monitor for other complications, such as infection and cardiac compromise.
- If the patient can't communicate because of paralysis, tracheostomy, or intubation, try to establish some form of communication, such as eye blinking to indicate yes or no.
- Provide diversions for the patient, such as television, family visits, or audiotapes.
- Support the patient and family members. Listen to their concerns. Stay with the patient during periods of severe stress.

Patient teaching
- Explain the syndrome, its signs and symptoms, and diagnostic tests that will be performed to the patient and his family.
- Discuss the treatments and their value. For example, if the patient loses his gag reflex, tell him tube feedings are necessary to maintain nutritional status.
- Advise family members to help the patient maintain mental alertness, fight boredom, and avoid depression by visiting frequently, reading books to the patient, and bringing him books on audiotape.
- Before discharge, prepare an appropriate home care plan. Teach the patient how to transfer from bed to wheelchair or from wheelchair to toilet or tub; also teach him how to walk short distances with a walker or a cane.
- Teach family members how to help the patient eat, compensating for facial weakness, and how to avoid skin breakdown.
- Emphasize the importance of establishing a regular bowel and bladder elimination routine.
- Tell the patient to schedule physical therapy sessions.

EVALUATION
Evaluation of patient outcomes determines the success of collaborative management. For the patient with Guillain-Barré syndrome, evaluation focuses on ability to maintain spontaneous respiration and effective airway clearance, vital signs and neurologic status within normal limits for the patient, effective communication technique, and completion of referrals for physical therapy and home care as needed.

Headache

Ninety percent of the time, this common neurologic symptom is caused by muscle contraction or vascular abnormalities. Occasionally, headaches indicate an underlying intracranial, systemic, or psychological disorder.

Throbbing vascular headaches called migraines affect 10% of Americans. They usually begin in childhood or adolescence and recur throughout adulthood. Migraines affect more females than males and have a strong familial incidence. They're usually heralded by fatigue, nausea, vomiting, sensitivity to light or noise, visual disturbances, sensory disturbances (tingling of face, lips, and hands), motor disturbances (staggering gait), extraocular muscle palsies, ptosis, partial vision loss, vertigo, ataxia, dysarthria, and tinnitus.

CAUSES
Most chronic headaches result from tension or muscle contraction stemming from emotional stress, fatigue, menstruation, or environmental stimuli (such as noise, crowds, and bright lights). Other causes include glaucoma; inflammation of the eyes or of the nasal or paranasal sinus mucosa; diseases of the scalp, teeth, extracranial arteries, or external or middle ear; and muscle spasms of the face, neck, or shoulders. Headaches may also be caused by vasodilators (such as nitrates, alcohol, or histamine), systemic disease, hypoxia, hypertension, head trauma or tumor, intracranial bleeding, abscess, or aneurysm.

The cause of migraine headaches is unknown, but these headaches may stem from the biochemical abnormalities that occur during an attack.

Headache pain may emanate from the pain-sensitive structures of the skin, scalp, muscles, arteries, and veins; from cranial nerves; and from cervical nerves. Intracranial mechanisms of headache include traction or displacement of arteries, venous sinuses, or venous tributaries and inflammation or direct pressure on the cranial nerves with afferent pain fibers.

DIAGNOSIS AND TREATMENT

Diagnosis is based on the patient's complaints and on the results of the physical examination. Various diagnostic tests, such as a computed tomography scan or magnetic resonance imaging, may be used to rule out underlying disorders such as a tumor.

Depending on the type of headache, analgesics may provide symptomatic relief and tranquilizers may help during acute attacks. Other measures include identifying and eliminating causative factors, psychotherapy for stress headaches, and muscle relaxants for chronic tension headaches.

One of the newest drugs for treating acute migraine attacks is sumatriptan. This drug can be taken any time during an attack but is not effective in preventing attacks. Another effective treatment for migraines is ergotamine alone or with caffeine; metoclopramide or naproxen is most effective when taken early in the attack. Propranolol and calcium channel blockers, such as verapamil and diltiazem, can help prevent migraines.

COLLABORATIVE MANAGEMENT

Care of the patient with a headache disorder focuses on relieving pain and teaching prevention.

ASSESSMENT

The patient's history may reveal precipitating factors, such as tension, menstruation, loud noises, menopause, or alcohol use. She may be taking oral contraceptives or show signs of prolonged fasting.

In pain associated with head injury or trauma, you may find neurologic deficits. Examination of the head and neck may reveal bruits, signs of infection, crepitus, or tender spots.

NURSING DIAGNOSES AND COLLABORATIVE PROBLEMS

Based on the following nursing diagnoses, you'll establish patient outcomes.

Pain related to headache. The patient will:
- demonstrate measures to control pain
- state that pain is lessened.

Anxiety related to chronic or acute discomfort. The patient will:
- use appropriate measures to decrease anxiety
- state that she feels relaxed.

Risk for fluid volume deficit related to nausea and vomiting. The patient will:
- exhibit electrolytes within normal limits
- demonstrate vital signs within her normal limits
- maintain weight within acceptable parameters.

PLANNING AND IMPLEMENTATION

These measures help the patient with headaches.
- Keep the patient's room quiet.
- Offer cool compresses or ice packs for her forehead.
- Administer pain medications and monitor for effectiveness.
- Administer antiemetics and monitor for effectiveness.
- Monitor serum laboratory studies, including electrolytes, for changes.
- Monitor intake and output and daily weight. Administer I.V. fluid replacement therapy as ordered; maintain I.V. line patency.
- Explain all treatments to the patient.
- Encourage the patient to verbalize her feelings and to participate in her care.

Patient teaching

- Help your patient understand the reason for her headaches so that she can avoid exacerbating factors; use her history as a guide.
- Advise her to lie down in a dark, quiet room during an attack and to place cool compresses or ice packs on her forehead or a cold cloth over her eyes.
- Teach the patient nonpharmacologic measures to relieve discomfort, such as relaxation, imagery, and deep breathing.

EVALUATION

Evaluation of patient outcomes determines the success of collaborative management. For the patient with a headache disorder, evaluation focuses on identifying the cause of the headaches, restoring fluid balance, and relieving discomfort, pain, and anxiety.

Herniated intervertebral disk

Also known as a herniated nucleus pulposus or a slipped disk, a herniated disk occurs when all or part of the nucleus pulposus—an intervertebral disk's gelatinous center—extrudes through the disk's weakened or torn outer ring (annulus fibrosus). The resultant pressure on spinal nerve roots or on the spinal cord itself causes back pain and other symptoms of nerve root irritation.

About 90% of herniations affect the lumbar and lumbosacral spine, 8% the cervical spine, and 1% to 2% the thoracic spine. The most common site for herniation is the L4-L5 disk space. Other sites include L5-S1, L2-L3, L3-L4, C6-C7, and C5-C6.

Lumbar herniation usually develops in people ages 20 to 45 and cervical herniation in those age 45 or older. Herniated disks affect more men than women.

Neurologic deficits (most common) and bowel and bladder problems (with lumbar herniations) are complications of herniated disk.

CAUSES

Herniated disks may result from severe trauma or strain, or they may be related to intervertebral joint degeneration. In an older adult with degenerative disk changes, minor trauma may cause herniation. A person with a congenitally small lumbar spinal canal or with osteophytes along the vertebrae may be more susceptible to nerve root compression and neurologic symptoms.

DIAGNOSIS AND TREATMENT

Diagnostic tests may include X-ray studies, myelography, computed tomography scan, magnetic resonance imaging, electromyography, and neuromuscular tests.

Unless neurologic impairment progresses rapidly, initial treatment is conservative, consisting of bed rest (possibly with pelvic traction) for 1 to 2 weeks, followed by physical therapy, use of supportive devices (such as a brace), heat or ice applications, and exercise. Nonsteroidal anti-inflammatory drugs reduce inflammation and edema at the injury site. Steroidal drugs, such as dexamethasone, may be prescribed for the same purpose. Muscle relaxants (diazepam or methocarbamol) also may help.

A herniated disk that fails to respond to conservative treatment may require surgery. The most common procedure, laminectomy, removes a portion of the lamina and the protruding nucleus pulposus. If that fails, too, the patient may undergo spinal fusion to stabilize the spine. Laminectomy and spinal fusion may be performed concurrently.

Chemonucleolysis, an enzyme injection to dissolve the nucleus pulposus, is performed rarely because of its limited success. In percutaneous automated diskectomy, another alternative, the doctor suctions out the disk portion that causes pain. Typically used for smaller, less severe disk abnormalities, this procedure succeeds about 50% of the time.

COLLABORATIVE MANAGEMENT

Care of the patient with a herniated intervertebral disk focuses on relieving pain and restoring mobility.

ASSESSMENT

Initially, the patient may seek relief for low back pain radiating to the buttocks, legs, and feet. He may report a previous traumatic injury or back strain. Look for:

■ reports of pain that began suddenly after a traumatic injury, subsided in a few days, and then recurred at shorter intervals and with progressive intensity

■ descriptions of sciatic pain that began as a dull ache in the buttocks and increased with Valsalva's maneuver, coughing, sneezing, or bending
■ complaints of accompanying muscle spasms and pain that subsides with rest
■ limited ability to bend forward and a posture favoring the affected side; in later stages, muscle atrophy and palpable tenderness over the affected region
■ radicular pain from straight-leg raising (with lumbar herniation) and increased pain from neck movement (with cervical herniation).

Thorough assessment of the patient's peripheral vascular status—including posterior tibial and dorsalis pedis pulses and skin temperature of the arms and legs—may help to rule out ischemic disease as the cause of leg pain or numbness.

NURSING DIAGNOSES AND COLLABORATIVE PROBLEMS

Based on the following nursing diagnoses, you'll establish patient outcomes.

Impaired physical mobility related to pain and neurologic impairment. The patient will:
■ maintain normal muscle strength and joint range of motion
■ avoid complications, such as contracture, venous stasis, thrombus formation, and skin breakdown
■ regain physical mobility with treatment.

Chronic pain related to nerve root irritation. The patient will:
■ express pain relief after analgesic administration
■ comply with prescribed treatments
■ become pain-free with treatment.

Impaired home maintenance management related to pain and physical limitations. The patient will:
■ report any home maintenance needs
■ seek assistance from available resources
■ regain the ability to perform self-care and home maintenance activities with treatment.

PLANNING AND IMPLEMENTATION

These measures help the patient with a herniated intervertebral disk.
■ Offer supportive care, careful patient teaching, and emotional encouragement to help the patient cope with the discomfort and frustration of chronic back pain and impaired mobility.
■ With the patient and doctor, plan a pain-control regimen, using such methods as relaxation, transcutaneous electrical nerve stimulation, distraction, heat or ice application, traction, bracing, or positioning. Give pain medications and muscle relaxants, as ordered.
■ Encourage the patient to express his concerns about his disorder. Include the patient and family members or friends in all phases of care. Answer questions as honestly as you can.

Preventing back injury

When you teach your patient how to prevent back injury, provide information about changes he'll need to make in the way he sits, drives, stands, walks, lifts, and exercises. Review the following:

- correct posture, including assessment technique
- for individuals prone to back injury, moving correctly to avoid more serious injuries
- proper body mechanics, such as bending the knees and hips (never the waist), standing straight, and carrying objects close to the body
- the need to lie down when he's tired and to sleep on his side (never his abdomen) on an extra-firm mattress or a bed board
- the need to maintain an ideal body weight to prevent lordosis caused by obesity
- relaxation techniques to promote rest and relaxation and the value of using the techniques on a regular schedule.

■ If the patient will undergo myelography, question him about allergies to iodides, iodine-containing substances, or seafood—indicating sensitivity to an agent used in the test. Monitor intake and output. Watch for seizures and an allergic reaction.

■ Before chemonucleolysis, make sure the patient is not allergic to meat tenderizers because the enzyme chymopapain is a similar substance and can produce severe anaphylaxis in a sensitive patient.

■ After chemonucleolysis, enforce bed rest, as ordered. Administer analgesics and apply heat, as needed. Urge the patient to cough and breathe deeply. Assist with special exercises.

■ Prepare the patient for a laminectomy or spinal fusion, as indicated.

■ After microdiskectomy, encourage the patient to increase activity quickly. If a blood drainage system (Hemovac) is in use, check the tubing frequently for patency and a secure vacuum seal. Empty the system at the end of each shift, as ordered, and record the amount and color of drainage. Immediately report colorless moisture on dressings (possible cerebrospinal fluid leakage) or excessive drainage. Administer analgesics as ordered, and assist the patient during his first attempt to walk. Provide a straight-backed chair and allow him to sit in it briefly.

■ During conservative treatment, watch for deterioration in neurologic status (especially in the first 24 hours after admission), which may indicate an urgent need for surgery.

■ Perform neurovascular checks of the patient's legs (color, motion, temperature, sensation).

■ Monitor vital signs, and check for bowel sounds and abdominal distention.

■ Urge the patient to perform, at his own pace, as much self-care as his immobility and pain allow; emphasize activities that promote rest and relaxation.

■ Use antiembolism stockings, as prescribed, and encourage leg movement. Provide high-topped sneakers or a footboard to prevent footdrop.

■ Work closely with the physical therapy department to ensure a consistent regimen of leg- and back-strengthening exercises.

■ Give plenty of fluids to prevent urinary stasis.

■ Remind the patient to cough, breathe deeply, or use an incentive spirometer to avoid pulmonary complications. Provide meticulous skin care.

Patient teaching

■ Teach the patient about conservative treatments and, if necessary, surgery (including preoperative and postoperative procedures).

■ Before myelography, explain the need for this test and tell the patient to expect some pain. Assure him that he'll receive a sedative before the test, if needed. After the test, urge him to remain in bed with his head elevated and to drink plenty of fluids.

■ Before discharge, teach proper body mechanics. (See *Preventing back injury*.)

■ Discuss all prescribed medications with the patient, including possible adverse effects, and when to contact the doctor. If the patient takes a prescribed muscle relaxant, caution him about effects such as drowsiness. Warn him to avoid activities that require alertness until his tolerance to the drug's sedative effect builds.

■ As necessary, refer the patient to an occupational therapist or a home health nurse.

EVALUATION

Evaluation of patient outcomes determines the success of collaborative management. For the patient with a herniated intervertebral disk, evaluation focuses on vital signs and neurologic status within acceptable limits; absence of signs or symptoms of complications; ability to control pain with oral analgesics and to maintain bowel and bladder function; ability to perform activities of daily living and ambulate independently or with minimal help; and referrals for physical therapy and home care as needed.

Huntington's disease

In this hereditary disease (also called Huntington's chorea), degeneration in the cerebral cortex and basal ganglia causes chronic progressive chorea (dancelike movements) and mental deterioration, ending in dementia.

Huntington's disease usually strikes people between ages 25 and 55 (the average age is 35); however, 2% of cases occur in children, and 5% as late as age 60. Death usually results 10 to 15 years after onset, from heart failure or pneumonia.

Potential complications include choking, aspiration, pneumonia, heart failure, and infections.

CAUSES

In 1993, after decades of research, scientists discovered the gene that causes Huntington's disease. Because the disease is transmitted as an autosomal dominant trait, either sex can transmit and inherit it. Each child of a parent with this disease has a 50% chance of inheriting it; however, the child who doesn't inherit it can't pass it on to his own children.

DIAGNOSIS AND TREATMENT

Positron emission tomography and deoxyribonucleic acid analysis can detect Huntington's disease, but no reliable confirming test exists. However, the recent discovery of the causative gene has opened the way for development of further tests to detect and predict the disease. Computed tomography scan, a secondary study, shows brain atrophy.

Because no cure currently exists for Huntington's disease, treatment is supportive, protective, and based on the patient's symptoms. Tranquilizers as well as chlorpromazine, haloperidol, or imipramine help control choreic movements, but they can't stop mental deterioration. They also alleviate discomfort and depression. However, tranquilizers increase patient rigidity. To control choreic movements without rigidity, choline may be prescribed.

Psychotherapy to decrease anxiety and stress may also be helpful. The patient may require institutionalization because of mental deterioration.

COLLABORATIVE MANAGEMENT

Care of the patient with Huntington's disease focuses on support and protection.

ASSESSMENT

Assessment findings vary, depending on disease progression. The patient history usually shows a family history of the disorder, along with emotional and mental changes.

The onset of Huntington's disease is insidious. The patient eventually becomes totally dependent through intellectual decline, emotional disturbances, and loss of musculoskeletal control. Look for:
- in early stages, reports of clumsiness, irritability, impatience, fits of anger, and periods of suicidal depression, apathy, or elation
- in later stages, reports of impaired judgment and memory; hallucinations, delusions, and paranoid thinking; gradual loss of intellectual ability
- ravenous appetite, especially for sweets; loss of bladder and bowel control
- choreic movements that are rapid, often violent, and purposeless; progressing from mild fidgeting to grimacing, tongue smacking, dysarthria, athetoid movements (especially of the hands), and torticollis
- in final stages, constant writhing and twitching, unintelligible speech, difficulty chewing and swallowing, inability to walk, emaciation, and exhaustion.

NURSING DIAGNOSES AND COLLABORATIVE PROBLEMS

Based on the following nursing diagnoses, you'll establish patient outcomes.

Altered health maintenance related to progressive physical and mental deterioration. The patient will:
- avoid injury resulting from a physical or mental deficit
- receive adequate care from a family member or caregiver.

Chronic low self-esteem related to physical and mental disabilities. The patient will:
- express his feelings about how the disease has affected his self-esteem
- describe at least two positive qualities about himself
- take steps to optimize his physical and emotional wellness.

Impaired physical mobility related to neurologic dysfunction. The patient will:
- use assistive devices and seek help when performing physical activities
- maintain normal muscle strength and joint range of motion
- avoid complications of impaired physical mobility, such as skin breakdown, contractures, venous stasis, or thrombus formation.

PLANNING AND IMPLEMENTATION

These measures help the patient with Huntington's disease.
- Provide psychological support to the patient and his family. Listen to their fears and concerns, and answer their questions honestly. Stay with the patient during especially stressful periods.

- Take suicide precautions as necessary. Control the patient's environment to protect him from self-inflicted injury.
- Administer medications as ordered, and watch for desired and adverse effects.
- Monitor the patient's temperature and white blood cell count to detect and correct infection early.
- Assess the patient for signs of neurologic deterioration.
- Identify his self-care deficits each time he's admitted to the hospital. Increase support as mental and physical deterioration make him increasingly immobile.
- Encourage the patient to remain as independent as possible by giving short, explicit directions; demonstrate and give the patient ample time to perform appropriate tasks.
- To help improve the patient's body image, allow him to participate in his care as much as possible. Encourage his efforts to adapt to the changes he's experiencing.
- Provide the incontinent patient with bladder elimination devices, such as an indwelling urinary catheter and body-worn drainage devices, as appropriate. If he has bowel incontinence, provide aids, such as pad and pants or bed protector pads.
- If necessary, provide a walker to help him maintain his balance. If his choreic movements are violent enough to cause injury, pad the bed rails and secure him in a chair or wheelchair.
- If the patient is confined to bed, turn him every 2 hours. Post a turning schedule at the bedside.
- Elevate the head of the bed whenever the patient eats to reduce the risk of aspiration. Stay with him while he's eating, and instruct him to eat only small amounts of food at one time.
- If the patient has difficulty speaking, provide communication aids, such as an alphabet board. Allow him sufficient time to communicate.

Patient teaching

- Teach the patient and family members about the disease and its genetic cause. Explain the diagnostic tests and any required treatments.
- Encourage them to receive genetic counseling. All affected family members should realize that each of their offspring has a 50% chance of inheriting this disease.
- Teach family members how to perform home care.
- Refer the patient and family members to appropriate community organizations, such as home health care agencies, the social services department, psychiatric counseling, and long-term care facilities.
- To obtain more information about this degenerative disease, refer them to the Huntington's Disease Society of America.

EVALUATION

Evaluation of patient outcomes determines the success of collaborative management. For the patient with Huntington's disease, evaluation focuses on vital signs and neurologic status within acceptable parameters; absence of complications; ability to manage bowel or bladder function, to perform activities of daily living, and to ambulate with minimal assistance; and completion of referrals for physical therapy and home care as needed.

Increased intracranial pressure

Intracranial pressure (ICP) is the pressure exerted by brain tissue, cerebrospinal fluid (CSF), and blood within the skull. ICP continually fluctuates. Healthy individuals experience transient elevations with such actions as sneezing, coughing, and straining during defecation. However, in patients with cranial insults or injuries, prolonged increases in ICP can diminish cerebral blood flow and cause irreversible brain damage or even death.

CAUSES

Increased ICP can result from injury to the brain due to trauma, infections, hypoxia, or any number of other conditions or surgeries that affect the brain.

DIAGNOSIS AND TREATMENT

Diagnostic testing may include computed tomography scan, magnetic resonance imaging, and ICP monitoring.

Because small increases in ICP can escape detection, the doctor may implant an ICP monitoring device. When caring for a patient with an ICP monitor, record pressure readings at least hourly, always correlating changes in ICP readings with assessment findings. Notify the doctor of any sudden increase.

The doctor may order one or more of the following treatments to reduce ICP:

- 100% oxygen, or controlled hyperventilation with mechanical ventilation, to reduce blood levels of carbon dioxide (constricts cerebral vessels and reduces perfusion, lowering ICP)
- I.V. barbiturates (usually pentobarbital or phenobarbital) to decrease the metabolic rate, cerebral blood flow, and ultimately ICP
- an intraventricular catheter, a subarachnoid screw, or an epidural probe to monitor ICP (the catheter also can drain CSF from the brain)
- an implanted ventricular shunt to drain excess CSF from the ventricular system, thereby lowering ICP.

COLLABORATIVE MANAGEMENT

Care of the patient with increased ICP focuses on monitoring his response to invasive diagnostic measures.

ASSESSMENT

A complete neurologic assessment will give you a clear picture of the patient's condition and a baseline for his neurologic status. Watch for changes in the patient's overall condition, rather than the onset of one specific symptom.

Because altered level of consciousness is often the earliest sign of elevated ICP, he may exhibit restlessness, confusion, or unresponsiveness. Watch closely for pupillary changes, such as unequal pupil size, constriction, dilation, or a brisk, sluggish, or absent response to light. Note that increased pressure on motor and sensory tracts may cause partial or total loss of function.

In monitoring vital signs hourly, you may see Cushing's triad: bradycardia, hypertension, and changes in respiratory pattern. Remember, increased ICP will first stimulate and then depress the patient's respiratory and circulatory function. Be alert for widening pulse pressure.

NURSING DIAGNOSES AND COLLABORATIVE PROBLEMS

Based on the following nursing diagnoses, you'll establish patient outcomes.

Risk for injury related to increased pressure. The patient will:
- maintain ICP within normal limits
- remain free from injury.

Altered cardiopulmonary tissue perfusion related to decreased cellular exchange. The patient will:
- maintain a patent airway
- exhibit tissue perfusion and oxygenation within normal limits for patient.

PLANNING AND IMPLEMENTATION

These measures help the patient with increased ICP.
- Keep resuscitation equipment on hand in case of a sudden deterioration in the patient's condition.
- Elevate the head of his bed 15 to 30 degrees to promote venous drainage from the brain.
- Don't place the patient in a jackknife position; this elevates intra-abdominal and intrathoracic pressure, which in turn raises ICP. Instead, place his head in a neutral position and support it with a cervical collar or neck rolls, especially when he's lying on his side.
- Institute seizure precautions, such as padding side rails.
- As ordered, administer a diuretic to reduce intracranial hypertension.

- To decrease cerebral edema, administer I.V. lidocaine (a new treatment that shows promise in some patients), as ordered.
- Monitor ICP and drain CSF as ordered. Notify the doctor of any changes.
- Observe CSF drainage and note the amount, color, clarity, and presence of any blood or sediment. If ordered, send daily drainage specimens to the laboratory for culture and sensitivity studies, white blood cell count, and protein, glucose, or chloride levels.
- Take measures to prevent further increases in ICP.
- If an ICP monitor is in place, perform regular neurologic checks.
- Be alert for early signs of increased ICP, such as headache, pupillary changes, vision disturbances, focal neurologic deficits, and changes in respiratory patterns.
- Carefully record fluid intake and output. If the patient is unresponsive or incontinent, insert an indwelling urinary catheter to obtain accurate measurements.
- Anticipate the need for a central venous line or a pulmonary artery catheter to aid in fluid management and an intra-arterial line to provide continuous blood pressure monitoring.
- Keep the patient's room softly lit and quiet.
- Enforce bed rest and limit activity that can increase ICP.
- Instruct the patient to exhale while moving or turning in bed.
- Give stool softeners, as ordered, to prevent straining.
- Provide help if the patient needs to sit up, and instruct him not to flex his neck or hips or to push against the footboard with his legs.
- If you need to suction him, give him oxygen before starting and proceed carefully.
- Watch for signs of infection, and use strict aseptic technique when caring for the insertion site and the equipment.
- Administer prophylactic antibiotics, if ordered, and periodically check the patient's temperature.
- Assist the doctor when he irrigates the insertion site. Don't use preservative-containing saline solutions because they cause cortical necrosis. And never use heparin, which increases the risk of bleeding.
- Carefully position the patient to prevent joint stiffness and neck pain, and turn him often.
- Assist with range-of-motion exercises.
- Watch for complications associated with bed rest, such as skin breakdown, constipation, and muscle weakness.
- Because increased ICP and frequent diagnostic tests can be frightening, provide emotional support and reassurance to the patient and family members.

Patient teaching

■ Teach the patient and his family about the disease and its effects. Explain diagnostic tests and treatments. Be sure to explain procedures to the patient, even if he's comatose.

■ Explain that behavior changes caused by encephalitis are usually transitory, but permanent problems sometimes occur. If a neurologic deficit is severe and appears permanent, refer the patient to a rehabilitation program as soon as the acute phase passes.

■ If the patient receives a shunt, teach family members about proper suture line care. Demonstrate how to mix a 1:1 hydrogen peroxide and saline solution and how to use sterile technique when cleaning the suture line. Tell them to report signs of infection or increased ICP immediately.

■ Advise the patient's family to make sure the patient doesn't lie over the catheter's course for a prolonged period.

■ Teach the patient and family members how to pump the shunt. As ordered, teach them to locate the pump by feeling for the soft center of the device under the skin behind the ear and to depress the center of the pump with a forefinger and then slowly release it. Advise the patient to pump only as many times as the doctor has ordered (usually between 25 and 50 times, once or twice a day). Warn that excessive pumping can lead to serious complications.

■ After shunt insertion, inform the patient and family members of the possible 6- to 12-month course of anticonvulsant drug therapy. If therapy is required, emphasize the importance of complying with the medication schedule to prevent seizures. Also discuss possible adverse effects (especially those affecting the central nervous and cardiovascular systems) and the need to inform the doctor of any such effects.

EVALUATION

Evaluation of patient outcomes determines the success of collaborative management. For the patient with increased ICP, evaluation focuses on maintenance of vital signs, neurologic status, fluid balance, and respiratory balance within acceptable parameters; maintenance of a safe environment, a clean and dry incision site (from shunt insertion), and a working shunt (if inserted); and absence of signs or symptoms indicating complications or deterioration in the patient's condition.

Intracranial hemorrhage

An epidural hemorrhage or hematoma is a rapid accumulation of blood between the skull and the dura mater. A subdural hemorrhage or hematoma is a slow accumulation of blood between the dura mater and the subarachnoid membrane. An intracerebral hemorrhage or hematoma occurs within the cerebrum itself.

CAUSES

An intracranial hemorrhage is usually caused by trauma from a fall or a blow to the head. It can also result from uncontrolled hypertension.

DIAGNOSIS AND TREATMENT

A computed tomography scan is imperative for any patient with a head injury to detect bleeding within the brain.

An intracranial hematoma (epidural, subdural, or intracerebral) usually requires lifesaving surgery to lower intracranial pressure (ICP). Even if the patient doesn't face an immediate threat to his life, he usually requires surgery to prevent irreversible damage from cerebral or brain stem ischemia.

For a solid clot, or for a liquid one that can't be completely aspirated through burr holes, the surgeon performs a craniotomy. After exposing the hematoma, he aspirates it with a small suction tip. He also may wash out parts of the clot with saline irrigation, then ligate any bleeding vessels in the hematoma cavity and close the bone and scalp flaps. (If cerebral edema is severe, he may leave the craniotomy site exposed and replace the flaps only after edema subsides.) Usually, he places a drain in the surgical site.

If the hematoma is fluid, the surgeon may use a twist drill to create burr holes through the skull, usually in the frontoparietal or temporoparietal areas. He drills at least two holes to delineate the extent of the clot and allow its complete aspiration. Once he reaches the clot, he inserts a small suction tip into the holes to aspirate the clot, then inserts drains that usually remain in place for 24 hours.

Hematoma aspiration carries the risk of severe infection and seizures as well as the physiologic problems associated with immobility during the prolonged recovery period. Even if hematoma removal proves successful, associated head injuries and complications, such as cerebral edema, can produce permanent neurologic deficits, coma, or even death.

COLLABORATIVE MANAGEMENT

Care of the patient with an intracranial hemorrhage focuses on monitoring for increased ICP and respiratory problems.

ASSESSMENT

A thorough neurologic examination may reveal disorientation, pupils unequal in reactivation to light, alteration in muscle strength, changes in level of consciousness (LOC), and history of trauma to the head.

Because altered LOC is often the earliest sign of elevated ICP caused by the intracranial bleeding, assess frequently for restlessness, confusion, or unresponsiveness. If the patient lapses into unconsciousness, turn him onto his side to maintain airway patency, and insert a nasogastric tube to prevent aspiration of vomitus and secretions.

Watch closely for pupillary changes, such as unequal pupil size, dilation, or a sluggish or absent response to light. If dilation occurs, particularly on the same side as the hematoma—a sign of impending brain herniation—notify the doctor immediately. Frequently assess the patient's motor and sensory function. Increased pressure on motor and sensory tracts may cause partial or total loss of function or posturing.

Monitor vital signs at least every hour. You may see Cushing's triad: bradycardia, hypertension, and changes in respiratory pattern. Remember, increased ICP will first stimulate and then depress the patient's respiratory and circulatory function. Be alert for widening pulse pressure.

NURSING DIAGNOSES AND COLLABORATIVE PROBLEMS

Based on the following nursing diagnoses, you'll establish patient outcomes.

Risk for injury related to increased pressure from bleeding into the brain. The patient will:
- exhibit ICP within normal limits
- remain free from injury.

Altered cardiopulmonary tissue perfusion related to decreased cellular exchange. The patient will:
- maintain a patent airway
- exhibit tissue perfusion and oxygenation within his normal limits.

PLANNING AND IMPLEMENTATION

These measures help the patient with an intracranial hemorrhage.
- Keep resuscitation equipment on hand in case of a sudden deterioration in the patient's condition.
- Elevate the head of his bed 15 to 30 degrees to promote venous drainage from the brain. Avoid a jackknife position; this elevates intra-abdominal and intrathoracic pressure, which in turn raises ICP. Place his head in a neutral position and support it with a cervical collar or neck rolls, especially when he's lying on his side.
- Institute seizure precautions, such as padding side rails.
- As ordered, administer a diuretic to reduce intracranial hypertension and perhaps a corticosteroid (controversial) or I.V. lidocaine (a new treatment that shows promise in some patients) to decrease cerebral edema.

- Monitor ICP and drain cerebrospinal fluid (CSF), as ordered. Notify the doctor of any changes.
- Observe CSF drainage and note the amount, color, clarity, and presence of any blood or sediment. If ordered, send daily drainage specimens to the laboratory for culture and sensitivity studies; white blood cell count; and protein, glucose, or chloride levels.
- Take measures to prevent further increases in ICP. For example, keep the patient's room softly lit and quiet. Enforce bed rest and raise the patient's head 30 to 45 degrees to promote drainage. Instruct him to exhale while moving or turning in bed. Give stool softeners, as ordered, to prevent straining. Provide help if he needs to sit up, and instruct him not to flex his neck or hips or to push against the footboard with his legs. If you need to suction him, give him oxygen before starting and proceed carefully.
- While the monitoring device is in place, perform regular neurologic checks. Be alert for early signs of increased ICP, such as headache, pupillary changes, vision disturbances, focal neurologic deficits, and changes in respiratory patterns.
- Watch for signs of infection, and use strict aseptic technique when caring for the insertion site and the equipment. Administer prophylactic antibiotics, if ordered, and periodically check the patient's temperature.
- Assist the doctor when he irrigates the insertion site. Don't use alcohol-containing saline solutions because they cause cortical necrosis. And never use heparin, which increases the risk of bleeding.
- Carefully record fluid intake and output. An unresponsive or incontinent patient may need an indwelling urinary catheter to allow accurate measurements.
- Anticipate the need for a central venous line or a pulmonary artery catheter to aid in fluid management and an intra-arterial line to provide continuous blood pressure monitoring.
- As ordered, maintain fluid restrictions and administer osmotic diuretics or corticosteroids to decrease cerebral edema.
- Regularly check the surgical dressing and area for excessive bleeding or drainage.
- Evaluate drain patency by noting the amount of drainage. Although the doctor may set guidelines, drainage usually shouldn't exceed 100 ml in the first 8 hours after surgery, 75 ml in the following 8 hours, and 50 ml in the next 8 hours. Report any abnormal drainage, and ensure that the drainage is tested for glucose to detect any leakage of CSF.
- Carefully position the patient to prevent joint stiffness and neck pain, and turn him often. Assist with range-of-motion exercises.

■ Watch for complications associated with bed rest, such as skin breakdown, constipation, and muscle weakness.

■ Because the illness and frequent diagnostic tests can be frightening, provide emotional support and reassurance to the patient and family members.

Patient teaching

■ Teach the patient and a family member or friend about the disorder and its effects. Explain diagnostic tests and treatments. Be sure to explain procedures to the patient even if he's comatose.

■ Teach the patient and family members how to perform proper suture care. Tell them to watch the suture line for signs of infection, such as redness and swelling, and to report such signs immediately. Also advise them to watch for and report any neurologic symptoms, such as altered LOC and sudden weakness.

■ Instruct the patient to continue taking prescribed anticonvulsants, as ordered, to minimize the risk of seizures. Have him report any adverse reactions, such as excessive drowsiness or confusion.

■ Advise him to wear a wig, hat, or scarf until hair grows back. Tell him to use a lanolin-based lotion to help keep the scalp supple and decrease itching. Caution against applying lotion to the suture line.

■ Instruct him to take acetaminophen or another mild nonnarcotic analgesic for headaches, if needed.

EVALUATION

Evaluation of patient outcomes determines the success of collaborative management. For the patient with an intracranial hemorrhage, evaluation focuses on vital signs, neurologic status, and ICP within acceptable parameters; a clean, dry wound; headaches relieved by analgesics; and adequate knowledge of the disorder, its treatment, and the need for follow-up care.

Meningitis

In meningitis, the brain and spinal cord meninges become inflamed. The inflammation may affect all three meningeal membranes—the dura mater, the arachnoid membrane, and the pia mater.

For most patients, meningitis follows respiratory symptoms. In about 50% of cases, it develops over a period of 1 to 7 days; in just under 20%, it follows respiratory symptoms by 1 to 3 weeks. Meningitis has an unheralded, sudden onset in about 25% of patients, who then become seriously ill within 24 hours.

Infants, children, and older people have the highest risk of developing meningitis. In addition to age, other risk factors include malnourishment, immunosuppression (as from radiation therapy, chemothera-

py, or long-term steroid therapy), and central nervous system trauma.

The prognosis is good and complications are rare, especially if the disease is recognized early and the infecting organism responds to antibiotics. However, mortality in untreated meningitis is 70% to 100%. The prognosis is poorer for infants and older people.

Depending on the cause and severity of the illness, potential complications of meningitis include visual impairment, optic neuritis, cranial nerve palsies, deafness, personality change, headache, paresis or paralysis, endocarditis, coma, vasculitis, and cerebral infarction. Other complications, seen primarily in children, include unilateral or bilateral sensory hearing loss, epilepsy, mental retardation, hydrocephalus, and subdural effusions.

CAUSES

Meningitis can be caused by various bacteria, viruses, protozoa, or fungi. It usually results from a bacterial infection with *Neisseria meningitidis, Haemophilus influenzae, Streptococcus pneumoniae,* or *Escherichia coli.* Occasionally, no causative organism can be found.

The infection that causes meningitis usually occurs secondary to another bacterial infection, such as bacteremia (especially from pneumonia, empyema, osteomyelitis, and endocarditis), sinusitis, otitis media, encephalitis, myelitis, or brain abscess. It may also follow a skull fracture, a penetrating head wound, lumbar puncture, or ventricular shunting procedures.

When meningitis is caused by a virus, it's known as aseptic viral meningitis. This benign syndrome is characterized by headache, fever, vomiting, and meningeal symptoms. It results from some form of viral infection, such as enterovirus (most common), arbovirus, herpes simplex virus, mumps virus, or lymphocytic choriomeningitis virus.

DIAGNOSIS AND TREATMENT

The following tests are useful for diagnosing meningitis:

■ Lumbar puncture shows typical cerebrospinal fluid (CSF) findings associated with meningitis (elevated CSF pressure, cloudy or milky white CSF, high protein level, positive Gram stain and culture that usually identifies the infecting organism—unless it's a virus—and depressed CSF glucose concentration).

■ Chest X-rays can reveal pneumonitis or lung abscess, tubercular lesions, or granulomas secondary to fungal infection.

■ Sinus and skull films may help identify cranial osteomyelitis, paranasal sinusitis, or skull fracture.

■ White blood cell count usually indicates leukocytosis; serum electrolyte levels often are abnormal.

■ Computed tomography scan can rule out cerebral hematoma, hemorrhage, or tumor.

Medical management of meningitis includes appropriate antibiotic therapy and vigorous supportive care. Usually, I.V. antibiotics are given for at least 2 weeks, followed by oral antibiotics, such as penicillin G, ampicillin, or nafcillin. However, if the patient is allergic to penicillin, tetracycline, chloramphenicol, or kanamycin may be used. Other drugs include a digitalis glycoside (such as digoxin) to control arrhythmias, mannitol to decrease cerebral edema, an anticonvulsant (usually given I.V.) or a sedative to reduce restlessness, and aspirin or acetaminophen to relieve headache and fever.

Supportive measures consist of bed rest, hypothermia, and fluid therapy to prevent dehydration. Isolation is necessary if nasal cultures are positive. Treatment includes appropriate therapy for any coexisting conditions, such as endocarditis or pneumonia.

To prevent meningitis, prophylactic antibiotics are sometimes used after ventricular shunting procedures, skull fracture, or penetrating head wounds, but this use is controversial.

Management of aseptic meningitis includes bed rest, maintenance of fluid and electrolyte balance, analgesics for pain, and exercises to combat residual weakness. Isolation isn't necessary. Careful handling of excretions and good hand-washing technique prevent the spread of the disease.

COLLABORATIVE MANAGEMENT
Care of the patient with meningitis focuses on monitoring antibiotic therapy and preventing spread of the disease.

ASSESSMENT
The patient history and your knowledge of seasonal epidemics are essential in differentiating among the many forms of aseptic viral meningitis. Negative bacteriologic cultures and CSF analysis showing pleocytosis and increased protein levels suggest the diagnosis; isolation of the virus from CSF confirms it. Look for:
- infection and increased intracranial pressure (ICP), the cardinal signs of meningitis
- a recent illness
- reports of headache, stiff neck and back, malaise, photophobia, chills and, in some patients, vomiting, twitching, and seizures
- fever; vomiting and fever more often in children (in infants, fretfulness and refusal to eat)
- in aseptic viral meningitis, reports that the disease began suddenly with a temperature up to 104° F (40° C); drowsiness, confusion, or stupor (signs of altered level of consciousness [LOC]; and neck or spinal stiffness (when bending forward) that is slight at first
- in pneumococcal meningitis, a recent lung, ear, or sinus infection or endocarditis; other conditions, such as alcoholism, sickle cell disease, basal skull fracture, recent splenectomy, or organ transplant

- in *H. influenzae* meningitis, recent respiratory tract or ear infection.

Physical findings vary, depending on the severity of the meningitis. Look for:
- opisthotonos (a spasm in which the back and extremities arch backward so that the body rests on the head and heels), a sign of meningeal irritation
- positive Brudzinski's and Kernig's signs; exaggerated and symmetrical deep tendon reflexes; altered LOC, ranging from confusion or delirium to deep stupor or coma
- diplopia and other visual problems; in rare cases, papilledema (another sign of increased ICP)
- in meningococcal meningitis, a purpuric, petechial, or ecchymotic rash on the lower part of the body
- in aseptic meningitis, headache, nausea, vomiting, abdominal pain, poorly defined chest pain, and sore throat.

NURSING DIAGNOSES AND COLLABORATIVE PROBLEMS
Based on the following nursing diagnoses, you'll establish patient outcomes.

Risk for injury related to increased ICP. The patient will:
- regain and maintain normal ICP
- avoid permanent neurologic deficits caused by increased ICP.

Hyperthermia related to infection caused by the organism responsible for meningitis. The patient will:
- exhibit a reduced temperature after antipyretic measures
- avoid complications associated with hyperthermia, such as dehydration and seizures
- regain and maintain a temperature within the normal range.

Pain related to meningeal irritation. The patient will:
- express relief of pain after analgesic administration
- become pain-free.

PLANNING AND IMPLEMENTATION
These measures help the patient with meningitis.
- Follow your facility's policy for infection control and isolation precautions. (Remember that discharges from the nose and the mouth are considered infectious.) Follow strict aseptic technique for patients with head wounds or skull fractures.
- Administer prescribed medications and monitor for desired and adverse effects.
- Continually assess neurologic function and vital signs. Monitor for changes in LOC and signs of increased ICP (plucking at the bedcovers, vomiting, seizures, and changes in motor function and vital signs). Also watch for signs of cranial nerve involvement (ptosis, strabismus, and diplopia).

- Watch for signs of deterioration, especially a temperature increase, deteriorating LOC, seizures, and altered respirations.
- Administer oxygen as required to maintain partial pressure of oxygen at desired levels. If necessary, provide mechanical ventilation and care for his endotracheal tube or tracheostomy.
- Monitor arterial blood gas measurements as ordered.
- Position the patient carefully to prevent joint stiffness and neck pain. Turn him often, according to a planned positioning schedule. Assist with range-of-motion exercises.
- Provide a laxative or stool softener, as ordered, to help avoid strain during defecation.
- Assess the patient's fluid volume. Measure and record central venous pressure, and document intake and output. Maintain adequate fluid intake to avoid dehydration, but avoid fluid overload and cerebral edema.
- Maintain adequate nutrition with small, frequent meals or with supplemental nasogastric tube or parenteral feedings.
- Provide mouth care regularly.
- Maintain a quiet environment; darken the room to decrease photophobia.
- Relieve headaches with a nonnarcotic analgesic, such as aspirin or acetaminophen, as ordered. (Narcotics interfere with accurate neurologic assessment.)
- Provide reassurance and support. The patient may be frightened by his illness and frequent lumbar punctures.
- If the patient is delirious or confused, frequently attempt to reorient him.
- Reassure family members that the delirium and behavior changes caused by meningitis usually disappear. However, if a severe neurologic deficit appears to be permanent, refer the patient to a rehabilitation program as soon as the acute phase of this illness has passed.

Patient teaching
- Inform the patient and his family members about the risks of contagion. Stress that people in close contact with the patient should receive preventive medications as well as immediate medical attention if fever or other signs of meningitis develop.
- To help prevent meningitis, teach patients with chronic sinusitis or other chronic infections the importance of proper medical treatment.

EVALUATION
Evaluation of patient outcomes determines the success of collaborative management. For the patient with meningitis, evaluation focuses on vital signs and neurologic status within acceptable parameters; ICP within normal limits; headache relieved by oral analgesics; adequate infection control; and absence of any complications.

Multiple sclerosis

Multiple sclerosis (MS), a major cause of disability in young adults ages 20 to 40, is caused by progressive demyelination of the white matter of the brain and spinal cord. (See *When myelin breaks down.*) This chronic disease is characterized by exacerbations and remissions. The prognosis varies. MS may progress rapidly, disabling the patient by early adulthood or causing death within months of onset. However, about 70% of patients lead active, productive lives with prolonged remissions.

The incidence of MS is highest in women, people in higher socioeconomic groups, those living in northern climates, and those in urban areas. A family history of MS also increases the risk.

Complications of MS include injuries from falls, urinary tract infections (UTIs), constipation, joint contracture, pressure ulcers, rectal distention, and pneumonia.

CAUSES
The exact cause of MS is unknown, but theories suggest a slow-acting viral infection, an autoimmune response, or an allergic response to an infectious agent. Other possible causes are trauma, anoxia, toxins, nutritional deficiencies, vascular lesions, and anorexia, all of which may contribute to destruction of axons and the myelin sheath. Sporadic patches of demyelination in various parts of the long conduction pathways of the central nervous system cause widespread and varied neurologic dysfunction.

Emotional stress, overwork, fatigue, pregnancy, and acute respiratory tract infections all have been known to precede the onset of this illness.

DIAGNOSIS AND TREATMENT
Because diagnosis is difficult, some patients may undergo years of periodic testing and close observation. Tests that are helpful in diagnosing MS include EEG, cerebrospinal fluid analysis, evoked potential studies, computed tomography scan, magnetic resonance imaging, and neuropsychological tests to rule out other disorders.

The aim of treatment is to shorten exacerbations and, if possible, to relieve neurologic deficits so that the patient can resume a normal lifestyle.

Because MS is thought to have allergic and inflammatory causes, corticotropin, prednisone, or dexamethasone is used to reduce associated myelin sheath edema during exacerbations. Corticotropin and corticosteroids seem to relieve symptoms and hasten remission, but they don't prevent future exacerbations. New drugs, such as interferon beta-1b (Betaseron), have been used to decrease relapses.

Other useful drugs include chlordiazepoxide to mitigate mood swings, baclofen or dantrolene to relieve spasticity, and bethanechol or oxybutynin to relieve urine retention and minimize urinary frequency and urgency.

During acute exacerbations, supportive measures include bed rest, comfort measures such as massages, prevention of fatigue and pressure ulcers, bowel and bladder training (if necessary), treatment of bladder infections with antibiotics, physical therapy, and counseling.

COLLABORATIVE MANAGEMENT

Care of the patient with MS focuses on avoiding complications, managing pain, and improving mobility.

ASSESSMENT

Clinical findings in MS correspond to the extent and site of myelin destruction, the extent of remyelination, and the adequacy of subsequent restored synaptic transmission. Symptoms may be transient or may last for hours or weeks. They may vary from day to day, with no predictable pattern, and be difficult for the patient to describe. Look for:
- initially, visual problems and sensory impairment, such as paresthesia
- subsequently, blurred vision or diplopia; dysphagia; speech difficulty; urinary problems, such as incontinence, frequency, urgency, and UTIs; and emotional lability, such as mood swings, irritability, euphoria, and depression
- muscle weakness of the involved area, such as an arm or leg, and spasticity, hyperreflexia, intention tremor, gait ataxia, and paralysis (ranging from monoplegia to quadriplegia)
- nystagmus, scotoma, optic neuritis, or ophthalmoplegia.

NURSING DIAGNOSES AND COLLABORATIVE PROBLEMS

Based on the following nursing diagnoses, you'll establish patient outcomes.

Altered urinary elimination related to neurologic dysfunction. The patient will:
- regain bladder control with bladder training
- avoid complications associated with urinary incontinence, such as infection and skin breakdown.

Impaired physical mobility related to neurologic dysfunction. The patient will:
- maintain muscle strength and joint range of motion

When myelin breaks down

Myelin plays a key role in speeding electrical impulses to the brain for interpretation. A lipoprotein complex formed of glial cells or oligodendrocytes, the myelin sheath protects the neuron's long nerve fiber (the axon), much like the insulation on an electrical wire. Its high electrical resistance and low capacitance allow the myelin sheath to permit sufficient conduction of nerve impulses from one node of Ranvier to the next.

However, myelin is susceptible to injury, for example, by hypoxemia, toxic chemicals, vascular insufficiency, and autoimmune responses. As a result, the myelin sheath becomes inflamed and the membrane layers break down into smaller components that become well-circumscribed plaques (filled with microglial elements, macroglia, and lymphocytes). This process is called demyelination.

The damaged myelin sheath impairs normal conduction, causing partial loss or dispersion of the action potential and consequent neurologic dysfunction.

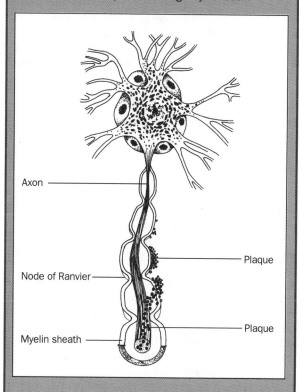

- avoid complications associated with impaired mobility, such as contractures, venous stasis, thrombus formation, and skin breakdown
- achieve the highest level of mobility possible with effective treatment of MS.

Sensory and perceptual alterations (visual, tactile, kinesthetic) related to neurologic deficits. The patient will:
■ compensate for visual, tactile, and kinesthetic loss by using adaptive devices
■ express feelings of safety, comfort, and security
■ regain at least part of lost sensory and perceptual functioning during remission.

PLANNING AND IMPLEMENTATION
These measures help the patient with MS.
■ Help the patient establish a daily routine to maintain her optimum level of activity. Encourage daily physical exercise and regular rest periods.
■ Assist with physical therapy. Increase the patient's comfort with massages and relaxing baths, avoiding too-hot water that may temporarily intensify symptoms. Assist with active, resistive, and stretching exercises to maintain muscle tone and joint mobility, decrease spasticity, improve coordination, and boost morale.
■ Administer medications, as ordered, and watch for adverse reactions. For instance, dantrolene may cause muscle weakness and decreased muscle tone.
■ Assess the patient's neurologic status for deficits, and monitor for exacerbations and remissions of MS.
■ Encourage adequate fluid intake and regular urination. Institute bowel and bladder training as indicated. Eventually, the patient may require urinary drainage by self-catheterization or, in men, condom catheter. Keep a bedpan or urinal accessible because the need to void is immediate.
■ Monitor bowel and bladder function during hospitalization.

Patient teaching
■ Educate the patient and family members about this chronic disease. Inform them of the need to avoid stress, infections, and fatigue and to maintain independence by developing new ways of performing daily activities.
■ Emphasize the importance of exercise. Tell the patient that walking exercise may improve her gait. If her motor dysfunction causes coordination or balance problems, teach her to walk with a wide base of support. If she has trouble with position sense, tell her to watch her feet while walking. If she's still in danger of falling, she may need a walker or a wheelchair.
■ Stress the importance of regular rest periods, preferably lying down.
■ Emphasize the importance of maintaining a nutritious, well-balanced diet that contains sufficient fiber to prevent constipation.
■ Teach the patient about bowel and bladder training, including how to use suppositories to establish a regular bowel elimination schedule.

■ Provide emotional and psychological support for the patient and family members, and answer their questions honestly. Stay with them during crisis periods. Encourage the patient by suggesting ways to help her cope with her disease.
■ Refer the patient to the social services department, when appropriate, and to a local chapter of the National Multiple Sclerosis Society.

EVALUATION
Evaluation of patient outcomes determines the success of collaborative management. For the patient with MS, evaluation focuses on adequate nutrition; absence of complications; ability to control muscle pain using oral analgesics, to manage bowel and bladder function, to perform activities of daily living, and to ambulate with minimal assistance; and referrals for physical therapy and home care as needed.

Myasthenia gravis

This disorder produces sporadic but progressive weakness and abnormal fatigability of striated (skeletal) muscles. Muscle weakness is exacerbated by exercise and repeated movement but improved by anticholinesterase drugs. Myasthenia gravis commonly starts with muscles that are innervated by the cranial nerves. Ptosis and diplopia are typical early signs. Eventually, muscle weakness affects the face, lips, tongue, neck, and throat. Generalized weakness occurs in about 85% of patients. When the disease involves the respiratory system, it may be life-threatening.

Myasthenia gravis follows an unpredictable course of recurring exacerbations and periodic remissions. No cure is known. However, drug treatment has improved the prognosis and allows patients to lead relatively normal lives, except during exacerbations.

Myasthenia gravis affects 2 to 20 people per 100,000. It can occur at any age, but incidence is highest in women ages 18 to 25 and in men ages 50 to 60. About three times as many women as men develop this disease.

Potential complications include respiratory distress, pneumonia, and chewing and swallowing difficulties that may lead to choking and food aspiration.

CAUSES
Myasthenia gravis is thought to be an autoimmune disorder. For an unknown reason, the patient's blood cells and thymus gland produce antibodies that block, destroy, or weaken the neuroreceptors that transmit nerve impulses, causing a failure in transmission of nerve impulses at the neuromuscular junction.

DIAGNOSIS AND TREATMENT

Diagnostic tests may include the tensilon test (confirms diagnosis), electromyography, nerve conduction studies, chest X-rays, and a computed tomography scan.

Anticholinesterase drugs, such as neostigmine and pyridostigmine, counteract fatigue and muscle weakness and allow about 80% of normal muscle function. However, they become less effective as the disease worsens. Corticosteroids may also help to relieve symptoms.

Some patients may undergo plasmapheresis if medications prove ineffective. This procedure removes acetylcholine-receptor antibodies and temporarily lessens the severity of symptoms.

Patients with thymomas require thymectomy, which, if done within 2 years of diagnosis, leads to remission in adult-onset myasthenia gravis in about 40% of patients.

Acute exacerbations that cause severe respiratory distress may signal the onset of myasthenic or cholinergic crisis and require emergency treatment. Myasthenic crisis is a sudden relapse of myasthenic symptoms in someone who has moderate to severe disease. Cholinergic crisis results from the toxic effects of anticholinesterase drugs. Tracheotomy, ventilation with a positive-pressure ventilator, and vigorous suctioning to remove secretions usually bring improvement in a few days. Because anticholinesterase drugs aren't effective in myasthenic crisis, they're discontinued until respiratory function begins to improve. Such a crisis requires immediate hospitalization and vigorous respiratory support.

COLLABORATIVE MANAGEMENT

Care of the patient with myasthenia gravis focuses on pain relief and lifestyle changes.

ASSESSMENT

Depending on the muscles involved and the severity of the disease, assessment findings may vary. Muscle weakness is progressive; eventually some muscles may lose function entirely. Look for:
- complaints of extreme muscle weakness and fatigue; ptosis and diplopia (the most common early findings); difficulty chewing and swallowing; jaw hanging open (especially when tired); bobbing head; and need to tilt head back to see properly
- weak arm or hand muscles (in about 15% of patients); rarely, leg weakness
- symptoms that are milder on awakening and worsen as the day progresses; muscle function that improves after short rest periods
- symptoms that become more intense during menses and after emotional stress, prolonged exposure to sunlight or cold, or infections
- sleepy, masklike expression (caused by involvement of facial muscles) and a drooping jaw (especially if the patient is tired)
- hypoventilation if the respiratory muscles are involved
- difficulty breathing due to decreased tidal volume (from respiratory muscle involvement); potential for pneumonia and other respiratory tract infections
- severe respiratory distress and myasthenic crisis due to progressive weakness of the diaphragm and the intercostal muscles.

NURSING DIAGNOSES AND COLLABORATIVE PROBLEMS

Based on the following nursing diagnoses, you'll establish patient outcomes.

Impaired gas exchange related to respiratory dysfunction. The patient will:
- maintain adequate gas exchange with mechanical assistance during myasthenic crisis
- perform bronchial hygiene correctly to keep airways clear
- regain normal gas exchange after myasthenic crisis, as evidenced by normal arterial blood gas values and normal respiratory function.

Impaired physical mobility related to muscle weakness. The patient will:
- maintain normal joint range of motion
- avoid complications associated with impaired mobility, such as contractures, venous stasis, thrombus formation, and skin breakdown
- achieve the highest level of mobility possible.

Impaired swallowing related to muscle weakness. The patient will:
- exhibit correct eating or feeding techniques to maximize her ability to swallow
- maintain an adequate nutritional intake
- avoid aspiration pneumonia.

PLANNING AND IMPLEMENTATION

These measures help the patient with myasthenia gravis.
- Provide psychological support. Listen to the patient's concerns, and answer her questions honestly. Encourage her to participate in her own care.
- After a severe exacerbation, try to increase social activity as soon as possible.
- Administer medications on time and at evenly spaced intervals, as ordered, to prevent relapses. Be prepared to give atropine for anticholinesterase overdose or toxicity.
- Plan exercise, meals, patient care, and activities to make the most of energy peaks. For example, administer medication 20 to 30 minutes before meals to facilitate chewing or swallowing.

- If surgery is scheduled, prepare the patient according to your facility's policy.
- When swallowing is difficult, provide soft, semisolid foods (applesauce, mashed potatoes) instead of liquids to lessen the risk of choking.
- Establish an accurate neurologic and respiratory baseline. Thereafter, regularly monitor the patient's tidal volume, vital capacity, and inspiratory force.
- Stay alert for signs of impending myasthenic crisis (increased muscle weakness, respiratory distress, and difficulty talking or chewing). The patient may need a ventilator and frequent suctioning to remove accumulated secretions.

Patient teaching
- Help the patient plan daily activities to coincide with energy peaks.
- Stress the need for frequent rest periods throughout the day. Emphasize that periodic remissions, exacerbations, and day-to-day fluctuations are common.
- Teach the patient to recognize adverse effects of anticholinesterase drugs (headaches, weakness, sweating, abdominal cramps, nausea, vomiting, diarrhea, excessive salivation, and bronchospasm) and corticosteroids (decreased or blurred vision, increased thirst, frequent urination, restlessness, depression, rectal bleeding, burning, or itching).
- Warn the patient to avoid strenuous exercise, stress, infection, and needless exposure to the sun or cold weather, all of which may worsen signs and symptoms. Wearing an eye patch or glasses with one frosted lens may help the patient with diplopia.
- Teach the patient who has trouble swallowing to eat semisolid foods and to avoid alcohol because it increases weakness. Tell her that eating warm (not hot) foods can help ease swallowing.
- If surgery is scheduled, provide preoperative teaching. Explain that her chest will be cleaned and she'll receive a general anesthetic. Tell her that, depending on where the surgeon makes the incision, she may awaken from surgery with a chest tube or a drain in place. Also tell her that she may require intubation and mechanical ventilation after surgery and that she'll receive antimyasthenic drugs I.V. or I.M. until she's well enough to take them orally. Explain that these medications will be progressively withdrawn so that the doctor can assess her muscle strength after surgery.
- For information and support, refer the patient to the Myasthenia Gravis Foundation.

EVALUATION
Evaluation of patient outcomes determines the success of collaborative management. For the patient with myasthenia gravis, evaluation focuses on adequate nutrition; absence of complications; vital signs and neurologic and respiratory status within normal limits; ability to control muscle pain with oral drugs, to manage bowel or bladder dysfunction, to perform activities of daily living, and to ambulate with minimal assistance; and completion of referrals for physical therapy and home care as needed.

Parkinson's disease

Named for the English doctor who first accurately described the disease in 1817, Parkinson's disease characteristically produces progressive muscle rigidity, akinesia, and involuntary tremors. Deterioration progresses for an average of 10 years, with death usually resulting from aspiration pneumonia or some other infection.

Also known as parkinsonism, paralysis agitans, or shaking palsy, Parkinson's disease is one of the most common crippling diseases in the United States. It affects more men than women and usually occurs in middle age or later, striking 1 in every 100 people over age 60. Because of increased longevity, this amounts to roughly 60,000 new cases diagnosed annually in the United States alone.

Common complications include injury from falls, food aspiration because of impaired voluntary movements, urinary tract infections, and skin breakdown as the patient becomes less mobile. (See *Recognizing parkinsonian characteristics*.)

CAUSES
The cause of Parkinson's disease is unknown in most cases. However, studies of the extrapyramidal brain nuclei (corpus striatum, globus pallidus, substantia nigra) have established that in this disease, a dopamine deficiency prevents affected brain cells from performing their normal inhibitory function within the central nervous system.

Some cases of Parkinson's disease are caused by exposure to toxins (such as manganese dust and carbon monoxide) that destroy cells in the substantia nigra.

DIAGNOSIS AND TREATMENT
Although urinalysis may reveal decreased dopamine levels, laboratory test results usually are of little value in identifying Parkinson's disease. Computed tomography scan or magnetic resonance imaging may be performed to rule out other disorders, such as intracranial tumors.

There is no cure for Parkinson's disease, so treatment aims to relieve symptoms and keep the patient functional as long as possible. Treatment consists of drugs, physical therapy and, when the disease is unresponsive to drugs, stereotaxic neurosurgery.

Recognizing parkinsonian characteristics

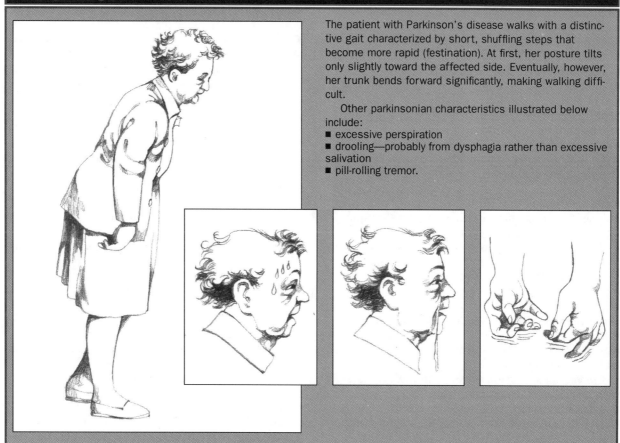

The patient with Parkinson's disease walks with a distinctive gait characterized by short, shuffling steps that become more rapid (festination). At first, her posture tilts only slightly toward the affected side. Eventually, however, her trunk bends forward significantly, making walking difficult.

Other parkinsonian characteristics illustrated below include:
- excessive perspiration
- drooling—probably from dysphagia rather than excessive salivation
- pill-rolling tremor.

Drug therapy usually includes levodopa, a dopamine replacement that is most effective for the first few years of use. The drug dosage is increased until signs and symptoms are relieved or adverse reactions appear. Because adverse reactions can be serious, levodopa is frequently given in combination with carbidopa (a dopa-decarboxylase inhibitor) to halt peripheral dopamine synthesis. The patient may receive bromocriptine as an additive to reduce the levodopa dose.

When levodopa proves ineffective or too toxic, alternatives include anticholinergics (such as trihexyphenidyl or benztropine) and antihistamines (such as diphenhydramine). Antihistamines may help decrease tremors because of their central anticholinergic and sedative effects. Anticholinergics may be used in combination with levodopa to control tremors and rigidity. Amantadine, an antiviral agent, is used early in treatment to reduce rigidity, tremors, and akinesia. Tricyclic antidepressants may be given to decrease the depression that often accompanies the disease.

Physical therapy complements drug treatment and neurosurgery to maintain the patient's normal muscle tone and function. Appropriate physical therapy includes both active and passive range-of-motion exercises, routine daily activities, walking, and baths and massage to help relax muscles.

COLLABORATIVE MANAGEMENT
Care of the patient with Parkinson's disease focuses on relieving symptoms, regaining self-esteem, and retaining function.

ASSESSMENT
The patient history reveals the cardinal symptoms of Parkinson's disease, which include muscle rigidity, akinesia, and an insidious tremor known as unilateral pill-roll tremor, which begins in the fingers. Although the patient often can't pinpoint exactly when the tremors began, he typically reports that they increase during stress or anxiety and decrease with purposeful

movement and sleep. He may also report dysphagia. Look for:

- complaints of fatigue after activities of daily living and muscle cramps of the legs, neck, and trunk
- reports of oily skin, increased perspiration, insomnia, and mood changes
- dysarthria and high-pitched, monotone speech
- drooling and a masklike facial expression
- difficulty walking (retropulsive or propulsive gait, loss of posture control, and walking with the body bent forward); tendency to pivot with difficulty and lose balance easily
- oculogyric crisis (eyes fixed upward, with involuntary tonic movements) or blepharospasm (eyelids closed); delayed movement to perform a purposeful action
- muscle rigidity that results in resistance to passive muscle stretching; may be either uniform (lead-pipe rigidity) or jerky (cogwheel rigidity).

As you assess this patient, keep in mind that Parkinson's disease itself doesn't impair the intellect but that a coexisting disorder, such as arteriosclerosis, may.

NURSING DIAGNOSES AND COLLABORATIVE PROBLEMS

Based on the following nursing diagnoses, you'll establish patient outcomes.

Chronic low self-esteem related to involuntary movement and drooling. The patient will:
- acknowledge feelings of low self-esteem
- seek help in raising self-esteem from appropriate sources
- demonstrate in words and behavior an increase in self-esteem.

Impaired home maintenance management related to self-care deficits caused by neuromuscular dysfunction. The patient will:
- describe changes needed to promote maximum health and safety at home
- seek and obtain assistance from family members, friends, and agencies to meet personal needs
- be able to live at home at the highest level of health possible within the disease limitations.

Impaired physical mobility related to involuntary movement. The patient will:
- have no fractures, burns, bruises, or other injuries caused by involuntary movement
- incorporate safety precautions into his everyday routine
- maintain functional mobility.

PLANNING AND IMPLEMENTATION

These measures help the patient with Parkinson's disease.
- Provide emotional and psychological support to the patient and family members. Listen to their concerns, and answer their questions.
- Encourage independence by helping the patient recognize the activities of daily living that he can perform.
- Provide assistive devices as appropriate. For example, to help the patient turn himself in bed, tie a rope to the foot of the bed so that he can pull himself to a sitting position.
- To help the patient who has severe tremors achieve partial control of his body, have him sit on a chair and use its arms to steady himself.
- Remember that fatigue may cause him to depend more on others, so provide rest periods between activities.
- Work with the physical therapist to develop a program of daily exercises, including stretching exercises, swimming, use of a stationary bicycle, and postural exercises.
- Provide frequent warm baths and massage to help relax muscles and relieve muscle cramps.
- Protect the patient from injury by using the bed's side rails and assisting him as necessary when he walks and eats.
- Monitor for complications caused by involuntary movement, such as aspiration or injury from falls.
- Evaluate the patient's nutritional intake, and weigh him regularly. Provide him with a semisolid diet, which is easier to swallow than a diet consisting of solids and liquids.
- Help the patient overcome problems related to eating and elimination. For example, offer supplementary feedings or small, frequent meals to increase caloric intake. Encourage him to drink at least 2 qt (2 L) of liquids daily and to eat high-fiber foods. He may need an elevated toilet seat.
- To decrease the possibility of aspiration, have the patient sit in an upright position when eating. Keep in mind that many Parkinson's patients are silent aspirators: Even they don't realize that they're aspirating.
- Monitor drug treatment so the dosage can be adjusted to minimize adverse reactions. Report adverse reactions.
- If the patient has surgery, be alert for signs of hemorrhage and increased intracranial pressure by frequently checking level of consciousness and vital signs.

Patient teaching

- Teach the patient and family members about the disease, its progressive stages, and treatments. Explain the actions of prescribed medications and their possible adverse effects.
- If appropriate, show family members how to prevent pressure ulcers and contractures by proper positioning.

- Instruct them in household safety measures, such as installing or using side rails in halls and stairs and removing throw rugs.
- Explain the importance of daily bathing to the patient who has oily skin and increased perspiration.
- To make dressing easier, advise the patient to wear clothing fitted with zippers or Velcro fasteners rather than buttons.
- To improve communication, instruct the patient to make a conscious effort to speak, to speak slowly, to take a few deep breaths before he speaks, and to think about what he wants to say before he begins.
- If appropriate, give the patient tips on how to eat. Tell him to place food on the tongue, close the lips, chew first on one side and then the other, then lift the tongue up and back and make a conscious effort to swallow. Because Parkinson's patients eat slowly, allow them plenty of time to eat.
- Refer the patient and family members to the National Parkinson Foundation, the American Parkinson Disease Association, or the United Parkinson Foundation for more information.

EVALUATION

Evaluation of patient outcomes determines the success of collaborative management. For the patient with Parkinson's disease, evaluation focuses on adequate nutrition; acceptable physiologic status; absence of complications; ability to manage bowel and bladder function, to control muscle pain with oral analgesics, to perform activities of daily living, and to ambulate with minimal assistance; and referrals for physical therapy and home care as needed.

Seizure disorders

Also known as epilepsy, seizure disorders are characterized by recurrent, paroxysmal events associated with abnormal electrical discharges of neurons in the brain. In most patients, this condition doesn't affect intelligence. Seizure disorders affect 0.5% to 2% of the population; they usually first appear under age 20. However, about 80% of patients have good seizure control with medication.

Associated complications include anoxia from airway occlusion by the tongue or vomitus and traumatic injury from a fall or from the rapid, jerking movements that occur during or after a generalized tonic-clonic seizure.

CAUSES

About half of all cases of seizure disorders are idiopathic. No specific cause can be found, and the patient has no other neurologic abnormalities. Nonidiopathic seizure disorders may be caused by:

- genetic abnormalities, such as tuberous sclerosis and phenylketonuria
- perinatal injuries
- metabolic abnormalities, such as hypocalcemia, hypoglycemia, and pyridoxine deficiency
- brain tumors or other space-occupying lesions
- infections, such as meningitis, encephalitis, or brain abscess
- traumatic injury, especially if the dura mater was penetrated
- ingestion of toxins, such as mercury, lead, or carbon monoxide
- cerebrovascular accident.

Researchers also have detected hereditary EEG abnormalities in some families, and certain seizure disorders appear to run in families.

DIAGNOSIS AND TREATMENT

Diagnostic tests may include EEG, computed tomography scan, magnetic resonance imaging, serum glucose and calcium studies, skull X-rays, lumbar puncture, brain scan, and cerebral angiography.

Typically, the first line of treatment is drug therapy specific to the type of seizure. The most commonly prescribed drugs include phenytoin, carbamazepine, phenobarbital, and primidone administered individually for generalized tonic-clonic seizures and complex partial seizures. Valproic acid, clonazepam, and ethosuximide are commonly prescribed for absence seizures.

If drug therapy fails, treatment may include surgical removal of a demonstrated focal lesion in an attempt to end seizures. Surgery is also performed when the seizures result from an underlying problem, such as intracranial tumors, brain abscess or cysts, or vascular abnormalities.

COLLABORATIVE MANAGEMENT

Care of the patient with a seizure disorder focuses on protecting him from injury and teaching him to manage his illness. (See *Monitoring a seizure disorder [phase 1, noninvasive]*, page 316.)

ASSESSMENT

Depending on the type and cause of the seizure, signs and symptoms vary. (See *Differentiating among seizure types*, page 317.) Look for:

- normal physical findings, if the patient isn't having a seizure and the cause is idiopathic
- signs and symptoms of an underlying problem
- a seizure as the only symptom of a brain tumor
- reports by the patient that the seizures are unpredictable and unrelated to activities
- reports of precipitating factors or events, such as seizures at a particular time (during sleep), or in a particular circumstance (exhaustion or emotional stress)

CLINICAL PATH

Monitoring a seizure disorder (phase 1, noninvasive)

CARE ELEMENT	Event 1 (Date:_____) Admission	Event 2 (Date:_____) (Seizure ≥3)	Event 3 (Date:_____) Discharge home
CARE UNIT	Neurology unit with monitoring capabilities		
CONSULTS	■ Physical therapy consult for exercise bike _____ (date) ■ Neuropsychology		
TESTS, LAB TESTS, RADIOLOGY	■ Drug levels: _____ _____ _____ ■ Other lab tests: _____ _____ _____ ■ Continuous EEG monitoring ⟶	■ Continuous EEG monitoring ⟶	■ Drug levels: _____ _____ _____
TREATMENTS Call doctor for:	■ Insertion of sphenoidal electrodes by doctor ■ Electrodes placed by EEG dept. ■ Medication-lock (ML) flush every shift ■ Exercise bike ■ Vital signs (VS) every shift ■ Full assessments every shift ■ Oxygen (O₂) and suction equipment in room ■ I.V. access maintained ■ No gum chewing or smoking ■ Fall and seizure precautions ■ Light left on in room ■ Sleep deprived on third night if no seizures	■ ML flush every shift ■ Bike ■ VS every shift ⟶ ■ Full assessments every shift ⟶ ■ O₂ and suction equipment in room ■ I.V. access maintained ⟶ ■ No gum chewing or smoking ⟶ ■ Fall and seizure precautions ⟶ ■ Light left on in room ⟶ ■ Sleep deprived on third night if no seizures	■ Electrodes discontinued ■ ML discontinued ■ Bike ■ VS every shift ⟶ ■ Full assessments every shift ⟶ ■ O₂ and suction equipment in room ■ I.V. access maintained ⟶ ■ No gum chewing or smoking ⟶ ■ Fall and seizure precautions ⟶
MEDICATIONS	■ Anticonvulsants	■ Anticonvulsants tapered	■ Anticonvulsants restarted
PAIN/SYMPTOM CONTROL	■ Tylenol 650 mg P.O. every 4 hr as needed (p.r.n.) ■ Tylenol #3 1 to 2 tablets P.O. every 4 hr p.r.n. ■ Ativan 1 to 2 mg I.V. p.r.n. for 1 general tonic-clonic (GTC) seizure or 2 complex partial (CP) seizures per 8-hr shift; call doctor when given ■ Benadryl 25 to 50 mg P.O. every 6 hr p.r.n. ■ Milk of Magnesia 30 ml every day p.r.n. for constipation	■ Tylenol 650 mg P.O. every 4 hr p.r.n. ■ Tylenol #3 1 to 2 tablets P.O. every 4 hr p.r.n. ■ Ativan 1 to 2 mg I.V. p.r.n. for 1 GTC seizure or 2 CP seizures per 8-hr shift; call doctor when given ■ Benadryl 25 to 50 mg P.O. every 6 hr p.r.n. ■ Milk of Magnesia 30 ml every day p.r.n. for constipation	■ Tylenol 650 mg P.O. every 4 hr p.r.n. ■ Tylenol #3 1 to 2 tablets P.O. every 4 hr p.r.n. ■ Ativan 1 to 2 mg I.V. p.r.n. for 1 GTC seizure or 2 CP seizures per 8-hr shift; call doctor when given ■ Benadryl 25 to 50 mg P.O. every 6 hr p.r.n. ■ Milk of Magnesia 30 ml every day p.r.n. for constipation
ACTIVITY	■ Bathroom privileges (BRP) ■ Exercise bike at bedside for use only when attended	■ BRP ⟶	■ As tolerated ⟶
NUTRITION	■ Regular ⟶	■ Regular ⟶	■ Regular ⟶
DISCHARGE PLANNING/TEACHING	■ Admission data base ■ Unit orientation ■ Seizure and fall precautions ■ Epilepsy program requirements per EEG protocol ■ Discharge needs assessment	■ Review fall and seizure precautions. ■ Provide sleep deprivation instructions. ■ Assess discharge needs.	■ Review discharge instructions. ■ Medication sheets: Anticonvulsants

RECIPIENT OF TEACHING: _____

Adapted with permission from Shands Hospital at the University of Florida, Gainesville.

Differentiating among seizure types

The hallmark of epilepsy is recurring seizures, which can be classified as partial or generalized. Some patients may be affected by more than one type.

Partial seizures

Arising from a localized area in the brain, these seizures cause specific symptoms. In some patients, partial seizure activity may spread to the entire brain, causing a generalized seizure. Partial seizures include simple partial (jacksonian motor-type and sensory-type), complex partial (psychomotor or temporal lobe), and secondarily generalized partial seizures.

Simple partial (jacksonian motor-type) seizure

This type begins as a localized motor seizure, which is characterized by a spread of abnormal activity to adjacent areas of the brain. Typically, the patient experiences a stiffening or jerking in one extremity, accompanied by a tingling sensation in the same area. For example, the seizure may start in the thumb and spread to the entire hand and arm. The patient seldom loses consciousness, although the seizure may progress to a generalized tonic-clonic seizure.

Simple partial (sensory-type) seizure

Perception is distorted in this type of seizure. Symptoms can include hallucinations, flashing lights, tingling sensations, a foul odor, vertigo, and a déja vu sensation.

Complex partial (psychomotor or temporal lobe) seizure

Symptoms of this seizure type are variable but usually include purposeless behavior. The patient may experience an aura and exhibit overt signs, including a glassy stare, picking at his clothes, aimless wandering, lip smacking or chewing motions, and unintelligible speech. The seizure may last for a few seconds or as long as 20 minutes. Afterward, mental confusion may last for several minutes; as a result, an observer may mistakenly suspect psychosis or intoxication with alcohol or drugs. The patient has no memory of his actions during the seizure.

Secondarily generalized partial seizure

This type of seizure can be either simple or complex and can progress to a generalized seizure. An aura may precede the progression. Loss of consciousness occurs immediately or within 1 to 2 minutes of the start of the progression.

Generalized seizures

As the term suggests, these seizures cause a generalized electrical abnormality within the brain. They include several distinct types.

Absence seizure

This type occurs most often in children, although it may affect adults as well. It usually begins with a brief change in level of consciousness, indicated by blinking or rolling of the eyes, a blank stare, and slight mouth movements. The patient retains his posture and continues preseizure activity without difficulty. The impairment is so brief that the patient is sometimes unaware of it. Typically, the seizure lasts from 1 to 10 seconds. If not properly treated, these seizures can recur as often as 100 times a day. An absence seizure may progress to a generalized tonic-clonic seizure.

Myoclonic seizure

Also called bilateral massive epileptic myoclonus, this seizure type is marked by brief, involuntary muscle jerks of the body or extremities, which may occur in a rhythmic manner, and a brief loss of consciousness.

Generalized tonic-clonic seizure

Typically, this seizure begins with a loud cry, precipitated by air rushing from the lungs through the vocal cords. The patient falls to the ground, losing consciousness. The body stiffens (tonic phase) and then alternates between episodes of muscle spasm and relaxation (clonic phase). Tongue biting, incontinence, labored breathing, apnea, and subsequent cyanosis may also occur. The seizure stops in 2 to 5 minutes, when abnormal electrical conduction of the neurons is completed. The patient then regains consciousness but is somewhat confused and may have difficulty talking. If he can talk, he may complain of drowsiness, fatigue, headache, muscle soreness, and arm or leg weakness. He may fall into a deep sleep after the seizure.

Akinetic seizure

Characterized by a general loss of postural tone and a temporary loss of consciousness, this type of seizure occurs in young children. Sometimes it's called a drop attack because it causes the child to fall.

■ reports of nonspecific changes, such as headache, mood changes, lethargy, and myoclonic jerking, up to several hours before the onset of a seizure

■ status epilepticus (See *Understanding status epilepticus,* page 318.)

■ with a generalized seizure, reports of an aura that precedes seizure onset by a few seconds or minutes. An aura, which represents the beginning of abnormal electrical discharges within a focal area of the brain, may consist of a pungent smell, nausea or indigestion, a rising or sinking feeling in the stomach, a

Understanding status epilepticus

A continuous seizure state, status epilepticus can occur in all seizure types and is considered an emergency. It can result from abrupt withdrawal of anticonvulsants, hypoxic or metabolic encephalopathy, acute head trauma, or septicemia secondary to encephalitis or meningitis.

Signs and symptoms

There are three types of status epilepticus. Patients with *generalized tonic-clonic status epilepticus*, the most life-threatening form, have continuous generalized tonic-clonic seizures with no intervening return of consciousness. Respiratory distress also occurs. In the second type, *petit mal status epilepticus*, the patient may exhibit 200 to 300 "absences" per day. In the third type, partial or focal status or *epilepsia continua*, focal seizures occur continuously or regularly, and the patient usually remains conscious unless generalization occurs.

Emergency interventions

- Notify the doctor immediately but don't leave the patient unattended.
- Ensure a patent airway.
- Draw blood for glucose, electrolyte, blood urea nitrogen, arterial blood gas, and creatine kinase levels to determine the possible cause, and establish an I.V. line.
- Be prepared to administer I.V. medication to stop seizure activity. The most commonly used I.V. drugs are diazepam, phenytoin, and phenobarbital; dextrose 50% (when seizures are secondary to hypoglycemia); and thiamine (for a patient with chronic alcoholism or one undergoing withdrawal).

dreamy feeling, an unusual taste, or a visual disturbance such as a flashing light.

If you observe the patient during a seizure, be sure to note the type of seizure he's experiencing. Otherwise, details obtained from a family member or friend may help to identify the seizure type.

NURSING DIAGNOSES AND COLLABORATIVE PROBLEMS

Based on the following nursing diagnoses, you'll establish patient outcomes.

Risk for aspiration related to absence of protective mechanisms. The patient will:
- maintain a patent airway
- exhibit tissue perfusion and oxygenation within normal limits for him
- show no signs of aspiration.

Risk for injury related to potential for seizures. The patient will:

- instruct family members, friends, and coworkers on how to protect him from injury during a seizure
- remain free from injury during a seizure.

Social isolation related to the stigma attached to behavior exhibited during a seizure. The patient will:
- express his negative feelings about seizures and communicate an understanding of his disorder
- recover from negative feelings associated with social isolation
- resume active participation in society.

PLANNING AND IMPLEMENTATION

These measures help the patient with a seizure disorder.

- During seizures, monitor the patient continuously; maintain a patent airway using a gentle chin-lift, jaw-thrust maneuver; suction the airway as needed; avoid placing sharp objects between his teeth; and administer oxygen as necessary.
- Protect the patient from injury by padding side rails as your facility directs and by keeping sharp objects and tubing out of reach.
- Administer anticonvulsants as prescribed, and monitor the patient continually for signs and symptoms of toxicity, such as slurred speech, ataxia, lethargy, dizziness, drowsiness, nystagmus, irritability, nausea, and vomiting. Also monitor him closely when administering I.V. phenytoin.
- Monitor the patient's compliance with anticonvulsant drug therapy.
- When administering phenytoin I.V., use a large vein, administer slowly (usually 50 mg/minute), and mix only with normal saline solution.
- Prepare the patient for surgery if necessary.
- Provide preoperative and postoperative care appropriate for the type of surgery he'll undergo.
- Encourage the patient and family members to express their fears and concerns. Suggest counseling to help them cope.

Patient teaching

- Teach the patient and family members about the seizure disorder and the myths and misconceptions surrounding it. Be sure to dispel the notion that seizures are contagious.
- Tell them that the disorder is controllable and, with medication, allows a normal lifestyle.
- Explain that anticonvulsants are safe when taken as ordered and that the patient must comply with the prescribed drug schedule.
- Reinforce dosage instructions; suggest reminders for taking medications regularly and maintaining an adequate drug supply.
- Teach the patient about possible adverse effects, such as drowsiness, lethargy, hyperactivity, confusion, visual and sleep disturbances (all indicate needed

dosage adjustment) and about the need to report them immediately.

■ Explain that phenytoin therapy may lead to hyperplasia of the gums, which may be relieved by conscientious oral hygiene.

■ Stress the importance of regularly checking anticonvulsant blood levels, even if the seizures are under control.

■ Advise the patient to eat regular meals and to check with his doctor before dieting. Explain that adequate glucose levels are necessary to fuel nervous system neurons for normal activity.

■ Tell him to limit alcohol intake and that the doctor may prohibit alcohol.

■ Teach seizure prevention measures, such as adequate sleep, stress control, and avoidance of trigger factors (flashing lights, hyperventilation, loud noises, heavy musical beats, video games and television).

■ Alert him to note and report odors associated with an attack.

■ Advise him to treat a fever early during an illness and to report any fever he can't reduce.

■ If the patient is a candidate for surgery, explain preoperative activities and postoperative care.

■ Refer him to appropriate local social agencies, the Epilepsy Foundation of America, and the state motor vehicle department for information about a driver's license.

■ Teach the patient's family members how to care for him during a seizure. This is especially important if the patient experiences generalized tonic-clonic seizures, which may require first aid. Instruct family members or a friend to:

– avoid restraining the patient during a seizure

– help him to a lying position, loosen any tight clothing, and place something flat and soft, such as a jacket or hand, under his head

– clear the area of hard objects

– avoid forcing anything into the patient's mouth if his teeth are clenched

– avoid using a tongue blade or spoon, which could lacerate the mouth and lips or displace teeth, precipitating respiratory distress

– protect the patient's tongue, if his mouth is open, by placing a soft object (such as folded cloth) between his teeth

– turn the patient's head to the side to provide an open airway

– reassure the patient after the seizure subsides by telling him that he's all right, orienting him to time and place, and informing him that he's had a seizure.

EVALUATION

Evaluation of patient outcomes determines the success of collaborative management. For the patient with a seizure disorder, evaluation focuses on identifying the cause of seizures, controlling seizures, maintaining neurologic and respiratory status within acceptable parameters, and ensuring adequate knowledge about therapy and the need for compliance.

Skull fracture

A skull fracture is always considered serious and at times may be life-threatening. Because the primary concern is possible damage to the brain, the injury is considered a neurosurgical condition.

Skull fractures are classified as simple (closed) or compound (open) and may displace bone fragments. They're also described as linear, comminuted, or depressed. A linear, or hairline, fracture doesn't displace structures and seldom requires treatment. A comminuted fracture splinters or crushes the bone into several fragments. A depressed fracture, which pushes the bone toward the brain, is considered serious only if it compresses underlying structures.

Skull fractures also are classified by location, such as cranial vault or basilar. A basilar fracture is located at the base of the skull and may involve the cribriform plate and the frontal sinuses. Because of the danger of cranial complications and meningitis, basilar fractures usually are considered far more serious than cranial vault fractures.

Skull fractures can lead to infection, intracerebral hemorrhage and hematoma, brain abscess, and increased intracranial pressure (ICP) from edema. Recovery from the injury can be further complicated by residual effects, such as seizure disorders, hydrocephalus, and organic mental syndrome.

CAUSES

A skull fracture can result from a blow to the head resulting from a fall, an object striking the head, or the person being thrown (for example, in a motor vehicle accident, where the victim is thrown or ejected onto a stationary object).

DIAGNOSIS AND TREATMENT

Diagnostic tests may include skull X-ray, computed tomography scan, and magnetic resonance imaging.

The type of treatment depends on the type of skull fracture. In general, if the patient hasn't lost consciousness, he should be observed in the emergency department for at least 4 hours. After this period, a patient with stable vital signs can be discharged with an instruction sheet for continuing with 24 to 48 hours of observation at home.

Although a simple linear skull fracture can tear an underlying blood vessel or cause a leak of cerebrospinal fluid (CSF), most require only supportive treatment. Such treatment includes mild analgesics (acetaminophen) and wound management (local injection of procaine, shaving the wound area, and cleaning and debriding the wound).

More severe vault fractures, especially depressed fractures, usually require a craniotomy to elevate or remove fragments that have been driven into the brain and to extract foreign bodies and necrotic tissue. This reduces the risk of infection and further brain damage. Cranioplasty may be necessary with the use of tantalum mesh or acrylic plates to replace the removed skull section. The patient commonly requires antibiotics and, in profound hemorrhage, blood transfusions.

A basilar fracture calls for immediate prophylactic antibiotics to prevent meningitis from CSF leakage. The patient also needs close observation for secondary hematomas and hemorrhages and may require surgery.

COLLABORATIVE MANAGEMENT

Care of the patient with a skull fracture will focus on maintaining his safety and comfort while monitoring his neurologic status.

ASSESSMENT

The patient's history (which may be obtained from a family member, an eyewitnesses, or emergency personnel) will reveal a traumatic injury to the head, possibly followed by a period of unconsciousness. An unconscious patient may appear pale and motionless. A conscious patient may appear drowsy or easily disturbed by any form of stimulation, such as noise or light.

You'll evaluate the patient's level of consciousness (LOC), pupillary responses, and strength of extremities. Vital signs aren't good indicators of neurologic status and don't correlate specifically with the type of injury, unless the brain stem is involved. With a skull fracture, look for:

- complaints of a persistent, localized headache; dazed, anxious, or agitated appearance
- scalp abrasions, contusions, lacerations, or avulsions
- if the scalp was lacerated or torn away, profuse bleeding, but rarely enough to induce shock
- in a severe head injury, a state of shock from other injuries or from medullary failure
- bleeding in the nose, pharynx, or ears; under the conjunctivae; under the periorbital skin (raccoon's eyes); and behind the eardrum
- Battle's sign (bruising behind the ear)
- CSF and brain tissue leakage from ears and nose (check pillowcase or bed linens), particularly with basilar fractures

- palpable fractures, areas of swelling, and possibly hematoma formation
- in a concussion, skull tenderness or hematomas
- in a vault fracture, soft-tissue swelling near the site, making other fractures hard to detect without X-rays
- altered LOC along with other classic signs of brain injury: agitation and irritability, abnormal deep tendon reflexes, altered pupillary and motor responses, hemiparesis, dizziness, seizures, and projectile vomiting. Loss of consciousness may last for hours, days, weeks, or indefinitely. Many findings, however, will vary with the location and severity of the fracture. For example, a linear fracture associated only with a concussion won't produce loss of consciousness; a sphenoidal fracture may produce vision loss; a temporal fracture may trigger unilateral hearing loss or facial paralysis.

NURSING DIAGNOSES AND COLLABORATIVE MANAGEMENT

Based on the following nursing diagnoses, you'll establish patient outcomes.

Risk for injury related to complications of head injury. The patient will:

- exhibit normal neurologic findings after the head injury heals
- avoid permanent neurologic deficit.

Pain related to altered brain or skull tissue. The patient will:

- maintain normal ICP
- express pain relief with treatment
- obtain complete pain relief after the head injury heals.

PLANNING AND IMPLEMENTATION

These measures help the patient with a skull fracture.

- Administer medications as ordered. However, don't administer narcotics or sedatives because they may depress respirations, raise partial pressure of arterial carbon dioxide, lead to increased ICP, and mask changes in neurologic status. Give acetaminophen for pain, as ordered.
- Speak calmly to the patient and explain your actions, even if he's unconscious.
- Don't make any sudden, unexpected moves. Touch the patient gently.
- Depending on the patient's condition, use side rails, assist him with walking, and stay with him while he uses the bathroom. If the patient is confused, place him where you can easily observe him.
- If the patient is unconscious, insert a nasogastric (NG) tube to prevent aspiration, but only after a basilar skull fracture has been ruled out. Otherwise, the tube might be inserted into the cranial vault. If the patient has a basilar fracture, a soft nasal airway may

be inserted first; then an NG tube may be inserted through the nasal airway.

■ Carefully observe the patient for CSF leakage. Check the bed sheets for a blood-tinged spot surrounded by a lighter ring (halo sign).

■ Position the patient so that secretions drain properly. If you detect CSF leakage from the nose, place a gauze pad under the nostrils. If CSF leaks from the ear, position him to drain naturally. Don't pack the ear or nose. If required, suction by mouth, not the nose, to avoid introducing bacteria.

■ If the patient has CSF leakage or is unconscious, elevate the head of the bed 30 degrees. Otherwise, leave it flat to avoid jugular compression, leading to increased ICP. Enforce bed rest.

■ After the patient is stabilized, clean and dress any superficial scalp wounds, wearing sterile gloves. (If the skin has been broken, he may need tetanus prophylaxis.) Assist with suturing if needed. Carefully cover scalp wounds with a sterile dressing; control any bleeding as necessary.

■ Check vital signs and neurologic status, including LOC and pupil size, every 15 minutes. If the patient's symptoms increase or LOC and vital signs change, arrange for a neurosurgical consultation.

■ Observe the patient for headache, dizziness, irritability, and anxiety. If these symptoms appear, perform a complete neurologic evaluation and notify the doctor.

■ Observe the patient for agitated behavior, which may stem from hypoxia or increased ICP.

■ Monitor the older patient especially closely. He may have brain atrophy and therefore more space for cerebral edema; ICP may increase, yet cause no signs.

■ If the patient remains stable after 4 or more hours of observation, he can be discharged in the care of a responsible adult. (See *After a skull fracture.*)

Patient teaching

■ If the patient is discharged from the emergency department, tell a family member or friend to observe his condition at home for the next 24 to 48 hours. An unaccompanied patient may be hospitalized briefly. Be sure to provide a head injury instruction sheet.

■ Tell the caregiver to wake the patient every 2 hours throughout the night to ask him his name, his location, and the caregiver's identity. Tell the caregiver to return the patient to the hospital if he is difficult to arouse, is disoriented, or has seizures.

■ Advise the caregiver to keep the sleep area quiet so the patient can sleep in the 2-hour intervals.

■ Tell the patient to return to the hospital immediately if he experiences a peristent or worsening headache, forceful or constant vomiting, blurred vision, abnormal eye movements, any change in personality, a staggering gait, or twitching.

DISCHARGE READY ▷ **After a skull fracture**

The skull fracture patient is ready for discharge if, after prolonged observation, he meets the following criteria:

■ Vital signs are stable and within normal limits for patient.
■ Neurologic function is stable; patient is awake, alert, and oriented to time, place, and person.
■ There is no evidence of neurologic deficit.
■ The scalp wound is clean and dry without signs of bleeding or increased size.
■ Temperature is within normal limits for patient.
■ The headache is controlled with oral analgesics.
■ Patient has a family member or friend who can observe him for the next 24 to 48 hours and report any changes in his condition and bring him back to the hospital if needed.

■ Instruct the patient not to take anything stronger than acetaminophen. Warn him that aspirin may heighten the risk of bleeding.

■ Instruct the patient who vomits to eat lightly until vomiting stops. (Occasional vomiting is normal after a concussion.)

■ Teach him to recognize symptoms of postconcussion syndrome: headache, dizziness, vertigo, anxiety, and fatigue. Tell him that this syndrome may persist for several weeks.

■ Teach the patient and a family member how to care for his scalp wound, if applicable. Emphasize the need to return for suture removal and follow-up evaluation.

EVALUATION

Evaluation of patient outcomes determines the success of collaborative management. For the patient with a skull fracture, evaluation focuses on maintaining vital signs and neurologic status within acceptable parameters, maintaining a clean and dry incision, controlling headaches with analgesics, and preventing any complications.

Spinal cord injury

Usually the result of trauma to the head or neck, spinal cord injuries (other than spinal cord damage) include fractures, contusions, and compressions of the vertebral column. Spinal injuries most commonly affect the twelfth thoracic, first lumbar, and fifth and sixth cervical areas. The real danger from such injuries lies in associated damage to the spinal cord, which may result in paralysis and even death.

CAUSES

Most serious spinal injuries result from motor vehicle accidents, falls, dives into shallow water, and gunshot wounds. Less serious injuries are caused by lifting heavy objects and minor falls. Spinal dysfunction also may result from hyperparathyroidism and neoplastic lesions.

DIAGNOSIS AND TREATMENT

Spinal X-rays, myelography, computed tomography scans, and magnetic resonance imaging are used to locate the fracture and site of the compression.

The primary treatment after a spinal injury is immediate immobilization to stabilize the spine and prevent further cord damage; other treatment is supportive.

Cervical injuries require immobilization, using sandbags on both sides of the patient's head, a plaster cast, a hard cervical collar, or skeletal traction with skull tongs (Crutchfield, Barton, Vinke) or a halo device.

Treatment of stable lumbar and dorsal fractures consists of bed rest on a firm surface (such as a bed board), analgesics, and muscle relaxants until the fracture stabilizes (usually in 10 to 12 weeks). Later treatment includes exercises to strengthen the back muscles and a back brace or corset to provide support while walking.

An unstable dorsal or lumbar fracture requires a brace; a severe fracture, laminectomy and spinal fusion.

With spinal cord trauma, high-dose methylprednisolone therapy is believed to decrease the risk of permanent damage to the cord. When damage results in compression of the spinal column, neurosurgery may relieve the pressure. Surface wounds that accompany the spinal injury require wound care and tetanus prophylaxis unless the patient has recently been immunized.

COLLABORATIVE MANAGEMENT

Care of the patient with a spinal cord injury focuses on avoiding cord damage and restoring mobility.

ASSESSMENT

The patient's history may reveal trauma. Look for:
- complaints of muscle spasm and back or neck pain that worsens with movement
- in cervical fractures, point tenderness
- in dorsal and lumbar fractures, pain radiating to other body areas such as the legs
- limitation of movement and activities that cause the patient pain

- surface wounds that occurred with the spinal injury; loss of sensation
- with spinal cord damage, effects that range from mild paresthesia to quadriplegia and shock.

NURSING DIAGNOSES AND COLLABORATIVE PROBLEMS

Based on the following nursing diagnoses, you'll establish patient outcomes.

Impaired gas exchange related to neurologic deficits. The patient will:
- maintain a patent airway
- demonstrate tissue perfusion and oxygenation as evidenced by blood studies within normal levels for patient.

Fear related to potential for permanent neurologic deficits. The patient will:
- identify and express feelings of fear
- use available support systems to cope with fear
- demonstrate healthy coping behaviors in managing fear.

Diversional activity deficit related to potential for prolonged inactivity. The patient will:
- express interest in using his leisure time meaningfully
- participate in activities provided
- report a decrease in boredom.

Impaired physical mobility related to neurologic dysfunction. The patient will:
- maintain muscle strength and joint range of motion (ROM)
- show no evidence of complications, such as contracture, venous stasis, or skin breakdown
- achieve the highest level of mobility possible following spinal injury.

PLANNING AND IMPLEMENTATION

As in all spinal injuries, suspect cord damage until proved otherwise. These measures help the patient with a spinal cord injury.
- During the initial assessment and X-rays, immobilize the patient on a firm surface, with sandbags on both sides of his head. Tell him not to move because hyperflexion can damage the cord. If you must move him, get at least one other member of the staff to help you logroll him so that you don't disturb his body alignment.
- If surgery is necessary, administer prophylactic antibiotics, as ordered. Catheterize the patient as ordered to avoid urine retention, and monitor defecation patterns to avoid impaction.
- If the patient has a halo or skull tong traction device, clean the pin sites daily, trim his hair short, and provide analgesics for headaches.
- During traction, turn the patient often to prevent pneumonia, embolism, and skin breakdown. Perform

passive ROM exercises to maintain muscle tone. If available, use a CircOlectric bed or Stryker frame to facilitate turning and to avoid spinal cord injury.

■ Help the patient walk as soon as the doctor allows.

■ Immediately report neurologic changes, such as alteration in skin sensation and loss of muscle strength. Either could point to pressure on the spinal cord from edema or shifting bone fragments.

■ If necessary, insert a nasogastric tube to prevent gastric distention.

■ To prevent aspiration, turn the patient on his side and create a relaxed atmosphere at mealtimes.

■ Measure tidal volumes daily as indicated, especially for higher spinal cord fractures, and alert the doctor to decreasing trends; suction the airway as necessary.

■ Suggest appropriate diversionary activities to fill the hours of immobility. Offer prism glasses for reading.

■ Offer comfort and reassurance to the patient, talking to him quietly and calmly. Remember, the fear of possible paralysis will be overwhelming. Allow a family member who isn't too distraught to stay with him.

Patient teaching

■ Explain traction methods to the patient and family, and reassure them that a halo traction device or skull tongs won't penetrate the brain.

■ Tell the patient about the prescribed regimen for home care.

■ Teach him exercises to maintain physical mobility.

■ Tell him about his medications, including adverse effects and the duration of treatment.

■ Stress the importance of follow-up examinations.

EVALUATION

Evaluation of patient outcomes determines the success of collaborative management. For the patient with a spinal cord injury, evaluation focuses on vital signs and neurologic and respiratory status within acceptable parameters; adequate nutrition; absence of complications; ability to control pain and perform activities of daily living and ambulate with minimal assistance; and completion of referrals for follow-up care as needed.

Trigeminal neuralgia

Also called tic douloureux, this painful disorder affects one or more branches of the fifth cranial (trigeminal) nerve, resulting in severe facial pain. Trigeminal neuralgia can subside spontaneously, with remissions lasting from several months to years.

CAUSES

The cause of trigeminal neuralgia is unknown. This disorder occurs mainly in people over age 40, in women more often than men, and on the right side of the face more often than the left. Upon stimulation of a trigger zone, the patient experiences paroxysmal attacks of excruciating facial pain.

DIAGNOSIS AND TREATMENT

The patient's pain history forms the basis for diagnosis. To rule out sinus or tooth infections and tumors, the patient may undergo skull X-rays or a computed tomography scan.

Oral administration of carbamazepine or phenytoin may temporarily relieve or prevent pain. Narcotics may prove helpful during painful episodes.

When these medical measures fail or attacks become increasingly frequent or severe, neurosurgical procedures may provide permanent relief. The preferred procedure is percutaneous electrocoagulation of nerve rootlets under local anesthesia. Percutaneous radiofrequency trigeminal gangliolysis and percutaneous retrogasserian glycerol rhizotomy also relieve pain. Microsurgery can treat vascular decompression of the trigeminal nerve.

COLLABORATIVE MANAGEMENT

Care of the patient with trigeminal neuralgia focuses on pain relief and coping strategies.

ASSESSMENT

Characteristically, the patient experiences searing or burning jabs of pain lasting from 1 to 15 minutes (usually 1 to 2 minutes), localized in an area innervated by one of the divisions of the trigeminal nerve and initiated by a light touch to a hypersensitive area, such as the tip of the nose, the cheeks, or the gums.

NURSING DIAGNOSES AND COLLABORATIVE PROBLEMS

Based on the following nursing diagnoses, you'll establish patient outcomes.

Pain related to nerve stimulation. The patient will:

■ demonstrate measures to alleviate pain

■ exhibit positive coping strategies

■ state relief of pain.

Altered nutrition: Less than body requirements, related to pain interfering with ability to eat. The patient will:

■ maintain adequate nutritional status

■ demonstrate weight within acceptable parameters.

PLANNING AND IMPLEMENTATION

These measures help the patient with trigeminal neuralgia.

■ Observe and record the characteristics of each attack, including the patient's protective mechanisms.

- Avoid stimulation of trigger zones (lips, cheeks, and gums) by air, heat, or cold.
- After surgical decompression of the root or partial nerve dissection, check neurologic and vital signs frequently.
- Provide adequate nutrition in small, frequent meals at room temperature. Ask the dietitian to help plan meals that take into account the patient's likes and dislikes and the nutritional value.
- Monitor intake and output and daily weight.
- Promote independence through self-care and maximum physical activity.
- Provide emotional support, and encourage the patient to express his fear and anxiety.

Patient teaching

- Warn the patient receiving carbamazepine to immediately report fever, sore throat, mouth ulcers, easy bruising, or petechial or purpuric hemorrhage; these symptoms may signal thrombocytopenia or aplastic anemia and may require discontinuation of drug therapy.
- After resection of the first branch of the trigeminal nerve, advise the patient to wear glasses or goggles outdoors, to blink often, and to avoid rubbing his eyes and using aerosol sprays.
- After surgery to sever the second or third branch, tell the patient to avoid hot foods and drinks, which could burn his mouth, and to chew carefully to avoid biting his mouth. Advise him to place food in the unaffected side of his mouth when chewing, to brush his teeth and rinse his mouth often, and to see the dentist twice a year to detect cavities. (Cavities in the area of the severed nerve will not cause pain.)

EVALUATION

Evaluation of patient outcomes determines the success of collaborative management. For the patient with trigeminal neuralgia, evaluation focuses on pain relief with oral analgesics, use of positive coping strategies, and adequate knowledge to minimize stimulating triggers and to comply with treatment.

Treatments and procedures

Various treatments and procedures can be used for patients with neurologic disorders. The most common include carotid endarterectomy, craniotomy, laminectomy, and spinal fusion.

CAROTID ENDARTERECTOMY

Carotid endarterectomy is a surgical procedure that removes atheromatous plaque from the inner lining of the carotid arteries. This improves intracranial perfusion by increasing blood flow through the carotid arteries.

This procedure may help patients with reversible ischemic neurologic deficit or a completed cerebrovascular accident (CVA). Patients who experience transient ischemic attacks, syncope, and dizziness and those who have high-grade asymptomatic or ulcerative lesions may also benefit from this procedure.

For patients with concurrent coronary artery disease (CAD), carotid endarterectomy may reduce CAD and prevent CVA in one operation (if the patient is neurologically stable and otherwise a good surgical candidate). Because carotid lesions commonly lead to CVA in both symptomatic and asymptomatic patients, some surgeons consider this operation a prophylactic treatment for CVA. However, many intraoperative and postoperative risks are associated with the procedure, making it unsuitable for some patients.

Carotid endarterectomy usually involves the use of cervical block anesthesia and sedatives, which allow the patient to be closely monitored. Alternatively, light general anesthesia may be used so that brain waves can be assessed.

PROCEDURE

An incision is made along the anterior border of the sternocleidomastoid or transversely in a skin crease in the neck. Once the incision is made, the common carotid artery, external carotid artery, and internal carotid artery are exposed and the carotid artery is clamped to evaluate perfusion. If cerebral perfusion is inadequate, a shunt is inserted to permit blood flow past the obstruction in the carotid artery and to ensure adequate cerebral circulation during surgery.

Once the carotid artery is stabilized, a heparin infusion is started to prevent thrombosis. The affected arteries are then incised and the plaque is dissected. Next, the artery is patched with an autogenous saphenous vein or prosthetic material and closed. If a shunt is in place, it's removed before complete closure.

COLLABORATIVE MANAGEMENT

Care of the patient undergoing carotid endarterectomy requires thorough preparation, close monitoring, and diligent patient teaching.

Preparation

- To reduce their anxiety, teach the patient and family members about the procedure and answer their questions.
- Explain all preoperative diagnostic tests, including periorbital ultrasonography, ocular pneumoplethysmography, carotid phonoangiography, computed tomography scan, and cerebral angiography. If the patient has concurrent CAD, also explain electrocardiography (ECG), coronary angiography, and the treadmill exercise stress test.

■ Give the patient and family members a tour of the intensive care unit.

■ Explain postoperative care, and warn the patient and family which I.V. lines, hemodynamic measuring devices, tubes, and machines will be connected to the patient.

■ Tell the patient that he'll have some postoperative discomfort or pain but that pain medication will be available.

■ Inform him that a nurse will check his neurologic status, including level of consciousness (LOC), orientation, extremity strength, speech, and fine hand movements, every hour after surgery. Explain that this is routine, not an indication that he isn't doing well.

■ Before surgery, help the doctor insert a radial arterial catheter to monitor arterial blood gas levels and blood pressure.

■ Ensure that a baseline EEG is done before the patient is anesthetized.

Monitoring and aftercare

■ Monitor vital signs every 15 minutes for the first hour until the patient is stable. Decreased blood pressure and elevated heart and respiratory rates could indicate cerebral ischemia.

■ Perform a neurologic assessment every hour for the first 24 hours. Check extremity strength, fine hand movements, speech, LOC, and orientation. Also check the patient's tongue strength and shoulder shrug (to test cranial nerves IX, X, and XII).

■ Monitor intake and output hourly for the first 24 hours.

■ Perform continuous cardiac monitoring for the first 24 hours. Perform an ECG if the patient has any chest pain or arrhythmias (many patients undergoing this procedure also have CAD).

Patient teaching

■ Teach the patient and a family member how to care for the surgical wound. Review the signs and symptoms of infection (fever, sore throat, or redness, swelling or drainage from the wound), and tell them to call the doctor immediately if these occur.

■ Teach the patient about risk factors for atherosclerosis, and encourage him to make necessary lifestyle changes, such as stopping smoking, reducing his fat intake, and losing weight.

■ Make sure the patient understands the dosage and possible adverse effects of all prescribed medications.

■ If he has had a CVA and needs follow-up care, refer him and his family to a home health care agency.

■ Teach the patient how to manage any neurologic, sensory, or motor deficits that occurred during surgery.

■ Tell him to contact the doctor immediately if any new neurologic symptoms occur (reocclusion may occur in up to 23% of patients).

■ Emphasize the importance of regular checkups.

COMPLICATIONS

The most common complication of carotid endarterectomy is blood pressure lability. Transient hypertension also commonly occurs from manipulation of the carotid body. Perioperative CVA, the most serious complication, may result from embolization of debris during dissection.

Temporary or permanent loss of carotid body function may occur. Blood pressure and ventilation normally increase in response to hypoxia; however, with the loss of carotid body function, blood pressure and ventilation decrease in response to hypoxia. Other possible complications include rethrombosis, postoperative respiratory distress caused by tracheal compression from a hematoma, and wound infection at the surgical site.

An uncommon complication is a sudden increase in cerebral blood flow, which can lead to ipsilateral vascular headaches, seizures, and intracerebral hemorrhage. Rarely, vocal cord paralysis may arise from manipulation of the vagus nerve.

CRANIOTOMY

This procedure involves an incision into the skull and exposure of the brain for treatments, such as ventricular shunting, excision of a tumor or abscess, hematoma aspiration, and aneurysm clipping.

PROCEDURE

The surgical approach to a supratentorial craniotomy can be frontal, parietal, temporal, or occipital or a combination of these areas. If structures below the tentorium are involved, the surgical approach to an infratentorial craniotomy involves an incision slightly above the neck in the back of the skull. In the operating room just before surgery, the anesthetist will start a peripheral I.V. line, a central venous pressure (CVP) line, and an arterial line. The CVP line provides access to remove air in case an air embolus occurs—a particular risk when posterior fossa surgery is performed.

After the patient receives a general anesthetic, the surgeon marks an incision line and cuts through the scalp to the cranium, forming a scalp flap that he folds to one side. He then bores four or five holes through the skull in the corners of the cranial incision and cuts out a bone flap. After pulling aside or removing the bone flap, he incises and retracts the dura, exposing the brain.

After surgery is completed, the surgeon reverses the incision procedure and covers the site with a sterile dressing.

COLLABORATIVE MANAGEMENT

Care of the patient undergoing a craniotomy requires thorough preparation, close monitoring, and diligent patient teaching.

Preparation

■ Help the patient and family members cope with the surgery by clarifying the doctor's explanation and by encouraging them to ask questions. Your answers should be informative and honest. Although you can't guarantee a complete and uncomplicated recovery, you can help instill a sense of confidence in the surgeon and in a successful outcome.

■ Explain preoperative procedures. Tell the patient that his hair will be washed with an antiseptic shampoo on the night before surgery. In the operating room, his head will be shaved and he'll receive steroids to reduce postoperative inflammation. He'll also have a peripheral I.V. line, a CVP line, and an arterial line inserted.

■ Explain that antiembolism stockings or pneumatic compression may be applied to his legs to improve venous return and reduce the risk of thrombophlebitis. And, because craniotomy is a lengthy procedure, tell him he may have an indwelling urinary catheter inserted.

■ Prepare him for postoperative recovery. Explain that he'll awaken with a large dressing on his head to protect the incision. He also may have a surgical drain implanted in his skull for at least 24 hours and will be receiving prophylactic antibiotics. Warn him to expect a headache and facial swelling for 2 to 3 days after surgery, and reassure him that he'll receive medication to reduce the pain.

■ Explain the importance of postoperative leg exercises and deep breathing. Tell him that he should be walking within 2 to 3 days after surgery and that the doctor will usually remove the sutures within 7 to 10 days.

■ Before surgery, perform a complete neurologic assessment. Carefully record your assessment data to use as a baseline for postoperative evaluation.

■ Because the patient will go to the intensive care unit after surgery, arrange a preoperative visit there for him and his family. Explain the equipment and introduce them to the staff.

Monitoring and aftercare

■ Check the patient's vital signs and neurologic status every 15 minutes for the first 4 hours, then once every 30 to 60 minutes for the next 24 to 48 hours.

■ If the patient's level of consciousness is decreased, place him on his side to help prevent increased intracranial pressure (ICP) and to protect his airway. Elevate his head 15 to 30 degrees to increase venous re-turn and to help him breathe more easily. With another nurse's help, turn him carefully every 2 hours.

■ Throughout postoperative care, observe the patient closely for signs of increased ICP. Notify the doctor at once if you observe worsening mental status, pupillary changes, or focal signs such as increasing weakness in an extremity.

■ Closely observe the patient's respiratory status, noting rate and pattern. Report any abnormalities at once. Encourage him to breathe deeply and cough, but not too strenuously. Suction gently as ordered.

■ Monitor and record intake and output. Administer fluids as prescribed to maintain normal fluid balance. Check urine specific gravity every 2 hours, and weigh the patient as ordered.

■ Check serum electrolyte levels every 24 hours, and watch for signs of imbalance. Low potassium levels may cause confusion and stupor; reduced sodium and chloride levels may produce weakness, lethargy, and even coma. Because fluid and electrolyte imbalance can precipitate seizures, report such signs at once.

■ Provide good wound care. Make sure the dressing stays dry and in place and is not too tight (from soft-tissue swelling). If the patient has a closed drainage system, periodically check drain patency and document the amount and characteristics of any discharge. Notify the doctor of excessive bloody drainage, which may indicate cerebral hemorrhage, or of clear or yellow drainage, which may indicate a cerebrospinal fluid leak. Also monitor the patient for signs of wound infection, such as fever and purulent drainage.

■ Finally, provide supportive care. Ensure a quiet, calm environment to minimize anxiety and agitation and help lower ICP. Administer anticonvulsants as ordered, and maintain seizure precautions. Provide other ordered medications, such as steroids to prevent or reduce cerebral edema, stool softeners to prevent increased ICP from straining during defecation, and analgesics to relieve pain.

■ Develop a discharge plan. (See *After craniotomy.*)

Patient teaching

■ Before discharge, teach the patient proper wound care techniques. Tell him to keep the suture line dry and to regularly clean the incision with hydrogen peroxide and normal saline solution.

■ Instruct him to evaluate the incision regularly for redness, warmth, or tenderness and to report any of these findings to the doctor.

■ If the patient is self-conscious about his appearance, suggest that he wear a wig, hat, or scarf until his hair grows back. Tell him to apply a lanolin-based lotion to his scalp (avoiding the suture line) to keep it supple and decrease itching.

- Remind the patient to continue taking prescribed anticonvulsants to minimize the risk of seizures. Depending on the type of surgery performed, he may need to continue anticonvulsant therapy for up to 12 months after surgery. Also remind him to report any adverse drug effects, such as excessive drowsiness or confusion.
- Teach the patient about prescribed steroids. Warn him that these drugs may cause weight gain and GI bleeding.

COMPLICATIONS

Craniotomy can cause many potential complications, including infection, vasospasm, hemorrhage, air embolism, respiratory compromise, increased ICP, diabetes insipidus, syndrome of inappropriate secretion of diuretic hormone, seizures, and cranial nerve damage; the degree of risk depends largely on the patient's condition and the surgery's complexity.

LAMINECTOMY AND SPINAL FUSION

In laminectomy, the surgeon removes one or more of the bony laminae that cover the vertebrae. Most commonly performed to relieve pressure on the spinal cord or spinal nerve roots from a herniated disk, laminectomy also may be done to treat compression fracture, dislocation of vertebrae, or a spinal cord tumor.

After removal of several laminae, spinal fusion—grafting bone chips between vertebral spaces—is commonly performed to stabilize the spine. It also may be done apart from laminectomy in some patients with vertebrae seriously weakened by trauma or disease. Usually, spinal fusion is done when more conservative treatments—including prolonged bed rest, traction, or the use of a back brace—prove ineffective.

PROCEDURE

The patient is given a general anesthetic and placed in a prone position. The surgeon makes a midline vertical incision and strips the fascia and muscles off the bony laminae. He then removes one or more sections of laminae to expose the spinal defect. For a herniated disk, the surgeon removes part or all of the disk. For a spinal cord tumor, he incises the dura and explores the cord for metastasis. He then dissects the tumor and removes it, using suction, forceps, or dissecting scissors.

To perform spinal fusion, the surgeon exposes the affected vertebrae, then inserts bone chips obtained from the patient's iliac crest, from a bone bank, or both. For optimum strength, he uses wire, spinal plates, rods, or screws to secure these bone grafts into several vertebrae surrounding the area of instability. Then he closes the incision and applies a dressing. Af-

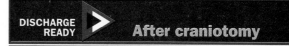

DISCHARGE READY ▷ **After craniotomy**

After undergoing a craniotomy, the patient should exhibit the following criteria before discharge:

- stable vital signs within normal limits
- stable neurologic function
- intracranial pressure within normal limits
- normal fluid and electrolyte balance
- a clean, dry healing incision
- headache controlled by oral analgesics
- absence of pulmonary, cardiovascular, or GI complications
- absence of fever or infection.

ter surgery, the patient may require a brace if surgery was performed on the lumbar region, or a hard cervical collar if surgery was performed on the neck.

COLLABORATIVE MANAGEMENT

Care of the patient undergoing laminectomy and spinal fusion requires thorough preparation, close monitoring, and diligent patient teaching.

Preparation

- Explain the procedure to the patient and his family. Try to ease their fears by answering their questions clearly.
- Discuss postoperative recovery and rehabilitation. Explain that surgery won't relieve back pain immediately and that pain may even worsen after the operation. Explain that relief will come only after chronic nerve irritation and swelling subside, which may take several weeks. Reassure the patient that analgesics and muscle relaxants will be available during recovery.
- Tell him that he'll return from surgery with a dressing over the incision and that he'll be kept on bed rest as prescribed by the doctor.
- Explain that he'll be turned often to prevent pressure sores and pulmonary complications. Show him the logrolling method of turning, and explain that he'll use this method later to get in and out of bed by himself.
- Just before surgery, perform a baseline assessment of motor function and sensation in the patient's lower trunk, legs, and feet as well as upper extremities and fingers for cervical involvement.

Monitoring and aftercare

- After surgery, monitor the patient's vital signs every 15 minutes until he's stable.
- Keep the head of the patient's bed flat or elevated no more than 45 degrees for at least 24 hours. Urge

the patient to remain in the supine position for the prescribed period to prevent any strain on the involved vertebrae.

■ When he's able to assume a side-lying position, make sure he keeps his spine straight, with his knees flexed and drawn up toward his chest. Insert a pillow between his knees to relieve pressure on the spine from hip adduction.

■ Inspect the dressing frequently for bleeding or cerebrospinal fluid leakage; report either immediately. The surgeon will probably perform the initial dressing change himself; you may be asked to perform subsequent changes.

■ Assess motor and neurologic function in the patient's trunk and lower extremities as well as upper extremities and fingers for cervical involvement, and compare the results with baseline findings. Also evaluate circulation in his legs and feet, and report any abnormalities. Give analgesics and muscle relaxants as ordered.

■ Every 2 to 4 hours, assess urine output and auscultate for the return of bowel sounds. If the patient doesn't void within 8 to 12 hours after surgery, notify the doctor and prepare to insert an indwelling urinary catheter to relieve urine retention.

■ If the patient can void normally, assist him in getting on and off a bedpan while maintaining proper alignment.

Patient teaching

■ Teach the patient and his caregiver proper incision care measures. Tell them to check the incision site often for signs of infection—increased pain and tenderness, redness, swelling, and changes in the amount and character of drainage—and to report any such signs immediately.

■ Instruct the patient to avoid soaking his stitches in a bathtub until healing is complete. Also advise him to shower with his back out of the stream of water.

■ Make sure he understands the importance of resuming activity gradually after surgery. As ordered, instruct him to start with short walks and to slowly progress to longer distances.

■ Review any prescribed exercises, such as pelvic tilts, leg raises, and toe pointing. Advise him to rest frequently and avoid overexertion.

■ Review any prescribed activity restrictions. Usually, the doctor will prohibit sitting for prolonged periods, lifting heavy objects or bending over, and climbing long flights of stairs. He may also impose other restrictions, depending on the patient's condition.

■ Teach the patient proper body mechanics to lessen strain and pressure on his spine. Instruct him to lie on his back, with his knees propped up with pillows, or on his side, with his knees drawn up and a pillow placed between his legs.

■ Warn him against lying on his stomach or on his back with legs flat. He should sit with his feet on a low stool to elevate his knees above hip level. He should use a firm, straight-backed chair and sit up straight with his lower back pressed flat against the chair back.

■ Tell the patient that, when standing for prolonged periods, he should alternate placing each foot on a low stool to straighten his lower back and relieve strain. When bending, he should keep his spine straight and bend at his knees and hips rather than at his waist.

■ Instruct the patient to sleep only on a firm mattress. If necessary, advise him to purchase a new one or to insert a bed board between his existing mattress and box spring.

COMPLICATIONS

This complex and delicate surgery carries the risk of several potentially serious complications. The most common are herniation relapse, arachnoiditis, chronic neuritis due to adhesions and scarring, and problems associated with prolonged immobility, such as urine retention, paralytic ileus, and pulmonary complications. Even though surgery may relieve pressure on the nerves, reducing pain and improving mobility, it can't reverse existing nerve or muscle damage from chronic disorders, which may lead to further complications.

Selected references

Crigger, N., and Forbes, W. "Assessing Neurologic Function in Older Patients," *AJN* 97(3):37-40, March 1997.

Diseases, 2nd ed. Springhouse, Pa.: Springhouse Corp., 1997.

Franges, E.Z. "Lumbar Punctures: Helping a 'Sticky' Procedure Go Smoothly," *Nursing96* 26(3):48-50, March 1996.

Huether, S.E., and McCance, K.L. *Understanding Pathophysiology.* St. Louis: Mosby–Year Book, Inc., 1996.

Illustrated Manual of Nursing Practice, 2nd ed. Springhouse, Pa.: Springhouse Corp., 1994.

Meissner, J.E. "Disease Review: Caring for Patients with Meningitis," *Nursing95* 25(7):50-51, July 1995.

Monahan, F.D., et al. *Nursing Care of Adults.* Philadelphia: W.B. Saunders Co., 1994.

Phipps, W.J., et al. *Medical-Surgical Nursing: Concepts and Clinical Practice,* 5th ed. St. Louis: Mosby–Year Book, Inc., 1995.

Polaski, A.L., and Tatro, S.E. *Luckmann's Core Principles and Practice of Medical-Surgical Nursing.* Philadelphia: W.B. Saunders Co., 1996.

Womack, C., and Thomas, J.D. "Easing the Way Through an MRI," *RN* 59(10):34-37, October 1996.

Eye and ear disorders

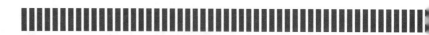

Because so much sensory information reaches the brain through the eyes and ears, eye and ear problems and resultant visual and hearing impairment interfere with your patient's ability to function independently, to perceive meaning in the world, to enjoy aesthetic pleasure, and to communicate. Although fewer people today lose their sight or hearing from infections or injuries, the incidence of blindness is rising. The main causes of new blindness in the United States are macular degeneration among older adults (16.8%), glaucoma (11.5%), diabetic retinopathy (10.1%), cataracts (9.8%), and optic atrophy (4.3%).

When left untreated, ear disorders can impair equilibrium and cause hearing loss. Hearing loss can also be congenital or noise- or drug-induced; it can occur suddenly or develop gradually as a result of aging.

Anatomy and physiology review of the eye

The sensory organ of sight, the eye transmits visual images to the brain for interpretation. The eyeball is about 1″ (2.5 cm) in diameter and occupies the bony orbit, a skull cavity formed anteriorly by the frontal, maxillary, zygomatic, acromial, sphenoid, ethmoid, and palatine bones. Nerves, adipose tissue, and blood vessels cushion and nourish the eye posteriorly.

Extraocular (external) and intraocular (internal) structures form the eye, and extraocular muscles and nerves control it.

EXTRAOCULAR STRUCTURES
Eyelids, also called the palpebrae, are loose folds of skin that cover the anterior eye. They protect the eye from foreign bodies, regulate entrance of light, and distribute tears. The palpebral fissure—the distance

between the lid margins—should be equal in both eyes.

The conjunctivae, which also protect the eye from foreign bodies, consist of transparent mucous membranes that extend from the lid margins. The meibomian glands secrete sebum onto the posterior lid margins to retain tears and keep the eye lubricated.

The lacrimal glands, punctum, lacrimal sac, and nasolacrimal duct constitute the lacrimal apparatus, which lubricates and protects the cornea and conjunctivae by producing and absorbing tears. The tears drain through the punctum into the lacrimal canals and lacrimal sac to the nasolacrimal duct into the nose.

EXTRAOCULAR MUSCLES AND NERVES
The extraocular muscles function together to hold both eyes parallel and create binocular vision. The superior and inferior rectus muscles move the eye up and down on a transverse axis; the medial and lateral rectus muscles move the eye toward the nose and toward the temple on an anteroposterior axis; and the superior and inferior oblique muscles move the eye to the right and left on a vertical axis.

Six cranial nerves—the optic, oculomotor, trochlear, trigeminal, abducens, and facial—innervate the eye, the ocular muscles, and the lacrimal apparatus. The coordinated action of six eye muscles—the superior, inferior, medial, and lateral rectus muscles, and the superior and inferior oblique muscles—controls eye movement.

INTRAOCULAR STRUCTURES
Easily visible anterior intraocular structures include the sclera, cornea, anterior chamber, iris, and pupil. Other intraocular structures are visible only with the use of an ophthalmoscope or another instrument. These include the aqueous humor, lens, ciliary body,

Reviewing intraocular structures

You can view some intraocular structures, such as the sclera, cornea, pupil, and anterior chamber, through inspection. However, others, such as the retina, must be viewed through an ophthalmoscope.

Sclera and cornea

The white sclera coats four-fifths of the outside of the eyeball, maintaining its size and form. It also coats the optic nerve. The cornea is continuous with the sclera at the limbus, revealing the pupil and the iris. The cornea is a smooth, avascular, transparent tissue whose epithelium merges with the bulbar conjunctiva at the limbus.

Iris, pupil, and anterior chamber

The iris is a circular contractile disk containing smooth and radial muscles and perforated in the center by the pupil. Eye color depends on the amount of pigment in the endothelial layers of the iris.

Pupils should be equal, round, and 3 to 7 mm in diameter, depending on the patient's age. The posterior portion of the iris contains involuntary dilator and sphincter muscles that regulate light entry by controlling pupil size.

The anterior chamber is filled with a clear, watery fluid called aqueous humor, which drains into canal of Schlemm.

Lens and ciliary body

Located directly behind the iris at the pupillary opening, the avascular lens refracts and focuses light onto the retina. The ciliary body (the three muscles and the iris, which make up the anterior part of the vascular uveal tract) controls the lens thickness and, together with the coordinated action of the iris's muscles, regulates the light focused through the lens onto the retina.

Posterior chamber, vitreous humor, and choroid

This small potential space directly posterior to the iris but anterior to the lens is filled with aqueous humor. Vitreous humor is a thick, gelatinous material that fills the area behind the lens, maintaining the placement of the retina and the spherical shape of the eyeball. The choroid lines the inner aspect of the eyeball beneath the retina (adjacent to the sclera) and contains many small arteries and veins.

Cross section of the eye

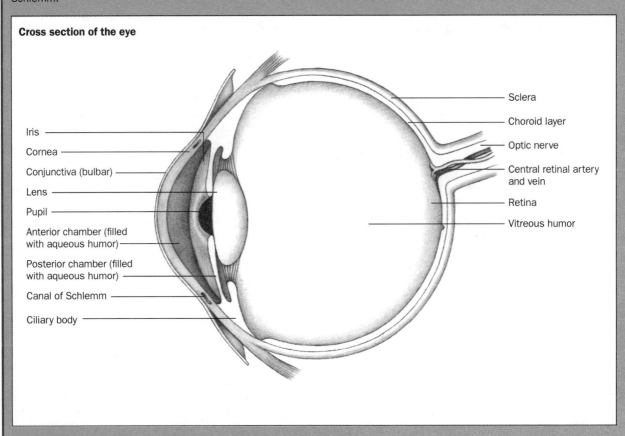

Retina

The main function of the retina, the innermost coat of the eyeball, is to receive visual stimuli and send them to the brain. Each of the four sets of retinal vessels contains a transparent arteriole and vein. The arterioles are smaller than the veins and brighter in color; both become progressively thinner as they leave the optic disk.

The optic disk is a well-defined, 1.5-mm round or oval area within the nasal portion of the retina. This creamy yellow to pink disk allows the optic nerve to enter the retina at a point called the nerve head. The physiologic cup is a light-colored depression within the optic disk on the temporal side; it covers one-third of the center of the disk.

The visual receptors of the retina consist of photoreceptor neurons called rods and cones. The rods respond to low-intensity light and shades of gray, and the cones respond to bright light and color. The macula, located laterally to the optic disk, is darker than the rest of the retina and contains no visible retinal vessels.

The fovea centralis is a slight depression in the center of the macula that appears as a bright reflection in ophthalmoscopic examination. Because it contains the heaviest concentration of cones, it's the main receiver of vision and color.

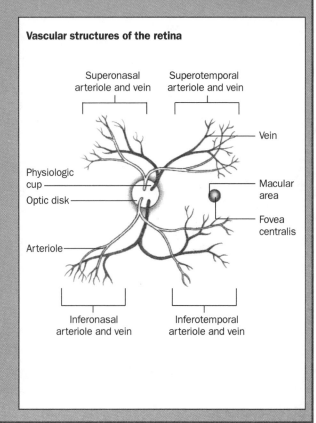

Vascular structures of the retina

Superonasal arteriole and vein

Superotemporal arteriole and vein

Vein

Physiologic cup

Optic disk

Macular area

Fovea centralis

Arteriole

Inferonasal arteriole and vein

Inferotemporal arteriole and vein

vitreous humor, retina, and choroid. The eye must be surgically rotated in order to see the posterior sclera.

The retina, the innermost eyeball layer, contains neural tissue to receive visual images. The reddish orange color of the retina comes from its deep pigment layers and the extensive vascular supply from the choroid. The color varies with the patient's complexion.

With ophthalmoscopic (funduscopic) examination of the posterior portion of the eye (the fundus), you can view the retinal blood vessels, the optic disk, the physiologic cup of the optic disk, the macula, and the fovea centralis. (See *Reviewing intraocular structures*.)

PHYSIOLOGY OF VISION

Every object reflects light. For an individual to perceive an object clearly, this reflected light must be intercepted by the eye and pass through numerous intraocular structures, including the cornea, anterior chamber, pupil, lens, and vitreous humor. The lens focuses the light into an upside-down and reversed image on the retina. Reacting to the light, specialized photoreceptor cells (rods and cones) in the retina send nerve impulses, via the optic nerve and optic tract, to the visual cortex of the occipital lobe, which then interprets the image.

Anatomy and physiology review of the ear

A sensory organ, the ear allows hearing and maintains equilibrium. It is conveniently divided into three main parts—the external ear, the middle ear, and the inner ear. The skin-covered cartilaginous auricle and the external auditory canal make up the external ear. The tympanic membrane (eardrum) separates the external ear from the middle ear at the proximal portion of the auditory canal. The middle ear, a small, air-filled cavity in the temporal bone, contains three small bones—the malleus, incus, and stapes. It leads to the inner ear, a bony and membranous labyrinth. (See *Reviewing ear structures and function*, pages 332 and 333.)

SOUND TRANSMISSION

The auricle picks up sound waves and channels them into the auditory canal. There, the waves strike the tympanic membrane, which vibrates and causes the handle of the malleus to vibrate as well. These vibrations travel from the malleus to the incus, to the stapes, through the oval window and the fluid in the cochlea, to the round window. The membrane covering the round window shakes the delicate hair cells in the organ of Corti, which stimulates the sensory endings of the cochlear branch of the acoustic nerve (cranial nerve VIII). The nerve sends the impulses to the

Reviewing ear structures and function

External ear
The cartilaginous anthelix, crux of the helix, lobule, tragus, and concha together form the auricle (pinna). Although not part of the external ear, the mastoid process is an important bony landmark behind the lower part of the auricle.

Thin, sensitive skin covers the cartilage that forms the outer third of the external auditory canal. The adult's external canal leads inward, downward, and forward to the middle ear.

Middle ear
The tympanic membrane separates the middle from the external ear at the proximal portion of the auditory canal. Composed of layers of skin, fibrous tissue, and mucous membranes, it appears pearly gray, shiny, and translucent.

The external canal leads into the middle ear—a small, air-filled cavity in the temporal bone. Within this cavity, three small bones called the malleus, incus, and stapes (the auditory ossicles) link together to transmit sound.

The stapes sits in an opening called the oval window (fenestra ovalis), through which sound vibrations travel to the inner ear. The eustachian tube, which connects the middle ear to the nasopharynx, equalizes pressure between the inner and outer surfaces of the tympanic membrane.

Inner ear
A bony labyrinth, the inner ear consists of the vestibule, the cochlea, and the semicircular canals. The semicircular canals contain sensory epithelium for maintaining a sense of position and equilibrium, and the cochlea contains the organ of Corti for transmitting sound to the cochlear branch of the acoustic nerve (cranial nerve VIII). The vestibular branch of the acoustic nerve contains peripheral

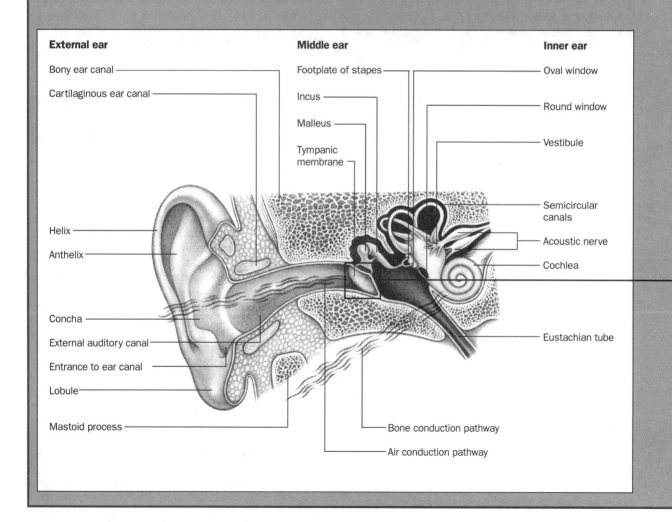

External ear

- Bony ear canal
- Cartilaginous ear canal
- Helix
- Anthelix
- Concha
- External auditory canal
- Entrance to ear canal
- Lobule
- Mastoid process

Middle ear

- Footplate of stapes
- Incus
- Malleus
- Tympanic membrane
- Bone conduction pathway
- Air conduction pathway

Inner ear

- Oval window
- Round window
- Vestibule
- Semicircular canals
- Acoustic nerve
- Cochlea
- Eustachian tube

nerve fibers that terminate in the epithelium of the semicircular canals, and the central branch terminates in the medulla at the vestibular nucleus.

Hearing pathways

For hearing to occur, sound waves travel through the ear by two pathways: air conduction and bone conduction. Air conduction occurs when sound waves travel in the air through the external and middle ear to the inner ear. Bone conduction occurs when sound waves travel through bone to the inner ear.

The vibrations transmitted through air and bone stimulate nerve impulses in the inner ear. The cochlear branch of the acoustic nerve transmits these vibrations to the auditory area of the cerebral cortex, where the temporal lobe of the brain interprets the sound.

Otoscopic view of right tympanic membrane

- Pars flaccida
- Short process of malleus
- Pars tensa
- Handle of malleus
- Umbo
- Light reflex
- Annulus

auditory area of the temporal lobe in the brain, which then interprets the sound.

Assessment of the eye

To obtain an accurate and complete patient history, adjust questions to the patient's specific complaint and compare the answers with the results of the physical assessment. You can adapt your questions to the patient's age. For example, ask a child if the writing on the school chalkboard is readable, or ask an older adult about peripheral vision, visual acuity, glaucoma testing, problems with glare, and abnormal tearing.

HISTORY

The patient history should focus on current and past health status, family history, and lifestyle patterns. Before the interview, determine whether the patient ordinarily wears glasses or contact lenses and adjust your questions accordingly. During the interview, observe the patient's eye movements and focusing ability for clues to visual acuity and eye muscle coordination.

CHIEF COMPLAINT

Carefully document the patient's chief complaint in his own words. Ask for a complete description of the current problem and any others. To investigate further, ask the following questions about eye function:
- Do you have any problems with your eyes? Besides indicating visual disturbances, eye problems can indicate other conditions, such as diabetes, hypertension, and neurologic disorders.
- Do you wear or have you ever worn corrective lenses? If so, for how long? This establishes how long the patient has had a vision disorder and his need to wear corrective lenses during the visual acuity check.
- If you wear corrective lenses, are they glasses or hard or soft contact lenses? Improperly fitted or prolonged wearing of contact lenses can cause eye inflammation and corneal abrasions. Those who wear soft lenses are especially vulnerable to conjunctival inflammation and infection because these lenses can irritate the eye if worn for long periods.
- For what eye condition do you wear corrective lenses? Besides providing information about any existing eye condition, the answer allows adjustment of the diopters for ophthalmoscopic examination of nearsightedness or farsightedness.
- If you wear corrective lenses, do you wear them all the time or just for certain activities, such as reading or driving? The answer provides information about the severity and type of visual disturbance.

■ When did you last have your lenses changed? A recent lens change with continued visual disturbances could indicate an underlying health problem such as a brain tumor.

■ If you once wore corrective lenses and have stopped wearing them, why and when did you stop? Eyestrain or excessive tearing may occur if the patient is not wearing necessary lenses.

MEDICAL HISTORY

Ask the following questions to gather additional information about the patient's eyes and general physical condition:

■ Have you ever had blurred vision? Blurred vision can indicate a need for corrective lenses or suggest a neurologic disorder, such as a brain tumor, or an endocrine disorder, such as diabetic retinopathy.

■ Have you ever seen spots, floaters, or halos around lights? If so, is this a sudden development or has it occurred for a while? The sudden appearance of flashing lights or floaters may indicate retinal detachment; halos are associated with glaucoma. Chronic appearance of spots or floaters is a common normal occurrence in older and myopic patients.

■ Do you suffer from frequent eye infections or inflammation? Frequent infections or inflammation can indicate low resistance to infection, eyestrain, allergies, or occupational or environmental exposure to an irritant.

■ Have you ever had eye surgery? A history of eye surgery may indicate glaucoma, cataracts, or injuries such as detached retina, which may appear as abnormalities on the ophthalmoscopic examination.

■ Have you ever had an eye injury? Injuries, such as those from a penetrating foreign body, can distort the ophthalmoscopic examination.

■ Do you often have sties? Sties, infected meibomian glands or glands of Zeis, tend to recur.

■ Do you have a history of high blood pressure? High blood pressure can cause arteriosclerosis of the retinal blood vessels and visual disturbances.

■ Do you have a history of diabetes? Diabetes causes noninflammatory changes in the retina that can lead to blindness.

■ Are you currently taking any prescription medications for your eyes? If so, which ones and how often? Prescription eye medications should alert you to an eye disorder. For example, a patient who's taking pilocarpine probably has glaucoma.

■ What other medications are you taking, including prescription and over-the-counter drugs and home remedies? Certain medications can cause visual disturbances.

FAMILY HISTORY

Next, investigate for familial eye disorders. Ask if anyone in the patient's family has ever been treated for myopia, cataracts, glaucoma, or loss of vision.

SOCIAL HISTORY

Explore the patient's daily habits that affect the eyes by asking the following questions:

■ Does your occupation require close use of your eyes, such as long-term reading or prolonged use of a video display terminal? These activities can cause eyestrain or dryness when the person forgets to blink.

■ Does the air where you work or live contain anything that causes you eye problems? Cigarette smoke, formaldehyde insulation, or occupational materials such as glues or chemicals can cause eye irritation.

■ Do you wear goggles when working with power tools, chain saws, or table saws or when engaging in sports that might irritate or endanger the eye, such as swimming, fencing, or playing racquetball? Serious eye irritation or injury can occur with these activities.

PHYSICAL EXAMINATION

Assessment of the eye includes testing the patient's vision and extraocular muscle function, inspecting and palpating external ocular structures, and inspecting internal structures with an ophthalmoscope. Test the patient's vision before inspecting and palpating, which can cause eye irritation. Also keep in mind that the eyes should never be manipulated if the patient has a history of (or suspected) traumatic eye injury.

For a basic eye assessment, obtain a Snellen eye chart, a piece of newsprint, an eye occluder or an opaque 3″ × 5″ card, a penlight, a wisp of cotton, a pencil or another narrow cylindrical article, and an ophthalmoscope. Wash your hands, and make sure the room is well lit and without glare. The patient usually remains seated for the eye assessment.

DISTANCE VISION

To test the distance vision of someone who can read English, use the Snellen alphabet chart containing various-sized letters. For patients who are illiterate or unable to speak English, use the Snellen E chart, which displays the letter E in varying sizes and positions. The patient indicates the position of the E by duplicating the position with his fingers.

Be certain to position the patient 20′ (6 m) from the chart. You'll record visual acuity as a fraction. The numerator will be 20 (the distance between the patient and the chart); the denominator, which will range from 10 to 200, indicates the distance from which a person with normal vision can read the chart. For example, if the patient reads a line identified by the numbers 20/20, this means that he can read from 20′ what a person with normal vision can also read from 20′. However, if he can only read a line identified by the numbers 20/100, this means that he can read from 20′ what a person with normal vision can read from 100′ (30 m). The greater the denominator, the poorer the vision.

Test each eye separately by covering the left eye first, and then the right, with the opaque card or an eye occluder. Afterward, test binocular vision by having the patient read the chart with both eyes uncovered. A patient who normally wears corrective lenses for distance vision should wear them for the test. Start with the line marked 20/40. Continue down the chart until the patient can read a line correctly with no more than two errors. That line indicates the patient's distance visual acuity. If he reads the 20/20 line correctly, this is considered normal visual acuity. Record the eye that was tested and whether vision was achieved with or without corrective lenses.

NEAR VISION

Test the patient's near vision by holding either a Snellen chart or a card with newsprint 12″ to 14″ (30 to 35 cm) in front of the patient's eyes. A patient who normally wears reading glasses should wear them for the test. As with distance vision, test both eyes separately and then together. Any patient who complains of blurring with the card at 12″ to 14″ or who can't read it accurately needs retesting and then referral to an ophthalmologist if necessary. Keep in mind that a patient who is illiterate may be too embarrassed to say so. If a patient seems to be struggling to read the type or stares at it without attempting to read, change to the Snellen E chart.

COLOR PERCEPTION

Congenital color blindness is usually a sex-linked recessive trait passed from mothers to male offspring. (Acquired color deficit is pathologic.) People with color blindness can't distinguish among red, green, and blue.

Of the many tests used to detect color blindness, the most common involves asking a patient to identify patterns of colored dots on colored plates. The patient who can't discern colors will miss the patterns. Early detection of color blindness allows the child to learn to compensate for the deficit and also alerts teachers to the student's special needs.

EXTRAOCULAR MUSCLE FUNCTION

To assess extraocular muscle function, first inspect the eyes for position and alignment, making sure they're parallel. Next, perform the six cardinal positions of gaze test, the cover-uncover test, and the corneal light reflex test.

The gaze test evaluates the function of each of the six extraocular muscles and tests the cranial nerves responsible for their movement (cranial nerves III, IV, and VI). Normal eye muscles work together so that when the right eye moves upward and inward, the left eye moves upward and outward.

The cover-uncover test assesses the fusion reflex, which makes binocular vision possible. The fusion reflex results from adequate extraocular muscle balance, which keeps the eyes parallel and on the same axis as the working muscles.

The corneal light reflex test assesses the ability of the extraocular muscles to hold the eyes steady, or parallel, when fixed on an object.

PERIPHERAL VISION

Assessment of peripheral vision tests the optic nerve (cranial nerve II) and measures the retina's ability to receive stimuli from the periphery of its field. You can grossly evaluate peripheral vision by assessing visual fields, which compares the patient's peripheral vision with your own. However, because this test assumes that you have normal vision, it can be subjective and inaccurate.

INSPECTION

After performing vision testing, inspect the eyelids, eyelashes, eyeball, and lacrimal apparatus. Also inspect the conjunctiva, sclera, cornea, anterior chamber, iris, and pupil. Using an ophthalmoscope, inspect the vitreous humor and retina.

Eyelids, eyelashes, eyeball, and lacrimal apparatus. Inspect these structures for general appearance. The eyes are normally bright and clear. The eyelids should close completely over the sclera; when opened, the margins of the upper eyelids should fall between the superior pupil margin and the superior limbus, covering a small portion of the iris. The eyelids should be free from edema, scaling, or lesions, and the eyelashes should curve outward and be equally distributed along the upper and lower eyelid margins. Eyelid color should be consistent with the patient's complexion. Inspect the palpebral folds for symmetry and the eyes for nystagmus (involuntary oscillations) and lid lag (unequal eyelid movement). Also inspect the eyes for excessive tearing or dryness and the puncta for inflammation and swelling.

Conjunctiva and sclera. Next, inspect the bulbar and palpebral portions of the conjunctiva for clarity. The conjunctiva should be free from hyperemic (engorged) blood vessels and drainage.

View the sclera through the bulbar portion of the conjunctiva. The sclera is normally white. However, many patients with dark complexions, such as blacks

Performing an ophthalmoscopic examination

An ophthalmoscopic examination can help identify inner eye abnormalities. This exam should be performed in a darkened or semidarkened room. Neither you nor the patient should wear glasses unless you're very myopic or astigmatic; however, both of you may wear contact lenses.

1. Sit or stand in front of the patient with your head about 18″ (46 cm) in front of and about 15 degrees to the right of the patient's line of vision in the right eye. Hold the ophthalmoscope in your right hand with the viewing aperture as close to your right eye as possible. Place your left thumb on the patient's right eyebrow to prevent hitting the patient with the ophthalmoscope as you move in close. Keep your right index finger on the lens selector to adjust the lens as necessary. To examine the left eye, perform these steps on the patient's left side.

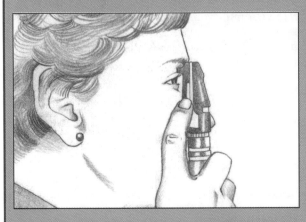

2. Instruct the patient to look straight ahead at a fixed point on the wall at eye level. Next, approaching from an oblique angle about 15″ (38 cm) out and with the diopter at 0, focus a small circle of light on the pupil, as shown below. Look for the orange-red glow of the red reflex, which should be sharp and distinct through the pupil. The red reflex indicates that the lens is free from opacity and clouding.

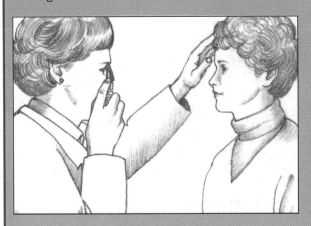

3. Move closer to the patient, changing the lens with your forefinger to keep the retinal structures in focus.

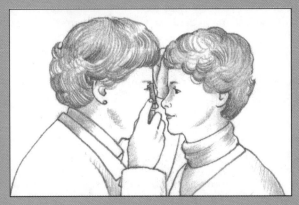

4. Change to a positive diopter to view the vitreous humor, observing for any opacity.

5. Next, view the retina, using a strong negative lens. Look for a retinal blood vessel, and follow that vessel toward the patient's nose, rotating the lens selector to keep the vessel in focus. Carefully examine all the retinal structures, including the retinal vessels, the optic disk, the retinal background, the macula, and the fovea.

6. Examine the vessels for their color, the size ratio of arterioles to veins, the arteriole light reflex, and the arteriovenous (AV) crossing. The crossing points should be smooth, without nicks or narrowings, and the vessels should be free of exudate, bleeding, and narrowing. Retinal vessels normally have an AV ratio of 2:3 or 4:5.

7. Evaluate the color of the retinal structures. The retina should be light yellow to orange and the background free from hemorrhages, aneurysms, and exudates. The optic disk, located on the nasal side of the retina, should be orange-red with distinct margins. The physiologic cup is normally yellow-white and readily visible.

8. Examine the macula last and as briefly as possible because it's very light-sensitive. The macula, which is darker than the rest of the retinal background, is free of vessels and located laterally to the optic disk. The fovea centralis is a slight depression in the center of the macula.

and those from the Middle East, have small, dark-pigmented spots on the sclera.

Cornea, anterior chamber, and iris. To inspect the cornea and anterior chamber, shine a penlight into the patient's eye from several side angles (tangentially). Normally, the cornea and anterior chamber are clear and transparent. Calculate the depth of the anterior chamber from the side by figuring the distance between the cornea and the iris. The iris should illuminate with the side lighting.

The surface of the cornea normally appears shiny and bright, without any scars or irregularities. The lids of both eyes should close when you touch either cornea.

Inspect the iris for shape and color. It should appear rather flat when viewed from the side.

Pupil. Examine the pupil of each eye for equality of size, shape, reaction to light, and accommodation. To test pupillary reaction to light, darken the room and, with the patient staring straight ahead at a fixed point, sweep a beam from a penlight from the side of the left eye to the center of its pupil. Both pupils should respond; the pupil receiving the direct light constricts directly, while the other pupil constricts simultaneously and consensually. Now test the pupil of the right eye. The pupils should react immediately, equally, and briskly (within 1 to 2 seconds). If the results are inconclusive, wait 15 to 30 seconds and try again. The pupils should be round and equal before and after the light flash.

To test for accommodation, ask the patient to stare at an object across the room. Normally, the pupils should dilate. Then ask him to stare at your index finger or at a pencil held about 2″ (5 cm) away. The pupils should constrict and converge equally on the object. To document a normal pupil assessment, use the abbreviation PERRLA (which stands for **p**upils **e**qual, **r**ound, **r**eactive to **l**ight, and **a**ccommodation) and the terms *direct* and *consensual*.

PALPATION
After inspection, palpate the eye and related structures. Begin by gently palpating the eyelids for swelling and tenderness. Then palpate the eyeball by placing the tips of both index fingers on the eyelids over the sclera while the patient looks down. The eyeballs should feel equally firm.

Next, palpate the lacrimal sac by pressing the index finger against the patient's lower orbital rim on the side closest to his nose. While pressing, observe the punctum for any abnormal regurgitation of purulent material or excessive tears, which could indicate blockage of the nasolacrimal duct.

OPHTHALMOSCOPIC EXAMINATION
An ophthalmoscopic examination can detect many disorders of the optic disk and retina, but the technique and the interpretation of abnormalities require skill, experience, and knowledge. Three of the major optic disk disorders detected by ophthalmoscopic examination are papilledema, optic atrophy, and glaucoma. (See *Performing an ophthalmoscopic examination.*)

Assessment of the ear

To obtain an accurate and complete history, adapt your questions to the patient's specific complaint and compare the answers with the results of the physical assessment.

HISTORY
Before the interview, determine whether the patient hears well. If not, look directly at him when asking questions and speak clearly.

CHIEF COMPLAINT
Document the patient's chief complaint in his own words. Ask relevant questions, such as whether he has recently noticed any difference in hearing in one or both ears. Does he have ear pain or trouble with earwax? If he has pain, is it unilateral or bilateral? What remedies has he tried?

Ask if he has frequent headaches, a nasal discharge, or a postnasal drip. Also ask about frequent or prolonged nosebleeds, difficulty swallowing or chewing, and hoarseness or changes in the sound of his voice.

MEDICAL HISTORY
Find out if the patient has had an ear injury. Ask if he has experienced ringing or crackling in his ears and whether he recently has had a foreign body in his ear. Does he suffer from frequent ear infections? Has he had drainage from his ears or problems with balance, dizziness, or vertigo? Also ask about sinus infections or tenderness, allergies that cause breathing difficulty, and sensations that his throat is closing.

Inquire about previous hospitalization, drug therapy, or surgery for an ear, nose, or throat disorder or any other relevant condition. Has anyone in the patient's family had hearing, sinus, or nasal problems? Does the patient work around loud equipment, such as printing presses, airguns, or airplanes? If so, does he wear ear protectors?

Determine if the patient smokes, chews tobacco, inhales cocaine, or drinks alcohol and, if so, to what extent.

Performing an otoscopic examination

Before inserting the speculum into the ear, inspect the canal opening for a foreign body or discharge. Palpate the tragus and pull up the auricle to assess for tenderness. If tenderness is present, the patient may have external otitis media; in such a case, don't insert the speculum because you'll probably cause pain. Also inspect the external auditory canal before proceeding.

1. Tip the adult patient's head to the side opposite the ear being assessed. Straighten the canal by pulling up and back on the superior posterior auricle (as shown below).

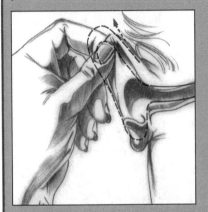

2. Hold the otoscope firmly against the patient's head to prevent jerking the speculum against the external canal. Examine the external canal, which should be free from inflammation and scaling. Note the color of cerumen.

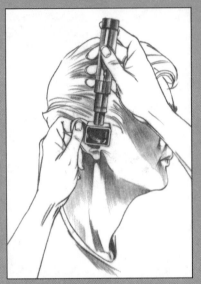

3. Because the inner two-thirds of the canal is sensitive to pressure, insert the speculum gently to avoid causing pain. Gently rotate the angle of the speculum as needed to gain a complete view of the tympanic membrane.

4. Examine the tympanic membrane; it should be pearly gray and glistening, with the annulus appearing white and denser than the rest of the membrane. The inferior edge is posterior to the outside, and the superior edge is anterior. Look for bulging, retraction, or perforations at the periphery of the tympanic membrane.

Next, check the light reflex, which is in the anterior inferior quadrant in the 5 o'clock position in the right tympanic membrane and in the 7 o'clock position in the left. The light reflex usually appears as a bright cone of light with its point directed at the umbo and its base at the periphery of the tympanic membrane.

Examine the malleus. The handle of the malleus originates in the superior hemisphere of the tympanic membrane and, when viewed through the membrane, looks like a dense whitish streak. The malleus attaches to the center of the tympanic membrane at the umbo.

PHYSICAL EXAMINATION

You'll primarily use inspection and palpation to assess the ears. If appropriate, you'll also perform an otoscopic examination.

Examine ear color and size. The ears should be similarly shaped, colored the same as the face, and sized in proportion to the head. Look for drainage, nodules, and lesions. Some ears normally drain large amounts of cerumen. Also, check behind the ears for inflammation, masses, or lesions.

Palpate the external ear and the mastoid process to discover any areas of tenderness, swelling, nodules, or lesions, and then gently pull the helix of the ear backward to determine if the patient feels pain or tenderness.

OTOSCOPIC EXAMINATION

Before examining the auditory canal and the tympanic membrane, become familiar with the function of the otoscope. (See *Performing an otoscopic examination*.)

Tympanic membranes vary slightly in size, shape, color, and clarity of landmarks. You may need to inspect numerous healthy tympanic membranes before you can recognize an abnormal one.

GROSS HEARING SCREENING

You can perform two gross screenings of hearing: the whispered or spoken voice test and the watch-tick test. For the voice test, have the patient plug one ear with a finger. To test the other ear, stand behind the patient at a distance of 1' to 2' (30 to 60 cm) and whisper a word or phrase. A patient with normal acuity should be able to repeat what was whispered.

The watch-tick test evaluates the patient's ability to hear high-frequency sounds. Gradually move a watch away from the patient's ear until he can no longer hear the ticking, which should occur when the watch is about 5″ (13 cm) away.

WEBER TEST

This test evaluates bone conduction. Perform it by placing a vibrating tuning fork on top of the patient's head at midline or in the middle of his forehead. The patient should perceive the sound equally in both ears. If he has a conductive hearing loss, he'll hear the sound in the ear that has the conductive loss because the sound is being conducted directly through the bone to the ear. If he has a sensorineural hearing loss in one ear, the sound will lateralize to the unimpaired ear because nerve damage in the impaired ear prevents hearing. Document a normal Weber test by recording a negative lateralization of sound.

RINNE TEST

This test compares bone conduction with air conduction in both ears. Assess bone conduction by placing the base of a vibrating tuning fork on the mastoid process, noting how many seconds pass before the patient can no longer hear it. Then quickly place the still-vibrating tuning fork, with the tines parallel to the patient's auricle, near the ear canal (to test air conduction). Hold the tuning fork in this position until the patient no longer hears the tone. Note how many seconds he can hear the tone. Repeat the test on the other ear.

Because sound traveling through air remains audible twice as long (a 2:1 ratio) as sound traveling through bone, a sound heard for 10 seconds by bone conduction should be heard for 20 seconds by air conduction. If the patient reports hearing the sound longer through bone conduction, he has a conductive loss. In a sensorineural loss, the patient will report hearing the sound longer through air conduction, but the ratio will not be the normal 2:1.

Acoustic neuroma

This benign, progressively enlarging tumor affects the ear's vestibular or acoustic nerve. It may be unilateral or bilateral and commonly affects the cerebellum because of its location.

CAUSES

The cause of acoustic neuroma is unknown, but researchers speculate that it may result from an autosomal dominant trait.

DIAGNOSIS AND TREATMENT

Diagnosis is based on computed tomography scanning. Audiograms can detect sensorineural hearing loss. Cerebrospinal fluid assays show increased pressure and the presence of proteins.

Treatment of an acoustic neuroma involves surgical excision and removal by a craniotomy. Hearing loss may occur when surgery is performed. Recurrence is rare once the tumor is surgically removed.

COLLABORATIVE MANAGEMENT

Care of the patient with an acoustic neuroma focuses on improving ability to hear and maintain communication with others and adequate knowledge about the disorder, its treatment, and measures taken to prevent further hearing loss.

ASSESSMENT

Signs and symptoms may vary, depending on the size and exact location of the lesion. The patient may have impaired hearing, facial movement, and facial sensation as well as increased intracranial pressure (ICP) because of the tumor's space-occupying nature. The pressure it places on the nerves causes tinnitus, gradual hearing loss, vertigo, and damage to adjacent nerves as the tumor progresses.

NURSING DIAGNOSES AND COLLABORATIVE PROBLEMS

Based on the following nursing diagnoses, you'll establish patient outcomes.

Sensory/perceptual alteration (auditory) related to hearing loss. The patient will:
- demonstrate measures to cope with altered hearing
- demonstrate ability to understand what is being said.

Risk for injury related to hearing loss. The patient will:
- demonstrate measures to ensure his safety
- remain free from injury.

PLANNING AND IMPLEMENTATION

These measures help the patient with an acoustic neuroma.
- When speaking to a patient with hearing loss who can read lips, stand directly in front of him, with the light on your face, and speak slowly and distinctly in a low tone; avoid shouting. Approach the patient within his visual range, and get his attention by raising your arm or waving; touching him may be unnecessarily startling.
- Alert other staff members and hospital personnel to your patient's handicap and his established method of communication.

- Make sure the patient with hearing loss is in an area where he can observe unit activities and people as they approach because such a patient depends totally on visual clues.
- Carefully explain all diagnostic tests and hospital procedures in a way the patient understands.
- Provide emotional support and encouragement to the patient learning to use a hearing aid.
- After a craniotomy, monitor the incision, level of consciousness, and ICP, as indicated.
- Refer a child with suspected hearing loss to an audiologist or otolaryngologist for further evaluation.

Patient teaching
- Teach the patient who just received a hearing aid how it works and how to maintain it.
- Teach the patient the signs and symptoms of a possible wound infection. Advise him to notify the doctor if any occur.
- Instruct family members in effective methods of communicating with the patient.

EVALUATION
Evaluation of patient outcomes determines the success of collaborative management. For the patient with an acoustic neuroma, evaluation focuses on improved ability to hear with assistive devices and to communicate as well as an adequate knowledge about the disorder, its treatment, and follow-up care.

Cataract

A common cause of gradual vision loss, a cataract is an opacity of the eye's lens or lens capsule. In this disorder, light shining through the cornea is blocked by the clouded lens. This, in turn, blurs the image cast onto the retina. As a result, the brain interprets a hazy image.

Cataracts commonly affect both eyes, but each cataract progresses independently. Exceptions are traumatic cataracts, which are usually unilateral, and congenital cataracts, which may remain stationary. Cataracts are most prevalent in people over age 70. Surgery restores vision in about 95% of patients. Without surgery, a cataract eventually leads to complete vision loss.

CAUSES
Cataracts are classified by their causes:
- *Senile cataracts* develop in older adults, probably because of chemical changes in lens proteins.
- *Congenital cataracts* occur in neonates from inborn errors of metabolism or from maternal rubella infec-

tion during the first trimester of pregnancy. These cataracts may also result from a congenital anomaly or from genetic causes. Transmission is usually autosomal dominant; however, recessive cataracts may be sex-linked.
- *Traumatic cataracts* develop after a foreign body injures the lens with sufficient force to allow aqueous or vitreous humor to enter the lens capsule.
- *Complicated cataracts* occur secondary to uveitis, glaucoma, retinitis pigmentosa, or retinal detachment. They can also occur with systemic diseases, such as diabetes, hypoparathyroidism, or atopic dermatitis, or from ionizing radiation or infrared rays.
- *Toxic cataracts* result from drug or chemical toxicity with ergot, dinitrophenol, naphthalene, or phenothiazines.

DIAGNOSIS AND TREATMENT
Indirect ophthalmoscopy reveals a dark area in the normally homogeneous red reflex. Slit-lamp examination confirms the diagnosis of a lens opacity. Visual acuity testing confirms the degree of vision loss. Surgical lens extraction and implantation of an intraocular lens to correct the visual deficit is the treatment for a cataract.

COLLABORATIVE MANAGEMENT
Care of the patient with a cataract focuses on maintaining safety and comfort while minimizing further visual damage and deficits.

ASSESSMENT
Typically, the patient complains of painless, gradual vision loss. He may also report a blinding glare from headlights when he drives at night, poor reading vision, and an annoying glare and poor vision in bright sunlight. If he has a central opacity, he may report seeing better in dim light than in bright light. That's because the cataract is nuclear, and as the pupil dilates, the patient can see around the opacity.

Inspection with a penlight may reveal a milky white pupil and, in an advanced cataract, a grayish white area behind the pupil.

NURSING DIAGNOSES AND COLLABORATIVE PROBLEMS
Based on the following nursing diagnoses, you'll establish patient outcomes.

Fear related to complete loss of vision caused by untreated cataracts. The patient will:
- identify and verbalize his fears
- request information about cataracts to diminish his fears
- state that his fears have been reduced.

Providing care after cataract surgery

Following are selected portions of the clinical practice guidelines for the rehabilitation of patients who've undergone cataract removal. The guidelines were developed by the Agency for Health Care Policy and Research of the U.S. Department of Health and Human Services.

■ Your careful preoperative assessment of the patient's and family members' ability to understand and comply with instructions is critical to ensure adequate postoperative care. If the patient can't read written instructions because of impaired vision or other physical or mental problems, refer him to a home health care agency for further education and evaluation.

■ Review instructions for infection control, signs and symptoms to report to the ophthalmologist, and protective and preventive measures with the patient both before discharge and again at home. This is to ensure that he'll follow the postoperative regimen at home, either independently or with the help of a caregiver.

■ Before discharge and during postoperative visits, teach the patient how to instill medications properly and safely.

■ As a nurse, you are one of the health care professionals best prepared to assess the patient's current and future health status because you're trained to do extensive patient interviewing and physical, psychological, and home assessments. Keep in mind that the patient living alone may need assessment for in-home support services, such as assistance with bathing, dressing, and preparing meals.

■ If your cataract patient who is considering surgery also functions as the primary caretaker for another individual, refer him to a home health care agency or a family service agency for interim help with that responsibility.

■ Assess the patient's emotional and spiritual needs and arrange the appropriate pastoral support.

■ If your patient doesn't speak English, arrange for an interpreter to ensure that he understands self-care instructions.

Risk for injury related to decrease in vision caused by the cataract. The patient will:
■ take precautions to protect himself from injury
■ sustain no injury.

Sensory/perceptual alterations (visual) related to diminishing ability to see properly as a result of the cataract. The patient will:
■ discuss how his vision loss affects his lifestyle and institute measures to compensate
■ resume a functional lifestyle
■ regain lost vision.

PLANNING AND IMPLEMENTATION

These measures help the patient with cataracts.
■ Provide a safe environment. For example, keep bed side rails raised and assist the patient with activities as needed.
■ Check the patient's vision regularly.
■ Allow the patient to express his fears and anxieties about his vision loss.
■ Keep the call bell and other necessary objects within reach.
■ Assist with activities of daily living as needed. (See *Providing care after cataract surgery.*)
■ Prepare the patient for cataract surgery as appropriate.

Patient teaching
■ Explain how and why cataracts form.

■ Stress the importance of regular ophthalmologic examinations to monitor the degree of visual impairment and to determine when surgery can be performed. Encourage the patient to have the cataract removed.
■ Advise the patient to take safety precautions, including no night driving, until the cataract can be removed.

EVALUATION
Evaluation of patient outcomes determines the success of collaborative management. For the patient with a cataract, evaluation focuses on maintaining safety and comfort while minimizing further visual damage and deficits.

CMV retinitis

Cytomegalovirus (CMV) is an opportunistic infection of the eye that occurs in many patients with human immunodeficiency virus (HIV) infection. In most cases, it begins unilaterally but eventually the other eye becomes infected by viremia.

CAUSES
Cytomegalovirus retinitis is caused by the virus for which it's named. CMV is a DNA, ether-sensitive virus

belonging to the herpes family. The infection occurs worldwide and is transmitted by human contact. CMV invades the cells of the retina directly, causing damage and necrosis. Deep, dense granular white dots appear on the retina close to major blood vessels. These lesions coalesce to form patches of opacification.

If untreated, the patches expand, affecting large portions of the retina. Atrophy and papilledema of the optic nerve occur as well as hemorrhaging. Vision is affected and the condition can progress to acute retinal necrosis.

DIAGNOSIS AND TREATMENT
Serologic testing confirms the presence of CMV. Indirect ophthalmoscopy may reveal hemorrhaging and retinal necrosis. Visual acuity tests determine the degree of vision loss.

The goal of treatment is to maintain functional vision and arrest the disease process. Ganciclovir is used to slow the proliferative nature of the disease, but it does not eradicate the virus. Trisodium phosphornoformate has also been approved to treat CMV retinitis.

COLLABORATIVE MANAGEMENT
Care of the patient with CMV retinitis focuses on improved vision, maintenance of safety, and adequate knowledge to ensure compliance and follow-up.

ASSESSMENT
Diagnosis is based on the patient history and ocular findings. The patient may be asymptomatic and complain of another unrelated ocular problem. He may complain of changes in vision and the appearance of flashes of light or floaters. Rapid detection is crucial because the disease progresses quickly.

Ophthalmoscopic examination may reveal areas of white granulation that appear as cotton wool spots.

NURSING DIAGNOSES AND COLLABORATIVE PROBLEMS
Based on the following nursing diagnoses, you'll establish patient outcomes.

Risk for injury related to decreased visual fields. The patient will:
- demonstrate measures to remain safe
- remain free from injury.

Sensory/perceptual alteration (visual) related to infection. The patient will:
- comply with treatment to ensure optimal vision
- maintain optimal visual function.

PLANNING AND IMPLEMENTATION
These measures help the patient with CMV retinitis.
- Assess the patient's vision, including vision changes, and document the degree of his peripheral vision.
- Administer medications as ordered.
- Orient the patient to the environment, provide a clear path for walking, and make sure his room is well lit.

Patient teaching
- For patients with HIV infection, explain the need for early detection and treatment of CMV retinitis.
- Teach the patient the proper use of prescribed medications, and explain how they prevent the spread of his infection.

EVALUATION
Evaluation of patient outcomes determines the success of collaborative management. For the patient with CMV retinitis, evaluation focuses on improved vision, safety, and adequate knowledge about complying with treatments and follow-up care.

Conjunctivitis

An inflammation of the conjunctiva commonly known as pinkeye, conjunctivitis is usually benign and self-limiting. It may also be chronic, possibly indicating degenerative changes or damage from repeated acute attacks.

In the Western hemisphere, conjunctivitis is probably the most common eye disorder. It's transmitted by contaminated towels, washcloths, or the patient's own hands, and it usually spreads rapidly from one eye to the other.

CAUSES
Common causes include bacterial, viral, and chlamydial infection. Less common causes are allergy, parasitic disease and, rarely, fungal infection or occupational irritants. An idiopathic form may be associated with certain systemic diseases, such as erythema multiforme and thyroid disease.

DIAGNOSIS AND TREATMENT
Stained smears of conjunctival scrapings reveal predominant monocytes if the cause is a virus, polymorphonuclear cells (neutrophils) if the cause is bacteria, and eosinophils if the cause is an allergy. Culture and sensitivity tests are done when a purulent discharge is evident to identify the causative bacterial organism and to indicate appropriate antibiotic therapy.

Treatment of conjunctivitis varies with the cause. Bacterial conjunctivitis requires topical application of the appropriate antibiotic or sulfonamide. Viral conjunctivitis resists treatment, but sulfonamide or broad-spectrum antibiotic eyedrops may prevent secondary infection. Herpes simplex keratitis usually responds to treatment with trifluridine drops, but the infection may persist for 2 to 3 weeks. Treatment of vernal (allergic) conjunctivitis includes administration of vasoconstrictor eyedrops such as naphazoline 0.1%, cold compresses to relieve itching and, occasionally, oral antihistamines.

Instillation of 1% silver nitrate prevents gonococcal infections in neonates. Erythromycin is preferred because it prevents chlamydial conjunctivitis.

COLLABORATIVE MANAGEMENT

Care of the patient with conjunctivitis focuses on resolving the infection and teaching prevention.

ASSESSMENT

Inspection reveals the characteristic signs and symptoms. These include hyperemia of the conjunctiva, possible discharge (mucopurulent with bacterial infection, watery with viral infection), as well as pain and photophobia in corneal involvement, itching and burning in allergy, and a foreign body sensation in the eye in acute bacterial infection. An accompanying sore throat or fever is possible in children.

NURSING DIAGNOSES AND COLLABORATIVE PROBLEMS

Based on the following nursing diagnoses, you'll establish patient outcomes.

Risk for injury related to decreased visual fields. The patient will:
■ demonstrate measures to ensure safety
■ remain safe.

Pain related to swelling and irritation. The patient will:
■ carry out measures to alleviate pain
■ state that pain is relieved.

Risk for infection related to communicability of conjunctivitis. The patient will:
■ demonstrate infection-control measures
■ experience no spread of infection to unaffected eye.

PLANNING AND IMPLEMENTATION

These measures help the patient with conjunctivitis.
■ Assess the patient's vision and document his degree of peripheral vision.
■ Orient the patient to the environment, ensure that he has a clear path to walk, and illuminate the room adequately.

■ Notify public health authorities if cultures show *Neisseria gonorrhoeae.*
■ Apply therapeutic ointment or drops, as ordered. Have the patient wash his hands before he uses the medication and use clean washcloths or towels so he doesn't infect his other eye.
■ Assess the effects of medications, compresses, and other treatments.

Patient teaching

■ Teach the patient about possible adverse effects of interventions, such as eyedrops and ointment.
■ Teach proper hand-washing technique because conjunctivitis can be highly contagious.
■ Tell the patient to avoid sharing washcloths, towels, and pillows with family members to minimize the risk of spreading the infection. Warn against rubbing the infected eye, which can spread the infection to the other eye and to other people.
■ Teach the patient to instill eyedrops and ointments correctly, without touching the bottle tip to his eye or lashes.
■ Stress the importance of wearing safety glasses for the patient who works near chemical irritants.

EVALUATION

Evaluation of patient outcomes determines the success of collaborative management. For the patient with conjunctivitis, evaluation focuses on resolution of the infection and adequate knowledge about infection-control measures and medication therapy.

Glaucoma

A group of eye disorders, glaucoma is characterized by high intraocular pressure (IOP) that damages the optic nerve. Glaucoma may occur as a primary or congenital disease or secondary to other causes, such as injury, infection, surgery, or prolonged use of topical corticosteroids.

Primary glaucoma has two forms: *open-angle* (also known as chronic, simple, or wide-angle) glaucoma and *angle-closure* (also known as acute or narrow-angle) glaucoma. Angle-closure glaucoma occurs suddenly and may cause permanent vision loss in 48 to 72 hours.

One of the leading causes of blindness in the United States, glaucoma affects about 2% of Americans over age 40 and accounts for about 12% of newly diagnosed cases of blindness. The incidence is highest among blacks. In the United States, the prognosis for preserving vision is good with early detection and effective treatment.

If untreated, glaucoma can progress from gradual vision loss to total blindness.

CAUSES

Open-angle glaucoma results from degenerative changes in the trabecular meshwork. These changes block the flow of aqueous humor from the eye, which causes IOP to increase. The result is optic nerve damage. Affecting about 90% of all patients who have glaucoma, open-angle glaucoma commonly occurs in families.

Angle-closure glaucoma results from obstructed outflow of aqueous humor caused by an anatomically narrow angle between the iris and the cornea. This causes IOP to increase suddenly. Angle-closure glaucoma attacks may be triggered by trauma, pupillary dilation, stress, or any ocular change that pushes the iris forward (a hemorrhage or a swollen lens, for example).

Secondary glaucoma can develop from such conditions as uveitis, trauma, venous occlusion, and diabetes or from the use of certain drugs (such as corticosteroids). In some instances, new blood vessels may form (neovascularization), blocking the passage of aqueous humor.

DIAGNOSIS AND TREATMENT

Diagnostic tests may include tonometry, slit-lamp examination, gonioscopy, ophthalmoscopy, perimetry or visual field tests, and fundus photography.

For open-angle glaucoma, initial treatment aims to reduce pressure by decreasing aqueous humor production with medications. These include beta blockers, such as timolol (used cautiously in asthmatic patients or patients with bradycardia) or betaxolol. Other drug treatments include epinephrine to decrease production of and increase outflow of aqueous humor (contraindicated in angle-closure glaucoma) and miotic eyedrops, such as pilocarpine, to promote aqueous humor outflow.

Patients who don't respond to drug therapy may benefit from argon laser trabeculoplasty or from a surgical filtering procedure called trabeculectomy.

In *argon laser trabeculoplasty,* the ophthalmologist focuses an argon laser beam on the trabecular meshwork of an open angle. This produces a thermal burn that changes the meshwork surface and facilitates the outflow of aqueous humor.

In *trabeculectomy,* the surgeon dissects a flap of sclera to expose the trabecular meshwork. He removes a small tissue block and performs a peripheral iridectomy, which produces an opening for aqueous outflow under the conjunctiva and creates a filtering bleb. After surgery, subconjunctival injections of fluorouracil may be given to maintain the fistula's patency.

An emergency, angle-closure glaucoma requires immediate treatment to lower high IOP. Initial drug therapy aims to lower IOP with acetazolamide, pilocarpine (which constricts the pupil, forces the iris away from the trabeculae, and allows fluid to escape), and I.V. mannitol or oral glycerin (which forces fluid from the eye by making the blood hypertonic).

If these medications fail to decrease the pressure, laser iridotomy or surgical peripheral iridectomy must be performed promptly to save the patient's vision. Both of these procedures relieve pressure by excising part of the iris to reestablish the outflow of aqueous humor—an iridotomy by use of a laser and an iridectomy by surgery. A few days after an iridectomy, the surgeon performs a prophylactic iridectomy on the other eye to prevent an acute glaucoma attack in that eye.

If the patient has severe pain, treatment may include narcotic analgesics. After peripheral iridectomy, treatment includes cycloplegic eyedrops to relax the ciliary muscle and decrease inflammation, thereby preventing adhesions.

COLLABORATIVE MANAGEMENT

Care of the patient with glaucoma focuses on normalization of IOP, maintenance of optimal vision, absence of complications, and adequate knowledge to comply with treatment and follow-up.

ASSESSMENT

Inspection may reveal unilateral eye inflammation, a cloudy cornea, and a moderately dilated pupil that fails to react to light. Palpation may also disclose increased IOP discovered by applying gentle fingertip pressure to the patient's closed eyelids. With angle-closure glaucoma, one eye may feel harder than the other.

NURSING DIAGNOSES AND COLLABORATIVE PROBLEMS

Based on the following nursing diagnoses, you'll establish patient outcomes.

Fear related to potential for blindness. The patient will:
- identify sources of fear
- seek knowledge about glaucoma from an appropriate source to help reduce his fears
- express an understanding that compliance with the prescribed treatment regimen can prevent further vision loss.

Risk for injury related to visual disturbances. The patient will:
- take precautions to prevent injury when visual disturbances occur during periods of elevated IOP
- sustain no injury from visual impairment.

Sensory/perceptual alteration (visual) related to increased IOP. The patient will:
- identify types of visual changes that can occur when his IOP increases beyond a safe level
- seek medical attention when visual changes occur
- regain and maintain normal vision with treatment.

PLANNING AND IMPLEMENTATION

These measures help the patient with glaucoma.
- For the patient with angle-closure glaucoma, give medications as ordered, and prepare him physically and psychologically for laser iridotomy or iridectomy.
- Remember to administer cycloplegic eyedrops *in the affected eye only.* In the unaffected eye, these drops may precipitate an attack of angle-closure glaucoma and threaten the patient's residual vision.
- Administer pain medication as ordered.
- Encourage the patient to express his concerns about having a chronic condition.
- After trabeculectomy, give medications, as ordered, to dilate the pupil. Also apply topical corticosteroids, as ordered, to rest the pupil.
- After surgery, protect the affected eye by applying an eye patch and eye shield, positioning the patient on his back or unaffected side, and following general safety measures.
- Monitor the patient's ability to see clearly. Question him regularly about the occurrence of visual changes.
- Monitor the patient's IOP regularly.
- Monitor his compliance with treatment and lifelong follow-up care.

Patient teaching
- Stress the importance of meticulous compliance with the prescribed drug regimen to maintain low IOP and prevent optic disk changes that cause vision loss.
- Explain all procedures and treatments, especially surgery, to help reduce the patient's anxiety.
- Inform the patient that lost vision can't be restored but that treatment can usually prevent further loss.
- Teach family members how to modify the patient's environment for safety. For example, suggest keeping pathways clear and reorienting the patient to room layouts, if necessary.
- Teach the patient the signs and symptoms that require immediate medical attention, such as a sudden vision change or eye pain.
- Discuss the importance of glaucoma screening for early detection and prevention. Point out that all people over age 35 should have an annual tonometric examination. (See *Preventing vision loss.*)

HEALTHY LIVING **Preventing vision loss**

The best way to prevent vision loss is through regular eye examinations. The recommended frequency for visual testing is every 2 years. Glaucoma testing should be done routinely, especially for individuals age 40 and older.

Further ways to prevent vision loss include the following:
- Protect your eyes from strain.
- Wear protective eyeware when performing hazardous tasks.

EVALUATION

Evaluation of patient outcomes determines the success of collaborative management. For the patient with glaucoma, evaluation focuses on maintenance of optimal vision, absence of complications, ability to carry out activities of daily living, and adequate knowledge about treatment and follow-up care.

Hearing loss

Hearing loss results from a mechanical or nervous system impediment to the transmission of sound waves. It can be classified as conductive, sensorineural, or mixed.

CAUSES

Congenital hearing loss may be transmitted as a dominant, an autosomal dominant, an autosomal recessive, or a sex-linked recessive trait. Hearing loss in neonates may also result from trauma, toxicity, or infection during pregnancy or delivery. Predisposing factors include a family history of hearing loss or known hereditary disorders (such as otosclerosis), maternal exposure to rubella or syphilis during pregnancy, use of ototoxic drugs during pregnancy, prolonged fetal anoxia during delivery, and congenital abnormalities of the ears, nose, or throat.

Premature or low-birth-weight infants are most likely to have structural or functional hearing impairment; those with serum bilirubin levels greater than 20 mg/dl also risk hearing impairment from bilirubin's toxic cerebral effects. Also, trauma during delivery may cause intracranial hemorrhage and damage the cochlea or acoustic nerve.

Sudden hearing loss in a person with no prior hearing impairment is considered a medical emergency because prompt treatment may restore full hearing. Its causes and predisposing factors may include:

■ acute infections, especially mumps (most common cause of unilateral sensorineural hearing loss in children); other bacterial and viral infections, such as rubella, rubeola, influenza, herpes zoster, and infectious mononucleosis; and mycoplasmal infections

■ metabolic disorders, such as diabetes mellitus, hypothyroidism, and hyperlipoproteinemia

■ vascular disorders, such as hypertension and arteriosclerosis

■ head trauma and brain tumors

■ ototoxic drugs, such as tobramycin, streptomycin, quinine, gentamicin, furosemide, and ethacrynic acid

■ neurologic disorders, such as multiple sclerosis and neurosyphilis

■ blood dyscrasias, such as leukemia and hypercoagulation.

Noise-induced hearing loss, whether transient or permanent, may follow prolonged exposure to loud noise (85 to 90 decibels [db]) or brief exposure to extremely loud noise (greater than 90 db). Such hearing loss is common in workers subjected to constant industrial noise and in military personnel, hunters, and rock musicians.

Presbycusis, an otologic effect of aging, results from a loss of hair cells in the organ of Corti. This disorder causes sensorineural hearing loss, usually of high-frequency tones.

In conductive hearing loss, transmission of sound impulses from the external ear to the junction of the stapes and oval window is interrupted. In sensorineural loss, impaired cochlear or acoustic nerve (cranial nerve VIII) function prevents transmission of sound impulses within the inner ear or brain. In mixed hearing loss, conductive hearing loss and sensorineural dysfunction are combined.

DIAGNOSIS AND TREATMENT

The Weber and Rinne tests and specialized audiologic tests differentiate between conductive and sensorineural hearing loss.

Therapy for congenital hearing loss that is refractory to surgery consists of teaching the patient to communicate through sign language, speech reading, or other effective means. Measures that can be taken to prevent congenital hearing loss include immunizing children against rubella to reduce the risk of maternal exposure during pregnancy; educating pregnant women about the dangers of exposure to drugs, chemicals, or infection; and careful monitoring during labor and delivery to prevent fetal anoxia.

To treat sudden deafness, the underlying cause must be promptly identified. Educating laymen and health care professionals about the many causes of

sudden deafness can greatly reduce the incidence of this problem.

In individuals whose hearing loss is induced by noise levels greater than 90 db for several hours, overnight rest usually restores normal hearing. However, hearing is not restored if the person was exposed to such noise repeatedly. As the patient's hearing deteriorates, speech and hearing rehabilitation must be provided because hearing aids are rarely helpful. To prevent noise-induced hearing loss, people must learn about the dangers of noise exposure and insist on using protective devices such as ear plugs against occupational exposure to noise.

Presbycusis usually requires the use of a hearing aid.

COLLABORATIVE MANAGEMENT

Care of the patient with hearing loss focuses on improved hearing, communication, and safety.

ASSESSMENT

Although congenital hearing loss may produce no obvious signs of hearing impairment at birth, a deficient response to auditory stimuli usually becomes apparent within 2 to 3 days. As the child grows older, hearing loss impairs speech development.

Because the sensorineural damage caused by noise depends on the duration and intensity of the noise, noise-induced hearing loss may be progressive. Initially, the patient loses perception of certain frequencies (around 4,000 Hz); with continued exposure, he eventually loses perception of all frequencies.

Presbycusis usually produces tinnitus and the inability to understand the spoken word.

The patient interview, family and occupational histories, and a complete audiologic examination usually provide ample evidence of hearing loss and suggest possible causes or predisposing factors.

NURSING DIAGNOSES AND COLLABORATIVE PROBLEMS

Based on the following nursing diagnoses, you'll establish patient outcomes.

Sensory/perceptual alteration (auditory) related to hearing loss. The patient will:

■ take measures to improve hearing

■ demonstrate comprehension of what is being said.

Risk for injury related to hearing loss. The patient will:

■ demonstrate measures to maintain safety

■ remain free from injury.

PLANNING AND IMPLEMENTATION

These measures help the patient with hearing loss.

- When speaking to a patient with hearing loss who can read lips, stand directly in front of him, with the light on your face, and speak slowly and distinctly in a low tone; avoid shouting. Approach the patient within his visual range, and get his attention by raising your arm or waving; touching him may be unnecessarily startling.
- Alert other staff members and hospital personnel to your patient's handicap and his established method of communication.
- Make sure a hearing-impaired patient is in an area where he can observe unit activities and people as they approach because such a patient depends totally on visual clues.
- Carefully explain all diagnostic tests and hospital procedures in a way that the patient understands.
- To help prevent hearing loss, watch for signs of hearing impairment in patients receiving ototoxic drugs.
- Provide emotional support and encouragement to the patient learning to use a hearing aid.
- Refer a child with suspected hearing loss to an audiologist or otolaryngologist for further evaluation.

Patient teaching
- Teach the patient who just received a hearing aid how it works and how to maintain it.
- Emphasize the danger of excessive exposure to noise, and encourage the use of protective devices in a noisy environment.
- Stress the danger of exposure to drugs, chemicals, and infection (especially rubella) to pregnant women. (See *Preventing hearing loss*.)

EVALUATION
Evaluation of patient outcomes determines the success of collaborative management. For the patient with hearing loss, evaluation focuses on improved hearing, ability to communicate and avoid injury, and adequate knowledge about the disorder, its treatment, and preventive measures.

Keratitis

An inflammation of the cornea, keratitis usually occurs unilaterally. It may be acute or chronic, and superficial or deep. Superficial keratitis is fairly common and may develop at any age. The prognosis is good with treatment. Untreated, recurrent keratitis may lead to blindness.

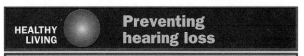

HEALTHY LIVING — **Preventing hearing loss**

Hearing loss may result from repeated exposure to excessively loud noises, such as high volume on stereos or headphones, live music concerts, or noisy work environments (jackhammers or other loud machinery).

To prevent injury to the ears and hearing loss, recommend the use of protective devices, especially when the patient can't avoid exposure. When possible, advise him to lower the volume on radios and to avoid areas where he can't control the decibel level.

Also stress the danger of exposure to drugs, chemicals, and infection—especially rubella—to pregnant women.

CAUSES
Infection by herpes simplex virus type 1 (dendritic keratitis) is the usual cause. Other causes include exposure of the cornea because of an inability to close the eyelids, bacterial or fungal infection (less common), or congenital syphilis, which causes interstitial keratitis.

DIAGNOSIS AND TREATMENT
Slit-lamp examination confirms keratitis. If the disorder is caused by the herpesvirus, staining the eye with a fluorescein strip reveals one or more small branchlike (dendritic) lesions. Vision testing may show decreased acuity if the lesion is in the pupillary region.

For acute keratitis caused by herpesvirus, treatment consists of trifluridine or acyclovir eyedrops. Trifluridine is used to treat recurrent herpetic keratitis. A broad-spectrum antibiotic may prevent secondary bacterial infection. Chronic dendritic keratitis may respond more quickly to vidarabine. Long-term topical therapy may be necessary. (Corticosteroid therapy is contraindicated in dendritic keratitis and in any other viral or fungal disease of the cornea.) Treatment of fungal keratitis consists of natamycin.

Keratitis caused by exposure requires application of moisturizing ointment to the exposed cornea and of a plastic bubble eye shield or eye patch. Treatment of severe corneal scarring may include keratoplasty (corneal transplantation).

COLLABORATIVE MANAGEMENT
Care of the patient with keratitis focuses on resolving the infection and teaching prevention.

ASSESSMENT

Typically, the patient with keratitis will exhibit opacities of the cornea, mild irritation, tearing, photophobia and, possibly, blurred vision.

NURSING DIAGNOSES AND COLLABORATIVE PROBLEMS

Based on the following nursing diagnoses, you'll establish patient outcomes.

Risk for injury related to decreased visual fields. The patient will:
- demonstrate appropriate safety measures
- remain free from injury.

Pain related to the effects of keratitis. The patient will:
- carry out measures to alleviate pain
- verbalize relief of pain.

Risk for infection related to communicability of keratitis. The patient will:
- demonstrate measures to control infection
- experience no spread of infection.

PLANNING AND IMPLEMENTATION

These measures help the patient with keratitis.
- Assess the patient's vision and document his degree of peripheral vision.
- Orient the patient to the environment, provide a clear path for him to walk, and make sure his room is well lit.
- Teach the patient the possible adverse effects of interventions.
- Protect the exposed corneas of an unconscious patient by cleaning the eyes daily, applying moisturizing ointment, or covering the eyes with an eye shield or taping them shut.

Patient teaching

- Explain that stress, trauma, fever, colds, and overexposure to the sun may trigger flare-ups of herpes keratitis.
- Teach the patient to instill eyedrops and ointments correctly, without touching the bottle tip to his eye or lashes.
- Teach the patient about proper hand-washing technique and the need to avoid sharing towels, washcloths, or pillows with family members.

EVALUATION

Evaluation of patient outcomes determines the success of collaborative management. For the patient with keratitis, evaluation focuses on resolution of the infection, adequate knowledge of infection-control measures and medication therapy and, if keratitis is due to exposure, protection of the cornea as directed.

Ménière's disease

Also known as endolymphatic hydrops, this labyrinthine dysfunction of the ear usually affects adults between ages 30 and 60, producing paroxysmal attacks of severe vertigo that last from 10 minutes to several hours. Afer multiple attacks over several years, Ménière's disease leads to residual tinnitus and hearing loss.

CAUSES

Ménière's disease may result from overproduction or decreased absorption of endolymph, the fluid within the cochlea and semicircular canals. Pressure from this excess fluid damages the sensory cells that transmit hearing and balance perception to the brain. The cause of this overproduction is unknown.

DIAGNOSIS AND TREATMENT

Audiometric studies indicate a sensorineural hearing loss and loss of discrimination and recruitment. Electronystagmography and X-rays of the internal meatus may be necessary for a differential diagnosis.

Treatment with atropine may stop an attack in 20 to 30 minutes. Epinephrine or diphenhydramine may be necessary in a severe attack. Dimenhydrinate, meclizine, diphenhydramine, or diazepam may relieve a milder attack.

Long-term management includes use of a diuretic or vasodilator and restricted sodium intake. Prophylactic antihistamines or mild sedatives (phenobarbital or diazepam) may also help. If Ménière's disease persists after more than 2 years of treatment or produces incapacitating vertigo, the patient may require surgical destruction of the affected labyrinth. This procedure permanently relieves symptoms but results in irreversible hearing loss.

COLLABORATIVE MANAGEMENT

Care of the patient with Ménière's disease focuses on relieving symptoms, using safety measures to prevent injury, and teaching about the medication regimen and follow-up care.

ASSESSMENT

Characteristic effects of Ménière's disease include severe vertigo, tinnitus, and sensorineural hearing loss. During severe attacks, other symptoms may include nausea, vomiting, sweating, giddiness, nystagmus, and loss of balance and falling to the affected side.

NURSING DIAGNOSES AND COLLABORATIVE PROBLEMS

Based on the following nursing diagnoses, you'll establish patient outcomes.

Risk for fluid volume deficit related to vomiting. The patient will:
■ exhibit vital signs within normal limits for patient
■ demonstrate signs and symptoms of adequate hydration.

Activity intolerance related to effects of the disease. The patient will:
■ experience decrease in symptoms
■ return to previous level of function as symptoms subside.

PLANNING AND IMPLEMENTATION

These measures help the patient with Ménière's disease.
■ Encourage the patient to move slowly, especially upon rising.
■ Make sure that he doesn't try to get up without assistance; keep the bed side rails up to prevent falls.
■ Before surgery, give prophylactic antibiotics and antiemetics, as ordered. If the patient is vomiting, record fluid intake and output and characteristics of vomitus. Give small amounts of fluid frequently.
■ After surgery, record intake and output carefully.
■ Encourage the patient to express his feelings, and offer support.
■ Help the patient resume his normal activities as symptoms subside.

Patient teaching

■ If the patient is in the hospital during an attack of Ménière's disease, advise him against reading and exposure to glaring lights.
■ Instruct him not to get out of bed or walk without assistance. Advise him to avoid sudden position changes and any tasks that vertigo makes hazardous.
■ Explain diagnostic tests and offer reassurance and emotional support.
■ If the patient will be undergoing surgery, tell him to expect dizziness and nausea for 1 to 2 days afterward.
■ Explain the adverse effects of antihistamine therapy (drowsiness and dry mouth).

EVALUATION

Evaluation of patient outcomes determines the success of collaborative management. For the patient with Ménière's disease, evaluation focuses on relief of symptoms (vertigo, tinnitus, nausea, and vomiting), absence of injuries, and adequate knowledge about the medication regimen and the need for follow-up care.

Otitis media

Otitis media, inflammation of the middle ear, may be suppurative or secretory, and acute or chronic. Acute otitis media occurs commonly in children. Its incidence rises during the winter, paralleling the seasonal rise in nonbacterial respiratory tract infections.

With prompt treatment, the prognosis for acute otitis media is excellent; however, prolonged accumulation of fluid within the middle ear cavity causes chronic otitis media.

CAUSES

This disorder is caused by disruption of eustachian tube patency. In the suppurative form, a respiratory tract infection, an allergic reaction, or positional changes (such as holding an infant supine during feeding) allow reflux of nasopharyngeal flora through the eustachian tube and colonization in the middle ear. In the secretory form, obstruction of the eustachian tube results in negative pressure in the middle ear that promotes transudation of sterile serous fluid from blood vessels in the membrane of the middle ear.

Acute suppurative otitis media is caused by pneumococci, beta-hemolytic streptococci, or gram-negative bacteria. In children under age 6, the most common cause is *Haemophilus influenzae;* in children over age 6, it's staphylococci.

Chronic suppurative otitis media results from inadequate treatment of acute infection as well as infection by resistant strains of bacteria.

Acute secretory otitis media may be caused by a viral infection, an allergy, or barotrauma (a pressure injury caused by an inability to equalize pressures between the environment and the middle ear).

Chronic secretory otitis media may be caused by adenoidal tissue overgrowth that obstructs the eustachian tube, edema due to allergic rhinitis or chronic sinus infection, or inadequate treatment of acute suppurative otitis media.

DIAGNOSIS AND TREATMENT

Diagnosis is based on the patient's complaints and the results of the physical examination.

In acute suppurative otitis media, ampicillin or amoxicillin is the antibiotic of choice for infants, children, and adults. For those who are allergic to penicillin derivatives, cefaclor or co-trimoxazole may be given. Aspirin or acetaminophen helps control pain and fever. Severe, painful bulging of the tympanic membrane usually necessitates myringotomy. Broad-spectrum antibiotics can help prevent acute suppurative otitis media in high-risk patients, such as children with recurring episodes of otitis. However, in patients with recurring otitis, antibiotics must be used sparingly and with discretion to prevent development of resistant strains of bacteria.

In acute secretory otitis media, performing Valsalva's maneuver several times a day to inflate the eustachian tube may be the only treatment required. Otherwise, nasopharyngeal decongestant therapy may be helpful. It should continue for at least 2 weeks and, sometimes, indefinitely, with periodic evaluation. If decongestant therapy fails, myringotomy and aspiration of middle ear fluid, followed by insertion of a polyethylene tube into the tympanic membrane, are necessary for immediate and prolonged equalization of pressure. The tube falls out spontaneously after 9 to 12 months. Concomitant treatment of the underlying cause (such as elimination of allergens, or adenoidectomy for hypertrophied adenoids) may also help.

Treatment of chronic otitis media includes antibiotics for exacerbations of acute infection, elimination of eustachian tube obstruction, treatment of otitis externa (when present), myringoplasty (tympanic membrane graft) and tympanoplasty to reconstruct middle ear structures when thickening and scarring are present and, possibly, mastoidectomy. Cholesteatoma (a cystlike mass in the middle ear) requires excision.

COLLABORATIVE MANAGEMENT
Care of the patient with otitis media focuses on relieving pain and fever, restoring hearing, and intense patient teaching.

ASSESSMENT
A patient with acute suppurative otitis media may be asymptomatic but usually experiences severe, deep, throbbing pain; signs of upper respiratory tract infection; mild to high fever; hearing loss (usually mild and conductive); dizziness; obscured or distorted bony landmarks of the tympanic membrane (evident on otoscopy); and nausea and vomiting. Other possible effects include bulging of the tympanic membrane, with concomitant erythema, and purulent drainage in the ear canal from tympanic membrane rupture.

The patient with acute secretory otitis media is commonly asymptomatic but may develop severe conductive hearing loss ranging from 15 to 35 decibels, depending on the thickness and amount of fluid in the middle ear cavity. Look for:
- reports of a sensation of fullness in the ear; popping, crackling, or clicking sounds with swallowing or jaw movement; hearing an echo when speaking; or experiencing a vague feeling of top-heaviness
- evidence of tympanic membrane retraction, which

causes the bony landmarks to appear more prominent (seen on otoscopy)
- clear or amber fluid behind the tympanic membrane
- blue-black tympanic membrane (seen on otoscopy if hemorrhage into the middle ear has occurred)
- in chronic otitis media (from childhood into adulthood), decreased or absent tympanic membrane mobility; cholesteatoma; and a painless, purulent discharge (in chronic suppurative otitis media).

Conductive hearing loss varies with the size and type of tympanic membrane perforation and ossicular destruction. Some patients develop thickening and scarring of the tympanic membrane (evident on otoscopy).

NURSING DIAGNOSES AND COLLABORATIVE PROBLEMS
Based on the following nursing diagnoses, you'll establish patient outcomes.

Sensory/perceptual alteration (auditory) related to otitis media. The patient will:
- verbalize measures to adequately cope with changes in hearing
- maintain optimum hearing.

Pain related to inflammation. The patient will:
- demonstrate measures to relieve pain
- state that pain is relieved with treatment.

PLANNING AND INTERVENTIONS
These measures help the patient with otitis media.
- Speak clearly and allow the patient time to answer.
- Include the patient's family in care decisions.
- After myringotomy, maintain drainage flow. Don't place cotton or plugs deep in the ear canal; however, you may place sterile cotton loosely in the external ear to absorb drainage.
- To prevent infection, change the cotton whenever it gets damp and wash your hands before and after providing ear care.
- Be alert for and report headache, fever, severe pain, or disorientation.
- After tympanoplasty, reinforce dressings and observe for excessive bleeding from the ear canal. Administer analgesics as needed.

Patient teaching
- Warn the patient against blowing his nose or getting the ear wet when bathing.
- Encourage him to complete the prescribed course of antibiotic treatment.
- If nasopharyngeal decongestants are ordered, teach correct instillation.
- Suggest applying heat to the ear to relieve pain.
- Advise the patient with acute secretory otitis media

to watch for and immediately report pain and fever—signs of secondary infection.

■ To promote eustachian tube patency, instruct the patient to perform Valsalva's maneuver several times daily.

■ Urge prompt treatment of otitis media to prevent perforation of the tympanic membrane (the disorder may also lead to the more benign otitis externa).

■ Instruct parents not to feed their infant in a supine position or put him to bed with a bottle. Head elevation prevents reflux of nasopharyngeal flora.

EVALUATION

Evaluation of patient outcomes determines the success of collaborative management. For the patient with otitis media, evaluation focuses on relief of pain and fever, restoration of hearing, and adequate knowledge about medication therapy, need to complete antibiotics, and prevention tips.

Otosclerosis

In this disorder, spongy bone slowly forms in the otic capsule, particularly at the oval window. The most common cause of conductive deafness, otosclerosis occurs in at least 10% of whites and twice as often in females, usually between ages 15 and 30. With surgery, the prognosis is good.

CAUSES

Otosclerosis results from a genetic factor transmitted as an autosomal dominant trait. Many patients with this disorder report a family history of hearing loss (excluding presbycusis). Pregnancy may trigger the onset.

DIAGNOSIS AND TREATMENT

A Rinne test that shows bone conduction lasting longer than air conduction (normally, the reverse is true) indicates otosclerosis. As the condition progresses, bone conduction also deteriorates. A Weber test detects sound lateralizing to the more affected ear.

Treatment usually consists of stapedectomy (removal of the stapes) and insertion of a prosthesis to restore partial or total hearing. This procedure is performed one ear at a time, beginning with the most damaged. Postoperative treatment includes hospitalization for 2 to 3 days and antibiotics to prevent infection. If stapedectomy is not possible, a hearing aid (air conduction aid with molded ear insert receiver) enables the patient to hear conversation in normal surroundings; however, a hearing aid is not as effective as stapedectomy.

COLLABORATIVE MANAGEMENT

Care of the patient with otosclerosis focuses on improved hearing, prevention of complications, and patient teaching about therapy and the need for follow-up care.

ASSESSMENT

Several signs and symptoms can indicate otosclerosis. They include a slowly progressive unilateral hearing loss, which may advance to bilateral deafness; tinnitus (low and medium pitch); and paracusis of Willis (hearing conversation better in a noisy environment than in a quiet one).

NURSING DIAGNOSES AND COLLABORATIVE PROBLEMS

Based on the following nursing diagnoses, you'll establish patient outcomes.

Sensory/perceptual alteration (auditory) related to impaired hearing conduction. The patient will:

■ verbalize improvement in ability to hear

■ demonstrate ability to hear what is being said.

Risk for injury related to hearing loss. The patient will:

■ demonstrate measures to maintain safety

■ remain free from injury.

PLANNING AND IMPLEMENTATION

These measures help the patient with otosclerosis.

■ Assess the patient's gross hearing ability. Perform the Rinne and Weber tests as indicated.

■ Determine how best to communicate with the patient, using gestures, lip reading, and written words as necessary.

■ When speaking to a partially hearing-impaired person, speak clearly and slowly in a normal to deep voice and offer concise explanations of procedures.

■ Make sure all staff members are aware of the patient's hearing impairment and respond to his call light as soon as possible.

■ Allow the patient to express feelings of concern and loss, and be available to answer questions. This enhances acceptance of the hearing loss, clears up misconceptions, and reduces anxiety.

Patient teaching

■ Review the course of treatment and expected effects.

■ Ensure that the patient understands all information given to promote self-care.

■ Provide written instructions to reinforce your teaching.

■ Encourage the patient to use assistive devices in the home to maintain his independence.

EVALUATION

Evaluation of patient outcomes determines the success of collaborative management. For the patient with otosclerosis, evaluation focuses on improved hearing, absence of complications, and adequate knowledge about therapy and the need for follow-up care.

Retinal detachment

In this eye disorder, separation of the retinal layers creates a subretinal space that fills with fluid. Twice as common in men as in women, retinal detachment may be primary or secondary. It usually involves only one eye but may occur in the other eye later. Rarely healing spontaneously, a detached retina can usually be reattached successfully with surgery. The prognosis depends on the area of the retina affected. Retinal detachment may result in severe vision impairment and, possibly, blindness.

CAUSES

A primary detachment occurs spontaneously because of a change in the retina or vitreous. A secondary detachment results from another problem, such as intraocular inflammation or trauma. The most common cause of retinal detachment is a hole or tear in the retina. This hole allows the liquid vitreous to seep between the retinal layers and separate the sensory retinal layer from its choroidal blood supply. In adults, retinal detachment usually results from degenerative changes related to aging (which cause a spontaneous tear). Predisposing factors include myopia, cataract surgery, and trauma.

Additionally, retinal detachment may result from fluid seeping into the subretinal space as an effect of inflammation, tumors, or systemic disease. It may also result from traction placed on the retina by vitreous bands or membranes (resulting from proliferative diabetic retinopathy, posterior uveitis, or a traumatic intraocular foreign body, for example). Retinal detachment can also be inherited, usually in association with myopia.

DIAGNOSIS AND TREATMENT

Diagnostic tests may include the following:
- Direct ophthalmoscopy, after full pupil dilation, shows folds or discoloration in the usually transparent retina.
- Indirect ophthalmoscopy can detect retinal tears.
- Ocular ultrasonography may be performed to examine the retina if the patient has an opaque lens.

Depending on the detachment's location and severity, treatment may consist of restricting eye movements to prevent further separation until surgical repair can be made.

A hole in the peripheral retina may be treated with cryotherapy. A hole in the posterior retina may respond to laser therapy.

To reattach the retina, scleral buckling may be performed. In this procedure, the surgeon places a silicone plate or sponge over the reattachment site and secures it in place with an encircling band. The pressure exerted gently pushes the choroid and retina together. Scleral buckling may be followed by replacement of the vitreous with silicone, oil, air, or gas.

COLLABORATIVE MANAGEMENT

Care of the patient with retinal detachment focuses on improved vision, absence of complications, a decrease in pain, and no signs or symptoms of infection.

ASSESSMENT

Initially, the patient may report that he sees floating spots and recurrent light flashes. As detachment progresses, he may report gradual, painless vision loss described as looking through a veil, curtain, or cobweb. He may relate that the "veil" obscures objects in a particular visual field.

NURSING DIAGNOSES AND COLLABORATIVE PROBLEMS

Based on the following nursing diagnoses, you'll establish patient outcomes.

Anxiety related to potential for loss of vision in affected eye. The patient will:
- identify and express feelings of anxiety
- cope with anxiety by being involved in decisions about his care
- display fewer physical symptoms of anxiety.

Diversional activity deficit related to activity restrictions used to prevent further retinal detachment. The patient will:
- identify activities that he can do safely
- express a positive attitude about activity restrictions
- report decreased feelings of boredom.

Sensory/perceptual alteration (visual) related to loss of vision. The patient will:
- discuss the impact of visual loss on his lifestyle
- compensate for visual loss by using adaptive devices
- remain safe in his environment.

PLANNING AND IMPLEMENTATION

These measures help the patient with retinal detachment.

- Provide encouragement and emotional support to decrease anxiety caused by vision loss.
- Prepare the patient for surgery by cleaning his face with a mild (no-tears) shampoo. Give antibiotics and cycloplegic or mydriatic eyedrops, as ordered.
- Postoperatively, position the patient as directed (the position will vary according to the surgical procedure). To prevent increasing intraocular pressure (IOP), administer antiemetics as indicated. Discourage any activities that would raise IOP.
- In macular involvement, keep the patient on bed rest (with or without bathroom privileges) to prevent further retinal detachment.
- To reduce edema and discomfort following laser therapy, apply ice packs and administer acetaminophen, as ordered, for headache.
- Assess the patient for persistent pain and report it if present. Give prescribed analgesics as needed.
- Watch for slight localized corneal edema and perilimbal congestion, which may follow laser therapy.
- If the patient receives a retrobulbar injection, apply a protective eye patch because the eyelid will remain partially open.
- After removing the protective patch, give cycloplegic and steroidal or antibiotic eyedrops, as ordered. Apply cold compresses to decrease swelling and pain.
- Monitor the patient's degree of visual loss.

Patient teaching
- Explain to the patient undergoing laser therapy that the procedure may be done in the same-day surgery unit. Forewarn him that he may have blurred vision for several days afterward.
- Instruct him to rest and to avoid driving, bending, heavy lifting, or any other activities that increase IOP for several days after eye surgery. Discourage activities that might cause the patient to bump his eye.
- Encourage leg and deep-breathing exercises to prevent complications of immobility.
- Show the patient who is having scleral buckling surgery how to instill eyedrops properly. After surgery, remind him to lie in the position recommended by the doctor.
- Advise the patient to wear sunglasses if photosensitivity occurs.
- Instruct him to take acetaminophen as needed for headaches and to apply ice packs to his eye to reduce swelling and alleviate discomfort.
- Review the signs of infection, emphasizing those that require immediate attention.

EVALUATION
Evaluation of patient outcomes determines the success of collaborative management. For the patient with a detached retina, evaluation focuses on improved vision, absence of complications (including signs or symptoms of infection), and decreased pain.

Treatments and procedures

Several surgical procedures are available to maintain or improve sight and hearing, two of the five human senses. These procedures include cataract removal, corneal transplant, iridectomy, myringotomy, and stapedectomy.

CATARACT REMOVAL
Lens opacities, called cataracts, can be removed by one of two techniques. In the first technique, intracapsular cataract extraction (ICCE), the entire lens is removed, usually with a cryoprobe. In the other technique, extracapsular cataract extraction (ECCE), the patient's anterior capsule, cortex, and nucleus are removed, leaving the posterior capsule intact. This technique involves manual extraction, irrigation and aspiration, or phacoemulsification. The patient may receive a local or general anesthetic.

ECCE is the primary treatment for congenital and traumatic cataracts. It's characteristically used to treat children and young adults because the posterior capsule adheres to the vitreous until about age 20. By leaving the posterior capsule undisturbed, ECCE avoids disruption and loss of vitreous matter.

Immediately after removal of the natural lens, many patients receive an intraocular lens implant. An implant is especially well suited for older adults who are unable to use eyeglasses or contact lenses (because of arthritis or tremors, for example).

PROCEDURE
In ICCE, the surgeon makes a partial incision at the superior limbus arc. He then removes the lens using specially designed forceps or a cryoprobe, which freezes and adheres to the lens to facilitate its removal.

In ECCE, the surgeon may use manual extraction, irrigation and aspiration, or phacoemulsification. With irrigation and aspiration, he makes an incision at the limbus, opens the anterior lens capsule with a cystotome, and exerts pressure from below to express the lens. He then irrigates and suctions the remaining lens cortex. In phacoemulsification, he uses an ultrasonic probe to break the lens into minute particles, which are aspirated by the probe.

After cataract removal, the surgeon may insert an intraocular lens implant. After enlarging the incision, he implants the lens into the capsular sac. If he implants the lens without sutures, he administers a miotic agent, such as pilocarpine, to prevent the iris from dilating too widely and causing the lens to slip.

In both ICCE and ECCE, the surgeon may also perform a peripheral iridectomy to reduce intraocular pressure (IOP) and may briefly instill alpha-chymotrypsin, a proteolytic enzyme, in the anterior chamber to dissolve resistant zonular fibers. After the procedure, the surgeon may administer a miotic agent to constrict the pupil. Then he closes the sutures, instills antibiotic drops or ointment, and places a patch and shield over the eye.

COLLABORATIVE MANAGEMENT

Care of the patient undergoing cataract removal requires thorough preparation, close monitoring, and intense patient teaching.

Preparation

■ Explain the planned surgical technique to the patient. Tell him that he'll receive mydriatics and cycloplegics to dilate the eye and facilitate cataract removal, osmotics and antibiotics to reduce the risk of infection, and possibly a sedative to help him relax.
■ Inform the patient that after surgery he'll have to wear an eye patch temporarily to prevent traumatic injury and infection.
■ Instruct him to call for help when getting out of bed, and tell him that he should sleep on the unaffected side to reduce IOP. Explain that he'll temporarily experience loss of depth perception and decreased peripheral vision on the operative side.
■ If ordered, perform an antiseptic facial scrub to reduce the risk of infection.

Monitoring and aftercare

■ Assess the patient's vital signs until stable.
■ After the patient returns to his room, notify the doctor if severe pain, bleeding, increased drainage, or fever occurs. Also report any increased IOP.
■ Because of the change in the patient's depth perception, keep the side rails of his bed raised, assist him with ambulation, and observe other safety precautions.
■ Maintain the eye patch and have the patient wear an eye shield, especially when sleeping. Tell him to continue wearing the shield during sleep for several weeks, as ordered.

Patient teaching

■ Warn the patient to immediately contact the doctor if he experiences sudden eye pain or visual changes, red or watery eyes, or photophobia.
■ Instruct him to avoid activities that raise IOP, including heavy lifting, bending, straining during defe-

cation, and vigorous coughing and sneezing, for as long as the doctor orders. Tell him not to exercise strenuously for 6 to 10 weeks.
■ Explain that follow-up appointments are necessary to monitor the results of the surgery and to detect any complications.
■ Teach the patient or a family member how to instill prescribed eyedrops and ointments and how to change the eye patch.
■ Suggest that the patient wear dark glasses in bright light to relieve the glare that he may experience.
■ If the patient is to wear eyeglasses, explain that changes in his vision can present safety hazards. To compensate for loss of depth perception, show him how to use up-and-down head movements to judge distances. To overcome the loss of peripheral vision on the operative side, teach him to turn his head fully in that direction to view objects to his side.
■ If the patient is to wear contact lenses, teach him how to insert, remove, and care for his lenses or have him arrange to visit a doctor routinely for removal, cleaning, and reinsertion of extended-wear lenses.

COMPLICATIONS

Cataract removal can cause numerous complications, most of which can be corrected. Complications include pupillary block, corneal decompensation, vitreous loss, hemorrhage, cystoid macular edema, lens dislocation, secondary membrane opacification, and retinal detachment.

CORNEAL TRANSPLANT

In a corneal transplant, or keratoplasty, healthy corneal tissue from a human donor replaces a damaged part of the cornea. Corneal transplants help restore corneal clarity lost through injury, inflammation, ulceration, or chemical burns. They may also correct corneal dystrophies such as keratoconus, the abnormal thinning and bulging of the central portion of the cornea.

A corneal transplant can take one of two forms: a full-thickness penetrating keratoplasty, involving excision and replacement of the entire cornea, or a lamellar keratoplasty, which removes and replaces a superficial layer of corneal tissue. The full-thickness procedure, the more common of the two, produces a high degree of clarity and restores vision in 95% of patients.

A lamellar transplant is used if damage is limited to the anterior stroma or if the patient is uncooperative and likely to exert pressure on the eye after surgery. The degree of clarity produced by a lamellar transplant rarely matches that of a full-thickness graft. As a treatment for dystrophies, its success depends on the type and extent of the abnormality.

Because the cornea is avascular and doesn't recover as rapidly as other parts of the body, healing may take up to a year. Usually, sutures remain in place and vision isn't completely functional until healing is complete.

PROCEDURE

In a full-thickness keratoplasty, the surgeon cuts a "button" from the donor cornea and a button from the host cornea, sized to remove the abnormality. Next, he anchors the donor button in place with extremely fine sutures. Finally, he patches the eye and tapes a shield in place over it.

In a lamellar, or partial-thickness, keratoplasty, the surgeon excises a shallower layer of corneal tissue in both the donor and host corneas. He then peels away the excised layers of tissue and sutures the donor graft in place. As in the full-thickness procedure, he patches the eye and applies a rigid shield.

COLLABORATIVE MANAGEMENT

Care of the patient undergoing a corneal transplant requires thorough preparation, close monitoring, and intense patient teaching.

Preparation

■ Explain the transplant procedure to the patient, and answer any questions he may have. Inform him that healing will be slow and that his vision may not be completely restored until the sutures are removed, in about a year.

■ Tell the patient that most corneal transplants are performed under local anesthesia and that he can expect momentary burning during injection of the anesthetic. Explain to him that the procedure will last for about an hour and that he must remain still until it has been completed.

■ Tell the patient that he can have analgesics after surgery because he may experience a dull aching. Inform him that the doctor will place a bandage and protective shield over the eye.

■ As ordered, administer a sedative or an osmotic agent to reduce intraocular pressure (IOP).

Monitoring and aftercare

■ Assess the patient's vital signs until stable.

■ After the patient recovers from anesthesia, assess for and immediately report sudden, sharp, or excessive pain; bloody, purulent, or clear viscous drainage; or fever.

■ As ordered, instill corticosteroid eyedrops or topical antibiotics to prevent inflammation and graft rejection.

Patient teaching

■ After the procedure, instruct the patient to lie on his back or on his unaffected side, with the bed flat or slightly elevated, as ordered. Tell him to avoid squinting and rubbing his eyes. Also have him avoid rapid head movements, hard coughing or sneezing, bending over, lifting or pushing heavy objects, straining during defecation, and other activities that could increase IOP.

■ Remind the patient to ask for help in standing or walking until he adjusts to changes in his vision. Make sure that all his personal items are within his field of vision.

■ Teach the patient and a family member or friend to recognize the signs of graft rejection (inflammation, cloudiness, drainage, and pain at the graft site.) Instruct them to immediately notify the doctor if any of these signs occur.

■ Emphasize that rejection can occur many years after surgery; stress the need for assessing the graft *daily* for the rest of the patient's life. Also remind the patient to keep regular appointments with his doctor.

■ Explain that photophobia, a common adverse effect, gradually decreases as healing progresses. Suggest that he wear dark glasses in bright light.

■ Teach the patient how to correctly instill prescribed eyedrops.

■ Remind him to wear an eye shield when sleeping.

COMPLICATIONS

Graft rejection occurs in about 15% of patients and may happen at any time during the patient's life. Uncommon complications include wound leakage, loosening of the sutures, dehiscence, and infection.

IRIDECTOMY

Performed by laser or standard surgery, an iridectomy reduces intraocular pressure (IOP) by facilitating the drainage of aqueous humor. This procedure is commonly used to treat acute angle-closure glaucoma. Because glaucoma is a bilateral disorder, preventive iridectomy is often performed on the unaffected eye. It may also help a patient with an anatomically narrow angle between the cornea and iris. Iridectomy is also used in chronic angle-closure glaucoma, in excision of tissue for biopsy or treatment, and sometimes with other eye surgeries, such as cataract removal, keratoplasty, and glaucoma-filtering procedures.

PROCEDURE

The doctor uses a laser to make a hole in the iris, creating an opening through which the aqueous humor can flow to bypass the pupil. Most iridectomies are performed in the superior peripheral area of the iris because the eyelid will cover the iridectomy. They're usually done under local anesthesia as an outpatient procedure.

COLLABORATIVE MANAGEMENT

Care of the patient undergoing iridectomy requires thorough preparation, close monitoring, and intense patient teaching.

Preparation

■ Make it clear to the patient that an iridectomy can't restore vision loss caused by glaucoma but may prevent further loss.
■ Administer miotics, topical beta blockers, and oral or I.V. osmotic agents, as ordered, to reduce IOP in the acute stages of angle-closure glaucoma.

Monitoring and aftercare

■ After an iridectomy, watch for hyphema with sudden, sharp eye pain or a small, half-moon-shaped blood speck in the anterior chamber. (Check with a flashlight.) If either occurs, have the patient rest quietly in bed, with his head elevated, and notify the doctor.
■ To decrease inflammation, administer topical corticosteroids and medication to dilate the pupil.
■ If the patient received osmotic therapy before the procedure, encourage him to increase his fluid intake to restore normal hydration and electrolyte balance.
■ To prevent elevated IOP due to increased venous pressure in the head, neck, and eyes, administer stool softeners to prevent constipation and straining during bowel movements, and advise the patient to refrain from coughing, sneezing, vigorous nose blowing, and rubbing or squeezing his eyes.

Patient teaching

■ Instruct the patient to report any sudden, sharp eye pain immediately because it may indicate increased IOP.
■ Tell him to refrain from strenuous activity, coughing, sneezing, and vigorous nose blowing for 3 weeks. Explain that these actions all increase venous pressure in the head, neck, and eyes, which can strain the suture line or the blood vessels in the affected area.
■ Instruct the patient to move slowly, keep his head raised, and sleep on two pillows.
■ Tell him to make a follow-up appointment with his ophthalmologist, and inform him that he'll need periodic tests to determine if his vision is being maintained.

COMPLICATIONS

Occasionally, spontaneous hemorrhage in the anterior chamber (hyphema) may occur, causing increased IOP and injuring the eye.

MYRINGOTOMY

This surgical incision of the tympanic membrane relieves pain and prevents membrane rupture by allowing drainage of pus or fluid from the middle ear. Myringotomy is most commonly performed on children with acute otitis media, typically when antibiotics, decongestants, or antihistamines fail to correct the causative infection or when the infection itself damages the middle ear mucosa or causes such severe pressure that the tympanic membrane may rupture. If the tympanic membrane does rupture, the doctor may perform myringoplasty, in which the ruptured tympanic membrane is repaired by a graft taken from the fascia of the temporalis muscle.

PROCEDURE

The doctor makes an incision in the tympanic membrane and removes fluid by suction. Myringotomy may be performed on one or both ears. After the procedure, the doctor may insert a pressure-equalizing tube through the incision to allow fluid drainage. In most cases, myringotomy provides almost instant symptomatic relief; the incision typically heals in 2 to 3 weeks. (If tubes have been inserted, they're usually expelled spontaneously after 6 to 12 months.)

COLLABORATIVE MANAGEMENT

Care of the patient undergoing myringotomy requires thorough preparation, close monitoring, and intense patient teaching.

Preparation

■ Inform the patient or parents whether surgery will involve one or both ears and whether it will be performed with a local or general anesthetic.
■ Mention that the doctor may insert a tube through the incision to allow drainage until the inflammation subsides.

Monitoring and aftercare

■ Assess the condition of the patient's ear. If fluid is draining from it, note the amount, type, color, and odor. If you see bright red blood in the drainage, notify the doctor immediately; this may indicate injury to the ear canal.
■ If needed, cover the ear with a gauze pad or lay cotton fluff gently over the ear's orifice to absorb drainage. Apply petroleum jelly or zinc oxide to the external ear to protect it from excoriation by drainage, and change dressings as needed. If exudate cakes on the outer ear, remove it by gently swabbing with a cotton-tipped applicator dipped in hydrogen peroxide. Don't attempt to clean the ear canal or allow peroxide to run into the ear.

Patient teaching

■ If the patient has a dressing in place to absorb ear drainage, tell him or his parents to wash their hands before and after changing it and to place old dressings in a small paper or plastic bag before throwing them in the trash.

■ Emphasize the need to notify the doctor if drainage lasts more than 1 week or changes in color or character—for example, from serous to purulent. Advise the patient to report any ear pain or fever, which may signal blocked tubing or reinfection.

■ Explain the importance of not allowing water to enter the ear canal until the tympanic membrane is intact. Show the patient or his parents how to roll absorbent cotton in petroleum jelly to form a plug and how to insert the plug in the outer part of the ear before showering or washing hair.

■ If the doctor permits swimming, advise inserting ear plugs first and avoid ducking beneath the water. Tell the patient to expect considerable drainage through the tubes. Emphasize the need to return for follow-up examinations and to notify the doctor if the tubes are expelled.

COMPLICATIONS

The patient may develop an infection from the procedure, or the tubes may dislodge prematurely.

STAPEDECTOMY

This surgery removes all or part of the stapes. It is the treatment of choice for otosclerosis, a hereditary condition in which new bone grows around the ear's oval window, limiting movement of the stapes and causing a conductive hearing loss. Because otosclerosis is often bilateral, the doctor usually performs stapedectomy twice: first in the ear with the greatest hearing loss and then, a year or so later, in the second ear.

PROCEDURE

A total stapedectomy involves removal of both the suprastructure and the footplate of the stapes, followed by the insertion of a graft and prosthesis to bridge the gap between the incus and the inner ear. A partial stapedectomy can involve severing and removing the anterior crus and the anterior portion of the footplate, or removing the entire suprastructure while leaving the footplate in place, drilling it, and fitting it with a piston.

Laser stapedectomy, a relatively new technique, is easier to perform but carries some risk of the laser beam penetrating the bone.

COLLABORATIVE MANAGEMENT

Care of the patient undergoing stapedectomy requires thorough preparation, close monitoring, and intense patient teaching.

Preparation

■ Inform the patient that improved hearing may not be evident for several weeks after surgery because ear packing and edema may mask any initial improvement. Tell him that the doctor usually removes the packing after a week.

Monitoring and aftercare

■ Monitor vital signs until stable. After surgery, position the patient as ordered. The doctor may prefer that the patient lie on his operated ear to facilitate drainage, on his opposite ear to avoid graft displacement, or simply in the most comfortable position.

■ Advise the patient to move slowly without bending when he changes position to help prevent vertigo and nausea. If he develops either of these symptoms, administer antiemetic drugs as ordered, and keep the bed's side rails up at all times. Help the patient when he first tries to walk because he may feel dizzy. Keep in mind that vertigo may also indicate labyrinthitis or an inner ear reaction. Provide pain medication, as ordered.

■ When you change the patient's dressings, use aseptic technique. Replace soiled or bloody pledgets in the ear canal as needed, and be sure to keep the ear dry.

■ Tell the patient to refrain from coughing, sneezing, or blowing his nose because these actions could dislodge his prosthesis and graft.

Patient teaching

■ Instruct the patient to call the doctor immediately if he develops fever, pain, changes in taste, prolonged vertigo, or a "sloshing" feeling in his ear. These symptoms may indicate infection or displacement of the prosthesis.

■ Tell him to protect his ear from cold drafts for 1 week and to avoid contact with people who have colds, influenza, or other contagious illnesses. Advise him to take his prescribed antibiotics and to report any respiratory infection to his doctor immediately.

■ Instruct the patient to postpone washing his hair for 2 weeks and, for the next 4 weeks, to avoid getting water in his ears when washing his hair. Instruct him not to swim for 6 weeks unless the doctor specifically allows it.

■ To avoid prosthesis dislodgment, warn him to avoid blowing his nose for at least 1 week after surgery and not to travel by airplane for 6 months.

COMPLICATIONS

Possible complications include fever, headache, ear pain, or persistent facial nerve paralysis. If facial paralysis results from the surgery, the patient may require facial nerve decompression or corticosteroid therapy.

Selected references

Diseases, 2nd ed. Springhouse, Pa.: Springhouse Corp., 1997.

Huether, S.E., and McCance, K.L. *Understanding Pathophysiology.* St. Louis: Mosby–Year Book, Inc., 1996.

Illustrated Manual of Nursing Practice, 2nd ed. Springhouse, Pa.: Springhouse Corp., 1994.

Monahan, F.D., et al. *Nursing Care of Adults.* Philadelphia: W.B. Saunders Co., 1994.

Phipps, W.J., et al. *Medical-Surgical Nursing: Concepts and Clinical Practice,* 5th ed. St. Louis: Mosby–Year Book, Inc., 1995.

Polaski, A.L., and Tatro, S.E. *Luckmann's Core Principles and Practice of Medical-Surgical Nursing.* Philadelphia: W.B. Saunders Co., 1996.

Professional Guide to Diseases, 5th ed. Springhouse Pa.: Springhouse Corp., 1995.

Renal and metabolic disorders

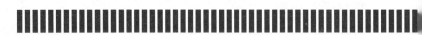

Anatomy and physiology review

The urinary system and the kidneys retain useful materials and excrete foreign or excessive materials and waste. Through this basic function, the kidneys profoundly affect other body systems and the patient's overall health.

The urinary system consists of two kidneys, two ureters, one bladder, and one urethra. Working together, these structures remove wastes from the body, regulate acid-base balance by retaining or excreting hydrogen ions, and regulate fluid and electrolyte balance.

The kidneys are bean-shaped, highly vascular organs that measure approximately 4½″ (11.5 cm) long and 2½″ (6.5 cm) wide. Located retroperitoneally, they lie on either side of the vertebral column, between the 12th thoracic and 3rd lumbar vertebrae. Here, the kidneys are protected, behind the abdominal contents and in front of the muscles attached to the vertebral column. A perirenal fat layer offers further protection.

Crowded by the liver, the right kidney extends slightly lower than the left. Atop each kidney (suprarenal) lies an adrenal gland. At the hilus—an indentation in the kidney's medial aspect—the renal artery, renal vein, lymphatic vessels, and nerves enter the kidney. The renal pelvis, a funnel-shaped ureter extension, also enters here.

A cross section of the kidney reveals the outer renal cortex, central renal medulla, internal calyces, and renal pelvis. At the microscopic level, the nephron serves as the kidney's functional unit. (See *Inside the normal kidney*, page 360.)

The ureters are ducts that carry urine from the kidneys to the bladder. Because the left kidney is higher than the right, the left ureter typically is slightly longer. Originating in the ureteropelvic junction of the kidneys, the ureters travel obliquely to the bladder, channeling urine via peristaltic waves that occur approximately one to five times per minute.

The bladder is a hollow, spherical, muscular organ in the pelvis that stores urine. It lies anterior and inferior to the pelvic cavity and posterior to the symphysis pubis. Bladder capacity ranges from 17 to 20 oz (500 to 600 ml) in a normal adult, less in children and older adults.

Urination results from involuntary (reflex) and voluntary (intentional) processes. When urine distends the bladder, the involuntary process begins: Parasympathetic nervous system fibers transmit impulses that make the bladder contract and the internal sphincter (located at the internal urethral orifice) relax. Then the cerebrum stimulates voluntary relaxation and contraction of the external sphincter (located about 3″ [7.5 cm] beyond the internal sphincter).

The urethra is a small duct that channels urine outside the body from the bladder. It has an exterior opening called the urethral (urinary) meatus. In the female the urethral meatus is located anterior to the vaginal opening; in the male, at the end of the glans penis. The male urethra serves as a passageway for semen as well as urine.

URINE FORMATION

Three processes—glomerular filtration, tubular reabsorption, and tubular secretion—take place in the nephrons, ultimately leading to urine formation.

The kidneys can vary the amount of substances reabsorbed and secreted in the nephrons, changing the composition of excreted urine. Normal urine constituents include sodium, chloride, potassium, calci-

Inside the normal kidney

These drawings show the gross structure of the kidney and its basic and functional unit, the nephron.

The kidney

Each kidney contains about 1.5 million nephrons, organized into 18 to 20 collection units, the renal pyramids, which channel their output into the renal pelvis for excretion. Protected by a fibrous capsule and by layers of perinephric fat, the renal parenchyma consists of an outer cortex and an inner medulla. The medulla contains the renal pyramids, composed mostly of tubular structures. The tapered portion of each pyramid empties into a cuplike calyx. The calyces channel urine from the pyramids into the renal pelvis.

This section of kidney tissue shows how the glomeruli and proximal and distal tubules of the nephrons are located in the cortex, while the long loops of Henle, together with their accompanying blood vessels and collecting tubules, are formed into renal pyramids in the medulla. Here, countercurrent multiplication maintains the relative osmolality of the urine and interstitial fluid. The tapered end of each pyramid forms a papilla, where the collecting tubules empty the urine into the renal pelvis.

Renal vascularization

Blood is supplied to the kidney by the renal artery, which subdivides into several branches. Some of these branches are responsible for distributing blood within the kidney, while others nourish the kidney cells themselves.

Of the blood brought to the kidney for filtration, about 99% returns to general body circulation through the renal vein. The remaining 1% is processed further, producing urine-containing waste products that flow to the calyx and renal pelvis. From the pelvis, the urine enters the ureter.

The nephron

The nephrons are the kidneys' structural units. They consist of a glomerulus (inside Bowman's capsule), a tubular apparatus, and a collecting duct.

The nephrons perform two main activities: mechanical filtration of fluids, wastes, electrolytes, acids, and bases into the tubular system; and selective reabsorption and secretion of ions.

Blood is brought to and carried away from the glomerular capillaries by two small blood vessels, the afferent and efferent arterioles. The glomerular capillaries act as bulk filters and pass protein-free and red blood cell–free filtrate to the proximal convoluted tubules.

Reabsorption and excretion

The proximal convoluted tubules have freely permeable cell membranes. This allows reabsorption of nearly all the filtrate's glucose, amino acids, metabolites, and electrolytes into nearby capillaries and the circulation. As these substances return to the circulation, they passively carry large amounts of water.

By the time the filtrate enters the descending limb of the loop of Henle, located in the medulla, its water content has been reduced by 70%. At this point, the filtrate contains a high concentration of salts, chiefly sodium. As the filtrate moves deeper into the medulla and into the loop of Henle, osmosis draws even more water into the extracellular spaces, further concentrating the filtrate.

Once the filtrate enters the ascending limb, its concentration is readjusted by transport of ions into the tubule. This transport continues until the filtrate enters the distal convoluted tubule.

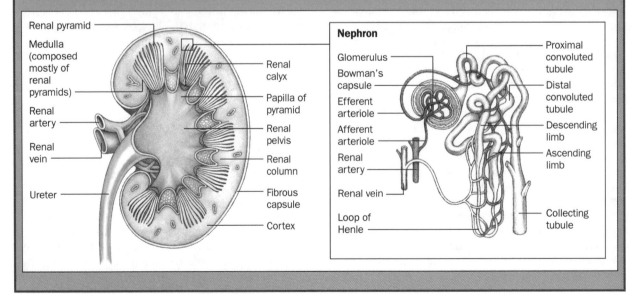

um, magnesium, sulfates, phosphates, bicarbonates, uric acid, ammonium ions, creatinine, and urobilinogen. A few leukocytes and red blood cells (RBCs) and in the male, some spermatozoa, may enter the urine as it passes from the kidney to the ureteral orifice. Urine also may contain drugs if the patient is receiving drugs excreted in urine.

Varying with fluid intake and climate, total daily urine output averages from 24 to 81 oz (720 to 2,400 ml). For example, after a patient drinks a large volume of fluid, urine output increases as the body rapidly excretes excess water. If a patient restricts water intake or has an excessive intake of such solutes as sodium, urine output declines as the body retains water to restore normal fluid concentration.

HORMONES AND THE KIDNEYS

Hormones help regulate tubular reabsorption and secretion. For example, antidiuretic hormone (ADH) acts in the distal tubule and collecting ducts to increase water reabsorption and urine concentration. ADH deficiency decreases water reabsorption, causing dilute urine. Aldosterone affects tubular reabsorption by regulating sodium retention and helping to control potassium secretion by tubular epithelial cells.

By secreting the enzyme renin, the kidneys play a crucial role in blood pressure and fluid volume regulation. Juxtaglomerular cells near each of the kidney's glomeruli secrete renin into the blood. A low sodium load and low perfusion pressure (in the renal afferent arteriole) such as in hypovolemia increase renin secretion; a high sodium load and high pressure decrease it. Renin circulates throughout the body. In the liver, renin converts angiotensinogen to angiotensin I. In the lungs, angiotensin I is converted to angiotensin II, a potent vasoconstrictor that acts on the adrenal cortex to stimulate production of the hormone aldosterone. Aldosterone acts on the juxtaglomerular cells in the nephron to increase sodium and water retention and to stimulate or depress further renin secretion, completing the feedback cycle that automatically readjusts homeostasis.

Other hormonal functions of the kidneys include secreting the hormone erythropoietin and regulating calcium and phosphorus balance. In response to low arterial oxygen tension, the kidneys produce erythropoietin, which travels to the bone marrow. There, it stimulates increased RBC production. To help regulate calcium and phosphorus balance, the kidneys filter and reabsorb approximately half of unbound serum calcium and activate vitamin D_3, which is metabolized to a compound that promotes intestinal calcium absorption and regulates phosphate excretion.

Assessment

Assessing the renal and urologic system may uncover clues to possible problems in any body system.

HISTORY

If the patient is reluctant to discuss urologic problems, help him relax and try to build rapport. Remember to use familiar terms and ask open-ended questions that encourage communication. If you use medical terms, such as *void* or *catheter,* make sure the patient understands them.

CHIEF COMPLAINT

Ask the patient a general question such as "What made you seek medical help?" If he mentions several complaints, ask which bothers him most. Document his responses in his own words.

As you gather information, remain objective. Don't let the patient's opinions about his condition distract you from a thorough investigation. For example, a patient with a history of abdominal aneurysm who is experiencing flank pain may assume that the aneurysm is to blame. But further investigation could reveal renal calculi. You usually can detect renal dysfunction by assessing other, related body symptoms. (See *Assessing associated systems*, page 362.)

Find out how the patient's symptoms developed and progressed. Ask how long he's had the problem, how it affects his daily routine, when and how it began, and how often it occurs. Also ask about related signs and symptoms, such as nausea or vomiting. If he's had pain, ask about its location, radiation, intensity, and duration. Does anything precipitate, exacerbate, or relieve it? Which, if any, self-help remedies or over-the-counter (OTC) medications has he used?

MEDICAL HISTORY

For clues to the patient's present condition, explore past medical problems, including any experienced as a child. If he ever had a serious condition, such as kidney disease or a tumor, find out what treatment he received and its outcome. Ask similar questions about traumatic injuries, surgery, or any condition that required hospitalization.

Next, obtain an immunization and allergy history, including a history of medication reactions. Also inquire about current medications (whether prescription or OTC), alcohol use, smoking habits, and recreational drug use.

For clues to risk factors, ask if any blood relatives have ever been treated for renal or cardiovascular disorders, diabetes, cancer, or any other chronic illness.

Assessing associated systems

The renal and urologic system affects many body functions. Generally you can detect renal dysfunction by assessing other, related body systems.

Neurologic system
First assess level of consciousness. In renal failure, accumulating nitrogenous waste can cause neurologic problems ranging from slight confusion to coma.

Eyes
Look for conjunctival pallor, indicating anemia (a common complication of chronic renal disease). Using an ophthalmoscope, examine the internal eye, especially if the patient has malignant hypertension.

Funduscopic examination may reveal arteriosclerotic changes typical of hypertension and diabetes that may affect the kidney, such as widening of the light reflex, increased tortuosity of vessels, and arteriovenous nicking.

Skin
Pallor may indicate anemia, whereas excoriation from scratching may accompany uremia. Large ecchymoses and petechiae—characteristic signs of clotting abnormalities and decreased platelet adhesion—may reflect chronic renal failure. Observe for uremic frost—white or yellow urate crystals on the skin—indicating late-stage renal failure.

Inspect the mucous membranes in the mouth. Dryness reflects mild dehydration; parched, cracked lips, with markedly dry mucous membranes, and sunken eyes suggest severe dehydration. Also, evaluate skin turgor by gently pinching the patient's forearm skin with your thumb and index finger, then releasing it. If the skin doesn't return to its normal position immediately, suspect advanced dehydration.

Also check for edema. Sometimes accompanying renal disease, edema may be systemic or local; local edema may be pitting or nonpitting.

Respiratory system
Auscultate the lungs for bibasilar crackles, which may reflect pulmonary edema. Pulmonary edema and fluid overload commonly complicate renal disease. Pleural effusion suggests nephrotic syndrome. Hypoxia and hemoptysis appear early in Goodpasture's syndrome.

Cardiovascular system
You may detect friction rubs in a uremic patient. Cardiac enlargement from hypertension or circulatory overload can accompany renal failure. Inspect the patient's neck veins for distention, which, when accompanied by pitting edema, means fluid overload.

Investigate psychosocial factors that may affect the way the patient deals with his condition. Marital problems, poor living conditions, job insecurity, and other such stresses can strongly affect how he feels.

Find out how the patient views himself. A disfiguring genital lesion or a sexually transmitted disease can alter self-image. Try to determine what concerns he has about his condition. For example, does he fear that the disease or therapy will affect his sex life? If he can express his fears and concerns, you can develop appropriate nursing interventions more easily.

A complete sexual history helps you identify your patient's knowledge deficits and expectations. This information may suggest a need for psychological or sexual therapy. It can also guide treatment decisions. For example, pain or discomfort associated with intercourse or diminished sexual desire may reflect disease progression or depression.

PHYSICAL EXAMINATION
Begin the physical examination by documenting baseline vital signs and weighing the patient. Comparing subsequent weight measurements to this baseline may reveal a developing problem, such as dehydration or fluid retention. Because the urinary system affects many body functions, a thorough assessment includes examining multiple related body systems in addition to using inspection, auscultation, percussion, and palpation techniques.

Ask the patient to urinate into a specimen cup. Assess the sample for color, odor, and clarity. Then have the patient undress, providing him with a gown and drapes, and proceed with a systematic physical examination.

INSPECTION
Urinary system inspection includes examination of the abdomen and urethral meatus.

Help the patient assume a supine position with his arms relaxed at his sides. Make sure he's comfortable and draped appropriately. Expose the patient's abdomen from the xiphoid process to the symphysis pubis, and inspect the abdomen for gross enlargements or fullness by comparing left and right sides, noting any asymmetrical areas. In a normal adult, the abdomen is smooth, flat or scaphoid (concave), and symmetrical. Abdominal skin should be free from scars, lesions, bruises, and discolorations.

Extremely prominent veins may accompany other vascular signs associated with renal dysfunction, such as hypertension and renal artery bruits. Distention, skin tightness and glistening, and striae (streaks or linear scars caused by rapidly developing skin tension) may signal fluid retention. If you suspect ascites, perform the fluid wave test. Ascites may suggest nephrotic syndrome.

Help the patient feel more at ease during your inspection by examining the urethral meatus last and by explaining beforehand how you'll assess this area. Be sure to wear gloves.

Urethral meatus inspection may reveal several abnormalities. In a male patient, a meatus deviating from the normal central location may represent a congenital defect. In any patient, inflammation and discharge may signal urethral infection. Ulceration usually indicates a sexually transmitted disease.

AUSCULTATION

Auscultate the renal arteries in the left and right upper abdominal quadrants by pressing the stethoscope bell lightly against the abdomen and instructing the patient to exhale deeply. Begin auscultating at the midline and work to the left. Then return to the midline and work to the right. Systolic bruits (whooshing sounds) or other unusual sounds are potentially significant abnormalities. For example, in a patient with hypertension, systolic bruits suggest renal artery stenosis.

PERCUSSION

After auscultating the renal arteries, percuss the patient's kidneys to detect any tenderness or pain, and percuss the bladder to evaluate its position and contents. Abnormal kidney percussion findings include tenderness and pain, suggesting glomerulonephritis or glomerulonephrosis. A dull sound heard on percussion in a patient who has just urinated may indicate urine retention, reflecting bladder dysfunction or infection.

PALPATION

Palpation of the kidneys and bladder is the next step in the physical examination. Through palpation, you can detect any lumps, masses, or tenderness. To achieve the best results, have the patient relax his abdomen by taking deep breaths through his mouth.

Bladder cancer

Bladder tumors are most prevalent in people over age 50, are more common in men, and cluster in densely populated industrial areas. Bladder cancer is the fourth most common cause of cancer deaths in men over age 75.

Despite treatment, the patient with superficial disease has up to an 80% chance for recurrence. Only about 10% of superficial bladder cancers develop into invasive disease; in invasive disease, however, the patient's chances for metastasis increase to 90%. With treatment, about 50% of patients with invasive cancer experience complete remission; 20% have partial remission.

If bladder cancer progresses, complications include bone metastases and problems from the tumor's invasion of contiguous viscera.

CAUSES

These benign or malignant tumors may develop on the bladder wall surface or grow within the wall itself and quickly invade underlying muscles. About 90% of bladder cancers are transitional cell carcinomas, arising from the transitional epithelium of mucous membranes. They're sometimes a malignant transformation of benign papillomas. Less common bladder tumors include adenocarcinomas and squamous cell carcinomas.

Certain substances—such as 2-naphthylamine, tobacco, nitrates, and coffee—may predispose a person to transitional cell tumors. This places certain industrial workers (including rubber workers, weavers, aniline dye workers, hairdressers, petroleum workers, spray painters, and leather finishers) at high risk for developing these tumors. The latency period between exposure to the carcinogen and development of signs and symptoms of a tumor is about 18 years.

DIAGNOSIS AND TREATMENT

To confirm a bladder cancer diagnosis, the patient typically undergoes cystoscopy and biopsy. If the test results show cancer cells, further studies will determine the cancer stage and treatment.

Cystoscopy is best performed when hematuria first appears. If the patient receives an anesthetic during the procedure, he also may undergo a bimanual examination to detect whether the bladder is fixed to the pelvic wall. More specific tests include excretory urography, urinalysis, retrograde cystogram, bone scan, computed tomography scan or magnetic resonance imaging, and ultrasonography. Laboratory tests, such as a complete blood count and chemistry profile, can evaluate conditions such as anemia, commonly associated with bladder cancer.

The cancer's stage and the patient's lifestyle, other health problems, and mental outlook will influence selection of therapy. Choices are surgery, chemotherapy, and radiation therapy.

Superficial bladder tumors are typically removed cystoscopically by transurethral resection and electrically by fulguration. This approach usually is effective treatment if the tumor hasn't invaded the muscle. Additional tumors may also develop, however, and fulguration may then have to be repeated every 3 months for years. Once the tumors penetrate the muscle layer or recur frequently, cystoscopy with fulguration is no longer an appropriate choice.

Intravesical chemotherapy is used to treat superficial tumors (especially tumors in several sites) and prevent recurrence. This approach directly washes the bladder with drugs that fight the cancer. Commonly used anticancer agents include thiotepa, doxorubicin, and mitomycin.

Intravesical administration of the live, attenuated *bacille Calmette-Guérin* vaccine has been effective in the treatment of superficial bladder cancers, particularly primary and relapsed carcinoma in situ.

Tumors too large for treatment by cystoscopy require segmental bladder resection. This surgical approach removes a full-thickness section of the bladder and is practical only if the tumor isn't near the bladder neck or ureteral orifices. Bladder instillation of thiotepa after transurethral resection also may help.

For patients with infiltrating bladder tumors, the treatment of choice is radical cystectomy.

Treatment of patients with advanced bladder cancer includes cystectomy to remove the tumor, radiation therapy, and combination systemic chemotherapy with cisplatin, the most active agent. Other agents include methotrexate, vinblastine, and doxorubicin. In some instances, this combined treatment successfully arrests the disease.

COLLABORATIVE MANAGEMENT

Care of the patient with bladder cancer focuses on improving urinary function, arranging for adequate support after discharge, and patient teaching.

ASSESSMENT

The patient typically reports gross, painless, intermittent hematuria (often with clots). He may complain of suprapubic pain after voiding (which suggests invasive lesions). Other signs and symptoms include bladder irritability, urinary frequency, nocturia, and dribbling. If the patient reports flank pain, he may have an obstructed ureter.

NURSING DIAGNOSES AND COLLABORATIVE PROBLEMS

Based on the following nursing diagnoses, you'll establish patient outcomes.

Altered urinary elimination related to changes in bladder function. The patient will:
■ maintain adequate urine elimination through natural or artificial means
■ recognize and report changes in urine elimination pattern to the doctor
■ adhere to the prescribed treatment plan used to eradicate cancer cells in the bladder.

Fear related to potential radical changes in body image and possibly death from bladder cancer. The patient will:
■ express his fears

■ seek help in coping with fears from support groups, family members, and friends
■ express reduced fear and demonstrate no physical signs of fear.

Pain related to urinary tract infection or cancer cell invasion to surrounding tissues. The patient will:
■ seek medical care for pain relief
■ express feelings of relief and comfort after analgesic administration or other therapy to treat complication responsible for the pain
■ become pain-free.

PLANNING AND IMPLEMENTATION

These measures help the patient with bladder cancer.
■ Listen to the patient's fears and concerns. Stay with him during episodes of severe stress and anxiety, and provide psychological support. As appropriate, encourage him to express typical feelings and concerns about the extent of the cancer, the surgical procedure, an altered body image (especially if he undergoes urinary diversion surgery), and sexual dysfunction.
■ Give ordered analgesics for pain as necessary. Implement comfort measures and provide distractions that will enable the patient to relax.
■ As appropriate, implement measures to prevent or alleviate complications of treatment.
■ If the patient is being given intravesical chemotherapy, watch closely for myelosuppression, chemical cystitis, or skin rashes.
■ If the patient is receiving chemotherapy, watch for complications from the particular drug regimen.
■ Monitor the patient's intake and output. Question him regularly about changes in his urine elimination pattern to detect changes in his condition.
■ Observe the patient's urine for signs of hematuria (reddish tint to gross bloodiness) or infection (cloudy, foul smelling, with sediment present).
■ Monitor the patient's laboratory tests, such as changes in white blood cell differential indicating possible bone marrow suppression from chemotherapy.

Patient teaching

■ Tell the patient what to expect from the diagnostic tests. For example, make sure he understands that he may have anesthesia before cystoscopy. After the test results are known, explain their implications to the patient and his family members.
■ Explain the types of treatment that are being planned for the patient.
■ Teach the patient and family members to recognize and manage adverse effects of chemotherapy.
■ Teach them how to care for urinary diversions, if performed; arrange for home care follow-up if necessary.

■ Stress the importance of notifying the doctor if the patient develops signs and symptoms of urinary tract infection or other sudden changes in his condition.

■ Refer the patient to the American Cancer Society as appropriate.

EVALUATION

Achievement of patient outcomes determines the success of collaborative management. For the patient with bladder cancer, evaluation focuses on improved urinary elimination, absence of fever, no evidence of infection or other complications, pain control with oral analgesics, ability to ambulate at the preoperative level, adequate knowledge of the disease and necessary treatment and follow-up, and an adequate support system for postdischarge assistance.

Electrolyte imbalances

Electrolytes play a part in numerous body functions, such as fluid and acid-base balance, neuromuscular activity, and enzyme reactions. The major electrolytes are sodium, potassium, calcium, and magnesium. Concentrations of intracellular and extracellular electrolytes differ: Sodium is more abundant in extracellular fluid, whereas potassium is concentrated in intracellular fluid.

Electrolyte imbalances occur when extracellular electrolyte concentrations fall outside normal levels. Any deviation from normal levels can have profound physiologic effects.

CAUSES

Besides deficient or excessive dietary intake, electrolyte imbalances can result from vomiting, diarrhea, fever, burns, or a variety of disorders and drugs.

Causes of sodium imbalance include adrenal gland disorders, hypothyroidism, heart failure, cirrhosis of the liver, syndrome of inappropriate antidiuretic hormone secretion, and thiazide diuretics.

Causes of potassium imbalance include renal disease, hyperglycemia, alkalosis, adrenal disorders, and potassium-wasting and potassium-sparing diuretics.

Causes of calcium imbalance include malabsorption syndromes, laxative abuse, renal failure, parathyroid disorders, certain cancers, multiple fractures with prolonged immobilization, and thiazide diuretics.

Causes of magnesium imbalance include chronic alcoholism, malabsorption syndromes, overuse of magnesium-containing antacids or laxatives, prolonged diuretic therapy, and therapy with cisplatin, amphotericin, tobramycin, or gentamicin.

DIAGNOSIS AND TREATMENT

Diagnostic tests may include serum levels of electrolytes, arterial blood gas measurements, and electrocardiogram (ECG) changes.

Treatment for an electrolyte balance aims to return the electrolyte level to within normal range. This is accomplished primarily by correcting the underlying cause of the imbalance. In addition, if the imbalance is an excess, treatment aims to reduce the serum level of the electrolyte. If the imbalance is a deficit, treatment is aimed at replacing the electrolyte, usually intravenously or orally. Caution is necessary because, in many cases, attempts to restore the balance of the electrolyte can cause the opposite imbalance to occur. In addition, in an attempt to correct the electrolyte imbalance, your treatment may affect other electrolytes.

COLLABORATIVE MANAGEMENT

Care of the patient with electrolyte imbalance focuses on restoring fluid and electrolyte balance, avoiding complications, and teaching the patient how to avoid the imbalance.

ASSESSMENT

An electrolyte imbalance reflects disturbances in body function. Signs and symptoms become more severe as electrolyte imbalances worsen. (See *Managing electrolyte imbalances*, page 366.)

NURSING DIAGNOSES AND COLLABORATIVE PROBLEMS

Based on the following nursing diagnoses, you'll establish patient outcomes.

Decreased cardiac output related to effect of electrolyte imbalance on cardiac muscle. The patient will:
■ maintain hemodynamic status
■ exhibit cardiac output within acceptable parameters
■ remain free from signs and symptoms of arrhythmias.

Risk for injury related to effects of electrolyte imbalance. The patient will:
■ identify and avoid factors that increase risk
■ remain free from injury.

Altered nutrition: Less than body requirements, related to inability to ingest or adequately absorb amounts of specific electrolytes. The patient will:
■ identify and consume electrolyte-rich foods.

Knowledge deficit related to electrolyte imbalance or treatment. The patient will:
■ explain measures to reduce or eliminate risk factors
■ identify foods to include or avoid
■ demonstrate understanding of signs and symptoms of electrolyte imbalance.

Managing electrolyte imbalances

Electrolyte imbalance	Causes	Assessment findings	Collaborative management
HYPONATREMIA Sodium (Na) <135 mEq/L	GI, skin, or renal losses; syndrome of inappropriate antidiuretic hormone; heart failure; oliguric renal failure; liver failure; inadequate sodium intake; excess water intake or retention; burns; hemorrhage	Abdominal and muscle cramps, anorexia, headache, postural hypotension, lethargy, confusion, seizures	Administer I.V. hypertonic saline solution (3% or 5% sodium chloride); initiate seizure precautions and other safety measures.
HYPERNATREMIA Sodium >145 mEq/L	Osmotic diuresis, diabetes insipidus, salt-water near drowning, inability to perceive thirst, high protein feedings; inadequate water intake	Low-grade fever; flushed skin; weakness; thirst; hypotension; pulmonary congestion; edema; dry, swollen tongue; disorientation	Administer water I.V. or by mouth to replace loss. Give diuretics and water I.V. or by mouth for sodium gain; correct slowly to prevent cerebral edema.
HYPOKALEMIA Potassium (K) < 3 mEq/L	GI or renal losses, hyperaldosteronism, increased diaphoresis, diuretics, diabetic ketoacidosis	Fatigue, nausea, vomiting, muscle weakness, decreased bowel motility, anorexia, hyporeflexia, cardiac arrhythmias	Administer K I.V. or by mouth for replacement; administer parenterally, not to exceed 40 mEq/2 hr; institute cardiac monitoring.
HYPERKALEMIA Potassium >5.5 mEq/L	Renal disease, potassium sparing diuretics, tissue breakdown, acidosis, insulin deficiency, excessive potassium replacement, lead poisoning, burns	Muscle weakness, nausea, diarrhea, hypotension, cardiac arrhythmias	Give ion exchange resin to exchange Na for K. Give I.V. glucose, insulin, and sodium bicarbonate ($NaHCO_3$) to drive K into cell temporarily. Give I.V. calcium gluconate to block neuromuscular and cardiac effects. Institute cardiac monitoring.
HYPOCALCEMIA Calcium (Ca) <8.5 mg/dl	Alkalosis, administration of banked citrated blood, impaired vitamin D absorption, hypoparathyroidism, decreased magnesium or phosphate, overuse of laxatives containing phosphates	Tetany, seizures, positive Chvostek's and Trousseau's signs, tingling of fingers and mouth, muscular twitching, memory impairment, seizures, cardiac arrhythmias	Give Ca I.V. or by mouth for replacement. Give vitamin D by mouth to increase GI absorption of Ca. Give aluminum hydroxide by mouth to promote binding with phosphate. Institute seizure precautions and cardiac monitoring.
HYPERCALCEMIA Calcium >10.5 mg/dl	Acidosis, renal failure, cancer or multiple myeloma, hyperparathyroidism, increased intestinal absorption, excessive calcium intake orally or in solution, immobility, osteoporosis	Muscle weakness, nausea, vomiting, anorexia, constipation, memory impairment, abdominal pain, cardiac arrhythmias	Administer normal saline solution I.V. to aid Ca excretion. Give phosphate I.V. to cause inverse drop in Ca. Encourage low-calcium diet. Administer steroids to alter vitamin D absorption. Promote weight bearing, if tolerated, to stimulate bone deposition. Give $NaHCO_3$ to treat acidosis. Institute cardiac monitoring.
HYPOMAGNESEMIA Magnesium (Mg) < 1.5 mEq/L	Alcoholism, GI loss, administration of banked citrated blood, osmotic diuresis, hypercalcemia, elevated aldosterone levels, hyperthyroidism, acute pancreatitis, diabetic ketoacidosis	Tremors, difficulty swallowing, tetany, positive Chvostek's and Trousseau's signs, seizures, mood swings, hyperreflexia, cardiac arrhythmias	Increase dietary intake of Ca. Administer magnesium sulfate I.V., and observe for signs of hypermagnesemia. Institute cardiac monitoring and seizure precautions.
HYPERMAGNESEMIA Magnesium >2.5 mEq/L	Renal failure, excessive Mg administration, untreated diabetic ketoacidosis, severe dehydration, excessive infusion of magnesium-containing fluids	Facial flushing, hypotension, respiratory depression, muscle, weakness, loss of deep tendon reflexes, cardiac arrhythmias, coma	Administer Ca I.V. Prepare for dialysis. Institute mechanical ventilation if respiratory depression is significant. Institute cardiac monitoring.

Fluid volume excess (or deficit) related to electrolyte imbalance. The patient will:
- tolerate restricted or increased intake without problems
- maintain urine output at least 1 to 2 oz (30 to 60 ml)/hr
- demonstrate vital signs and weight within acceptable parameters
- regain normal fluid balance.

PLANNING AND IMPLEMENTATION
These measures help the patient with electrolyte imbalance.
- Monitor intake and output to assess fluid status.
- Obtain daily weights using same scale at the same time each day.
- Monitor vital signs; note any changes.
- Review patient's diet and include or restrict foods containing the electrolyte in question.
- Monitor the ECG to observe for signs of continuing changes in cardiac rhythm or complexes.
- Be alert for the need of emergency intervention or mechanical ventilation if the patient develops respiratory depression from hypermagnesemia.
- Carefully reposition the patient with hypercalcemia because he may have brittle bones, prone to fracture.
- Assess the patient with hypercalcemia for signs and symptoms of kidney stone formation, such as hematuria, intermittent low back pain, and nausea or vomiting.
- Ensure that the patient with hypomagnesemia can swallow, before giving oral drugs or foods.
- Evaluate the patient with hypermagnesemia for changes in deep tendon reflexes.
- Watch for signs of opposite electrolyte imbalance during treatment.

Patient teaching
- Teach the patient to avoid over-the-counter medications that contribute to electrolyte imbalance.
- Teach him the signs and symptoms of electrolyte imbalances and when to notify the doctor.
- Warn the patient taking a diuretic other than a potassium-sparing diuretic to increase intake of foods high in potassium.
- Instruct the patient to maintain adequate hydration.

EVALUATION
Achievement of patient outcomes determines the success of collaborative management. For the patient with an electrolyte imbalance, evaluation focuses on restoration of fluid and electrolyte balance, absence of complications, and adequate knowledge of the disorder and preventive measures.

Glomerulonephritis

Glomerulonephritis, a bilateral inflammation of the glomeruli, follows a Streptococcaceae infection elsewhere in the body. Also called acute poststreptococcal glomerulonephritis, the disorder is relatively common. Usually found in boys ages 3 to 7, it can affect people of any age. Up to 95% of children and 70% of adults recover fully; the rest, especially older adults, may progress to chronic renal failure within months.

CAUSES
Acute poststreptococcal glomerulonephritis is caused by the entrapment and collection of antigen-antibody complexes (an immunologic mechanism in response to a group A beta-hemolytic streptococcus) in the glomerular capillary membranes, inducing inflammatory damage and impeding glomerular function. Sometimes the immune complement further damages the glomerular membrane. The damaged and inflamed glomeruli lose the ability to be selectively permeable, allowing red blood cells (RBCs) and proteins to filter through, as the glomerular filtration rate (GFR) falls. Uremic poisoning may result.

Renal function progressively deteriorates in 33% to 50% of adults who contract sporadic acute poststreptococcal glomerulonephritis, usually in the form of glomerulosclerosis accompanied by hypertension. The more severe the disorder, the more likely it is that complications will follow.

DIAGNOSIS AND TREATMENT
Kidney-ureter-bladder X-rays show bilateral kidney enlargement. After blood tests and urinalysis, the patient may require a renal biopsy to confirm the diagnosis or assess renal tissue status.

Therapy aims to relieve symptoms and prevent complications. Vigorous supportive care includes bed rest, fluid and dietary sodium restrictions, and correction of electrolyte imbalances (possibly with dialysis, although this seldom is necessary).

Treatment may include loop diuretics, such as metolazone or furosemide, to reduce extracellular fluid overload, and vasodilators, such as hydralazine, nifedipine, or propranolol. If the patient has a documented staphylococcal infection, antibiotics are recommended for 7 to 10 days; otherwise, their use is controversial.

COLLABORATIVE MANAGEMENT
Care of the patient with glomerulonephritis focuses on restoring renal function and preventing complications.

ASSESSMENT

In most cases, acute poststreptococcal glomerulonephritis begins within 1 to 3 weeks after an untreated streptococcal infection in the respiratory tract. Look for:

- reports of decreased urination, dark brown or rust-colored urine, and fatigue
- complaints of shortness of breath, dyspnea, and orthopnea; symptoms of pulmonary edema, pointing to heart failure resulting from hypervolemia
- evidence of oliguria (with output less than 13½ oz [400 ml]/24 hours) and mild to moderate periorbital edema
- findings of mild to severe hypertension, resulting from either sodium or water retention (caused by decreased GFR) or inappropriate renin release
- in an older adult, complaints of vague, nonspecific symptoms, such as nausea, malaise, and arthralgia
- apparent bibasilar crackles if heart failure is present.
- abnormal blood values: elevated electrolyte, blood urea nitrogen (BUN), and creatinine levels and decreased serum protein levels
- RBCs, white blood cells, mixed cell casts, and protein in the urine, indicating renal failure
- high levels of fibrin-degradation products and C3 protein in the urine
- elevated antistreptolysin-O titers (in 80% of patients), elevated streptozyme and anti-DNase B titers, and low serum complement levels, verifying recent streptococcal infection
- throat culture showing group A beta-hemolytic streptococci.

NURSING DIAGNOSES AND COLLABORATIVE PROBLEMS

Based on the following nursing diagnoses, you'll establish patient outcomes.

Altered urinary elimination related to changes in renal function. The patient will:

- identify abnormal changes in his urine elimination pattern and seek medical attention
- communicate an understanding of the treatment prescribed to restore renal function
- regain and maintain his normal urine elimination pattern.

Fluid volume excess related to inability of kidneys to excrete fluid adequately. The patient will:

- not show signs and symptoms of severe fluid retention such as heart failure
- adhere to fluid and sodium restrictions to minimize fluid retention
- regain and maintain normal kidney function and normal fluid balance.

Powerlessness related to illness-related regimen. The patient will:

- express an understanding of the prescribed treatment and the need for compliance to minimize or prevent kidney damage
- regain and maintain normal kidney function or demonstrate ability to plan for controllable factors.

PLANNING AND IMPLEMENTATION

These measures help the patient with glomerulonephritis.

- Check the patient's vital signs and electrolyte values.
- Assess renal function daily through serum creatinine and BUN levels and urine creatinine clearance tests.
- Immediately report signs of acute renal failure (oliguria, azotemia, and acidosis).
- Monitor intake and output and daily weight. Report peripheral edema or the formation of ascites.
- Provide bed rest during the acute phase. Perform passive range-of-motion exercises for the patient on bed rest; allow resumption of normal activities gradually as symptoms subside.
- Consult the dietitian about a diet high in calories and low in protein, sodium, potassium, and fluids.
- Protect the debilitated patient against secondary infection by providing good nutrition and good hygienic technique and preventing contact with infected persons.
- Provide emotional support for the patient and family members.
- Encourage the patient to verbalize his concerns about his inability to perform in his expected role. Assure him that the activity restrictions are temporary.

Patient teaching

- Stress to the patient or his parents that follow-up examinations are necessary to detect chronic renal failure.
- Emphasize the need for regular blood pressure, urine protein, and renal function assessments during the convalescent months to detect recurrence.
- Explain that after acute poststreptococcal glomerulonephritis, gross hematuria may recur during nonspecific viral infections and abnormal urinary findings may persist for years.
- If the patient is scheduled for dialysis, explain the procedure fully.
- Advise a patient with a history of chronic upper respiratory tract infections to report signs and symptoms of infection, such as fever and sore throat, immediately.
- Encourage a pregnant patient with a history of acute poststreptococcal glomerulonephritis to have frequent medical evaluations because pregnancy further stresses the kidneys and increases the risk of chronic renal failure.

- Explain to the patient taking diuretics that he may experience orthostatic hypotension and dizziness when he changes positions quickly.

EVALUATION

Achievement of patient outcomes determines the success of collaborative management. For the patient with glomerulonephritis, evaluation focuses on restoration of urinary elimination (renal function) and fluid balance within acceptable parameters, absence of infection, and adequate knowledge of the disorder and measures to prevent recurrence.

Hydronephrosis

An abnormal dilation of the renal pelvis and the calyces of one or both kidneys, hydronephrosis is caused by an obstruction of urine flow in the genitourinary tract. Although a partial obstruction and hydronephrosis may not produce symptoms initially, the pressure built up behind the area of obstruction eventually results in symptoms of renal dysfunction.

CAUSES

Almost any type of obstructive uropathy can lead to hydronephrosis. The most common causes are benign prostatic hyperplasia, urethral strictures, and calculi. Less common causes include strictures or stenosis of the ureter or bladder neck, congenital abnormalities, and abdominal tumors.

If the obstruction is in the urethra or bladder, hydronephrosis usually is bilateral; if the obstruction is in a ureter, hydronephrosis usually is unilateral. Obstructions distal to the bladder cause the bladder to dilate and act as a buffer zone, delaying hydronephrosis. Total and prolonged obstruction of urine flow with dilation of the collecting system ultimately causes complete cortical atrophy and cessation of glomerular filtration.

Prolonged pressure of retained urine damages renal tubules, limiting their ability to concentrate urine. Removing the obstruction relieves the pressure, but tubular function may not significantly improve for days or weeks, depending on the patient's condition.

The most common complication of an obstructed kidney is life-threatening infection (pyelonephritis) caused by urinary stasis that exacerbates renal damage. If hydronephrosis results from acute obstructive uropathy, the patient may develop paralytic ileus. Untreated bilateral hydronephrosis can lead to renal failure, a life-threatening condition.

DIAGNOSIS AND TREATMENT

Diagnostic tests may include the following: excretory urography, retrograde pyelography, and renal function studies confirm the diagnosis. Visualization tests show concave (early-stage) or convex (later-stage) calyces as dilation progresses.

If the disease is extensive, tests will show atrophied distal and proximal tubules and obstructions. Urine studies will confirm the inability to concentrate urine, a decreased glomerular filtration rate and, possibly, pyuria if infection is present.

Treatment should preserve renal function and prevent infection by surgical removal of the obstruction. Surgery includes dilatation for a urethral stricture or prostatectomy for benign prostatic hyperplasia.

If renal function has already been affected, therapy may include a diet low in protein, sodium, and potassium. This diet is designed to stop the progression of renal failure before surgery.

Inoperable obstructions may necessitate decompression and drainage of the kidney, using a nephrostomy tube placed temporarily or permanently in the renal pelvis. Concurrent infection requires appropriate antibiotic therapy.

COLLABORATIVE MANAGEMENT

Care of the patient with hydronephrosis focuses on stabilizing vital signs and patient teaching of self-care measures.

ASSESSMENT

The patient's history and chief complaint will vary, depending on the cause of the obstruction. For example, a patient may have no symptoms or complain of only mild pain and slightly decreased urine flow. Or he may report severe, colicky renal pain or dull flank pain that radiates to the groin and gross urinary abnormalities, such as hematuria, pyuria, dysuria, alternating oliguria and polyuria, and anuria.

A patient with hydronephrosis also may report nausea, vomiting, abdominal fullness, pain on urination, dribbling, and urinary hesitancy. Pain on only one side, usually in the flank area, may signal a unilateral obstruction.

NURSING DIAGNOSES AND COLLABORATIVE PROBLEMS

Based on the following nursing diagnoses, you'll establish patient outcomes.

Altered urinary elimination related to urinary tract obstruction. The patient will:
- recognize and report changes in his urine elimination pattern
- seek immediate medical attention if his urine elimination pattern changes
- avoid complications of urinary tract obstruction

Understanding postobstructive diuresis

Polyuria—urine output that exceeds 2,000 ml in an 8-hour period—and excessive electrolyte losses characterize postobstructive diuresis. Although usually self-limiting, this condition can cause vascular collapse, shock, and death if not treated with fluid and electrolyte replacement.

Although diuresis typically abates in a few days, it persists if serum creatinine levels remain high. When these levels approach the normal range (0.7 to 1.4 mg/dl), diuresis usually subsides.

■ show how to safely manage catheters placed to relieve or bypass the obstruction
■ regain a normal urine elimination pattern with treatment.

Risk for infection related to urinary stasis. The patient will:
■ maintain a normal temperature and normal serum and urine white blood cell counts
■ exhibit clear urine with no foul odor
■ avoid urinary tract or kidney infection.

Pain related to urinary tract irritation and inflammation caused by obstruction. The patient will:
■ express pain relief after analgesic administration
■ become pain-free once the obstruction and disease resolve.

PLANNING AND IMPLEMENTATION

These measures help the patient with hydronephrosis.
■ Give prescribed pain medication as needed.
■ Allow the patient to express his fears and anxieties, and help him find effective coping strategies.
■ Remember that postobstructive diuresis may cause the patient to lose excessive dilute urine over hours or days. If this occurs, give I.V. fluids at a constant rate, as ordered, and in an amount equal to a percentage of hourly urine, to safely replace intravascular volume. (See *Understanding postobstructive diuresis.*)
■ Consult with a dietitian to provide a diet consistent with the treatment plan.
■ Check renal function studies daily, including blood urea nitrogen, serum creatinine, and serum potassium levels. As appropriate, arrange for specific gravity tests at the bedside.
■ Prepare the patient for surgery, as indicated.
■ Postoperatively, closely monitor intake and output, vital signs, and fluid and electrolyte status. Watch for a rising pulse rate and cold, clammy skin, which may signal impending hemorrhage and shock.

■ If a nephrostomy tube has been inserted, check it frequently for bleeding and patency. Irrigate the tube only as ordered, and don't clamp it. If a nephrostomy tube is placed percutaneously and is small, irrigation may be dangerous and done only if the tube isn't draining. Give meticulous skin care to the area around the tube; if urine leaks, provide a protective skin barrier to decrease excoriation. Use sterile technique in care of nephrostomy tubes.
■ Observe for signs of infection.
■ Monitor vital signs and urinary studies carefully.

Patient teaching

■ Explain hydronephrosis to the patient and his family. Also explain the purpose of diagnostic tests and how they're performed.
■ If the patient is scheduled for surgery, explain the procedure and postoperative care.
■ If he'll be discharged with a nephrostomy tube in place, teach him how to care for it, including how to thoroughly clean the skin around the insertion site.
■ If the patient must take antibiotics after discharge, tell him to take all of the prescribed medication, even if he feels better.
■ To prevent the progression of hydronephrosis to irreversible renal disease, urge an older male patient (especially a patient with a family history of benign prostatic hyperplasia or prostatitis) to have routine medical checkups.
■ Teach him to recognize and report symptoms of hydronephrosis, such as colicky pain or hematuria, or urinary tract infection.

EVALUATION

Achievement of patient outcomes determines the success of collaborative management. For the patient with hydronephrosis, evaluation focuses on vital signs and urine studies within normal limits for the patient, urine intake and output comparable and returning to normal, and adequate knowledge of the disease and self-care measures.

Metabolic acidosis

Produced by an underlying disorder, metabolic acidosis is a physiologic state of excess acid accumulation and deficient base bicarbonate. Symptoms are caused by the body's attempts to correct the acidotic condition through compensatory mechanisms in the lungs, kidneys, and cells. Severe or untreated metabolic acidosis may lead to coma, arrhythmias, and cardiac arrest.

CAUSES

Metabolic acidosis usually relates to excessive burning of fats in the absence of usable carbohydrates. The disorder is caused by diabetic ketoacidosis, chronic alcoholism, malnutrition, or a low-carbohydrate, high-fat diet—all of which produce more keto acids than the metabolic process can handle. Other causes include anaerobic carbohydrate metabolism (as occurs with pulmonary or hepatic disease, shock, or anemia), renal insufficiency and failure (renal acidosis), diarrhea and intestinal malabsorption, massive rhabdomyolysis (excess of organic acids from cell breakdown causes high anion gap acidosis), poisoning and drug toxicity, and hypoaldosteronism or use of potassium sparing diuretics.

DIAGNOSIS AND TREATMENT

Diagnostic tests may include the following: arterial blood gas (ABG) analysis, urinalysis, and blood tests for serum potassium levels, blood glucose levels, serum ketone body levels, and plasma lactic acid levels.

For acute metabolic acidosis, treatment may include I.V. administration of sodium bicarbonate (when arterial pH is less than 7.2) to neutralize blood acidity. For chronic metabolic acidosis, you may give oral bicarbonate. Other treatment measures include careful evaluation and correction of electrolyte imbalances and, ultimately, correction of the underlying cause. For example, diabetic ketoacidosis requires insulin administration and fluid replacement.

Your patient may require mechanical ventilation to ensure adequate respiratory compensation.

COLLABORATIVE MANAGEMENT

Care of the patient with metabolic acidosis focuses on restoring acid-base balance, avoiding complications, and thorough patient teaching.

ASSESSMENT

The history of a patient with metabolic acidosis may point to the presence of risk factors, including associated disorders or the use of medications that contain alcohol or aspirin. Information about the patient's urine output, fluid intake, and dietary habits (including any recent fasting) may help to establish the underlying cause and severity of metabolic acidosis. Look for:
- a history of central nervous system symptoms, such as changes in level of consciousness (LOC) that range from lethargy, drowsiness, and confusion to stupor and coma
- Kussmaul's respirations (as the lungs attempt to compensate by "blowing off" carbon dioxide)
- with underlying diabetes mellitus, a fruity breath odor from catabolism of fats and excretion of accumulated acetone through the lungs
- cold and clammy skin
- as acidosis grows more severe, warm and dry skin, indicating ensuing shock
- hypotension and arrhythmias
- diminished muscle tone and deep tendon reflexes.

NURSING DIAGNOSES AND COLLABORATIVE PROBLEMS

Based on the following nursing diagnoses, you'll establish patient outcomes.

Altered thought processes related to neurologic dysfunction. The patient will:
- remain safe and free from injury
- exhibit orientation to time, place, and person.

Decreased cardiac output related to arrhythmias. The patient will:
- remain hemodynamically stable
- avoid manifestations of profoundly decreased cardiac output, such as shock or ischemia
- regain a normal sinus rhythm and normal cardiac output.

Ineffective breathing pattern related to pulmonary dysfunction. The patient will:
- regain a normal respiratory rate and pattern
- avoid signs and symptoms of hypoxia
- maintain adequate ventilation.

PLANNING AND IMPLEMENTATION

These measures help the patient with metabolic acidosis.
- Provide care to eliminate the underlying cause. For example, give insulin and I.V. fluids, as ordered, to reverse diabetic ketoacidosis.
- Give sodium bicarbonate, as prescribed, and keep sodium bicarbonate ampules handy for emergency administration.
- Position the patient to promote chest expansion. If he's stuporous, turn him frequently.
- Frequently assess vital signs, laboratory test results, and LOC because changes can occur rapidly.
- Monitor the patient's respiratory function. Check his ABG values frequently.
- If the patient has diabetic acidosis, watch for secondary changes caused by hypovolemia such as decreasing blood pressure.
- Record intake and output accurately to monitor renal function. Watch for signs and symptoms of excessive serum potassium, such as weakness, flaccid paralysis, and arrhythmias (which may lead to cardiac arrest). After treatment, check for overcorrection of hypokalemia.

■ Orient the patient frequently, as needed. Reduce unnecessary environmental stimulation. Ensure a safe environment if he's confused. Keep the bed in the lowest position, with the side rails raised.

■ Provide good oral hygiene. Use sodium bicarbonate washes to neutralize mouth acids, and lubricate the patient's lips with lemon and glycerin swabs.

Patient teaching

■ To prevent diabetic ketoacidosis, teach the patient with diabetes how to test blood glucose levels or urine for glucose and acetone. Encourage strict adherence to hypoglycemic therapy, and reinforce the need to follow the prescribed dietary therapy.

■ As needed, teach the patient and family members about prescribed medications, their actions, and possible adverse effects. Provide verbal and written instructions.

EVALUATION

Achievement of patient outcomes determines the success of collaborative management. For the patient with metabolic acidosis, evaluation focuses on restoration of acid-base balance, absence of complications, and adequate knowledge of the disorder's underlying causes and measures to prevent recurrence.

Metabolic alkalosis

Always secondary to an underlying cause, metabolic alkalosis is a clinical state marked by decreased amounts of acid or increased amounts of base bicarbonate. It's usually associated with hypocalcemia and hypokalemia, which may account for signs and symptoms. With early diagnosis and prompt treatment, the prognosis is good. However, untreated metabolic alkalosis may result in coma, atrioventricular arrhythmias, and death.

CAUSES

Metabolic alkalosis is caused by the loss of acid or the increase of base.

Causes of acid loss include vomiting, nasogastric (NG) tube drainage or lavage without adequate electrolyte replacement, fistulas, and the use of steroids and certain diuretics (furosemide, thiazides, and ethacrynic acid).

Hyperadrenocorticism is another cause of severe acid loss. Cushing's disease, primary hyperaldosteronism, and Bartter's syndrome, for example, all lead to retention of sodium and chloride and urinary loss of potassium and hydrogen.

Excessive retention of base may follow excessive intake of bicarbonate of soda or other antacids (usually for treatment of gastritis or peptic ulcer), excessive intake of absorbable alkali (as in milk-alkali syndrome, seen in many patients with peptic ulcers), administration of excessive amounts of I.V. fluids with high concentrations of bicarbonate or lactate, massive blood transfusions, or respiratory insufficiency.

DIAGNOSIS AND TREATMENT

Diagnostic tests may include arterial blood gas analysis, serum electrolyte studies, and electrocardiogram (ECG).

Correcting the underlying cause of metabolic alkalosis is the goal of treatment. Mild metabolic alkalosis generally requires no treatment. Rarely, therapy for severe alkalosis includes cautious I.V. administration of ammonium chloride to release hydrogen chloride and restore concentration of extracellular fluid (ECF) and chloride levels. Potassium chloride and normal saline solution (except with heart failure) are usually sufficient to replace losses from gastric drainage.

Electrolyte replacement with potassium chloride and discontinuation of diuretics correct metabolic alkalosis resulting from potent diuretic therapy.

Oral or I.V. acetazolamide, which enhances renal bicarbonate excretion, may correct metabolic alkalosis without rapid volume expansion. Because acetazolamide also enhances potassium excretion, you may give potassium before giving this drug.

COLLABORATIVE MANAGEMENT

Care of the patient with metabolic alkalosis focuses on restoring acid-base balance, avoiding complications, and patient teaching.

ASSESSMENT

The patient's history (obtained from a family member, if necessary) may disclose such risk factors as excessive ingestion of alkali antacids. The history may include ECF volume depletion, which is commonly associated with conditions leading to metabolic alkalosis (for example, vomiting or NG tube suctioning). Look for:

■ reports of irritability, belligerence, and paresthesia

■ tetany, if serum calcium levels are borderline or low

■ decreased rate and depth of respirations, as a compensatory mechanism (mechanism may be limited by hypoxemia, which stimulates ventilation)

■ altered level of consciousness (LOC), such as apathy, confusion, seizures, stupor, or coma, if alkalosis is severe

■ hyperactive reflexes and muscle weakness, if serum potassium is markedly low

■ cardiac arrhythmias, with hypokalemia.

NURSING DIAGNOSES AND COLLABORATIVE PROBLEMS

Based on the following nursing diagnoses, you'll establish patient outcomes.

Altered thought processes related to neurologic dysfunction. The patient will:
- remain safe and protected from injury
- become oriented to time, place, and person with effective treatment.

Decreased cardiac output related to atrioventricular arrhythmias. The patient will:
- maintain hemodynamic stability
- avoid manifestations of profoundly decreased cardiac output, such as shock and tissue ischemia
- exhibit correction of arrhythmia and improved cardiac output with treatment.

Risk for injury related to tetany. The patient will:
- maintain a normal calcium level
- avoid signs and symptoms of tetany.

PLANNING AND IMPLEMENTATION

These measures help the patient with metabolic alkalosis.

- When giving I.V. solutions containing potassium salts, dilute potassium with the prescribed I.V. solution and use an I.V. infusion pump. Infuse ammonium chloride 0.9% I.V. no faster than 1 qt (1 L) over 4 hours; faster administration may cause hemolysis of red blood cells (RBCs).
- Avoid giving excessive amounts of these solutions because this could cause overcorrection leading to metabolic acidosis. Don't give ammonium chloride to a patient who has signs of hepatic or renal disease.
- Observe seizure precautions, and provide a safe environment for the patient with altered thought processes. Orient the patient as needed, and assess LOC often.
- Irrigate the patient's NG tube with normal saline solution instead of plain water to prevent loss of gastric electrolytes.
- Monitor I.V. fluid concentrations of bicarbonate or lactate. Observe the infusion rate of I.V. solutions containing potassium salts to prevent damage to blood vessels.
- Monitor I.V. solutions containing ammonium chloride to prevent hemolysis of RBCs. Watch for signs of phlebitis.
- Assess the patient's laboratory values, including pH, serum bicarbonate, serum potassium, and serum calcium levels. Notify the doctor if you detect significant changes or if the patient responds poorly to treatment.
- Observe the ECG for arrhythmias.
- Watch closely for signs of muscle weakness, tetany, or decreased activity.

- Check the patient's vital signs frequently, and record intake and output to evaluate respiratory, fluid, and electrolyte status. Remember that the respiratory rate usually slows in an effort to compensate for alkalosis. Tachycardia may indicate electrolyte imbalance, especially hypokalemia.

Patient teaching

- To prevent metabolic alkalosis, warn the patient not to overuse alkaline agents.
- If he has an ulcer, teach him how to recognize signs of milk-alkali syndrome, including a distaste for milk, anorexia, weakness, and lethargy.
- If potassium wasting diuretics or potassium chloride supplements are prescribed, make sure the patient understands the medication regimen, including the purpose, dosage, and possible adverse effects.

EVALUATION

Achievement of patient outcomes determines the success of collaborative management. For the patient with metabolic alkalosis, evaluation focuses on restoration of acid-base balance, absence of complications, and adequate knowledge of the disorder's underlying causes and measures to prevent recurrence.

Nephrotic syndrome

Although not a disease in itself, nephrotic syndrome is characterized by marked proteinuria, hypoalbuminemia, hyperlipidemia, and edema. It arises from a glomerular defect that affects the vessels' permeability and indicates renal damage. The prognosis is highly variable, depending on the underlying cause, but age plays no part in progression or prognosis. Some forms of nephrotic syndrome may eventually progress to end-stage renal failure.

CAUSES

About 75% of nephrotic syndrome cases result from primary (idiopathic) glomerulonephritis. Up to 20% of adults with nephrotic syndrome develop focal glomerulosclerosis. This condition can develop spontaneously at any age, can occur after kidney transplantation, or can result from heroin injection. Lesions initially affect some of the deeper glomeruli, causing hyaline sclerosis. Involvement of the superficial glomeruli occurs later. These lesions usually cause slowly progressive deterioration in renal function, although remissions may occur in children.

Membranous glomerulonephritis is the most common lesion in adult idiopathic nephrotic syndrome. It's characterized by the appearance of immune complexes, seen as dense deposits, within the glomerular basement membrane and by the uniform thickening of the basement membrane. It eventually progresses to renal failure.

Membranous glomerulonephritis may also follow infection, particularly streptococcal infection, and occurs primarily in children and young adults.

Additional causes of nephrotic syndrome include metabolic diseases such as diabetes mellitus; collagen-vascular disorders, such as systemic lupus erythematosus and periarteritis nodosa; circulatory diseases, such as heart failure, sickle cell anemia, and renal vein thrombosis; nephrotoxins, such as mercury, gold, and bismuth; infections, such as tuberculosis and enteritis; allergic reactions; pregnancy; hereditary nephritis; and certain neoplastic diseases such as multiple myeloma.

All of these diseases increase glomerular protein permeability, which leads to increased urinary excretion of protein (especially albumin) and subsequent hypoalbuminemia.

Edema, often seen in nephrotic syndrome, results from a decrease in protein and albumin, which allows fluid to shift from the vascular compartments into the interstitial spaces. The development of hyperlipidemia is associated with lipiduria and proteinuria. Hyperlipidemia usually worsens as the disease progresses.

Major complications of nephrotic syndrome include malnutrition, infection, coagulation disorders, thromboembolic vascular occlusion (especially in the lungs and legs), and accelerated atherosclerosis. Hypochromic anemia can develop from excessive urinary excretion of transferrin. Acute renal failure may occur.

DIAGNOSIS AND TREATMENT

Consistently heavy proteinuria (levels > 3.5 mg/dl/ 24 hours) strongly suggests nephrotic syndrome. Urine examination reveals an increased number of hyaline, granular, and waxy, fatty casts along with oval fat bodies. Supportive serum values include increased cholesterol, phospholipid, and triglyceride levels and decreased albumin levels. After blood tests and urinalysis, histologic identification of the lesion necessitates a renal biopsy.

Effective treatment of nephrotic syndrome requires correction of the underlying cause, if possible. Supportive treatment consists of a nutritious diet of 0.6 g of protein/kg of body weight, with restricted sodium intake, diuretics for edema, and antibiotics for infection.

Some patients respond to an 8-week course of a corticosteroid such as prednisone, followed by maintenance therapy. Others respond better to a combination of prednisone and azathioprine or cyclophos-

phamide. Treatment for hyperlipidemia generally is unsuccessful.

COLLABORATIVE MANAGEMENT

Care of the patient with nephrotic syndrome focuses on restoring renal function and fluid balance, preventing complications, and teaching about the disease and its treatment.

ASSESSMENT

The patient may complain of lethargy and depression. Your assessment may reveal two common problems: periorbital edema, which occurs primarily in the morning, and mild to severe dependent edema of the ankles or sacrum. Look for orthostatic hypotension, ascites, swollen external genitalia, signs of pleural effusion, anorexia, and pallor.

NURSING DIAGNOSES AND COLLABORATIVE PROBLEMS

Based on the following nursing diagnoses, you'll establish patient outcomes.

Altered nutrition: Less than body requirements, related to loss of protein in urine. The patient will:
- consume a nutritionally balanced diet
- avoid signs and symptoms of malnutrition.

Fluid volume excess related to edema. The patient will:
- comply with prescribed sodium restrictions and diuretic therapy to minimize edema
- avoid complications associated with edema, such as skin breakdown and impaired mobility
- regain a normal fluid balance.

Risk for infection related to nephrotic syndrome. The patient will:
- maintain a normal temperature and white blood cell (WBC) count
- maintain a urine output that is clear, odorless, and free from WBCs
- avoid infection.

PLANNING AND IMPLEMENTATION

These measures help the patient with nephrotic syndrome.
- Give medications, such as diuretics, antibiotics, and corticosteroids, as ordered. Assess the patient's response, desired and adverse.
- Ask the dietitian to plan a low-sodium diet with moderate amounts of protein.
- Frequently check the patient's urine for protein, indicated by a frothy appearance.
- Monitor plasma albumin and transferrin concentrations to evaluate his overall nutritional status.
- Provide meticulous skin care to combat the edema that usually occurs with nephrotic syndrome. Use a

reduced-pressure mattress or padding to help prevent pressure ulcers.

■ Monitor and document the location and character of edema. (See *Evaluating edema.*)

■ Measure blood pressure, both supine and standing. Immediately report any drop in systolic or diastolic pressure that exceeds 20 mm Hg.

■ Monitor intake and output, and weigh the patient each morning after he voids and before he eats.

■ To avoid thrombophlebitis, encourage activity and exercise; provide antiembolism stockings, as ordered, and teach their safe use.

■ After a renal biopsy, watch for bleeding and signs of shock.

■ Offer the patient and family member reassurance and support, especially during the acute phase, when edema is severe and the patient's body image changes.

Patient teaching

■ If the patient is taking immunosuppressants, teach him and family members to report even mild signs of infection.

■ If he's undergoing long-term corticosteroid therapy, teach them to report muscle weakness and mental changes.

■ To prevent GI complications, suggest steroids with an antacid or with cimetidine or ranitidine.

■ Explain that adverse effects of steroids will subside when therapy stops, but warn the patient not to discontinue the drug abruptly or without a doctor's consent.

■ Stress the importance of adhering to the special diet.

EVALUATION

Achievement of patient outcomes determines the success of collaborative management. For the patient with nephrotic syndrome, evaluation focuses on restoration of renal function and fluid balance, adequate nutrition, absence of complications, and adequate knowledge of the disease and its treatment.

Neurogenic bladder

All types of bladder dysfunction linked to an interruption of normal bladder innervation by the nervous system are referred to as neurogenic bladder. (Other names are neuromuscular dysfunction of the lower urinary tract, neurologic bladder dysfunction, and neuropathic bladder.) Neurogenic bladder can be hyperreflexic (hypertonic, spastic, or automatic) or flaccid (hypotonic, atonic, or autonomous).

Evaluating edema

To assess pitting edema, press firmly for 5 to 10 seconds over a bony surface, such as the subcutaneous part of the tibia, fibula, sacrum, or sternum. Then remove your finger and note how long the depression remains. Document your observation on a scale from +1 (barely detectable depression) to +4 (persistent pit as deep as 1" [2.5 cm]).

In severe edema, tissue swells so much that fluid can't be displaced, making pitting impossible. The surface feels rock-hard, and subcutaneous tissue becomes fibrotic. Brawny edema eventually may develop.

+1 pitting edema

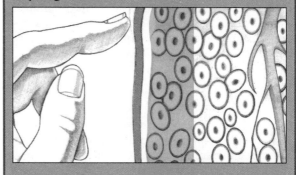

+4 pitting edema

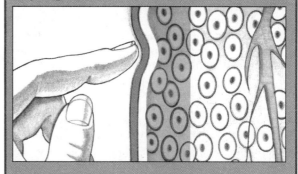

Brawny edema

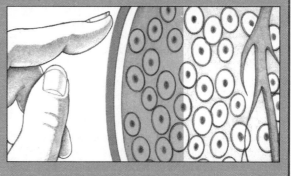

CAUSES

At one time, neurogenic bladder was thought to result primarily from spinal cord injury; now it appears to stem from a host of underlying conditions, including:
- cerebral disorders, such as cerebrovascular accident, brain tumor (meningioma and glioma), Parkinson's disease, multiple sclerosis, dementia, and incontinence associated with aging
- spinal cord disease or trauma, such as spinal stenosis (causing cord compression) or arachnoiditis (causing adhesions between the membranes covering the cord), cervical spondylosis, spina bifida, myelopathies from hereditary or nutritional deficiencies and, rarely, tabes dorsalis
- disorders of peripheral innervation, including autonomic neuropathies resulting from endocrine disturbances such as diabetes mellitus (most common)
- metabolic disturbances, such as hypothyroidism, porphyria, or uremia (infrequent)
- acute infectious diseases, such as Guillain-Barré syndrome and transverse myelitis
- heavy metal toxicity
- chronic alcoholism
- collagen diseases such as systemic lupus erythematosus
- vascular diseases such as atherosclerosis
- distant effects of certain cancers such as primary oat cell carcinoma of the lung
- herpes zoster
- sacral agenesis.

An upper motor neuron lesion (at or above the second to fourth sacral vertebrae) causes spastic neurogenic bladder, with spontaneous contractions of detrusor muscles, increased intravesical voiding pressure, bladder wall hypertrophy with trabeculation, and urinary sphincter spasms. A lower motor neuron lesion (below the second to fourth sacral vertebrae) causes flaccid neurogenic bladder, with decreased intravesical pressure, increased bladder capacity and residual urine retention, and poor detrusor contraction.

Incontinence, residual urine retention, urinary tract infection (UTI), calculus formation, and renal failure can complicate neurogenic bladder.

DIAGNOSIS AND TREATMENT

These diagnostic tests will help assess bladder function: voiding cystourethrography, urodynamic studies (urine flow, cystometry, urethral pressure profile, and sphincter electromyelography), and retrograde urethrography.

The goals of treatment are to maintain the integrity of the upper urinary tract; control infection; and prevent urinary incontinence through evacuation of the bladder, drug therapy, surgery or, less commonly, nerve blocks and electrical stimulation.

Techniques for bladder evacuation include Valsalva's maneuver and intermittent self-catheterization.

The patient can perform Valsalva's maneuver himself by sitting on the toilet and forcefully exhaling (while keeping his mouth closed). This helps the bladder release urine and promotes complete emptying.

Intermittent self-catheterization—more effective than Valsalva's maneuver—is a major advance in treatment because it completely empties the bladder without the risks of an indwelling urinary catheter. A male can perform this procedure more easily, but a female can learn self-catheterization with the help of a mirror. Intermittent self-catheterization, along with a bladder retraining program, is especially useful in patients with flaccid neurogenic bladder. Anticholinergics and alpha-adrenergic stimulators can help the patient with hyperreflexic neurogenic bladder until intermittent self-catheterization is performed.

Drug therapy for neurogenic bladder may include bethanechol and phenoxybenzamine to facilitate bladder emptying and propantheline, methantheline, flavoxate, dicyclomine, imipramine, and pseudoephedrine to facilitate urine storage.

When conservative treatment fails, surgery may correct the structural impairment through transurethral resection of the bladder neck, urethral dilatation, external sphincterotomy, or urinary diversion procedures. The patient may require implantation of an artificial urinary sphincter, if permanent incontinence follows surgery.

COLLABORATIVE MANAGEMENT

Care of the patient with neurogenic bladder focuses on regaining bladder control, preventing infection, and thorough patient teaching.

ASSESSMENT

The patient's history will include a condition or disorder that can cause neurogenic bladder. He'll have some degree of incontinence and will experience changes in initiation or interruption of micturition or an inability to completely empty his bladder. He also may have a history of frequent UTIs. Other assessment findings may depend on the site and extent of the spinal cord lesion.

NURSING DIAGNOSES AND COLLABORATIVE PROBLEMS

Based on the following nursing diagnoses, you'll establish patient outcomes.

Risk for infection related to urinary stasis. The patient will:
- maintain a temperature and white blood cell count within the normal range
- avoid complications associated with UTI, such as sepsis and dehydration

■ demonstrate normal urinalysis results and produce odorless urine with a normal appearance.

Reflex incontinence related to neurologic dysfunction. The patient will:

■ comply with conservative measures and drug therapy prescribed to control incontinence

■ avoid complications caused by incontinence, such as skin breakdown and UTI

■ achieve bladder control with effective management of neurogenic bladder.

Urinary retention related to neurogenic bladder caused by a lower motor neuron lesion. The patient will:

■ demonstrate complete bladder emptying through such methods as self-catheterization, Credé's or Valsalva's maneuver, and bladder retraining

■ avoid UTIs caused by urine retention.

PLANNING AND IMPLEMENTATION

These measures help the patient with neurogenic bladder.

■ Use strict aseptic technique during insertion of an indwelling urinary catheter (a temporary measure to drain the incontinent patient's bladder). Don't interrupt the closed drainage system for any reason. Obtain urine specimens with a syringe and small-bore needle inserted through the aspirating port of the catheter itself (below the junction of the balloon instillation site). Irrigate in the same manner, if ordered.

■ Clean the catheter insertion site with soap and water at least twice daily. Don't allow the catheter to become encrusted. Keep the drainage bag below the tubing and below the level of the bladder. Clamp the tubing or empty the bag before transferring the patient to a wheelchair or stretcher, to prevent accidental urine reflux if the drainage container doesn't have an antireflux valve. If urine output is considerable, empty the bag more often than every 8 hours because bacteria can multiply in standing urine and migrate up the catheter and into the bladder.

■ When the patient is on an intermittent self-catheterization and bladder retraining program, regulate fluid intake at 1 qt (1 L)/day to maintain sufficient amounts of urine. For females, the goal is urine retention because no acceptable urinary incontinence devices are available. Males can use an external device when bladder function returns. Reevaluate the patient when urine volume, returned with catheterization, is 10 oz (300 ml) between independent voidings; at that point, you may need to reduce the frequency of the catheterizations. In a patient with neurogenic bladder, catheterization can end when the amount of postvoiding residual urine is consistently less than 3 oz (100 ml).

■ If the patient will undergo a urinary diversion procedure, such as catheter drainage or suprapubic

catheter insertion, consult with an enterostomal therapist and coordinate the plans of care.

■ Monitor the patient's urine output. Palpate and percuss his bladder regularly to check for urine retention.

■ Watch for signs of UTI (fever, cloudy or foul-smelling urine) and other complications, such as incontinence, renal calculi, and renal failure.

■ Monitor the effectiveness of drugs and procedures, and remain alert for adverse reactions.

■ Try to keep the patient as mobile as possible, or perform passive range-of-motion exercises if necessary.

■ Neurogenic bladder can produce emotional turmoil. Suggest a support group at a local rehabilitation center or health care facility.

Patient teaching

■ Explain all diagnostic tests clearly so that the patient understands the procedure, the time involved, and the possible results. Assure him that the lengthy diagnostic process is necessary to identify the most effective treatment plan. After the treatment plan is chosen, explain it to him in detail.

■ Encourage the patient to drink plenty of fluids to prevent calculus formation and infection from urinary stasis.

■ Before discharge, teach the patient and family members evacuation techniques as necessary (for example, Valsalva's maneuver or intermittent self-catheterization). Also teach him how to care for the catheter, if appropriate.

■ Discuss sexual activities. The patient with neurogenic bladder will feel embarrassed and worried about sexual function, so provide emotional support.

■ Demonstrate good hand-washing technique, and encourage meticulous cleaning of the drainage site.

■ Teach the patient the signs of UTI, and warn him to report them immediately.

EVALUATION

Achievement of patient outcomes determines the success of collaborative management. For the patient with neurogenic bladder, evaluation focuses on control of urinary elimination, infection prevention, ability to perform self-care, and adequate knowledge of measures to promote urinary elimination.

Polycystic kidney disease

Polycystic kidney disease affects males and females equally. It has an insidious onset but usually becomes obvious between ages 30 and 50; rarely, it may not cause symptoms until the patient is in his 70s.

View of the polycystic kidney

The kidney shown in the cross section below has multiple areas of cystic damage. Each indentation represents a cyst.

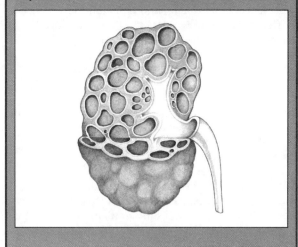

CAUSES

This inherited disorder is genetically transmitted as an autosomal dominant trait. It's characterized by multiple, bilateral, grapelike clusters of fluid-filled cysts that enlarge the kidneys, compressing and eventually replacing functioning renal tissue. (See *View of the polycystic kidney.*) Renal deterioration is gradual, and the disease progresses relentlessly to fatal uremia.

The prognosis is extremely variable. Progression may be slow, even after symptoms of renal insufficiency appear. Once uremic symptoms develop, polycystic kidney disease usually is fatal within 4 years, unless the patient receives dialysis.

This disease may cause recurrent hematuria, life-threatening retroperitoneal bleeding from cyst rupture, proteinuria, and colicky abdominal pain from the ureteral passage of clots or calculi. In most cases, progressive compression of kidney structures by the enlarging mass produces renal failure about 10 years after symptoms appear.

DIAGNOSIS AND TREATMENT

In a patient with polycystic disease, these laboratory tests are typical: excretory or retrograde urography, ultrasonography, computed tomography scan, radioisotopic scans, magnetic resonance imaging, urinalysis, and creatinine clearance tests.

Diagnosis must rule out renal tumors.

Polycystic kidney disease is incurable. The primary goal of treatment is to preserve renal parenchyma and prevent pyelonephritis. Progressive renal failure requires treatment similar to that for other types of renal disease, including dialysis or, rarely, kidney transplantation.

When polycystic kidney disease is discovered in the asymptomatic stage, careful monitoring is required, including urine cultures and creatinine clearance tests every 6 months. When urine culture detects infection, the patient needs prompt and vigorous antibiotic treatment, even if he has no symptoms.

As renal impairment progresses, selected patients may undergo dialysis, transplantation, or both. Cystic abscess or retroperitoneal bleeding may necessitate surgical drainage; intractable pain (an uncommon symptom) also may require surgery. Nephrectomy usually isn't recommended because this disease occurs bilaterally and the infection could recur in the remaining kidney.

COLLABORATIVE MANAGEMENT

Care of the patient with polycystic kidney disease focuses on restoring function, stabilizing weight, and teaching about maintenance treatments.

ASSESSMENT

The patient with polycystic kidney disease commonly is asymptomatic while in his 30s and 40s, but he may report polyuria, urinary tract infections (UTIs), and other nonspecific symptoms. Your assessment may show hypertension.

Later assessment reveals overt symptoms caused by the enlarging kidney mass, such as lumbar pain, widening girth, and a swollen or tender abdomen. The patient states that abdominal pain usually is worsened by exertion and relieved by lying down. In advanced stages, palpation easily reveals grossly enlarged kidneys.

NURSING DIAGNOSES AND COLLABORATIVE PROBLEMS

Based on the following nursing diagnoses, you'll establish patient outcomes.

Altered urinary elimination related to progressive renal failure. The patient will:
■ maintain fluid balance with or without dialysis or transplantation
■ demonstrate skill in managing urinary elimination problems caused by renal failure.

Risk for infection related to predisposition to UTI. The patient will:
■ maintain a normal temperature and white blood cell count
■ maintain a normal urine color and odor
■ show no signs or symptoms of UTI, such as dysuria and hematuria.

Pain related to enlarging kidney mass. The patient will:
■ express feelings of comfort following analgesic administration
■ avoid or seek help with activities that precipitate or heighten pain.

PLANNING AND IMPLEMENTATION
These measures help the patient with polycystic kidney disease.
■ Provide supportive care to minimize any associated symptoms.
■ Encourage the patient to rest, and help with activities of daily living when the patient has abdominal pain. Offer analgesics as needed.
■ Allow the patient to verbalize his fears and concerns about this progressive disorder.
■ Carefully evaluate the patient's lifestyle and physical and mental state. Determine how rapidly the disease is progressing. Use this information to plan individualized patient care.
■ Acquaint yourself with all aspects of end-stage renal disease, including dialysis and transplantation, so that you can provide appropriate care and patient teaching as the disease progresses.
■ Give antibiotics, as ordered, for UTI. Provide adequate hydration during antibiotic therapy.
■ Observe standard precautions when handling all blood and body fluids.
■ Prepare the patient for peritoneal dialysis or hemodialysis, as indicated.
■ Monitor the patient's renal function regularly, as ordered. Measure his intake and output.
■ Screen urine for blood, cloudiness, and calculi or granules. Report any of these findings immediately.
■ Before beginning excretory urography and other procedures that use an iodine-based contrast medium, ask the patient if he's ever had an allergic reaction to iodine or shellfish. Even if he says no, watch for a possible allergic reaction after the procedures.
■ Monitor the patient for complications associated with polycystic kidney disease.

Patient teaching
■ Discuss the patient's prognosis honestly, including such possible treatments as dialysis or transplantation; answer any questions.
■ Explain all diagnostic procedures to the patient and family members or friends. Review any treatments such as dialysis.
■ Discuss prescribed medications and their possible adverse effects. Stress the need to take medications exactly as prescribed, even if symptoms are minimal or absent.

■ Discuss signs and symptoms of urinary tract infection.

EVALUATION
Achievement of patient outcomes determines the success of collaborative management. For the patient with polycystic kidney disease, evaluation focuses on vital signs and physiologic function within normal parameters, minimal symptoms of renal malfunction (such as edema and electrolyte imbalance), moist and clean mucous membranes, steady weight, and maintenance of treatments such as peritoneal dialysis, as applicable.

Renal cancer

About 85% of renal cancers—also called kidney cancer, nephrocarcinoma, renal cell carcinoma, and hypernephroma—originate in the kidneys. Others are metastases from various primary-site cancers.

The incidence of renal cancer is rising, possibly from exposure to environmental carcinogens and increased longevity. Even so, renal cancer accounts for only about 2% of all adult cancers. Twice as common in men as in women, renal cancer typically strikes after age 40, with peak incidence between ages 50 and 60. Renal pelvic tumors and Wilms' tumors occur most commonly in children.

Renal cancer divides histologically into clear cell, granular cell, and spindle cell types. Sometimes the prognosis is considered better for the clear cell type than for the others; in general, however, the prognosis depends more on the cancer's stage than on its type.

Overall prognosis has improved considerably, with the 5-year survival rate at about 50% and the 10-year survival rate at 18% to 23%. Left untreated, renal cancer is fatal.

Hemorrhage, respiratory problems from metastasis to the lungs, neurologic problems from brain metastasis, and GI problems from liver metastasis are possible complications.

CAUSES
Although the cause of renal cancer is unknown, some studies implicate particular factors, including heavy cigarette smoking. Patients who receive regular hemodialysis also may be at increased risk.

Most kidney tumors are large, firm, nodular, encapsulated, unilateral, and solitary. They may affect either kidney; occasionally they're bilateral or multifocal.

DIAGNOSIS AND TREATMENT

Renal ultrasonography and a computed tomography scan can distinguish between simple cysts and renal cancer. In many cases, these tests eliminate the need for renal angiography. Other tests that aid diagnosis and help in staging include excretory urography, nephrotomography, and kidney-ureter-bladder radiography.

Additional relevant tests include liver function studies, which show increased alkaline phosphatase, bilirubin, and transaminase levels and prolonged prothrombin time. Such results may point to liver metastasis. If the tumor hasn't metastasized, these abnormal values reverse after tumor resection.

Radical nephrectomy, with or without regional lymph node dissection, offers the only chance of cure. It's the treatment of choice in localized cancer or with tumor extension into the renal vein and vena cava. Nephrectomy won't help in disseminated disease.

Because this disease resists radiation, this treatment is used only when the cancer has spread into the perinephric region or the lymph nodes or when surgery can't completely excise the primary tumor or metastatic sites. Then, the patient usually needs high radiation doses.

Chemotherapy and hormonal therapy have no effect on renal cancer. Immunotherapy with lymphokine-activated killer T cells plus recombinant interleukin-2 shows promise but is expensive and causes many adverse reactions. Interferon is somewhat effective in treating advanced disease.

COLLABORATIVE MANAGEMENT

Care of the patient with renal cancer focuses on improving renal function, avoiding complications, and patient teaching.

ASSESSMENT

The patient may complain of hematuria and commonly a dull, aching flank pain. He also may report weight loss, although this is uncommon. Rarely, his temperature is elevated. Palpation may reveal a smooth, firm, nontender abdominal mass.

NURSING DIAGNOSES AND COLLABORATIVE PROBLEMS

Based on the following nursing diagnoses, you'll establish patient outcomes.

Fear related to the diagnosis of renal cancer. The patient will:
- verbalize his feelings about having cancer
- use available support systems to help him cope with his renal cancer
- manifest no physical signs or symptoms of fear.

Risk for injury related to lung, brain, or liver metastasis. The patient will:
- agree to have a nephrectomy
- demonstrate no signs or symptoms of lung, brain, or liver dysfunction.

Pain related to tumor pressure in the kidney. The patient will:
- express relief from pain following analgesic administration
- employ distraction techniques to minimize pain
- become pain-free after a nephrectomy is performed.

PLANNING AND IMPLEMENTATION

These measures help the patient with renal cancer.
- Give prescribed analgesics as necessary.
- Monitor the patient's degree of pain, and assess the effectiveness of prescribed analgesics.
- Provide comfort measures, such as positioning and distractions, to help the patient cope with his discomfort.
- Prepare the patient for a nephrectomy.
- Encourage the patient to express his anxieties and fears, and remain with him during periods of severe stress and anxiety.
- Watch for adverse effects of radiation or chemotherapy and provide symptomatic treatment.
- Be alert for signs and symptoms of pulmonary, neurologic, and liver dysfunction.
- Monitor laboratory test results for anemia, polycythemia, and abnormal blood chemistry values that may point to bone or hepatic involvement or may result from radiation therapy or chemotherapy.

Patient teaching
- Tell the patient what to expect from surgery and other treatments.
- Explain the possible adverse effects of radiation and drug therapy. Teach the patient how to prevent or minimize these problems.
- Stress the importance of compliance with any prescribed outpatient treatment. This includes an annual follow-up chest X-ray to rule out lung metastasis and excretory urography every 6 to 12 months to check for contralateral tumors.
- If appropriate, refer the patient and family members or friends to health care and community services, such as cancer support groups and hospice care.

EVALUATION

Achievement of patient outcomes determines the success of collaborative management. For the patient with renal cancer, evaluation focuses on improved renal function, absence of complications, pain relief,

Causes of acute renal failure

Acute renal failure can be classified as prerenal, intrarenal, or postrenal. All conditions that lead to prerenal failure impair renal perfusion, resulting in decreased glomerular filtration rate and increased proximal tubular reabsorption of sodium and water. Intrarenal failure is caused by damage to the kidneys themselves; postrenal failure, by obstruction of urine flow.

Prerenal failure

Cardiovascular disorders
- Arrhythmias
- Cardiac tamponade
- Cardiogenic shock
- Heart failure
- Myocardial infarction

Hypovolemia
- Burns
- Dehydration
- Diuretic abuse
- Hemorrhage
- Hypovolemic shock
- Trauma

Peripheral vasodilation
- Antihypertensive drugs
- Sepsis

Renovascular obstruction
- Arterial embolism
- Arterial or venous thrombosis
- Tumor

Severe vasoconstriction
- Disseminated intravascular coagulation
- Eclampsia
- Malignant hypertension
- Vasculitis

Intrarenal failure

Acute tubular necrosis
- Ischemic damage to renal parenchyma from unrecognized or poorly treated prerenal failure
- Nephrotoxins—analgesics (such as phenacetin), anesthetics (such as methoxyflurane), antibiotics (such as gentamicin), heavy metals (such as lead), radiographic contrast media, organic solvents
- Obstetric complications—eclampsia, postpartum renal failure, septic abortion, uterine hemorrhage
- Pigment release—crush injury, myopathy, sepsis, transfusion reaction

Other parenchymal disorders
- Acute glomerulonephritis
- Acute interstitial nephritis
- Acute pyelonephritis
- Bilateral renal vein thrombosis
- Malignant nephrosclerosis
- Papillary necrosis
- Periarteritis nodosa
- Renal myeloma
- Sickle cell disease
- Systemic lupus erythematosus
- Vasculitis

Postrenal failure

Bladder obstruction
- Anticholinergic drugs
- Autonomic nerve dysfunction
- Infection
- Tumor

Ureteral obstruction
- Blood clots
- Calculi
- Edema or inflammation
- Necrotic renal papillae
- Retroperitoneal fibrosis or hemorrhage
- Surgery (accidental ligation)
- Tumor
- Uric acid crystals

Urethral obstruction
- Prostatic hyperplasia or tumor
- Strictures

---

positive adjustment to the diagnosis, and adequate knowledge of the disorder, treatment, and prognosis.

Renal failure, acute

About 5% of all hospitalized patients develop acute renal failure—the sudden interruption of renal function resulting from obstruction, reduced circulation, or renal parenchymal disease. This condition is classified as prerenal, intrarenal, or postrenal and is usually reversible with medical treatment. If not treated, it may progress to end-stage renal disease, uremia, and death.

CAUSES

Each of the three types of acute renal failure has a separate cause. (See *Causes of acute renal failure*.) Prerenal failure is linked to conditions that diminish blood flow to the kidneys. Between 40% and 80% of all cases of acute renal failure are caused by prerenal azotemia. Intrarenal failure (also called intrinsic or parenchymal renal failure) results from damage to the kidneys themselves, usually from acute tubular necrosis. Postrenal failure is caused by bilateral obstruction of urine outflow.

Ischemic acute tubular necrosis can lead to renal shutdown. Electrolyte imbalance, metabolic acidosis, and other severe effects follow as the patient becomes increasingly uremic and renal dysfunction disrupts other body systems. If left untreated, the patient will die. Even with treatment, an older adult is particularly susceptible to volume overload, precipitating acute pulmonary edema, hypertensive crisis, hyperkalemia, and infection.

DIAGNOSIS AND TREATMENT

Diagnostic tests may include blood tests (showing elevated blood urea nitrogen, serum creatinine, and potassium levels and low blood pH, bicarbonate, and hemoglobin levels and hematocrit) and urinalysis (showing casts, cellular debris, decreased specific gravity and, in glomerular diseases, proteinuria and urine osmolality close to serum osmolality). The urine sodium level is under 20 mEq/L if oliguria results from decreased perfusion and above 40 mEq/L if it results from an intrarenal problem. Creatinine clearance tests decrease as renal failure progresses.

Other studies that help determine the cause of renal failure include kidney ultrasonography, plain films of the abdomen, kidney-ureter-bladder radiography, excretory urography, renal scan, retrograde pyelography, computed tomography scans, and nephrotomography.

An electrocardiogram (ECG) shows tall, peaked T waves, a widening QRS complex, and disappearing P waves if hyperkalemia is present.

Supportive measures include a diet high in calories and low in protein, sodium, and potassium, with supplemental vitamins and restricted fluids. Meticulous electrolyte monitoring is essential to detect hyperkalemia. If your patient develops hyperkalemia, acute therapy may include hypertonic glucose-and-insulin infusions and sodium bicarbonate—all given I.V.—and sodium polystyrene sulfonate by mouth or enema to remove potassium from the body.

If measures fail to control uremic symptoms, the patient may require hemodialysis or peritoneal dialysis. Early initiation of diuretic therapy during the oliguric phase may help.

COLLABORATIVE MANAGEMENT

Care of the patient with acute renal failure focuses on improving renal function, avoiding complications, restoring fluid and electrolyte balance, and patient teaching.

ASSESSMENT

The patient's history may include a disorder that can cause renal failure, and he may have a recent history of fever; chills; GI problems, such as anorexia, nausea, vomiting, diarrhea, or constipation; and central nervous system (CNS) problems such as headache. Look for:

- alterations in level of consciousness, such as irritability, drowsiness, and confusion
- in advanced stages, seizures and coma
- depending on the stage of renal failure, urine output of less than 400 ml/24 hours (oliguric) or less than 100 ml/24 hours (anuric)
- evidence of bleeding abnormalities, such as petechiae and ecchymoses; hematemesis may occur
- dry, pruritic skin and, rarely, uremic frost (white, powdery coating on the skin)
- dry mucous membranes, breath with a uremic odor
- hyperkalemia, muscle weakness
- tachycardia and, possibly, an irregular rhythm
- bibasilar crackles, with heart failure
- abdominal pain, with pancreatitis or peritonitis
- peripheral edema, with heart failure.

NURSING DIAGNOSES AND COLLABORATIVE PROBLEMS

Based on the following nursing diagnoses, you'll establish patient outcomes.

Fluid volume excess related to decreased ability of the kidneys to excrete water and sodium. The patient will:
- adhere to fluid restrictions
- not exhibit signs and symptoms of heart failure
- regain and maintain normal fluid volume with alleviation of acute renal failure.

Risk for infection related to renal dysfunction. The patient will:
- maintain a normal temperature and white blood cell count
- demonstrate appropriate infection-control measures
- show no signs and symptoms of an infection.

Risk for injury related to potential for hyperkalemia. The patient will:
- adhere to a potassium-restricted diet
- maintain a normal serum potassium level
- not show signs and symptoms of hyperkalemia.

PLANNING AND IMPLEMENTATION

These measures help the patient with acute renal failure.
- Use infection control measures during care because the patient with acute renal failure is highly susceptible to infection. Don't allow staff members or visitors with upper respiratory tract infections to come into contact with the patient. Also use standard precautions when handling all blood and body fluids.
- Prevent complications of immobility by encouraging frequent coughing and deep breathing and by performing passive range-of-motion exercises.

- Help the patient walk as soon as possible.
- Add lubricating lotion to his bath water to combat skin dryness.
- Provide meticulous perineal care to reduce the risk of ascending urinary tract infection in women and to protect skin integrity caused by frequent loose, irritating stools, particularly when sodium polystyrene sulfonate is used.
- Provide mouth care frequently to lubricate dry mucous membranes. If stomatitis occurs, use an antibiotic solution, if ordered, and have the patient swish it around in his mouth before swallowing.
- Give medications carefully, especially antacids and stool softeners.
- Use appropriate safety measures, such as side rails and restraints, because the patient with CNS involvement may become dizzy or confused.
- Replace blood components as ordered. Use packed red blood cells instead of whole blood so the patient doesn't get volume overloaded and develop heart failure and worsening renal failure.
- Maintain proper electrolyte balance. Avoid giving drugs that contain potassium.
- Maintain nutritional status. Provide a diet high in calories and low in protein, sodium, and potassium, with vitamin supplements. Give the anorexic patient small, frequent meals.
- Measure and record intake and output of all fluids, including wound drainage, nasogastric tube output, and diarrhea.
- Weigh the patient daily. You also may need to measure abdominal girth every day, marking the skin with indelible ink to measure the same place.
- Monitor renal function studies, electrolytes (especially potassium), hemoglobin level, and hematocrit regularly, as ordered.
- Monitor vital signs. Watch for and report signs of pericarditis (pleuritic chest pain, tachycardia, and pericardial friction rub), inadequate renal perfusion (hypotension), and acidosis.
- Prepare the patient for hemodialysis or peritoneal dialysis, as indicated.
- Give any prescribed drugs after hemodialysis is completed. Many medications are removed from the blood during treatment.
- Watch for symptoms of hyperkalemia (malaise, anorexia, paresthesia, muscle weakness, and ECG changes), and report them immediately.
- Assess the patient frequently, especially during emergency treatment to lower potassium levels. If he receives hypertonic glucose-and-insulin infusions, monitor potassium and glucose levels. If you give sodium polystyrene sulfonate rectally, make sure the patient doesn't retain it and become constipated. This can lead to bowel perforation.
- Monitor for GI bleeding by testing all stools for occult blood, using the guaiac test.
- Provide emotional support to the patient and family members.
- Assess the patient's ability to resume normal activities of daily living, and plan for gradual resumption.

Patient teaching

- Reassure the patient and family members or friends by clearly explaining all diagnostic tests, treatments, and procedures.
- Tell the patient about his prescribed medications, diet, and fluid allowance and stress the importance of complying with the regimen.
- Instruct the patient to weigh himself daily and report changes of 3 lb (1.5 kg) or more immediately.
- Advise against overexertion. If he becomes dyspneic or short of breath during normal activity, tell him to report it to his doctor.
- Teach him to recognize edema, and to report it to the doctor.

EVALUATION

Achievement of patient outcomes determines the success of collaborative management. For the patient with acute renal failure, evaluation focuses on improved renal function, absence of complications, restoration of fluid and electrolyte balance, and adequate knowledge of the disorder, treatment, and need for compliance.

Renal failure, chronic

Usually, chronic renal failure is the end result of a gradually progressive loss of renal function. Occasionally it is caused by a rapidly progressive disease of sudden onset that gradually destroys the nephrons and eventually causes irreversible renal damage. Few symptoms develop until after more than 75% of glomerular filtration is lost; then, the remaining normal parenchyma deteriorates progressively, and symptoms worsen as renal function decreases. This syndrome is fatal without treatment, but maintenance dialysis or a kidney transplant can sustain life.

CAUSES

Chronic renal failure may be caused by:
- chronic glomerular disease such as glomerulonephritis
- chronic infections, such as chronic pyelonephritis or tuberculosis
- congenital anomalies such as polycystic kidney disease

- vascular diseases, such as renal nephrosclerosis or hypertension
- obstructive processes such as calculi
- collagen diseases such as systemic lupus erythematosus
- nephrotoxic agents such as long-term aminoglycoside therapy
- endocrine diseases such as diabetic neuropathy.

Chronic renal failure may progress through the following stages:
- reduced renal reserve (glomerular filtration rate [GFR] 35% to 50% of normal)
- renal insufficiency (GFR 20% to 35% of normal)
- renal failure (GFR 20% to 25% of normal)
- end-stage renal disease (GFR less than 20% of normal).

If this condition continues unchecked, uremic toxins accumulate and produce potentially fatal physiologic changes in all major organ systems. Even if the patient can tolerate life-sustaining maintenance dialysis or a kidney transplant, he may still have anemia, peripheral neuropathy, cardiopulmonary and GI complications, sexual dysfunction, and skeletal defects.

DIAGNOSIS AND TREATMENT

Laboratory findings aid in the diagnosis and monitoring of chronic renal failure. Blood studies, arterial blood gas analysis, urine specific gravity, and urinalysis may show proteinuria, glycosuria, red blood cells (RBCs), leukocytes, and casts and crystals, depending on the cause. X-ray studies, renal biopsy, and EEG also aid in diagnosis.

Conservative treatment aims to correct specific symptoms. A low-protein diet reduces the production of end products of protein metabolism that the kidneys can't excrete. (However, a patient receiving continuous peritoneal dialysis should have a high-protein diet.) A high-calorie diet prevents ketoacidosis and the negative nitrogen balance that results in catabolism and tissue atrophy. The diet also should restrict sodium and potassium.

Maintaining fluid balance requires careful monitoring of vital signs, weight changes, and urine volume (if not anuric). You may reduce fluid retention with loop diuretics such as furosemide (if some renal function remains) and with fluid restriction. Digitalis glycosides in small doses may mobilize the fluids causing the edema; antihypertensives may control blood pressure and associated edema.

Antiemetics taken before meals may relieve nausea and vomiting, and cimetidine or ranitidine may decrease gastric irritation. Methylcellulose or docusate can help prevent constipation.

Anemia requires iron and folate supplements; severe anemia requires infusion of fresh frozen packed cells or washed packed cells. Transfusions relieve anemia only temporarily. Synthetic erythropoietin (epoetin alfa) stimulates the division and differentiation of cells within the bone marrow to produce RBCs.

Drug therapy commonly relieves associated symptoms. An antipruritic, such as trimeprazine or diphenhydramine, can relieve itching, and aluminum hydroxide gel can lower serum phosphate levels. The patient also may benefit from supplementary vitamins (particularly B vitamins and vitamin D) and essential amino acids.

Careful monitoring of serum potassium levels is necessary to detect hyperkalemia. Emergency treatment for severe hyperkalemia includes dialysis therapy and administration of 50% hypertonic glucose I.V., regular insulin, calcium gluconate I.V., sodium bicarbonate I.V., and cation exchange resins such as sodium polystyrene sulfonate. Cardiac tamponade resulting from pericardial effusion may require emergency pericardial tap or surgery.

Intensive dialysis and thoracentesis can relieve pulmonary edema and pleural effusion.

Hemodialysis or peritoneal dialysis (particularly the newer techniques of continuous ambulatory peritoneal dialysis and continuous cyclic peritoneal dialysis) can help control most manifestations of end-stage renal disease. Altering the dialysate can correct fluid and electrolyte disturbances. However, maintenance dialysis itself may produce complications, including serum hepatitis (hepatitis B) from numerous blood transfusions, protein wasting, refractory ascites, and dialysis dementia.

COLLABORATIVE MANAGEMENT

Care of the patient with chronic renal failure focuses on improving renal function, avoiding complications, and teaching the patient how to handle the disorder.

ASSESSMENT

The patient's history may include a disease or condition that can cause renal failure; however, he may not have any symptoms for a long time. Symptoms usually occur by the time the GFR is 20% to 35% of normal and almost all body systems are affected.

NURSING DIAGNOSES AND COLLABORATIVE PROBLEMS

Based on the following nursing diagnoses, you'll establish patient outcomes.

Altered nutrition: Less than body requirements, related to adverse GI effects. The patient will:
- regain his weight and maintain it within the normal range with no further weight loss
- tolerate oral feedings and obtain an adequate caloric intake
- not develop malnutrition.

Fluid volume excess related to inability of the kidneys to regulate water balance. The patient will:

- communicate an understanding of the importance of fluid and sodium restrictions
- adhere to fluid and sodium restrictions
- exhibit no signs or symptoms of excessive fluid retention.

Risk for injury related to adverse effects of chronic renal failure on all major organ systems. The patient will:

- recognize and report early signs of organ dysfunction
- comply with the prescribed treatment regimen to minimize or prevent complications
- take precautions in daily life to minimize or prevent injury caused by organ dysfunction.

PLANNING AND IMPLEMENTATION

These measures help the patient with chronic renal failure.

- Provide good skin care. Bathe the patient daily, using superfatted soaps, oatmeal baths, and skin lotion to ease pruritus. Give good perineal care, using mild soap and water.
- Pad side rails to guard against ecchymoses. Turn the patient often, and use a convoluted foam or low-pressure mattress to prevent skin breakdown.
- Prevent pathologic fractures by turning the patient carefully and ensuring his safety. Perform passive range-of-motion exercises for the bedridden patient.
- Provide good oral hygiene. Brush the patient's teeth often with a soft brush or sponge tip to reduce breath odor. Hard candy and mouthwash minimize metallic taste in the mouth and alleviate thirst.
- Infuse sodium bicarbonate for acidosis and sedatives or anticonvulsants for seizures, as ordered. Keep an oral airway and suction setup at the bedside.
- Give loop diuretics and restrict fluid and sodium intake to alleviate excess fluid retention, as ordered.
- Prepare the patient for hemodialysis or peritoneal dialysis, as indicated.
- Carefully assess the patient's hydration status. Check for jugular vein distention, and auscultate the lungs for crackles, rhonchi, and decreased lung sounds. Be alert for clinical signs of pulmonary edema (such as dyspnea and restlessness).
- Carefully measure daily intake and output, including all drainage, emesis, diarrhea, and blood loss. Record daily weight, presence or absence of thirst, axillary sweat, tongue dryness, hypertension, and peripheral edema.
- Carefully observe and document seizure activity. Periodically assess neurologic status, and check for Chvostek's and Trousseau's signs, indicators of low serum calcium levels.

- Watch for signs and symptoms of hyperkalemia: a weak pulse rate, cramping of the legs and abdomen, and diarrhea.
- Be sure the sodium polystyrene sulfonate enema is expelled; otherwise, it will cause constipation and won't lower potassium levels.
- Monitor the electrocardiogram for tall, peaked T waves, a widening QRS complex, a prolonged PR interval, and the disappearance of P waves.
- Observe for signs of bleeding: prolonged bleeding at puncture sites and vascular access site.
- Monitor hemoglobin level and hematocrit and check stool, urine, and vomitus for blood.
- Offer small, palatable, nutritious meals, including favorites within dietary restrictions, and encourage intake of high-calorie foods.
- Schedule medication administration carefully. Give iron before meals, aluminum hydroxide gels after meals, and antiemetics (as necessary) a half hour before meals. Give antihypertensives at appropriate intervals.
- Recommend antacid cookies as an alternative to aluminum hydroxide gels needed to bind GI phosphate. Don't give magnesium products because poor renal excretion can lead to toxic levels.
- Encourage deep breathing and coughing to prevent pulmonary congestion.
- Maintain strict aseptic technique. Use a micropore filter during I.V. therapy.
- Warn the outpatient to avoid contact with infected persons during the cold and flu season.
- Monitor for bone or joint complications.
- Watch for signs of infection (listlessness, high fever, and leukocytosis).
- Report signs or symptoms of pericarditis, such as a pericardial friction rub and chest pain. Also watch for the disappearance of friction rub, with a drop of 15 to 20 mm Hg in blood pressure during inspiration (paradoxical pulse), an early sign of pericardial tamponade.

Patient teaching

- Teach the patient how to take his medications and what adverse effects to watch for. Suggest that he take diuretics in the morning to avoid disturbing his sleep.
- Tell the anemic patient to conserve energy by resting frequently.
- Tell the patient to report leg cramps or excessive muscle twitching. Stress the importance of follow-up appointments to monitor electrolyte levels.
- Warn against high-sodium and high-potassium foods, reinforce fluid and protein restrictions, and stress the value of exercise and dietary fiber to prevent constipation.
- If the patient is having dialysis, remember that he and his family are under extreme stress. If the health care facility doesn't offer them a course on dialysis, you'll need to provide the information.

DISCHARGE READY > **After renal failure**

After treatment for chronic renal failure, the patient will meet the following criteria before discharge:

- ability to care for shunt or fistula
- vital signs within acceptable parameters
- nutritional intake and weight within acceptable parameters
- no evidence of complications

- fluid and electrolyte levels within acceptable limits
- ability to comply with and tolerate any nutritional or fluid restrictions
- ability to tolerate activity and manage activities of daily living
- understanding of medications and other treatments
- adequate home support to ensure compliance with therapy and referrals for follow-up care.

- Refer them for counseling, if needed.
- Suggest that the patient wear a medical identification bracelet or carry pertinent information with him.

EVALUATION

Achievement of patient outcomes determines the success of collaborative management. For the patient with chronic renal failure, evaluation focuses on improved renal function, absence of complications, restoration of fluid and electrolyte balance, and adequate knowledge of the disorder, treatment, and need for compliance. (See *After renal failure.*)

Urinary calculi

Although they may form anywhere in the urinary tract, urinary calculi (sometimes called kidney stones) most commonly develop in the renal pelvis or calyces.

About 1 in 1,000 Americans develops renal calculi. They're more common in men (especially those ages 30 to 50) than in women and rare in blacks and children.

CAUSES

Although the cause of renal calculi isn't known, predisposing factors include:
- dehydration; decreased water excretion concentrates calculus-forming substances.
- infection; infected, scarred tissue provides a site for calculus development. In addition, infected calculi (usually magnesium ammonium phosphate or staghorn calculi) may develop if bacteria serve as the nucleus in calculus formation. Struvite calculus formation commonly results from *Proteus* infections, which may lead to destruction of renal parenchyma.

- changes in urine pH; consistently acidic or alkaline urine may provide a favorable medium for calculus-formation, especially for magnesium ammonium phosphate or calcium phosphate calculi.
- obstruction; urinary stasis allows calculus constituents to collect and adhere, forming calculi. Obstruction also encourages infection, which compounds the obstruction.
- immobilization; immobility from spinal cord injury or other disorders allows release of calcium into the circulation and, eventually, filtration by the kidneys.
- metabolic factors; hyperparathyroidism, renal tubular acidosis, elevated uric acid (usually with gout), defective metabolism of oxalate, a genetically caused defect in metabolism of cystine, and excessive intake of vitamin D or dietary calcium may predispose a person to renal calculi.

Urinary calculi are particularly prevalent in certain geographic areas, such as the southeastern United States (called the "stone belt"), possibly because a hot climate promotes dehydration and concentrates calculus-forming substances or because of regional dietary habits.

Calculi form when substances that normally dissolve in the urine (calcium oxalate, calcium phosphate, magnesium ammonium phosphate [struvite] and, occasionally, urate or cystine) precipitate. Calculi vary in size and may be solitary or multiple.

Calculi may remain in the renal pelvis and damage or destroy renal parenchyma, or they may enter the ureter. (See *Variations in urinary calculi.*) Large calculi in the kidneys cause pressure necrosis. In certain locations, calculi cause obstruction, with resultant hydronephrosis, and tend to recur. They can cause intractable pain and serious bleeding.

DIAGNOSIS AND TREATMENT

Diagnosis is based on clinical features and the following tests: kidney-ureter-bladder radiography, excretory urography, kidney ultrasonography, urine culture, 24-

hour urine collection, calculus analysis, serial blood calcium and phosphorus levels, blood protein levels, and blood uric acid levels.

Appendicitis, cholecystitis, peptic ulcer, and pancreatitis must be ruled out as potential sources of pain before the diagnosis can be confirmed.

Because 90% of renal calculi are smaller than ¼″ (6 mm) in diameter, treatment usually involves encouraging their natural passage through vigorous hydration (more than 3 qt [3 L] per day). Other treatments include administration of antimicrobial agents for infection (varying with the cultured organism); analgesics, such as meperidine or morphine, for pain; and diuretics to prevent urinary stasis and further calculus formation (thiazides decrease calcium excretion into the urine). Methenamine mandelate is given to suppress calculus formation when infection is present.

Measures to prevent recurrence include a low-calcium diet, generally combined with oxalate-binding cholestyramine, for absorptive hypercalciuria; parathyroidectomy for hyperparathyroidism; administration of allopurinol for uric acid calculi; and daily oral doses of ascorbic acid to acidify the urine.

Calculi too large for natural passage may require removal. To remove a calculus lodged in the ureter, a cystoscope is inserted through the urethra. It manipulates the calculus with catheters or retrieval instruments. Extraction of calculi from other areas, such as the kidney calyx or renal pelvis, may take a flank or lower abdominal approach. Two other methods, percutaneous ultrasonic lithotripsy and extracorporeal shock-wave lithotripsy, shatter the calculus into fragments for removal by suction or natural passage.

Cystine calculi are difficult to treat without surgical intervention or invasive procedures. If electrohydraulic ultrasound isn't effective, the calculi are surgically removed.

COLLABORATIVE MANAGEMENT
Care of the patient with urinary calculi focuses on improving urinary elimination, relieving pain, and preventing or controlling infection.

ASSESSMENT
Assessment findings vary with the size, location, and cause of the calculi. The key symptom of renal calculi is severe pain, usually from obstruction by large, rough calculi occluding the opening to the ureteropelvic junction and increasing the frequency and force of peristaltic contractions. The patient usually reports that the pain travels from the costovertebral angle to the flank and then to the suprapubic region and external genitalia (classic renal colic pain). Pain intensity fluctuates and may be excruciating at its peak.

Variations in urinary calculi

Urinary calculi vary in size and type. Small calculi may remain in the renal pelvis or pass down the ureter. A staghorn calculus (a cast of the calyceal and pelvic collecting system) may develop from a stone that stays in the kidney.

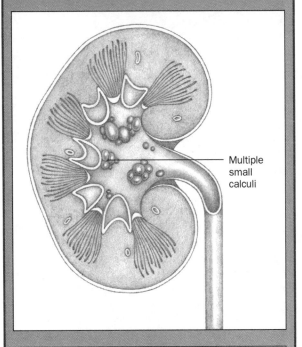

Multiple small calculi

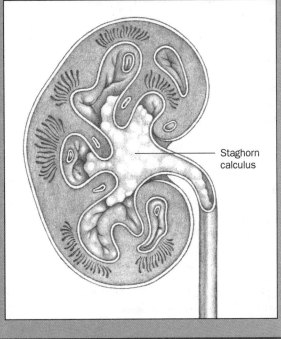

Staghorn calculus

DISCHARGE READY ▷ After urinary calculi

After treatment for urinary calculi, the patient will meet the following criteria before discharge:
• temperature within acceptable parameters
• improved urinalysis, including absence of gross hematuria
• absence of complications
• ability to strain urine (if indicated)
• incision (if applicable) that's clean, dry and intact.

The patient with calculi in the renal pelvis and calyces may complain of more constant, dull pain. He also may report back pain (from calculi causing obstruction within a kidney) and severe abdominal pain (from calculi traveling down a ureter). The patient with severe pain also typically complains of nausea, vomiting and, possibly, fever and chills.

You may note hematuria (when calculi abrade a ureter), abdominal distention and, rarely, anuria (from bilateral obstruction or, in the patient with one kidney, unilateral obstruction).

NURSING DIAGNOSES AND COLLABORATIVE PROBLEMS
Based on the following nursing diagnoses, you'll establish patient outcomes.

Altered urinary elimination related to increased output from high oral fluid intake and potential for calculi to lodge in urinary tract and interfere with urine flow. The patient will:
■ recognize the need for medical attention and seek it if his oral intake becomes greater than his urine output or anuria occurs
■ maintain an oral intake greater than 3 qt (3 L) per day until calculi have passed
■ regain and maintain a normal urinary elimination pattern with eradication of renal calculi.

Risk for infection related to abrasive nature of renal calculi as they pass through the urinary tract. The patient will:
■ maintain a normal temperature and white blood cell count
■ exhibit no signs and symptoms of a urinary tract infection, such as dysuria, hematuria, or cloudy, foul-smelling urine
■ remain free from urinary tract infections.

Pain related to presence of renal calculi. The patient will:
■ express feelings of comfort after analgesic administration
■ comply with the prescribed treatment to remove renal calculi and thus alleviate pain

■ become pain-free with the passage or removal of renal calculi.

PLANNING AND IMPLEMENTATION
These measures help the patient with urinary calculi.
■ To facilitate spontaneous passage of calculi, encourage the patient to walk, if possible. Also force fluids to maintain a urine output of 3 to 4 qt (3 to 4 L) per day (urine should be dilute and colorless).
■ If the patient can't drink the required amount of fluid, give supplemental I.V. fluids.
■ To help acidify urine, offer fruit juices, especially cranberry juice.
■ Record intake and output and daily weight to assess fluid status and renal function.
■ Monitor the patient's urine for evidence of renal calculi. To aid diagnosis, maintain a 24- to 48-hour record of urine pH, using nitrazine pH paper. Strain all urine through gauze or a tea strainer, and save all solid material for analysis.
■ Prepare the patient for lithotripsy or surgery, as indicated.
■ If the patient had calculi surgically removed, he'll probably have an indwelling urinary catheter or a nephrostomy tube. Unless the affected kidney was removed, expect bloody drainage from the catheter. Never irrigate the catheter without a doctor's order. Use sterile technique when changing dressings or providing catheter care.
■ Check dressings regularly for bloody drainage and ask the doctor how much drainage to expect. Immediately report excessive drainage or a rising pulse rate, symptoms of hemorrhage.
■ Watch for signs and symptoms of infection, such as a rising temperature or chills.
■ If the patient had lithotripsy, medicate him generously for pain when he's passing a calculus.
■ Monitor the patient's response to pain medication and other drugs. Also observe for adverse reactions.
■ Give antibiotics and other medications, as ordered.

Patient teaching
■ Encourage increased fluid intake. If appropriate, show the patient how to check his urine pH, and instruct him to keep a daily record. Tell him to immediately report symptoms of acute obstruction, such as pain or an inability to void.
■ Urge the patient to follow a prescribed diet and comply with drug therapy to prevent recurrence of calculi. For example, if a hyperuricemic condition caused the patient's calculi, teach him which foods are high in purine.
■ If surgery is necessary, supplement and reinforce the doctor's teaching. The patient may be fearful, especially if he needs a kidney removed, so emphasize

Correcting urinary incontinence

The following practice guidelines from the U.S. Department of Health and Human Services' Agency for Health Care Policy and Research outline the partial management of urinary incontinence.

Behavioral interventions
- Offer routine or scheduled toileting on a consistent schedule to an incontinent patient who can't participate in independent toileting.
- Institute habit training—toileting scheduled to match the patient's voiding habits—for a patient with an apparent voiding pattern.
- Use prompted voiding for a patient who can learn to recognize some degree of bladder fullness or the need to void, or who can ask for assistance or respond when prompted to void.
- For a patient with urge and mixed incontinence, provide bladder training, the systematic ability to delay voiding through the use of urge inhibition.
- Teach your patient pelvic muscle exercises—planned, active exercises of pelvic muscles to increase periurethral muscle strength. It may decrease the incidence of urge incontinence, and it can help a male who develops urinary incontinence following prostatectomy.
- For a patient with stress, urge, and mixed urinary incontinence, teach pelvic muscle rehabilitation and bladder inhibition, using biofeedback therapy.

Pharmacologic treatment
- Expect to give anticholinergic agents, such as oxybutynin, dicyclomine, and propantheline to a patient with detrusor instability. They're the first-line pharmacologic therapy because they block contraction by the normal bladder (probably the unstable bladder as well).
- Expect to give alpha-adrenergic agonist drugs, such as phenylpropanolamine and pseudoephedrine, to a female patient with stress incontinence. They're the first-line therapy because they may increase bladder outlet resistance.
- Be aware that estrogen (oral or vaginal) may be considered as an adjunctive pharmacologic agent for a postmenopausal woman with stress or mixed incontinence because it may increase bladder outlet resistance.

---

that the body can adapt well to one kidney. If he's having an abdominal or flank incision, teach deep-breathing and coughing exercises.

EVALUATION
Achievement of patient outcomes determines the success of collaborative management. For the patient with urinary calculi, evaluation focuses on improved urinary elimination, adequate intake and output, pain relief, infection control and prevention, and adequate knowledge of self-care. (See *After urinary calculi.*)

Urinary incontinence

Urinary incontinence is the uncontrollable passage of urine. Transient or permanent, it may involve large volumes of urine or scant dribbling.

Urinary incontinence takes several forms. Stress incontinence refers to intermittent leakage caused by a sudden physical strain, such as a cough, sneeze, or quick movement. Overflow incontinence is a dribble resulting from urine retention, which fills the bladder and prevents it from contracting with sufficient force to expel a urine stream. Urge incontinence refers to the inability to suppress a sudden urge to urinate. To-tal incontinence is continuous leakage, when the bladder can't retain any urine.

CAUSES
Urinary incontinence is caused by bladder abnormalities or neurologic disorders. A long list of conditions may set it off: benign prostatic hyperplasia, bladder calculus, bladder cancer, cerebrovascular accident, diabetic neuropathy, Guillain-Barré syndrome, multiple sclerosis, prostatic cancer, chronic prostatitis, spinal cord injury, and urethral stricture. It may also follow prostatectomy as a result of urethral sphincter damage. Diuretics, sedatives, hypnotics, antipsychotics, anticholinergics and alpha antagonists are also associated with urinary incontinence.

DIAGNOSIS AND TREATMENT
If the problem is due to weak musculature, the doctor may prescribe Kegel exercises to strengthen the pelvic floor. Bladder retraining programs also may help. In some cases, treatment may include surgery.

COLLABORATIVE MANAGEMENT
Care of the patient with urinary incontinence focuses on ending incontinence, preventing any infection, and teaching self-care. (See *Correcting urinary incontinence.*)

ASSESSMENT

Ask the patient about his voiding and incontinence history. Obtain a medical history, especially noting urinary tract infections and medication history. After the patient voids, inspect the urethral meatus for obvious inflammation or anatomic defect. Have a female patient bear down; note any urine leakage. Gently palpate the abdomen for bladder distention, which signals urine retention. Perform a complete neurologic assessment, noting motor and sensory function and muscle atrophy.

After diagnosis by assessment and history, voiding studies may evaluate the patient's status.

NURSING DIAGNOSES AND COLLABORATIVE PROBLEMS

Based on the following nursing diagnoses, you'll establish patient outcomes.

Altered urinary elimination related to underlying cause of incontinence. The patient will:
- maintain adequate urinary elimination through natural or artificial means
- recognize and report changes in urinary elimination pattern to the doctor
- adhere to the prescribed treatment plan.

Risk for infection related to inadequate voiding patterns. The patient will:
- remain free from signs and symptoms of infection
- develop regular voiding patterns.

Self-esteem disturbance related to urinary incontinence. The patient will:
- verbalize feelings
- develop positive attitude toward dealing with his condition.

PLANNING AND IMPLEMENTATION

These measures help the patient with urinary incontinence.
- Encourage adequate intake of fluids.
- Maintain accurate intake and output records.
- Institute a bladder regimen training pattern, such as catheterization, voiding schedule, and exercises, as established.
- Include family members in the training program.
- Encourage positive self-attitude and allow your patient to express his feelings about the disorder.
- Discuss sexual activities. The incontinent patient will feel embarrassed and worried about sexual function, so provide emotional support.
- Enlist the aid of support groups and counseling.

Patient teaching
- Reinforce bladder training program instructions and scheduling.
- Prepare the patient for diagnostic tests and workups.
- Teach him how to perform intermittent self-catheterization, if appropriate.
- If surgery is required, teach him about self-care for after the procedure.

EVALUATION

Achievement of patient outcomes determines the success of collaborative management. For the patient with urinary incontinence, evaluation focuses on control of incontinence with return to urinary elimination patterns within acceptable parameters, absence of infection, ability to perform self-care, and adequate knowledge of measures to promote urinary elimination.

Urinary tract infection, lower

Cystitis (infection of the bladder) and urethritis (infection of the urethra) are the two forms of lower urinary tract infection (UTI). They're nearly 10 times more common in females than in males (except in older males) and affect 10% to 20% of all females at least once.

In males, lower UTIs typically are associated with anatomic or physiologic abnormalities and therefore need close evaluation. Most UTIs respond readily to treatment, but recurrence and resistant bacterial flare-up during therapy are possible.

If untreated, chronic UTI can seriously damage the urinary tract lining. Pyelonephritis and other infections of adjacent organs and structures are possible. When this happens, the prognosis is poor.

CAUSES

Most lower UTIs result from ascending infection by a single gram-negative, enteric bacterium, such as *Escherichia coli, Klebsiella, Proteus, Enterobacter, Pseudomonas,* and *Serratia.* In a patient with neurogenic bladder, an indwelling urinary catheter, or a fistula between the intestine and bladder, a lower UTI may result from simultaneous infection with multiple pathogens.

In almost all patients, recurrent lower UTIs result from reinfection by the same organism or by some new pathogen. In the remaining patients, recurrence reflects persistent infection, usually from renal calculi, chronic bacterial prostatitis, or a structural anomaly that's a source of infection. The high rate of lower UTI among females probably relates to natural anatomic features that foster infection.

Studies suggest that infection results from a breakdown in local defense mechanisms in the bladder that allows bacteria to invade the bladder mucosa and multiply. These bacteria aren't readily eliminated by normal urination.

Bacterial flare-up during treatment usually is caused by the pathogen's resistance to the prescribed antimicrobial therapy. Even a small number of bacteria (fewer than 10,000/ml) in a midstream urine specimen obtained during treatment casts doubt on the effectiveness of treatment.

DIAGNOSIS AND TREATMENT
The following tests are used to diagnose lower UTI: microscopic urinalysis, clean-catch urinalysis, sensitivity testing, and voiding cystoureterography or excretory urography.

Appropriate antimicrobials are the treatment of choice for most initial lower UTIs. A 7- to 10-day course of antibiotics is standard, but studies suggest that a single dose or a 3- to 5-day regimen may be sufficient to render the urine sterile. (Older adults may still need the longer course to fully benefit from antibiotics.) If a culture shows that urine still isn't sterile after 3 days of antibiotic therapy, the bacteria probably are resistant, and require a different antimicrobial.

A single dose of amoxicillin or co-trimoxazole may succeed for females with acute, uncomplicated UTI. A urine culture taken 1 to 2 weeks later will show whether the infection has been eradicated. Recurrent infections from infected renal calculi, chronic prostatitis, or structural abnormalities may require surgery. Prostatitis also requires long-term antibiotic therapy. In patients without these predisposing conditions, long-term, low-dose antibiotic therapy is the treatment of choice.

COLLABORATIVE MANAGEMENT
Care of the patient with a lower UTI focuses on eliminating the infection and teaching prevention.

ASSESSMENT
The patient may complain of urinary urgency and frequency, dysuria, bladder cramps or spasms, itching, a feeling of warmth during urination, nocturia, and urethral discharge (in men). Other complaints include low back pain, malaise, nausea, vomiting, pain or tenderness over the bladder, chills, and flank pain. Inflammation of the bladder wall also causes hematuria and fever.

NURSING DIAGNOSES AND COLLABORATIVE PROBLEMS
Based on the following nursing diagnoses, you'll establish patient outcomes.

Altered urinary elimination related to inflammation of the lower urinary tract. The patient will:
■ comply with antibiotic therapy
■ report that signs and symptoms of abnormal urinary elimination are diminishing
■ regain and maintain normal urinary elimination.
Risk for infection related to high incidence of recurrence of UTI. The patient will:
■ take precautions to prevent recurrence of UTI
■ communicate an understanding of the early signs and symptoms of UTI that should be reported
■ remain free from recurrent UTIs, as exhibited by a normal urinalysis and the absence of signs and symptoms of UTI.
Pain related to bladder spasms and cramps. The patient will:
■ report a decrease in perineal discomfort after taking sitz baths or applying warm compresses
■ describe when and how to use a topical antiseptic correctly for pain relief
■ become pain-free when the UTI is eliminated.

PLANNING AND IMPLEMENTATION
These measures help your patient with UTI.
■ If ordered, give nitrofurantoin macrocrystals with milk or meals, to prevent GI distress.
■ Collect all urine specimens for culture and sensitivity testing carefully and promptly.
■ Monitor the patient for GI disturbances from antimicrobial therapy and for other possible adverse reactions.
■ Assess for complications of UTI.
■ Evaluate the patient's voiding pattern.
■ If sitz baths don't relieve perineal discomfort, apply warm compresses sparingly to the perineum, but be careful not to burn the patient.
■ Apply topical antiseptics to the urethral meatus, as necessary.

Patient teaching
■ Incorporate knowledge of risk factors into your teaching plan. (See *UTI risk factors,* page 392.)
■ Explain the nature and purpose of antimicrobial therapy. Emphasize the importance of completing the prescribed course of therapy or, with long-term prophylaxis, of strictly adhering to the ordered dosage.
■ Familiarize the patient with prescribed medications and their possible adverse effects. If antibiotics cause GI distress, explain that taking nitrofurantoin macrocrystals with milk or a meal can help prevent such problems. If therapy includes phenazopyridine, warn the patient that this drug turns urine red-orange.
■ Explain that an uncontaminated midstream urine specimen is essential for accurate diagnosis. Before collection, teach the female patient to clean the per-

UTI risk factors

Certain factors increase the risk of urinary tract infections (UTIs). They include natural anatomic variations, trauma or invasive procedures, urinary tract obstructions, and urine reflux.

Natural anatomic variations

Females are more prone to UTI than males because the female urethra is shorter than the male urethra (about 1″ to 2″ [2.5 to 5 cm] compared with 7″ to 8″ [18 to 20 cm]). It's also closer to the anus than the male urethra. This proximity allows bacteria to enter the urethra from the vagina, perineum, or rectum or from a sexual partner.

Pregnant women are especially prone to UTIs because of hormonal changes and because the enlarged uterus exerts greater pressure on the ureters. This restricts urine flow, allowing bacteria to linger longer in the urinary tract.

In men, release of prostatic fluid serves as an antibacterial shield. Men lose this protection around age 50 when the prostate gland begins to enlarge. This enlargement, in turn, may promote urine retention.

Trauma or invasive procedures

Fecal matter, sexual intercourse, and instruments, such as catheters and cystoscopes, can introduce bacteria into the urinary tract to trigger infection.

Obstructions

A narrowed ureter or calculi lodged in the ureters or the bladder can obstruct urine flow. Slowed urine flow allows bacteria to remain and multiply, risking damage to the kidneys.

Reflux

Vesicourethral reflux results when pressure inside the bladder (caused by coughing or sneezing) pushes a small amount of urine from the bladder into the urethra. When the pressure returns to normal, the urine flows back into the bladder, bringing bacteria from the urethra with it.

In vesicoureteral reflux, urine flows from the bladder back into one or both ureters. The vesicoureteral valve normally shuts off reflux. However, damage can prevent the valve from doing its job.

Other risk factors

Urinary stasis can promote infection, which, if undetected, can spread to the entire urinary system. And because urinary tract bacteria thrive on sugars, diabetes also is a risk factor.

ineum by wiping from front to back and to keep the labia separated during urination.

■ Suggest warm sitz baths for relief of perineal discomfort.

■ To prevent recurrent lower UTIs, teach a female patient to carefully wipe the perineum from front to back and to thoroughly clean it with soap and water after bowel movements. If she's infection-prone, she should urinate immediately after sexual intercourse. Tell her never to postpone urination and to empty her bladder completely.

■ Tell the male patient that prompt treatment of predisposing conditions such as chronic prostatitis will help prevent recurrent UTIs.

■ Urge the patient to drink at least eight glasses (about 2 qt [2 L]) of fluids a day during treatment. More or less than this amount may alter the antimicrobial's effect. Be aware that an older adult may resist this suggestion because it requires frequent trips, possibly up and down the stairs, to urinate.

■ Explain that fruit juices, especially cranberry juice, and oral doses of vitamin C may help acidify urine and enhance the medication's action.

EVALUATION

Achievement of patient outcomes determines the success of collaborative management. For the patient with a lower UTI, evaluation focuses on absence of signs and symptoms of infection, relief of discomfort and infection, and adequate knowledge of signs and symptoms of infection and measures to prevent recurrence.

Treatments and procedures

Renal and metabolic disorders can adversely affect almost every body system. Treatments and procedures are performed to improve metabolic function and prevent additional complications.

CYSTECTOMY

Cystectomy is partial or total removal of the urinary bladder and surrounding structures. It's sometimes necessary to treat advanced bladder cancer or, rarely, other bladder disorders such as interstitial cystitis. Cystectomy may be partial, involving resection of a portion of the bladder wall; simple or total, involving resection of the entire bladder; or radical, involving muscle-invasive primary bladder carcinoma (extensive).

PROCEDURE
In a partial cystectomy, the surgeon makes a midline incision from the umbilicus to the symphysis pubis. He then opens the bladder and removes the tumor along with a small portion of healthy tissue. To complete the procedure, he closes the wound, leaving a Penrose drain and suprapubic catheter in place.

In a simple cystectomy, the surgeon first makes a midline abdominal incision. In this procedure, though, he removes the entire bladder, leaving only a portion of the urethra.

In a radical cystectomy, the surgeon additionally removes the seminal vesicles and prostate in male patients and the uterus, ovaries, fallopian tubes, and anterior vagina in female patients. Depending upon the extent of the cancer, the surgeon may also remove the urethra and surrounding lymph nodes.

To complete either a simple or radical cystectomy, the surgeon provides for urinary diversion by attaching the ureters to an external collection device, such as a cutaneous ureterostomy, ileal conduit, or continent urinary neobladder.

COLLABORATIVE MANAGEMENT
Care of the patient undergoing cystectomy requires thorough preparation, close monitoring, and intense patient teaching.

Preparation
- Review the surgery with the patient and family members or friends. Pay special attention to the patient's emotional state. Help allay his fears by listening to his concerns and answering his questions.
- If the patient is undergoing simple or radical cystectomy, he'll probably worry about the effects of a urinary diversion on his lifestyle. Reassure him that such diversion needn't interfere with his normal activities.
- Arrange for a visit by an enterostomal therapist, who can provide additional information.
- If the patient is scheduled for radical cystectomy, remember to address concerns about the inevitable loss of sexual or reproductive function.
- Explain that he will awaken in an intensive care unit (ICU) after a radical cystectomy. He will return to his own hospital room following a partial cystectomy unless complications occur in the perioperative period.
- Mention that he will have a nasogastric (NG) tube, a central venous catheter, and an indwelling urinary catheter in place and a drain at the surgical site. Tell him that he can't eat or drink until the return of bowel function and that he'll receive I.V. fluids during this period. After bowel function returns, he can resume oral fluids and eventually progress to solids.
- If possible, arrange for the patient and family members to visit the ICU before surgery to familiarize themselves with the unit and meet the staff.
- Perform a standard bowel preparation as ordered. Antibiotics given orally (such as neomycin) or parenterally (such as cefazolin) are used prophylactically to reduce colonic microbial flora. To further clean the bowel, high colonic enemas (given until they run clear) or oral polyethylene glycol-electrolyte solution (PEG-ES), a nonabsorbable osmotic agent, are given. Large amounts of PEG-ES (4 qt [4 L]) are given over 3 to 4 hours; diarrhea begins within 1 hour.

Monitoring and aftercare
Monitor the amount and character of urine drainage every hour. Report output of less than 1 oz (30 ml)/hour, which may indicate retention. (Other signs of retention include bladder distention and spasms in a partial cystectomy.) If output is low, check the patency of the indwelling urinary catheter or stoma, as appropriate, and irrigate as ordered.

Monitor vital signs closely. Watch especially for signs of hypovolemic shock: increased pulse and respiratory rate, hypotension, diaphoresis, and pallor. (Be especially alert for hemorrhage if the doctor has ordered anticoagulant therapy to reduce the risk of pulmonary embolism.) Periodically, inspect the stoma (if present) and incision site for bleeding and observe urine drainage for frank hematuria and clots. Slight hematuria normally occurs for several days after surgery but should clear thereafter. Test all drainage from the NG tube, abdominal drains, indwelling urinary catheter, and urine collection appliance for blood, and notify the doctor of positive findings.

Observe the wound site and all drainage for signs of infection. Change abdominal dressings frequently, using sterile technique.

Periodically ask the patient about incision pain and, if he has had a partial cystectomy, about bladder spasms as well. Provide analgesics as ordered. You may also be asked to give an antispasmodic such as oxybutynin.

To prevent pulmonary complications associated with prolonged immobility, encourage frequent position changes, coughing, deep breathing and, if possible, early ambulation. Assess respiratory status regularly.

Continue to offer the patient emotional support throughout the recovery period to help him accept changes in body image and, if appropriate, sexual function. If possible, refer the patient and family members for psychological and sexual counseling to further aid this adjustment.

Patient teaching

■ Explain to the patient that incision pain and fatigue will probably last for several weeks after discharge. Tell him to notify the doctor if these effects persist or worsen.

■ Tell him to watch for and report any signs or symptoms of urinary tract infection (UTI) (fever, chills, flank pain, and decreased urine volume) or wound infection (redness, swelling, and purulent drainage at the incision site).

■ Tell him to report persistent hematuria.

■ Make sure the patient or a family member understands how to care for his type of urinary diversion and where to obtain needed supplies.

■ If needed, arrange for visits by a home care nurse who can reinforce urinary diversion care measures and provide emotional support.

■ Consider referring him to a support group, such as a local chapter of the United Ostomy Association, if a stoma is present.

■ Stress the importance of follow-up examinations to evaluate healing and recurrence of cancer.

COMPLICATIONS

Immediately after surgery, potential complications include bleeding, hypotension, and nerve injury (such as to the genitofemoral or peroneal nerve). Later complications include anuria, stoma stenosis, UTI, pouch leakage, electrolyte imbalance, stenosis of the ureteroileal junction, and vascular compromise. Radical and simple cystectomy may also cause psychological problems relating to changes in the patient's body image and loss of sexual or reproductive function.

HEMODIALYSIS

Hemodialysis, a procedure to remove impurities from the blood, can be performed in an emergency in acute renal failure or as chronic long-term therapy in end-stage renal disease. In chronic renal failure, the frequency and duration of treatments depend on the patient's condition. Rarely, hemodialysis is done to treat acute poisoning or drug overdose.

Specially trained nurses usually perform the procedure in a kidney center or satellite unit. Home dialysis, another option, is more convenient for the patient and allows greater flexibility and comfort. However, only 30% of patients needing dialysis meet the medical and training requirements to undergo the procedure at home.

PROCEDURE

This procedure removes toxic wastes and other impurities from the blood of a patient with renal failure. In hemodialysis, blood is removed from the body through a surgically created access site, pumped through a filtration unit to remove toxins, and then returned to the body. The extracorporeal dialyzer works through a combination of osmosis, diffusion, and filtration.

Within the dialyzer, the patient's blood flows between coils, plates, or hollow fibers of semipermeable material, depending on the machine being used. Simultaneously, the dialysis solution is pumped around the other side under hydrostatic pressure.

Pressure and concentration gradients between blood and the dialysis solution remove toxic wastes and excess water. Because blood has higher concentrations of hydrogen ions and electrolytes other than those in the dialysis solution, these solutes diffuse across the semipermeable material into the solution. Conversely, glucose and acetate are more highly concentrated in the dialysis solution and so diffuse back across the semipermeable material into the blood. Through this mechanism, hemodialysis removes excess water and toxins, reverses acidosis, and corrects electrolyte imbalances.

By extracting by-products of protein metabolism—notably urea and uric acid—as well as creatinine and excess water, hemodialysis helps restore or maintain acid-base and electrolyte balance and prevent complications associated with uremia.

Hemodialysis begins with connection of the blood lines from the dialyzer to needles placed in the patient's venous access site. After all connections have been made, blood samples are drawn for laboratory analysis.

When the pump is switched on, hemodialysis begins at a blood flow rate of 3 to 4 oz (90 to 120 ml)/minute. If heparin is used to prevent blood coagulation problems, a loading dose of 1,000 to 3,000 U is injected in the port on the arterial line. Blood pressure and vital signs are checked periodically; if stable, the blood flow rate is gradually increased to about 10 oz (300 ml)/minute and maintained at this level, unless there are complications. Depending on the patient's condition, dialysis continues for 3 to 5 hours.

To end the treatment, new blood samples are checked, the blood remaining in the dialyzer is returned to the patient, and the needles are removed from the venous access site.

COLLABORATIVE MANAGEMENT

Care of the patient undergoing hemodialysis requires thorough preparation, close monitoring, and intense patient teaching.

Preparation

If this is the patient's first hemodialysis session, help him understand the purpose of the treatment and what to expect during and after the procedure. Explain that he'll undergo surgery first to create vascular access. (See *Hemodialysis access sites.*)

Hemodialysis access sites

Hemodialysis requires vascular access. The site and type will vary, depending on the expected duration of dialysis, the surgeon's preference, and the patient's condition.

Arteriovenous fistula

To create a fistula, the surgeon makes an incision into the patient's wrist, then a small incision in the side of an artery and another in the side of a vein. He sutures the edges of these incisions together to make a common opening 1″ to 3″ (2.5 to 7.5 cm) long.

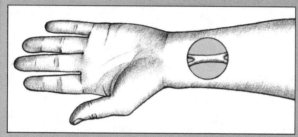

Arteriovenous shunt

To create a shunt, the surgeon makes an incision in the patient's wrist or (rarely) an ankle. He then inserts a 6″ to 10″ (15 to 25.5 cm) transparent Silastic cannula into an artery and another into a vein. Finally, he tunnels the cannulas out through incisions and connects them with a short piece of Teflon tubing.

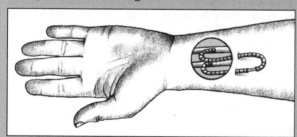

Arteriovenous graft

To create a graft, the surgeon makes an incision in the patient's forearm, upper arm, or thigh. He then tunnels a natural or synthetic graft under the skin and sutures the distal end to an artery and the proximal end to a vein.

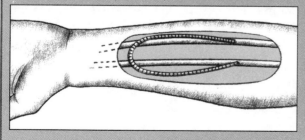

Subclavian vein catheterization

Using the Seldinger technique, the surgeon inserts an introducer needle into the subclavian vein. He then inserts a guide wire through the introducer needle and removes the needle. Using the guide wire, he then threads a 5″ to 12″ (12.5 to 30.5 cm) plastic or Teflon catheter (with a Y-hub) into the vein.

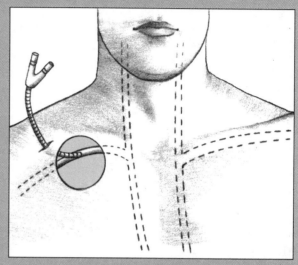

Femoral vein catheterization

Using the Seldinger technique, the surgeon inserts an introducer needle into the left or right femoral vein. He then inserts a guide wire through the introducer needle and removes the needle. Using the guide wire, he threads a 5″ to 12″ plastic or Teflon catheter into the vein. He may use a single catheter with a Y-hub or two catheters, one for inflow and another placed about 1″ (2.5 cm) distal to the first for outflow.

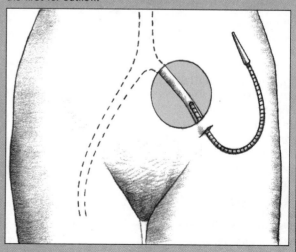

After vascular access has been created and the patient is ready for dialysis, weigh him and take his vital signs. Remember to measure blood pressure in the other arm while he's both in a supine position and standing.

As ordered, prepare the hemodialysis equipment, following the manufacturer's guidelines and the facility's protocol. Maintain strict aseptic technique to avoid introducing pathogens into the patient's bloodstream.

Place the patient in a supine position and make him as comfortable as possible. Keep the venous access site well supported and resting on a sterile drape or sterile barrier shield.

Monitoring and aftercare

Follow Occupational Safety and Health Administration guidelines by wearing appropriate gloves and protective eye shields throughout the procedure.

Once every 30 minutes, check and record vital signs to detect possible complications. Fever may indicate infection from pathogens in the dialysate or equipment; notify the doctor, who may prescribe an antipyretic, an antibiotic, or both. Hypotension may indicate hypovolemia or decreased hematocrit; give blood or I.V. fluid supplements, as ordered. Rapid respirations may signal hypoxemia; give supplemental oxygen, as ordered.

Approximately every hour, draw a blood sample for analysis of clotting time. Using the dialyzing unit's bed scale or a portable scale, weigh the patient regularly to ensure adequate ultrafiltration during treatment. Also periodically check the dialyzer's blood lines to make sure all connections are secure, and monitor the lines for clotting.

Assess the patient for headache, muscle twitching, backache, nausea or vomiting, and seizures, which may indicate disequilibrium syndrome caused by rapid fluid removal and electrolyte changes. If this syndrome occurs, notify the doctor immediately; he may reduce the blood flow rate or stop dialysis. Muscle cramps also may result from rapid fluid and electrolyte shifts. As ordered, relieve cramps by injecting normal saline solution into the venous return line.

Observe for signs of internal bleeding: apprehension; restlessness; pale, cold, clammy skin; excessive thirst; hypotension; rapid, weak, thready pulse; increased respirations; and decreased body temperature. Report these signs immediately and prepare to decrease heparinization. The doctor also may order blood transfusions.

Be especially alert for signs of air embolism—a potentially fatal complication characterized by sudden hypotension, dyspnea, chest pain, cyanosis, and a weak, rapid pulse. If these signs or symptoms develop, turn the patient onto his left side and lower the head of the bed (to help keep air bubbles on the right side of his body, where they're absorbed by the pulmonary artery); call the doctor immediately.

Monitor the venous access site for bleeding. If bleeding is excessive, maintain pressure on the site and notify the doctor. To prevent clotting and other blood flow problems, make sure the arm used for venous access isn't used for any other procedure, including I.V. line insertion, blood pressure monitoring, and venipuncture. At least four times a day, assess circulation at the access site by auscultating for bruits and palpating for thrills.

Remember to record the patient's food and fluid intake, and encourage him to comply with prescribed restrictions, such as limited protein, potassium, and sodium intake; increased caloric intake; and decreased fluid intake.

Patient teaching

■ Teach the patient how to care for the venous access site, cleaning the incision daily with hydrogen peroxide solution and drying it to prevent infection.

■ Tell him to notify the doctor of pain, swelling, redness, or drainage in the accessed arm. Teach him how to use a stethoscope to auscultate for bruits.

■ Explain that once the access site has healed (usually 10 to 14 days), he may use the arm freely.

■ Remind him not to allow any treatments or procedures on the accessed arm, including blood pressure measurement and needle punctures.

■ Warn him to avoid putting excessive pressure on the arm; for instance, don't sleep on it, wear constricting clothing, or lift heavy objects.

■ Instruct him to avoid showering, bathing, or swimming for several hours after dialysis.

■ Teach him exercises for the affected arm to promote venous dilation and enhance blood flow. One week after surgery, he should squeeze a small rubber ball or other soft object for 15 minutes, four times daily. Two weeks after surgery, he should apply a tourniquet to the upper arm, above the fistula site, making sure it's snug but not tight. Then, he should squeeze the rubber ball for 5 minutes, four times daily. After the incision has healed completely, he should perform the exercise with the arm submerged in warm water.

■ If the patient will perform hemodialysis at home, reinforce all aspects of the procedure. Give him the phone number of the dialysis center and encourage him to call if he has any questions. Also encourage him to arrange for a companion during dialysis in case any problems arise.

■ Encourage him to contact the American Association of Kidney Patients or the National Kidney Foundation for information and support.

COMPLICATIONS

Life-threatening complications may occur during or after hemodialysis, such as dialysis disequilibrium syndrome, air embolism, excessive bleeding, infections (sepsis, hepatitis), and acquired immunodeficiency syndrome. More common but less serious complications include hypotension, headache, nausea, malaise, vomiting, dizziness, fever, muscle cramps, and chronic anemia. Complications of chronic hemodialysis include arteriosclerotic cardiovascular disease, heart failure, stroke, gastric ulcers, and bone problems secondary to altered calcium metabolism.

ILEAL CONDUIT

Ileal conduit or uteteroileal urinary conduit is a type of urinary diversion that provides an alternate route for urine excretion when pathology impedes normal flow through the bladder. Most commonly done in patients who've undergone a cystectomy, diversion surgery also helps patients with a congenital urinary tract defect; a severe, unmanageable urinary tract infection that threatens renal function; an injury to the ureters, bladder, or urethra; an obstructive malignancy; or a neurogenic bladder.

PROCEDURE

The most common urinary diversion, ileal conduit involves anastomosis of the ureters to a small portion of the ileum excised especially for the procedure, followed by the creation of a stoma from one end of the ileal segment. (See *View of the ileal conduit.*) Because the ileum makes a much larger stoma than a ureter, an ileal conduit is generally easier to care for than a ureterostomy. Like the cutaneous ureterostomy, the patient will wear an external collection device at all times.

After the patient is anesthetized, the surgeon makes a midline or paramedial abdominal incision. To construct an ileal conduit, the surgeon excises a 6″ to 8″ (15- to 20.5-cm) segment of the ileum (also taking its mesentery to help preserve tissue viability) and then anastomoses the remaining ileal ends to maintain intestinal integrity. Next, he dissects the ureters from the bladder and implants them in the ileal segment. He then sutures one end of the ileal segment closed and brings the other end through the abdominal wall to form a stoma.

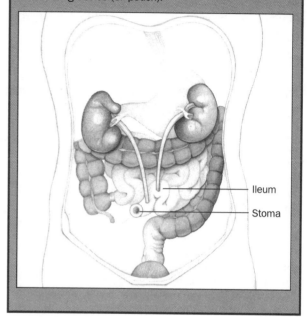

View of the ileal conduit

This procedure diverts urine through a segment of the ileum to a stoma on the abdomen (as shown). Because urine empties continuously, the patient will need to wear a collecting device (or pouch).

Ileum
Stoma

COLLABORATIVE MANAGEMENT

Care of the patient undergoing the ileal conduit procedure requires thorough preparation, close monitoring, and intense patient teaching.

Preparation

Review the planned surgery with the patient, reinforcing the doctor's explanations with simple anatomic diagram. Explain to the patient that he'll receive a general anesthetic and have a nasogastric (NG) tube in place after surgery.

If appropriate, prepare the patient for the appearance and general location of the stoma. For example, for an ileal conduit, explain that the stoma will sit in the lower abdomen, probably below the waistline.

Ensure that the patient having a continent internal ileal reservoir understands that his "new bladder" won't function identically to the natural bladder. If the reservoir is to attach to the external skin, explain that the stoma sits flush with the skin of the anterior abdominal wall, and that its exact location is generally decided during surgery.

Review the enterostomal therapist's explanation of the urine collection device or catheterization procedure planned for after surgery. Reassure the patient that he'll receive complete training on how to manage urine drainage after he returns from surgery.

If possible, arrange a visit by a well-adjusted patient who's undergone a similar procedure. He can provide a firsthand account of the operation and offer some insight into the realities of ongoing care of urinary drainage. Include family members in all aspects of preoperative teaching—especially if they'll be providing much of the routine care after discharge.

Before surgery, prepare the bowel to reduce the risk of postoperative infection from intestinal flora. As ordered, maintain the patient on a low-residue or clear liquid diet and give a cleansing enema and an antimicrobial drug, such as erythromycin or neomycin. Other possible measures may include total parenteral nutrition (TPN) or fluid replacement therapy for debilitated patients and prophylactic I.V. antibiotics.

Monitoring and aftercare

After surgery, monitor the patient's vital signs hourly, until they're stable. Carefully check and record urine output; report any decrease, which could indicate obstruction from postoperative edema or ureteral stenosis. Observe urine drainage for pus and blood; keep in mind that urine is often blood-tinged initially but should rapidly clear.

Record the amount, color, and consistency of drainage from the incision or stoma drain, ureteral stents (if present), and NG tube. Notify the doctor of any urine leakage from the drain or suture line—an indicator of developing complications such as hydronephrosis. Watch for signs or symptoms of peritonitis (fever, abdominal distention and pain), which can develop from intraperitoneal urine leakage.

Check dressings frequently and change them at least once each shift. (The doctor will probably perform the first dressing change.) When changing dressings, check the suture line for redness, swelling, and drainage.

Maintain fluid and electrolyte balance and continue I.V. replacement therapy, as ordered. Provide TPN, if necessary, to ensure adequate nutrition.

Perform routine ostomy maintenance, as indicated. Make sure the collection device fits tightly around the stoma; allow no more than a ⅛" (0.3-cm) margin of skin between the stoma and the device's faceplate. Regularly check the appearance of the stoma and peristomal skin. The stoma should appear bright red; if it becomes deep red or bluish, suspect a problem with blood flow and notify the doctor. It should also be smooth; report any dimpling or retraction, which may point to stenosis. Check the peristomal skin for irritation or breakdown. Remember that the main cause of irritation is urine leakage around the edges of the collection device's faceplate. If you detect leakage, change the device, taking care to properly apply the skin sealer to ensure a tight fit. Enlist the aid of the enterostomal therapist to help with skin care.

If the patient has a continent internal ileal reservoir, irrigate the drainage tube as ordered (usually every 2 to 8 hours) with about 2 oz (60 ml) of normal saline solution to maintain its patency. To avoid abdominal distention during the postoperative period and allow suture lines to heal, perform irrigations gently. Discontinue them when mucus evacuation stops and return is clear.

If the patient's skin shows signs of breakdown, clean the area with warm water and pat it dry; apply a light dusting of karaya powder and a thin layer of protective dressing. If you detect severe excoriation, notify the doctor.

Provide emotional support throughout the recovery period to help the patient adjust to the stoma and collection pouch or to self-catheterization, as indicated. Assure him that the pouch shouldn't interfere with his lifestyle and that he can eventually resume all of his former activities.

Patient teaching

■ Make sure the patient and family members or friends understand and can properly perform stoma care and change the ostomy pouch.
■ With a continent internal ileal reservoir, be sure they can care for the pouch drainage tube until it's removed (usually 3 weeks postoperatively) and then empty the pouch correctly, using either passive emptying or intermittent self-catheterization.
■ Tell them to watch for and report signs or symptoms of complications, such as fever, chills, flank or abdominal pain, and pus or blood in the urine.
■ Tell the patient that he probably can return to work soon after discharge, unless he does heavy lifting and the doctor advises waiting.
■ Explain that he can safely participate in most sports, even such strenuous ones as skiing, skydiving, and scuba diving. Exceptions are contact sports, such as football and wrestling.
■ If the patient expresses doubts or insecurities about his sexuality, related to the stoma and collection device, refer him for sexual counseling.
■ Assure the female ostomy patient that pregnancy should cause her no special problems, but urge her to consult with her doctor before she becomes pregnant.
■ Stress the importance of follow-up appointments with the doctor and enterostomal therapist to evaluate reservoir function and stoma care and make any necessary changes in equipment. For instance, stoma shrinkage, which normally occurs within 8 weeks af-

ter surgery, may require a change in pouch size to ensure a tight fit.

■ Refer the patient to a support group such as the United Ostomy Association.

COMPLICATIONS

Complications, such as tumor recurrence in the urethra and frequent nocturnal enuresis, can affect up to 50% of patients and are major drawbacks of the procedure. Postoperative complications of urinary diversion surgery include skin breakdown around the stoma site, wound infection or wound dehiscence, urinary extravasation, ureteral obstruction, small bowel obstruction, peritonitis, hydronephrosis, and stomal gangrene.

Delayed complications include ureteral obstruction, stomal stenosis, pyelonephritis, renal calculi, and electrolyte disturbances (from contact between the urine and the absorptive intestinal mucosa), especially hypokalemia. If chronic pyelonephritis occurs over a period of years, end-stage renal disease is possible.

In addition, the patient with a continent internal ileal reservoir may experience incontinence and, if the reservoir is connected to the urethra, frequent urinary tract infections and tumor recurrence (if cystectomy was performed because of bladder cancer).

Patients also commonly suffer psychological problems, such as depression and anxiety, related to altered body image and concern about lifestyle changes associated with the stoma and urine drainage. Even patients with a continent urinary reservoir attached to the urethra may still have a grief reaction to the loss of their natural bladder.

LITHOTRIPSY

Extracorporeal shock wave lithotripsy (ESWL), stone cracking by shock wave, is performed as a preventive measure in a patient with potentially obstructive calculi or as an emergency treatment for an acute obstruction. Because ESWL is noninvasive, the procedure generally is done in the outpatient department, and the patient can resume normal activities immediately after discharge. ESWL also minimizes many of the potentially serious complications associated with invasive methods of calculi removal, such as infection and hemorrhage.

ESWL isn't suitable for all patients, however. For instance, it may be contraindicated during pregnancy or in a patient with a pacemaker (risks electrical interference), with urinary or biliary tract obstruction distal to the calculi (blocks passage of fragments), with renal or gallbladder cancer, or with calculi that are fixed to the kidney, ureter, or gallbladder or located below the level of the iliac crest. Large or multiple calculi may require repeat treatments.

PROCEDURE

A noninvasive procedure for removing obstructive renal calculi or gallstones, ESWL uses high-energy shock waves to break up the calculi and allow their normal passage. The patient is anesthetized and placed in a water tank. His affected kidney or the area containing the gallstone is positioned over an electric spark generator that creates the shock waves that shatter calculi without damaging surrounding tissue. Afterward, the patient is easily able to excrete the fine gravel-like remains of the calculi through the urinary tract or biliary ductal system.

Percutaneous ultrasonic lithotripsy (PUL) may replace ESWL or follow it to remove residual fragments. In this technique, an ultrasonic probe inserted through a nephrostomy tube into the renal pelvis generates ultrahigh-frequency sound waves to shatter calculi, while continuous suctioning removes the fragments. PUL is particularly useful for radiolucent calculi lodged in the kidney, which aren't treatable by ESWL.

Some doctors prefer to perform PUL in two stages, with nephrostomy tube insertion on the first day followed by lithotripsy a day or two later, after intrarenal bleeding has subsided and the calculi are more visible. The day before treatment, the patient will have an I.V. pyelography or lower abdominal X-rays to locate the calculi.

Before undergoing ESWL, the patient receives a general or epidural anesthetic and has an I.V. line and indwelling urinary catheter inserted and electrocardiogram (ECG) electrodes attached. He's then placed in a semireclining position on the machine's hydraulic stretcher and lowered into the water tank. In the tank, the patient's position is adjusted so that the shock-wave generator focuses directly on the calculi. Biplane fluoroscopy confirms proper positioning.

To prevent disruption of the patient's cardiac rhythm, the shock waves are synchronized to the patient's R waves and fired during diastole. The number of waves fired depends on the size and composition of the stone—500 to 2,000 shocks during a treatment. After the shocks are delivered, the patient is removed from the tub and the ECG electrodes are removed.

COLLABORATIVE MANAGEMENT

Care of the patient undergoing lithotripsy requires thorough preparation, close monitoring, and intense patient teaching.

Preparation

Review the doctor's explanation of ESWL with the patient, if needed, and answer any questions. Explain who will perform the treatment and where, and that it should take 30 minutes to 1 hour. Tell him that he'll receive a general or epidural anesthetic, depending on the doctor's preference, and that he probably won't feel pain. However, if the patient is to receive ESWL for gallstones, warn him that he may experience mild pain if his gallbladder spasms trying to expel the stone fragments. Tell the patient that he'll have an I.V. line and indwelling urinary catheter in place for a short time after ESWL.

Ideally, arrange for the patient to see the ESWL device before his first scheduled treatment. Explain its components and how they work.

Monitoring and aftercare

Check the patient's vital signs regularly and notify the doctor of any abnormal findings.

Maintain indwelling urinary catheter and I.V. line patency and closely monitor intake and output. Strain all urine for calculi fragments for analysis. Note urine color and test pH. Remember that slight hematuria normally appears for several days after ESWL. However, notify the doctor of any frank or persistent bleeding.

Increase fluids and encourage ambulation as early as possible after treatment to help him pass calculi fragments. To help remove any particles lodged in gravity-dependent kidney pockets, tell the patient to lie face down with his head and shoulders over the edge of the bed for about 10 minutes. Have him perform this maneuver twice a day. To help it work, encourage fluids 30 to 45 minutes in advance.

Assess for pain on the treated side and give analgesics, as ordered. Remember that severe pain may indicate biliary or ureteral obstruction from new calculi; promptly report such findings to the doctor.

Patient teaching

■ Tell the patient to drink 3 to 4 qt (3 to 4 L) of fluid each day for about a month after treatment. Explain that this will help him pass fragments and avoid new ones.

■ Teach him how to strain his urine for fragments. Tell him to strain all urine for the first week after treatment, and bring all fragments to his first follow-up appointment, in the container you've provided.

■ Discuss expected adverse effects of ESWL, including pain in the treated side as fragments pass, slight redness or bruising, blood-tinged urine (for days, after removal of renal calculi), and mild GI upset. Reassure him that these effects are normal. However, tell him to report severe unremitting pain, persistent hema-

turia, inability to void, fever and chills, or recurrent nausea and vomiting.

■ Encourage him to resume normal activities, including exercise and work, as soon as he feels able (unless the doctor countermands). Explain that physical activity will help him pass calculi fragments.

■ Stress compliance with any special dietary or drug regimen designed to reduce the risk for new calculi formation.

COMPLICATIONS

Complications associated with ESWL include hemorrhage and hematoma formation.

NEPHRECTOMY

The surgical removal of a kidney, nephrectomy is the treatment of choice for advanced renal cell carcinoma that's refractory to chemotherapy and radiation. The procedure also is used to harvest a healthy kidney for transplantation. And when conservative treatments fail, nephrectomy treats renal trauma, infection, hypertension, hydronephrosis, and inoperable renal calculi.

PROCEDURE

Nephrectomy is unilateral or bilateral. Unilateral nephrectomy, the more commonly performed procedure, usually doesn't interfere with renal function as long as one healthy kidney remains. However, bilateral nephrectomy (removal of both kidneys) requires lifelong dialysis or transplantation to support renal function.

Four major types of nephrectomy are performed: partial nephrectomy removes only a portion of the kidney; simple nephrectomy removes the entire kidney; radical nephrectomy removes the entire kidney and the surrounding fat tissue; and nephroureterectomy removes the entire kidney, the perinephric fat, and the entire ureter. Except for variations in the extent of tissue removed, the surgical approach is basically the same.

To perform a unilateral nephrectomy, the surgeon makes a flank incision to expose the kidney. (Alternatively, he may make a thoracicoabdominal or transthoracic incision if extensive renovascular repair or radical excision of the kidney and surrounding structures is necessary, or if the patient has respiratory or cardiac dysfunction.) He then mobilizes the kidney, frees it of fat and adhesions, releases the lower pole, and locates the ureter and frees its upper third. He orders the ureter double-clamped, then cuts between the clamps and ligates both ends. Next, he frees and double-clamps the vascular pedicle. The renal artery is clamped first, followed by clamping of the renal vein. The kidney is then removed distal to the clamps. After resecting surrounding perinephric fat and the ureter, if necessary, he inserts a flank catheter and Penrose drain and sutures the wound closed.

COLLABORATIVE MANAGEMENT
Care of the patient undergoing nephrectomy requires thorough preparation, close monitoring, and intense patient teaching. (See *Managing nephrectomy care*, pages 402 and 403.)

Preparation
As with any organ excision, the patient will have many concerns and questions. He'll probably want to know how the surgery will affect his kidney function. If he's having unilateral nephrectomy, reassure him that one healthy kidney is all he'll need for adequate function. If he's scheduled for bilateral nephrectomy or removal of his only kidney, prepare him for radical changes in his lifestyle, most notably the need for regular dialysis. If appropriate, discuss the possibility of a future kidney transplant to restore normal function.

Describe postoperative measures. Tell him that he'll return from surgery with an indwelling urinary catheter in place to allow precise measurement of urine output and a nasogastric (NG) tube in place to prevent abdominal pain, distention, and vomiting. Explain that he won't receive food or fluids by mouth until bowel sounds have returned, but that he'll receive I.V. fluids. He'll also have a dressing and possibly a drain at the incision site. Prepare him for frequent dressing changes.

Stress the need for postoperative deep breathing and coughing to prevent pulmonary complications. Demonstrate these exercises, and have him practice them before surgery.

Ensure that the patient or a responsible family member has signed a consent form.

Monitoring and aftercare
Provide routine I.V. line, NG tube, and indwelling urinary catheter care. Carefully monitor the rate, volume, and type of I.V. fluids. Remember that mistakes in fluid therapy can be particularly devastating for a patient with only one kidney. Measure and record urine output, and notify the doctor if it falls below 50 ml/hour. Assess for signs of electrolyte imbalance and fluid overload.

Check the patient's dressing and drain every 4 hours for the first 24 to 48 hours, then once every shift to assess the amount and nature of drainage. Maintain drain patency.

The doctor probably will perform the first dressing change after surgery. Thereafter, you'll change the dressing whenever it becomes wet or once a day, using sterile technique and taking care not to dislodge the drain. During dressing changes, assess the suture line for swelling, redness, and purulent drainage.

Maintain food and fluid restrictions, as ordered. Periodically auscultate for bowel sounds. When they return and the patient is able to pass flatus (usually by the fourth day), notify the doctor and prepare to resume oral feedings. When oral intake is permitted, encourage fluids—up to 3 qt (3 L)/day.

Encourage coughing, deep breathing, incentive spirometry, and position changes. Regularly assess the patient's respiratory status. Be alert for signs of pulmonary embolism, especially 5 to 10 days after surgery. Watch for dyspnea, tachypnea, pleuritic chest pain, and hemoptysis. If any of these problems develops, immediately notify the doctor, raise the head of the patient's bed at least 30 degrees, and give oxygen.

To reduce the risk of deep vein thrombosis, encourage early and regular ambulation and apply antiembolism stockings, as ordered. Assess for signs and symptoms of deep vein thrombosis, such as leg pain, edema, and erythema.

Monitor for signs of hemorrhage and shock. Keep in mind that the risk of hemorrhage is greatest 8 to 12 days after surgery, owing to tissue sloughing.

Patient teaching
■ Teach the patient how to monitor intake and output at home, and explain how this helps assess renal function.
■ Instruct him to call the doctor immediately if he detects a significant decrease in urine output, a reliable sign of renal failure.
■ Tell him to notify the doctor if he experiences fever, chills, hematuria, or flank pain. Explain that these signs and symptoms may indicate urinary tract infection, a potentially serious complication.
■ If the patient has undergone nephrectomy to treat renal cell carcinoma, convey the importance of reporting any weight loss, bone pain, altered mental status, and paresthesia in the extremities—possible signs or symptoms of tumor metastasis.
■ Emphasize the importance of following the doctor's guidelines on fluid intake and dietary restrictions.
■ Inform the patient that he may experience incision pain and fatigue for several weeks after discharge; reassure him that these are normal postoperative effects.
■ Encourage him to refrain from strenuous exercise, heavy lifting, and sexual activity until his doctor grants permission.
■ Stress the need for regular follow-up examinations to evaluate kidney function and to assess for possible complications.

(Text continues on page 404.)

CLINICAL PATH

Managing nephrectomy care

	Day 1 (Surgery)	Day 2 (Postop Day 1)	Day 3 (Postop Day 2)	Day 4 (Postop Day 3)
CONSULTS	■ Social Service as needed (p.r.n.)			
TESTS	■ Complete blood count (CBC) ■ Blood chemistries	■ CBC ■ Blood chemistries	■ CBC ■ Blood chemistries ■ Chest X-ray p.r.n.	
TREATMENTS	■ I.V. ■ Incentive spirometer, leg exercises, coughing and deep breathing (C & DB) ■ Indwelling urinary catheter ■ Chest tube p.r.n. ■ Pneumatic antiembolism stockings (PAS) ■ Strict intake and output (I & O) ■ Vital signs (VS) every 4 hr	■ I.V. ■ Incentive spirometer, leg exercises, C & DB ■ Indwelling urinary catheter ■ Chest tube p.r.n. ■ PAS ■ Strict I & O ■ VS every 8 hr	■ I.V. ■ Incentive spirometer, leg exercises, C & DB ■ Indwelling urinary catheter ■ Chest tube discontinued p.r.n. ■ PAS ■ Strict I & O ■ VS every 8 hr	■ I.V. ■ Incentive spirometer ■ Indwelling urinary catheter discontinued ■ PAS discontinued; change to antiembolism stockings ■ Strict I & O ■ VS every 8 hr
MEDICATION	■ Patient-controlled analgesia (PCA) ■ I.V. antibiotics as ordered	■ PCA ■ I.V. antibiotics as ordered	■ PCA ■ I.V. antibiotics discontinued	■ PCA discontinued ■ I.M. or oral pain medication
DIET	■ Nothing by mouth (NPO)	■ NPO	■ NPO	■ As ordered
ACTIVITY	■ As ordered	■ As ordered	■ As ordered	■ As ordered
TEAM PROCESS	■ Patient history and assessment ■ Systems assessment ■ Assessment of dressing, incision, and drainage	■ Systems assessment	■ Systems assessment	■ Systems assessment
TEACHING	■ Pain management ■ Postop care instructions ■ Orientation to unit routine and policies ■ Review of plan of care ■ Fall prevention	■ Pain management ■ Postop care instructions ■ Fall prevention	■ Pain management ■ Postop care instructions ■ Fall prevention	■ Pain management ■ Postop care instructions
DISCHARGE PLANNING	■ Assess support network. ■ Reinforce length of stay.	■ Assess support network.		
NEEDS AND OUTCOMES	■ Patient's dressing is dry and moist. ■ Patient verbalizes relief of pain with medications given. ■ Patient and family verbalize understanding of fall-prevention plan. ■ Patient demonstrates proper use of incentive spirometer, leg exercises, and splinting. ■ Patient demonstrates proper use of PCA pump. ■ Patient and family verbalize understanding of plan of care and unit routine.	■ Patient's incision shows no redness, swelling, or drainage. ■ Patient demonstrates ability to get out of bed to chair with assistance. ■ Patient and family verbalize concerns about illness and hospitalization. ■ Patient and family verbalize understanding of diet regimen.	■ Patient's incision shows no redness, swelling, or drainage. ■ Patient is afebrile.	■ Patient voids clear urine without complaints. ■ Patient has no nausea, vomiting, or abdominal distention after eating. ■ Patient verbalizes relief of pain with medication. ■ Patient and family verbalize basic understanding of nature of the illness.
	Date met _____ Not met _____ Initials_____	Date met _____ Not met _____ Initials_____	Date met _____ Not met _____ Initials_____	Date met ___ Not met ___ Initials_____

Adapted with permission from North Shore University Hospital, NYU School of Medicine, Manhasset, N.Y. Courtesy of Center for Case Management, Inc., South Natick, Mass.

Day 5 (Postop Day 4)	Day 6 (Postop Day 5)	Day 7 (Postop Day 6)	Day 8 (Postop Day 7)
▪ Home care p.r.n.		▪ Home care p.r.n.	
▪ Blood chemistries			
▪ I.V. discontinued ▪ Antiembolism stockings ▪ VS every 8 hr ▪ I & O	▪ Antiembolism stockings ▪ VS every 8 hr ▪ I & O	▪ Antiembolism stockings ▪ Staples removed; changed to Steri-Strips ▪ I & O ▪ VS every 8 hr	▪ Antiembolism stockings discontinued ▪ VS every 8 hr
▪ Oral medication	▪ Oral medication ▪ Stool softener p.r.n. ▪ Sleep medication p.r.n.	▪ Oral medication ▪ Stool softener p.r.n. ▪ Sleep medication p.r.n.	▪ Prescription medications
▪ As ordered	▪ As ordered	▪ As ordered	▪ As ordered
▪ As ordered	▪ As ordered	▪ As ordered	▪ As ordered
▪ Systems assessment	▪ Systems assessment	▪ Systems assessment	▪ Systems assessment
▪ Postop care instructions	▪ Pain management ▪ Postop care instructions	▪ Postop care instructions ▪ Preprinted general surgery discharge instruction sheet given and reviewed	▪ Preprinted general surgery discharge instruction sheet and medication sheet reviewed with patient and family
▪ Assess support network.	▪ Assess support network.	▪ 24-hour written discharge notice given	▪ Discharge by 11 a.m. ▪ Follow-up appointment with doctor ▪ Written discharge instructions
▪ Patient's skin integrity is maintained. ▪ Patient can ambulate independently.	▪ Patient's incision is intact without redness, swelling, or drainage. ▪ Patient is afebrile. ▪ Patient and family verbalize signs and symptoms that are reportable and suggestive of complications.	▪ Patient participates in activities of daily living within limitations. ▪ Patient and family verbalize understanding of discharge instructions.	▪ Patient is afebrile. ▪ Patient and family verbalize understanding of discharge instructions.
Date met _____ *Not met* _____ *Initials*_____	*Date met* _____ *Not met* _____ *Initials*_____	*Date met* _____ *Not met* _____ *Initials*_____	*Date met* _____ *Not met* _____ *Initials*_____

COMPLICATIONS

Nephrectomy can cause serious complications. The most common are infection, hemorrhage, atelectasis, pneumonia, deep vein thrombosis, and pulmonary embolism.

PERITONEAL DIALYSIS

As a method of removing toxins from the blood, peritoneal dialysis has several advantages over hemodialysis—it's simpler, less costly, and less stressful. What's more, it's nearly as effective as hemodialysis, while posing fewer risks.

PROCEDURE

Like hemodialysis, peritoneal dialysis removes toxins from the blood of a patient with acute or chronic renal failure who doesn't respond to other treatments. But unlike hemodialysis, it uses the patient's peritoneal membrane as a semipermeable dialyzing membrane. In this technique, a hypertonic dialyzing solution is instilled through a catheter inserted into the peritoneal cavity. Then, by diffusion, excessive concentrations of electrolytes and uremic toxins in the blood move across the peritoneal membrane and into the dialysis solution. Next, by osmosis, excessive water in the blood does the same. After an appropriate dwelling time, the dialysis solution is drained, taking toxins and wastes with it.

Peritoneal dialysis is performed manually, by an automatic or semiautomatic cycler machine, or as continuous ambulatory peritoneal dialysis (CAPD). In manual dialysis, the nurse, the patient, or a family member instills dialyzing solution through the catheter into the peritoneal cavity, allows it to dwell for a specified time, and then drains it. Typically, this process is repeated for 6 to 8 hours at a time, five or six times a week.

The cycler machine requires sterile setup and connection technique, and then it automatically completes dialysis.

CAPD is performed by the patient himself. He fills a special plastic bag with dialyzing solution and then instills the solution through a catheter into his peritoneal cavity. While the solution remains in the peritoneal cavity, he can roll up the empty bag, place it under his clothing, and go about his normal activities. After 6 to 8 hours of dwelling time, he drains the spent solution into the bag, removes and discards the full bag, and attaches a new bag and instills a new batch of dialyzing solution. He repeats the process to ensure continuous dialysis 24 hours a day, 7 days a week. As its name implies, CAPD allows the patient to move around during dialysis and thus only minimally disrupts his lifestyle.

Some patients use CAPD in combination with an automatic cycler, in a treatment called continuous-cycling peritoneal dialysis (CCPD). In CCPD, the cycler performs dialysis at night while the patient sleeps and the patient performs CAPD in the daytime.

To begin dialysis, open the clamps on the infusion lines and infuse the prescribed amount of dialyzing solution over a period of 5 to 10 minutes. When the bottle is empty, immediately close the clamps to prevent air from entering the tubing.

Allow the solution to dwell in the peritoneal cavity for the prescribed length of time (usually between 10 minutes and 4 hours) so that excess water, electrolytes, and accumulated wastes can move from the blood through the peritoneal membrane and into the solution. At the completion of the prescribed dwelling time, open the outflow clamps and allow the solution to drain from the peritoneal cavity into the collection bag.

Repeat the infusion-dwell-drainage cycle, using new solution each time, for the prescribed solution amount and cycles. When dialysis is completed, put on sterile gloves and clamp the catheter with a small, sterile plastic clamp. Disconnect the inflow line from the catheter, taking care not to dislodge or pull on the catheter, and place a sterile protective cap over the catheter's distal end. Apply povidone-iodine or antibiotic ointment to the catheter insertion site with a sterile gauze sponge, then place two split-drain sponges around the site and secure them with tape.

COLLABORATIVE MANAGEMENT

Care of the patient undergoing peritoneal dialysis requires thorough preparation, close monitoring, and intense patient teaching.

Preparation

For the first-time peritoneal dialysis patient, explain the purpose of the treatment and what he can expect during and after the procedure. Tell him that first the doctor will insert a catheter into his abdomen to allow instillation of dialyzing solution; explain the appropriate insertion procedure.

Before catheter insertion, record the patient's baseline vital signs and weight. (Be sure to check blood pressure in both the supine and standing positions.) Ask him to urinate to reduce the risk of bladder perforation and increase comfort during catheter insertion. If he can't urinate, perform straight catheterization, as ordered, to drain the bladder.

While the patient is undergoing peritoneal catheter insertion, warm the dialysate to body temperature. The dialysate may be a 1.5%, 2.5%, or 4.25% dextrose solution, usually with heparin added to prevent clotting in the catheter. The dialysate should be clear and colorless. Add any prescribed drug at this time.

Next, put on a surgical mask and prepare the dialysis administration set. Place the drainage bag below the patient for gravity drainage, and connect the outflow tubing to it. Then, connect the dialysis infusion lines to the bags or bottles of dialyzing solution and hang the containers on an I.V. pole at the patient's bedside. Maintain sterile technique during solution and equipment preparation to avoid introducing pathogens into the patient's peritoneal cavity.

When the equipment and solution are ready, place the patient in a supine position, have him put on a surgical mask, and tell him to relax. Prime the tubing with solution, keeping the clamps closed, and connect one infusion line to the abdominal catheter. To test the catheter's patency, open the clamp on the infusion line and rapidly instill 17 oz (500 ml) of dialyzing solution into the patient's peritoneal cavity. Immediately unclamp the outflow line and let fluid drain into the collection bag; outflow should be brisk. Once you've established catheter patency, you're ready to start dialysis.

Monitoring and aftercare
During dialysis, monitor the patient's vital signs every 10 minutes until they stabilize, then every 2 to 4 hours or as ordered. Report any abrupt or significant changes.

Watch closely for developing complications. Peritonitis may manifest itself as fever, persistent abdominal pain and cramping, slow or cloudy dialysis drainage, swelling and tenderness around the catheter, and an increased white blood cell count. If you detect these signs and symptoms, notify the doctor and send a dialysate specimen to the laboratory for smear and culture.

Observe the outflow drainage for blood. Keep in mind that drainage is commonly blood tinged after catheter placement but should clear after a few fluid exchanges. Notify the doctor of bright red or persistent bleeding.

Watch for respiratory distress, which may indicate fluid overload or leakage of dialyzing solution into the pleural space. If it's severe, drain the patient's peritoneal cavity and call the doctor.

Periodically check the outflow tubing for clots or kinks that might obstruct drainage. If you cannot clear an obstruction, notify the doctor.

Have the patient change position frequently. Provide passive range-of-motion exercises, and encourage deep breathing and coughing. This will improve patient comfort, reduce the risk of skin breakdown and respiratory problems, and enhance dialysate drainage.

Periodically check the patient's weight, and report any gain. Using aseptic technique, change the catheter dressing every 24 hours or whenever it becomes wet or soiled.

To help prevent fluid imbalance, calculate the patient's fluid balance at the end of each dialysis session or after every 8-hour period in a longer session. Include both oral and I.V. fluid intake as well as urine output, wound drainage, and perspiration. Record and report any significant imbalance, either positive or negative.

Maintain adequate nutrition, following any prescribed diet. Keep in mind that the patient loses protein through the dialysis procedure and so requires protein replacement.

Patient teaching
■ If the patient will perform CAPD or CCPD at home, make sure he thoroughly understands and can do each step of the procedure. Normally, he'll go through a 2-week training program before beginning treatment on his own.
■ Warn the patient to wear a medical identification bracelet or carry a card identifying him as a dialysis patient and to keep the phone number of the dialysis center with him.
■ Tell him to watch for and report signs of infection and fluid imbalance. Make sure he knows how to take his vital signs to provide a record of response to treatment.
■ Stress the importance of follow-up appointments with the doctor and dialysis team to evaluate the success of treatment and detect any problems.
■ If possible, introduce him to other patients on peritoneal dialysis, to help him develop a support system.
■ Arrange for periodic visits by a home care nurse to assess his adjustment to CAPD or CCPD.

COMPLICATIONS
Peritoneal dialysis can lead to severe complications, most seriously peritonitis, when bacteria enters the peritoneal cavity through the catheter or the insertion site. Other complications include catheter obstruction from clots, lodgment against the abdominal wall, or kinking; hypotension; and hypovolemia from excessive plasma fluid removal.

RENAL TRANSPLANTATION
Ranking among the most commonly performed and most successful of all organ transplants, renal transplantation represents an alternative to dialysis for many patients with otherwise unmanageable end-stage renal disease. It also may sustain life in a patient who has suffered traumatic loss of renal function or in whom dialysis is contraindicated.

Renal transplantation, with a healthy organ from a living relative or cadaver donor, however, isn't performed on all patients who seemingly could benefit. For instance, severely debilitated, diabetic, elderly, or young patients generally aren't considered good candidates.

PROCEDURE

In this transplantation, the healthy kidney is implanted in the recipient's iliac fossa and anastomosed in place. The recipient's own kidneys usually aren't removed unless they're chronically infected, greatly enlarged, cancerous, or causing intractable hypertension. Because the recipient's own kidneys may secrete erythropoietin fluid, they're left in place to increase circulating hematocrit, to ease dialysis management, and to reduce blood transfusion requirements in case of transplant rejection.

With the patient under general anesthesia, the surgeon makes a curvilinear incision in the right or left lower quadrant, extending from the symphysis pubis to the anterior superior iliac spine and up to just below the thoracic cage. He exposes the iliac fossa with a self-retaining retractor, then performs segmental separation, ligature, and division of perivascular tissue. Next, he clamps the iliac vein and artery in preparation for anastomosis to the donor kidney's renal vein and artery.

Meanwhile, the donor kidney is prepared for transplantation. If a cadaver kidney is being used, it's removed from cold storage or a perfusion preparation machine. If the kidney is from a living donor, it's harvested in an adjacent operating room and placed in cold lactated Ringer's solution. Before transplantation, the donor kidney's renal artery is flushed with cold heparinized lactated Ringer's solution to prevent clogging. Then, the surgeon positions the kidney in a sling over the implantation site. (He never holds the kidney in his hands because this would warm it and possibly cause necrosis.)

The surgeon then implants the kidney in the retroperitoneal area of the iliac fossa, where it's protected by the hip bone. If a donor's left kidney is being used, the surgeon implants it in the recipient's right side; conversely, he implants a donor's right kidney in the recipient's left side. Doing so permits the renal pelvis to rest anteriorly and allows the new kidney's ureter to rest in front of the iliac artery, where the ureter is more accessible.

Once the kidney is in place, the surgeon anastomoses its renal vein to the recipient's iliac vein and the renal artery to the recipient's internal iliac artery. He then removes the venous and arterial clamps and checks for patency of the anastomoses. Next, he attaches the donor kidney's ureter to the recipient's

bladder, taking care to ensure a watertight closure. When the transplantation is complete, the surgeon sutures the incision and sends the patient to the recovery room.

COLLABORATIVE MANAGEMENT

Care of the patient undergoing renal transplantation requires thorough preparation, close monitoring, and intense patient teaching.

Preparation

Prepare the patient thoroughly for transplantation and a prolonged recovery period, and offer him ongoing emotional support. Encourage him to express his feelings. If he's concerned about rejection of the donor kidney, explain that if this happens and is irreversible, he will resume dialysis and wait for another suitable donor organ. Reassure him that transplant rejection is common and normally isn't life-threatening.

Describe routine preoperative measures, such as a thorough physical examination and a battery of laboratory tests to detect any infection (followed by antibiotic therapy to clear it up), electrolyte studies, abdominal X-rays, an electrocardiogram (ECG), a cleansing enema, and shaving of the incision site.

Tell the patient that he'll undergo dialysis the day before surgery to clean his blood of unwanted fluid and electrolytes. Also point out that he may need dialysis for a few days after surgery if his transplanted kidney doesn't start functioning immediately.

Review the transplantation procedure, supplementing the doctor's explanation as necessary. Tell the patient that he'll receive a general anesthetic before surgery and that the procedure should take about 4 hours. Next, explain what he can expect after he awakens from anesthesia, including the presence of I.V. lines, an indwelling urinary catheter, an arterial line, and possibly a ventilator. Describe routine postoperative care, including frequent checks of vital signs, monitoring of intake and output, and respiratory therapy. Prepare him for postoperative pain, and reassure him he can have analgesics. If possible, arrange for him to tour the postanesthesia and intensive care units.

Teach the patient the proper methods for coughing, turning, deep breathing and, if ordered, incentive spirometry.

Discuss the immunosuppressant drugs that he'll take, their possible adverse effects, and his increased susceptibility to infection. As ordered, begin giving immunosuppressants, such as azathioprine, cyclosporine, and corticosteroids. You may begin oral azathioprine as early as 5 days before surgery. In contrast, you'll usually begin slow I.V. infusion of cyclosporine 4 to 12 hours before surgery; when doing so, closely monitor the patient for anaphylaxis, especially during the first 30 minutes of administration. If anaphylaxis occurs, give epinephrine, as ordered.

Give blood transfusions as ordered.

Monitoring and aftercare

Remember that your patient's immune system has been suppressed by drugs. Take precautions to reduce infection risk. For instance, use strict aseptic technique when changing dressings and performing catheter care. Also, limit the patient's contact with staff, other patients, and visitors and have all persons in the patient's room wear surgical masks for the first 2 weeks after surgery. Monitor the patient's white blood cell (WBC) count; if it drops precipitously, notify the doctor, who may order isolation.

Throughout the recovery period, watch for signs and symptoms of tissue rejection. Observe the transplant site for redness, tenderness, and swelling. Does the patient have a fever or an elevated WBC count? Decreased urine output with increased proteinuria? Sudden weight gain or hypertension? Elevated serum creatinine and blood urea nitrogen (BUN) levels? Report any of these adverse effects immediately.

If he's in pain, provide analgesics as ordered. Look for a significant decrease in pain after 24 hours.

Carefully monitor urine output; promptly report output of less than 100 ml per hour. In a living-donor transplant, urine flow generally begins immediately after revascularization and connection of the ureter to the recipient's bladder. In a cadaver-kidney transplant, anuria may persist for anywhere from 2 days to 2 weeks; dialysis will be necessary during this period.

Connect the patient's indwelling urinary catheter to a closed drainage system to prevent bladder overextension. Observe his urine color; it is slightly blood tinged for several days and then gradually clears. Irrigate the catheter as ordered, using strict aseptic technique.

Review daily the results of renal function tests, such as creatinine clearance and BUN, hematocrit, and hemoglobin levels. Also review results of tests that assess renal perfusion, such as urine creatinine, urea, sodium, potassium, pH, and specific gravity. Monitor for hematuria and proteinuria.

Assess the patient's fluid and electrolyte balance. Watch particularly for signs and symptoms of hyperkalemia, such as weakness and pulse irregularities and peaked T waves on ECG. If these signs develop, notify the doctor and give calcium carbonate I.V. as ordered. Weigh the patient daily, and report any rapid gain—a possible sign of fluid retention.

Periodically auscultate for bowel sounds, and notify the doctor when they return. He'll order gradual resumption of a normal diet, perhaps with some restrictions. For instance, he may order a low-sodium diet if the patient is receiving corticosteroids, to prevent fluid retention.

Patient teaching

■ Instruct the patient to carefully measure and record intake and output to monitor renal function. Teach him how to collect 24-hour urine specimens and tell him to notify the doctor if output falls below 20 oz (590 ml) during any 24-hour period. Tell him to drink at least 1 qt (1 L) of fluid a day unless the doctor says otherwise.

■ Have the patient weigh himself at least twice a week and report any rapid gain, which could indicate fluid retention.

■ Direct the patient to watch for and promptly report signs and symptoms of infection or transplant rejection, including redness, warmth, tenderness, or swelling over the kidney; temperature exceeding 100 °F (37.8 °C); decreased urine output; and elevated blood pressure.

■ Because he's vulnerable to infection, advise him to avoid crowds and contact with persons with known or suspected infections for at least 3 months after surgery.

■ Stress the need for strict compliance with the prescribed medication regimen. Remind the patient that he must continue immunosuppressant therapy for as long as he has the transplanted kidney, to prevent rejection.

■ If ordered, teach him to take an antacid immediately before a corticosteroid, to combat its ulcerogenic effects, and to report any adverse reactions.

■ Encourage a gradually building program of regular, moderate exercise.

■ Recommend that he avoid excessive bending, heavy lifting, or contact sports for at least 3 months or until the doctor allows such activities.

■ Also warn against activities or positions that place pressure on the new kidney—long car trips and lap-style seat belts.

■ Advise the patient to wait at least 6 weeks before resuming sexual relations. Because pregnancy poses an added risk to a new kidney, provide the female patient with information on birth control.

■ Stress the importance of regular follow-up doctor's visits to evaluate renal function and transplant acceptance.

COMPLICATIONS

The major impediment to successful transplantation is the body's rejection of the donated organ. However, careful tissue matching between donor and recipient decreases this risk.

In hyperacute rejection, the patient's circulating antibodies attack the donor kidney several minutes to hours after transplantation. Renal perfusion plummets, and the organ rapidly becomes ischemic and dies.

If the patient experiences hyperacute rejection, prepare him for removal of the rejected kidney. Provide emotional support to help lessen his disappointment. Also provide support for the donor, if possible, who may feel dejected.

Acute rejection can occur 1 week to 6 months after transplantation of a living-donor kidney or 1 week to 2 years after transplantation of a cadaver kidney (7 to 14 days is most common). This form of rejection is caused by an antigen-antibody reaction, which produces acute tubular necrosis.

Most transplantation patients have at least one or two episodes of acute rejection, which are stopped with early recognition and immediately increased dosages of immunosuppressant drugs. If that fails, the transplanted kidney eventually stops functioning.

Be alert for the characteristics of acute rejection: signs of infection (fever, rapid pulse, elevated WBC count, lethargy), oliguria or anuria, hypertension, or a weight gain of more than 3 lb (1.4 kg) in a day. If the patient displays these signs, reassure him that this is common and often reversible. As ordered, prepare him for dialysis.

Chronic rejection is an irreversible complication that can start several months or even years after transplantation. It's caused by long-term antibody destruction of the donor kidney. Typically, it's detected by serial laboratory studies that show a declining glomerular filtration rate with rising BUN and serum creatinine levels.

If the patient is experiencing chronic rejection, tell him that complete destruction of the donor kidney may take several years. Prepare him for a renal scan, renal biopsy, and other tests, as ordered. Give increased dosages of immunosuppressant drugs and adjust his dietary and fluid regimen, as ordered. When necessary, prepare him for dialysis or another transplantation, as ordered.

Renal transplantation is associated with vascular complications—stenosis of the renal artery, vascular leakage, and thrombosis at the surgical site—or genitourinary tract complications—ureteral leakage, ureteral fistula, ureteral obstruction, calculus formation, bladder neck contracture, scrotal swelling, and graft rupture. Other potential complications include infection, hematomas, abscesses, and lymphoceles.

Selected references

Black, J., and Matassarin-Jacobs, E., eds. *Luckmann and Sorensen's Medical-Surgical Nursing: A Psychophysiologic Approach,* 5th ed. Philadelphia: W.B. Saunders Co., 1997.

Illustrated Handbook of Nursing Care. Springhouse, Pa.: Springhouse Corp., 1998.

Kelly, M. "Acute Renal Failure," *AJN* 97(3):32-33, March 1997.

Lewis, S.M., et al. *Medical-Surgical Nursing: Assessment and Management of Clinical Problems,* 4th ed. St. Louis: Mosby–Year Book, Inc., 1996.

Nursing98 Drug Handbook. Springhouse, Pa.: Springhouse Corp., 1998.

Peschman, P. "Renal Physiology," in *Critical Care Nursing,* 2nd ed. Edited by Clochesy, J.M., et al. Philadelphia: W.B. Saunders Co., 1996.

Phipps, W.J., et al. *Medical-Surgical Nursing: Concepts and Clinical Practice,* 5th ed. St. Louis: Mosby–Year Book, Inc., 1995.

Professional Guide to Signs and Symptoms, 2nd ed. Springhouse, Pa.: Springhouse Corp., 1997.

Whittaker, A. "Patients with Acute Renal Failure," in *Critical Care Nursing,* 2nd ed. Edited by Clochesy, J.M., et al. Philadelphia: W.B. Saunders Co., 1996.

Endocrine disorders

Anatomy and physiology review

Common disorders of the endocrine system are classified as hypofunction and hyperfunction, inflammation, and tumor. While diagnostic tests are needed to confirm endocrine disorders, clinical data usually provide the first clues to these disorders. Nursing assessment can reveal common signs and symptoms of endocrine dysfunction, such as excessive or delayed growth, wasting, weakness, polydipsia, polyuria, and mental changes.

The endocrine system consists of three major components: glands, hormones, and receptors. The glands are specialized cell clusters or organs. Hormones are chemical substances secreted by glands in response to stimulation, whereas receptors are protein macromolecules that initiate activity in a target cell in response to hormonal stimulation.

GLANDS
The major glands of the endocrine system, which collectively weigh less than 7 oz (198.5 g), include the hypothalamus, pituitary, thyroid, parathyroid, pineal, and adrenal glands; the gonads (ovaries and testes); and selected areas of the pancreas known as the islets of Langerhans. Endocrine glands release hormones into the bloodstream for transport to specific target sites. At each target site, hormones combine with specific receptors to trigger specific physiologic changes. (See *Understanding endocrine anatomy,* pages 410 and 411.)

HORMONES
Structurally, hormones are classified into three types: polypeptides, steroids, and amines.

Polypeptides, proteins with a defined, genetically coded structure, include anterior pituitary hormones (growth hormone, thyroid-stimulating hormone [TSH], corticotropin, follicle-stimulating hormone, luteinizing hormone [LH], interstitial-cell-stimulating hormone, and prolactin); posterior pituitary hormones (antidiuretic hormone [ADH] and oxytocin); parathyroid hormone (PTH); and pancreatic hormones (insulin and glucagon).

Steroids, derived from cholesterol, include the adrenocortical hormones secreted by the adrenal cortex (aldosterone and cortisol), and the sex hormones (estrogen and progesterone in females and testosterone in males) secreted by the gonads.

Amines are derived from tyrosine (an essential amino acid found in most proteins). They include the thyroid hormones (thyroxine [T_4] and triiodothyronine [T_3]) and the catecholamines (epinephrine, norepinephrine, and dopamine).

Although all hormone release is caused by endocrine gland stimulation, release patterns vary greatly. For example, corticotropin and cortisol are released in irregular spurts in response to body rhythm cycles, with levels peaking in the morning. In contrast, secretion of PTH and prolactin proceeds fairly evenly throughout the day. Insulin has both steady and sporadic release patterns. Pancreatic beta cells secrete small amounts of insulin continuously but secrete additional insulin in response to food intake. (See *Understanding hormone storage and release,* pages 412 and 413.)

After release into the bloodstream, thyroid and steroid hormones circulate, bound to plasma proteins, whereas catecholamines and most polypeptides circulate "free" (not protein bound).

HORMONAL ACTION
Once a hormone reaches its target site, it binds to a specific receptor on the cell membrane or within the

Understanding endocrine anatomy

The endocrine glands secrete hormones directly into the bloodstream to regulate body function. The illustration locates the endocrine glands, which are described below.

Pituitary gland
Also known as the hypophysis, the pituitary gland rests in the sella turcica—a depression in the sphenoid bone at the base of the brain. The pea-sized gland weighs less than 0.75 g and has two regions. The largest, the anterior pituitary lobe (adenohypophysis), produces at least six hormones: somatotropin, or growth hormone; thyrotropin, or thyroid-stimulating hormone; corticotropin, or adrenocorticotropic hormone; follicle-stimulating hormone; luteinizing hormone; and prolactin, or mammotropin.

The posterior pituitary lobe makes up about 25% of the gland. It stores and releases oxytocin and antidiuretic hormones, which are produced by the hypothalamus.

Thyroid gland
The thyroid lies directly below the larynx, partially in front of the trachea. Two lobes, one on either side of the trachea, join with a narrow tissue bridge called the isthmus to give the thyroid its butterfly-like shape. The lobes function as one unit to produce the hormones thyroxine (T_4), triiodothyronine (T_3), and thyrocalcitonin. T_4 and T_3 are referred to collectively as thyroid hormone.

Parathyroid glands
Four parathyroid glands lie embedded on the posterior surface of the thyroid, one in each corner. Like the thyroid lobes, the parathyroid glands work together as a single gland, producing parathyroid hormone.

Adrenal glands
The two adrenal glands sit atop the two kidneys. Each gland contains two distinct endocrine glands with separate functions. The inner portion—the medulla—produces the catecholamines epinephrine and norepinephrine. Because these hormones play important roles in the autonomic nervous system, the adrenal medulla is also considered a neuroendocrine structure.

The much larger outer adrenal portion—the cortex—has three zones. The outermost zone, the zona glomerulosa, produces mineralocorticoids, primarily aldosterone. The zona fasciculata, the middle and largest zone, produces the glucocorticoids cortisol (hydrocortisone), cortisone, and corticosterone as well as small amounts of the sex hormones androgen and estrogen. The inner zone, the zona reticularis, produces mainly glucocorticoids and some sex hormones.

Pancreas
The pancreas lies across the posterior abdominal wall, in the left upper quadrant behind the stomach. The islets of Langerhans, which perform the endocrine function of this gland, contain alpha, beta, and delta cells. Alpha cells produce glucagon; beta cells produce insulin; and delta cells produce somatostatin.

Thymus
Located below the sternum, the thymus contains lymphatic tissue. Although it produces the hormones thymosin and thymopoietin, its major role seems related to the immune system—producing T cells, important in cell-mediated immunity.

Pineal gland
The tiny pineal—only about ¼" (6 mm) in diameter—lies at the back of the third ventricle of the brain and is a neuroendocrine gland. The pineal gland produces the hormone melatonin, which may have a role in the neuroendocrine reproductive axis as well as other widespread actions.

Hypothalamus
The hypothalamus is the ventral part of the diencephalon that forms the floor and part of the lateral wall of the third ventricle. The hypothalamus synthesizes antidiuretic hormone and oxytocin—which travel to the posterior pituitary for storage—as well as many releasing and inhibiting hormones and factors. With these, it exerts control over functions of the anterior pituitary gland (adenohypophysis).

cell. Polypeptides and some amines bind to membrane receptor sites; the smaller, more lipid-soluble steroids and thyroid hormones diffuse through the cell membrane and bind to intracellular receptors.

After binding, each hormone produces unique physiologic changes, depending on its target site and its specific action at that site. A particular hormone may have different effects at different target sites.

HORMONAL REGULATION
To maintain the body's delicate homeostatic balance, a feedback mechanism involving hormones, blood chemicals and metabolites, and the nervous system regulates hormone synthesis and secretion. Feedback refers to information sent to endocrine glands that signals the need for changes in hormone levels, either increasing or decreasing hormone production and release. Four basic mechanisms control hormone release: the pituitary-target gland axis, the hypothalam-

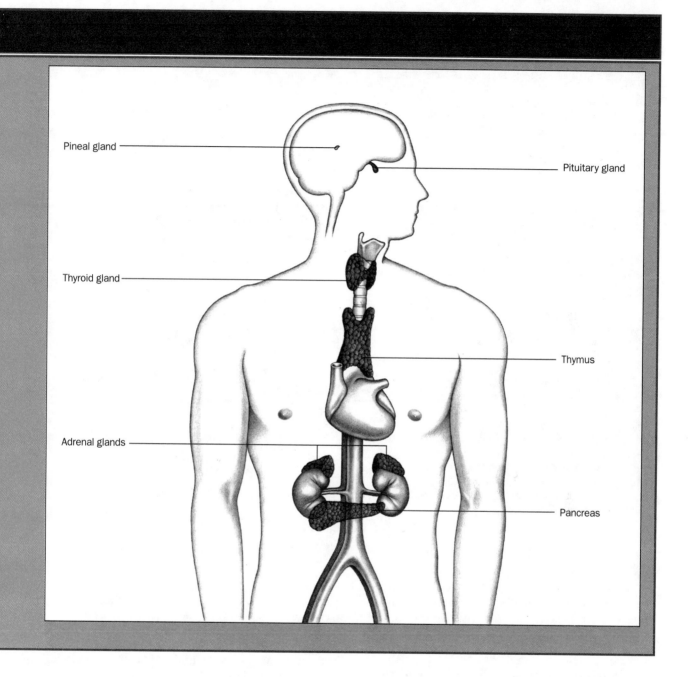

ic-pituitary-target gland axis, chemical regulation, and nervous system regulation.

Pituitary-target gland axis. The pituitary gland regulates other endocrine glands—and their hormones—through secretion of trophic hormones, including corticotropin, TSH, and LH. Corticotropin regulates the adrenal cortex hormones; TSH regulates the thyroid hormones T_4 and T_3; and LH regulates gonadal hormones. The pituitary gets feedback about target glands by continuously monitoring levels of hormones produced by these glands. If a change occurs, the pituitary corrects it in one of two ways: It increases trophic hormones, which stimulates the target gland and increases target gland hormones, or it decreases trophic hormones, which decreases target gland stimulation and target gland hormones.

The pituitary increases or decreases its trophic hormones from moment to moment, by continuously monitoring its target gland hormone and changing its

Understanding hormone storage and release

Endocrine cells manufacture and release their hormones in several ways, as shown here.

Pancreas

Many endocrine cells have receptors on their membranes that respond to stimuli. For example, neural stimulation of this pancreatic beta cell synthesizes the hormone precursor, preproinsulin, and converts it to proinsulin in beadlike ribosomes located on the endoplasmic reticulum.

Proinsulin is transferred to the Golgi complex, which collects it into secretory granules and cleaves it to insulin. The granules fuse with the plasma membrane and disperse insulin into the bloodstream. Hormonal release by membrane fusion is called exocytosis.

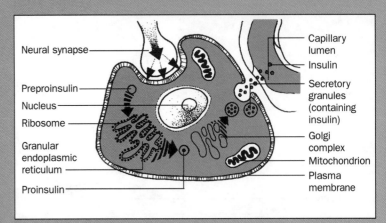

Thyroid

Thyroid cells store a hormone precursor, colloidal iodinated thyroglobulin, which contains iodine and thyroglobulin. When stimulated by thyroid stimulating hormone (TSH), a follicular cell takes up some stored thyroglobulin by endocytosis—the reverse of exocytosis. The cell membrane extends fingerlike projections into the colloid, then pulls portions of it back into the cell. Lysosomes fuse with the colloid, which is then degraded by proteolysis into triiodothyronine (T_3) and thyroxine (T_4), which are released into the circulation and lymphatic system by exocytosis.

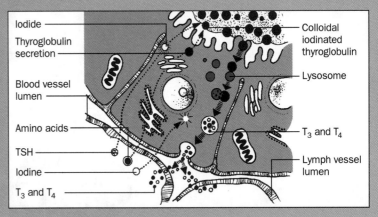

own level in the opposite direction. For instance, if the cortisol level rises, corticotropin levels decline and so reduce adrenal cortex stimulation, which in turn decreases cortisol secretion. Conversely, if the cortisol level drops, corticotropin levels rise, stimulating the adrenal cortex to produce and secrete more cortisol.

Hypothalamic-pituitary-target gland axis. The hypothalamus, in the diencephalon of the brain, also produces trophic hormones. These releasing and inhibiting hormones regulate anterior pituitary hormones. By controlling anterior pituitary hormones, which control the target gland hormones, the hypothalamus affects target glands as well.

Chemical regulation. Endocrine glands not controlled by the pituitary gland may be controlled by specific substances that trigger gland secretions. For

example, serum glucose is a major regulator of glucagon and insulin release. An elevated serum glucose level stimulates the pancreas to increase insulin secretion and suppress glucagon secretion. Conversely, a depressed serum glucose level triggers increased glucagon secretion and suppresses insulin secretion.

Sodium and potassium indirectly regulate aldosterone secretion. Decreased extracellular sodium levels and increased serum potassium levels stimulate formation of angiotensin II, which stimulates the adrenal cortex to release more aldosterone.

ADH regulation occurs mainly through changes in plasma osmolality (the osmotic pressure of a solution expressed in milliosmols representing the concentration of particles in a solution), although other factors also affect ADH levels. Elevated plasma osmolality (indicating dehydration) stimulates ADH to promote water retention; diminished osmolality (indicating fluid

Hypothalamus and pituitary

Anterior and posterior pituitary secretions are controlled by hypothalamic signals. On the left side of this drawing, the hypothalamic neuron produces antidiuretic hormone (ADH), which travels down the axon and is stored in secretory granules in nerve endings in the posterior pituitary for later release.

The right side of the drawing shows how the anterior pituitary is stimulated to produce its many hormones. Here, a hypothalamic neuron manufactures inhibitory and stimulatory hormones and secretes them into a capillary of the portal system; the hormones travel down the pituitary stalk to the anterior pituitary. There, they cause inhibition or release of many pituitary hormones, including adrenocorticotropic hormone (ACTH), TSH, growth hormone (GH), follicle-stimulating hormone (FSH), luteinizing hormone (LH), and prolactin.

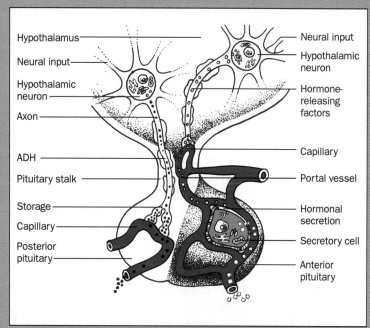

overload) suppresses ADH secretion to promote diuresis.

Nervous system regulation. The central nervous system (CNS) helps regulate hormone secretion in several ways. The hypothalamus controls pituitary hormones, as described earlier. Because hypothalamic nerve cells produce the posterior pituitary hormones ADH and oxytocin, these hormones are controlled directly by the CNS. Stimuli, such as hypoxia, nausea, pain, stress, and certain drugs, also affect ADH levels. The autonomic nervous system controls catecholamine secretion by the adrenal medulla.

The relationship between the hypothalamus and the pituitary underscores the interdependence of the nervous system and endocrine function. The nervous system also modifies other endocrine hormones. For example, stress, which leads to sympathetic stimula-tion, causes the pituitary to release corticotropin. The nervous and endocrine systems share other regulatory mechanisms, as part of the fight-or-flight reaction and other stress responses.

HORMONAL IMBALANCE

Endocrine dysfunction takes one of two forms: hyperfunction, resulting in excessive hormone effects, or hypofunction, resulting from relative or absolute hormone deficiency. Hormonal imbalance also is classified according to disease site. Primary dysfunction results from disease within an endocrine gland—for example, Addison's disease (adrenal hypofunction); secondary dysfunction from disease in a tissue that secretes hormones that affect the target tissue; and functional hyperfunction or hypofunction, from disease in a nonendocrine tissue or organ.

Assessment

As with other body systems, to thoroughly assess the endocrine system, you must take an accurate health history and conduct a physical examination.

HISTORY

Because of the endocrine system's interrelationships with all other body systems, remember to ask patients about their overall patterns of health and illness.

CHIEF COMPLAINT

Ask the patient to describe his chief complaint. Common chief complaints associated with endocrine disorders include fatigue, weakness, weight changes, mental status changes, polyuria, polydipsia, and abnormalities of sexual maturity and function.

MEDICAL HISTORY

By asking pertinent questions, you may identify insidious and vague symptoms of endocrine dysfunction that otherwise could go unreported. Some of these questions are: At what age did puberty start? Have you ever had a fracture of the skull or other bone? Have you ever had surgery, and if so, were there any complications? Have you ever had a brain infection, such as meningitis or encephalitis?

Conduct a complete body systems review, adding questions such as: Have you noticed any changes in your skin? Do you bruise more easily than you used to? Have you noticed any change in the amount or distribution of your body hair? Do your eyes burn or feel "gritty" when you close them? How good is your sense of smell?

FAMILY HISTORY

Take a thorough family history because certain endocrine disorders are inherited or have strong familial tendencies. Ask the patient if any family member has diabetes mellitus, thyroid disease, hypertension, or elevated serum lipid levels.

PHYSICAL EXAMINATION

Remember to include an evaluation of all body systems, including a complete neurologic assessment because of the role the hypothalamus plays in regulating endocrine function through the pituitary gland.

As usual, to obtain the most objective findings, you'll inspect, palpate, and auscultate the patient. Before you begin, remember to gather a tape measure, a scale with a height-measuring device, a stethoscope, a watch with a second hand, a glass of water with a straw, a gown, and drapes. The examination room should be warm and well lit.

VITAL SIGNS, HEIGHT, AND WEIGHT

Begin with the patient's vital signs, height, and weight. Compare the findings with normal expected values and the patient's baseline measurements, if available.

INSPECTION

Continue your physical assessment by systematically inspecting the patient's overall appearance and examining all areas of his body.

General appearance. Assess the patient's physical appearance and mental and emotional status. Note such factors as overall affect, speech, level of consciousness and orientation, appropriateness and neatness of dress and grooming, and activity level. Evaluate general body development, including posture, body build, proportionality of body parts, and distribution of body fat.

Skin, hair, and nails. Note the patient's overall skin color, and inspect the skin and mucous membranes for any lesions or areas of increased, decreased, or absent pigmentation. As you do so, remember to consider racial and ethnic variations. In a dark-skinned patient, color variations are best assessed in the sclera, conjunctiva, mouth, nail beds, and palms. Next, assess skin texture and hydration.

Inspect the patient's hair for amount, distribution, condition, and texture. Assess scalp and body hair, looking for abnormal patterns of growth or loss. Again, remember to consider normal racial and ethnic—as well as sexual—differences in hair growth and texture. Then, check the patient's fingernails for cracking, peeling, separation from the nail bed (onycholysis), and clubbing, and the toenails for fungal infection, ingrown nails, discoloration, length, and thickness.

Head and neck. Assess the patient's face for overall color and presence of erythematous areas, especially in the cheeks. Note facial expression. Is it pained and anxious, dull and flat, or alert and interested? Note the shape and symmetry of the eyes and look for eyeball protrusion, incomplete eyelid closure, or periorbital edema. Have the patient extend his tongue, and inspect it for color, size, lesions, positioning, and any tremors or unusual movements.

Standing in front of the patient, examine the neck—first, as he holds it straight, then slightly extended, and finally while the patient swallows water. Check neck symmetry and midline positioning as well as symmetry of the trachea.

Chest. Evaluate the overall size, shape, and symmetry of the patient's chest, noting any deformities. In females, assess the breasts for size, shape, symmetry, pigmentation (especially on the nipples and in skin creases), and nipple discharge (galactorrhea). In males, observe for bilateral or unilateral breast enlargement (gynecomastia) and nipple discharge.

Genitalia. Inspect the patient's external genitalia—particularly the testes and clitoris—for normal development.

Extremities. Inspect the patient's arms and hands for tremors. Have the patient hold both arms outstretched in front with the palms down and fingers separated. Then place a sheet of paper on the outstretched fingers and watch for any trembling. Note any muscle wasting, especially in the upper arms, and have the patient grasp your hands to assess the strength and symmetry of his grip.

Next, inspect the legs for muscle development, symmetry, color, and hair distribution. Then, assess muscle strength by having the patient sit on the edge of the examination table and extend the legs horizontally. A patient who can maintain this position for 2 minutes usually exhibits normal strength. Examine the feet for size, and note any lesions, corns, calluses, or marks made from socks or shoes. Inspect the toes and the spaces between them for maceration and fissures.

PALPATION
Use the following guidelines to palpate the thyroid gland and testes, the only endocrine glands accessible to palpation.

In many patients, though, you may be unable to palpate the thyroid gland. But if you can, the gland should feel smooth, finely lobulated, nontender, and either soft or firm. You should feel the gland's sections.

Use tangential lighting to aid visualization. An enlarged thyroid may appear diffuse and asymmetrical. Thyroid nodules feel like a knot, a protuberance, or a swelling; a firm, fixed nodule may be a tumor. Remember not to confuse thick neck musculature with an enlarged thyroid or a goiter.

If you suspect that a patient has hypocalcemia (low serum calcium levels) related to deficient or ineffective parathyroid hormone secretion from hypoparathyroidism or surgical removal of the parathyroid glands, attempt to elicit Chvostek's sign and Trousseau's sign. To elicit Chvostek's sign, tap the facial nerve in front of the ear with a finger; if the facial muscles contract toward the ear, the test is positive for hypocalcemia. To elicit Trousseau's sign, place a blood pressure cuff on the arm and inflate it above the patient's systolic pressure. In a positive test, the patient will exhibit carpal spasm (ventral contraction of the thumb and digits) within 3 minutes.

AUSCULTATION
If you palpate an enlarged thyroid, auscultate the gland for systolic bruits. Such bruits, caused by vibrations produced by accelerated blood flow through the thyroid arteries, may indicate hyperthyroidism. To auscultate for bruits, place the bell of the stethoscope over one of the lateral lobes of the thyroid, then listen carefully for a low, soft, rushing sound. To ensure that tracheal sounds don't obscure any bruits, have the patient hold his breath while you auscultate.

To distinguish a bruit from a venous hum, listen for the rushing sound, then gently occlude the jugular vein with your fingers on the side you're auscultating and listen again. A venous hum (produced by jugular blood flow) disappears during venous compression; a bruit doesn't.

Addison's disease

Also called adrenal insufficiency, this disorder has primary and secondary forms. Primary adrenal hypofunction (Addison's disease) originates within the adrenal gland itself and is characterized by decreased mineralocorticoid, glucocorticoid, and androgen secretion. A relatively uncommon disorder, Addison's disease is diagnosed in persons between ages 30 and 50 and in both sexes.

Adrenal hypofunction can also occur secondary to a disorder outside the gland (such as pituitary tumor with corticotropin deficiency), but aldosterone secretion may continue intact. With early diagnosis and adequate replacement therapy, the prognosis for both primary and secondary adrenal hypofunction is good.

CAUSES
Addison's disease occurs when more than 90% of the adrenal gland is destroyed. Such massive destruction usually results from an autoimmune process in which circulating antibodies react specifically against the adrenal tissue.

Other causes include tuberculosis; bilateral adrenalectomy; hemorrhage into the adrenal gland; metastatic cancers, such as lung and breast cancer; infections, such as histoplasmosis, human immunodeficiency virus, and cytomegalovirus; and, rarely, a familial tendency toward autoimmune disease.

Secondary adrenal hypofunction that leads to glucocorticoid deficiency can stem from hypopituitarism (causing decreased corticotropin secretion), from abrupt withdrawal of long-term corticosteroid therapy (long-term exogenous corticosteroid stimulation sup-

How adrenal crisis develops

The most serious complication of adrenal hypofunction, adrenal crisis can occur gradually or with catastrophic suddenness, making prompt emergency treatment essential.

Also known as acute adrenal insufficiency, this potentially lethal condition usually develops in a patient who doesn't respond to hormone replacement therapy, who undergoes marked stress without adequate glucocorticoid replacement, or who abruptly stops hormonal therapy. It can also result from trauma, bilateral adrenalectomy, or

adrenal gland thrombosis after a severe infection (Waterhouse-Friderichsen syndrome).

Signs and symptoms include profound weakness, fatigue, nausea, vomiting, hypotension, dehydration and, occasionally, high fever followed by hypothermia. If untreated, this condition can ultimately cause vascular collapse, renal shutdown, coma, and death.

The flowchart below summarizes what happens in adrenal crisis and pinpoints its warning signs and symptoms.

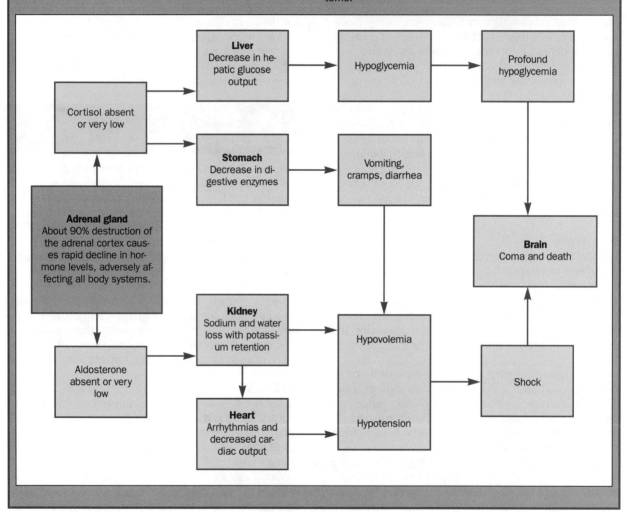

presses pituitary corticotropin secretion and causes adrenal gland atrophy), or from removal of a nonendocrine, corticotropin-secreting tumor.

Adrenal crisis strikes a patient with adrenal hypofunction when trauma, surgery, or other physiologic

stress exhausts his body's stores of glucocorticoids. (See *How adrenal crisis develops*.)

DIAGNOSIS AND TREATMENT
Diagnosis requires demonstration of decreased corticosteroid concentrations in plasma or urine and an

accurate classification of adrenal hypofunction as primary or secondary. Baseline plasma and urine steroid testing is followed by a metyrapone test to confirm secondary adrenal hypofunction, a corticotropin stimulation test, and a rapid corticotropin test.

In a patient with typical symptoms of Addison's disease, laboratory findings strongly suggest acute adrenal insufficiency. In addition, X-rays may show a small heart and adrenal calcification.

Lifelong glucocorticoid replacement is the main treatment for all patients with primary or secondary adrenal hypofunction. In general, cortisone or hydrocortisone is given. Patients with Addison's disease may also need fludrocortisone to prevent dangerous dehydration and hypotension. Patients with secondary adrenocortical insufficiency require fludrocortisone treatment. Women with Addison's disease who have muscle weakness and decreased libido may benefit from testosterone injections, but risk unfortunate masculinizing effects.

Treatment for adrenal crisis is prompt I.V. bolus administration of 100 mg of hydrocortisone, followed by hydrocortisone diluted with dextrose in normal saline solution or 5% dextrose in saline and given I.V. until the patient's condition stabilizes. The patient may need up to 300 mg/day of hydrocortisone and 3 to 5 L of I.V. normal saline solution during the acute stage. With proper treatment, the crisis usually subsides quickly, with blood pressure stabilizing and water and sodium levels returning to normal. After the crisis, maintenance doses of hydrocortisone preserve physiologic stability.

COLLABORATIVE MANAGEMENT

Care of the patient with Addison's disease focuses on returning hormonal levels to normal, avoiding complications, and teaching about treatment.

ASSESSMENT

The patient may report synthetic steroid use, adrenal surgery, or recent infection. Look for:
- complaints of muscle weakness, fatigue, light-headedness when rising from a chair or bed
- reports of weight loss, cravings for salty food, decreased tolerance for even minor stress, and various GI disturbances
- complaints of anxiety, irritability, and confusion
- reduced urine output and other symptoms of dehydration
- in women, decreased libido, due to reduced androgen production, and amenorrhea
- poor coordination
- dry skin and mucous membranes, related to dehydration
- decreased axillary and pubic hair in women

- conspicuous bronze coloration of the skin, especially in the creases of the hands and over joints, elbows, and knees
- darkening of scars, areas of vitiligo (absence of pigmentation), and increased pigmentation of the mucous membranes, especially the buccal mucosa
- in secondary adrenal hypofunction, no hyperpigmentation
- weak, irregular pulse
- blood pressure revealing hypotension.

NURSING DIAGNOSES AND COLLABORATIVE PROBLEMS

Based on the following nursing diagnoses, you'll establish patient outcomes.

Altered protection related to decreased ability to produce and release adrenocorticoid hormones as needed. The patient will:
- experience no hypotension, tachycardia, nausea and vomiting, restlessness, or other signs or symptoms of adrenal crisis
- demonstrate protective measures, including compliance with adrenocorticoid replacement therapy, use of stress-reduction techniques, and early recognition and treatment of adrenal insufficiency.

Risk for infection related to suppressed inflammatory response caused by steroid therapy. The patient will:
- maintain a normal temperature and white blood cell count and differential
- remain free from infection
- take precautions to avoid or decrease the risk of infection.

Knowledge deficit related to inadequate understanding of adrenal hypofunction and steroid therapy. The patient will:
- express a need to know about adrenal hypofunction and steroid therapy
- express an understanding of what he has learned about adrenal hypofunction and steroid therapy
- state his intentions to seek help from health professionals, when needed, and adhere to the prescribed medical treatment.

PLANNING AND IMPLEMENTATION

These measures help the patient with Addison's disease.
- Give a corticosteroid as ordered. Until the onset of the mineralocorticoid effect, force fluids to replace excessive fluid loss.
- Control the patient's environment to prevent stress. Encourage him to use relaxation techniques. Plan periods of rest during the day, and gradually increase activities depending upon his tolerance.
- Encourage him to dress in layers to retain body heat, and adjust room temperature if possible.

- Consult a dietitian to plan a diet that maintains sodium and potassium balances and provides adequate proteins and carbohydrates. If the patient is anorexic, suggest six small meals a day to increase calorie intake. Keep a late-morning and evening snack available in case he becomes hypoglycemic.

- If the patient also has diabetes mellitus, check blood glucose levels periodically because steroid replacement may necessitate adjustment of the insulin dosage.

- Observe the patient for cushingoid signs such as fluid retention around the eyes and face. Check fluid and electrolyte balance, especially if he is receiving mineralocorticoids. Monitor weight, blood pressure, and intake and output to assess body fluid status. Remember, steroids given in the late afternoon or evening may cause central nervous system stimulation and insomnia in some patients. Check for petechiae because the patient may bruise easily.

- If the patient receives only glucocorticoids, observe for orthostatic hypotension or electrolyte abnormalities, which may indicate a need for mineralocorticoid therapy.

- In women receiving testosterone injections, watch for and report facial hair growth and other signs of masculinization. She may need a dosage adjustment.

- In adrenal crisis, monitor vital signs carefully, especially for hypotension, volume depletion, and other signs of shock. Check for decreased level of consciousness and reduced urine output, which may also signal shock. Monitor for hyperkalemia before treatment and for hypokalemia afterward (from excessive mineralocorticoid effect). Check for cardiac arrhythmias.

- Provide good skin care. Use alcohol-free skin care products and an emollient lotion after bathing. Turn and reposition the bedridden patient every 2 hours. Avoid pressure over bony prominences.

- Use protective measures to minimize the risk of infection. Provide the patient with a private room and reverse isolation if necessary. Limit visitors, especially those with infectious conditions. Use meticulous hand-washing technique.

- Encourage the patient to verbalize his feelings about body image changes and sexual dysfunction. Discuss fear of rejection by others, and offer emotional support. Help him to develop coping strategies. Refer him to a mental health professional for additional counseling if necessary.

Patient teaching

- Explain that lifelong steroid therapy is necessary. Teach the patient and family members or friends to identify and report signs and symptoms of drug overdose (weight gain and edema) or underdose (fatigue, weakness, and dizziness).

- Tell the patient that he may need to increase the dosage during times of stress (when he has a cold, for example). Warn that infection, injury, or profuse sweating in hot weather may precipitate adrenal crisis. Caution him not to withdraw the drug suddenly because this may also cause adrenal crisis.

- Instruct the patient always to carry a medical identification card. Teach him and family members how to inject hydrocortisone, and advise them to keep on hand a prepared syringe of hydrocortisone for use in times of stress.

- Instruct the patient to take steroids with antacids or meals to minimize gastric irritation. Suggest taking two-thirds of the dosage in the morning and the remaining one-third in the early afternoon to mimic diurnal adrenal secretion.

- Remind the patient and family members that the disease causes mood swings and changes in mental status, which steroid replacement therapy can correct.

- Review protective measures to decrease stress and help prevent infections.

EVALUATION

Achievement of patient outcomes determines the success of collaborative management. For the patient with Addison's disease, evaluation focuses on return of hormonal levels to within acceptable parameters, absence of complications, and adequate knowledge to comply with treatment.

Cushing's syndrome

Cushing's syndrome is a syndrome of adrenal hyperfunction. It reflects excessive levels of adrenocortical hormones (particularly cortisol) or related corticosteroids and, to a lesser extent, androgens and aldosterone. Cushing's syndrome is more common in females than in males.

CAUSES

Cushing's syndrome is most commonly iatrogenic, resulting from chronic glucocorticoid therapy.

Spontaneous Cushing's syndrome is caused by pituitary or adrenal abnormalities or corticotropin secretion by nonpituitary tumors. In about 70% of patients, excess production of corticotropin-releasing hormone and consequent hyperplasia of the adrenal cortex cause the syndrome. Corticotropin overproduction may stem from pituitary hypersecretion (Cushing's disease), a corticotropin-producing tumor in another organ (particularly bronchogenic or pancreatic carcinoma), or administration of synthetic glucocorticoids or corticotropin. In the remaining 30% of patients, Cushing's syndrome is caused by a cortisol-secreting adrenal tumor, which is usually benign.

The stimulating and catabolic effects of cortisol produce the complications of Cushing's syndrome.

Increased calcium resorption from bone may lead to osteoporosis and pathologic fractures. Peptic ulcer may result from increased gastric secretions, pepsin production, and decreased gastric mucus. Increased hepatic gluconeogenesis and insulin resistance can cause impaired glucose tolerance. Overt diabetes mellitus occurs in fewer than 20% of patients.

A patient may have frequent infections or slow wound healing due to decreased lymphocyte production and suppressed antibody formation. Suppressed inflammatory response may mask even a severe infection.

Hypertension due to sodium and water retention is common and may lead to ischemic heart disease and heart failure. Menstrual disturbances and sexual dysfunction also occur. Decreased ability to handle stress may result in psychiatric problems, ranging from mood swings to frank psychosis.

Adrenal crisis, a critical deficiency of mineralocorticoids and glucocorticoids, is the most serious complication. It requires immediate, vigorous treatment.

DIAGNOSIS AND TREATMENT

Diagnosis of Cushing's syndrome depends on a demonstrated increase in cortisol production and the failure to suppress endogenous cortisol secretion after administration of dexamethasone. Initial screening may consist of a 24-hour urine test to determine free cortisol excretion rate in addition to the tests described below. Failure to suppress plasma and urine cortisol levels confirms the diagnosis of Cushing's syndrome.

A high-dose dexamethasone suppression test can determine if Cushing's syndrome results from pituitary dysfunction (Cushing's disease). In this diagnostic test, dexamethasone suppresses plasma cortisol levels, and urine 17-hydroxycorticosteroid and 17-ketosteroid levels fall to 50% or less of basal levels. Failure to suppress these levels indicates that the syndrome results from an adrenal tumor or a nonendocrine, corticotropin-secreting tumor. This test can produce false-positive results.

In a stimulation test, administration of metyrapone, which blocks cortisol production by the adrenal glands, evaluates the ability of the pituitary gland and the hypothalamus to detect and correct low levels of plasma cortisol by increasing corticotropin production.

Radiologic evaluation for Cushing's syndrome seeks to locate the causative tumor in the pituitary gland or the adrenals. Tests include ultrasonography, a computed tomography scan, and magnetic resonance imaging enhanced with gadolinium.

Management to restore hormone balance and reverse Cushing's syndrome may require radiation, drug therapy, or surgery.

Pituitary-dependent Cushing's syndrome with adrenal hyperplasia may require bilateral adrenalectomy, hypophysectomy, or pituitary irradiation. Nonendocrine corticotropin-producing tumors require excision of the tumor, followed by drug therapy with mitotane, metyrapone, or aminoglutethimide. Aminoglutethimide and cyproheptadine decrease cortisol levels and have helped many cushingoid patients. Aminoglutethimide alone, or in combination with metyrapone, can help in metastatic adrenal carcinoma.

Before surgery, the patient with cushingoid symptoms requires management to control hypertension, edema, diabetes, and cardiovascular manifestations and to prevent infection. Glucocorticoid administration the morning of surgery can help prevent acute adrenal insufficiency during surgery. Cortisol therapy is essential during and after surgery to help the patient tolerate the physiologic stress imposed by removal of the pituitary or adrenal glands. If normal cortisol production resumes, steroid therapy may gradually be tapered and eventually discontinued. However, bilateral adrenalectomy or total hypophysectomy mandates lifelong steroid replacement therapy to correct hormonal deficiencies.

COLLABORATIVE MANAGEMENT

Care of the patient with Cushing's syndrome focuses on restoring acceptable cardiopulmonary status, avoiding complications, and teaching about the disease, treatment, and care.

ASSESSMENT

The patient may report using synthetic steroids. She may complain of fatigue, muscle weakness, sleep disturbances, water retention, amenorrhea, decreased libido, irritability, and emotional lability. Additionally, she may list signs and symptoms similar to those of hypoglycemia.

Inspection may reveal a spectrum of characteristic signs and symptoms, including thin hair, a moon-shaped face from fluid retention, hirsutism, acne, a buffalo-humplike back, and thin extremities from muscle wasting. Other observable features are petechiae, ecchymoses, and purplish striae; delayed wound healing; and swollen ankles. Assessment typically reveals hypertension. (See *Cushing's syndrome: An assessment guide,* page 420.)

NURSING DIAGNOSES AND COLLABORATIVE PROBLEMS

Based on the following nursing diagnoses, you'll establish patient outcomes.

Body image disturbance related to changes in physical appearance caused by Cushing's syndrome. The patient will:

■ verbalize her feelings about her changed body image

Cushing's syndrome: An assessment guide

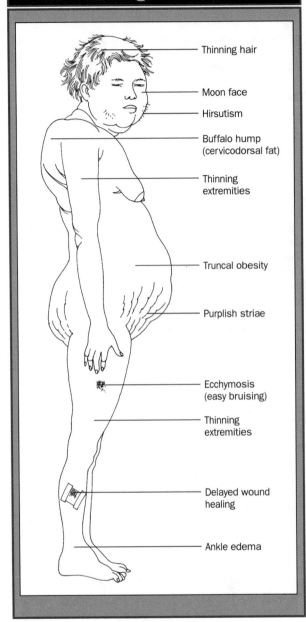

- Thinning hair
- Moon face
- Hirsutism
- Buffalo hump (cervicodorsal fat)
- Thinning extremities
- Truncal obesity
- Purplish striae
- Ecchymosis (easy bruising)
- Thinning extremities
- Delayed wound healing
- Ankle edema

Risk for injury related to the stimulating and catabolic adverse effects of excessive corticosteroid production on body tissue. The patient will:

- identify the early signs and symptoms of complications associated with Cushing's syndrome and state the importance of seeking medical attention if they appear
- express an understanding of measures to prevent complications, such as obtaining adequate rest, eating a well-balanced diet, complying with the treatment regimen, and taking precautions against infection
- remain free from injury.

PLANNING AND IMPLEMENTATION

These measures help the patient with Cushing's syndrome.

- Consult a dietitian to plan a diet high in protein and potassium but low in calories, carbohydrates, and sodium.
- Schedule activities around the patient's rest periods to avoid fatigue. Gradually increase activity as tolerated.
- Institute safety precautions to minimize the risk for injury from falls. Help her walk to avoid bumps and bruises.
- Help the bedridden patient turn and reposition herself every 2 hours. Use extreme caution while moving the patient to minimize skin trauma and bone stress. Inspect her skin regularly for signs of breakdown. Provide frequent skin care, especially over bony prominences. Provide support with pillows and a convoluted foam mattress.
- Prepare the patient for surgery, as indicated.
- Monitor her vital signs, intake and output, weight, and daily serum electrolyte levels.
- Monitor her nutritional intake, and assess her for nutritional imbalances.
- Assess her for signs and symptoms of diabetes mellitus, such as polyuria, polyphagia, polydipsia, fatigue, weight loss, and an elevated serum glucose level.
- Watch her for other complications of Cushing's syndrome, such as a peptic ulcer, osteoporosis, fluid and electrolyte imbalances, psychiatric disorders, and infection.
- Use standard precautions to reduce the risk for infection. If necessary, provide a private room and institute reverse isolation precautions. Use meticulous hand-washing technique.
- Encourage the patient to verbalize her feelings about body image changes and sexual dysfunction. Offer emotional support and a positive, realistic assessment of her condition. Help her to develop coping strategies. Include family members or friends as a support system, and help them to develop positive coping mechanisms to deal with the patient. Refer her

- express positive feelings about herself.

Risk for infection related to suppressed inflammatory response caused by excessive corticosteroid production. The patient will:

- maintain a normal temperature and white blood cell count and differential
- remain free from infection
- take precautions to avoid, or decrease her risk for, infection.

to a mental health professional for additional counseling, if necessary.

Patient teaching

- Encourage the patient to wear a medical identification bracelet and carry her drugs with her at all times.
- Teach her protective measures to decrease stress and infections. For example, she should get adequate rest and avoid fatigue, eat a balanced diet, and avoid people with infections. Also teach her relaxation and stress-reduction techniques.
- Stress the importance of lifelong follow-up care.

EVALUATION

Achievement of patient outcomes determines the success of collaborative management. For the patient with Cushing's syndrome, evaluation focuses on cardiopulmonary status within acceptable parameters, restoration of hormonal levels, absence of complications, and adequate knowledge of disease, treatment, and care.

Diabetes insipidus

A deficiency of vasopressin (also called antidiuretic hormone) causes this metabolic disorder, characterized by excessive fluid intake and hypotonic polyuria. The disorder may start in childhood or early adulthood (the median age is 21), and it occurs more commonly in men than in women.

In uncomplicated diabetes insipidus, with adequate water replacement, the prognosis is good, and patients usually lead normal lives. However, in patients with an underlying disorder such as cancer, the prognosis varies.

Untreated diabetes insipidus can produce hypovolemia, hyperosmolality, circulatory collapse, unconsciousness, and central nervous system (CNS) damage. These complications are most likely to occur if the patient has an impaired (or absent) thirst mechanism.

A prolonged increase in urine flow may produce chronic complications, such as bladder distention, enlarged calyces, hydroureter, and hydronephrosis. Complications may also result from underlying conditions, such as metastatic brain lesions, head trauma, and infections.

CAUSES

The most common cause of diabetes insipidus is failure of vasopressin secretion in response to normal physiologic stimuli (pituitary or neurogenic diabetes insipidus). A less common cause is failure of the kidneys to respond to vasopressin (congenital nephrogenic diabetes insipidus).

Two types of pituitary diabetes insipidus exist: primary and secondary. The primary form affects about 50% of patients. Familial or idiopathic in origin, this form may occur in neonates as a result of congenital malformation of the CNS, infection, trauma, or tumor.

Secondary pituitary diabetes insipidus is linked to intracranial neoplastic or metastatic lesions, hypophysectomy or other types of neurosurgery, a skull fracture, or head trauma—which damages the neurohypophyseal structures. This disease also is caused by infection, granulomatous disease, and vascular lesions.

A transient form of diabetes insipidus strikes during pregnancy, usually after the fifth or sixth month of gestation. The condition usually reverses spontaneously after delivery.

DIAGNOSIS AND TREATMENT

To distinguish diabetes insipidus from other types of polyuria, the doctor may order urinalysis, a dehydration test (which measures urine osmolality after a period of dehydration with urine osmolality after subcutaneous [S.C.] injection of vasopressin), and plasma and urinary vasopressin evaluations (expensive, time-consuming, last-resort tests). In critically ill patients, the doctor may base the diagnosis on the following laboratory values only:

- urine osmolality—below 200 mOsm/kg
- urine specific gravity—below 1.005
- serum osmolality—above 300 mOsm/kg
- serum sodium—above 147 mEq/L.

Until the cause of diabetes insipidus is identified and eliminated, administration of vasopressin or a vasopressin stimulant can control fluid balance and prevent dehydration.

Aqueous vasopressin is a replacement agent given by S.C. injection in doses of 5 to 10 U with a duration of action of 3 to 6 hours. It's used in the initial management of diabetes insipidus after head trauma or a neurosurgical procedure.

Vasopressin tannate (in oil), an I.M. preparation in a 1.5 to 5 U/ml suspension, is given in doses of 0.3 to 1 ml, as required. Duration is 24 to 72 hours.

Desmopressin acetate, a synthetic vasopressin analogue, exerts prolonged antidiuretic activity and has no pressor effects. It's given intranasally in doses of 0.1 to 0.4 ml or S.C. in doses of 2 to 4 mcg. Duration of action is 12 to 24 hours, making it the drug of choice.

Lypressin is a synthetic vasopressin replacement given as a short-acting nasal spray. It has significant disadvantages: variable absorption rate, nasal congestion and irritation, ulcerated nasal passages (with repeated use), substernal chest tightness, coughing, and dyspnea (after accidental inhalation of large doses).

Chlorpropamide, an oral antidiabetic agent used in patients who have residual release of vasopressin, stimulates or potentiates the action of submaximal amounts of vasopressin on the renal tubules and reduces polyuria. It may be given with clofibrate.

COLLABORATIVE MANAGEMENT

Care of the patient with diabetes insipidus focuses on returning fluid and electrolyte balance to normal, avoiding complications, and teaching about the disease and its treatment.

ASSESSMENT

The patient's history shows an abrupt onset of extreme polyuria (usually 4 to 16 L/day of dilute urine, but sometimes as much as 30 L/day), extreme thirst, and consumption of extraordinary volumes of fluid. Look for:
- reports of weight loss, dizziness, weakness, constipation, slight to moderate nocturia
- in severe cases, fatigue from inadequate rest caused by frequent voiding and excessive thirst
- signs of dehydration, such as dry skin and mucous membranes, fever, and dyspnea
- urine that is pale and voluminous
- poor skin turgor, tachycardia, and decreased muscle strength
- hypotension.

NURSING DIAGNOSES AND COLLABORATIVE PROBLEMS

Based on the following nursing diagnoses, you'll establish patient outcomes.

Altered urinary elimination related to polyuria. The patient will:
- express an understanding of how the prescribed drug can control polyuria
- recover and maintain normal urine output volume with drug therapy.

Fluid volume deficit related to polyuria. The patient will:
- recover and maintain normal fluid volume as evidenced by equal intake and output
- exhibit normal serum osmolality and sodium levels
- not have complications related to fluid volume deficit.

Knowledge deficit related to diabetes insipidus and the prescribed treatment. The patient and caregiver will:
- express a desire to learn about his condition and therapy
- communicate an understanding of how his prescribed treatment can control the symptoms of diabetes insipidus
- correctly administer vasopressin nasally or S.C.

PLANNING AND IMPLEMENTATION

These measures help the patient with diabetes insipidus.
- Make sure the patient has easy access to the bathroom or bedpan, and answer his call signals promptly.
- Institute safety precautions if the patient complains of dizziness or weakness.
- Provide meticulous skin and mouth care. Use a soft toothbrush and mild mouthwash to avoid trauma to the oral mucosa, and apply petroleum jelly, as needed, to cracked or sore lips. Use alcohol-free skin care products and apply emollient lotion after baths.
- Give vasopressin cautiously to a patient with coronary artery disease (CAD) because the drug may cause vasoconstriction. If the patient is receiving vasopressin, monitor for electrocardiogram changes and exacerbation of angina.
- If the patient is taking chlorpropamide, provide adequate caloric intake, and keep orange juice or another carbohydrate handy to treat hypoglycemic episodes. Monitor for signs of hypoglycemia. Watch for decreasing urine output and increasing urine specific gravity between doses. Check laboratory values for hyponatremia and hypoglycemia.
- Keep accurate records of hourly fluid intake and urine output, vital signs, and daily weight.
- Monitor urine specific gravity and serum electrolyte and blood urea nitrogen levels.
- During dehydration testing, watch for signs of hypovolemic shock. Monitor blood pressure, pulse rate, body weight, and changes in mental or neurologic status.
- Monitor serum osmolality and sodium levels with drug therapy.
- Urge the patient to verbalize his feelings. Offer encouragement and a realistic assessment of his situation. Identify his strengths for use in developing coping strategies. Refer him to a mental health professional for counseling, if necessary.

Patient teaching
- Encourage the patient to maintain adequate fluid intake during the day to prevent severe dehydration, but to limit fluids in the evening to prevent nocturia.
- Teach the patient and family members or friends to identify and report signs of severe dehydration and impending hypovolemia.
- Tell the patient to record his weight daily, and teach him and a family member how to monitor intake and output and how to use a hydrometer to measure urine specific gravity.
- Tell them about long-term hormone replacement therapy: that the patient must take the drug as prescribed and never stop it abruptly or without the doctor's advice. Teach them how to give S.C. or I.M. injections and how to use nasal applicators. Dis-

cuss the drug's adverse effects and when to report them.

■ Advise the patient to wear a medical identification bracelet and to carry his medication with him at all times.

EVALUATION

Achievement of patient outcomes determines the success of collaborative management. For the patient with diabetes insipidus, evaluation focuses on fluid and electrolyte balance, urinary elimination and renal function within normal limits, absence of injury and complications, and adequate knowledge to deal with disease and treatment.

Diabetes mellitus

A chronic disease of absolute or relative insulin deficiency or resistance, diabetes mellitus is characterized by disturbances in carbohydrate, protein, and fat metabolism. Insulin transports glucose into the cells for use as energy and storage as glycogen; it also stimulates protein synthesis and free fatty acid storage in the adipose tissues. Insulin deficiency compromises the body tissues' access to essential nutrients for fuel and storage.

Diabetes mellitus is thought to affect about 3.1% of the U.S. population (7.8 million diagnosed cases). About half of those affected are undiagnosed. Incidence is equal in males and females and rises with age.

CAUSES

The disorder occurs in two primary forms: type I, insulin-dependent diabetes mellitus, and the more prevalent type II, non-insulin-dependent diabetes mellitus. Several secondary forms also exist.

Type I diabetes is caused by destruction of the beta cells in the pancreas. By the time the disorder becomes apparent, about 80% of the beta cells have been destroyed. This destruction almost certainly results from an autoimmune process, although details are obscure. The genes that predispose a person to type I diabetes are found in the human leukocyte antigen region of chromosome 6, which contains genes that control immune response. Patients with autoantibodies to islet cell antigens, insulin, or glutamic acid decarboxylase are most likely to develop type I diabetes. Although viruses have been suggested to cause type I diabetes, their mechanism of action hasn't been proven. Further studies of risk factors and their interactions are needed to provide details about the cause and management of type I diabetes.

Type II diabetes may arise from abnormal insulin secretion and resistance to insulin action in target tissues. This may be caused by primary islet cell abnormality. Acquired insulin resistance, usually obesity-related, is probably required for hyperglycemia to develop.

Secondary forms of diabetes mellitus result from such conditions as pancreatic disease, pregnancy, hormonal or genetic syndromes, or ingestion of certain drugs, chemicals, agents, or toxins. Physiologic or emotional stress may trigger prolonged elevation of stress hormone levels (cortisol, epinephrine, glucagon, and growth hormone), which raises blood glucose and places increased demands on the pancreas. Pregnancy causes weight gain and increased estrogen and placental hormone levels. Certain drugs, including thiazide diuretics, adrenal corticosteroids, and oral contraceptives, antagonize the effects of insulin.

Two acute metabolic complications of diabetes are diabetic ketoacidosis (DKA) and hyperosmolar hyperglycemic nonketotic syndrome (HHNS). These life-threatening conditions require immediate medical intervention.

Patients with diabetes mellitus also have a higher risk of various systemic chronic illnesses. The most common chronic complications include cardiovascular and peripheral vascular disease, retinopathy, nephropathy, diabetic dermopathy, and peripheral and autonomic neuropathy.

Peripheral neuropathy usually affects the hands and feet and may cause numbness or pain. Autonomic neuropathy may manifest itself as gastroparesis (leading to delayed gastric emptying and a feeling of nausea and fullness after meals), nocturnal diarrhea, impotence, and postural hypotension.

Hyperglycemia impairs the patient's resistance to infection because the glucose content of the epidermis and urine encourages bacterial growth. The patient is, therefore, susceptible to skin and urinary tract infections and vaginitis.

In insulitis, the islets are infiltrated with activated T lymphocytes, and the beta cells are mistaken as foreign by the immune system. Cytotoxic antibodies develop and act in conjunction with cell-mediated immune mechanisms to destroy the beta cells.

DIAGNOSIS AND TREATMENT

For critical test values, in nonpregnant adults, one of the following findings confirms a diagnosis of diabetes mellitus: symptoms of uncontrolled diabetes and a glucose level of 200 mg/dl or higher in a random sample of blood, a fasting plasma glucose level of 126 mg/dl or higher on at least two occasions, an oral glucose tolerance test result showing the glucose level above 200 mg/dl at 2 hours and on at least one other occasion during the test (despite normal results

Revised guidelines for diagnosing diabetes

The American Diabetes Association (ADA) recently proposed new guidelines for diagnosing diabetes that lower the acceptable level of fasting glucose in the blood. The guidelines also call for earlier testing of healthy people and more frequent testing of high-risk groups.

Blood glucose level guidelines
The ADA now classifies blood glucose levels as follows:
- *Provisional diabetes:* 126 mg/dl or more, confirmed by repeat test done on another day (previous guidelines: 140 mg/dl or more)
- *Impaired:* 110 to 125 mg/dl
- *Normal:* less than 110 mg/dl.

Testing guidelines
The ADA recommends routine testing every 3 years for people age 45 and older without symptoms. People with classic symptoms—abnormal thirst, frequent urination, and unexplained weight loss—should be tested immediately.

More frequent testing is recommended for the following high-risk groups:
- Blacks, Hispanics, and Native Americans
- those who are obese (more than 20% over ideal body weight)
- those who have a close relative with diabetes
- those with high blood pressure (140/90 mm Hg or higher)
- those with high levels of high-density lipoprotein cholesterol (35 mg/dl or higher) or triglycerides (250 mg/dl or higher)
- those who on previous tests had impaired glucose tolerance or impaired fasting glucose
- women who have delivered a baby weighing more than 9 lb or who have been diagnosed with gestational diabetes.

during the fasting phase of the test). (See *Revised guidelines for diagnosing diabetes.*)

An ophthalmologic examination may show diabetic retinopathy. Other tests include urinalysis for acetone and blood testing for glycosylated hemoglobin (hemoglobin A), which reflects recent glucose control.

Treatment of diabetes normalizes the blood glucose level and reduces complications. In type I diabetes, goals are achieved with insulin replacement, diet, and exercise. Current forms of insulin replacement therapy include single-dose, mixed-dose, split-mixed-dose, and multiple-dose regimens. The multiple-dose regimens are commonly given with an insulin pump.

Insulin may be rapid-acting (lispro), short-acting (regular), intermediate-acting (NPH), long-acting (Ultralente), or a combination of rapid-acting and intermediate-acting (Mixtard). Insulin types are standard or purified, and derived from beef, pork, or human sources. Purified human insulin is used commonly today. Pancreas transplantation, another type of therapy, remains experimental.

Treatment of both types also requires strict adherence to a diet carefully planned to meet nutritional needs, control blood glucose levels, and reach and maintain appropriate body weight. An estimate is made of the total energy intake needed daily based on the patient's ideal body weight. Then a decision is made regarding carbohydrate, fat, and protein content, and an appropriate diet is constructed.

For the obese patient with type II diabetes, weight reduction is a dietary goal. In type I, the calorie allotment may be high, depending on the patient's growth

stage and activity level. The successful patient will follow the diet consistently and eat at regular times.

Exercise along with weight reduction and proper diet has proven useful in managing type II diabetes. Physical activity increases insulin sensitivity, improves glucose tolerance, and promotes weight loss. Patients with type II diabetes may also need oral antidiabetic drugs to stimulate endogenous insulin production and, possibly, increase insulin sensitivity at the cellular level.

Treatment of long-term complications may include dialysis or kidney transplantation for renal failure, photocoagulation or vitrectomy for retinopathy, and vascular surgery for large vessel disease. Precise blood glucose control is essential. (See *Managing uncontrolled diabetes mellitus,* pages 426 and 427.)

COLLABORATIVE MANAGEMENT
Care of the patient with diabetes mellitus focuses on achieving adequate blood glucose level control, avoiding complications, and teaching him how to comply with treatment.

ASSESSMENT
The patient with type I diabetes usually reports rapidly developing symptoms. With type II diabetes, the patient's symptoms are usually vague and long-standing and develop gradually. Patients with type II diabetes generally report a family history of diabetes mellitus, gestational diabetes or the delivery of a baby weighing more than 9 lb (4 kg), severe viral infection, autoimmune dysfunction, other endocrine disease, re-

cent stress or trauma, or use of drugs that increase blood glucose levels. In both types, look for:

- symptoms related to hyperglycemia, such as polyuria, polydipsia, polyphagia, weight loss, and fatigue
- complaints of weakness; vision changes; frequent skin infections; dry, itchy skin; sexual problems; and vaginal discomfort—all symptoms of complications.
- apparent retinopathy or cataract formation
- skin changes—especially on the legs and feet—representing impaired peripheral circulation
- in type I, muscle wasting and loss of subcutaneous fat
- in type II, thin, muscular limbs and fat deposits around the face, neck, and abdomen
- poor skin turgor and dry mucous membranes related to dehydration
- decreased peripheral pulses, cool skin temperature, and decreased reflexes
- orthostatic hypotension
- with DKA, a characteristic "fruity" breath odor because of increased acetone production.

NURSING DIAGNOSES AND COLLABORATIVE PROBLEMS

Based on the following nursing diagnoses, you'll establish patient outcomes.

Risk for injury related to complications. The patient will:

- comply with treatment as evidenced by a normal glycosylated hemoglobin level
- recognize the signs and symptoms of hypoglycemia and hyperglycemia quickly and take appropriate action to achieve a normal blood glucose level—or seek emergency help if such measures fail
- exhibit no signs or symptoms of chronic complications, such as retinopathy, neuropathy, and nephropathy
- experience no injury from diabetes.

Impaired adjustment related to chronicity of disease and complexity of treatment. The patient will:

- identify an inability to cope adequately
- seek help with coping and make use of available resources and support groups to adjust to diabetes
- accept the prescribed diabetic treatment.

Knowledge deficit related to diabetes mellitus and the complex treatment regimen. The patient will:

- identify the need to learn about diabetes and its management and obtain this information from a reputable source
- express an understanding of his prescribed treatment regimen and demonstrate skill in managing it.

PLANNING AND IMPLEMENTATION

These measures help the patient with diabetes mellitus.

- Consult a dietitian to plan a diet with the recommended amounts of calories, protein, carbohydrates, and fats.
- Give insulin or an oral antidiabetic drug as prescribed.
- Have the patient participate in a supervised exercise program.
- Keep accurate records of vital signs, weight, fluid intake, urine output, and caloric intake. Monitor serum glucose and urine acetone levels.
- Monitor the patient's compliance with his prescribed diabetic regimen.
- Monitor for acute complications of diabetic therapy, especially hypoglycemia. Also watch for signs of ketoacidosis (acetone breath, dehydration, weak and rapid pulse, and Kussmaul's respirations) and HHNS (polyuria, thirst, neurologic abnormalities, and stupor).
- Treat hypoglycemic reactions promptly by giving carbohydrates in the form of fruit juice, hard candy, honey or, if the patient is unconscious, glucagon or I.V. dextrose. Treat hyperglycemic crises with I.V. fluids, insulin and, possibly, potassium replacement, as ordered.
- Monitor diabetic effects on the cardiovascular system, such as cerebrovascular, coronary artery, and peripheral vascular impairment, and on the peripheral and autonomic nervous systems.
- Observe for signs of urinary tract and vaginal infections, and monitor the patient's urine for protein, an early sign of nephropathy.
- Look for signs and symptoms of diabetic neuropathy (numbness or pain in the hands and feet, footdrop, and neurogenic bladder).
- Provide meticulous skin care, especially to the feet and legs. Refer the patient to a podiatrist.
- Encourage the patient to verbalize his feelings about diabetes and its effects on lifestyle and life expectancy. Offer emotional support and a realistic assessment of his condition. Stress that, with proper treatment, he can have a near-normal life.
- Help him develop coping strategies. Refer him and family members or friends to a counselor, if necessary, and encourage them to join a support group.

Patient teaching

- Stress the importance of strictly complying with the prescribed therapy.
- Tailor your teaching to the patient's needs, abilities, and age. Discuss diet, drugs, exercise, monitoring techniques, hygiene, and how to prevent and recognize hypoglycemia and hyperglycemia.
- To encourage compliance with lifestyle changes, emphasize how blood glucose control affects long-term health.
- Teach the patient how to care for his feet: He should wash them daily, carefully dry between his

Managing uncontrolled diabetes mellitus

Initiation
Average length of stay (LOS): 6 days (Goal: 4 days)
Actual LOS:

	Day 1	Days 2 to 3

MEDICAL INTERVENTIONS	■ History and physical
	■ Order the following:
	  –Fingersticks before meals and at bedtime
	  –American Diabetes Association (ADA) diet
	  –Intake and output (I & O)
	  –No dextrose in routine I.V. fluids
	  –Hypoglycemic therapy
	■ Initiate assessment for precipitating factors.
		■ Complete assessment for precipitating factors.
		■ Reassess need for ongoing glycemic control.
		■ Assess need for home glucose monitoring.
		■ Day before discharge: Post "Tentative discharge in a.m." order on chart; order discharge medications and supplies.

NURSING INTERVENTIONS	■ Do complete data base assessment. ■ Document patient's self-care ability. ■ Obtain fingersticks as ordered and as needed (p.r.n.). ■ Administer glycemic medications as ordered. ■ Assess learning ability. ■ Obtain I & O as ordered.	■ Fingersticks, I & O as ordered ■ Glycemic medications as ordered ■ Initiate educational activities. ■ Facilitate patient participation in diabetes classes.
SOCIAL WORK	■ Respond to assessed need if patient has inadequate support systems or needs assistance with discharge.	■ Assess support systems.
NUTRITION	■ Dietary screening ■ ADA diet	■ Individualized caloric assessment ■ Instruction in diet
TESTS	■ Urinalysis ■ Blood chemistries: Sodium, potassium, CO_2, glucose, creatinine	■ Continue to document glucose monitoring.
CONSULTS	■ Dietitian ■ Endocrinologist	■ Dietitian consult in progress
ACTIVITY	■ Screen ability to perform activities of daily living (ADLs).	■ Assess ability to perform ADLs.
PATIENT EDUCATION	■ Screen ability to learn. ■ Initiate teaching protocol.	■ Distribute educational literature. ■ Discuss disease process, self-care, and home glucose monitoring. ■ Demonstrate medication administration; observe return demonstration.
DISCHARGE PLANNING	■ Identify support system: Family involvement. ■ Identify lifestyle and health habits prior to admission.	■ Order glucometer, if applicable. ■ Initiate referral for home care, if applicable.
KEY PATIENT OUTCOMES	■ Initiation of assessment for presence or absence of precipitating factors *Date met_____ Not met_____ Initials _____*	■ Random blood glucose >60 and <300 *Date met_____ Not met_____ Initials _____* ■ Fasting blood glucose >60 and <240 *Date met_____ Not met_____ Initials _____* ■ Therapy for precipitating factors initiated, if applicable *Date met_____ Not met_____ Initials _____*
	Signature _____	Signature _____

Adapted with permission from Veterans Affairs Maryland Health Care System at Baltimore.

Day 4

- Address need for home health referral.
- Complete discharge instructions; discuss with patient.
- Dictate discharge summary.
- Post discharge order on order sheet.

- Reinforce self-care activities.
- Reinforce medication information.

- Caloric assessment completed
- Diet reinforcement

- Follow-up with ophthalmology; podiatry and diabetic management class arranged, if applicable
- Follow-up arranged with endocrine clinic within 4 weeks

- Document ability to perform ADLs.

- Address use of home glucose monitor.
- Reinforce medication administration.

- Stress importance of maintaining medical regimen and clinic appointments.
- Discuss and review discharge instructions.
- Review procedure for mail-in renewal for supplies.
- Provide telephone numbers for clinic, doctor, and support groups.

- Random blood glucose >60 and <280

Date met——— Not met——— Initials ———

- Fasting blood glucose >60 and <180

Date met——— Not met ———Initials ———

- Home glucose monitoring initiated, if applicable

Date met——— Not met——— Initials ———

- Patient and family able to verbalize understanding of self-care, knowledge of follow-up, and medication renewal.

Date met——— Not met——— Initials ———

Signature ———

toes, and inspect for corns, calluses, redness, swelling, bruises, and breaks in the skin. He should report any skin changes to the doctor. Advise him to wear comfortable, nonconstricting shoes and never to walk barefoot.

- Recommend regular ophthalmologic examinations for early detection of diabetic retinopathy.
- Describe the signs and symptoms of diabetic neuropathy, and emphasize the need for safety precautions because decreased sensation can mask injuries.
- Teach the patient how to manage his diabetes when he has a minor illness, such as a cold, flu, or upset stomach.
- Teach the patient and family members how to monitor the patient's diet and use food exchange lists. Show them how to read labels in the supermarket to identify fat, carbohydrate, protein, and sugar content.
- Encourage them to contact the Juvenile Diabetes Foundation, the American Association of Diabetes Educators, and the American Diabetes Association for more information.

EVALUATION
Achievement of patient outcomes determines the success of collaborative management. For the patient with diabetes mellitus, evaluation focuses on adequate control of blood glucose levels with diet, exercise, and drugs; absence of injury and complications; and adequate knowledge of the disease to comply with treatment.

Diabetic ketoacidosis

Diabetic ketoacidosis (DKA) is an acute complication of hyperglycemic crisis. It usually affects people with type I diabetes; in fact, it may be the first evidence of previously unrecognized type I diabetes. (See *Understanding DKA and HHNS*, pages 428 and 429.)

CAUSES
Acute insulin deficiency from illness, stress, infection, or failure to take insulin can precipitate DKA. The resulting buildup of glucose in the blood produces the signs and symptoms of DKA and hyperosmolar hypoglycemic nonketotic syndrome: soaring glucose levels, fluid loss, dehydration, shock, coma, and death. Keep in mind the patient with DKA also shows evidence of metabolic acidosis. (See "Diabetes mellitus" and "Hyperosmolar hyperglycemic nonketotic syndrome" in this chapter.)

DIAGNOSIS AND TREATMENT
Diagnostic tests will show the patient's blood sugar is above normal, serum sodium and potassium are nor-

Understanding DKA and HHNS

Diabetic ketoacidosis (DKA) and hyperglycemic nonketotic syndrome (HHNS) are acute complications of hyperglycemic crisis that may occur in the diabetic patient. If not treated properly, either may result in coma or death.

DKA usually occurs in patients with type I diabetes; in fact, it may be the first evidence of previously unrecognized type I diabetes. HHNS usually occurs in patients with type II diabetes. But HHNS may also occur in anyone whose insulin tolerance is stressed and in patients who've undergone certain therapeutic procedures—such as peritoneal dialysis, hemodialysis, tube feedings, or total parenteral nutrition.

Acute insulin deficiency (absolute in DKA; relative in HHNS) precipitates both conditions. Causes include ill-ness, stress, infection, and failure to take insulin (*only* in a patient with DKA).

Buildup of glucose

Inadequate insulin hinders glucose uptake by fat and muscle cells. Because the cells can't take in glucose to convert to energy, glucose accumulates in the blood. At the same time, the liver responds to the demands of the energy-starved cells by converting glycogen to glucose and releasing glucose into the blood, *further* increasing the blood glucose level. When this level exceeds the renal threshold, excess glucose is excreted in the urine.

Still, the insulin-deprived cells can't utilize glucose. Their response is rapid metabolism of protein, which results in loss of intracellular potassium and phosphorus

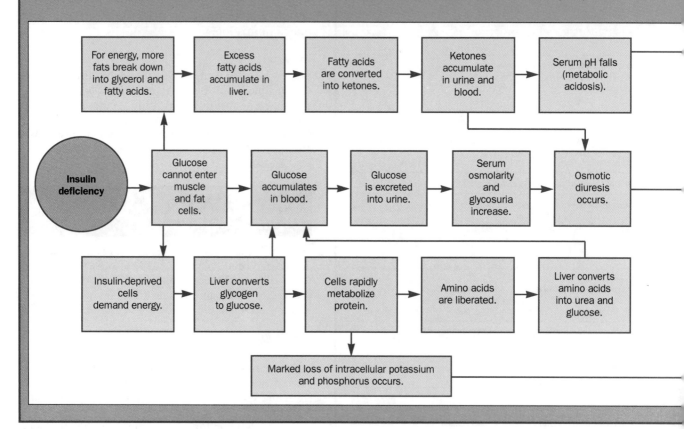

mal (potassium may also be above normal), ketones are largely positive, and serum osmolarity is above normal but usually less than 330 mOsm/L. Hematocrit may be above normal. The patient may have metabolic acidosis with compensatory respiratory alkalosis. Urine glucose level is above normal. Urine output is initially polyuric and later becomes oliguric.

Treatment involves administration of insulin, fluid replacement, electrolyte replacement and, possibly, antiacidosis therapy.

COLLABORATIVE MANAGEMENT

Care of the patient with diabetic ketoacidosis focuses on restoring blood glucose control, avoiding compli-

and in excessive liberation of amino acids. The liver converts these amino acids into urea and glucose.

As a result of these processes, blood glucose levels are grossly elevated. The aftermath is increased serum osmolarity and glycosuria (higher in HHNS than in DKA because blood glucose levels are higher in HHNS), leading to osmotic diuresis.

A deadly cycle
The massive fluid loss from osmotic diuresis causes fluid and electrolyte imbalances and dehydration. Water loss exceeds electrolyte loss, contributing to hyperosmolarity. This, in turn, perpetuates dehydration, decreasing the glomerular filtration rate and reducing the amount of glucose excreted in the urine. This leads to a deadly cycle:

Diminished glucose excretion *further* raises blood glucose levels, producing severe hyperosmolarity and dehydration and finally causing shock, coma, and death.

Further DKA complication
All these steps hold true for both DKA and HHNS. But DKA has an additional simultaneous process that leads to metabolic acidosis. The *absolute* insulin deficiency causes cells to convert fats into glycerol and fatty acids for energy. The fatty acids can't be metabolized as quickly as they're released, so they accumulate in the liver, where they're converted into ketones (ketoacids). These ketones accumulate in the blood and urine and cause *acidosis*. Acidosis leads to more tissue breakdown, more ketosis, more acidosis, and eventually shock, coma, and death.

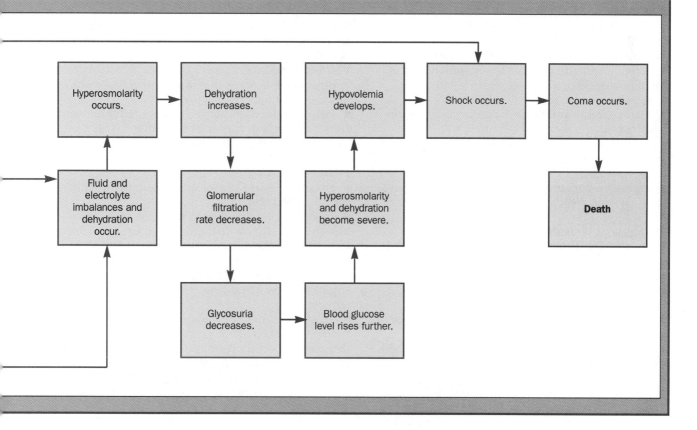

cations, and teaching him how to participate actively in disease-control planning.

ASSESSMENT
The patient's skin is usually warm, flushed, and dry. He may be confused and lethargic with diminished reflexes or coma. Look for:

- weak muscles
- reports of anorexia, nausea, vomiting, diarrhea and abdominal tenderness, or pain
- a fever or hypothermia
- mildly tachycardic, weak pulse
- subnormal blood pressure
- initially, deep and fast respirations

- later, Kussmaul's sign; fruity, acetone-smelling breath
- complaints of thirst.

NURSING DIAGNOSES AND COLLABORATIVE PROBLEMS

Based on the following nursing diagnoses, you'll establish patient outcomes.

Risk for injury related to complications. The patient will:
- comply with treatment as evidenced by a normal glycosylated hemoglobin level
- recognize the signs and symptoms of hypoglycemia and hyperglycemia quickly and take appropriate action to achieve a normal blood glucose level—or seek emergency help if such measures fail
- exhibit no signs or symptoms of chronic complications, such as retinopathy, neuropathy, and nephropathy
- not experience injury from diabetes.

Altered thought processes related to physiologic symptoms. The patient will:
- recognize and verbalize the need for assistance
- accept treatment, resulting in restoration of thought processes
- remain safe and free from injury.

Knowledge deficit related to diabetes mellitus and the complex treatment regimen. The patient will:
- identify the need to learn about diabetes and its management and obtain this information from a reputable source
- express an understanding of his prescribed treatment regimen and demonstrate skill in managing it.

PLANNING AND IMPLEMENTATION

These measures help the patient with diabetic ketoacidosis.
- Carefully monitor serum glucose levels, as ordered.
- Provide initial rehydration with normal saline solution or lactated Ringer's solution, as ordered.
- Institute measures to reduce blood glucose levels, give insulin I.V., as ordered.
- Prepare to administer bicarbonate for severe acidosis that does not respond to insulin.
- Treat hypoglycemic reactions promptly by giving carbohydrates in the form of fruit juice, hard candy, honey or, if the patient is unconscious, glucagon or I.V. dextrose. Treat hyperglycemic crises with I.V. fluids, insulin and, possibly, potassium replacement, as ordered.
- Keep accurate records of vital signs, weight, fluid intake, urine output, and caloric intake. Monitor serum glucose and urine acetone levels.
- Consult a dietitian to plan a special diet with the recommended amounts of calories, protein, carbohydrates, and fats.

- Have the patient participate in a supervised exercise program.
- Continue to monitor for acute complications of diabetic therapy, especially hypoglycemia.
- Monitor diabetic effects on the cardiovascular system, such as cerebrovascular, coronary artery, and peripheral vascular impairment, and on the peripheral and autonomic nervous systems.
- Observe for signs of urinary tract and vaginal infections, and monitor the patient's urine for protein, an early sign of nephropathy.
- Look for signs and symptoms of diabetic neuropathy (numbness or pain in the hands and feet, footdrop, and neurogenic bladder).
- Monitor the patient's compliance with his prescribed diabetic regimen.
- Provide meticulous skin care, especially to the feet and legs. Treat all injuries, cuts, and blisters promptly. Avoid constricting hose, slippers, or bed linens. Refer the patient to a podiatrist.
- Encourage the patient to verbalize his feelings about diabetes and its effects on lifestyle and life expectancy.
- Offer emotional support and a realistic assessment of his condition. Stress that, with proper treatment, he can have a near-normal life.
- Help him develop coping strategies. Refer him and family members or friends to a counselor, if necessary, and encourage them to join a support group.

Patient teaching

- Stress the importance of strictly complying with the prescribed therapy.
- Tailor your teaching to the patient's needs, abilities, and age. Discuss diet, drugs, exercise, monitoring techniques, hygiene, and how to prevent and recognize hypoglycemia and hyperglycemia.
- To encourage compliance with lifestyle changes, emphasize how blood glucose control affects long-term health.
- Teach the patient how to care for his feet: He should wash them daily, carefully dry between his toes, and inspect for corns, calluses, redness, swelling, bruises, and breaks in the skin. He should report any skin changes to the doctor. Advise him to wear comfortable, nonconstricting shoes and never to walk barefoot.
- Recommend regular ophthalmologic examinations for early detection of diabetic retinopathy.
- Describe the signs and symptoms of diabetic neuropathy, and emphasize the need for safety precautions because decreased sensation can mask injuries.
- Teach the patient how to manage his diabetes when he has a minor illness, such as a cold, flu, or upset stomach.

- Teach the patient and family members how to monitor the patient's diet and use food exchange lists. Show them how to read labels in the supermarket to identify fat, carbohydrate, protein, and sugar content.
- Teach the patient and family members the signs and symptoms of DKA (acetone breath; Kussmaul respirations; weak, rapid pulse; and dehydration).
- Encourage them to contact the Juvenile Diabetes Foundation, the American Association of Diabetes Educators, and the American Diabetes Association for more information.

EVALUATION
Achievement of patient outcomes determines the success of collaborative management. For the patient with DKA, evaluation focuses on restoration of blood glucose control, laboratory study levels within acceptable parameters, absence of injury and complications, and adequate knowledge to participate actively in disease control planning.

Hyperosmolar hyperglycemic nonketotic syndrome

Hyperosmolar hyperglycemic nonketotic syndrome (HHNS) is an acute complication of hyperglycemic crisis in people with diabetes mellitus. It usually strikes patients with type II diabetes. But HHNS may also affect anyone whose insulin tolerance is stressed and who's undergone certain therapeutic procedures—such as peritoneal dialysis or tube feedings.

CAUSES
Acute insulin deficiency may precipitate the condition. Additional causes include illness, stress, infection, certain drugs and medical procedures, and severe burns treated with high glucose concentrations.

DIAGNOSIS AND TREATMENT
Diagnostic tests will show your patient's blood glucose level markedly above normal; serum sodium and potassium may be normal or above normal. Serum ketones are usually negative or small. Serum osmolarity is markedly above normal (350 to 450 mOsm/L). Hematocrit is above normal. Arterial blood gas levels are normal or show slight metabolic acidosis. Urine glucose is markedly above normal. Urine output is initially above normal; later, oliguria occurs.

When you recognize the signs and symptoms of this condition, notify the doctor immediately and prepare to transfer the patient to the intensive care unit. Treatment begins with I.V. fluid replacement therapy as soon as possible. Expect to give an injection of regular insulin immediately—either I.M. or I.V.—followed by a continuous I.V. insulin drip.

You'll provide supportive care as indicated by the patient's condition (for example, treatment for arrhythmias caused by electrolyte imbalance and intubation or mechanical ventilation for severe respiratory depression).

COLLABORATIVE MANAGEMENT
Care of the patient with HHNS focuses on restoring blood glucose control, avoiding complications, and teaching disease control.

ASSESSMENT
A buildup of glucose in the blood causes HHNS signs and symptoms: soaring glucose levels, fluid loss, dehydration, shock, coma, and death. The patient's skin may be warm, flushed, and dry. He'll have weak muscle strength, fever, rapid pulse, subnormal blood pressure, rapid respirations, normal breath odor, and thirst.

NURSING DIAGNOSES AND COLLABORATIVE PROBLEMS
Based on the following nursing diagnoses, you'll establish patient outcomes.

Risk for injury related to complications. The patient will:
- comply with treatment as evidenced by a normal glycosylated hemoglobin level
- recognize the signs and symptoms of hypoglycemia and hyperglycemia quickly and take appropriate action to achieve a normal blood glucose level—or seek emergency help if such measures fail
- exhibit no signs or symptoms of chronic complications, such as retinopathy, neuropathy, and nephropathy
- experience no injury from diabetes.

Altered thought processes related to physiologic symptoms. The patient will:
- recognize and verbalize the need for assistance
- accept treatment, resulting in restoration of thought processes
- remain safe and free from injury.

Knowledge deficit related to diabetes mellitus and the complex treatment regimen. The patient will:
- identify the need to learn about diabetes and its management and obtain this information from a reputable source
- express an understanding of his prescribed treatment regimen and demonstrate skill in managing it.

PLANNING AND IMPLEMENTATION
These measures help the patient with HHNS.
- Consult a dietitian to plan a special diet with the recommended amounts of calories, protein, carbohydrates, and fats.

DISCHARGE READY > **After HHNS**

After treatment for hyperosmolar hypoglycemic nonketotic syndrome (HHNS), the patient will meet the following criteria before discharge:

- vital signs within acceptable parameters
- blood glucose levels returning to acceptable levels with minimal fluctuations
- knowledge of the factors that precipitate HHNS
- ability to comply with diabetic management regimen
- absence of complications.

■ Give insulin or an oral antidiabetic drug as prescribed.

■ Have the patient participate in a supervised exercise program.

■ Monitor for acute complications of diabetic therapy, especially hypoglycemia. Also watch for signs and symptoms of ketoacidosis (acetone breath, dehydration, weak and rapid pulse, and Kussmaul's respirations) and HHNS (polyuria, thirst, neurologic abnormalities, and stupor).

■ Treat hypoglycemic reactions promptly by giving carbohydrates in the form of fruit juice, hard candy, honey or, if the patient is unconscious, glucagon or I.V. dextrose.

■ Treat hyperglycemic crises with I.V. fluids, insulin and, possibly, potassium replacement, as ordered.

■ Keep accurate records of vital signs, weight, fluid intake, urine output, and caloric intake. Monitor serum glucose and urine acetone levels.

■ Monitor diabetic effects on the cardiovascular system, such as cerebrovascular, coronary artery, and peripheral vascular impairment, and on the peripheral and autonomic nervous systems.

■ Observe for signs of urinary tract and vaginal infections, and monitor the patient's urine for protein, an early sign of nephropathy.

■ Look for signs and symptoms of diabetic neuropathy (numbness or pain in the hands and feet, footdrop, and neurogenic bladder).

■ Monitor the patient's compliance with his prescribed diabetic regimen.

■ Provide meticulous skin care, especially to the feet and legs. Treat all injuries, cuts, and blisters promptly. Avoid constricting hose, slippers, or bed linens. Refer the patient to a podiatrist.

■ Encourage the patient to verbalize his feelings about diabetes and its effects on lifestyle and life expectancy. Offer emotional support and a realistic assessment of his condition.

■ Stress that, with proper treatment, he can have a near-normal lifestyle and life expectancy.

■ Assist the patient to develop coping strategies. Refer him and family members or friends to a counselor, if necessary, and encourage them to join a support group.

Patient teaching

■ Stress the importance of strict compliance with the prescribed therapy.

■ Tailor your teaching to the patient's needs, abilities, and age. Discuss diet, drugs, exercise, monitoring techniques, hygiene, and how to prevent and recognize hypoglycemia and hyperglycemia.

■ To encourage compliance with lifestyle changes, emphasize how blood glucose control affects long-term health.

■ Teach the patient how to care for his feet: He should wash them daily, carefully dry between his toes, and inspect for corns, calluses, redness, swelling, bruises, and breaks in the skin. He should report any skin changes to the doctor. Advise him to wear comfortable, nonconstricting shoes and never to walk barefoot.

■ Teach the patient and family members the signs and symptoms of HHNS (polyuria, thirst, neurologic abnormalities, and stupor).

■ Recommend regular ophthalmologic examinations for early detection of diabetic retinopathy.

■ Describe the signs and symptoms of diabetic neuropathy, and emphasize the need for safety precautions because decreased sensation can mask injuries.

■ Teach the patient how to manage his diabetes when he has a minor illness, such as a cold, flu, or upset stomach.

■ Teach the patient and family members how to monitor the patient's diet and use food exchange lists. Show them how to read labels in the supermarket to identify fat, carbohydrate, protein, and sugar content.

■ Encourage them to contact the Juvenile Diabetes Foundation, the American Association of Diabetes Educators, and the American Diabetes Association for more information.

EVALUATION

Achievement of patient outcomes determines the success of collaborative management. For the patient with HHNS, evaluation focuses on restoration of blood glucose control, laboratory study levels within acceptable parameters, absence of injury and complications, and adequate knowledge to participate actively in disease-control planning. (See *After HHNS*.)

Hyperparathyroidism

Characterized by overactivity of one or more of the four parathyroid glands, hyperparathyroidism is two to four times more common in women than in men and increases dramatically in both men and women after age 50. The disorder is classified as primary or secondary, based on its etiology.

CAUSES

In primary hyperparathyroidism, one or more of the parathyroid glands enlarges, increasing parathyroid hormone (PTH) secretion and elevating serum calcium levels. The cause of primary hyperparathyroidism is unknown. Agenetic factors may be involved. Also, patients with thyroid carcinoma who've had neck irradiation have developed primary hyperparathyroidism.

In secondary hyperparathyroidism, excessive compensatory production of PTH stems from a hypocalcemia-producing abnormality outside the parathyroid gland, which causes a resistance to the metabolic action of PTH. Rickets, chronic renal failure, vitamin D deficiency, osteomalacia due to laxative abuse or phenytoin, or an excessive intake of thiazide diuretics, vitamin D, and calcium supplements may cause hypocalcemia.

Hyperparathyroidism results in excessive secretion of PTH. Increased PTH levels act directly on the bone and kidney tubules, causing an increase of calcium in the extracellular fluid that can't be compensated for by renal excretion or uptake into the soft tissues or skeleton.

Untreated hyperparathyroidism damages the skeleton and kidneys from hypercalcemia. The patient may develop bone and articular problems, such as chondrocalcinosis; occasional severe osteopenia, especially of the vertebrae; erosions of the juxta-articular surface; subchondral fractures; traumatic synovitis; and pseudogout.

Renal complications include renal calculi, renal colic, nephrolithiasis, urinary tract infections, renal insufficiency and, eventually, renal failure. Other possible complications include peptic ulcers, cholelithiasis, pancreatitis, cardiac arrhythmias, vascular damage, hypertension, and heart failure. Severe hypercalcemia may cause parathyroid poisoning, which includes central nervous system (CNS) changes, renal failure, rapid precipitation of calcium throughout the soft tissues and, possibly, coma.

DIAGNOSIS AND TREATMENT

The diagnostic tests most commonly used to detect hyperparathyroidism are serum PTH, calcium, and phosphorus levels and urine cyclic adenosine monophosphate determinations. Radioimmunoassay confirms the diagnosis and X-rays reveal bone changes. Esophagography, thyroid scan, parathyroid thermography, ultrasonography, thyroid angiography, computed tomography scan, and magnetic resonance imaging can help locate parathyroid lesions.

Supportive laboratory tests reveal decreased serum phosphorus; elevated urine and serum calcium, chloride, uric acid, creatinine, alkaline phosphatase, and basal acid secretion; and serum immunoreactive gastrin levels.

In diagnosing secondary hyperparathyroidism, laboratory test findings show normal or slightly decreased serum calcium levels and variable serum phosphorus levels, especially when hyperparathyroidism is due to rickets, osteomalacia, or renal disease. Other laboratory values and physical examination findings identify the cause of secondary hyperparathyroidism.

Primary hyperparathyroidism may be treated by surgical removal of the adenoma or, depending on the extent of hyperplasia, all but half of one gland (the remaining part is necessary to maintain normal PTH levels). Although surgery may relieve bone pain within 3 days, renal damage may be irreversible.

Preoperatively—or if surgery isn't feasible or necessary—other treatments can decrease calcium levels. Such treatments include forcing fluids; limiting dietary intake of calcium; promoting sodium and calcium excretion through forced diuresis using normal saline solution (up to 6 L in life-threatening circumstances), furosemide, or ethacrynic acid; and giving oral sodium or potassium phosphate, calcitonin, or plicamycin.

To prevent postoperative magnesium and phosphate deficiencies, the patient receives I.V. magnesium and phosphate or sodium phosphate solution given orally or by retention enema. In addition, during the first 4 to 5 days after surgery, when serum calcium falls to low-normal levels, supplemental calcium may be necessary; vitamin D or calcitriol also can raise serum calcium levels.

Treatment of secondary hyperparathyroidism aims to correct the underlying cause of parathyroid hypertrophy and includes vitamin D therapy or, in the patient with renal disease, aluminum hydroxide for hyperphosphatemia. The patient with renal failure requires dialysis—possibly for the rest of her life—to lower calcium levels. In the patient with chronic secondary hyperparathyroidism, the enlarged glands may not revert to normal size and function, even after calcium levels have been controlled.

Glucocorticoids are effective inhibitors of bone resorption and may be particularly useful in treating hypercalcemia associated with hematologic malignant neoplasms.

COLLABORATIVE MANAGEMENT

Care of the patient with hyperparathyroidism focuses on returning her vital signs to within acceptable parameters and teaching her about the disease, treatment, and care.

ASSESSMENT

Patients with primary hyperparathyroidism are usually asymptomatic or have nonspecific symptoms, such as weakness and low stamina. When symptoms occur, they are attributed to two causes: hypercalcemia, with associated hypercalciuria, or osteitis fibrosa cystica.

On inspection, you may note marked muscle weakness and atrophy, particularly in the legs, and joint hyperextensibility. With CNS involvement, alterations in level of consciousness, such as disorientation, stupor, and coma, may appear. Skeletal deformities of the long bones are visible. Palpation may detect hyporeflexia, and auscultation of blood pressure may reveal hypertension.

NURSING DIAGNOSES AND COLLABORATIVE PROBLEMS

Based on the following nursing diagnoses, you'll establish patient outcomes.

Activity intolerance related to bone pain and neuromuscular deficits. Based on this nursing diagnosis, you'll establish these patient outcomes. The patient will:
- regain and maintain normal muscle mass and strength
- maintain maximum joint range of motion
- perform self-care activities as tolerated.

Risk for injury related to the effects of hypercalcemia. The patient will:
- express an understanding of how hypercalcemia affects her body
- comply with prescribed treatments, as shown by normal serum calcium levels, to minimize organ damage
- maintain normal body functions.

Pain related to musculoskeletal changes caused by persistently elevated serum calcium levels. The patient will:
- express pain relief after analgesic administration
- use comfort measures to relieve pain
- become pain-free when calcium levels return to normal.

PLANNING AND IMPLEMENTATION

These measures help the patient with hyperparathyroidism.
- Obtain baseline serum potassium, calcium, phosphate, and magnesium levels before treatment because these values may change abruptly once treatment begins.
- Monitor the patient's serum potassium, calcium, phosphate, and magnesium levels regularly.

- Provide at least 3 qt (3 L) of fluid a day, including cranberry or prune juice, to increase urine acidity and help prevent calculus formation.
- During hydration aimed at reducing the serum calcium level, monitor and record intake and output and strain urine to check for renal calculi.
- Take safety precautions to minimize the risk of injury from a fall. Help the patient walk, keep the bed in the lowest position, and raise the side rails. Lift the immobilized patient carefully to minimize bone stress.
- Give antacids, as appropriate, to prevent peptic ulcers. Consult a dietitian to plan a diet with adequate calories.
- Auscultate the lungs regularly. Check for signs of pulmonary edema in the patient receiving large amounts of normal saline solution, especially if she has pulmonary or cardiac disease.
- Assess the patient for parathyroid poisoning, musculoskeletal changes, and renal impairment.
- Schedule care to allow the patient with muscle weakness as much rest as possible.
- Gradually increase activity according to her tolerance. Moderate weight-bearing activities are more beneficial than exercising in a bed or chair.
- Provide comfort measures to alleviate bone pain. Help the patient turn, and reposition her every 2 hours. Support the affected extremities with pillows. Use extreme care when lifting her. Provide analgesics as ordered.
- Observe for signs of pain and monitor for the effectiveness of analgesics and comfort measures.
- Encourage her to verbalize her feelings about body image changes and rejection by others. Offer emotional support, and help her develop coping strategies. Refer her to a mental health professional for additional counseling, if necessary.

Patient teaching
- Before discharge, advise the patient of possible adverse reactions to drug therapy.
- Teach the patient and family members to identify and report signs of tetany, respiratory distress, and renal dysfunction.
- Emphasize the need for periodic blood tests.
- If the patient didn't have surgery to correct her hyperparathyroidism, warn her to avoid calcium-containing antacids and thiazide diuretics.
- Encourage her to wear a medical identification bracelet.

EVALUATION

Achievement of patient outcomes determines the success of collaborative management. For the patient with hyperparathyroidism, evaluation focuses on physiologic status within acceptable parameters, return of laboratory studies to acceptable parameters, improved energy level and activity status, and adequate knowledge of the disease, treatment, and care.

Hyperpituitarism

Also called gigantism, hyperpituitarism is a chronic, progressive disease marked by hormonal dysfunction and startling skeletal overgrowth. Although the prognosis depends on the cause, this disease usually reduces life expectancy.

Hyperpituitarism appears in two forms: acromegaly (rare) and gigantism. Acromegaly occurs after epiphyseal closure, causing bone thickening and transverse growth and visceromegaly. This form of hyperpituitarism occurs equally among men and women, usually between ages 30 and 50.

Gigantism begins before epiphyseal closure and causes proportional overgrowth of all body tissues. It affects infants and children, causing them to grow to as much as three times the normal height for their age. As adults, they may eventually reach a height of more than 8′ (2.4 m).

CAUSES

In most patients, the source of excessive growth hormone (GH) secretion is a GH-producing adenoma of the anterior pituitary gland, usually macroadenoma (eosinophilic or mixed-cell). However, the etiology of the tumor itself is unclear. Occasionally, hyperpituitarism occurs in more than one family member, suggesting a genetic cause.

Prolonged effects of excessive GH secretion include arthritis, carpal tunnel syndrome, osteoporosis, kyphosis, hypertension, arteriosclerosis, heart enlargement, and heart failure.

As hyperpituitarism progresses, loss of other trophic hormones, such as thyroid-stimulating hormone, luteinizing hormone, follicle-stimulating hormone, and corticotropin, may cause dysfunction of the target organs.

Acromegaly may lead to blindness and severe neurologic disturbances due to tumor compression of surrounding tissues. Both gigantism and acromegaly may also cause signs of glucose intolerance and clinically apparent diabetes mellitus because of the insulin-antagonistic character of GH.

DIAGNOSIS AND TREATMENT

A diagnosis of hyperpituitarism is supported by GH radioimmunoassay, showing intermittently increased plasma GH levels; glucose suppression tests, more reliably showing a high GH level; skull X-ray, computed tomography scan, magnetic resonance imaging, or pneumoencephalography, locating the pituitary tumor; and bone X-rays, showing abnormalities.

Treatment aims to curb overproduction of GH by removing the underlying tumor. Removal occurs by cranial or transsphenoidal hypophysectomy or pituitary radiation therapy. In acromegaly, surgery is mandatory when a tumor is compressing surrounding healthy tissue. Postoperative therapy commonly requires replacement of thyroid, cortisone, and gonadal hormones. Adjunctive treatment may include bromocriptine, which inhibits GH synthesis, and a long-acting analogue of somatostatin, which lowers GH levels in at least two-thirds of patients with acromegaly.

COLLABORATIVE MANAGEMENT

Care of the patient with gigantism or acromegaly focuses on hormonal control, improved body image, absence of injury and complications, and adequate knowledge to comply with treatment and follow-up.

ASSESSMENT

Gigantism develops abruptly, producing some of the same skeletal abnormalities seen in acromegaly. In infants, inspection reveals a highly arched palate, muscular hypotonia, slanting eyes, and exophthalmos. On palpation, patients commonly exhibit a characteristic moist, doughy, weak handshake.

The onset of acromegaly is gradual. The patient may report soft-tissue swelling and hypertrophy of the face and extremities at first. Then as the disease progresses, he may complain of diaphoresis, oily skin, fatigue, heat intolerance, weight gain, headaches, decreased vision, decreased libido, impotence, oligomenorrhea, infertility, joint pain (possibly from osteoarthritis), hypertrichosis, and sleep disturbances (related to obstructive sleep apnea). Look for:
■ an enlarged jaw, thickened tongue, enlarged and weakened hands, coarsened facial features, oily or leathery skin, and a prominent supraorbital ridge
■ a deep, hollow-sounding voice, caused by laryngeal hypertrophy, and enlarged paranasal sinuses and tongue
■ irritability, hostility, and other psychological disturbances
■ cartilaginous and connective tissue overgrowth, causing a characteristic hulking appearance and thickened ears and nose
■ prognathism (projection of the jaw) becomes marked and may interfere with chewing
■ fingers that are thick, with tips that appear on X-ray as "tufted" or shaped like arrowheads

NURSING DIAGNOSES AND COLLABORATIVE PROBLEMS

Based on the following nursing diagnoses, you'll establish patient outcomes.

Altered growth and development related to abnormal increase in growth and development. The patient will:
- seek medical treatment early to minimize the effects of hyperpituitarism
- stop excessive growth with treatment.

Body image disturbance related to physical changes. The patient will:
- acknowledge how his body image has changed
- express positive feelings about himself
- exhibit an ability to cope with his altered body image.

Risk for injury related to long-term effects of excessive GH. The patient will:
- comply with prescribed medical or surgical treatment to reduce his GH level
- avoid complications of hyperpituitarism.

PLANNING AND IMPLEMENTATION

These measures help the patient with hyperpituitarism:
- Prepare the patient for surgery or radiation, as indicated. Provide supportive care if adverse effects occur.
- Evaluate GH levels regularly to assess the effectiveness of therapy.
- Check the strength of the patient's hand clasp to assess muscle weakness, especially in late-stage acromegaly.
- Assess the patient for complications of hyperpituitarism, and report any suggestive findings.
- Monitor serum glucose levels. Observe for signs of hyperglycemia, such as sweating, fatigue, polyuria, and polydipsia.
- If the patient has skeletal manifestations, such as arthritis of the hands or osteoarthritis of the spine, give analgesics and provide comfort measures. To preserve joint function, perform or assist with range-of-motion exercises. Apply heat or cold as ordered. Use pillows and splints to support painful extremities.
- If the patient suffers muscle weakness, help him walk and perform such tasks as cutting food. Also take other safety precautions to prevent injury.
- Provide meticulous skin care. Keep the skin dry, and use oil-free skin cleansers and lotions.
- Remember that the tumor may cause visual problems. If the patient has hemianopia, stand where he can see you. Use soft lighting if the patient has photophobia.
- The grotesque body changes and sexual dysfunction that come with this disorder can cause severe psychological stress. Provide emotional support to help the patient cope with an altered body image.

- Encourage him to verbalize his feelings, and discuss fear of rejection by others. Provide a positive, but realistic, assessment of his situation.
- Encourage him to develop other interests that support a positive self-image and de-emphasize appearance. Refer him and family members or friends for counseling to help them deal with body image changes and sexual dysfunction.
- Be sensitive to any mood changes the patient may experience. Reassure him and family members that these changes are caused by hormonal imbalances linked to the disease and can lessen with treatment.

Patient teaching
- If the patient is scheduled for surgery or radiation therapy, teach him about the procedure.
- If the patient is taking bromocriptine, explain that nausea, light-headedness, and postural hypotension are common at the beginning of therapy but will usually subside. Other adverse effects include constipation and nasal congestion.
- Advise the patient to wear a medical identification bracelet at all times.
- Tell the patient he'll always need annual follow-up examinations because of the slight chance that the tumor may recur.

EVALUATION

Achievement of patient outcomes determines the success of collaborative management. For the patient with hyperpituitarism, evaluation focuses on hormonal control; improved body image; absence of injury and complications; a clean, dry, healing incision (if surgery was performed); and adequate knowledge to comply with treatment and follow-up.

Hyperthyroidism

Thyroid hormone overproduction causes a metabolic imbalance in this disorder. Forms of the disorder include Graves' disease, toxic adenoma (Plummer's disease), thyrotoxicosis factitia, functioning metastatic thyroid carcinoma, thyroid-stimulating hormone-secreting pituitary tumor, and subacute thyroiditis.

The most common form of hyperthyroidism is Graves' disease, which increases thyroxine (T_4) production, enlarges the thyroid gland (goiter), and causes multiple systemic changes. The incidence of Graves' disease is highest between ages 30 and 40; only 5% of hyperthyroid patients are younger than age 15. The disorder is more common in females and in persons with family histories of thyroid abnormalities. With treatment, most patients can lead normal lives. However, thyrotoxic crisis or thyroid storm—an acute exacerbation of hyperthyroidism clinically manifested by a marked hypermetabolism and excessive adrenergic response (flushing, fever, and sweating)—is a medical emergency that may lead to life-threatening cardiac, hepatic, or renal failure. (See *Surveying hyperthyroid disorders*.)

CAUSES

The origin of hyperthyroidism is unclear, but in view of its various manifestations, it may not have a single cause. For example, many experts believe that Graves' disease results from genetic and immunologic factors. Increased incidence in monozygotic twins points to an inherited factor, probably an autosomal recessive gene. Graves' disease occasionally coexists with abnormal iodine metabolism and other endocrine abnormalities, such as diabetes mellitus, thyroiditis, and hyperparathyroidism. It's also associated with production of autoantibodies (long-acting thyroid stimulator [LATS], LATS-protector, and human thyroid adenylate cyclase stimulators), possibly caused by a defect in suppressor-T-lymphocyte function that allows the formation of these autoantibodies.

In a patient with latent hyperthyroidism, excessive intake of iodine and, possibly, stress can precipitate clinical hyperthyroidism. Similarly, in a patient with inadequately treated hyperthyroidism, stressful conditions (such as surgery, infection, toxemia of pregnancy, and diabetic ketoacidosis) can precipitate thyrotoxic crisis.

Thyroid hormones have widespread effects on almost all body tissues, so the complications of hypersecretion may be far-reaching and varied. Cardiovascular complications are most common in older adult patients and include arrhythmias, especially atrial fibrillation; cardiac insufficiency; cardiac decompensation; and resistance to the usual therapeutic dose of digitalis glycosides. Additional complications include muscle weakness and atrophy; paralysis; osteoporosis; vitiligo and skin hyperpigmentation; corneal ulcers; myasthenia gravis; impaired fertility; decreased libido; and gynecomastia.

DIAGNOSIS AND TREATMENT

The following laboratory test results confirm the diagnosis of hyperthyroidism:

■ Radioimmunoassay shows increased serum triiodothyronine (T_3) and T_4 concentrations. (This test is contraindicated in pregnant patients.)

■ Thyroid scan reveals increased uptake of radioactive iodine (^{131}I).

■ Thyrotropin-releasing hormone (TRH) stimulation test indicates hyperthyroidism if thyroid-stimulating hormone (TSH) level fails to rise within 30 minutes after administration of TRH.

Surveying hyperthyroid disorders

Besides Graves' disease, other forms of hyperthyroidism include toxic adenoma, thyrotoxicosis factitia, functioning metastatic thyroid carcinoma, thyroid stimulating hormone (TSH)—secreting pituitary tumor, and subacute thyroiditis.

Toxic adenoma
A small, benign nodule in the thyroid gland, toxic adenoma secretes thyroid hormone and is the second most common cause of hyperthyroidism. The cause of toxic adenoma is unknown; its incidence is highest in older adults.

Clinical effects are similar to those of Graves' disease except that toxic adenoma doesn't induce ophthalmopathy, pretibial myxedema, or acropachy. The presence of adenoma is confirmed by ^{131}I uptake and thyroid scan, which show a single hyperfunctioning nodule suppressing the rest of the gland.

Treatment includes ^{131}I therapy or surgery to remove the adenoma after antithyroid drugs achieve a euthyroid state.

Thyrotoxicosis factitia
This form of hyperthyroidism is caused by chronic ingestion of thyroid hormone for thyrotropin suppression in patients with thyroid carcinoma. It may also follow thyroid hormone abuse by persons trying to lose weight.

Functioning metastatic thyroid carcinoma
A rare disease, this carcinoma causes excess production of thyroid hormone.

TSH-secreting pituitary tumor
In this disorder, a TSH-secreting pituitary tumor causes overproduction of thyroid hormone.

Subacute thyroiditis
A virus-induced granulomatous inflammation of the thyroid, subacute thyroiditis produces transient hyperthyroidism associated with fever, pain, pharyngitis, and tenderness of the thyroid gland.

Other supportive test results show increased serum protein-bound iodine and decreased serum cholesterol and total lipid levels. Ultrasonography confirms subclinical ophthalmopathy.

In hyperthyroidism, treatment consists of drugs, radioiodine, and surgery. Antithyroid drug therapy is used for children, young adults, pregnant women, and patients who refuse surgery or radioiodine treatment. Thyroid hormone antagonists include propylthiouracil and methimazole, which block thyroid hormone synthesis. Although hypermetabolic symptoms subside in 4 to 8 weeks, the patient must continue the drugs for 6 months to 2 years. In many patients, concomitant propranolol is used to manage tachycardia and other peripheral effects of excessive hypersympathetic activity.

During pregnancy, antithyroid drugs should be kept at the minimum dosage required to maintain normal maternal thyroid function and to minimize the risk of fetal hypothyroidism—even though most infants of hyperthyroid mothers are born with mild and transient hyperthyroidism. (Neonatal hyperthyroidism may even require treatment with antithyroid drugs and propranolol for 2 to 3 months.) Because exacerbation of hyperthyroidism sometimes occurs in the puerperium, continuous control of maternal thyroid function is essential. About 3 to 6 months postpartum, antithyroid drugs can be gradually decreased and thyroid function reassessed (drugs may be discontinued at that time). Mothers shouldn't breast-feed during treatment with antithyroid drugs because this may cause neonatal hypothyroidism.

Treatment with ^{131}I consists of a single oral dose and is the treatment of choice for women past reproductive age or men and women planning to have no children. (Patients of reproductive age must give informed consent for this treatment because small amounts of ^{131}I concentrate in the gonads.) During treatment, the thyroid gland picks up the radioactive element as it would regular iodine. Subsequently, the radioactivity destroys some of the cells that normally concentrate iodine and produce thyroxine, thus decreasing thyroid hormone production and normalizing thyroid size and function. In most patients, hypermetabolic symptoms diminish in 6 to 8 weeks after such treatment. However, some patients may require a second dose. The most common complication is hypothyroidism.

Subtotal (partial) thyroidectomy is indicated for the patient under age 40 who has a large gland or multinodular goiter and whose hyperthyroidism has repeatedly relapsed after drug therapy. This surgery removes part of the thyroid gland, decreasing its size and capacity for hormone production. Preoperatively, the patient may receive iodides (Lugol's or potassium iodide oral solution), antithyroid drugs, or high doses of propranolol, to help prevent thyroid storm. If euthyroidism isn't achieved, delay surgery and give propranolol to decrease cardiac arrhythmias that are caused by hyperthyroidism.

Therapy for hyperthyroid ophthalmopathy includes local applications of topical medications but may require high doses of corticosteroids. A patient with severe exophthalmos that causes pressure on the optic nerve may require surgical decompression to lessen pressure on the orbital contents.

Treatment of thyrotoxic crisis includes administration of an antithyroid drug such as propylthiouracil, I.V. propranolol to block sympathetic effects, a corticosteroid to inhibit the conversion of T_3 to T_4 and to replace depleted cortisol, and an iodide to block release of the thyroid hormones. Supportive measures include nutrients, vitamins, fluid administration, and sedatives, as necessary.

COLLABORATIVE MANAGEMENT

Care of the patient with hyperthyroidism focuses on restoring thyroid levels, avoiding complications, and teaching the patient about the disorder.

ASSESSMENT

The patient may report that the onset of symptoms followed a period of acute physical or emotional stress. A family history of Graves' disease is also common. The patient may report classic symptoms of nervousness, heat intolerance, weight loss despite increased appetite, excessive sweating, diarrhea, tremor, and palpitations. Symptoms suggesting nervous system involvement generally dominate in younger patients, whereas cardiovascular and myopathic symptoms are more common in older patients. Look for:
- complaints of difficulty concentrating, trouble climbing stairs, dyspnea on exertion and possibly at rest, anorexia, nausea and vomiting, and menstrual abnormalities
- anxious and restless behavior
- a fine tremor of the fingers and tongue, shaky handwriting, clumsiness, emotional instability, and mood swings (occasional outbursts to overt psychosis)
- flushed skin and fine, soft hair
- premature graying and increased hair loss, in both sexes
- nails that appear fragile, and the distal nail separated from the nail bed (onycholysis).
- pretibial myxedema over the dorsum of the legs or feet, which produces raised, thickened skin that may be itchy, hyperpigmented, and usually well demarcated from normal skin
- lesions that typically look plaquelike or nodular
- generalized or localized muscle atrophy and acropachy (soft-tissue swelling with underlying bone changes where new bone formation occurs)
- infrequent blinking, a characteristic stare, and lid lag, resulting from sympathetic overstimulation
- exophthalmos, which results from accumulated mucopolysaccharides and fluids in the retro-orbital tissues that force the eyeball outward
- reddened conjunctiva and cornea; an impaired upward gaze; convergence; and strabismus due to ocular muscle weakness (exophthalmic ophthalmoplegia)

- a thyroid gland that feels asymmetrical, lobular, and enlarged to three or four times its normal size
- an enlarged liver
- warm, moist skin with a velvety texture
- tachycardia with a full bounding pulse
- hyperreflexia
- paroxysmal supraventricular tachycardia and atrial fibrillation (especially in older patients)
- occasionally, a systolic murmur at the left sternal border
- wide pulse pressures, audible when taking blood pressure readings
- increased bowel sounds
- in Graves' disease, an audible bruit over the thyroid gland, indicating thyrotoxicity (occasionally, other disorders associated with a hyperplastic thyroid).

NURSING DIAGNOSES AND COLLABORATIVE PROBLEMS
Based on the following nursing diagnoses, you'll establish patient outcomes.

Altered nutrition: Less than body requirements, related to hypermetabolism. The patient will:
- eat a nutritionally balanced diet containing enough calories to prevent further weight loss
- regain lost weight and maintain weight within a normal range
- have no signs and symptoms of malnutrition or nutritional deficits.

Altered thought processes related to emotional lability. The patient will:
- remain safe and protected in his environment
- receive emotional support and understanding from his family members and friends
- regain emotional stability with hyperthyroidism treatment.

Decreased cardiac output related to supraventricular tachycardia. The patient will:
- regain and maintain a normal heart rate and electrocardiogram (ECG) pattern with hyperthyroidism treatment
- maintain adequate cardiac output, as shown by normal blood pressure, alertness, and orientation to time, place, and person.

PLANNING AND IMPLEMENTATION
These measures help the patient with hyperthyroidism.
- Prepare the patient for surgery, as indicated.
- Give prescribed antithyroid drugs, as ordered.
- Avoid excessive palpation of the thyroid—this can precipitate thyroid storm. (See *Understanding thyrotoxic crisis*, page 440.)
- Monitor and record the patient's vital signs, weight, fluid intake, and urine output. Measure neck circumference daily to check for progression of thyroid enlargement.
- Evaluate serum electrolyte levels, and check for hyperglycemia and glycosuria. Monitor the ECG for arrhythmias and ST-segment changes.
- Assess the patient for signs of heart failure, such as dyspnea, jugular vein distention, pulmonary crackles, and peripheral or sacral edema.
- Check for signs and symptoms of hypotension (dizziness and decreased urine output) if the patient is taking propranolol.
- If the patient is taking propylthiouracil and methimazole, monitor complete blood count results periodically to detect leukopenia, thrombocytopenia, and agranulocytosis.
- Monitor the patient for thyrotoxic crisis and report any suspicious signs or symptoms to the doctor immediately.
- If iodide is part of the treatment, mix it with milk, juice, or water to prevent GI distress, and give it through a straw to prevent tooth discoloration.
- Give antidiarrheal preparations, as ordered. Provide meticulous skin care to minimize perianal skin breakdown.
- Consult a dietitian to ensure a nutritious diet with adequate calories and fluids. Offer frequent, small meals.
- Check stools for frequency and characteristics.
- If the patient has exophthalmos or other ophthalmopathy, moisten the conjunctivae often with isotonic eyedrops.
- Minimize physical and emotional stress. Try to balance rest and activity periods. Keep the patient's room cool and quiet and the lights dim. Encourage him to dress in loose-fitting, cotton clothing.
- Reassure the patient and family members that mood swings and nervousness will probably subside with treatment.
- Encourage the patient to verbalize feelings about changes in body image. Help him identify and develop coping strategies. Offer emotional support. Refer him and family members to a mental health counselor, if necessary.

Patient teaching
- Stress the importance of regular medical follow-up because hypothyroidism may develop 2 to 4 weeks postoperatively and after ^{131}I therapy.
- Tell the patient he'll need lifelong thyroid hormone replacement. Encourage him to wear a medical identification bracelet and to carry his drugs with him at all times.
- Tell the patient who has had ^{131}I therapy not to expectorate or cough freely because his saliva is radioactive for 24 hours. Stress the need for repeated mea-

Understanding thyrotoxic crisis

Also known as thyroid storm, thyrotoxic crisis is an acute manifestation of hyperthyroidism, usually affecting patients with preexisting (though often unrecognized) thyrotoxicosis. Left untreated, it's invariably fatal.

Causes

Onset is almost always abrupt, evoked by a stressful event, such as trauma, surgery, or infection. Other, less common, precipitators include:

- insulin-induced hypoglycemia or diabetic ketoacidosis
- cerebrovascular accident
- myocardial infarction
- pulmonary embolism
- sudden discontinuation of antithyroid drug therapy
- initiation of ^{131}I therapy
- preeclampsia
- subtotal thyroidectomy with excess intake of synthetic thyroid hormone.

Pathophysiology

The thyroid gland secretes the thyroid hormones triiodothyronine (T_3) and thyroxine (T_4). When it overproduces them in response to any of the above factors, systemic adrenergic activity increases. This results in epinephrine overproduction and severe hypermetabolism, leading rapidly to cardiac, GI, and sympathetic nervous system decompensation.

Assessment findings

Initially, the patient may have marked tachycardia, temperature above 100.4° F (38° C), vomiting, and stupor. Untreated, he may experience vascular collapse, hypotension, coma, and death. Other findings include irritability and restlessness, visual disturbance such as diplopia, tremor and weakness, angina, or shortness of breath, a cough, and swollen extremities. Palpation may disclose warm, moist flushed skin and a high fever (beginning insidiously and rising rapidly to a lethal level).

Emergency interventions

If you suspect your patient may be experiencing thyrotoxic crisis, take these steps:

- Notify the patient's doctor immediately and prepare to transfer the patient to the intensive care unit.
- Monitor the patient's vital signs, electrocardiogram pattern, and cardiopulmonary status continuously.
- Expect to administer an antithyroid drug such as propylthiouracil or beta blockers such as propranolol to block sympathetic effects; a corticosteroid to inhibit the conversion of T_3 to T_4 and to replace depleted cortisol; and an iodide to block the release of the thyroid hormones.
- Closely monitor the patient's temperature. If indicated, employ cooling measures and administer acetaminophen, as ordered. Never administer aspirin because it may further increase the patient's metabolic rate.
- Provide supportive care, such as administering vitamins, nutrients, fluids, and sedatives, as necessary.

surement of serum T_4 levels. Assure that he understands he mustn't resume antithyroid drug therapy.

- Instruct the patient taking propylthiouracil and methimazole to take these drugs with meals to minimize GI distress, and to avoid over-the-counter cough preparations because many contain iodine.
- Tell the patient taking propranolol to rise slowly after sitting or lying down to prevent a feeling of faintness.
- Instruct the patient taking antithyroid drugs or radioisotope therapy to identify and report symptoms of hypothyroidism.
- Advise the patient with exophthalmos or other ophthalmopathy to wear sunglasses or eye patches to protect his eyes from light. If he has severe lid retraction, warn him to avoid sudden physical movements that might cause the lid to slip behind the eyeball. Tell him to report signs of decreased visual acuity.

EVALUATION

Achievement of patient outcomes determines the success of collaborative management. For the patient with hyperthyroidism, evaluation focuses on restoration of thyroid levels, physiologic status within acceptable parameters, absence of complications, and adequate knowledge of the disorder, treatment, and care.

Hypoglycemia

Potentially dangerous, hypoglycemia is an abnormally low blood glucose level. It's classified as reactive, pharmacologic, or fasting. Reactive hypoglycemia links the patient's reaction to the disposition of meals. Blood glucose levels typically fall 2 to 4 hours after a meal.

Pharmacologic hypoglycemia is a response to a drug that does one of the following: increases the amount of insulin circulating in the blood, enhances insulin action, or impairs the liver's glucose-producing capacity. Blood glucose levels may fall slowly or rapidly.

Fasting hypoglycemia causes discomfort during periods of fasting. Blood glucose levels fall gradually. Signs and symptoms don't appear until 5 hours or more after a meal. This rare type of hypoglycemia usually occurs during the night.

CAUSES

Reactive hypoglycemia may take several forms. Most commonly, it results from alimentary hyperinsulinism caused by dumping syndrome. Fructose or galactose ingestion may cause hypoglycemia in patients with fructose intolerance or galactosemia. Reactive hypoglycemia may also occur secondary to imminent onset of type II diabetes mellitus or impaired glucose tolerance. In some patients, reactive hypoglycemia may have no known cause (idiopathic reactive).

Pharmacologic hypoglycemia most commonly results from the use of insulin or oral sulfonylureas. Other causes include the use of beta blockers and excessive alcohol ingestion.

Fasting hypoglycemia most commonly results from hepatic disease or a tumor. Insulinomas, small islet cell tumors in the pancreas, secrete excessive amounts of insulin, which inhibits hepatic glucose production. These tumors are usually benign (in 90% of patients). Extrapancreatic tumors, though uncommon, can also cause hypoglycemia by increasing glucose utilization and inhibiting glucose output. Such tumors occur primarily in the mesenchyma, liver, adrenal cortex, GI system, and lymphatic system. They may be benign or malignant.

Among nonendocrine causes of fasting hypoglycemia are severe hepatic diseases, including hepatitis, cancer, cirrhosis, and liver congestion associated with heart failure. All of these conditions reduce the uptake and release of glycogen from the liver.

Some endocrine causes include destruction of pancreatic islet cells; adrenocortical insufficiency, which contributes to hypoglycemia by reducing the production of cortisol and cortisone needed for gluconeogenesis; and pituitary insufficiency, which reduces corticotropin and growth hormone levels.

Hypoglycemia occurs when glucose burns up too rapidly, when the glucose release rate falls behind tissue demands, or when excessive insulin enters the bloodstream. When the brain is deprived of glucose, as with oxygen deprivation, its functioning becomes deranged. With prolonged glucose deprivation, tissue damage—or even death—may result.

Manifestations of hypoglycemia tend to be vague and depend on how quickly the patient's glucose levels drop. Gradual onset of hypoglycemia produces predominantly central nervous system (CNS) signs and symptoms; a more rapid decline in plasma glucose levels results predominantly in adrenergic signs and symptoms.

Acute hypoglycemia initially causes signs and symptoms of mild cerebral dysfunction, such as headache, dizziness, restlessness, and decreased mental capacity. If left untreated, the blood glucose level continues to drop, producing such adrenergic signs and symptoms as hunger, weakness, diaphoresis, tachycardia, pallor, anxiety, tremor, and possibly rebound hyperglycemia. If hypoglycemia continues, any beneficial effects of rebound hyperglycemia quickly dissipate and coma, seizures, and permanent brain damage or even death may follow.

Prolonged or severe hypoglycemia (blood glucose levels of 20 mg/dl or less) can cause permanent brain damage and death.

DIAGNOSIS AND TREATMENT

Glucometer readings provide quick screening methods for determining blood glucose levels. Laboratory testing confirms the diagnosis by showing decreased blood glucose values of less than 40 mg/dl before a meal or less than 50 mg/dl after a meal.

In addition, the patient may take a 5-hour glucose tolerance test to provoke reactive hypoglycemia. Following a 12-hour fast, laboratory testing to detect plasma insulin and plasma glucose levels may identify fasting hypoglycemia.

A C-peptide assay helps diagnose fasting hypoglycemia. It also differentiates fasting hypoglycemia caused by an insulinoma from fasting hypoglycemia caused by insulin injections.

For severe hypoglycemia (producing confusion or coma), initial treatment is usually I.V. administration of a bolus of 25 or 50 g of glucose as a 50% solution. This is followed by a constant infusion of glucose until the patient can eat a meal. A patient who experiences adrenergic reactions without CNS symptoms may receive oral carbohydrate (parenteral therapy is not required).

Reactive hypoglycemia requires dietary modification to help delay glucose absorption and gastric emptying. Usually, this includes small, frequent meals; avoidance of simple carbohydrates; and ingestion of high-protein meals with added fiber. The patient may also receive anticholinergic drugs to slow gastric emptying and intestinal motility and to inhibit vagal stimulation of insulin release.

Fasting hypoglycemia may require surgery and drug therapy. In patients with insulinoma, removal of the tumor is the treatment of choice. Drug therapy may include diazoxide or octreotide for inoperable insulinomas. A patient may need hormone replacement therapy for pituitary or adrenal gland insufficiency. In many cases of recurrent hypoglycemia, the only treatment needed is avoidance of fasting.

COLLABORATIVE MANAGEMENT

Care of the patient with hypoglycemia focuses on restoring blood glucose control, avoiding complications, and teaching him how to participate actively in disease-control planning.

ASSESSMENT

The history of a patient with suspected hypoglycemia should note the pattern of food intake for the preceding 24 hours as well as drug and alcohol use. The medical or surgical history may note the existence of causative factors, such as gastrectomy or hepatic disease.

A patient with reactive hypoglycemia may report adrenergic symptoms, such as diaphoresis, anxiety, hunger, nervousness, and weakness, indicating a rapid decline in his blood glucose levels.

A patient with fasting hypoglycemia may report signs and symptoms of CNS disturbance, such as dizziness, headache, clouding of vision, restlessness, and mental status changes, indicating a slow decline in blood glucose levels. With prolonged glucose deprivation, the patient's history (obtained from family or friends, if necessary) may reveal seizures, decreasing level of consciousness (LOC), and coma. A patient with pharmacologic hypoglycemia may experience a rapid or slow decline in blood glucose levels.

Inspection may reveal adrenergic signs, such as diaphoresis, pallor, and tremor; or CNS signs, such as restlessness, loss of fine-motor skills, and altered LOC. Palpation may detect tachycardia.

NURSING DIAGNOSES AND COLLABORATIVE PROBLEMS

Based on the following nursing diagnoses, you'll establish patient outcomes.

Anxiety related to frequent or severe hypoglycemic episodes. The patient will:
- identify and express his feelings of anxiety
- request information about hypoglycemia
- exhibit fewer physical signs of anxiety.

Risk for injury related to neurologic damage from a hypoglycemic episode. The patient will:
- comply with treatments to prevent hypoglycemia-induced injury
- exhibit normal neurologic function after hypoglycemic episodes
- avoid neurologic damage.

Knowledge deficit related to hypoglycemia and its treatment. The patient will:
- express a need for information about hypoglycemia and its treatment

- participate in learning situations that address hypoglycemia and its treatment
- articulate an understanding of hypoglycemia and its treatment.

PLANNING AND IMPLEMENTATION

These measures help the patient with hypoglycemia.
- Give drugs, as prescribed.
- Avoid delays in meal times and provide a proper diet. Arrange to have a dietitian visit the patient to teach him about proper diet.
- Correct hypoglycemic episodes quickly. If possible, measure blood glucose before correcting hypoglycemia to verify its severity. Implement measures to protect the unconscious patient, such as maintaining a patent airway.
- Prepare the insulinoma patient for surgery, if indicated. Provide the same preoperative and postoperative care as for a patient undergoing abdominal surgery.
- Monitor any infusion of hypertonic glucose to avoid hyperglycemia, circulatory overload, and cellular dehydration.
- Measure blood glucose levels, as ordered.
- Assess the effects of drug therapy, and watch for adverse reactions.
- Encourage the patient to verbalize his feelings.
- Help him improve self-care and independence.

Patient teaching

- Explain the purpose, preparation, and procedure for any diagnostic tests.
- Emphasize the importance of preventing or promptly treating hypoglycemic episodes to avoid severe complications. (See *Reducing the number of hypoglycemic incidents.*)
- Be sure the patient understands the key danger with hypoglycemia: Once it occurs, he may quickly lose his ability to think clearly. If this should happen while he's driving a car or operating machinery, a serious accident could result.
- Inform the patient that he should note what early symptoms he typically experiences with hypoglycemia. Family, friends, and coworkers should also be trained to recognize the warning signs so that they can immediately begin treatment.
- Review with the patient and family members the treatment measures they should follow if the patient has a hypoglycemic episode. If the patient is conscious, he should consume a readily available source of glucose, such as five to six pieces of hard candy; 4 to 6 oz (118 to 177 ml) of apple juice, orange juice, cola, or other soft drink; or 1 tbs of honey or grape jelly. If the patient is unconscious, he should be given a subcutaneous injection of glucagon.
- Teach them how to give a glucagon injection.

■ Tell them to notify the doctor if hypoglycemic episodes don't respond to treatment or if they occur frequently.
■ Emphasize the importance of carefully following the prescribed diet to prevent a rapid drop in blood glucose levels. Advise the patient to eat small meals throughout the day, and mention that he may require bedtime snacks to keep blood glucose at an even level. Tell him to avoid alcohol and caffeine because they may trigger severe hypoglycemic episodes.
■ If the patient is obese and has impaired glucose tolerance, suggest ways he can restrict his caloric intake and lose weight. If necessary, help him find a weight-loss support group.
■ Warn the patient with fasting hypoglycemia not to postpone or skip meals and snacks. Tell him to call his doctor for instructions if he doesn't feel well enough to eat.
■ Discuss lifestyle and personal habits to help the patient identify precipitating factors, such as poor diet, stress, or noncompliance with diabetes mellitus treatment. Explain ways that he can change or avoid each precipitating factor identified. If necessary, teach him stress-reduction techniques, and encourage him to join a support group.
■ Teach the patient about precautions to take when exercising; for example, tell him to consume extra calories and not to exercise alone or when his blood glucose level is likely to drop.
■ Tell him that he should carry a source of fast-acting carbohydrate, such as hard candy, with him at all times. Advise him to wear a medical identification bracelet or to carry a medical identification card that describes his condition and its emergency treatment measures.
■ For the patient with pharmacologic hypoglycemia from insulin or oral antidiabetic agents, review the essentials of managing diabetes mellitus, if indicated.

■ If warranted, teach the patient about prescribed drug therapy or surgery.
■ Because hypoglycemia is a chronic disorder, encourage the patient to see his doctor regularly.
■ Encourage the patient and family to discuss their concerns about the patient's condition and treatment.

EVALUATION
Achievement of patient outcomes determines the success of collaborative management. For the patient with hypoglycemia, evaluation focuses on restoration of blood glucose control, laboratory study levels within acceptable parameters, absence of injury and complications, and adequate knowledge to participate actively in disease control planning.

Hypoparathyroidism

A deficiency in parathyroid hormone (PTH) secretion by the parathyroid glands or decreased action of peripheral PTH creates hypoparathyroidism.

Hypoparathyroidism is acute or chronic and classified as idiopathic, acquired, or reversible. The idiopathic and reversible forms are most common in children, and the clinical effects are usually correctable with replacement therapy. The acquired form, which is irreversible, is most common in older patients who've undergone thyroid gland surgery.

CAUSES
Idiopathic hypoparathyroidism may be caused by an autoimmune genetic disorder or the congenital absence of the parathyroid glands.

Acquired hypoparathyroidism typically results from accidental removal of or injury to one or more parathyroid glands during thyroidectomy or other neck surgery. It may also follow ischemic infarction of the parathyroid glands during surgery, hemochromatosis, sarcoidosis, amyloidosis, tuberculosis, neoplasms, trauma, or massive thyroid irradiation (rare).

Reversible hypoparathyroidism may result from hypomagnesemia-induced impairment of hormone synthesis, from suppression of normal gland function due to hypercalcemia, or from delayed maturation of parathyroid function.

Because the parathyroid glands primarily regulate calcium balance, hypoparathyroidism causes hypocalcemia, which produces neuromuscular symptoms ranging from paresthesia to tetany. PTH normally maintains serum calcium levels by increasing bone resorption and GI absorption of calcium. It also maintains the inverse relationship between serum calcium and phosphate levels by inhibiting phosphate reabsorption in the renal tubules. Abnormal PTH production in hypoparathyroidism disrupts this delicate balance.

In hypoparathyroidism, complications are related to long-standing hypocalcemia. Decreased calcium levels can cause reduced contractility and, eventually, heart failure. Lens calcification leads to cataract formation that persists despite calcium replacement therapy. Papillary edema from increased intracranial pressure, irreversible calcification of basal ganglion, and bone deformity also occur. Laryngospasm, respiratory stridor, anoxia, paralysis of the vocal cords, and death may occur in severe cases of tetany. Hypoparathyroidism that develops during childhood results in mental retardation, stunted growth, and malformed teeth.

DIAGNOSIS AND TREATMENT
Diagnostic tests may include radioimmunoassay, blood and urine tests, X-rays, and electrocardiograms (ECGs).

Because calcium absorption from the small intestine depends on the presence of activated vitamin D, treatment initially includes vitamin D, with or without supplemental calcium. Such therapy is usually lifelong, except in patients with reversible hyperthyroidism. If the patient can't tolerate the pure form of vitamin D, alternatives include dihydrotachysterol if renal function is adequate, and calcitriol if renal function is severely compromised.

COLLABORATIVE MANAGEMENT
Care of the patient with hypoparathyroidism focuses on cardiopulmonary status, safety, and patient teaching.

ASSESSMENT
The patient's history may reveal recent neck surgery or irradiation or long-term hypomagnesemia from GI malabsorption or alcoholism. Look for:
- reports of symptoms that reflect altered neuromuscular irritability (see *Dealing with acute tetany*)
- complaints of personality changes, ranging from irritability and anxiety to depression, delirium, and frank psychosis
- dry skin, brittle hair, alopecia, transverse and longitudinal ridges in the fingernails, loss of eyelashes and fingernails, and stained, cracked, and decayed teeth from weakened enamel
- Chvostek's and Trousseau's signs, which indicate latent tetany (Chvostek's sign may appear in other disorders, but only a hypocalcemic patient exhibits Trousseau's sign.)
- deep tendon reflexes resulting from neuromuscular irritability
- with auscultation of the apical pulse, cardiac arrhythmias.

NURSING DIAGNOSES AND COLLABORATIVE PROBLEMS
Based on the following nursing diagnoses, you'll establish patient outcomes.

Risk for injury related to acute and long-term calcium deficiency. The patient will:
- regain and maintain normal serum calcium and phosphorus levels
- exhibit no signs and symptoms of tetany
- avoid complications of long-term hypocalcemia.

Ineffective breathing pattern related to hyperventilation caused by neuromuscular irritability. The patient will:
- receive appropriate respiratory support to maintain adequate ventilation
- maintain adequate gas exchange, as shown by normal arterial blood gas values
- avoid hyperventilation once serum calcium levels return to normal.

Altered thought processes related to hypocalcemia-induced neurologic dysfunction. The patient will:
- remain safe and protected in his environment
- regain and maintain normal thought patterns through hypoparathyroidism treatment.

PLANNING AND IMPLEMENTATION
These measures help the patient with hypoparathyroidism.
- Maintain a patent I.V. line. Keep emergency equipment available, including I.V. calcium gluconate and calcium chloride, an airway, a tracheotomy tray, and an endotracheal tube. Maintain seizure precautions.
- Remember that hyperventilation, which may result from anxiety during a tetany episode, can worsen tetany. So can recent blood transfusions because anti-

Dealing with acute tetany

Acute (overt) tetany results from a sudden or severe drop in the serum calcium level. Remember that a calcium deficit increases neuronal membrane permeability and allows sodium to enter cells more easily than usual. In turn, this promotes spontaneous depolarization, causing neuromuscular irritability. The more severe the calcium deficit, the greater the neuromuscular irritability.

Signs and symptoms
In acute tetany, the patient may report tingling that begins in the fingertips, around the mouth and, occasionally, in the feet. Tingling spreads and becomes more severe, causing muscle tension and spasms. Pain varies with the degree of muscle tension, but rarely affects the face, legs, and feet. The patient may also complain of throat constriction and dysphagia. Smooth-muscle hyperactivity leads to GI upset, exhibited as nausea, vomiting, abdominal pain, or constipation or diarrhea.

During a tetany episode, you may note that the patient's hands, forearms and, less commonly, feet contort in a specific pattern, with thumb adduction followed by metacarpophalangeal joint flexion, interphalangeal joint extension, and wrist and elbow joint flexion. In severe cases, he may also have signs of laryngospasm, respiratory stridor, anoxia, and convulsions.

Emergency interventions
If you suspect acute tetany, take the following steps:
- Notify the doctor at once and have another staff member bring emergency equipment to the bedside.
- Maintain a patent airway, and have a tracheotomy tray and an endotracheal tube available. Take seizure precautions.
- Insert an I.V. line and prepare to administer 10% calcium gluconate or 10% calcium chloride I.V., stat, to raise the serum ionized calcium level.
- If the patient can do so, have him breathe into a paper bag so that he inhales his own carbon dioxide.
- Be prepared to administer anticonvulsant agents, such as phenytoin or phenobarbital, to control seizures until the serum calcium level rises. Avoid use of phenothiazine drugs because of possible inducement of severe dyskinesia.
- Monitor serum calcium and phosphorus levels closely.
- Be aware that hyperventilation, which may result from anxiety, can worsen tetany. Keep the patient calm, and give a sedative, if prescribed.
- Monitor the electrocardiogram in a patient taking a digitalis glycoside because calcium potentiates the drug's action on the heart.

coagulant in stored blood binds calcium. Keep the patient calm, and give a sedative, if prescribed. Help the patient with mild tetany rebreathe his own exhaled air by breathing into a paper bag.
- Check the patient's serum calcium and phosphorus levels regularly.
- Monitor his ECG for increasing QT-interval changes, heart block, and signs of decreasing cardiac output.
- Closely observe the patient who is receiving both digitalis glycosides and calcium because calcium potentiates the effect of digitalis glycosides. Stay alert for signs of digitalis toxicity (arrhythmias, nausea, fatigue, and visual changes).
- Assess the patient for tetany and long-term complications of chronic hypocalcemia.
- Provide meticulous skin care. Use alcohol-free skin care products and an emollient lotion after bathing.
- Institute safety precautions to minimize the risk of injury from falls. Provide support for walking.
- Encourage the patient to verbalize his feelings about body image changes and rejection by others.
- Offer emotional support, and help him identify his strengths and use them to develop coping strategies.

Refer him to a mental health professional for additional counseling, if necessary.

Patient teaching
- Discuss the importance of long-term management and follow-up care, especially periodic checks of the patient's serum calcium levels.
- Advise the patient that he'll need long-term replacement therapy. Instruct him to take the drugs as ordered and never discontinue them abruptly.
- Tell him to take calcium supplements with or after meals and to chew the tablets well.
- Encourage him to wear a medical identification bracelet and to carry his drugs with him at all times.
- Teach the patient and family members to identify and report signs and symptoms of hypercalcemia, tetany, and respiratory distress.
- Teach the patient protective measures to decrease stress and to avoid fatigue and infection.
- Tell him to follow a high-calcium, low-phosphorus diet. Discuss foods high in calcium, such as dairy products, salmon, egg yolks, shrimp, and green, leafy vegetables. Caution him to avoid high-phosphate foods, such as spinach, rhubarb, and asparagus.

EVALUATION

Achievement of patient outcomes determines the success of collaborative management. For the patient with hypoparathyroidism, evaluation focuses on cardiopulmonary status within acceptable parameters, return of laboratory studies to acceptable limits, absence of injury and complications, and adequate knowledge of disease, treatment, and care.

Hypothyroidism

In this disorder, metabolic processes slow because of a deficiency of the thyroid hormones triiodothyronine (T_3) or thyroxine (T_4) or thyroid-stimulating hormone (TSH). Hypothyroidism is classified as primary or secondary. Primary hypothyroidism stems from a disorder of the thyroid gland. Secondary hypothyroidism is caused by a failure to stimulate normal thyroid function or by a failure of target tissues to respond to normal blood levels of thyroid hormones. Either type may progress to myxedema, which is clinically much more severe and considered a medical emergency.

The disorder is most prevalent in women. In the United States, incidence is rising significantly in people ages 40 to 50.

CAUSES

Hypothyroidism is linked to a variety of abnormalities that lead to insufficient synthesis of thyroid hormones. Common causes include thyroid gland surgery (thyroidectomy), inflammation from irradiation therapy, chronic autoimmune thyroiditis (Hashimoto's disease), or inflammatory conditions, such as amyloidosis and sarcoidosis.

The disorder may also result from pituitary failure to produce TSH, hypothalamic failure to produce thyrotropin-releasing hormone, inborn errors of thyroid hormone synthesis, or inability to synthesize thyroid hormones because of iodine deficiency (usually dietary) or the use of antithyroid drugs such as propylthiouracil.

Thyroid hormones affect almost every organ system in the body, so complications of hypothyroidism vary according to organs involved as well as to the duration and severity of the condition.

Cardiovascular complications may include hypercholesterolemia with associated arteriosclerosis and ischemic heart disease. Poor peripheral circulation, heart enlargement, heart failure, and pleural and pericardial effusions may also occur. In addition, the patient may have poor pulmonary function, displayed as shallow, slow respirations and impaired ventilatory response to hypercapnia and hypoxia.

GI complications include achlorhydria, pernicious anemia, and adynamic colon, resulting in megacolon and intestinal obstruction.

Anemia due to the generalized suppression of erythropoietin may foster bleeding tendencies and iron deficiency anemia. Other complications include conductive or sensorineural deafness, psychiatric disturbances, carpal tunnel syndrome, benign intracranial hypertension, and impaired fertility.

DIAGNOSIS AND TREATMENT

A diagnosis of hypothyroidism is confirmed when radioimmunoassay with radioactive iodine (^{131}I) shows low serum levels of thyroid hormones and when a thorough history and physical examination show characteristic signs and symptoms. A differential diagnosis requires additional tests of serum TSH levels, serum antithyroid antibodies, and ectopic thyroid tissue. Skull X-ray, computed tomography scan, and magnetic resonance imaging help locate pituitary or hypothalamic lesions, a likely underlying cause of hypothyroidism.

In hypothyroidism, treatment consists of gradual thyroid hormone replacement with synthetic hormone or thyroprotein derived from animal thyroids. Synthetic hormones include levothyroxine (T_4), liothyronine (T_3), desiccated thyroid USP, liotrix (T_3 and T_4), and thyroglobulin (T_3 and T_4). Levothyroxine is available in a pure, stable, inexpensive form. It is converted to T_3 intracellularly, so both hormones become available even though only one is given. It usually takes about 2 months to reach equilibrium on a full dosage of levothyroxine.

Rapid treatment may be necessary for patients with myxedema coma and those about to undergo emergency surgery (because of sensitivity to central nervous system depression). In these patients, both I.V. administration of levothyroxine and hydrocortisone therapy are warranted. (See *Dealing with myxedema coma.*)

In underdeveloped areas, prophylactic iodine supplements have successfully lowered the incidence of iodine-deficient goiter.

COLLABORATIVE MANAGEMENT

Care of the patient with hypothyroidism focuses on returning vital signs and cardiopulmonary status to acceptable parameters, stabilizing weight, and teaching the patient about the disorder.

ASSESSMENT

The patient history may reveal vague and varied symptoms that developed slowly over time. The patient may report energy loss, fatigue, forgetfulness, sensitivity to cold, unexplained weight gain, and constipation. As the disorder progresses, signs and symp-

toms may include anorexia, decreased libido, menor-rhagia, paresthesia, joint stiffness, and muscle cramping. Look for:
- decreased mental stability (slight mental slowing to severe obtundation)
- a thick, dry tongue, causing hoarseness and slow, slurred speech
- dry, flaky, inelastic skin; puffy face, hands, and feet; periorbital edema; drooping upper eyelids; and puffy, coarse facial features
- dry, sparse hair, with patchy hair loss and loss of the outer third of the eyebrow
- thick, brittle nails, with visible transverse and longitudinal grooves
- ataxia, intention tremor, and nystagmus
- rough, doughy skin that feels cool
- a weak pulse and bradycardia; muscle weakness
- sacral or peripheral edema
- delayed reflex relaxation time (especially in the Achilles tendon)
- thyroid tissue that's not easily palpable unless a goiter is present
- absent or decreased bowel sounds
- hypotension (or decreased systolic and increased diastolic blood pressure)
- a gallop or distant heart sounds
- adventitious breath sounds
- abdominal distention or ascites.

NURSING DIAGNOSES AND COLLABORATIVE PROBLEMS

Based on the following nursing diagnoses, you'll establish patient outcomes.

Activity intolerance related to slow metabolism and low energy level. The patient will:
- express an understanding of the need to increase his activity level gradually
- maintain blood pressure and heart and respiratory rates within prescribed limits whenever he's active
- regain and maintain his normal activity level.

Altered cardiopulmonary tissue perfusion related to arteriosclerosis and myocardial ischemic changes. The patient will:
- have no chest pain when he's at rest
- maintain a normal heart rate and rhythm and avoid ischemic changes on an electrocardiogram
- maintain adequate cardiopulmonary tissue perfusion.

Body image disturbance related to changes in weight, skin, and hair. The patient will:
- express his feelings about body image changes
- comply with treatments to improve his body image
- regain a positive body image and express positive feelings about himself.

Dealing with myxedema coma

A medical emergency, myxedema coma commonly has a fatal outcome. Progression is usually gradual, but when stress aggravates severe or prolonged hypothyroidism, coma may develop abruptly. Examples of severe stress are infection, exposure to cold, and trauma. Other precipitating factors include thyroid medication withdrawal and the use of sedatives, narcotics, or anesthetics.

Signs and symptoms
Patients in myxedema coma have significantly depressed respirations, so their partial pressure of arterial carbon dioxide may rise. Decreased cardiac output and worsening cerebral hypoxia may also occur. The patient is stuporous and hypothermic, and his vital signs reflect bradycardia and hypotension.

Emergency interventions
If your patient becomes comatose, begin these interventions as soon as possible:
- Maintain airway patency with ventilatory support if necessary.
- Maintain circulation through I.V. fluid replacement.
- Provide continuous electrocardiogram monitoring.
- Monitor arterial blood gas measurements to detect hypoxia and metabolic acidosis.
- Warm the patient by wrapping him in blankets. Don't use a warming blanket because it might increase peripheral vasodilation, causing shock.
- Monitor body temperature until stable with a low-reading thermometer.
- Replace thyroid hormone by administering large I.V. levothyroxine doses, as ordered. Monitor vital signs because rapid correction of hypothyroidism can cause adverse cardiac effects.
- Monitor intake and output and daily weight. With treatment, urine output should increase and body weight decrease; if not, report this to the doctor.
- Replace fluids and other substances such as glucose. Monitor serum electrolyte levels.
- Administer corticosteroids, as ordered.
- Check for possible sources of infection, such as blood, sputum, or urine, which may have precipitated coma. Treat infections or any other underlying illness.

PLANNING AND IMPLEMENTATION

These measures help the patient with hypothyroidism.
- Give thyroid hormone therapy, as prescribed.
- Increase the patient's activity level gradually, and provide frequent rest periods to avoid fatigue and decrease myocardial oxygen demand.

- Provide a high-bulk, low-calorie diet, and encourage activity to combat constipation and promote weight loss. Give cathartics and stool softeners, as needed.
- Provide extra clothing and blankets for a patient with decreased cold tolerance. Dress the patient in layers, and adjust room temperature, if possible.
- Monitor the patient for constipation. Auscultate bowel sounds, check for abdominal distention, and check bowel movement frequency.
- Observe the patient's mental and neurologic status. Check for disorientation, decreased level of consciousness, and hearing loss.
- During thyroid replacement therapy, watch for signs and symptoms of hyperthyroidism, such as restlessness, sweating, and excessive weight loss.
- Assess the patient's cardiovascular status. Auscultate heart and breath sounds, and watch for chest pain or dyspnea. Observe for dependent and sacral edema.
- Apply antiembolism stockings and elevate the patient's legs to assist venous return.
- Encourage the patient to cough and breathe deeply to prevent pulmonary complications. Maintain fluid restrictions and a low-sodium diet.
- Monitor and record vital signs, fluid intake, urine output, and daily weight.
- If needed, reorient the patient to time, place, and person, and use alternative communication techniques if he has impaired hearing. Explain all procedures slowly and carefully, and avoid sedation, if possible.
- Provide meticulous skin care. Turn and reposition the patient every 2 hours if he's on extended bed rest. Use alcohol-free skin care products and an emollient lotion after bathing.
- Provide a consistent environment to decrease confusion and frustration. Offer support and encouragement to the patient and his family.
- Encourage the patient to verbalize his feelings and fears about changes in body image and possible rejection by others. Help him identify his strengths and use them to develop coping strategies, and encourage him to develop interests that foster a positive self-image and de-emphasize appearance.

Patient teaching
- Help the patient and family members understand the patient's physical and mental changes (such as mood changes and altered thought processes). Stress that these problems will probably subside with proper treatment. Urge family members to encourage and accept the patient and to help him adhere to his treatment regimen. If necessary, refer them to a mental health professional for additional counseling.
- Teach them to identify the signs and symptoms of life-threatening myxedema. Stress the importance of obtaining prompt medical care for respiratory problems and chest pain.
- Explain long-term hormone replacement therapy. Emphasize that the patient needs lifelong administration if this drug is necessary, that he should take it exactly as prescribed, and that he should never abruptly discontinue it.
- Advise the patient to always wear a medical identification bracelet and carry his drugs with him.
- Tell the patient and a family member to keep accurate records of daily weight and intake and output.
- Instruct the patient to eat a well-balanced diet that's high in fiber and fluids to prevent constipation, to restrict sodium to prevent fluid retention, and to limit calories to minimize weight gain.
- Tell him to schedule activities to avoid fatigue and to get adequate rest.

EVALUATION
Achievement of patient outcomes determines the success of collaborative management. For the patient with hypothyroidism, evaluation focuses on vital signs and cardiopulmonary status within acceptable parameters; return of metabolic and laboratory studies to within acceptable parameters; improved intake, output, and daily weight; improved activity tolerance; and improved participation in self-care.

Syndrome of inappropriate antidiuretic hormone secretion

A potentially life-threatening condition, syndrome of inappropriate antidiuretic hormone (SIADH) secretion is marked by excessive release of antidiuretic hormone (ADH), which disturbs fluid and electrolyte balance. SIADH follows diseases that affect the osmoreceptors (supraoptic nucleus) of the hypothalamus. The prognosis depends on the underlying disorder and the patient's response to treatment.

Without prompt treatment, SIADH may lead to water intoxication, cerebral edema, and severe hyponatremia, with resultant coma and death.

CAUSES
Usually, SIADH is linked to oat cell carcinoma of the lung, which secretes excessive ADH or vasopressor-like substances. Other neoplastic diseases (such as pancreatic and prostatic cancers, Hodgkin's disease, and thymoma) may also trigger SIADH. Additional causes include central nervous system (CNS) disorders, pulmonary disorders, endocrine disorders (such as adrenal insufficiency and myxedema), drugs (for example, chlorpropamide, tolbutamide, vincristine, cyclophosphamide, haloperidol, carbamazepine, clofibrate, morphine, and thiazides), and miscellaneous conditions (such as psychosis).

DIAGNOSIS AND TREATMENT

Diagnostic tests may reveal serum osmolality levels of less than 280 mOsm/kg of water in conjunction with serum sodium levels less than 123 mEq/L. Urine sodium levels may reach more than 20 mEq/L without the use of diuretics. Renal function tests are normal with no evidence of dehydration in SIADH.

Based primarily on the patient's symptoms, treatment begins with restricted water intake (17 to 34 oz [500 to 1,000 ml]/day). Some patients who continue to have symptoms are given a high-salt, high-protein diet or urea supplements to enhance water excretion. Or they may receive demeclocycline or lithium to help block the renal response to ADH.

Rarely, with severe water intoxication, 7 to 10 oz (200 to 300 ml) of 3% to 5% sodium chloride solution may be needed to raise the serum sodium level. The doctor may prescribe a loop diuretic to reduce the risk of heart failure after the excess fluid load and the administration of the hypertonic sodium chloride solution. When possible, treatment should include correction of the underlying cause of SIADH. If SIADH is due to cancer, surgery, irradiation, or chemotherapy may alleviate water retention.

COLLABORATIVE MANAGEMENT

Care of the patient with SIADH focuses on improving fluid balance and neurologic status, avoiding injury and complications, and teaching about the disease, treatment, and care.

ASSESSMENT

The patient's medical and medication histories may provide a clue to the cause of SIADH. A history of cerebrovascular disease, cancer, pulmonary disease, or recent head injury is especially significant. Look for:

- complaints of anorexia, nausea, vomiting and, paradoxically, weight gain
- reports of CNS symptoms, such as lethargy, headaches, and emotional and behavioral changes
- a lack of expected edema, because much of the free water excess is within cellular boundaries
- tachycardia associated with increased fluid volume
- disorientation, which may progress to seizures and coma
- sluggish deep tendon reflexes and muscle weakness.

NURSING DIAGNOSES AND COLLABORATIVE PROBLEMS

Based on the following nursing diagnoses, you'll establish patient outcomes.

Altered thought processes related to neurologic dysfunction. The patient will:
- remain safe within his environment
- regain and maintain his orientation to time, place, and person.

Fluid volume excess related to cellular fluid retention. The patient will:
- adhere to fluid restriction
- show no evidence of complications from excess fluid retention
- regain and maintain normal serum osmolality and sodium levels.

Knowledge deficit related to causes and treatment of SIADH. The patient will:
- identify and express the need to learn about SIADH
- seek and obtain correct information about the causes and treatment of SIADH
- communicate an understanding of the causes and treatment of SIADH.

PLANNING AND IMPLEMENTATION

These measures help the patient with SIADH.
- Closely monitor and record the patient's intake and output, vital signs, and daily weight.
- Restrict fluids, and provide comfort measures for thirst, including ice chips, mouth care, lozenges, and staggered water intake.
- Monitor the patient's serum osmolality and serum and urine sodium levels.
- Observe for signs and symptoms of heart failure, which may occur as a result of fluid overload.
- Reduce unnecessary environmental stimuli and orient the patient, as needed.
- Provide a safe environment for the patient with an altered level of consciousness (LOC). Take seizure precautions as needed.
- Perform frequent neurologic checks, depending on the patient's status. Look for and report early changes in LOC.

Patient teaching

- If SIADH hasn't resolved by the time of discharge, explain to the patient and family members why he must restrict his fluid intake. Review ways to decrease his discomfort from thirst.
- If drug therapy is prescribed, teach the patient and family members about the regimen, including dosage, action, and possible adverse effects.
- Discuss self-monitoring techniques for fluid retention, including measurement of intake and output and daily weight. Teach the patient to recognize signs and symptoms that require immediate medical intervention.

EVALUATION

Achievement of patient outcomes determines the success of collaborative management. For the patient with SIADH, evaluation focuses on fluid balance and neurologic status within acceptable parameters, absence of injury and complications, and adequate knowledge of disease, treatment, and care.

Treatments and procedures

A variety of surgical procedures—including hypophysectomy, parathyroidectomy, and thyroidectomy—may be used to treat endocrine disorders.

HYPOPHYSECTOMY

New microsurgical methods have dramatically reversed the high mortality once associated with removal of pituitary and sella turcica tumors. Hypophysectomy is now the treatment of choice for pituitary tumors, which can cause acromegaly, gigantism, and Cushing's disease. And it's used as a palliative measure for patients with metastatic breast or prostate cancer to relieve pain and reduce the hormonal secretions that spur neoplastic growth.

Hypophysectomy is performed transfrontally (approaching the sella turcica through the cranium) or transsphenoidally (entering from the inner aspect of the upper lip through the sphenoid sinus). The transfrontal approach carries a high risk of mortality and such complications as smell and taste loss and permanent, severe diabetes insipidus. For these reasons, this approach is rarely used. In the commonly used transsphenoidal approach, powerful microscopes and improved radiologic techniques allow microadenoma removal. (See *Transsphenoidal hypophysectomy*.) Laser surgery, an alternative approach, is experimental.

PROCEDURE

In transsphenoidal hypophysectomy, with the patient under general anesthesia, the doctor makes an incision in the superior gingival tissue of the maxilla. After dissecting membranes and tissues, he places a speculum blade in the developed space, slightly anterior to the sphenoid sinus to avoid lateral compression of the opened anterior walls of the sinus. (Some doctors prefer the septal passage for the speculum.) Then he evaluates the deeper anatomy using an operating microscope with binocular vision and high-power lighting.

Using a microdrill, the doctor penetrates the sphenoid bone to visualize the anterior sella floor. He can then resect and aspirate a soft tumor downward. Before wound closure, he may apply hemostatic agents, such as oxidized cellulose cotton. Or he may use the patient's own subcutaneous fat or a muscle plug from the thigh as intrasellar graft tissue. The sella floor may be sealed off with a small piece of bone or cartilage.

Finally, the doctor inserts nasal catheters with petroleum gauze packed around them. He closes the initial incision with stitches inside the inner lip.

COLLABORATIVE MANAGEMENT

Care of the patient undergoing hypophysectomy requires thorough preparation, close monitoring, and intense patient teaching.

Preparation

Explain to the patient that this surgery will remove a tumor from his pituitary gland. Tell him he will receive a general anesthetic and, after surgery, will remain in the intensive care unit for 48 hours for careful monitoring. Mention that he'll have a nasal catheter and packing in place for 1 to 2 days after surgery, as well as an indwelling urinary catheter.

Arrange for appropriate tests and examinations, as ordered. For example, if the patient has acromegaly, he'll need a thorough cardiac evaluation because he's at risk for incipient myocardial ischemia. If he has Cushing's disease, he'll need blood pressure checks and serum potassium determinations. For any patient, arrange visual field tests to serve as a baseline.

Review the patient's preoperative drug regimen, if appropriate. If he develops hypothyroidism, he may need hormone replacement therapy. If he has a prolactin-secreting tumor, find out if he's been taking bromocriptine for 6 weeks before surgery to help shrink the tumor.

Monitoring and aftercare

Monitor vital signs until stable. Keep the patient on bed rest for 24 hours, then encourage ambulation. Keep the head of his bed elevated to avoid placing tension or pressure on the suture line. Tell him not to sneeze, cough, blow his nose, or bend over for several days to avoid disturbing the muscle graft.

Give mild analgesics, as ordered, for headache caused by cerebrospinal fluid (CSF) loss during surgery or for paranasal pain. Paranasal pain typically subsides when the catheters and packing are removed—usually 24 to 48 hours after surgery.

Expect the patient to develop transient diabetes insipidus, usually within 24 hours after surgery. Watch for increased thirst and greater urine volume with a low specific gravity. If diabetes insipidus occurs, replace fluids and give aqueous vasopressin, as ordered. Or give sublingual desmopressin acetate, as ordered. With these measures, diabetes insipidus usually resolves within 72 hours.

Arrange for visual field testing as soon as possible because visual defects may signal hemorrhage. Collect a serum sample to measure pituitary hormone levels and evaluate the need for hormone replacement. As ordered, give prophylactic antibiotics.

Patient teaching

■ Teach the patient how to recognize diabetes insipidus, and advise him to report signs and symptoms

Transsphenoidal hypophysectomy

When a pituitary tumor is confined to the sella turcica, the doctor will perform a transsphenoidal hypophysectomy. For this procedure, the patient is placed in a semirecumbent position and given a general anesthetic.

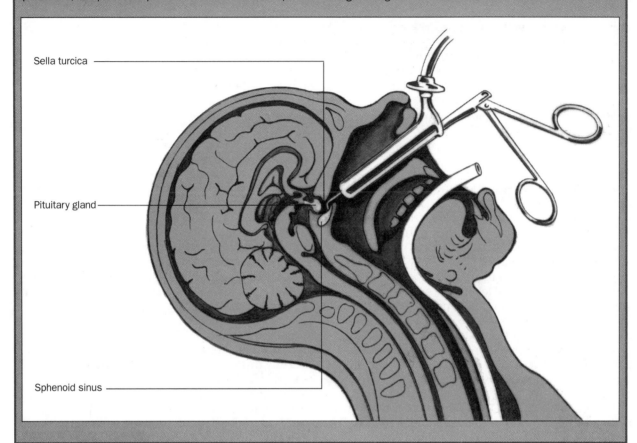

Sella turcica

Pituitary gland

Sphenoid sinus

immediately. Explain that he may need to limit fluid intake or take prescribed drugs.

■ If ordered, tell the patient not to brush his teeth for 2 weeks to avoid suture line disruption. Mention that he can use a mouthwash.

■ The patient may need hormonal replacement therapy because of decreased pituitary secretion of thyroid-stimulating hormone. If he needs cortisol or thyroid hormone replacement, teach him to recognize the signs of excessive or insufficient dosage. Advise him to wear a medical identification bracelet.

■ Tell the patient with hyperprolactinemia that he'll need follow-up visits for several years because relapse is possible. Explain that he may take bromocriptine if he has a relapse.

COMPLICATIONS

Transient diabetes insipidus is a common postsurgical problem; in some cases, it's followed by transient syn-

drome of inappropriate antidiuretic hormone, which requires careful patient monitoring for 24 to 48 hours. Other potential complications include infection, CSF leakage, hemorrhage, and visual defects. Total pituitary gland removal causes a hormonal deficiency that calls for close monitoring and replacement therapy; usually, though, the anterior pituitary is preserved.

PARATHYROIDECTOMY

Parathyroidectomy, the surgical removal of one or more of the four parathyroid glands, treats primary hyperparathyroidism. In this disorder, the parathyroids secrete excessive amounts of parathyroid hormone (PTH), causing high serum calcium and low serum phosphorus levels.

The number of glands removed depends on the underlying cause of excessive PTH secretion. For example, if the patient has a single adenoma, removing the affected gland corrects the problem. If more than one gland is enlarged, subtotal parathyroidectomy (removing the three largest glands and part of the fourth) can correct hyperparathyroidism. The remaining glandular segment decreases the risk of postoperative hypoparathyroidism and resulting hypocalcemia because it resumes normal function.

Total parathyroidectomy is necessary when cancer causes glandular hyperplasia. In this case, the patient will require lifelong treatment for hypoparathyroidism. The doctor may also perform subtotal thyroidectomy along with parathyroidectomy if he can't locate the abnormal tissue or adenoma and suspects an intrathyroid lesion.

Serum calcium levels typically decrease within 24 to 48 hours after surgery and become normal within 4 to 5 days.

PROCEDURE

After the patient is anesthetized, the doctor makes a cervical neck incision and exposes the thyroid gland. He then locates the four parathyroids (usually just above or below the point where the recurrent laryngeal nerve and the inferior thyroid artery cross) and identifies and tags them.

If he can't find one of them, he'll do a cervical thymectomy and thyroid lobectomy on the side where the gland is missing and send a sample for an immediate frozen section. If the missing gland isn't found in the removed tissue, the doctor may stop the procedure and order localization studies before a second surgery. Or, he may continue surgery by opening the sternum and exploring the mediastinum for the missing gland.

Once he has found all four glands, he examines them for hyperplasia and removes the affected ones. Before he sutures the incision, he inserts a Penrose drain or a closed-wound drainage device.

COLLABORATIVE MANAGEMENT

Care of the patient undergoing parathyroidectomy requires thorough preparation, close monitoring, and intense patient teaching.

Preparation

Tell the patient that this surgery will remove diseased parathyroid tissue. Explain that he'll receive a general anesthetic and that the doctor will make a neck incision, explore the area, and remove parathyroid tissue as necessary. Explain that the doctor may perform a subtotal thyroidectomy if he can't find diseased tissue.

Show the patient how to support his neck and perform coughing and deep-breathing exercises after surgery. Warn him that talking and swallowing will hurt for the first few days.

As ordered, take measures to bring the patient's calcium levels to near normal before surgery. For example, maintain calcium restrictions and provide plenty of fluids to dilute excess calcium. Also give such drugs as diuretics, mithramycin (an antihypercalcemic agent), and inorganic phosphates, as ordered, to lower calcium levels.

Monitoring and aftercare

Monitor vital signs until stable. Keep the patient in high Fowler's position after surgery to promote venous return from the head and neck and to decrease oozing into the incision. As soon as he begins to awaken from anesthesia, check for laryngeal nerve damage by asking him to speak.

Check the patient's dressing, and palpate the back of his neck, where drainage tends to flow. Expect about 50 ml of drainage in the first 24 hours; if you find no drainage, check for drain kinking or the need to reestablish suction. Expect only scant drainage after 24 hours.

Keep a tracheotomy tray nearby for the first 24 hours after surgery, and assess the patient frequently for signs of respiratory distress, such as dyspnea and cyanosis. Upper airway obstruction may result from tracheal collapse, mucus accumulation in the trachea, laryngeal edema, or vocal cord paralysis.

Expect the patient to complain of a sore neck (from hyperextension during surgery), a sore throat (from manipulation), and hoarseness and swallowing difficulty (from anesthesia and intubation). Give mild analgesics, as ordered.

Because transient hypoparathyroidism with resulting hypocalcemia is possible 1 to 4 days after surgery, watch closely for signs of increased neuromuscular excitability. Check for positive Chvostek's and Trousseau's signs, and tell the patient to report numbness and tingling of his fingers and toes or around his mouth (early signs of hypocalcemia) as well as muscle cramps. Keep I.V. calcium on hand in case tetany occurs.

Patient teaching

■ Tell the patient to keep his incision site clean and dry, and explain that the doctor will check it at follow-up appointments.

■ Explain that he'll need periodic serum calcium determinations to help evaluate the surgery's outcome.

■ Advise him not to take any nonprescription drugs without consulting his doctor. In particular, tell him to avoid magnesium-containing laxatives and antacids, mineral oil, and vitamins A and D.

■ If the patient has had a total parathyroidectomy, tell him to follow a high-calcium, low-phosphorus diet, as ordered, and to take his calcium drugs. If he's to receive dihydrotachysterol and calciferol, tell him not to take vitamins without consulting his doctor.

■ Tell him to call his doctor if he develops signs of hypercalcemia, such as excessive thirst, headache, vertigo, tinnitus, and anorexia.

COMPLICATIONS
Complications are rare, but may include hemorrhage, damage to the recurrent laryngeal nerve, and hypoparathyroidism.

THYROIDECTOMY
The surgical removal of part or all of the thyroid gland, thyroidectomy allows treatment of hyperthyroidism, respiratory obstruction from goiter, and thyroid cancer. Subtotal thyroidectomy, used to correct hyperthyroidism when drug therapy fails or radiation therapy is contraindicated, reduces secretion of thyroid hormone. It also effectively treats diffuse goiter. After surgery, the remaining thyroid tissue usually supplies enough thyroid hormone for normal function.

Total thyroidectomy is chosen for certain types of thyroid cancers, such as papillary, follicular, medullary, or anaplastic neoplasms. After this surgery, the patient requires lifelong thyroid hormone replacement therapy.

PROCEDURE
After the patient is anesthetized, the surgeon extends the neck fully and determines the incision line by measuring bilaterally from each clavicle. Then he cuts through the skin, fascia, and muscle and raises skin flaps from the strap muscles. He separates these muscles midline, revealing the thyroid's isthmus, and ligates the thyroid artery and veins to help prevent bleeding. Next, he locates and visualizes the laryngeal nerves and parathyroid glands and then begins dissection and removal of thyroid tissue, trying not to injure these nearby structures.

Before the surgeon sutures the incision, he may insert a Penrose drain or a closed-wound drainage device such as a Hemovac drain.

COLLABORATIVE MANAGEMENT
Care of the patient undergoing a thyroidectomy requires thorough preparation, close monitoring, and intense patient teaching.

Preparation
Explain to the patient that thyroidectomy will remove diseased thyroid tissue or, if necessary, the entire gland. Tell him that he'll have an incision in his neck; that he'll have a dressing and, possibly, a drain in place after surgery; and that he may experience some hoarseness and a sore throat from intubation and anesthesia. Reassure him that he'll receive analgesics to relieve his discomfort.

If your patient's thyroidectomy is to treat hyperthyroidism, ensure that he's followed his preoperative drug regimen, which renders the gland euthyroid and prevents thyroid storm during surgery. He's probably had either propylthiouracil or methimazole, usually starting 4 to 6 weeks before surgery. He'll probably get iodine as well for 10 to 14 days before surgery to reduce the gland's vascularity and prevent excess bleeding. He may also be receiving propranolol to block adrenergic effects. Notify the doctor immediately if the patient has failed to follow his drug regimen.

Collect samples for serum thyroid hormone determinations to check for euthyroidism. If necessary, arrange for an electrocardiogram to evaluate cardiac status.

Monitoring and aftercare
Monitor vital signs until stable and remember to keep the patient in high Fowler's position to promote venous return from the head and neck and to decrease oozing into the incision. Check for laryngeal nerve damage by asking the patient to speak as soon as he awakens from anesthesia.

Watch for signs of respiratory distress. Tracheal collapse, tracheal mucus accumulation, laryngeal edema, and vocal cord paralysis can all cause respiratory obstruction, with sudden stridor and restlessness. Keep a tracheotomy tray at the patient's bedside for 24 hours after surgery, and be prepared to assist with emergency tracheotomy, if necessary.

Remember to check for signs of hemorrhage, which may cause shock, tracheal compression, and respiratory distress. Check the patient's dressing and palpate the back of his neck, where drainage tends to flow. Expect about 50 ml of drainage in the first 24 hours; if you find no drainage, check for drain kinking or the need to reestablish suction. Expect only scant drainage after 24 hours.

Assess for hypocalcemia, which is a threat when the parathyroid glands are damaged. Test for Chvostek's and Trousseau's signs, indicators of neuromuscular irritability from hypocalcemia. Keep calcium gluconate available for emergency I.V. administration. Stay alert for signs of thyroid storm, a rare but serious complication.

As ordered, give him a mild analgesic to relieve a sore neck or throat. Reassure the patient that his discomfort should resolve within a few days.

If the patient doesn't have a drain in place, prepare him for discharge the day following surgery, as indicated. However, if he has a drain, the doctor will usually remove it, along with half of the surgical clips, on the second day after surgery; the remaining clips come off the following day, before discharge.

Patient teaching

■ If the patient is discharged the day after surgery, tell him to report any signs of respiratory distress or bleeding.

■ If he had a total thyroidectomy, explain the importance of regularly taking his prescribed thyroid hormone replacement. Teach him to recognize and report signs of hypothyroidism and hyperthyroidism.

■ If his parathyroid was damaged during surgery, explain that he'll need calcium supplements. Teach him to recognize the warning signs of hypocalcemia.

■ Tell him to keep the incision site clean and dry. Help him cope with concerns about its appearance. Suggest loosely buttoned collars, high-necked blouses, jewelry, or scarves, which can hide the incision until it has healed. The doctor may recommend using a mild body lotion to soften the healing scar and improve its appearance.

■ Arrange follow-up appointments, as necessary, and explain to the patient that the doctor needs to check the incision and serum thyroid hormone levels.

COMPLICATIONS

Usually performed under general anesthesia, thyroidectomy has a low incidence of complications if the patient is properly prepared with thyroid hormone antagonist. Potential complications include hemorrhage; parathyroid damage, causing postoperative hypocalcemia, which can lead to tetany; and laryngeal nerve damage, causing vocal cord paralysis. This last complication can cause hoarseness, if only one vocal cord is damaged, and respiratory distress (requiring tracheotomy), if both cords are affected. Thyroid storm is a potential problem, when a thyroidectomy is to treat hyperthyroidism. It's preventable, if the patient is properly prepared with antithyroid drug.

Selected references

DeGroot, L.J., ed. *Endocrinology*, 3rd ed. Philadelphia: W.B. Saunders Co., 1995.

Greenspan, F., and Strewler, G. *Basic and Clinical Endocrinology*, 5th ed. Stamford, Conn.: Appleton & Lange, 1997.

Illustrated Guide to Diagnostic Tests, 2nd ed. Springhouse, Pa.: Springhouse Corp., 1998.

Lavin, N. *Manual of Endocrinology and Metabolism*, 2nd ed. Boston: Little, Brown & Co., 1994.

McEwen, D. "Transphenoidal Adenectomy," *AORN Journal* 61(2):321-37. February 1995.

Meeker, M., and Rothrock, J. *Alexander's Care of the Patient in Surgery*, 10th ed. St. Louis: Mosby–Year Book, Inc., 1995.

Nursing98 Drug Handbook. Springhouse, Pa.: Springhouse Corp., 1998.

Professional Guide to Signs and Symptoms, 2nd ed. Springhouse, Pa.: Springhouse Corp., 1997.

Roberts, A., "The Anterior Pituitary," *Nursing Times* 91(24):41-43, June 14-20, 1995.

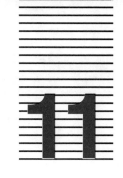

Reproductive disorders

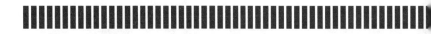

Because misinformation and cultural taboos may affect your patient's knowledge of the reproductive system, these disorders present a formidable nursing challenge. Difficulties such as impotence, abnormal uterine bleeding, and infertility threaten an individual's self-confidence at the deepest level. Besides requiring expert health care, each patient will need sensitive counseling and straightforward teaching. In many cases, you may have to help the patient overcome feelings of vulnerability, guilt, and embarrassment.

Anatomy and physiology review

The following review of male and female reproductive systems will help you meet your patients' needs and and answer their questions.

MALE REPRODUCTIVE SYSTEM
The two major organs of the male reproductive system are the penis and testes. (See *Reviewing the male reproductive system,* page 456.) The system supplies male sex cells (spermatogenesis) and is involved in male sex hormone secretion. The penis also eliminates urine.

PENIS
Internally, the cylindrical penile shaft is made up of three columns of erectile tissue bound together by heavy fibrous tissue. Two corpora cavernosa form the major part of the penis; on the underside, the corpus spongiosum encases the urethra. The penile shaft terminates distally in the glans penis, a cone-shaped expansion of the corpus spongiosum that is highly sensitive to sexual stimuli. The expanded lateral margin of the glans forms a ridge of tissue known as the coro-

na. Thin, loose skin covers the penile shaft. In an uncircumcised male, a skin flap—the foreskin, or prepuce—covers the corona and much of the glans. The urethral meatus opens through the glans to allow urination and ejaculation.

SCROTUM
The penis meets the scrotum, or scrotal sac, at the penoscrotal junction. The scrotum consists of a thin layer of skin overlying a tighter, musclelike layer, which in turn overlies the tunica vaginalis, a serous membrane covering the internal scrotal cavity. Externally, the median raphe (seam of union of the two halves) continues from the penis to superficially bisect the scrotal skin. Internally, a septum divides the scrotum into two sacs, each containing a testis, an epididymis, and a spermatic cord. Each testis measures about 2″ (5 cm) long by 1″ (2.5 cm) wide and weighs about ½ oz (14 g). The testes contain the seminiferous tubules, where spermatogenesis takes place.

A complex duct system conveys sperm from the testes to the ejaculatory ducts near the bladder. From the seminiferous tubules, newly formed sperm travel to the epididymis—a tubular reservoir for sperm storage and maturation that curves over the posterolateral surface and upper end of the testes. Mature sperm then move from the epididymis to the vas deferens. This duct begins at the end of the epididymis, passes up through the external inguinal canal, and descends near the bladder fundus, where it enters the ejaculatory duct inside the prostate gland. The vas deferens is enclosed within the spermatic cord, a compact bundle of vessels, nerves, and muscle fibers.

PROSTATE GLAND
Lying under the bladder and surrounding the urethra, the walnut-sized (approximately 1½″ [4 cm] in diameter) prostate gland consists of three lobes—the left

◆◆◆ **455**

Reviewing the male reproductive system

The male reproductive system consists of the penis, the scrotum and its contents, the prostate gland, and the inguinal structures.

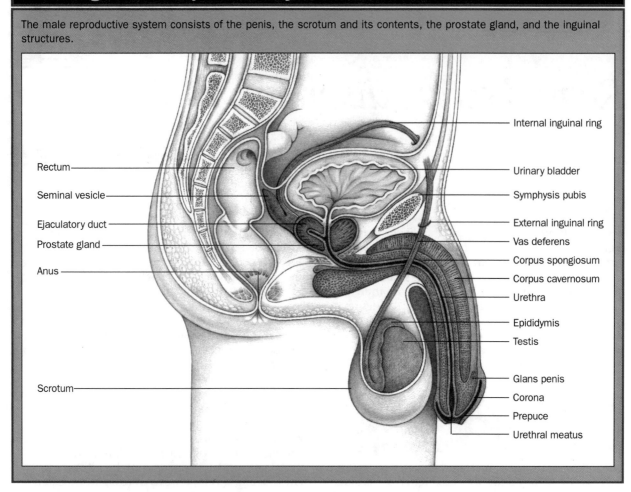

Rectum
Seminal vesicle
Ejaculatory duct
Prostate gland
Anus
Scrotum

Internal inguinal ring
Urinary bladder
Symphysis pubis
External inguinal ring
Vas deferens
Corpus spongiosum
Corpus cavernosum
Urethra
Epididymis
Testis
Glans penis
Corona
Prepuce
Urethral meatus

and right lateral lobes and the median lobe. The prostate continuously secretes prostatic fluid, a thin, milky alkaline fluid. During sexual activity, prostatic fluid adds volume to the semen and enhances sperm motility and possibly fertility by neutralizing the acidity of the urethra and the woman's vagina.

INGUINAL STRUCTURES
The spermatic cord travels from the testis through the inguinal canal, exiting the scrotum through the external inguinal ring and entering the abdominal cavity through the internal inguinal ring. The external inguinal ring is located just above and lateral to the pubic tubercle; the internal ring, about ½″ (1.3 cm) above the midpoint of the inguinal ligament, between the pubic tubercle of the symphysis pubis and the anterior superior iliac spine. Between the two rings lies the inguinal canal. Lymph nodes from the

penis, scrotal surface, and anus drain into the inguinal lymph nodes. Lymph nodes from the testes drain into the lateral aortic and preaortic lymph nodes in the abdomen.

SPERMATOGENESIS
Sperm formation begins when a male reaches puberty and normally continues throughout life. Stimulated by male sex hormones, mature sperm cells are formed continuously within the seminiferous tubules.

Sperm is formed in several stages:
■ Spermatogonia, the primary germinal epithelial cells, grow and develop into primary spermatocytes. Both spermatogonia and primary spermatocytes contain 46 chromosomes, which consist of 44 autosomes and the 2 sex chromosomes, X and Y.
■ Primary spermatocytes divide to form secondary spermatocytes. No new chromosomes are formed in

this stage—the pairs only divide. Each secondary spermatocyte contains half the number of autosomes (22); 1 secondary spermatocyte contains an X chromosome; the other, a Y chromosome.

■ Each secondary spermatocyte then divides again to form spermatids.

■ Finally, the spermatids undergo a series of structural changes that transform them into mature spermatozoa, or sperm. Each spermatozoon has a head, neck, body, and tail. The head contains the nucleus; the tail, a large amount of adenosine triphosphate, which provides energy for sperm motility.

Newly mature sperm pass from the seminiferous tubules through the vasa recta into the epididymis, where they mature. The epididymis can store only a few sperm; most of them move into the vas deferens, where they're stored until sexual stimulation triggers emission. Sperm cells retain their potency in storage for many weeks. After ejaculation, sperm survive for 24 to 72 hours at body temperature.

The number and motility of sperm affect fertility. A low sperm count (less than 20 million/ml of ejaculated semen) or poor sperm motility may cause infertility.

HORMONAL CONTROL AND SEXUAL DEVELOPMENT

The male sex hormones (androgens) are produced in the testes and the adrenal glands. Located in the testes between the seminiferous tubules, Leydig's cells secrete testosterone, the most significant male sex hormone. These cells proliferate during puberty and remain abundant throughout life. Testosterone is responsible for the development and maintenance of male sex organs and secondary sex characteristics. Its presence is required for spermatogenesis.

Male sexuality is also affected by other hormones. Two of these—luteinizing hormone (LH) and follicle-stimulating hormone (FSH)—directly affect testosterone secretion.

Testosterone secretion begins in utero. Starting at approximately the second month of gestation, release of chorionic gonadotropins from the placenta stimulates Leydig's cells in the male fetus to secrete testosterone. The presence of fetal testosterone directly affects fetal sexual differentiation. With testosterone, fetal genitalia develop into a penis, scrotum, and testes; without testosterone, the genitalia develop into a clitoris, vagina, and other female organs.

During the last 2 months of fetal life in utero, testosterone normally causes the testes to descend into the scrotum. If the testes don't descend after birth, exogenous testosterone may correct the problem.

During early childhood, a boy does not secrete gonadotropins and thus has little circulating testosterone. Pituitary secretion of gonadotropins—which usually starts between ages 11 and 14—stimulates testicular function and testosterone secretion and marks the onset of puberty. During puberty, the penis and testes enlarge and the male reaches full adult sexual and reproductive capability. Puberty also marks the development of male secondary sexual characteristics: distinct body hair distribution, skin changes such as increased secretion by sweat and sebaceous glands, deepening of the voice from laryngeal enlargement, increased musculoskeletal development, and other intracellular and extracellular changes.

After full physical maturity is reached—usually by age 20—sexual and reproductive function remain fairly consistent throughout life. Although a man does not lose the ability to reproduce, he may experience subtle changes in sexual function with aging. For example, an older man may require more time to achieve an erection, may experience less firm erections, and may have reduced ejaculatory volume. After ejaculation, he may take longer to regain an erection.

FEMALE REPRODUCTIVE SYSTEM

Female external genitalia include the mons pubis, clitoris, labia majora, labia minora, and adjacent structures (Bartholin's glands, Skene's glands, and the urethral meatus). Internal genitalia include the vagina, uterus, ovaries, and fallopian tubes. (See *Reviewing the female reproductive system*, page 458.)

Hormonal influences determine the development and function of external and internal female genitalia and also affect fertility, childbearing, and the ability to experience sexual pleasure.

EXTERNAL GENITALIA

The vulva contains the external female genitalia that are visible on inspection. The mons pubis is the cushion of adipose and connective tissue covered by skin and coarse, curly hair over the symphysis pubis (the joint formed by union of the pubic bones anteriorly). The labia majora border the vulva laterally from the mons pubis to the perineum (muscle, fascia, and ligaments between the anus and vulva). The labia minora, two moist lesser mucosal folds that are dark pink to red, lie within and alongside the labia majora.

The clitoris is the small, protuberant organ located just beneath the arch of the mons pubis. The clitoris contains erectile tissue, venous cavernous spaces, and specialized sensory corpuscles that are stimulated during coitus.

When the labia are spread, the introitus (vaginal orifice) and the urethral meatus are visible. Less visible are the multiple orifices of Skene's glands, mucus-producing glands located on both sides of the urethral opening. Openings of the two mucus-producing Bartholin's glands are located laterally and posteriorly

Reviewing the female reproductive system

The illustrations below highlight the major female internal genitalia.

Lateral view of internal genitalia

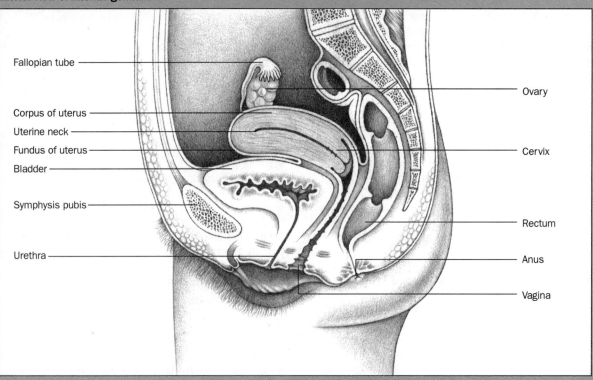

- Fallopian tube
- Corpus of uterus
- Uterine neck
- Fundus of uterus
- Bladder
- Symphysis pubis
- Urethra
- Ovary
- Cervix
- Rectum
- Anus
- Vagina

Anterior cross-sectional view of internal genitalia

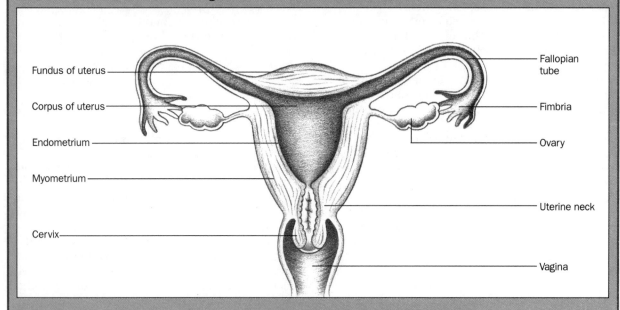

- Fundus of uterus
- Corpus of uterus
- Endometrium
- Myometrium
- Cervix
- Fallopian tube
- Fimbria
- Ovary
- Uterine neck
- Vagina

on either side of the inner vaginal orifice. The hymen, a tissue membrane varying in size and thickness, may completely or partially cover the vaginal orifice. A disrupted hymen appears as remnants of uneven mucosal tissue tags, called myrtiform caruncles.

INTERNAL GENITALIA

The vagina, a highly elastic muscular tube, is located between the urethra and the rectum. Approximately 2½" to 2¾" (6.5 to 7 cm) long anteriorly and 3½" (9 cm) long posteriorly, the vagina lies at a 45-degree angle to the long axis of the body.

The uterus, a small, firm, pear-shaped, muscular organ, rests between the bladder and the rectum. It usually lies at almost a 90-degree angle to the vagina, but other locations may be normal. The mucous membrane lining the uterus is called the endometrium; the muscular layer, the myometrium. In pregnancy, the elastic, upper uterine portion (the fundus) accommodates most of the growing fetus until term. The uterine neck (isthmus) joins the fundus to the cervix, the uterine part extending into the vagina. The fundus and the isthmus make up the corpus, the main uterine body.

Two fallopian tubes attach to the uterus at the upper angles of the fundus. Usually nonpalpable, these 2¾" to 5½" (7- to 14-cm) long, narrow tubes of muscle fibers have fingerlike projections, called fimbriae, on the free ends that partially surround the ovaries. The ovum is usually fertilized in the outer third of the fallopian tube.

Palpable almond-shaped organs approximately 1¼" to 1½" (3 to 4 cm) long, ¾" (2 cm) wide, and ¼" to ½" (0.6 to 1.3 cm) thick, the ovaries usually lie near the lateral pelvic walls, a little below the anterosuperior iliac spine.

DEVELOPMENT OF THE UTERUS AND CERVIX

Over a woman's lifetime, the sizes of the uterine corpus and cervix change, as does the percentage of space these parts occupy. For example, of the space filled by the whole uterus in a premenarchal female, one-third is uterine corpus, and two-thirds is cervix. In the adult multiparous female, the uterine corpus may occupy two-thirds of the space available, whereas the cervix may fill one-third. The central opening of the cervix (the external os), visible by speculum, is round and closed in a nulliparous woman. In a parous woman, the opening is an irregularly shaped slit.

HORMONAL FUNCTION AND THE MENSTRUAL CYCLE

The hypothalamus, ovaries, and pituitary gland secrete hormones that affect the buildup and shedding of the uterine lining during the menstrual cycle. (See *Understanding the menstrual cycle.*) Ovulation occurs

Understanding the menstrual cycle

The average menstrual cycle is 28 days, although the normal cycle may range from 22 to 34 days. The cycle is regulated by fluctuating hormone levels that, in turn, are regulated by negative and positive feedback mechanisms.

Menstrual phase
The cycle starts with menstruation (preovulatory, cycle day 1), which usually lasts 5 days. As the cycle begins, low estrogen and progesterone levels in the bloodstream stimulate the hypothalamus to secrete gonadotropin-releasing hormone (GnRH). In turn, this substance stimulates the anterior pituitary to secrete follicle-stimulating hormone (FSH) and luteinizing hormone (LH). When the FSH level rises, LH output increases.

Proliferative phase and ovulation
The proliferative (follicular) phase lasts from cycle days 6 to 14. During this phase, LH and FSH act on the ovarian follicle (mature ovarian cyst containing the ovum), causing estrogen secretion, which in turn stimulates the buildup of the endometrium. Late in the proliferative phase, estrogen levels peak, FSH secretion declines, and LH secretion increases, surging at midcycle (around day 14). Then, estrogen production decreases, the follicle matures, and the woman ovulates. Normally, one follicle matures during the ovulatory process and is released from the ovary during each cycle.

Luteal phase
During the luteal (secretory) phase, which lasts about 14 days, FSH and LH levels drop. Estrogen levels decline initially, then increase along with progesterone levels as the corpus luteum (progesterone-producing yellow structure that develops after the follicle ruptures) begins functioning. During this phase, the endometrium responds to progesterone stimulation by becoming thick and secretory in preparation for implantation of a fertilized ovum.

About 10 to 12 days after ovulation, the corpus luteum begins to diminish, as do estrogen and progesterone levels, until the hormone levels are insufficient to sustain the endometrium in a fully developed secretory state. Then the endometrial lining is shed (menses). Decreasing estrogen and progesterone levels stimulate the hypothalamus to produce GnRH, and the cycle begins again.

through a network of positive and negative feedback loops that run from the hypothalamus to the pituitary and to the ovaries and back to the hypothalamus and pituitary.

The menstrual cycle goes through three different phases: menstrual, proliferative (estrogen-dominated), and secretory (progesterone-dominated). These phases correspond to the phases of ovarian function.

MENOPAUSE

Cessation of menses usually begins between ages 40 and 55, with the average about age 51. Menstrual periods cease because of exhaustion of ovarian follicles that respond to FSH and LH released by the pituitary gland. The term *menopause* applies if menses are absent for 1 year. *Climacteric* refers to the transitional years from reproductive fertility to infertility during which several physiologic changes, including menopause, take place.

During menopause, estrogen and progesterone levels decrease and testosterone secretion increases. However, the woman does not become totally estrogen-deficient because a weaker form of estrogen, estrone, is produced in the peripheral tissues by a weak androgen (androstenedione). Uninhibited by ovarian estrogen and progesterone, the pituitary increases FSH and LH production.

Predominant reproductive system changes caused by the decline in estrogen include vasomotor symptoms such as hot flashes, and urogenital tissue atrophy, which causes decreased elasticity and thinning of the vaginal walls and increased urinary frequency. Estrogen loss also affects the integumentary system, as shown by sparse, gray pubic hair; the cardiovascular system, where it increases the risk of heart disease; and the musculoskeletal system, where it may cause osteoporosis.

Assessment

Gathering thorough information can prove crucial because many common reproductive disorders carry potentially serious physiologic and psychological consequences. For example, sexual or reproductive dysfunction can severely damage the patient's quality of life. Sexually transmitted diseases—the most common communicable diseases in the United States—can produce devastating complications if not detected and treated early.

HISTORY

Begin your assessment by obtaining a detailed health history. Establish a good rapport to help the patient relax and confide in you.

MALE PATIENTS

Most men are sensitive when questioned about sexual problems; they tend to equate sexual and reproductive functioning with manhood and may view sexual problems as signs of diminished masculinity. Older men may view declining sexual ability as a sign of lost youth and declining health. Although you'll focus your questions on the reproductive system, maintain a holistic approach by inquiring about other physical and psychological concerns. Keep in mind that reproductive system problems may affect other aspects of the patient's life, including self-image and overall wellness.

Chief complaint. Ask the patient why he's seeking medical care. Document the answer using his own words. If he can't identify a single chief complaint, ask more specific questions about his current health status, such as the following:
- Have you noticed any changes in the color of the skin on your penis or scrotum?
- If you're uncircumcised, can you retract and replace the foreskin easily?
- Have you noticed any sores, lumps, or ulcers on your penis?
- Have you noticed any discharge or bleeding from the opening where urine comes out?
- Have you noticed any swelling in your scrotum?
- Are you experiencing any pain in the penis, testes, or scrotal sac? If so, where? Does the pain radiate? If so, to where? When does it occur? What measures aggravate or relieve it?
- Have you felt a lump, a painful sore, or tenderness in the groin?
- Do you get up during the night to urinate? Do you have urinary frequency, hesitancy, or dribbling? Pain in the area between your rectum and penis, hips, or lower back?
- Do you have any difficulty achieving and maintaining an erection during sexual activity? If so, do you have erections at other times, such as on awakening?
- Do you have any difficulty with ejaculation?
- Do you ever experience pain from erection or ejaculation?
- What medications (prescribed, over-the-counter) do you take? At what dosage and for what reason? Have you ever taken drugs for recreational purposes?

Many drugs affect the male reproductive system. For example, impotence may be caused by anticonvulsants, antidepressants, antihypertensives, beta blockers, antipsychotics, anticholinergics, and androgenic steroids. Changes in libido are linked to use of antidepressants, antihypertensives, antipsychotics, beta blockers, benzodiazepines, and androgenic steroids. Ejaculatory failure may be caused by antidepressants and beta blockers. Priapism may be caused by antidepressants, antihypertensives, and antipsychotics.

Medical history. This information is important; past reproductive system problems or dysfunctions in other body systems may affect present reproductive function. Important questions include:
- Have you fathered any children? If so, how many and what are their ages? Have you ever had a problem with infertility? Is it a current concern?
- Have you ever had surgery on the genitourinary tract? If so, where, when, and why? Did you experience any postoperative complications?
- Have you ever experienced trauma to the genitourinary tract? If so, what happened, when did it occur, and what symptoms—if any—have developed as a result?
- Have you ever seen blood in your urine, had difficulty urinating, felt an excessive urge to urinate, or had dribbling or difficulty maintaining the urine stream?
- Have you ever been diagnosed with a sexually transmitted disease or any other infection in the genitourinary tract? If so, what was the specific problem? How long did it last? What treatment was provided? Did any associated complications develop? Have you ever been tested for human immunodeficiency virus, the virus that causes acquired immunodeficiency syndrome (AIDS)?
- Have you had diabetes mellitus, cardiovascular disease, neurologic disease, or cancer of the genitourinary tract?
- Do you have a history of undescended testes or an endocrine disorder? Have you ever had mumps? If so, did the disease affect your testes?
- Do you examine your testes periodically? Have you been taught the proper procedure?

Family history. Questions about family health history can provide clues to disorders with known familial tendencies. Ask the patient if anyone in his family has had infertility problems or a hernia. Also ask him if anyone in his family ever had cancer of the reproductive tract.

Social history. Gather information about the patient's lifestyle and relationships with others. Ask the following questions:
- If you are sexually active, do you have more than one partner? How many partners have you had during the last month?
- Are your sexual practices homosexual, bisexual, or heterosexual?

- Do you take any precautions to prevent contracting a sexually transmitted disease or AIDS? If so, what do you do?
- What is your job?
- Are you now or have you ever been exposed to radiation or toxic chemicals?
- Do you engage in sports or any activity that requires heavy lifting or straining? If so, do you wear any protective or supportive devices, such as a jock strap, protective cup, or truss?
- Would you describe yourself as being under a lot of stress?
- What is your self-image? Do you consider yourself attractive to others?
- What is your cultural and religious background? Do any cultural or religious factors affect your beliefs or practices regarding sexuality and reproduction?
- Do you have a supportive relationship with another person?
- If you are experiencing sexual difficulty, is it affecting your emotional and social relationships?

FEMALE PATIENTS

Conduct your interview in a comfortable environment that protects the patient's privacy. Avoid rushing her; let important details come out. Use terms that the patient understands and explain technical terms. Remember that in some cultures, such as Asian, discussing female physiologic function or problems is taboo.

Ideally, the patient remains seated and dressed until you begin the physical assessment. Always ask your health history questions before the patient is in the lithotomy position. In many busy medical practices or health clinics, the patient is asked to undress, get on the examination table, and wait for the doctor to come in and begin the examination and interview. Some women find this demeaning as well as stressful.

Although you'll focus your questions on the reproductive system, maintain a holistic approach by inquiring about other physical and psychological concerns. Keep in mind that reproductive system problems may affect other aspects of the patient's life, including self-image and overall wellness.

Chief complaint. Ask the patient why she's seeking medical care. Document the answer in her own words. Guide her with more specific questions if she has trouble focusing on a single complaint.

Using the PQRST method, help the patient completely describe the main complaint and any other concerns. The following questions cover the menstrual and contraceptive history:
- How old were you when you began menstruating?
- When was the first day of your last menstrual period?

- Was that period normal compared with your previous periods?
- When was the first day of your previous menstrual period?
- How often do your periods occur?
- How long do your periods normally last?
- How would you describe your menstrual flow? How many pads or tampons do you use on each day of your period?
- Are your sexual practices bisexual, homosexual, or heterosexual?
- Are you currently using an oral contraceptive? If so, what do you use? How long have you used it?
- If you don't use an oral contraceptive, what method of contraception do you use? How long have you used it? If it's a device, is it in good condition?
- How much alcohol do you drink? How long have you been drinking?
- Do you smoke? If so, how much do you smoke? How long have you smoked?
- What prescription or over-the-counter medications are you currently taking? At what dosage and for what reason? Have you ever taken drugs for recreational purposes?

Many drugs can affect the female reproductive system. For example, amenorrhea can stem from use of androgens, antihypertensives, antipsychotics, cytotoxic drugs, estrogens, progestins, and steroids. Other menstrual irregularities may result from use of antidepressants and thyroid hormones. Changes in libido are linked to use of antidepressants, antihypertensives, beta blockers, and estrogens. Vaginal candidiasis is caused by estrogens, and infertility is linked to some cytotoxic drugs.

Reproductive history. To obtain data about the patient's reproductive history, ask the following questions:

- Do you have any signs or symptoms of infection, such as discharge, itching, painful intercourse, sores or lesions, fever, chills, or swelling of the vagina or vulva?
- Do you ever miss your period? If so, how much exercise do you normally engage in?
- Do you ever bleed between periods? If so, how much and for how long?
- Do you ever have vaginal bleeding after intercourse?
- Have you had any uncomfortable signs and symptoms before or during your periods?
- How often do you visit the gynecologist?
- Has anyone ever told you that something is wrong with your womb or other female organs? Have you ever had a positive Papanicalaou (Pap) test? When was your last Pap test?

- Have you ever had a sexually transmitted disease or another genital or reproductive system infection?
- Have you ever had surgery for a reproductive system problem?
- Have you ever been pregnant?
- Have you ever had problems conceiving?
- Have you ever had an abortion or a miscarriage?

Because some reproductive problems seem familial, ask about family reproductive history. Ask the patient if she or anyone in her family has ever had reproductive problems, hypertension, diabetes mellitus, gestational diabetes, obesity, heart disease, or gynecologic surgery. Next, ask her if she's having any problems that she believes are related to her reproductive system or any other problems not yet covered during the interview.

Ask her if she is sexually active. If so, ask when she had intercourse last and if she's sexually active with more than one partner. Ask if her sexual partner has any signs or symptoms of infection, such as genital sores, warts, or penile discharge. Finally, answer any questions the patient may have about her reproductive organs or sexual activity.

PHYSICAL EXAMINATION

For the male patient, physical assessment involves inspecting and palpating the groin, penis, and scrotum. If the patient is over age 50 or has a high likelihood of prostate problems, you'll also palpate the prostate gland. For the female patient, assessment may involve the external genitalia only or a complete gynecologic examination.

EXAMINING THE MALE PATIENT

Before beginning the physical assessment, wash your hands and gather gloves, water-soluble lubricant, and a flashlight.

Instruct the patient to urinate before the examination (to reduce discomfort from a full bladder) and to undress. Allow him to don a gown to prevent unnecessary exposure.

Because the physical examination requires exposure and handling of the genitalia, the patient may feel anxious and embarrassed. Explain each assessment step before performing it, and expose only the necessary areas. Also, maintain a calm, professional demeanor. If the patient realizes you're uncomfortable, he will be, too.

If the patient objects to being examined by a female, a male nurse or doctor should perform the examination. The patient may attempt to relieve feelings of embarrassment by using offensive language. If so, continue the assessment in a professional manner. If you feel threatened, have a male nurse or doctor finish the assessment.

Inspection. To begin physical assessment of the male reproductive system, inspect the patient's genitalia and inguinal area. Be sure to put on gloves before starting.

Begin penis inspection by evaluating the color and integrity of the penile skin. This should appear loose and wrinkled over the shaft and taut and smooth over the glans penis. The skin should appear pink to light brown in whites and light to dark brown in blacks; it should be free from scars, lesions, ulcers, or breaks of any kind.

Ask an uncircumcised patient to retract his prepuce to expose the glans penis. Normally, he can do this easily to reveal a glans with no ulcers or lesions, and then replace it as easily over the glans after inspection.

The urethral meatus, a slitlike opening, usually is located at the tip of the glans. Inspection of the urethral meatus should reveal no discharge.

To inspect the scrotum, first evaluate the amount, distribution, color, and texture of pubic hair. Hair should cover the symphysis pubis and scrotum.

Next, inspect the scrotal skin for obvious lesions, ulcerations, induration, or reddened areas, and evaluate the scrotal sac for symmetry and size. The scrotal skin should be coarse and more deeply pigmented than the body skin. The left testis usually hangs slightly lower than the right.

Check the inguinal area for obvious bulges—a sign of hernias. Then ask the patient to bear down as you inspect again. This maneuver increases intra-abdominal pressure, which pushes any herniation downward and makes it more easily visible. Also check for enlarged lymph nodes, a sign of infection.

Palpation. After inspection, palpate the penis and scrotum for structural abnormalities; then palpate the inguinal area for hernias.

To palpate the penis, gently grasp the shaft between your thumb and first two fingers and palpate along its entire length, noting any indurated, tender, or lumpy areas. The flaccid penis should feel soft and free from nodules.

Like the penis, the scrotum is palpated using the thumb and first two fingers. Begin by feeling the scrotal skin for nodules, lesions, or ulcers. Next, palpate the scrotal sac. Normally, the right and left halves of the sac have identical contents and feel the same. You should feel the testes as separate, freely movable oval masses low in the scrotal sac. Their surface should feel smooth and even in contour. Slight compression of the testes should elicit a dull, aching sensation that radiates to the patient's lower abdomen. He shouldn't feel this pressure-pain sensation when the other structures are compressed or any other pain or tenderness.

The absence of a testis may result from temporary migration. The cremaster muscle surrounding the testes contracts in response to such stimuli as cold air, cold water, or touching the inner thigh. This contraction raises the contents of the scrotum toward the inguinal canal. When the muscle relaxes, the scrotal contents resume their normal position. This temporary migration is normal and may occur at any time during the assessment.

Palpate the epididymis on the posterolateral surface by grasping each testis between the thumb and forefinger and feeling from the epididymis to the spermatic cord or vas deferens up to the inguinal ring. The epididymis should feel like a ridge of tissue lying vertically on the testicular surface. The vas deferens should feel like a smooth cord that is freely movable. The arteries, veins, lymph vessels, and nerves, which are located next to the vas deferens, may feel like indefinite threads.

Any swellings, lumps, or nodular areas should be transilluminated. For this technique, darken the room; then hold a flashlight behind the scrotum and direct its beam through the tissue. If the swollen area contains serous fluid, it will glow orange-red; otherwise, it will be opaque. Describe a lump or mass anywhere in the scrotal sac according to its placement, size, shape, consistency, tenderness, and response to the flashlight.

Finally, palpate the inguinal area for hernias.

EXAMINING THE FEMALE PATIENT

You may either assist a doctor or nurse practitioner with a gynecologic assessment or perform the assessment yourself. This section describes how to prepare for and perform a complete gynecologic assessment.

Before beginning the assessment, gather the necessary equipment and supplies. This includes gloves, several different sizes and types of specula, a lubricant, a spatula, swabs, an endocervical brush, glass slides and cover slips, a cytologic fixative, culture bottles or plates, a sponge, forceps, a mirror, and a light source.

Because a full bladder produces discomfort and interferes with accurate palpation, tell the patient to empty her bladder before the examination begins.

Assist the patient to the lithotomy position for the assessment. Secure her heels in the stirrups, and position her knees comfortably in the knee supports if they are used. Adjust the foot or knee supports so that her legs are equally and comfortably separated and symmetrically balanced.

If the patient can't assume the lithotomy position because of age, arthritis, back pain, or other reasons, place her in Sims' (left lateral) position instead. To assume this position, the patient should lie on her left side almost prone, with her buttocks close to the edge of the table, her left leg straight, and her right leg slightly bent in front of her left leg.

Inspection. Sometimes, you need inspect only the patient's external genitalia to determine the origin of sores or itching. Wash your hands; then follow these steps.

Place the patient in a supine position with the pubic area uncovered, and begin the assessment by determining sexual maturity. Inspect pubic hair for amount and pattern. It usually is thick and appears on the mons pubis as well as the inner aspects of the upper thighs. Using a gloved index finger and thumb, gently spread the labia majora and look for the labia minora. The labia should appear pink and moist with no lesions. Normal cervical discharge varies in color and consistency; it's clear and stretchy before ovulation, white and opaque after ovulation, and usually odorless and nonirritating to the mucosa. You should see no other discharge.

Gynecologic assessment. If you practice in a facility specializing in women's health care, you may perform complete gynecologic assessments. As part of this assessment, obtain a Pap smear after inspecting the cervix. (Collect the smear before touching the cervix in any manner.) Also get other specimens if an abnormal cervical or vaginal discharge indicates infection.

Benign prostatic hyperplasia

Most men over age 50 have some prostatic enlargement, known as benign prostatic hyperplasia (BPH). This condition produces symptoms when the prostate gland enlarges sufficiently to compress the urethra and cause some overt urinary obstruction. Depending on the size of the enlarged prostate, the age and health of the patient, and the extent of the obstruction, BPH is treated surgically or symptomatically. (See *Treating BPH.*)

CAUSES
The cause of BPH is unknown. What's known is that circulating androgens (specifically testosterone) and aging are necessary for BPH to develop.

As the prostate enlarges, it may extend toward the bladder and obstruct urine outflow by compressing or distorting the prostatic urethra. BPH also may cause a weakening of the detrusor musculature that retains urine when the rest of the bladder empties.

Because BPH causes urinary obstruction, a patient may have one or more of the following complications:

- urine retention or incomplete bladder emptying, leading to urinary tract infection (UTI) or calculi
- bladder wall trabeculation
- detrusor muscle hypertrophy
- bladder diverticuli and saccules
- urethral stenosis
- hydronephrosis
- overflow incontinence
- acute or chronic renal failure
- acute postobstructive diuresis.

DIAGNOSIS AND TREATMENT
The following tests help to confirm a diagnosis of BPH: excretory urography, blood urea nitrogen and serum creatinine levels, urinalysis and urine culture, and prostate-specific antigen levels (routinely drawn to rule out prostate cancer).

When symptoms are severe, cystourethroscopy is the definitive diagnostic measure and helps to determine the best surgical procedure. It can show prostate enlargement, bladder wall changes, calculi, and a raised bladder.

Medications can help relieve symptoms of urethral obstruction caused by BPH. Alpha blockers, such as terazosin and doxazosin, relax the bladder neck and prostatic urethra; adverse effects include hypotension, dizziness, headaches, and nasal congestion. Finasteride blocks the conversion of testosterone to dihydrotestosterone within the prostate, preventing the continued progression of BPH. One of its few adverse effects is a slight decrease in sexual potency during the first part of therapy, but this effect is transient. Symptoms improve after 6 to 12 months of treatment.

Surgery is the only effective therapy for relief of acute urine retention, hydronephrosis, severe hematuria, and recurrent UTI or for palliative relief of intolerable symptoms. Continuous drainage with an indwelling urinary catheter alleviates urine retention in high-risk patients. The doctor may do a transurethral resection if the prostate weighs under 2 oz (56.7 g). Weight is approximated by digital examination.

Other procedures involve open surgical removal of the prostate (prostatectomy). One of the following operations may be appropriate:
- Suprapubic (transvesical) prostatectomy is the most common and is especially useful when prostatic enlargement is confined to the bladder area.
- Perineal prostatectomy usually is performed for a large gland in an older patient. The operation commonly results in impotence and incontinence.
- Retropubic (extravesical) prostatectomy allows direct visualization; potency and continence usually are maintained in about 50% of patients.

COLLABORATIVE MANAGEMENT

Care of the patient with BPH focuses on achieving urinary elimination and teaching catheter care, if needed, and ways of dealing with the disease.

ASSESSMENT

Clinical features of BPH depend on the extent of prostatic enlargement and the lobes affected. Characteristically, the patient complains of obstructive voiding symptoms: decreased urine stream caliber and force, an interrupted stream, urinary hesitancy, and difficulty starting urination, which results in straining and a feeling of incomplete voiding.

As the obstruction increases, the patient may report irritative voiding symptoms: frequent urination with nocturia, dribbling, urine retention, incontinence and, possibly, hematuria.

Physical examination may reveal a visible midline mass above the symphysis pubis, indicating an incompletely emptied bladder. The distended bladder can be palapated, and rectal examination discloses an enlarged prostate.

NURSING DIAGNOSES AND COLLABORATIVE PROBLEMS

Based on the following nursing diagnoses, you'll establish patient outcomes.

Altered urinary elimination related to obstruction of the urethra. The patient will:
- identify signs and symptoms of urine retention and seek medical attention
- be able to empty the bladder effectively.

The patient and family member or caretaker will:
- demonstrate skill in managing urine elimination problems.

Risk for infection related to potential for urine retention. The patient will:
- have clear, yellow urine that's odorless, sediment-free, and bacteria-free
- experience no signs or symptoms of UTI.

Urge incontinence related to obstruction of the urethra. The patient will:
- experience no complications of urinary incontinence, such as skin breakdown
- seek medical or surgical treatment
- regain continence.

PLANNING AND IMPLEMENTATION

The following measures help the patient with BPH.
- Prepare the patient for diagnostic tests and surgery, as appropriate.
- If he's retaining urine, insert an indwelling urinary catheter. This is difficult in a patient with BPH; if you can't pass the catheter transurethrally, assist with suprapubic cystostomy (using local anesthesia).

CLINICAL PRACTICE GUIDELINES ▐▐▐ **Treating BPH**

The following are selected portions of the clinical practice guidelines for treating benign prostatic hyperplasia (BPH) developed by the Agency for Health Care Policy and Research of the U.S. Department of Health and Human Services.

- Watchful waiting is an appropriate treatment strategy for the majority of patients with BPH. Patients should be monitored periodically by reassessment of symptom level, physical findings, routine laboratory testing, and optional urologic diagnostic procedures. Though no studies define the optimal interval, annual follow-up is reasonable.
- Of all treatment options, prostate surgery offers the best chance for symptom improvement. However, surgery also has the highest rates of significant complications. Transurethral resection of the prostate is the most common and useful surgical treatment.
- Balloon dilatation of the prostatic urethra is less effective than surgery for relieving symptoms but produces fewer complications. Recent studies suggest that improvement may be temporary, with symptoms returning within 2 years. At present, balloon dilatation is a reasonable treatment option for patients with smaller prostates and no middle lobe enlargement.
- Transurethral incision of the prostate, a procedure limited to patients whose prostates weigh an estimated 30 g or less, can be performed in ambulatory settings or during a 1-day hospitalization.
- Alpha-$_1$-adrenergic receptor blockers, such as doxazosin, prazosin, and terazosin, relax smooth muscle of the bladder neck and prostate. In the average patient, they cause a small increase in peak urinary flow rate and a small but perceptible reduction in symptoms.
- Finasteride is a 5-alpha reductase inhibitor that blocks conversion of testosterone to dihydrotestosterone, the major intraprostatic androgen in men. This treatment takes 6 months or more to achieve its maximum effect.

- Avoid giving decongestants, tranquilizers, alcohol, antidepressants, or anticholinergics because these drugs can worsen obstruction.
- Observe the patient for signs and symptoms of UTI, such as dysuria or changes in urine appearance.
- Obtain a urine culture if UTI is suspected. Give antibiotics, as ordered, for UTI, urethral procedures that involve instruments, and cystoscopy.
- Monitor and record the patient's vital signs, intake and output, and daily weight. Watch closely for signs of postobstructive diuresis (such as increased urine output and hypotension), which may lead to serious

dehydration, lowered blood volume, shock, electrolyte losses, and anuria.

Patient teaching

- If the patient has had an indwelling urinary catheter to maintain urine flow before surgery, he may experience urinary frequency, dribbling and, occasionally, hematuria after the catheter has been removed. Reassure him and his family members that he'll gradually regain urinary control.
- Teach the patient to recognize the signs of UTI and to report these signs to the doctor immediately because infection can worsen obstruction.
- Tell the patient to follow the prescribed oral antibiotic regimen, and inform him of the indications for using gentle laxatives.
- Urge the patient to seek medical care immediately if he can't urinate, passes bloody urine, or develops a fever.
- Tell him that it may take several months of medical therapy before symptoms improve; emphasize the importance of regular follow-up appointments.

EVALUATION

Achievement of patient outcomes determines the success of collaborative management. For the patient with BPH, evaluation focuses on absence of urinary obstruction and urine retention, urinary elimination within acceptable parameters, ability to perform catheter care if needed, and adequate knowledge of the disease, treatment, and care.

Cervical cancer

The third most common cancer of the female reproductive system, cervical cancer is classified as either preinvasive or invasive.

Preinvasive cancer ranges from minimal cervical dysplasia, in which the lower third of the epithelium contains abnormal cells, to carcinoma in situ, in which the full thickness of epithelium contains abnormally proliferating cells (also known as cervical intraepithelial neoplasia). Preinvasive cancer is curable in 75% to 90% of patients with early detection and proper treatment. If untreated, it may progress to invasive cervical cancer, depending on the form.

In invasive disease, cancer cells penetrate the basement membrane and can spread directly to contiguous pelvic structures or disseminate to distant sites via lymphatic routes. Invasive cancer of the uterine cervix accounts for 4,900 deaths annually in the United States. In 95% of cases, the histologic type is squamous cell carcinoma, which varies from well-differentiated cells to highly anaplastic spindle cells. Only 5%

of cases are adenocarcinomas. Invasive cancer typically occurs between ages 40 and 50; rarely, under age 20. (Dysplasia commonly occurs in women in their 30s.) Women age 65 or older account for 24% of new cases and 40% of deaths.

Disease progression can cause flank pain from sciatic nerve or pelvic wall invasion and hematuria and renal failure associated with bladder involvement.

CAUSES

Although the cause is unknown, several predisposing factors have been associated with cervical cancer: frequent intercourse at a young age (under 16), multiple sexual partners, multiple pregnancies, and human papillomavirus or other bacterial or viral venereal infections.

Other risk factors include low socioeconomic status, smoking, exposure to diethylstilbestrol, vitamin A and C deficiency, and possibly oral contraceptives.

DIAGNOSIS AND TREATMENT

Diagnostic tests may include a Papanicolaou (Pap) test and cone biopsy. Additional studies, such as lymphangiography, cystography, and major organ and bone scans, can detect metastasis.

Accurate clinical staging will determine the type of treatment. The doctor may treat preinvasive lesions with total excisional biopsy, loop electrosurgical excision, cryosurgery, laser destruction, conization (followed by frequent Pap tests) or, rarely, hysterectomy. Therapy for invasive squamous cell carcinoma may include radical hysterectomy and radiation therapy (internal, external, or both). Rarely, the doctor performs pelvic exenteration for recurrent cervical cancer. (See *Managing pelvic exenteration.*)

COLLABORATIVE MANAGEMENT

Care of the patient with cervical cancer focuses on restoring sexual and childbearing function, if possible, and teaching about the disease, prognosis, treatment, care, and follow-up.

ASSESSMENT

Preinvasive cancer produces no symptoms or other clinical changes. In early invasive cervical cancer, the patient's history will include abnormal vaginal bleeding, such as a persistent vaginal discharge that's yellowish, blood-tinged, and foul-smelling; postcoital pain and bleeding; and bleeding between menstrual periods or unusually heavy menstrual periods. The patient's history may suggest one or more of the predisposing factors for this disease.

If the cancer has advanced into the pelvic wall, the patient may report gradually increasing flank pain, which can indicate sciatic nerve involvement. Leakage of urine may point to metastasis into the bladder

Managing pelvic exenteration

Provide the following teaching and preoperative and postoperative care for the patient who's undergoing pelvic exenteration. Offer emotional support as needed.

Before pelvic exenteration
■ Teach the patient about ileal conduit and possible colostomy, and make sure she understands that her vagina will be removed.
■ To minimize the risk of infection, supervise a rigorous bowel and skin preparation procedure. Decrease the residue in the patient's diet for 48 to 72 hours; then maintain a diet ranging from clear liquids to nothing by mouth. Administer oral antibiotics, as ordered, and prepare the skin daily with antibacterial soap.
■ Instruct the patient about postoperative procedures: I.V. therapy, an arterial or central venous catheter, a blood drainage system, and an unsutured perineal wound with gauze packing.

After pelvic exenteration
■ Check the stoma, incision, and perineal wound for drainage. Be especially careful to check the perineal wound for bleeding after the packing is removed. Expect red or serosanguineous drainage, but notify the doctor immediately if drainage is excessive, continuously bright red, foul-smelling, or purulent or if there's bleeding from the conduit.
■ Provide excellent skin care because of draining urine and feces. Use warm water and normal saline solution to clean the skin, because soap may be too drying and may increase skin breakdown.
■ Teach the patient the self-care steps she'll need to know.

---

with fistula formation. Leakage of feces may indicate metastasis to the rectum with fistula formation.

NURSING DIAGNOSES AND COLLABORATIVE PROBLEMS
Based on the following nursing diagnoses, you'll establish patient outcomes.

Fear related to potential for cervical cancer to become invasive. The patient will:
■ identify and verbalize her fears
■ use at least one fear-reducing coping mechanism daily, such as asking questions about treatment progress
■ experience no physical signs or symptoms of fear and state that her fears have diminished.

Impaired tissue integrity related to changes in cervical tissue caused by cervical cancer. The patient will:
■ understand the treatment regimen and verbalize the need for adequate fluid and nutritional intake to promote tissue healing
■ experience a cessation of vaginal discharge
■ exhibit, upon physical examination, healing cervical tissue.

Pain related to invasive cervical cancer. The patient will:
■ obtain pain relief with analgesics
■ become free from pain through therapy.

PLANNING AND IMPLEMENTATION
These measures help the patient with cervical cancer.
■ Listen to the patient's fears and concerns, and offer reassurance when appropriate.

■ Encourage her to use relaxation techniques to promote comfort during the diagnostic procedures.
■ If a biopsy or laser therapy is planned, drape and prepare the patient as for a routine pelvic examination. Assist the doctor as needed, and provide support for the patient throughout the procedure.
■ For a biopsy, have a container of formaldehyde ready to preserve the specimen during transfer to the pathology laboratory.
■ Prepare the patient for surgery or internal radiation therapy, if indicated. With radiation therapy, explain why you may need to limit your exposure time. (See *Safe time for implant exposure,* page 468.)
■ Institute measures to prevent or alleviate complications, as indicated.
■ Monitor the patient's response to therapy through frequent Pap tests and cone biopsies, as ordered.
■ Watch for complications related to therapy by listening to and observing the patient, monitoring laboratory studies, and obtaining frequent vital signs.

Patient teaching
■ Explain to the patient who's having a biopsy performed that she may feel pressure, minor abdominal cramps, or a pinch from the punch forceps. Reassure her that biopsy pain is minimal because the cervix has few nerve endings.
■ Explain any surgical or therapeutic procedure to the patient, including what to expect both before and after the procedure.
■ After excisional biopsy or laser therapy, tell the patient to expect a discharge or spotting for about 1

Safe time for implant exposure

Your distance from the implant defines your safe exposure time to cesium.

Rolling shield

110 hours

42 hours,
30 minutes

6 hours,
40 minutes

3'

6'

Implant:
Cesium
70 mg in
Fletcher
afterloader

---

week. Advise her not to douche, use tampons, or engage in sexual intercourse during this time.
- After biopsy or laser therapy, caution her to report signs of infection.
- Review the possible complications of the type of therapy ordered. Remind the patient to watch for and report uncomfortable adverse reactions.
- Reassure her that cervical cancer and its treatment shouldn't radically alter her lifestyle or prohibit sexual intimacy.
- Stress the need for a follow-up Pap test and a pelvic examination 3 to 4 months after biopsy or therapy and periodically thereafter.
- Explain the importance of complying with follow-up visits to the gynecologist and oncologist to detect disease progression or recurrence.

EVALUATION
Achievement of patient outcomes determines the success of collaborative management. For the patient with cervical cancer, evaluation focuses on physiologic status within acceptable parameters, positive coping skills, and adequate knowledge of the disease, prognosis, treatment, care, and follow-up.

Dysfunctional uterine bleeding

Dysfunctional uterine bleeding (DUB) is abnormal endometrial bleeding without recognizable organic lesions. The prognosis varies with the cause. DUB is the reason for almost 25% of all gynecologic surgeries.

CAUSES

The bleeding usually is caused by an imbalance in the hormonal-endometrial relationship whereby estrogen persistently and unopposedly stimulates the endometrium. Sustained high estrogen levels are linked to polycystic ovary syndrome, obesity, immaturity of the hypothalamic-pituitary-ovarian mechanism (in post-pubertal teenagers and perimenopausal women), and anovulation from vigorous exercise, stress, malnutrition, and use of certain medications.

The endometrium usually shows no pathologic changes. But in chronic unopposed estrogen stimulation (for example from a hormone-producing ovarian tumor), the endometrium may exhibit hyperplastic or malignant changes.

DUB may lead to anemia, and it may have social consequences, affecting work or school performance.

DIAGNOSIS AND TREATMENT

Initial tests are performed to rule out pregnancy, coagulation disorders, genital tract lesions, and endocrine imbalances. They include:
- transvaginal ultrasound to provide an anatomic evaluation
- hysteroscopy to view the endocervix and the endometrial cavity and to obtain tissue specimens for biopsy
- dilatation and curettage (D&C) and endometrial tissue analyses to confirm the diagnosis by revealing endometrial hyperplasia
- hemoglobin levels and hematocrit to determine the need for blood or iron replacement.

High-dose estrogen-progestin combination therapy (oral contraceptives), the primary treatment, is designed to control endometrial growth and reestablish a normal menstrual cycle. These drugs are usually given four times daily for 5 to 7 days, even though bleeding usually stops in 12 to 24 hours. (The patient's age and the cause of bleeding help determine the drug choice and dosage.)

In patients over age 35, endometrial biopsy is required before the start of estrogen therapy, to rule out endometrial adenocarcinoma. Progestin therapy for 10 days each month is a necessary alternative in some women, such as those susceptible to the adverse effects of estrogen (thrombophlebitis, for example).

If drug therapy fails, D&C serves as a supplementary treatment by removing a large portion of the bleeding endometrium. This procedure can also help determine the original cause of hormonal imbalance and can aid in planning further therapy.

Regardless of the primary therapy, the patient may need iron replacement and transfusions of packed cells or whole blood because of anemia caused by recurrent bleeding.

COLLABORATIVE MANAGEMENT

Care of the patient with DUB focuses on controlling bleeding and teaching about the disorder, treatment, and care.

ASSESSMENT

The patient with DUB typically reports episodes of vaginal bleeding between menses (metrorrhagia), heavy or prolonged menses lasting longer than 8 days (hypermenorrhea), or a menstrual cycle lasting fewer than 18 days (chronic polymenorrhea).

NURSING DIAGNOSES AND COLLABORATIVE PROBLEMS

Based on the following nursing diagnoses, you'll establish patient outcomes.

Altered sexuality patterns related to DUB. The patient will:
- express feelings about changes in sexual activity
- resume normal sexual activity when DUB subsides.

Anxiety related to DUB as a possible cancer sign. The patient will:
- express feelings of anxiety
- verbalize an understanding of necessary diagnostic tests to evaluate her condition
- use support systems to assist with coping
- show fewer physical signs and symptoms of anxiety.

Fatigue related to DUB-induced anemia. The patient will:
- identify measures to prevent or modify fatigue
- recover and retain normal hemoglobin levels and hematocrit
- regain a normal energy level.

PLANNING AND IMPLEMENTATION

These measures help the patient with DUB.
- Encourage the patient and her partner to verbalize their feelings about DUB and its effect on their relationship. Offer emotional support and reassurance.
- Help the patient identify her strengths and use them to develop coping strategies.
- Monitor the patient's bleeding pattern, including the duration and amount of bleeding.
- Monitor the patient's response to therapy.
- Monitor hemoglobin counts and administer transfusions as indicated.
- Monitor vital signs for tachycardia, decreased blood pressure, increased respiratory rate, and decreased urine output.

Patient teaching
- Explain the normal menstrual cycle. Ask the patient to keep a menstrual calendar to help with diagnosis and to document the effectiveness of treatment.

- Explain the benefits of adhering to the prescribed hormonal therapy. Instruct the patient to take her medication exactly as ordered and to avoid abruptly discontinuing it.
- Explain all procedures and treatment options to the patient to allay anxiety.
- Urge the patient to schedule regular checkups to assess treatment effectiveness.

EVALUATION
Achievement of patient outcomes determines the success of collaborative management. For the patient with DUB, evaluation focuses on vital signs and blood studies within acceptable parameters, control of bleeding, and adequate knowledge of the disorder, treatment, and care.

Dysmenorrhea

Dysmenorrhea is a painful menstrual flow that's classified as primary or secondary. Primary dysmenorrhea is unrelated to other disorders, but the secondary type may be linked to underlying diseases, such as pelvic inflammatory disease, endometriosis, and uterine tumors.

CAUSES
Primary dysmenorrhea is linked to increased production and release of uterine prostaglandins, which are produced by the endometrium during the luteal phase of the menstrual cycle. Prostaglandin levels rise during the luteal phase of the menstrual cycle and peak at the onset of menses. These levels stimulate the myometrium and cause severe spasms that constrict the uterine blood flow and may result in ischemia and pain.

DIAGNOSIS AND TREATMENT
Diagnostic tests, such as blood studies, X-rays, and ultrasound, are performed to rule out any underlying conditions.

Prostaglandin synthetase inhibitors (ibuprofen, naproxen sodium, and mefenamic acid) may be prescribed. Other treatments include ovulation inhibitors to decrease prostaglandin activity, oral contraceptives, and pain-relieving measures, such as acupressure, sedatives, opioids, exercise, swimming, yoga, application of heat or cold, massage, biofeedback, relaxation techniques, and nutritional measures (increasing intake of vitamin B_6, calcium, magnesium, and protein and decreasing intake of sodium).

COLLABORATIVE MANAGEMENT
Care of the patient with dysmenorrhea focuses on relieving pain and teaching about the disorder and its treatment.

ASSESSMENT
A thorough history will include the patient's age at menarche, characteristics of menstruation, obstetric history, contraceptive history, and instances of pain and previous therapy.

The patient may also have associated signs and symptoms, including headache, syncope, nervousness, fatigue, diarrhea, bloating, and breast tenderness.

NURSING DIAGNOSES AND COLLABORATIVE PROBLEMS
Based on the following nursing diagnoses, you'll establish patient outcomes.

Pain related to pathophysiology of the disease. The patient will:
- demonstrate measures to control pain
- verbalize a decrease in pain.

Altered role performance related to pain. The patient will:
- demonstrate measures to control pain and engage in activities
- return to previous level of functioning with control of symptoms.

PLANNING AND IMPLEMENTATION
These measures help the patient with dysmenorrhea.
- Administer prescribed medications.
- Assess the patient's degree of pain. Encourage her to take medication before her pain gets too severe. Monitor the effectiveness of pain medications.
- Let the patient choose alternative measures of pain relief, and assess their effectiveness.
- Encourage the patient to verbalize her feelings and to assist in her own care.

Patient teaching
- Explain all procedures and treatments.
- Teach the patient about her prescribed medications, including proper dosage. Tell her about the drugs' adverse effects and which symptoms to report to her doctor.

EVALUATION
Achievement of patient outcomes determines the success of collaborative management. For the patient with dysmenorrhea, evaluation focuses on pain relief and adequate knowledge of the disorder, treatment, and care.

Endometriosis

When endometrial tissue appears outside the lining of the uterine cavity, endometriosis results. Such ectopic tissue is generally confined to the pelvic area, most commonly around the ovaries, uterovesical peritoneum, uterosacral ligaments, and cul-de-sac, but it can appear anywhere in the body. During menstruation, the ectopic tissue bleeds, which causes inflammation of the surrounding tissues. This inflammation causes fibrosis, leading to adhesions, which produce pain and infertility.

Active endometriosis usually occurs between ages 30 and 40, especially in women who postpone childbearing; it's uncommon before age 20. Severe symptoms of endometriosis may have an abrupt onset or may develop over many years. This disorder usually becomes progressively severe during the menstrual years but tends to subside after menopause.

The primary complication of endometriosis is infertility. Other complications include spontaneous abortion, anemia due to excessive bleeding, and emotional problems due to infertility.

CAUSES

The direct cause of endometriosis is unknown, but familial susceptibility or recent hysterotomy may be predisposing factors. Research has focused on the following possible causes:

■ transportation (retrograde menstruation)—During menstruation, the fallopian tubes expel endometrial fragments that implant outside the uterus.
■ formation in situ—Inflammation or a hormonal change triggers metaplasia.
■ induction (a combination of transportation and formation in situ)—The endometrium chemically induces undifferentiated mesenchyma to form endometrial epithelium (the most likely cause).
■ immune system defects—Endometriosis may be caused by a specific defect in cell-mediated immunity. Researchers have documented higher titers of antibodies to endometrial antigens in patients with this disorder.

DIAGNOSIS AND TREATMENT

Laparoscopy confirms the diagnosis and identifies the stage of the disease. A scoring and staging system created by the American Fertility Society grades endometrial implants according to size, character, and location. Stage I (1 to 5 points) signifies minimal disease; stage II (6 to 15 points), mild disease; stage III (16 to 40 points), moderate disease; and stage IV (more than 40 points), severe disease. Barium enema rules out bowel disease.

The stage of the disease and the patient's age and desire to have children determine the course of treatment. Conservative therapy for young women who want to have children includes androgens such as danazol, which produce a temporary remission in stages I and II. Progestins and oral contraceptives are also useful in relieving symptoms. A newer treatment involves use of gonadotropin-releasing analogues to suppress estrogen production. This causes atrophic changes in the ectopic endometrial tissue, which allows healing.

Laparoscopy can also be used to lyse adhesions, remove small implants, cauterize implants, and permit laser vaporization of implants. This surgery is usually followed with hormonal therapy to suppress the return of endometrial implants.

If the patient has ovarian masses, she may need surgery to rule out cancer. Conservative surgery is possible, but the treatment of choice for women who don't want to bear children or for those with extensive disease (stages III and IV) is a total abdominal hysterectomy with bilateral salpingo-oophorectomy.

Minor gynecologic procedures are contraindicated immediately before and during menstruation.

COLLABORATIVE MANAGEMENT

Care of the patient with endometriosis focuses on emotional well-being, coping strategies, and patient teaching.

ASSESSMENT

The patient may complain of infertility or acquired dysmenorrhea that may produce constant pain in the lower abdomen, vagina, posterior pelvis, and back. This pain usually begins 5 to 7 days before menses, reaches a peak, and lasts for 2 to 3 days. It differs from primary dysmenorrheal pain, which is more cramplike and concentrated in the abdominal midline. However, the severity of pain doesn't necessarily indicate the extent of the disease.

Other clinical features depend on the location of the ectopic tissue. Look for:
■ a history of infertility and profuse menstrual bleeding (oviducts and ovaries)
■ deep-thrust dyspareunia (ovaries and cul-de-sac)
■ suprapubic pain, dysuria, and hematuria (bladder)
■ painful defecation, rectal bleeding with menses, and pain in the coccyx or sacrum (rectovaginal septum and colon)
■ nausea and vomiting that worsen before menses, and abdominal cramps (small bowel and appendix)
■ palpable multiple tender nodules on uterosacral ligaments or in the rectovaginal septum (that enlarge and become more tender during menses)

- ovarian enlargement in the presence of endometrial cysts on the ovaries or thickened, nodular adnexa (as in pelvic inflammatory disease).

NURSING DIAGNOSES AND COLLABORATIVE PROBLEMS
Based on the following nursing diagnoses, you'll establish patient outcomes.

Chronic pain related to cyclic inflammation of surrounding tissue resulting in fibrosis. The patient will:
- use diversionary activities to help relieve pain
- express comfort after administration of analgesics.

Fatigue related to anemia caused by excessive bleeding. The patient will:
- pace her activities of daily living and take frequent rests to minimize fatigue
- seek assistance with activities that cause fatigue
- regain and maintain normal hemoglobin levels.

Ineffective individual coping related to infertility. The patient will:
- express an understanding of the relationship between her emotional state and behavior
- identify effective and ineffective coping techniques
- use available support systems, such as family members, friends, or a mental health professional, to develop and maintain effective coping skills.

PLANNING AND IMPLEMENTATION
These measures help the patient with endometriosis.
- Encourage the patient and her partner to verbalize their feelings about the disorder and its effect on their relationship.
- Offer emotional support. Stress the need for open communication before and during intercourse to minimize discomfort and frustration.
- Help the patient develop effective coping strategies. Encourage her to contact a support group such as the Endometriosis Association. Refer her and her partner to a mental health professional for counseling, if necessary.
- Give analgesics as ordered for pain, and monitor their effectiveness.
- Encourage the patient to balance exercise and rest.
- Monitor for signs and symptoms of anemia. Check hemoglobin levels as ordered.
- Provide adequate nutrition, including iron supplements if anemia develops.
- Monitor the patient's response to therapy.

Patient teaching
- Explain all procedures and treatment options. Clarify any misconceptions about the disorder, associated complications, and fertility.

- Advise adolescents to use sanitary napkins instead of tampons. This can help prevent retrograde flow in girls with a narrow vagina or a small vaginal meatus.
- Because infertility is a possible complication, counsel the patient who wants children not to postpone childbearing.
- Recommend annual pelvic examinations and Papanicolaou tests.

EVALUATION
Achievement of patient outcomes determines the success of collaborative management. For the patient with endometriosis, evaluation focuses on physiologic status within acceptable parameters, positive coping strategies, and adequate knowledge of the disorder, treatment, and required care.

Erectile dysfunction

A man with erectile dysfunction can't attain or maintain a penile erection sufficient to complete intercourse. The patient with primary impotence has never achieved a sufficient erection. In secondary impotence (more common and less serious), the patient has succeeded in completing intercourse in the past. Transient periods of impotence are not considered dysfunctional and probably happen to half of adult males.

Erectile dysfunction affects all age-groups but increases in frequency with age. The prognosis depends on the severity and duration of impotence and on the underlying cause.

CAUSES
Psychogenic factors cause approximately 50% to 60% of all cases of erectile dysfunction; organic factors underlie the rest. In some patients, psychogenic and organic factors coexist, hampering isolation of the primary cause.

Psychogenic causes may be intrapersonal, reflecting personal sexual anxieties, or interpersonal, reflecting a disturbed sexual relationship. Intrapersonal factors usually involve guilt, fear, depression, or feelings of inadequacy resulting from a previous traumatic sexual experience, rejection by parents or peers, exaggerated religious orthodoxy, abnormal mother-son intimacy, or homosexual experiences.

Interpersonal factors often are linked to differences in sexual preferences between partners, lack of communication, insufficient knowledge of sexual function, or nonsexual personal conflicts. Situational impotence, a temporary condition, may develop in response to stress.

Organic causes include chronic disorders, such as cardiopulmonary disease, hypertension, diabetes, multiple sclerosis, or renal failure; spinal cord trauma; complications of surgery; drug- or alcohol-induced dysfunction; and, rarely, genital anomalies or central nervous system defects.

DIAGNOSIS AND TREATMENT

Diagnosis must rule out chronic diseases, such as diabetes, and other vascular, neurologic, or urogenital problems.

Sex therapy, largely directed at reducing performance anxiety, may cure psychogenic impotence. Such therapy should include both partners. Its course and content depend on the specific cause of the dysfunction and the nature of the male-female relationship. Sex therapy usually includes sensate focus techniques and may also include improving verbal communication skills, eliminating unreasonable guilt, and reevaluating attitudes toward sex and sexual roles.

Treatment of organic impotence focuses on reversing the cause, if possible. If that's not possible, psychological counseling may help the couple deal realistically with their situation and explore alternatives for sexual expression. Certain patients with organic impotence may benefit from surgically inserted inflatable or noninflatable penile implants; others with low testosterone levels benefit from testosterone injections. In drug- or alcohol-induced dysfunction, treatment of the substance abuse may solve the problem.

COLLABORATIVE MANAGEMENT

Care of the patient with erectile dysfunction focuses on improving erectile function, relieving fears, and patient teaching.

ASSESSMENT

The patient's personal sexual history is the key in differentiating between organic and psychogenic factors and between primary and secondary impotence. Secondary erectile dysfunction is classified as follows:
- partial—the patient can't achieve a full erection
- intermittent—the patient is sometimes potent with the same partner
- selective—the patient is potent only with certain partners.

Some patients lose erectile function suddenly; others lose it gradually. If the cause isn't organic, masturbation may achieve an erection.

Patients with psychogenic impotence may appear anxious, with sweating and palpitations, or they may become totally disinterested in sexual activity. Patients with psychogenic or drug-induced impotence may suffer extreme depression, which may cause the impotence or result from it.

Specific interview questions include the following:
- Do you have intermittent, selective, nocturnal, or early-morning erections?
- Can you achieve erections through other sexual activity, such as masturbation or fantasizing?
- When did your problem begin, and what was your life situation at that time? Did it occur suddenly or gradually?
- Are you taking large quantities of prescription or over-the-counter drugs? What is your alcohol intake?

NURSING DIAGNOSES AND COLLABORATIVE PROBLEMS

Based on the following nursing diagnoses, you'll establish patient outcomes.

Body image disturbance related to negative self-image. The patient will:
- verbalize one positive body feature
- ask questions about surgical options for treating impotence
- achieve improved self-image.

Anxiety related to impotence. The patient will:
- express his concerns about sexual function
- ask questions and obtain information to alleviate anxiety.

Altered sexuality patterns related to erectile dysfunction. The patient will:
- discuss alternatives with partner
- report an improvement in sexual function
- reestablish a satisfying sexual relationship.

PLANNING AND IMPLEMENTATION

These measures help the patient with erectile dysfunction.
- Help the patient with impotence or with a condition that may cause impotence feel comfortable about discussing his sexuality.
- Assess his sexual health during your initial nursing history.
- When appropriate, refer him for further evaluation or treatment.
- Discuss possible treatment options, and include the patient's partner in the discussion. Encourage the patient to share his feelings with his partner.

Patient teaching
- After penile implant surgery, instruct the patient to avoid intercourse until the incision heals, usually in 6 weeks.
- If your patient has just had surgery or has a condition that requires modification of daily activities, such as cardiac disease, diabetes, hypertension, or chronic obstructive pulmonary disease, provide information about resuming sexual activity.

EVALUATION

Achievement of patient outcomes determines the success of collaborative management. For the patient with erectile dysfunction, evaluation focuses on improvement in erectile function, relief of anxiety and fears, satisfaction with sexual relationships, and adequate knowledge of the disease, treatment, and care.

Ovarian cancer

After cancers of the lung, breast, and colon, primary ovarian cancer ranks as the most common cause of cancer-related death among American women. In women with previously treated breast cancer, the ovaries are the most common site of metastasis. Incidence is higher in women between the ages of 20 and 54, especially those of upper socioeconomic status. However, the disease may strike during childhood or even pregnancy.

The three main types of ovarian cancer are primary epithelial tumors (90% of all ovarian cancers), germ cell tumors, and sex cord (stromal) tumors. Primary epithelial tumors arise in the müllerian epithelium; germ cell tumors, in the ovum itself; and sex cord tumors appear in the ovarian stroma. Ovarian tumors rapidly spread intraperitoneally by local extension or surface seeding and, occasionally, through the lymphatics and the bloodstream. In most cases, extraperitoneal spread occurs through the diaphragm into the chest cavity, which may cause pleural effusions.

The prognosis varies with the histologic type and stage of the disease, but it's usually poor because ovarian tumors are difficult to diagnose and progress rapidly. Early ovarian cancer rarely causes symptoms. As the disease progresses and spreads, pelvic pain, bowel dysfunction, or continuous urinary tract infections or incontinence may occur. Although about 40% of women with ovarian cancer survive for 5 years, the overall survival rate has not improved in the past 30 years.

Fluid and electrolyte imbalance, leg edema, ascites, and intestinal obstruction (causing nausea, malnutrition, and hunger) are common complications of progressive disease. The patient may experience profound cachexia and recurrent malignant effusions such as pleural effusions.

CAUSES

Environmental and lifestyle factors seem to play a role in ovarian cancer. Women who live in industrialized nations and those whose diet is high in saturated fat are at greater risk. Other risk factors include infertility problems or nulliparity, celibacy, exposure to asbestos and talc, a history of breast or uterine cancer, and a family history of ovarian cancer.

DIAGNOSIS AND TREATMENT

Many diagnostic tests are ordered to help assess the patient's condition, including a complete blood count, blood studies, and electrocardiography. Exploratory laparotomy, including lymph node evaluation and tumor resection, is required for accurate diagnosis and staging. Other tests check obstructions, metastasis sites, and tumor size. Laboratory tumor marker studies, such as ovarian carcinoma antigen, carcinoembryonic antigen, and human chorionic gonadotropin, are also evaluated.

Depending on the cancer stage and the patient's age, treatment requires varying combinations of surgery, chemotherapy and, possibly, radiation therapy. Occasionally, in girls or young women with a unilateral encapsulated tumor who wish to maintain fertility, the following conservative approach works:
- resection of the involved ovary with exploration of the abdomen
- biopsies of the omentum and the uninvolved ovary
- peritoneal washings for cytologic examination of pelvic fluid
- careful follow-up, including periodic X-rays, to rule out metastasis.

However, ovarian cancer usually requires more aggressive treatment, including total abdominal hysterectomy and bilateral salpingo-oophorectomy with tumor resection, omentectomy, appendectomy, lymph node palpation with probable lymphadenectomy, tissue biopsies, and peritoneal washings. Complete tumor resection is impossible if the tumor has matted around other organs or if it involves organs that the doctor can't resect. Bilateral salpingo-oophorectomy in a prepubertal girl is followed by hormonal replacement therapy, beginning at puberty, to induce the development of secondary sex characteristics.

Chemotherapy after surgery extends survival time in most patients but is largely palliative in advanced disease—although some patients have prolonged remissions. Drugs used include melphalan, chlorambucil, thiotepa, methotrexate, cyclophosphamide, doxorubicin, vincristine, vinblastine, dactinomycin, bleomycin, and cisplatin. These drugs are usually given in combination. Intraperitoneal administration of cisplatin is under investigation, but the technique hasn't slowed disease progression or prolonged survival.

Radiation therapy isn't commonly used because it causes myelosuppression, which limits chemotherapy.

Radioisotopes have been used as adjuvant therapy but cause small-bowel obstructions and stenosis.

Investigational immunotherapy consists of I.V. injection of *Corynebacterium parvum* or bacille Calmette-Guérin vaccine, lymphokine-activated killer cells, and interleukin-2.

COLLABORATIVE MANAGEMENT

Care of the patient with ovarian cancer focuses on controlling pain, avoiding complications, and teaching the patient about the disease, treatment, prognosis, and required care.

ASSESSMENT

Because ovarian cancer produces no obvious signs, it's seldom diagnosed early. Usually, it has metastasized before a diagnosis is made. Signs and symptoms vary with the tumor's size and the extent of metastasis.

In later stages, the patient's history may disclose urinary frequency, constipation, pelvic discomfort, distention, and weight loss. She may complain of pain, possibly associated with tumor rupture, torsion, or infection. In a young patient, the pain may mimic that of appendicitis.

You may see a patient who is alert but gaunt. She may have a grossly distended abdomen accompanied by ascites—typically the sign that prompts her to seek treatment.

Palpation of the abdominal organs and peritoneum may disclose masses. An ovarian tumor may feel hard, rubbery, or cystlike. Postmenopausal women whose ovaries are palpable require further evaluation for an ovarian tumor.

NURSING DIAGNOSES AND COLLABORATIVE PROBLEMS

Based on the following nursing diagnoses, you'll establish patient outcomes.

Altered nutrition: Less than body requirements, related to malnutrition. The patient will:
- eat a well-balanced diet high in calories and protein
- take supplements as needed to gain weight and alleviate malnutrition
- regain any lost weight, then maintain weight within a normal range.

Anticipatory grieving related to the threat of death. The patient and family will:
- express their feelings about the diagnosis and prognosis
- use healthy coping mechanisms to deal with grief
- demonstrate control over the situation by participating in decisions about care.

Fluid volume excess related to ascites. The patient will:

- comply with prescribed sodium and fluid restrictions to minimize fluid retention
- ambulate and carry out activities of daily living as tolerated
- describe the signs and symptoms of worsening fluid retention and seek medical treatment if they occur.

PLANNING AND IMPLEMENTATION

These measures help the patient with ovarian cancer.
- If the patient is in pain, make her as comfortable as possible. Give her prescribed analgesics as necessary, provide diversionary activities, and have her perform relaxation techniques.
- Listen to her concerns and fears, and answer her questions honestly. Provide support for the patient and her family.
- If the patient is a young woman who must undergo surgery and lose her childbearing ability, help her and her family overcome feelings of despair. If the patient is a child, find out whether her parents have told her she has cancer and respond to her questions accordingly.
- Provide supportive care for the adverse effects of therapy. If the patient is undergoing intraperitoneal chemotherapy, help alleviate her discomfort by infusing the fluid at a slower rate and repositioning her in an attempt to distribute the fluid evenly.
- If the patient develops flulike symptoms with immunotherapy, give her aspirin or acetaminophen. Cover her with blankets and provide warm liquids to relieve chills. Give her an antiemetic as needed.
- Prepare the patient for surgery, as indicated.
- If the patient has effusions and must undergo paracentesis and thoracentesis, assist with the procedure as necessary. Help her find a comfortable position during the procedure; then help her maintain it, using pillows. After the procedure, encourage her to drink fluids.
- Monitor the patient's fluid status, and measure intake and output. If she has ascites, measure her abdominal girth daily.
- Monitor her nutritional status and weight daily.
- Give the malnourished patient supplementary enteral or parenteral nutrition, as ordered. If her GI tract is intact, offer her frequent, small meals. If her GI tract is obstructed, discuss the possibility of a gastrostomy or jejunostomy tube with the doctor and the patient.
- Assess the patient's response to therapy and comfort measures.

Patient teaching
- Teach the patient relaxation techniques and other measures that may help ease her discomfort.

- Stress the importance of preventing infection, emphasizing good hand-washing technique.
- Explain measures that may help maintain adequate nutrition, such as eating small, frequent meals.
- If the patient will undergo drug therapy or radiation therapy, explain the possible adverse effects and suggest ways to alleviate and prevent them.
- Before surgery, thoroughly explain all preoperative tests, the expected course of treatment, and surgical and postoperative procedures.
- In premenopausal women, explain that bilateral oophorectomy induces early menopause. Such patients may experience hot flashes, headaches, palpitations, insomnia, depression, and excessive perspiration.
- As appropriate, refer the patient and family members to the social services department, home health care agencies, hospices, and support groups such as the American Cancer Society.

EVALUATION
Achievement of patient outcomes determines the success of collaborative management. For the patient with ovarian cancer, evaluation focuses on physiologic status within acceptable parameters, adequate fluid balance, pain control, absence of complications, positive coping strategies, and adequate knowledge of the disease, treatment, prognosis, and required care.

Pelvic inflammatory disease

An umbrella term, pelvic inflammatory disease (PID) refers to any acute, subacute, recurrent, or chronic infection of the oviducts and ovaries, with adjacent tissue involvement. It includes inflammation of the cervix (cervicitis), uterus (endometritis), fallopian tubes (salpingitis), and ovaries (oophoritis), which can extend to the connective tissue lying between the broad ligaments (parametritis).

Possible complications of PID include potentially fatal septicemia from a ruptured pelvic abscess, pulmonary emboli, infertility, and shock. Early diagnosis and treatment and well-planned nursing care help prevent damage to the reproductive system. Untreated PID can be fatal.

CAUSES
About 60% of PID cases are caused by overgrowth of one or more of the common aerobic or anaerobic bacteria found in the cervical mucus. *Neisseria gonorrhoeae* and *Chlamydia trachomatis* are the most common causes because they most readily penetrate the bacteriostatic barrier of cervical mucus.

Other common bacteria found in cervical mucus include staphylococci, streptococci, diphtheroids, chlamydiae, and coliforms (including *Pseudomonas* and *Escherichia coli*).

Uterine infection can result from any one or several of these organisms, or it may follow the multiplication of normally nonpathogenic bacteria in an altered endometrial environment. Bacterial multiplication is most common during parturition because the endometrium is atrophic, quiescent, and not stimulated by estrogen.

Risk factors for PID include:
- any sexually transmitted infection
- multiple sex partners
- conditions or procedures that alter or destroy cervical mucus, allowing bacteria to ascend into the uterine cavity, such as conization or cauterization of the cervix
- any procedure that risks transfer of contaminated cervical mucus into the endometrial cavity by an instrument (such as a biopsy curet or an irrigation catheter) or by tubal insufflation or abortion
- infection during or after pregnancy
- infectious foci within the body, such as drainage from a chronically infected fallopian tube, a pelvic abscess, a ruptured appendix, or diverticulitis of the sigmoid colon.

DIAGNOSIS AND TREATMENT
Diagnostic tests for PID include Gram stain, culture and sensitivity testing and culdocentesis to select an antibiotic, and ultrasonography, computed tomography scan, and magnetic resonance imaging to identify and locate an adnexal or uterine mass. (See *Forms of pelvic inflammatory disease.*)

To prevent progression of PID, antibiotic therapy begins as soon as culture specimens are obtained. The choice of antibiotic will be reevaluated as soon as laboratory results are available (usually within 24 to 48 hours). Infection may become chronic if treated inadequately.

The preferred antibiotic therapy for PID includes I.V. doxycycline and cefoxitin for 4 to 6 days (or alternatively, clindamycin and gentamicin), followed by oral doxycycline for another 10 to 14 days. Outpatient therapy may consist of I.M. cefoxitin, I.M. procaine penicillin G, oral amoxicillin, or oral ampicillin (each with probenecid), followed by oral doxycycline for 10 to 14 days. The patient may also require therapy for syphilis. Supplemental measures include bed rest, analgesics, and I.V. fluids as needed.

Development of a pelvic abscess requires adequate drainage. A ruptured pelvic abscess is a life-threatening condition that may require a total abdominal hysterectomy with bilateral salpingo-oophorectomy.

Forms of pelvic inflammatory disease

Clinical features	Test results
CERVICITIS ■ *Acute:* purulent, foul-smelling vaginal discharge; vulvovaginitis, with itching or burning; red, edematous cervix; pelvic discomfort; sexual dysfunction; metrorrhagia; infertility; spontaneous abortion ■ *Chronic:* cervical dystocia, laceration or eversion of the cervix, ulcerative vesicular lesion (when cervicitis results from herpes simplex virus 2)	■ Cultures for *N. gonorrhoeae* are positive in more than 90% of patients. ■ Cytologic smears may reveal severe inflammation. ■ If cervicitis isn't complicated by salpingitis, white blood cell (WBC) count is normal or slightly elevated; erythrocyte sedimentation rate (ESR) is elevated. ■ In *acute* cervicitis, cervical palpation reveals tenderness. ■ In *chronic* cervicitis, causative organisms are usually *Staphylococcus* or *Streptococcus.*
ENDOMETRITIS (GENERALLY POSTPARTUM OR POSTABORTION) ■ *Acute:* mucopurulent or purulent vaginal discharge oozing from the cervix; edematous, hyperemic endometrium, possibly leading to ulceration and necrosis (with virulent organisms); lower abdominal pain and tenderness; fever; rebound pain; abdominal muscle spasm; thrombophlebitis of uterine and pelvic vessels (in severe forms) ■ *Chronic:* recurring acute episodes (increasingly common because of widespread use of intrauterine devices)	■ In severe infection, palpation may reveal a boggy uterus. ■ Uterine and blood samples are positive for a causative organism, usually *Staphylococcus.* ■ WBC count and ESR are elevated.
SALPINGO-OOPHORITIS ■ *Acute:* sudden onset of lower abdominal and pelvic pain, usually following menses; increased vaginal discharge; fever; malaise; lower abdominal pressure and tenderness; tachycardia; pelvic peritonitis ■ *Chronic:* recurring acute episodes	■ Blood studies show leukocytosis or a normal WBC count. ■ X-rays may show ileus. ■ Pelvic examination reveals extreme tenderness. ■ Smear of cervical or periurethral gland exudate shows gram-negative intracellular diplococci.

COLLABORATIVE MANAGEMENT

Care of the patient with PID focuses on restoring vital signs, eliminating infection, and providing thorough patient teaching.

ASSESSMENT

The patient with PID may complain of profuse, purulent vaginal discharge, sometimes accompanied by low-grade fever and malaise (particularly if gonorrhea is the cause). She may also describe lower abdominal pain and vaginal bleeding. Vaginal examination may reveal pain during movement of the cervix or palpation of the adnexa.

NURSING DIAGNOSES AND COLLABORATIVE PROBLEMS

Based on the following nursing diagnoses, you'll establish patient outcomes.

Altered sexuality patterns related to infection of the reproductive system. The patient will:
■ abstain from sexual activity until the infection is cured

■ identify and avoid sexual risk factors that increase the chance of reinfection
■ resume normal sexual activity when the infection is cured.

Risk for injury related to inflammation of reproductive structures. The patient will:
■ comply with the prescribed therapy to minimize the risk of permanent damage to reproductive structures
■ demonstrate normal reproductive function following PID.

Pain related to inflammation caused by PID. The patient will:
■ use diversionary activities to minimize pain perception
■ express relief of pain after analgesic administration
■ become pain-free when PID is cured.

PLANNING AND IMPLEMENTATION

These measures help the patient with PID.
■ Give antibiotics and analgesics, as ordered.
■ Monitor the patient's level of pain and the effectiveness of analgesics.

- Check for adverse reactions to drugs and other complications.
- Provide frequent perineal care if vaginal drainage occurs.
- Use meticulous hand-washing technique; follow standard and contact precautions if necessary.
- Monitor vital signs for fever and fluid intake and output for signs of dehydration. Watch for abdominal rigidity and distention, possible signs of developing peritonitis.
- Encourage the patient to discuss her feelings, offer her emotional support, and help her develop effective coping strategies.

Patient teaching

- Explain the disease and its severity. To prevent recurrence, encourage compliance with the treatment regimen.
- Stress that the patient's sexual partner should undergo an examination and may need treatment for infection.
- Discuss the use of condoms to prevent the spread of sexually transmitted diseases.
- Because PID may cause dyspareunia, advise the patient to consult with her doctor about sexual activity.
- To prevent infection after minor gynecologic procedures such as dilatation and curettage, tell the patient to immediately report any fever, increased vaginal discharge, or pain. After such procedures, instruct her to avoid douching or intercourse for at least 7 days.

EVALUATION

Achievement of patient outcomes determines the success of collaborative management. For the patient with PID, evaluation focuses on vital signs within acceptable parameters, resolution of infection, absence of complications, positive coping strategies, and adequate knowledge of the disease, treatment, and prevention.

Premenstrual syndrome

Effects of premenstrual syndrome (PMS) range from minimal discomfort to severe, disruptive behavioral and somatic changes. Symptoms appear 7 to 14 days before menses and usually subside with its onset. Incidence seems to rise with age and parity.

CAUSES

Although its direct cause is unknown, PMS may result from a progesterone deficiency in the luteal phase of the menstrual cycle or from an increased estrogen-progesterone ratio. About 10% of patients with PMS have elevated prolactin levels.

DIAGNOSIS AND TREATMENT

Evaluation of estrogen and progesterone blood levels may help rule out hormonal imbalance. Psychological evaluation may rule out or detect an underlying psychiatric disorder.

Primarily symptomatic, treatment may include lifestyle changes (diet, exercise, and stress management) as well as tranquilizers, sedatives, antidepressants, nonsteroidal anti-inflammatory drugs, and progestins. The patient may require a diet that is low in simple sugars, caffeine, and salt, with adequate amounts of protein, high amounts of complex carbohydrates and, possibly, vitamin supplements formulated for PMS.

COLLABORATIVE MANAGEMENT

Care of the patient with PMS focuses on relieving pain and teaching about the disorder and its treatment.

ASSESSMENT

Behavioral changes in PMS include mild to severe personality changes, nervousness, hostility, irritability, agitation, sleep disturbances, fatigue, lethargy, and depression.

Somatic changes include breast tenderness or swelling, abdominal tenderness or bloating, joint pain, headache, edema, and diarrhea or constipation. The patient may also experience exacerbations of skin problems, such as acne or rash; respiratory problems such as asthma; and neurologic problems such as seizures.

NURSING DIAGNOSES AND COLLABORATIVE PROBLEMS

Based on the following nursing diagnoses, you'll establish patient outcomes.

Pain related to premenstrual syndrome. The patient will:
- demonstrate measures to control pain
- verbalize an understanding of medication therapy
- verbalize a decrease in pain.

Risk for injury related to weakness and fatigue. The patient will:
- demonstrate use of appropriate safety measures
- remain free from injury.

Altered role performance related to discomfort. The patient will:
- demonstrate measures to control discomfort and engage in normal activities
- return to previous level of functioning with control of symptoms.

Altered nutrition: Less than body requirements, related to irritability, anxiety, and bloating. The patient will:
- express feelings of anxiety
- identify foods that contribute to her condition

- initiate recommended changes in diet
- verbalize diminished bloating.

PLANNING AND IMPLEMENTATION
These measures help the patient with PMS.
- Encourage the patient to verbalize her feelings.
- Give the patient prescribed medications, and monitor their effectiveness.
- Evaluate the use of palliative treatments, such as warm compresses and ice.
- Obtain a complete patient history to help identify any emotional problems that may contribute to PMS.
- Review the patient's dietary history for possible intake of stimulants.
- Work with the patient to identify foods that may be contributing to her signs and symptoms.
- If the patient has weakness and fatigue, help her walk; warn her not to get up by herself. Keep all her personal objects within reach.

Patient teaching
- Inform the patient about support groups for women with PMS. If appropriate, help her contact such a group.
- Discuss lifestyle changes—such as avoiding stimulants—that might help alleviate symptoms by reducing stress and anxiety.
- Explain the value of further medical consultation if severe symptoms disrupt the patient's normal lifestyle.
- If necessary, refer the patient for psychological counseling.

EVALUATION
Achievement of patient outcomes determines the success of collaborative management. For the patient with PMS, evaluation focuses on pain relief and adequate knowledge of the disorder, treatment, and care.

Prostatic cancer

The most common neoplasm in men over age 50, prostatic cancer is a leading cause of cancer-related death in men. Incidence is highest in Blacks and lowest in Asians; it appears unaffected by socioeconomic status or fertility. Adenocarcinoma is the most common form of prostatic cancer; sarcoma is rare. About 85% of prostatic cancers originate in the posterior prostate gland, with the rest growing near the urethra.

Slow-growing prostatic cancer seldom produces signs and symptoms until it's well advanced. Typically, when primary prostatic lesions spread beyond the prostate gland, they invade the prostatic capsule and then spread along the ejaculatory ducts in the space between the seminal vesicles or perivesicular fascia. The primary site of metastasis is bone. When prostatic cancer is treated in its localized form, the 5-year survival rate is 70%; after metastasis, it's under 35%. Death is usually caused by widespread bone metastasis.

Progressive disease can lead to spinal cord compression, deep vein thrombosis, pulmonary emboli, and myelophthisis.

CAUSES
The exact cause of prostatic cancer is unknown. Risk factors include age (the cancer seldom develops in men under age 40) and infection. Endocrine factors may also have a role, leading researchers to suspect that a majority of prostatic cancers are caused by androgens that speed tumor growth. Malignant prostatic tumors seldom result from the benign hyperplastic enlargement that commonly develops around the prostatic urethra in older men.

DIAGNOSIS AND TREATMENT
Diagnostic tests may include a digital rectal examination, the standard screening test; blood tests for elevated prostate-specific antigen; transrectal prostatic ultrasonography; bone scan and excretory urography to determine the disease's extent; and magnetic resonance imaging and computed tomography scanning to help define the tumor's boundaries.

Therapy depends on the cancer stage and whether treatment is curative or palliative. It may include radiation, prostatectomy, orchiectomy (removal of the testes) to reduce androgen production, cryosurgery, and hormonal therapy with synthetic estrogen (diethylstilbestrol) or agonistic analogues of luteinizing hormone–releasing hormone (such as triptorelin, leuprolide, and goserelin). Radical prostatectomy is usually effective for localized lesions without metastasis. The doctor may perform a transurethral resection of the prostate to relieve an obstruction.

Radiation therapy may cure locally invasive lesions in early disease and may relieve bone pain from metastatic skeletal involvement. It's also used prophylactically for patients with tumors in regional lymph nodes. Alternatively, internal beam radiation may be used because it permits increased radiation to reach the prostate but minimizes the surrounding tissues' exposure to radiation.

If hormonal therapy, surgery, and radiation therapy aren't feasible or successful, the doctor may try chemotherapy. Combinations of cyclophosphamide, doxorubicin, fluorouracil, cisplatin, and vindesine offer limited benefits. Research continues to seek the most effective chemotherapeutic regimen.

COLLABORATIVE MANAGEMENT
Care of the patient with prostatic cancer focuses on restoring urinary elimination and providing thorough patient teaching.

ASSESSMENT
The patient usually has no signs or symptoms in early disease. Later, he may report urinary problems, such as dysuria, frequency, complete urine retention, back or hip pain, and hematuria. When these signs and symptoms appear, the disease is usually advanced. What's more, back or hip pain may signal bone metastasis.

Inspection may reveal edema of the scrotum or leg in advanced disease. During rectal examination, palpation of the prostate may detect a nonraised, firm, nodular mass with a sharp edge (in early disease) or a hard lump (in advanced disease).

NURSING DIAGNOSES AND COLLABORATIVE PROBLEMS
Based on the following nursing diagnoses, you'll establish patient outcomes.

Altered urinary elimination related to functional changes in the lower urinary tract. The patient will:
- express feelings of increased comfort when urinating
- avoid or minimize complications, such as urinary tract infection or obstruction
- regain a normal urinary elimination pattern with eradication of prostatic cancer.

Anxiety related to diagnosis. The patient will:
- identify and express his feelings of anxiety
- identify and perform activities that decrease anxiety
- cope with the diagnosis without showing signs of severe anxiety.

Pain related to metastasis of prostatic cancer to bone. The patient will:
- express feelings of comfort after analgesic administration
- identify and carry out appropriate interventions for pain relief
- become pain-free with eradication of prostatic cancer.

PLANNING AND IMPLEMENTATION
These measures help the patient with prostatic cancer.
- Encourage the patient to express his fears and concerns, including those about changes in his sexual identity. Offer reassurance when possible.
- Give ordered analgesics as necessary, and provide comfort measures to reduce pain. Encourage the patient to identify care measures that promote his comfort and relaxation.
- Evaluate the patient's pain level and the effectiveness of analgesics.
- Provide supportive care for adverse effects of hormonal therapy or chemotherapy.
- Measure intake and output, and monitor for urinary system dysfunction.
- Prepare the patient for orchiectomy or prostatectomy, as indicated.
- Encourage the patient undergoing radiation to drink at least eight 8-oz (240-ml) glasses of fluid daily. Give him analgesics and antispasmodics to decrease his discomfort.
- Watch for the common adverse effects of radiation to the prostate: proctitis, diarrhea, bladder spasms, and urinary frequency. Internal radiation of the prostate almost always results in cystitis in the first 2 to 3 weeks of therapy.
- If the patient is receiving diethylstilbestrol, watch for adverse reactions (gynecomastia, fluid retention, nausea, and vomiting) and for indications of thrombophlebitis (pain, tenderness, swelling, warmth, and redness in the calf).

Patient teaching
- If surgery is planned, teach the patient about his particular procedure.
- If appropriate, discuss the adverse effects of radiation therapy. All patients who receive pelvic radiation therapy will develop such signs and symptoms as diarrhea, urinary frequency, nocturia, bladder spasms, rectal irritation, and tenesmus.
- Encourage the patient to maintain as nearly normal a lifestyle as possible during recovery.
- When appropriate, refer him to the social services department, local home health care agencies, hospices, and other support organizations.

EVALUATION
Achievement of patient outcomes determines the success of collaborative management. For the patient with prostatic cancer, evaluation focuses on absence of urinary obstruction and urine retention, urinary elimination within acceptable parameters, ability to perform catheter care if needed, and adequate knowledge of the disease, treatment, prognosis, and care.

Rape trauma syndrome

Rape trauma syndrome refers to a victim's short-term and long-term reactions after a rape or an attempted rape and to the methods she uses to cope with this trauma.

Known victims of rape range from age 2 months to 97 years. The age-group most affected is 10 to 19; the average age of the victim is 13$\frac{1}{2}$. Most rapists are 15 to 24 years old. More than 50% of rapes occur in the home; about one-third of these involve a male intruder who has usually planned the attack. About half all rape victims have at least a casual acquaintance with their attacker.

In most cases, the rapist is a man and the victim is a woman. However, rapes do occur between persons of the same sex, especially in prisons, schools, hospitals, and other institutions. Many children are also victims of rape; these cases usually involve a member of the child's family having manual, oral, or genital contact with the child's genitals. In rare instances, a man or child is sexually abused by a woman.

The prognosis is good if the rape victim receives treatment for physical injuries and emotional support and counseling to help her deal with her feelings.

DIAGNOSIS AND TREATMENT

A physical examination can detect signs of physical trauma, and specimen collection from body orifices can provide further evidence of rape.

Treatment consists of supportive measures and protection against sexually transmitted diseases (STDs) and, if the patient wishes, against pregnancy. Give ordered antibiotics (spectinomycin 2 g I.M. or ceftriaxone 250 mg I.M.) to prevent STDs. Cultures can't detect gonorrhea for 5 to 6 days after a rape or syphilis for 6 weeks or more. Urge the patient to return for follow-up STD evaluation because other STDs, such as genital herpes, may develop.

If she wishes to prevent possible pregnancy as a result of the rape, she may be given two pills of Ovral (ethinyl estradiol 50 mg and norgestrel 0.5 mg) within the first 72 hours and two pills 12 hours later. Inserting an intrauterine device immediately may prevent pregnancy but may also cause an infection. Or the patient may wait 3 to 4 weeks and have a dilatation and curettage or a vacuum aspiration to abort a pregnancy.

If the victim has vulvar and perineal lacerations, the doctor will clean the area and repair the lacerations after all the evidence of rape is obtained.

COLLABORATIVE MANAGEMENT

Care of the patient with rape trauma syndrome focuses on promoting recovery from physical injuries and helping the patient express her feelings about the rape and use available support systems.

ASSESSMENT

First, remember that the victim must consent to examination and treatment as well as to collection and release of evidence to authorities. Be sure to follow state law for collecting evidence.

Signs and symptoms of rape trauma syndrome vary widely. Assess first for physical injuries. X-rays may be needed to rule out fractures. If the patient isn't seriously injured, allow her to remain clothed and take her to a private room where she can talk. Remember never to leave the patient alone because many rape victims are extremely fragile emotionally after the trauma.

Obtain a history, especially the date of the patient's last menstrual period and whether she was pregnant before the attack. Before the examination, ask the patient whether she douched, bathed, or washed before coming to the hospital. Place her clothes in paper bags—never use plastic because secretions and seminal stains will become moldy, destroying valuable evidence.

If the patient is wearing a tampon, be sure to wrap it and label it as evidence. The victim may urinate but not clean her perineal area before the examination. She'll need a thorough physical examination, including a pelvic examination by a gynecologist.

Note the following signs and symptoms:
- signs of physical trauma, especially if the assault was prolonged
- depending on specific body areas attacked, reports of a sore throat, mouth irritation, difficulty swallowing, ecchymoses, or rectal pain and bleeding
- hematomas, lacerations, bleeding, severe internal injuries, hemorrhage, and exposure if the attack was outdoors.

During the assessment, assist in collection of appropriate specimens (semen, specimens for gonorrhea culture). Carefully label all specimens with the patient's name, the doctor's name, and the body location from which the specimen was obtained. List all specimens in your notes. If the case comes to trial, all of your notes and the specimens will be used for evidence, so objectivity and accuracy are vital.

Carefully collect and label fingernail scrapings and foreign material obtained by combing the victim's pubic hair. Note to whom all specimens are given.

For a male victim, be especially alert for injury to the mouth, perineum, and anus. Obtain a pharyngeal specimen for a gonorrhea culture and rectal aspirate for acid phosphatase or sperm analysis.

NURSING DIAGNOSES AND COLLABORATIVE PROBLEMS

Based on the following nursing diagnoses, you'll establish patient outcomes.

Powerlessness related to trauma of rape. The patient will:
- verbalize feelings about the attack

- develop adequate coping mechanisms.
  Risk for infection related to assault and exposure to potential organisms. The patient will:
- state the signs and symptoms of possible infections
- demonstrate knowledge of need for follow-up
- remain free from infection and STDs.
  Pain related to assault and injuries. The patient will:
- exhibit healing of injuries without complications
- use measures to control pain
- experience relief of pain.

PLANNING AND IMPLEMENTATION

These measures help the patient with rape trauma syndrome.

- Arrange to have someone—ideally a family member or friend—remain with the victim at all times in a quiet, private, nonthreatening environment.
- Arrange for immediate patient counseling; put the patient in contact with a local rape hot line or rape crisis center.
- Encourage the patient to verbalize her feelings about the attack, and help her develop adequate coping skills.
- Obtain cultures as ordered.
- Apply ice packs topically to reduce vulvar swelling.
- Give analgesics as ordered and monitor their effectiveness.
- Give prophylactic antibiotics and treatments as ordered, including tetanus prophylaxis for any open and contaminated wounds.

Patient teaching

- Provide all instructions and follow-up information in writing so the patient will be able to remember them after the emotional crisis.
- Explain to the patient that recovery from rape may be prolonged, consisting of an acute phase (immediate reaction) and a reorganization phase. Tell her that during the acute phase, she'll probably experience physical reactions (such as pain, loss of appetite, and wound healing) and emotional reactions (such as shaking, crying, and mood swings).
- Tell the patient that the reorganization phase usually begins a week after the rape and may last months or years; assist her as necessary with restructuring her life.
- Warn the patient that, initially, she may have nightmares about feeling powerless, followed later by dreams in which she gradually gains control. Tell her that when she's alone, she may also suffer from "daymares"—frightening thoughts about the rape.
- Alert the patient that feelings of grief, anger, fear, or revenge may color her social interactions.
- Tell her she may have reduced sexual desire and may develop fear of intercourse or mistrust of men.

- Urge her to keep counseling appointments to help her identify coping mechanisms.
- To help her cope, encourage her to write her thoughts, feelings, and reactions in a daily diary.
- Refer her to organizations such as Women Organized Against Rape or a local rape crisis center.

EVALUATION

Achievement of patient outcomes determines the success of collaborative management. For the patient with rape trauma syndrome, evaluation focuses on recovery from physical injuries, expression of feelings about the rape, and use of available support systems to aid coping.

Sexually transmitted diseases

Sexually transmitted diseases (STDs) include gonorrhea, chlamydial infections, genital herpes, and syphilis (including prenatal syphilis).

CAUSES

STDs are transmitted through direct contact during sexual intercourse. Each disease has a specific bacterium or virus through which infection occurs. The agent that causes gonorrhea is *Neisseria gonorrhoeae*. The infecting organism for chlamydial infections is *Chlamydia trachomatis*. The herpes simplex type II virus is the cause of genital herpes and the spirochete *Treponema pallidum* causes syphilis. Since the early 1960s, the incidence of STDs has increased. Treatment today is difficult because many of the infecting agents are resistant to antibiotics. Multiple recurrences and drug-resistant STDs can cause infertility.

DIAGNOSIS AND TREATMENT

Diagnosis and treatment vary according to the infection, its progress, and the general health of the patient.

COLLABORATIVE MANAGEMENT

Care of the patient with an STD focuses on resolving the infection and teaching the patient to avoid reinfection.

ASSESSMENT

Signs and symptoms vary according to the infection. (See *Reviewing common STDs*, pages 483 to 485.)

NURSING DIAGNOSES AND COLLABORATIVE PROBLEMS

Based on the following nursing diagnoses, you'll establish patient outcomes.

(Text continues on page 486.)

Reviewing common STDs

Below you'll find a summary of current information about four common types of sexually transmitted diseases (STDs).

Gonorrhea

Gonorrhea is transmitted almost exclusively through sexual contact with an infected person. The infective organism is *Neisseria gonorrhoea.*

This common venereal disease infects the genitourinary tract (especially the urethra and cervix) and may occasionally infect the rectum, pharynx, and even the eyes. After adequate treatment, the prognosis in both males and females is excellent, although reinfection is common. Gonorrhea is especially prevalent among unmarried persons and young people, particularly between ages 19 and 25. Severe disseminated infection affects more women than men.

Left untreated, gonorrhea can spread through the blood to the joints, tendons, meninges, and endocardium. Children and adults with gonorrhea can contract gonococcal conjunctivitis by touching their eyes with contaminated hands. Children born of infected mothers can contract gonococcal ophthalmia neonatorum during passage through the birth canal. Other possible results of untreated disease include gonococcal septicemia (more common in females than in males), sterility, corneal ulceration and blindness, and arthritis.

Assessment findings

Most females remain asymptomatic, but inflammation and a greenish yellow discharge from the cervix are the most common symptoms. Males may be asymptomatic, but after a 3- to 6-day incubation period, they may manifest signs and symptoms of urethritis, including dysuria, purulent urethral discharge, and redness and swelling at the infection site.

Other findings vary according to the site involved:
- urethra—dysuria, urinary frequency and incontinence, purulent discharge, itching, red and edematous meatus
- vulva—occasional itching, burning, and pain caused by exudate from an adjacent infected area; vulval symptoms tend to be more severe before puberty or after menopause
- vagina (most common site in children over age 1)—engorgement, redness, swelling, and profuse purulent discharge
- pelvis—severe pelvic and lower abdominal pain, muscle rigidity, tenderness, and abdominal distention; as infection spreads, nausea, vomiting, fever, and tachycardia may develop in patients with salpingitis or pelvic inflammatory disease (PID)
- liver—right upper quadrant pain in patients with perihepatitis

- eyes—adult conjunctivitis (most common in men), with unilateral conjunctival redness and swelling; and gonococcal ophthalmia neonatorum, with lid edema, bilateral conjunctival infection, and abundant purulent discharge 2 to 3 days after birth.

Other possible signs and symptoms include pharyngitis, tonsillitis, rectal burning, itching, and bloody, mucopurulent discharge.

Diagnostic tests

Culture from the site of infection usually establishes the diagnosis by isolating the organism. A Gram stain showing gram-negative diplococci supports the diagnosis and may be sufficient to confirm gonorrhea in males.

Confirmation of gonococcal arthritis requires identification of gram-negative diplococci in smears of joint fluid and skin lesions. Complement fixation and immunofluorescent assays of serum reveal antibody titers four times higher than normal. Culture of conjunctival scrapings confirms gonococcal conjunctivitis.

Treatment

For uncomplicated gonorrhea in adults, recommended treatment is 250 mg of ceftriaxone given I.M. in a single dose plus 100 mg of doxycycline hyclate given twice daily by mouth for 7 days. As an alternative to the doxycycline—which helps combat gonorrhea and treats the commonly coexisting chlamydial or mycoplasmal infection—the patient can be given 500 mg of oral tetracycline four times daily for 7 days. For pregnant patients or others who can't take doxycycline or tetracycline, the regimen is 500 mg of oral erythromycin for 7 days.

When the infection is passed on by a person with susceptible non-penicillinase-producing gonorrhea, the patient can be given 1 g of probenecid by mouth (to block penicillin excretion) plus either 3.5 g of oral ampicillin in a single dose or 3 g of oral amoxicillin in a single dose. This is followed by a 7-day course of doxycycline or tetracycline. Disseminated gonococcal infection requires 1 g of ceftriaxone given I.M. or I.V. every 24 hours for 7 days. Adult gonococcal ophthalmia requires 1 g of ceftriaxone given I.M. in a single dose.

Because many strains of antibiotic-resistant gonococci exist, follow-up cultures are necessary 4 to 7 days after treatment and again in 6 months. (For a pregnant patient, final follow-up must occur before delivery.)

Routine instillation of 1% silver nitrate or erythromycin ointment into the eyes of neonates has greatly reduced the incidence of gonococcal ophthalmia neonatorum.

(continued)

Reviewing common STDs (continued)

Chlamydial infections

Chlamydial infections are almost always transmitted by sexual contact with an infected person. The infecting agent is *Chlamydia trachomatis,* a bacterium.

The most common sexually transmitted disorders in the United States, chlamydial infections include urethritis in men, cervicitis in women, and lymphogranuloma venereum (LGV) in both. Because many of these infections produce no symptoms until late in their development, sexual transmission usually occurs unknowingly.

Left untreated, chlamydial infections can lead to such complications as acute epididymitis, salpingitis, PID and, eventually, sterility. In pregnant women, chlamydial infections are also associated with spontaneous abortion, premature delivery, and neonatal death, although a direct link with *C. trachomatis* has not been established. Children born of infected mothers may contract trachoma, otitis media, and pneumonia during passage through the birth canal. Trachoma—a chronic, contagious form of conjunctivitis—is caused by a chlamydial infection that occurs rarely in the United States but is a leading cause of blindness in Third World countries.

Assessment findings

Clinical features vary with the specific type of infection:
- In LGV, the primary lesion is a painless vesicle or nonindurated ulcer, ⅟₁₆″ to ⅛″ (2 to 3 mm) in diameter (commonly unnoticed). The patient develops regional lymphadenopathy after 1 to 4 weeks and inguinal lymph node swelling about 2 weeks later. Systemic symptoms include myalgia, headache, fever, chills, backache, and weight loss.
- In proctitis, infection in the rectum may produce diarrhea, tenesmus, pruritus, bloody or mucopurulent discharge, or diffuse or discrete ulceration in the rectosigmoid colon.
- In cervicitis, clinical features may include cervical erosion, mucopurulent discharge, pelvic pain, or dyspareunia.
- In urethral syndrome, clinical features include dysuria, pyuria, or urinary frequency.
- In epididymitis, infection of the epididymis produces painful scrotal swelling and urethral discharge.
- In prostatitis, the patient may develop lower back pain, urinary frequency, dysuria, nocturia, urethral discharge, or painful ejaculation.
- In urethritis, clinical features may include dysuria, erythema and tenderness of the urethral meatus, urinary frequency, pruritus, or urethral discharge.

Diagnostic tests

A swab culture from the infection site (urethra, cervix, or rectum) usually establishes the diagnosis of urethritis, cervicitis, salpingitis, endometritis, or proctitis.

Culture of aspirated blood, pus, or cerebrospinal fluid establishes the diagnosis of epididymitis, prostatitis, or LGV.

Direct visualization of cell scrapings or exudate with Giemsa stain or fluorescein-conjugated monoclonal antibodies may be attempted if the site is accessible, but tissue cell cultures are more sensitive and specific.

Serologic tests to determine previous exposure to *C. trachomatis* include complement fixation and microimmunofluorescence tests.

Treatment

The recommended first-line treatment is 100 mg of doxycycline four times daily for 7 to 21 days or 500 mg of erythromycin four times daily for 7 days. Or, you can give the patient 300 mg of ofloxacin every 12 hours for 7 days. LGV requires extended treatment. A pregnant woman infected with *Chlamydia* should receive erythromycin stearate.

Genital herpes

The infecting agent is the herpes simplex virus type 2. Also known as herpes simplex virus type 2 or venereal herpes, this acute, inflammatory infection is one of the most common recurring disorders of the genitalia. The prognosis varies according to the patient's age, the strength of his immune system, and the infection site. Primary genital herpes is usually self-limiting but may cause painful local or systemic disease. In neonates, in patients with a weak immune system, and in those with disseminated disease, genital herpes is commonly severe, with complications and a high mortality.

Usually transmitted by sexual contact, genital herpes may also be spread (rarely) by contaminated toilet seats, towels, and bathtubs. In addition, pregnant women may transmit the infection to their neonates during vaginal delivery. Such transmitted infection may be localized (for instance, in the eyes) or disseminated and may be associated with central nervous system (CNS) involvement.

Complications are rare and usually arise from extragenital lesions. These include hepatic keratitis, which may lead to blindness, and potentially fatal herpes simplex encephalitis.

Assessment findings

Fluid-filled, painless vesicles appear after a 3- to 7-day incubation period. In women, they occur on the cervix (the primary infection site) and possibly on the labia, perianal skin, vulva, or vagina; in men, on the glans penis, foreskin, or penile shaft.

Extragenital lesions may occur in the mouth or anus. In both men and women, the vesicles will rupture and develop into extensive, shallow, painful ulcers. The patient will also have marked edema and tender inguinal lymph nodes. Other features of initial mucocutaneous infection include fever, malaise, dysuria and, in the female, leukorrhea.

Diagnostic tests
Demonstration of herpes simplex virus type 2 in vesicular fluid, using tissue culture techniques, confirms genital herpes. Other helpful but nondiagnostic measures include laboratory data showing increased antibody titers and atypical cells in smears of genital lesions.

Treatment
Acyclovir (Zovirax) is the treatment of choice for genital herpes. Each of the three available drug forms has a specific indication. I.V. administration may be required for patients who are hospitalized with severe genital herpes or who are immunocompromised and have potentially life-threatening herpes infections. The doctor may order oral acyclovir for patients suffering from first-time infections or from recurrent outbreaks. Patients experiencing outbreaks more often than every 6 weeks may require suppressive therapy consisting of 200 mg of acyclovir three to five times a day for 6 months.

Syphilis
The infecting agent is the spirochete *Treponema pallidum.* This chronic, infectious venereal disease begins in the mucous membranes and quickly becomes systemic, spreading to nearby lymph nodes and the bloodstream. The disorder spreads by sexual contact during the primary, secondary, and early latent stages of infection; it may also be spread to the neonate through the placenta.

Syphilis is the third most prevalent reportable infectious disease in the United States. Incidence is highest among urban populations, especially in persons between ages 15 and 39. Untreated syphilis leads to crippling or death, but the prognosis is excellent with early treatment.

Assessment findings
Clinical features vary with the stage of the disease:
- In primary syphilis (3 weeks after contact), the patient may develop chancres—small, fluid-filled lesions on genitalia, anus, fingers, lips, tongue, nipples, tonsils, or eyelids that eventually erode and develop indurated, raised edges and clear bases. Regional lymphadenopathy (unilateral or bilateral) may also appear during this stage.
- In secondary syphilis (from a few days to 8 weeks after the onset of initial chancres), look for a rash (macular, papular, pustular, or nodular) and for symmetrical mucocutaneous lesions. Macules commonly erupt between rolls of fat on the trunk and, proximally, on the arms, palms, soles, face, and scalp. In warm, moist areas (perineum,

scrotum, vulva, between rolls of fat), the lesions enlarge and erode, producing highly contagious, pink or grayish white lesions (condylomata lata).

Assess also for general lymphadenopathy, mild constitutional symptoms (headache, malaise, anorexia, weight loss, nausea, vomiting, and sore throat), brittle and pitted nails, possible low-grade fever, and possible alopecia.
- Latent syphilis is characterized by an absence of symptoms.
- The late syphilis stage includes three subtypes: late benign syphilis, cardiovascular syphilis, and neurosyphilis. Any or all may be present. In late benign syphilis, the typical lesion is a gumma—a chronic, superficial nodule or deep, granulomatous lesion that is solitary, asymmetrical, painless, and indurated. Other possible symptoms of this subtype include liver involvement, causing epigastric pain, tenderness, enlarged spleen, and anemia, and upper respiratory involvement with potential perforation of the nasal septum or palate.
- In cardiovascular syphilis, the patient may develop aortitis, aortic insufficiency, or aortic aneurysm, or he may experience no symptoms at all.
- In neurosyphilis, meningitis and widespread CNS damage typically occur. Symptoms of CNS damage include general paresis, personality changes, and arm and leg weakness.

Diagnostic tests
Culture of a lesion identifying *T. pallidum* confirms the diagnosis in primary, secondary, and prenatal syphilis.

The fluorescent treponemal antibody absorption test identifies antigens of *T. pallidum* in tissue, ocular fluid, cerebrospinal fluid (CSF), tracheobronchial secretions, and exudates from lesions in all stages of syphilis.

The Venereal Disease Research Laboratory (VDRL) slide test and rapid plasma reagin test detect nonspecific antibodies.

CSF examination identifies neurosyphilis when the total protein level is above 40 mg/dl, the VDRL slide test is reactive, and the cell count exceeds 5 mononuclear cells/µl.

Treatment
The treatment of choice is penicillin I.M. For early syphilis, treatment may consist of a single injection of penicillin G benzathine I.M. (2.4 million U). Syphilis of more than 1 year's duration should be treated with penicillin G benzathine I.M. (2.4 million U/week for 3 weeks).

Patients allergic to penicillin may be treated successfully with tetracycline or erythromycin (in either case, 500 mg P.O. four times a day for 15 days for early syphilis; 30 days for late infections). Tetracycline is contraindicated in pregnant females.

HEALTHY LIVING — **Avoiding STDs**

You can promote the health of patients infected with sexually transmitted diseases (STDs) by teaching them how to reduce the risk of transmission and reinfection. Instruct patients with syphilis, gonorrhea, genital herpes, or *Chlamydia* on the following:

- signs and symptoms of the diseases and possible complications
- use of condoms
- sexual abstinence versus safe sex
- need for completing all treatments
- Relationship of acquired immunodeficiency syndrome to STDs.

Decisional conflict related to sexual activity. The patient will:
- state the risks involved in unprotected sexual activity
- discuss conflicts between personal values and social pressure to be sexually active
- demonstrate measures to control infection and prevent transmission.

Pain related to infection. The patient will:
- demonstrate measures to promote comfort
- state that pain is diminished.

PLANNING AND IMPLEMENTATION

These measures help the patient with an STD.

- Follow standard precautions. Double-bag all soiled dressings and contaminated instruments, and wear gloves when handling contaminated material and giving patient care. Isolate the patient with a gonococcal eye infection.
- Routinely instill erythromycin in the eyes of all neonates immediately after birth to prevent gonococcal ophthalmia neonatorum.
- Check the neonates of mothers infected with gonorrhea or *Chlamydia* for signs of infection. Take specimens for culture from the infant's eyes, pharynx, and rectum. Remember that positive rectal cultures for *Chlamydia* will peak by 5 to 6 weeks postpartum.
- Urge the patient to inform sexual contacts of the infection so that they can seek treatment. Report all cases to public health authorities for follow-up on sexual contacts.
- Encourage the patient to get adequate rest and nutrition.
- Keep genital herpes lesions dry, except for applying prescribed medications (using aseptic technique).

- Make sure the pregnant patient with genital herpes understands the risk of transmitting the infection to her neonate during vaginal delivery. Most doctors will perform a cesarean section if cultures are positive at the due date.
- Check any patient with syphilis for a history of drug sensitivity before giving any drug.
- Make sure the patient clearly understands the drug dosage schedule.
- In secondary syphilis, keep lesions clean and dry.
- In late syphilis, provide symptomatic care during prolonged treatment.
- In cardiovascular syphilis, check for signs of decreased cardiac output (decreased urine output, hypoxia, or decreased sensorium) and pulmonary congestion.
- In neurosyphilis, regularly check level of consciousness, mood, and coherence. Watch for signs of ataxia.
- Give analgesics as ordered and monitor for effectiveness.
- To ease pain in the patient with gonococcal arthritis, apply moist heat to affected joints.
- Allow the patient to verbalize feelings and fears.

Patient teaching

- Warn the patient with gonorrhea that until cultures prove negative, he can still transmit gonococcal infection.
- If the patient is being treated as an outpatient, advise family members to take precautions against infection.
- To prevent the spread of gonorrhea, tell the patient to use condoms during intercourse, and to avoid sharing washcloths or douche equipment. (See *Avoiding STDs*.)
- Make sure the patient understands dosage requirements of prescribed drugs. Stress the importance of completing the course of drug therapy even after symptoms subside.
- To prevent reinfection, urge the patient to abstain from intercourse or use a condom.
- Advise the patient to continue condom use unless he's in a mutually monogamous relationship with a partner who has tested negative for *Chlamydia trachomatis*.
- For the patient with genital herpes, focus your teaching on helping him avoid subsequent infection and preventing the spread of the disease. Encourage him to avoid sexual intercourse during the active stage of the disease (while lesions are present).
- Advise the female patient to have a Papanicolaou test every 6 months.
- Encourage good nutrition, adequate rest, and stress reduction to help reduce subsequent outbreaks.

- Refer the patient to the Herpes Resource Center, an American Social Health Association group, for support.
- Advise the patient with syphilis to seek retesting after 3, 6, 12, and 24 months to detect a possible relapse.
- Advise the patient treated for latent or late syphilis to get blood tests at 6-month intervals for 2 years.
- Urge the patient with any STD to inform sexual partners of his infection so that they can get treatment.

EVALUATION

Achievement of patient outcomes determines the success of collaborative management. For the patient with an STD, evaluation focuses on resolution of the infection, absence of its signs and symptoms (such as lesions, discharges, pain, fever, or enlarged lymph nodes), effective self-management of signs and symptoms, infection control, and adequate knowledge to prevent recurrence or complications.

Testicular cancer

Malignant testicular tumors are the most prevalent solid tumors in men ages 20 to 40. Rare in nonwhite men, testicular cancer accounts for less than 1% of all cancer-related deaths in men.

With few exceptions, testicular tumors originate from germ cells. About 40% become seminomas, which are characterized by uniform, undifferentiated cells that resemble primitive gonadal cells. Other tumors—nonseminomas—show various degrees of differentiation.

The prognosis in testicular cancer depends on the cell type and stage. When treated with surgery, chemotherapy, and radiation therapy, all patients with stage I or stage II seminomas and 90% of those with stage I nonseminomas survive beyond 5 years. The prognosis is poor, however, if the disease advances beyond stage II. When the cancer extends beyond the testes, it typically spreads through the lymphatic system to the iliac, para-aortic, and mediastinal nodes and metastasizes to the lungs, liver, viscera, and bone.

Disease progression may induce back or abdominal pain (from retroperitoneal adenopathy), dyspnea, cough, hemoptysis from lung metastasis, and ureteral obstruction.

CAUSES

Although researchers don't know the immediate cause of testicular cancer, they suspect that cryptorchidism (even when surgically corrected) plays a role in the developing disease. A history of mumps orchitis, inguinal hernia in childhood, or maternal use of diethylstilbestrol (DES) or other estrogen-progestin combinations during pregnancy also increases the risk of developing this disease.

DIAGNOSIS AND TREATMENT

Diagnostic tests may include serum analyses and computed tomography scanning to detect metastasis; excretory urography to detect ureteral displacement; chest X-rays, lymphangiography, ultrasonography, and magnetic resonance imaging to find more metastases; and biopsy to confirm the diagnosis, help stage the disease, and plan treatment.

Treatment includes surgery, radiation therapy, and chemotherapy. Treatment intensity varies with the tumor cell type and stage. Surgical options include orchiectomy and retroperitoneal node dissection to prevent disease extension and assess its stage. Most surgeons remove just the testis, not the scrotum. The patient may need hormonal replacement therapy after bilateral orchiectomy.

Treatment of seminomas involves postoperative radiation to the retroperitoneal and homolateral iliac nodes. Patients whose disease extends to retroperitoneal structures may be given prophylactic radiation to the mediastinal and supraclavicular nodes. Treatment of nonseminomas includes radiation directed to all cancerous lymph nodes.

Chemotherapy is most effective for late-stage seminomas and for most nonseminomas when used for recurrent cancer after orchiectomy and removal of the retroperitoneal lymph nodes.

Autologous bone marrow transplantation is usually reserved for patients who don't respond to standard therapy. It involves giving high-dose chemotherapy, removing and treating the patient's bone marrow to kill remaining cancer cells, and returning the processed bone marrow to the patient.

COLLABORATIVE MANAGEMENT

Care of the patient with testicular cancer focuses on responding to the psychological impact of the disease, preventing postoperative complications, and minimizing and controlling the complications of radiation therapy and chemotherapy.

ASSESSMENT

The patient history may disclose previous injuries to the scrotum, viral infections (such as mumps), or the use of DES or other estrogen-progestin drugs by the patient's mother during pregnancy. Look for:

Sex after testicular cancer surgery

A patient with testicular cancer typically fears loss of sexual function after surgery (orchiectomy). To help him face his fear, provide support and a clear explanation of how orchiectomy affects sexual activity.

After unilateral orchiectomy
Unilateral orchiectomy doesn't cause sterility or impotence. And because most surgeons remove only the diseased testicle and leave the scrotum, later reconstructive surgery can be done. This involves implanting a gel-filled testicular prosthesis, which weighs the same as and feels like a normal testicle. The patient can resume sexual activity after the incision heals.

After bilateral orchiectomy
Bilateral testicular cancer is uncommon. However, if the patient will lose both testes, he'll be sterile. And if nerve or vascular damage (or both) occur with surgery, he'll also be impotent.

Be as positive and supportive as possible. Clearly express that a loss of fertility doesn't mean a loss of masculinity. Typically, the patient will take synthetic hormones to replace or supplement depleted male hormone levels. Surgical insertion of a penile implant can correct impotence.

■ reports of swollen testes or a painless lump found while performing testicular self-examination (usually the first sign)
■ reports of a feeling of heaviness or a dragging sensation in the scrotum
■ gynecomastia (a sign that the tumor is producing chorionic gonadotropins or estrogen)
■ in late disease stages, complaints of weight loss, a cough, hemoptysis, shortness of breath, lethargy, and fatigue; a lethargic, thin, and pallid appearance; a firm, smooth testicular mass; and enlarged lymph nodes in surrounding areas.

NURSING DIAGNOSES AND COLLABORATIVE PROBLEMS
Based on the following nursing diagnoses, you'll establish patient outcomes.

Anxiety related to sexual impairment and disfigurement caused by treatment. The patient will:
■ identify and express feelings of anxiety
■ communicate an understanding of how testicular cancer and its treatment affects sexuality and appearance

■ demonstrate healthy coping behaviors to reduce anxiety.

Body image disturbance related to removal of testis or testes and scrotum. The patient will:
■ acknowledge the change in body image
■ use available resources to cope with body image change
■ express positive feelings about himself.

Sexual dysfunction related to impotence caused by bilateral testicular cancer treatment. The patient will:
■ communicate an understanding of the reason for impotence
■ express acceptance of impotence
■ seek sexual counseling to learn alternative methods for sexual gratification.

PLANNING AND IMPLEMENTATION
These measures help the patient with testicular cancer.
■ Listen to the patient's fears and concerns. Remember that the patient with testicular cancer typically fears sexual impairment and disfigurement. (See *Sex after testicular cancer surgery.*) When possible, provide reassurance and stay with the patient during periods of severe anxiety and stress.
■ Encourage the patient to ask questions. Establish a trusting relationship so that he feels comfortable expressing his concerns.
■ Prepare the patient for orchiectomy, as indicated.
■ During radiation therapy, implement appropriate comfort and safety measures. For example, avoid rubbing the skin near radiation target sites to prevent or minimize pain, skin breakdown, and infection.
■ Monitor the patient for adverse reactions to radiation therapy.
■ During chemotherapy, know what problems to expect and how to prevent or ease them.
■ Give antiemetics, as ordered, to prevent severe nausea and vomiting. Offer the patient small, frequent feedings to maintain oral intake despite anorexia. Devise a mouth care regimen, and check regularly for stomatitis.
■ If the patient receives vinblastine, monitor for signs and symptoms of neurotoxicity (peripheral paresthesia, jaw pain, muscle cramps). If he receives cisplatin, check for ototoxicity.
■ To prevent renal damage during cisplatin therapy, encourage increased fluid intake. To maximize hydration, give I.V. fluids, as ordered, with a potassium supplement. Provide diuresis by giving furosemide or mannitol, as ordered.
■ Monitor the patient for adverse reactions to chemotherapy.

Patient teaching
- Explain tests and possible treatments, their purpose, possible complications, and the care required during and after the treatment.
- Provide reassurance that sterility and impotence usually don't follow unilateral orchiectomy.
- Explain that synthetic hormones can supplement depleted hormone levels.
- Inform the patient that most surgeons don't remove the scrotum. Also explain that a testicular prosthetic implant can correct disfigurement.
- As suitable, review sperm-banking procedures before the patient begins treatment, especially if infertility and impotence may result from surgery.
- Teach the patient how to perform testicular self-examination. Tell him that this is the best way to detect a new or recurrent tumor.
- Refer the patient to organizations that offer information and support during and after treatment, such as the American Cancer Society.

EVALUATION
Achievement of patient outcomes determines the success of collaborative management. For the patient with testicular cancer, evaluation focuses on physiologic status within acceptable parameters, absence of urinary problems, and adequate knowledge of the disease, treatment, prognosis, and care.

Toxic shock syndrome

An acute bacterial infection, toxic shock syndrome is usually associated with continuous use of tampons, especially the superabsorbent type, during menstruation. The incidence of this infection continues to rise, and the recurrence rate is about 30%. Although most patients recover fully, some can develop persistent neurologic and psychological abnormalities, renal failure, a rash, dehydration, and peripheral cyanosis.

CAUSES
Toxic shock syndrome is caused by penicillin-resistant *Staphylococcus aureus*. Although tampons are clearly implicated in this infection, their exact role is uncertain. They may contribute to the infection by:
- introducing *S. aureus* into the vagina during insertion
- absorbing toxin from the vagina
- traumatizing the vaginal mucosa during insertion, thus leading to infection
- providing a favorable environment for growth of *S. aureus*.

When toxic shock syndrome is unrelated to menstruation, it seems linked to *S. aureus* infection in the form of an abscess, osteomyelitis, or postoperative infection.

DIAGNOSIS AND TREATMENT
Isolation of *S. aureus* from vaginal discharge or lesions helps support the diagnosis, but confirmation must follow the criteria set by the Centers for Disease Control and Prevention. These criteria require the presence of at least three of the following:
- GI effects, including vomiting and profuse diarrhea
- muscular effects, with severe myalgia or a fivefold or greater increase in serum creatine kinase levels
- mucous membrane effects such as frank hyperemia
- renal involvement, with blood urea nitrogen or serum creatinine levels at least double the norm
- hepatocellular damage, with levels of serum bilirubin, alanine aminotransferase, and aspartate aminotransferase at least double the norm
- blood involvement, with signs of thrombocytopenia and a platelet count of less than 100,000/μl
- central nervous system effects such as disorientation without focal signs.

Negative results on blood tests for Rocky Mountain spotted fever, leptospirosis, and measles help rule out these disorders.

You'll probably treat the patient with I.V. antistaphylococcal antibiotics that are beta-lactamase resistant, such as oxacillin, cloxacillin, nafcillin, and methicillin. To reverse shock, the patient will need fluid replacement with saline solution and colloids. Other measures may include supportive treatment for diarrhea, nausea, and vomiting.

COLLABORATIVE MANAGEMENT
Care of the patient with toxic shock syndrome focuses on stabilizing vital signs, maintaining fluid balance and neurologic status, and providing patient teaching.

ASSESSMENT
The patient commonly reports that she consistently uses tampons—especially the superabsorbent type—throughout menstruation and changes them infrequently. Look for:
- complaints of intense myalgia, vomiting, diarrhea, and headache
- a temperature of over 104° F (40° C)
- rigors, conjunctival hyperemia, vaginal hyperemia, and vaginal discharge
- a deep-red rash, especially on the palms and soles, appearing within a few hours of the onset of infection and later peeling off

- listlessness and confusion
- palpable signs of shock (a rapid, thready pulse and hypotension).

NURSING DIAGNOSES AND COLLABORATIVE PROBLEMS

Based on the following nursing diagnoses, you'll establish patient outcomes.

Altered thought processes related to neurologic dysfunction. The patient will:
- remain safe in her environment
- regain normal thought processes with eradication of toxic shock syndrome.

Diarrhea related to infectious process. The patient will:
- control her diarrhea with medication
- show no signs or symptoms of complications associated with diarrhea, such as skin breakdown or electrolyte imbalance.

Fluid volume deficit related to diarrhea and shock. The patient will:
- regain and maintain normal vital signs
- regain and maintain normal fluid balance
- produce an adequate urine volume.

PLANNING AND IMPLEMENTATION

These measures help the patient with toxic shock syndrome.
- Obtain specimens of vaginal and cervical secretions for culture of *S. aureus*.
- Use standard precautions for any vaginal discharge and lesion drainage.
- Give I.V. antibiotics over a 15-minute period to ensure peak levels that destroy microorganisms. Watch for signs of penicillin allergy.
- Check neurologic status and vital signs every 4 to 8 hours.
- Monitor intake, output, and weight daily to assess fluid balance and to prevent dehydration and renal failure. Replace fluids I.V., as ordered.
- Assess the degree of diarrhea, and watch for signs of dehydration. Inspect the perianal area for signs of breakdown if the patient has diarrhea.
- Monitor serum electrolyte levels for changes indicating possible imbalances.
- Reorient the patient as needed. Use appropriate safety measures to prevent injury.
- Give analgesics cautiously because of the risk of hypotension and liver failure.

Patient teaching
- Tell the patient to avoid using tampons, particularly the superabsorbent type, because of the risk of recurrence.

EVALUATION

Achievement of patient outcomes determines the success of collaborative management. For the patient with toxic shock syndrome, evaluation focuses on vital signs, fluid balance, and neurologic status within acceptable parameters; absence of complications; and adequate knowledge of the disorder, treatment, care, and prevention.

Trichomoniasis

Trichomoniasis is a protozoal infection of the lower genitourinary tract that affects about 15% of sexually active females and 10% of sexually active males. Usually spread by sexual contact, trichomoniasis also is spread by contaminated douche equipment or moist washcloths or, if the mother is infected, by vaginal delivery. In females, the condition is either acute or chronic. Recurrence of trichomoniasis is minimized when sexual partners are treated concurrently.

CAUSES

Trichomoniasis is caused by the organism *Trichomonas vaginalis*. Risk factors for infection include pregnancy, bacterial overgrowth, exudative vaginal or cervical lesions, frequent douching, and use of oral contraceptives.

DIAGNOSIS AND TREATMENT

Direct microscopic examination of vaginal or seminal discharge is diagnostic when it reveals *T. vaginalis*. Urine specimens that are clear may also reveal *T. vaginalis*. A cytologic cervical smear may be abnormal in untreated trichomoniasis.

Oral metronidazole given simultaneously to both sexual partners cures trichomoniasis. The recommended dosage is 250 mg given three times a day for 7 days or one 2-g dose. Oral metronidazole hasn't been proven safe during the first trimester of pregnancy. A pregnant patient in the first trimester may insert a clotrimazole vaginal tablet at bedtime for 7 days for symptomatic relief. Sitz baths may also help relieve symptoms.

After treatment, both sexual partners require a follow-up examination for residual signs of infection.

COLLABORATIVE MANAGEMENT

Care of the patient with trichomoniasis focuses on curing the infection and teaching the patient how to avoid reinfection.

ASSESSMENT

Approximately 70% of infected females—including those with chronic infections—and most infected males are asymptomatic. Acute infection may produce variable signs and symptoms. Women may develop a vaginal discharge (gray or greenish yellow and possibly profuse, frothy, and malodorous), "strawberry spots" on the cervix, severe itching, redness, swelling, tenderness, dyspareunia, dysuria, and urinary frequency. They may also experience postcoital spotting, menorrhagia, or dysmenorrhea.

Men with trichomoniasis may develop transient, mild to severe urethritis, dysuria, or urinary frequency.

NURSING DIAGNOSES AND COLLABORATIVE PROBLEMS

Based on the following nursing diagnoses, you'll establish patient outcomes.

Risk for infection related to high communicability. The patient will:
- demonstrate proper infection-control measures
- exhibit negative cytology results when testing is repeated.

Pain related to infection. The patient will:
- demonstrate measures to control pain and increase comfort
- state that pain is decreased.

Anxiety related to diagnosis and treatment. The patient will:
- use positive coping strategies
- demonstrate signs of decreased anxiety.

PLANNING AND IMPLEMENTATION

These measures help the patient with trichomoniasis.
- To prevent neonates from contracting trichomoniasis, make sure that infected pregnant women receive adequate treatment before delivery.
- Encourage good hand washing and perineal hygiene.
- Assess the patient's degree of pain; give drugs as ordered and monitor their effectiveness.
- Encourage the patient to perform self-care measures that relieve her symptoms, such as frequent perineal care.
- Encourage the patient to verbalize her feelings about the disease and its treatment.

Patient teaching
- Tell the patient not to douche before being examined for trichomoniasis to avoid washing away evidence of the infection.
- To help prevent reinfection during treatment, advise the patient to abstain from intercourse or use condoms.
- Warn the patient to abstain from alcoholic beverages while taking metronidazole because alcohol may provoke a disulfiram-type reaction (confusion, headache, cramps, vomiting, and seizures).

- Tell the patient that metronidazole may turn urine dark brown.
- Caution a female patient to avoid reinfection by contaminated douche equipment.
- Advise a female patient that chronic douching can alter vaginal pH. Tell her she can reduce the risk of genitourinary bacterial growth by wearing loose-fitting, cotton underwear that allows ventilation; bacteria flourish in a warm, dark, moist environment.

EVALUATION

Achievement of patient outcomes determines the success of collaborative management. For the patient with trichomoniasis, evaluation focuses on resolution of the infection, absence of symptoms, and adequate knowledge of the disease, treatment, follow-up, and prevention.

Uterine cancer

The most common gynecologic cancer, uterine cancer (cancer of the endometrium) typically affects postmenopausal women between ages 50 and 60. It's uncommon between ages 30 and 40 and rare before age 30. Most premenopausal women who develop uterine cancer have a history of anovulatory menstrual cycles or another hormonal imbalance. About 33,000 new cases of uterine cancer are reported annually; of these, roughly 5,500 are eventually fatal.

In most patients, uterine cancer is an adenocarcinoma that metastasizes late, usually from the endometrium to the cervix, ovaries, fallopian tubes, and other peritoneal structures. It may spread to distant organs, such as the lungs and the brain, by way of the blood or the lymphatic system. Lymph node involvement can also occur. Less common uterine tumors include adenoacanthoma, endometrial stromal sarcoma, lymphosarcoma, mixed mesodermal tumors (including carcinosarcoma), and leiomyosarcoma.

Intestinal obstruction, ascites, increasing pain, and hemorrhage can result from disease progression.

CAUSES

Uterine cancer appears linked to several predisposing factors:
- history of infertility, anovulation, or nulliparity
- history of uterine polyps or endometrial hyperplasia
- abnormal uterine bleeding
- obesity, hypertension, or diabetes
- prolonged estrogen therapy without use of progesterone
- familial tendency.

Using a dilator

After undergoing intracavitary radiation, the patient may need to use a dilator to relieve vaginal narrowing resulting from scar tissue. Tell the patient to insert the dilator once or twice a day and leave it in her vagina for about 5 minutes. Also, note the following:

- The dilator should feel smooth. If it has flaws or rough spots, the patient should use another one.
- Before and after each insertion, she should wash the dilator with soap and water.
- She should apply a water-soluble lubricant (such as K-Y Jelly) to the tip of the dilator before insertion.
- To properly insert the dilator, the patient should lie on her back with her knees slightly apart and then insert the dilator into the vagina as far as possible without causing pain.
- Dilator use may cause mild discomfort or a pink or slightly bloody discharge. Significant, menstrual-like bleeding should not occur.

DIAGNOSIS AND TREATMENT

Diagnostic tests may include endometrial, cervical, or endocervical biopsy to confirm cancer cells and fractional dilatation and curettage (D&C) when the disease is suspected but the endometrial biopsy is negative.

Positive diagnosis requires the following tests to provide baseline data and permit staging: multiple cervical biopsies and endocervical curettage to pinpoint cervical involvement; Schiller's test, where cancerous tissues resist a stain; computed tomography scanning or magnetic resonance imaging to detect metastasis to other organs; excretory urography and, possibly, cystoscopy to evaluate the urinary system; proctoscopy or barium enema studies if bladder and rectal involvement are suspected; and blood studies, urinalysis, and electrocardiography.

Depending on the cancer's extent, treatment may include surgery, radiation therapy, hormonal therapy, and chemotherapy (when other treatments have failed).

COLLABORATIVE MANAGEMENT

Care of the patient with uterine cancer focuses on restoring function and providing patient teaching.

ASSESSMENT

The patient history may reflect one or more predisposing factors. A younger patient may report spotting and protracted, heavy menstrual periods. A post-menopausal woman may report that bleeding began 12 or more months after menses had stopped. In either case, the patient may describe the discharge as watery at first, then blood-streaked, and gradually becoming bloodier.

In more advanced stages, palpation may disclose an enlarged uterus.

NURSING DIAGNOSES AND COLLABORATIVE PROBLEMS

Based on the following nursing diagnoses, you'll establish patient outcomes.

Fear related to possible metastasis. The patient will:
- express fears related to uterine cancer
- use available support systems to assist in coping with fear
- report reduced feelings of fear.

Risk for infection related to immunosuppression caused by radiation therapy or chemotherapy. The patient will:
- incorporate infection-control measures into everyday life
- maintain a normal body temperature and white blood cell (WBC) count
- show no signs or symptoms of infection.

Sexual dysfunction related to surgical procedure. The patient will:
- express feelings about changes in sexuality
- use available support systems to cope with changes in sexual function
- reestablish sexual activity at her pre-illness level.

PLANNING AND IMPLEMENTATION

These measures help the patient with uterine cancer.
- Listen to the patient's fears and concerns. She may fear for her survival and be concerned that treatment will alter her lifestyle or prevent sexual intimacy.
- Encourage her to use available support systems to cope with loss of fertility, if applicable.
- Remain with the patient during periods of severe stress and anxiety.
- Give ordered pain medications as necessary, and evaluate their effectiveness. Many patients who require drugs for this disease are in the late stages.
- Encourage the patient to identify actions that promote comfort, and then remember to perform them as often as possible. Provide distractions and help her perform relaxation techniques that may ease her discomfort.
- Prepare the patient for surgery, as indicated.
- Find out whether she will have internal or external radiation or both. Usually, internal radiation therapy is used first. (See *Using a dilator.*) Provide supportive care for adverse effects of radiation therapy or chemotherapy.

Protecting yourself from radiation exposure

There are three cardinal rules in internal radiation therapy:
- *Time.* Wear a radiosensitive badge to keep track of your total dose. Remember, your exposure increases with time, and the effects are cumulative. Therefore, carefully plan the time you spend with the patient to prevent overexposure. (However, don't rush procedures, ignore the patient's psychological needs, or give the impression you can't get out of the room fast enough.)
- *Distance.* Radiation loses its intensity with distance. Avoid standing at the foot of the patient's bed, where you're in line with the radiation source.
- *Shield.* Lead shields reduce radiation exposure. Use them whenever possible.

   In internal radiation therapy, remember that the patient is radioactive while the radiation source is in place, usually 48 to 72 hours. Also, note the following:
- If you're pregnant, you should not be assigned to care for a patient undergoing radiation therapy.
- Check the position of the source applicator every 4 hours. If it appears dislodged, notify the doctor immediately. If it's completely dislodged, remove the patient from the bed; then pick up the applicator with long forceps, place it on a lead-shielded transport cart, and notify the doctor immediately.

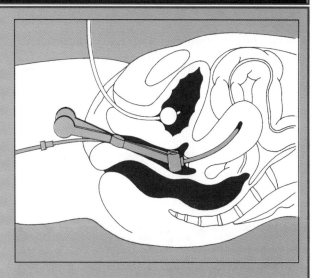

- *Never* pick up the radiation source with your bare hands. Notify the doctor and radiation safety officer whenever an accident occurs, and keep a lead-shielded transport cart on the unit as long as the patient has a radiation source in place.

- Monitor the patient's complete blood count (including differential) regularly for signs of immunosuppression caused by radiation therapy and chemotherapy.
- Monitor vital signs and watch for signs and symptoms of infection, bleeding, and anemia.
- Assess the patient for other adverse effects of uterine cancer or its treatments.

Patient teaching
- Discuss the tests used to diagnose and stage the disease, and explain potential treatments.
- Emphasize that prompt treatment significantly improves the patient's chances of survival.
- If your patient is premenopausal, explain that removal of her ovaries will induce menopause.
- As appropriate, explain that except in total pelvic exenteration, the vagina remains intact and that sexual intercourse will be possible once she recovers.
- Describe the procedure for radiation therapy. Answer questions, explain why you may need to limit your exposure, and counsel her about radiation's adverse effects. Tell her to rest frequently and maintain a well-balanced diet during radiation treatment. (See *Protecting yourself from radiation exposure.*)

- To minimize skin breakdown and reduce the risk of skin infection, tell her to keep the treatment area dry, to avoid wearing clothes that rub against the area, and to avoid using heating pads, alcohol rubs, or irritating skin creams.
- Because radiation therapy increases susceptibility to infection (possibly by lowering the WBC count), encourage her to avoid people with colds or other infections.
- Explain chemotherapy or immunotherapy to the patient and her family, and make sure they know what adverse effects to expect and how to alleviate them.
- If the patient is receiving a synthetic form of progesterone, such as hydroxyprogesterone, medroxyprogesterone, or megestrol, tell her to watch for depression, dizziness, backache, swelling, breast tenderness, irritability, and abdominal cramps.
- Instruct her to report symptoms of thrombophlebitis, such as pain in the calves, numbness, tingling, or loss of leg function.
- Advise the patient receiving chemotherapy to have her WBC count checked weekly, and reinforce the importance of preventing infection. Assure her that hair loss is temporary.

■ If the patient undergoing chemotherapy is employed, point out that continuing to work during this period may offer an important diversion. Advise her to try to arrange a flexible work schedule with her employer.

■ Refer the patient to the social services department and to community services that offer psychological support and information, such as the American Cancer Society.

EVALUATION
Achievement of patient outcomes determines the success of collaborative management. For the patient with uterine cancer, evaluation focuses on physiologic status within acceptable parameters, positive coping skills, and adequate knowledge of the disease, prognosis, treatment, care, and follow-up.

Uterine fibroid tumors

Also known as myomas, fibromyomas, and leiomyomas, these neoplasms are the most common benign tumors in women, affecting approximately 20% of all women over age 35. They are three times more common in blacks than whites and become malignant (leiomyosarcoma) in only 0.1% of patients.

CAUSES
The cause of uterine fibroids is unknown, but excessive levels of estrogen and human growth hormone (HGH) probably influence tumor formation by stimulating susceptible fibromuscular elements. Large doses of estrogen and the later stages of pregnancy increase both tumor size and HGH levels. Conversely, uterine leiomyomas usually shrink or disappear after menopause, when estrogen production decreases.

Uterine fibroids usually grow in multiples in the uterine corpus, although they may appear on the cervix or on the round or broad ligament.

DIAGNOSIS AND TREATMENT
Blood studies showing anemia support the diagnosis. Dilatation and curettage or submucosal hysterosalpingography detects submucosal leiomyomas, and laparoscopy visualizes subserous leiomyomas on the uterine surface.

Appropriate intervention depends on the severity of symptoms, the size and location of the tumors, and the patient's age, parity, pregnancy status, desire to have children, and general health.

The traditional treatment for a young woman who wants to have children is surgical removal of small fi-

broids that have caused problems in the past or that appear likely to threaten a future pregnancy.

A new outpatient procedure called myolyosis also preserves the uterus and childbearing potential. Usually after pretreatment with the fibroid-shrinking drug leuprolide, the surgeon performs a regular ambulatory laparoscopy and inserts a specially designed needle through a small puncture site in the lower abdomen. He repeatedly punctures the fibroids with this needle and coagulates them with an electrical current. The coagulation reduces fibroid size, and the devascularized tissue remains in place. Myolyosis is recommended for fibroids under 10 cm in diameter, but not for precancerous or cancerous conditions of the uterus or ovaries.

Tumors that twist or grow large enough to cause intestinal obstruction require a hysterectomy, with preservation of the ovaries if possible. Other surgical alternatives to hysterectomy include submucous resection of small fibroids; myomectomy, which usually leaves the uterus intact; and supercervical hysterectomy, which leaves the cervix intact.

If a pregnant patient has a uterus no larger than a 6-month normal uterus by the sixteenth week of pregnancy, the outcome for the pregnancy remains favorable, and surgery is usually unnecessary. However, if a pregnant woman has a leiomyomatous uterus the size of a 5- to 6-month normal uterus by the ninth week of pregnancy, spontaneous abortion will probably occur, especially with a cervical leiomyoma. If surgery is necessary, a hysterectomy is usually performed 5 to 6 months after delivery (when involution is complete), with preservation of the ovaries if possible.

COLLABORATIVE MANAGEMENT
Care of the patient with uterine fibroids focuses on improving blood study values and providing patient teaching.

ASSESSMENT
Clinical signs and symptoms include submucosal hypermenorrhea (the cardinal sign) and possibly other forms of abnormal endometrial bleeding, dysmenorrhea, and pain. If the tumor is large, the patient may develop a feeling of heaviness in the abdomen along with pain, intestinal obstruction, constipation, urinary frequency or urgency, and irregular uterine enlargement.

NURSING DIAGNOSES AND COLLABORATIVE PROBLEMS
Based on the following nursing diagnoses, you'll establish patient outcomes.

Anxiety related to diagnosis. The patient will:
■ demonstrate positive coping strategies

■ state that anxiety is diminished.
Risk for fluid volume deficit related to bleeding. The patient will:
■ exhibit vital signs and laboratory counts within normal limits
■ demonstrate a balance of fluid intake and output
■ maintain a stable weight.

PLANNING AND IMPLEMENTATION
These measures help the patient with uterine fibroids.
■ Monitor her vital signs, hemoglobin levels, and intake and output.
■ In a patient with severe anemia due to excessive bleeding, give iron and blood transfusions, as ordered.
■ Encourage the patient to verbalize her feelings about the condition. Reassure her and answer her questions honestly.
■ Encourage her to identify and use effective coping mechanisms.
■ Give antianxiety medications as ordered, and monitor their effectiveness.

Patient teaching
■ Tell the patient to report any abnormal bleeding or pelvic pain immediately.
■ If a hysterectomy or an oophorectomy is indicated, explain the effects of the operation on menstruation, menopause, and sexual activity. Reassure the patient that she won't experience premature menopause if her ovaries are left intact.
■ If she must undergo a multiple myomectomy, make sure she understands that pregnancy is still possible. However, if the surgeon must enter the uterine cavity, explain that she may need a cesarean delivery.

EVALUATION
Achievement of patient outcomes determines the success of collaborative management. For the patient with uterine fibroid tumors, evaluation focuses on hemodynamic status within acceptable parameters, positive coping strategies, absence of postoperative complications (if appropriate), and adequate knowledge of the disorder, treatment, and care.

Treatments and procedures

Various surgical procedures may be peformed to treat reproductive disorders. These include dilatation and curettage, hysterectomy, myomectomy, orchiectomy, and prostatectomy.

DILATATION AND CURETTAGE
Dilatation and curettage (D&C) is used to treat an incomplete abortion, to control abnormal uterine bleeding, and to obtain an endometrial or endocervical tissue specimen for cytologic study. A similar procedure, dilatation and evacuation (D&E), may be used to perform a therapeutic abortion, usually within the first trimester of pregnancy but occasionally as late as 16 weeks.

PROCEDURE
In these most common gynecologic procedures, the doctor expands or dilates the cervix to access the endocervix and uterus. In D&C, he uses a curette to scrape endometrial tissue; in D&E, he applies suction to extract the uterine contents.

COLLABORATIVE MANAGEMENT
Care of the patient undergoing D&C requires thorough preparation, close monitoring, and intense patient teaching.

Preparation
■ Confirm that the patient has followed preoperative directions for fasting and has used an enema to empty her colon before admission.
■ Remind her that she'll feel groggy after the procedure and won't be able to drive. Make sure that she has arranged transportation home.
■ Ask the patient to void before you give her any preoperative drugs, such as meperidine or diazepam.
■ Start I.V. fluids (either dextrose 5% in water or normal saline solution), as ordered, to facilitate administration of the anesthetic.
■ For D&C or D&E, the patient may receive a general anesthetic, a regional paracervical block, or a local anesthetic.

Monitoring and aftercare
■ Monitor the patient's vital signs until she's stable, and assess bleeding.
■ After surgery, give analgesics as ordered. Inform the patient that she'll probably have moderate cramping and pelvic and low back pain but that she should report any continuous, sharp abdominal pain that does not respond to analgesics—an indicator of a perforated uterus.
■ Monitor the patient for hemorrhage and signs of infection, such as purulent, foul-smelling vaginal drainage and hematuria. Report any of these signs immediately.
■ Give her fluids as tolerated, and allow her to eat if she requests food.
■ Keep the bed's side rails raised, and help her walk to the bathroom if appropriate.

Patient teaching

■ Tell the patient to report any signs of infection. Advise her to avoid using tampons and bathing in a tub because these actions increase the infection risk.

■ Tell her to use analgesics to control pain but to report any unrelenting sharp pain. Spotting and discharge may last a week or longer (up to 4 weeks after an abortion procedure). Tell her to report any bright red blood.

■ Advise the patient to schedule a follow-up appointment with the doctor.

■ Tell her to resume activity as tolerated but to follow her doctor's instructions for avoiding vigorous exercise and sexual intercourse (usually until 2 weeks after the follow-up visit).

■ Encourage her to seek birth control counseling, if needed, and refer her to an appropriate center.

COMPLICATIONS

Potential complications of D&C or D&E include uterine perforation, hemorrhage, and infection. If the patient suffers cervical trauma during these procedures, subsequent pregnancies may be affected. Rarely, such trauma can lead to spontaneous abortion, cervical incompetence, or premature birth. Neither D&C nor D&E is appropriate if the patient has an acute infection.

HYSTERECTOMY

A hysterectomy is a surgical procedure that involves removal of the uterus. Common indications for the procedure include malignant or benign tumors in or on the uterus, cervix, or adnexa; uterine bleeding and hemorrhage; uterine rupture or perforation; life-threatening pelvic infection; endometriosis that's unresponsive to conservative treatment; and pelvic floor relaxation or prolapse. (See *Managing total radical hysterectomy*, pages 498 and 499.)

PROCEDURE

The surgeon may perform a hysterectomy abdominally, vaginally, or through a laparoscope. In a laparoscopic hysterectomy, the surgeon uses the laparoscope to perform preparatory steps before removing the uterus through the vagina.

A hysterectomy is classified as either subtotal, total, panhysterectomy, or radical. Rarely performed today, a subtotal hysterectomy is the removal of the entire uterus except for the cervix. In a total hysterectomy, both the uterus and the cervix are removed. In a panhysterectomy, the entire uterus as well as the ovaries and the fallopian tubes are removed. And in a radical hysterectomy, the uterus, ovaries, fallopian tubes, adjoining ligaments and lymph nodes, upper one-third of the vagina, and surrounding tissues are all removed. Because of the extensiveness of the procedure, a radical hysterectomy requires an abdominal approach.

After the patient has been given general anesthesia, the surgeon makes the incision. For an abdominal approach, he makes a midline vertical incision from the umbilicus to the symphysis pubis or a horizontal incision in the lower abdomen. He then excises and removes the uterus and necessary accompanying structures. Afterward, he closes the incision and applies a dressing and perineal pad.

For a vaginal approach, the surgeon makes an incision inside the vagina above, but near, the cervix. After excising the uterus, he removes it through the vaginal canal. He then closes the opening to the peritoneal cavity with sutures and applies a perineal pad.

In a laparoscopic approach, the surgeon makes an incision in the umbilicus. He then infuses nitrous oxide or carbon dioxide into the abdominal cavity. This lifts the abdominal wall away from the abdominal organs, making viewing easier. The patient is then placed in the Trendelenburg position, which causes the small intestine to fall out of the pelvis, thus creating room for the instruments. The surgeon then inserts the laparoscope, which allows him to view the pelvic cavity. If he's using an operative laparoscope, no other incisions are required because this device contains a channel through which he can pass instruments. Otherwise, he'll make several other small abdominal incisions through which he'll pass the instruments to excise the uterus. After excising the uterus and any accompanying structures, the surgeon removes them vaginally. He then closes the incision and applies a dressing and perineal pad.

COLLABORATIVE MANAGEMENT

Care of the patient undergoing a hysterectomy requires thorough preparation, close monitoring, and intense patient teaching.

Preparation

■ Discuss the patient's expectations about menstrual and reproductive status after surgery, and answer any questions she may have about the procedure and her physical recovery.

■ Review the surgical approach and the extent of the excision. Tell her to expect a cleansing enema the evening before surgery and prophylactic antibiotics as ordered.

■ Make sure that preoperative laboratory tests have been performed and review the results.

■ Tell the patient about postoperative care measures. Explain that you'll ask her to turn, cough, and perform deep-breathing exercises often. Show her how to use an incentive spirometer.

- Tell her that after surgery she'll lie in a supine or other position to prevent pelvic congestion.
- Tell her that you'll encourage her to get out of bed and walk as soon as possible to prevent venous stasis.
- If she's having an abdominal hysterectomy, explain that she may require an indwelling urinary catheter or a suprapubic tube after surgery to prevent urine retention. Also explain that a nasogastric or rectal tube may be in place to prevent abdominal distention.
- Tell the patient that she'll probably have abdominal cramping and moderate amounts of drainage postoperatively and that she'll have a perineal pad in place.

Monitoring and aftercare

- Encourage the patient to cough, breathe deeply, and turn frequently (at least every 2 hours). Monitor her respiratory status for abnormalities that suggest complications such as pneumonia.
- Keep the patient in a supine position or a low Fowler's or semi-Fowler's position, but remember to change her position every 2 hours.
- Provide and regulate I.V. fluids as ordered until the patient can resume oral intake. Monitor intake and output and vital signs regularly.
- Auscultate for bowel sounds regularly. Give the patient nothing by mouth until peristalsis has returned and the doctor has said she can eat.
- Provide analgesics to relieve cramps or abdominal pain.
- Help her to begin walking as soon as ordered. Encourage her to perform the prescribed exercises to prevent venous stasis.
- Provide indwelling urinary catheter or suprapubic catheter care, if appropriate.
- Assess the patient's vaginal drainage and change her perineal pad frequently. Notify the doctor if she saturates more than one pad every 4 hours.
- If the patient has had an abdominal or laparoscopic hysterectomy, assess the abdominal incisions for drainage and bleeding.
- If she has had a vaginal or laparoscopic hysterectomy, provide perineal care.
- Assist with suture or clip removal (usually by the fifth postoperative day) in the patient with an abdominal or laparoscopic hysterectomy. Reassure the patient with a vaginal hysterectomy that vaginal sutures are usually absorbed.

Patient teaching

- If the patient has had a vaginal or laparoscopic hysterectomy, instruct her to report severe cramping, heavy bleeding, or hot flashes to her doctor immediately.

- If she's had an abdominal hysterectomy, tell her to avoid heavy lifting, rapid walking, or dancing, which can cause pelvic congestion. Encourage her to walk a little more each day and to avoid sitting for a prolonged period. Tell her that swimming is permissible but that she should avoid tub baths, douching, and sexual activity until after her 6-week checkup.
- Tell her to eat a high-protein, high-residue diet to avoid constipation, which may increase abdominal pressure. Her doctor may also order increased fluids (3 qt [3 L]/day).
- Advise the patient to express her feelings about her altered body image and to contact the doctor if she has questions about any changes.
- Explain to the patient and family members that she may temporarily feel depressed or irritable because of abrupt hormonal fluctuations. Encourage family members to respond calmly and with understanding.
- If the patient has had a panhysterectomy or radical hysterectomy, instruct her to discuss the potential for hormonal and calcium supplementation with her doctor.

COMPLICATIONS

Potential complications include wound infection, urine retention, abdominal distention, thromboembolism, atelectasis, pneumonia, hemorrhage, and ureteral or bowel injury. After an abdominal hysterectomy, the patient may also experience wound dehiscence, pulmonary embolism, or a paralytic ileus. Vaginal or laparoscopic hysterectomy usually causes fewer complications.

Regardless of the type of hysterectomy performed, the patient may also experience psychological complications, such as depression (the most common), loss of libido, and a perceived loss of femininity.

MYOMECTOMY

Myomectomy is the surgical removal of uterine fibroid tumors, preserving the uterus. This procedure is indicated for a woman of childbearing years who wants to have children, regardless of the size, number, or location of the fibroids. In 25% of the patients undergoing myomectomy, fibroids recur and may require a hysterectomy.

PROCEDURE

The surgeon uses a laser to remove the fibroids during the proliferative phase of the menstrual cycle to minimize blood loss and avoid interrupting an unknown pregnancy.

(Text continues on page 500.)

Managing total radical hysterectomy

CARE ELEMENT	Pre-admission	Day 1 (Surgery)	Day 2 (Postop Day 1)
CARE UNIT	■ Women's clinic	■ Post-anesthesia care unit ■ Postoperative unit	■ Postoperative unit
CONSULTS			
LAB TESTS	■ Per anesthesia guidelines ■ Urinalysis		■ Complete blood count @ 0600
ASSESSMENTS	Call doctor for: ■ Urine output <120 ml/4 hr ■ Jackson-Pratt (JP) drainage >____ ■ Temperature >38.5 ■ Heart rate >120 <60 ■ Systolic BP >180 <90 ■ Diastolic BP >105 <50 ■ Resp >30 <10	■ Routine nursing assessment ■ Vital signs (VS) check every 2 hr x 4, then every 4 hr ■ Empty: – Nasogastric (NG) tube every 4 hr – JP drains every 4 hr – Urethral catheter and suprapubic (SP) catheter every 4 hr) ■ Monitor: – Dressing every 4 hr – Intake and output (I&O) every 4 hr.	■ Routine nursing assessment ■ VS check every 4 hr. ■ Empty: JP and SP drain every 4 hr. ■ Monitor: – Incision every 4 hr – I&O every 4 hr
TREATMENTS		■ Incentive spirometer (IS) every 1 hr x 10 breaths between 0800 and 2200 ■ Turn every 2 hr ■ Pneumatic compression device ■ NG tube to low intermittent suction; flush with 100 ml tap water every shift and as needed (p.r.n.)	■ IS every 1 hr x 10 breaths between 0800 and 2200 ■ Turn every 2 hours while in bed ■ Pneumatic compression device ■ Discontinue NG if ordered ■ Discontinue urethral catheter only if SP catheter functioning well ■ JP dressing change every shift p.r.n. ■ SP site care every shift
ACTIVITY		■ Bed rest	■ Walk in hallway 2 times/shift days and evening with assistance.
MEDICATIONS	■ 1 bottle magnesium citrate evening before surgery	■ D₅ ½ NS +20 mEq KCL @ 125 ml/hr ■ Pepcid 20 mg I.V. every 12 hr	■ D₅ ½ NS +20 mEq KCL @ 125 ml/hr ■ Pepcid 20 mg I.V. every 12 hr
PAIN SYMPTOM CONTROL	Patient-controlled analgesia (PCA): morphine sulfate (MSO₄)	■ PCA: MSO₄ 1 mg with 6-min lockout (L/O); 10 mg max/hr ■ Phenergan 12.5 to 25 mg I.V. every 4 to 6 hr p.r.n.	■ PCA: MSO₄ 1 mg with 6 min L/O; 10 mg max/hr ■ Phenergan 12.5 to 25 mg I.V. every 4 to 6 hr p.r.n.
NUTRITION		■ Nothing by mouth (NPO) ■ Chips & sips (while NG tube in place)	■ NPO ■ Chips & sips (while NG tube in place)
DISCHARGE PLANNING AND TEACHING	■ Clinics distribute: –Adult health questionnaire (AHQ) –Patient clinical path and booklet.	■ Orient to: – Unit – IS – Pneumatic compression device – Turning every 2 hr – PCA use – NPO; ice only. ■ AHQ by family if patient unable	■ Complete AHQ (if not done). ■ Reinforce postop routine. ■ Review clinical path. ■ Discuss suprapubic site care with patient during process.

Adapted with permission from Shands Hospital at the University of Florida, Gainesville.

Day 3 (Postop Day 2)	Day 4 (Postop Day 3)	Day 5 (Postop Day 4)
■ Postoperative unit	■ Postoperative unit	■ Discharge
■ Routine nursing assessment ■ VS check every 4 hr ■ Empty JP and SP drains ■ Monitor: – Incision every shift – I&O every 4 hr.	■ Routine nursing assessment ■ VS check every 4 hr ■ Empty JP and SP drains every shift. ■ Assess for flatus/bowel movement (BM). ■ Monitor: – Incision every shift – I&O every 4 hr.	■ Routine nursing assessment ■ VS check every shift ■ Assess JP and SP drains. ■ Assess for flatus/BM.
■ IS every 1 hr x 10 breaths between 0800 and 2200 ■ Turn every 2 hr while in bed. ■ Pneumatic compression device ■ Discontinue NG tube if ordered. ■ Discontinue urethral catheter only if SP catheter functioning well ■ JP dressing change every shift ■ SP site care every shift ■ SP to large leg bag between 0800 and 2200; monitor and empty every 2 hr (switch to bedside drain bag [Foley bag] at night)	■ IS every 1 hr x 10 breaths between 0800 and 2200 ■ Encourage patient to turn every 2 hr. ■ Pneumatic compression device (discontinue if ambulating t.i.d. each shift) ■ I.V. site change/care ■ JP dressing change every shift ■ SP to large leg bag between 0800 and 2200; monitor and empty every 2 hr (switch to bedside drain bag [Foley bag] at night)	■ SP site care by patient
■ Walk in hallway 3 times/shift and evenings with assistance	■ Out of bed in chair for meals ■ Walk in hallway 4 times/shift days & evening with assistance.	■ Walk as tolerated with restrictions.
■ D$_5$½ NS +20 mEq KCL @ 125 ml/hr ■ Pepcid 20 mg I.V. every 12 hr	■ Medlock I.V. as per order ■ Discontinue Pepcid if tolerating clears.	■ Discontinue Medlock.
■ PCA: MSO$_4$ 1 mg with 6-min lockout; 10 mg max/hr ■ Phenergan 12.5 to 25 mg I.V. every 4 to 6 hr p.r.n.	■ Switch from PCA to Tylox 1 to 2 every 4 hr p.r.n. for pain per doctor's order. ■ Phenergan 12.5 to 25 mg I.V. every 4 to 6 hr p.r.n.	■ Tylox 1 to 2 every 4 hr p.r.n. for pain
■ NPO ■ Chips & sips (while NG tube in place)	■ Diet per doctor's order	■ Diet per doctor's order
■ Patient demonstration of SP site care with assistance ■ Leg bag instructions with demonstration by nurse	■ Patient demonstration of SP site care ■ Leg bag instructions with demonstration by nurse ■ Patient return demonstration of leg bag in p.m.	■ Review discharge instructions: – Discharge medications – Activity restrictions – Nothing in vagina for 6 to 8 weeks – Take temperature twice/day. Notify if >101° F., increased pain, or bleeding. – SP care. ■ Provide discharge instruction sheet.

DISCHARGE READY ▶ **After orchiectomy**

After undergoing orchiectomy, the patient will meet the following criteria before discharge:

- temperature within his normal limits
- vital signs within his normal limits
- no evidence of complications
- pain controlled with oral analgesics
- voiding within his normal limits
- healing incisions
- knowledge of follow-up care.

COLLABORATIVE MANAGEMENT

Care of the patient undergoing myomectomy requires thorough preparation, close monitoring, and intense patient teaching.

Preparation

- Review the options for surgery with the patient, including advantages and risks, preoperative and postoperative procedures, and convalescence needs.
- Prepare the patient for surgery, for example, by giving her a douche and an enema and shaving her abdomen or perineum.
- Confirm that results of laboratory tests, such as blood tests, chest X-ray, electrocardiogram, and urinalysis, are on the chart.
- Expect to give the patient diazepam, atropine, and prophylactic antibiotics.

Monitoring and aftercare

- Monitor the patient's vital signs until she's stable.
- Assess the amount of vaginal bleeding.
- Check the incision site for intactness.
- Maintain and monitor the patient's indwelling urinary catheter for 24 to 48 hours.
- Give her analgesics as ordered, and assess their effectiveness.
- Help prevent atelectasis and pneumonia by encouraging the patient to cough and breathe deeply.

Patient teaching

- Tell the patient to avoid or limit stair climbing for 1 month.
- Advise her to avoid tub baths and sitting for long periods because these activities pool blood in the pelvic vessels.
- Tell the patient to avoid strenuous activity or lifting anything weighing more than 10 lbs (4.5 kg).
- Tell her that she shouldn't drive a vehicle for at least 1 week.

COMPLICATIONS

Bleeding and recurrent fibroids are potential complications.

ORCHIECTOMY

Orchiectomy, surgical removal of one or both testes, is the surgery indicated for testicular cancer. Although orchiectomy is a relatively minor surgical procedure, it can have significant psychological impact on the patient and his family. Orchiectomy itself doesn't affect potency, but it threatens body image for many men. Bilateral orchiectomy and postsurgical radiation and chemotherapy threaten fertility.

PROCEDURE

The testis is removed through a high inguinal incision. At the time of surgery, the doctor performs a biopsy and then plans further treatments (radiation, chemotherapy, lymphadenectomy). The surgeon may perform a retroperitoneal lymphadenectomy through an abdominal incision several weeks after orchiectomy if the retroperitoneal nodes still show evidence of metastasis following radiation treatment.

COLLABORATIVE MANAGEMENT

Care of the patient undergoing orchiectomy requires thorough preparation, close monitoring, and intense patient teaching.

Preparation

- Explain to the patient that the surgeon will perform a biopsy on the diseased testis and base further treatment on those results.
- Review anatomy and physiology with the patient to give him a clear understanding of the location and function of the testes.
- Listen to the patient's concerns about body image, sexual function, and fertility.
- Explain that testicular prostheses are available to maintain physical appearance of the scrotum and that unless he's had a retroperitoneal lymphadenectomy, he should retain his potency and ability to ejaculate and experience orgasm.

Monitoring and aftercare

- Monitor vital signs until stable.
- Following orchiectomy, check inguinal incisions for drainage and use aseptic technique for wound care. Monitor abdominal dressing frequently for signs of hemorrhage. Give analgesics as needed. (See *After orchiectomy*.)
- Following transabdominal retroperitoneal lymphadenectomy, give the patient nothing by mouth until bowel sounds return, and monitor I.V. infusion and urine output.

Patient teaching

■ Inform the patient that sexual relations can begin when he feels able. Encourage him to share his feelings and concerns about sexuality and fertility with his partner and to report sexual dysfunction to his doctor.

■ Advise the patient to eat a balanced diet of nutritious foods to prepare himself for further therapy (radiation or chemotherapy).

COMPLICATIONS

Hemorrhage is a common complication of retroperitoneal lymphadenectomy. The patient may also lose the ability to ejaculate.

PROSTATECTOMY

When chronic prostatitis, benign prostatic hyperplasia, or prostate cancer fails to respond to drug therapy or other treatments, total or partial prostatectomy removes diseased or obstructive tissue and restores urine flow through the urethra. Depending on the disease, the surgeon uses one of several approaches. Transurethral resection of the prostate (TURP), the most common approach, involves insertion of a resectoscope into the urethra. Open surgical approaches include suprapubic, retropubic, and radical perineal prostatectomy. A new technique involving cryosurgery also may be performed.

PROCEDURE

In TURP, the patient is placed in a lithotomy position and anesthetized. The surgeon then introduces a resectoscope into the urethra and advances it to the prostate. After instilling a clear irrigating solution and viewing the obstruction, he uses the resectoscope's cutting loop to resect prostatic tissue and restore the urethral opening.

In suprapubic prostatectomy, the patient is given a general anesthetic and placed in a supine position. The surgeon begins by making a horizontal incision just above the pubic symphysis. After instilling fluid into the bladder to distend it, he makes a small incision in the bladder wall to expose the prostate. He then shells the obstructing prostatic tissue out of its bed with his finger. After clearing the obstruction and ligating all bleeding points, he usually inserts a suprapubic drainage tube and a Penrose drain.

In retropubic prostatectomy, the patient is anesthetized and placed in a supine position. The surgeon makes a horizontal suprapubic incision and approaches the prostate from between the bladder and the pubic arch. He then makes another incision in the prostatic capsule and removes the obstructing tissue. After controlling any bleeding, he usually inserts a suprapubic tube and a Penrose drain.

In radical perineal prostatectomy, the patient is anesthetized and placed in the perineal position, an exaggerated lithotomy position in which the knees are drawn up against the chest and the buttocks are slightly elevated. The surgeon makes an inverted U-shaped incision in the perineum, then removes the entire prostate and the seminal vesicles. He anastomoses the urethra to the bladder and closes the incision, leaving a Penrose drain in place.

In cryosurgery, liquid nitrogen is used to freeze the prostate gland.

COLLABORATIVE MANAGEMENT

Care of the patient undergoing prostatectomy requires thorough preparation, close monitoring, and intense patient teaching.

Preparation

■ Review the planned surgery and its aftermath with the patient, and encourage him to ask questions. Give straightforward answers to help clear up any misconceptions he may have.

■ Encourage the patient to express his fears. Reassure him by emphasizing the positive aspects of the surgery, such as improved urination and prevention of further complications.

■ Because some types of prostatectomy cause impotence, you may need to arrange for sexual counseling to help the patient and his partner cope with this devastating loss.

■ If the patient is scheduled for TURP, explain that this procedure may cause retrograde ejaculation, but otherwise doesn't impair sexual function.

■ Before surgery, shave and clean the surgical site if ordered. Give the patient a cleansing enema. Explain that he may have a catheter in place for days to weeks to ensure proper urine drainage and healing.

Monitoring and aftercare

■ Monitor the patient's vital signs closely, looking for indications of possible hemorrhage and shock.

■ Frequently check any incision site for signs of infection, and change dressings as necessary.

■ Watch for and report signs and symptoms of epididymitis: fever, chills, groin pain, and a tender, swollen epididymis.

■ Record the amount and nature of urine drainage.

■ Maintain indwelling urinary catheter patency through intermittent or continuous irrigation, as ordered. Watch for catheter blockage from kinking or clot formation.

■ Maintain the patency of any suprapubic tube, and monitor the amount and character of drainage. Drainage should appear amber or slightly blood tinged; report any abnormalities. Keep the collection container below the patient's bladder level to promote drainage, and keep the skin around the tube insertion site clean and dry.

■ Expect and report frank bleeding the first day after surgery. If bleeding is venous, the doctor may increase the traction on the catheter or increase the pressure in the catheter's balloon end. If bleeding is arterial (bright red, with numerous clots and increased viscosity), the doctor may control it surgically.

■ As ordered, give antispasmodics to control painful bladder spasms and analgesics to relieve incision pain.

■ Offer sitz baths to reduce perineal discomfort. Never give drugs rectally in a patient with a perineal prostatectomy.

■ Watch for signs of dilutional hyponatremia: altered mental status, muscle twitching, and seizures. If you see these signs, raise the bed's side rails to prevent injury, notify the doctor, draw blood for serum sodium determination, and prepare hypertonic saline solution for possible I.V. infusion.

■ Offer emotional support to the patient with a radical perineal prostatectomy because this procedure usually causes impotence. Try to arrange for psychological and sexual counseling during the recovery period.

Patient teaching

■ Tell the patient to drink ten 8-oz (237-ml) glasses of water a day, to urinate at least every 2 hours and, if he has trouble urinating, to notify the doctor immediately.

■ Explain that after catheter removal, he may have transient urinary frequency and dribbling. Reassure him that he'll gradually regain control over urination.

■ Teach him Kegel exercises to tighten the perineum and speed the return of sphincter control. Suggest that he avoid caffeine-containing beverages, which cause mild diuresis.

■ Reassure the patient that slightly blood-tinged urine is normal for the first few weeks after surgery. But tell him to report bright red urine or persistent hematuria.

■ Tell the patient to immediately report any signs of infection, such as fever, chills, and flank pain.

■ Warn him to avoid sexual relations, lifting anything heavier than 10 lb (4.5 kg), strenuous exercise (short walks are usually permitted), long car trips, or driving a car until the doctor gives permission. Explain that performing these activities too soon after surgery can cause bleeding.

■ Tell the patient to take his prescribed medications as ordered. Suggest sitz baths for perineal discomfort.

■ Urge the patient to keep all follow-up appointments and to have a yearly prostate examination (unless he's had a radical prostatectomy). Tell men who've had radical prostatectomies to have a prostate-specific antigen test every year.

COMPLICATIONS

Hemorrhage, infection, urine retention, impotence, and incontinence are potential complications of prostatectomy.

Selected references

Bran, D.F., et al. "Outpatient Vaginal Hysterectomy as a New Trend in Gynecology," *AORN Journal* 62(5):810-14, November 1995.

Haslett, S. "Hysterectomy," *Nursing Standard* 10(38):49-55, June 12, 1996.

Illustrated Guide to Diagnostic Tests, 2nd ed. Springhouse, Pa.: Springhouse Corp., 1998.

Keetch, D.W., et al. "Cryosurgical Ablation of the Prostate," *AORN Journal* 61(5):807-13, May 1995.

Meeker, M.H., and Rothrock, J.C. *Alexander's Care of the Patient in Surgery,* 10th ed. St. Louis: Mosby–Year Book, Inc., 1995.

Nursing98 Drug Handbook. Springhouse, Pa.: Springhouse Corp., 1998.

Professional Guide to Signs and Symptoms, 2nd ed. Springhouse, Pa.: Springhouse Corp., 1997.

Breast disorders

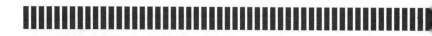

In both sexes, the breasts are similar until puberty, when estrogen and progesterone cause breast enlargement in females. Estrogen causes duct tissue growth and fat deposits. Progesterone stimulates glandular development. The male breast isn't stimulated by these hormones and retains its preadolescent characteristics.

Breast size and composition change with age. The breast on the female's dominant side is usually larger because she develops larger pectoral muscles under the breast on that side.

Female breasts are significantly associated with sexuality. Consequently, any threat to the breast can threaten a woman's body image and feelings of personal worth.

Anatomy and physiology review

Normally developing in pairs, the breasts are mammary glands located between the second and sixth ribs on the anterior chest wall over the pectoralis major and serratus anterior muscles. Horizontally, they lie between the sternal border and midaxillary line.

The nipple rises from the center of the breast and is surrounded by Montgomery's glands (round sebaceous glands), which appear as bumps or elevations. These glands secrete a fatty substance that protects the nipple during breast feeding. Cooper's suspensory ligaments attach to pectoral muscles and support the breast. (See *Reviewing breast anatomy*, page 504.)

The breasts may become slightly larger, tender, and nodular during the premenstrual period because of the increasing levels of estrogen and progesterone (3 to 4 days prior to menses). After menstruation, the cellular growth decreases, ducts recess, and water retention subsides.

The internal mammary and lateral thoracic arteries supply the breast with blood. Venous blood drains into the superior vena cava. Lymph drains through an extensive system near the axilla, via the jugular and subclavian veins. This system can spread cancerous cells deeply into the chest, abdomen, pelvis, vertebrae, brain, or opposite breast, depending on the location of the lesion.

PREGNANCY-RELATED CHANGES
During pregnancy, tremendous amounts of estrogen cause the ductal system to grow and branch. The stroma increase in quantity and large quantities of fat are added. Growth hormone, prolactin, adrenal glucocorticoids, and insulin also play a role in the functional development of the breast. During nursing, prolactin assists in lactation production and oxytocin assists in milk secretion.

Assessment

Discussing the breasts may be embarrassing and difficult for women and men alike. Remember to provide a comfortable environment for the patient history—one that offers privacy and freedom from interruption.

CHIEF COMPLAINT
Ask the patient if she has a particular complaint, such as a change or lump in her breast. If she reports a change, find out when she first noticed it and whether she's had any associated breast pain or tenderness or nipple discharge. In addition, find out about any drugs she's taking, such as oral contraceptives, hormonal replacements, or antidepressants.

◆◆◆ 503

Reviewing breast anatomy

The illustration below identifies the major breast structures.

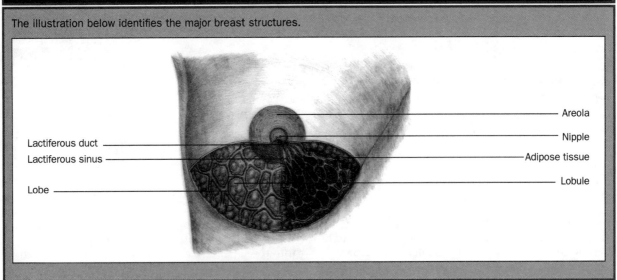

Lactiferous duct

Lactiferous sinus

Lobe

Areola

Nipple

Adipose tissue

Lobule

MEDICAL HISTORY

Ask the patient about any history of breast cancer or breast surgery. Note symptoms, including their onset, chronicity, location, radiation, severity, and duration. Ask about factors that precipitate or relieve symptoms. Has she had any surgery or other treatment for any conditions? Any laboratory tests, X-rays, or computed tomography scans? Does she have a relevant family history (especially for cancer of the breast) or social history (such as exposure to chemicals)? In addition, obtain information about her reproductive history. (See Chapter 11, Reproductive disorders.)

PHYSICAL EXAMINATION

Use a calm, relaxed approach, and be sure to provide privacy.

INSPECTION

Inspect the breasts with the patient in the following positions: sitting with arms relaxed at the sides, sitting with hands on the hips and pectoralis major muscles contracted, sitting with arms over the head, and lying in a position supine with the arm behind the head and a pillow under the shoulder being examined. Observe the breasts for symmetry, size, contour, integrity, edema, erythema, and any obvious venous patterns. Note any nipple irregularities. Look for any discharge. Note whether breast development is appropriate for the patient's age.

PALPATION

Using your finger pads, palpate the breasts while the patient is in a supine position. Remember to use an organized approach, such as following concentric circles or a wheel-spokes pattern. Be sure to examine all four quadrants, over the areolae, in the axilla, and in the supraclavicular and infraclavicular areas. Check for lymph nodes, masses, and tenderness. Note any masses, including location, size, shape, consistency, tenderness, mobility, borders, and retraction of any overlying skin. Squeeze the nipples and watch for a discharge. If you detect a discharge, note the amount and color and whether it appears bilaterally or unilaterally. Also, use this opportunity to teach the patient about breast self-examination.

Breast cancer

Breast cancer is the most common cancer in women, affecting about 10% of all women. It seldom strikes men.

Breast cancer may develop any time after puberty, but most cases are diagnosed in women ages 60 to 79. Five-year survival rates have been improving because of earlier diagnosis and better treatment. Mortality rates, however, haven't changed in the past 50 years.

The most reliable breast cancer detection method is regular breast self-examination, followed by immediate professional evaluation of any abnormality noticed. Mammography is another important detection method and is probably responsible for the increase in the number of reported cases. (See *Teaching about mammography*.)

Following are selected portions of the clinical practice guidelines for mammography developed by the Agency for Health Care Policy and Research of the U.S. Department of Health and Human Services.

Screening mammography
■ Inform women that they should have both a clinical breast examination and mammography as part of the breast cancer screening process.
■ Be aware that mammography is the most sensitive and specific screening test for breast cancer currently available.
■ If possible, women should be scheduled for screening mammography when they are not experiencing cyclic breast tenderness or conditions that increase breast density.
■ Remember that screening and diagnostic mammography differ in terms of purpose, views taken, and presence of the interpreting site. When referring women for mammography, specify whether screening or diagnostic mammography is requested.

Diagnostic mammography
■ Tell women whether they are being referred for screening or diagnostic mammography and how they will be informed of the results. If the referral is for diagnostic purposes, tell the patient why it is needed, what to expect during the procedure, and the necessity of follow-up.
■ Inform women who have had breast-conserving surgery that they should have regular clinical breast examinations and diagnostic mammography.
■ Women with breast signs or symptoms, such as a breast mass, skin changes, or unilateral spontaneous nip-
ple discharge, should be scheduled for diagnostic rather than screening mammography.
■ Be aware that although breast pain is a relatively uncommon presentation of breast cancer, its presence does not exclude the diagnosis of malignancy.

Mammography in women of different ages
■ Remember that the incidence of breast cancer increases with age. There is general consensus that screening mammography decreases mortality from breast cancer in women age 50 and over.
■ Know that opinion differs about the value of screening mammography in asymptomatic women ages 40 to 49.
■ Remember the risks and limitations of mammography for women under age 40 as well as special indicators for mammography in this age-group.

Possible problems
■ Be aware of the possible adverse consequences of mammography, such as excessive biopsies.
■ Understand that women may have substantial anxiety when they have to return for additional or repeat views. These extra views should be done as soon as possible to reduce fear.
■ Tell patients that the risk of breast cancer induction from annual screening mammography beginning at age 40 or 50 is negligible. The estimated risk of breast cancer induction increases in women who are younger at the time of exposure.
■ Know that in the process of detecting as many early breast cancers as possible, a certain number of biopsies will be done for benign mammographic abnormalities.

About half of all breast cancers develop in the upper outer quadrant, the section containing the most glandular tissue. The second most common site is the nipple, where all the breast ducts converge. The next most common site is the upper inner quadrant, followed by the lower outer quadrant and, finally, the lower inner quadrant.

Growth rates vary. A slow-growing breast tumor may take up to 8 years to become palpable at ⅜″ (1-cm) diameter. Breast cancer spreads by way of the lymphatic system and the bloodstream, through the right side of the heart to the lungs and to the other breast, chest wall, liver, bone, and brain. Survival time is based on tumor size and the number of involved lymph nodes.

Breast cancers are classified as:
■ adenocarcinoma (ductal)—arising from the epithelium
■ intraductal—developing within the ducts (includes Paget's disease)
■ infiltrating—occurring in the breast's parenchymal tissue
■ inflammatory (rare)—growing rapidly and causing overlying skin to become edematous, inflamed, and indurated
■ lobular carcinoma in situ—involving the lobes of glandular tissue
■ medullary or circumscribed—enlarging tumor with rapid growth rate.

Staging helps to determine the cancer's extent. The most common system for staging, both before and after surgery, is the tumor, node, metastasis (TNM) system.

Disease progression and metastasis lead to site-specific complications, including infection, decreased mobility if breast cancer metastasizes to the bone, central nervous system effects if the cancer metastasizes to the brain, and respiratory problems if the disease spreads to the lung.

CAUSES
The causes of breast cancer remain elusive. Significant risk factors include a family history of breast cancer (mother, sister, grandmother, aunt) and being a woman over age 45. Other possible risk factors include a long menstrual cycle, early onset of menses, or late menopause; first pregnancy after age 35; a high-fat diet; a history of endometrial or ovarian cancer or fibrocystic disease; radiation exposure; estrogen or antihypertensive therapy; and alcohol or tobacco use.

DIAGNOSIS AND TREATMENT
Mammography is the essential test for breast cancer because it can detect a tumor too small to palpate. Other tests include fine-needle aspiration and excisional biopsy to confirm the diagnosis; ultrasonography to distinguish between a fluid-filled cyst and a solid mass; chest X-ray, scans, and laboratory tests to detect distant metastases; and a hormonal receptor assay to determine whether the tumor is estrogen- or progesterone-dependent (this may affect the choice of treatment).

The type of treatment used for breast cancer usually reflects the disease's stage and type, the woman's age and menopausal status, and the disfiguring effects of the surgery. Appropriate therapy may include any combination of surgery, radiation, chemotherapy, and hormonal therapy.

Surgical options include lumpectomy, partial mastectomy, total mastectomy, and modified radical mastectomy. Modified radical mastectomy has replaced radical mastectomy as the most widely used surgical procedure for treating breast cancer.

Before or after tumor removal, primary radiation therapy may be effective for a patient who has a small tumor in early stages without distant metastases. Radiation therapy can also prevent or treat local recurrence. Furthermore, preoperative breast irradiation helps to "sterilize" the field, making the tumor more manageable surgically—especially in inflammatory breast cancer.

Chemotherapy, which can be used as either adjuvant or primary therapy, consists of a combination of drugs, such as cyclophosphamide, fluorouracil, methotrexate, doxorubicin, vincristine, and prednisone. A typical regimen is cyclophosphamide, methotrexate, and fluorouracil, which is used for both premenopausal and postmenopausal women.

Hormonal therapy blocks the uptake of estrogen and other hormones that may nourish breast cancer cells. For example, anti-estrogen therapy (specifically tamoxifen) is effective against tumors identified as estrogen-receptor-positive in postmenopausal women.

Alternatively, the patient may be treated with antiandrogens (aminoglutethimide), androgens (fluoxymesterone), estrogens (diethylstilbestrol), or progestins (megestrol).

COLLABORATIVE MANAGEMENT
Care of the patient with breast cancer focuses on regaining strength, controlling pain, and teaching self-care.

ASSESSMENT
The patient usually reports that she detected a painless lump or mass in her breast or that she noticed a thickening of breast tissue. Otherwise, the disease typically appears on a mammogram before a lesion becomes palpable. The patient's health history may indicate several significant risk factors for breast cancer.

Inspection of the patient's breast may reveal a clear, milky, or bloody nipple discharge, nipple retraction, scaly skin around the nipple, and such skin changes as dimpling, peau d'orange, or inflammation. Arm edema, which is also identified on inspection, may indicate advanced nodal involvement.

Palpation may identify a hard lump, a mass, or thickening of breast tissue. Palpation of the cervical supraclavicular and axillary nodes may also disclose lumps or enlargement.

NURSING DIAGNOSES AND COLLABORATIVE PROBLEMS
Based on the following nursing diagnoses, you'll establish patient outcomes.

Decisional conflict related to treatment options. The patient will:
- be well informed about the pros and cons of each treatment option
- seek a second opinion
- make a well-informed decision about her breast cancer treatment choice.

Fear related to potential for metastatic breast disease. The patient will:
- express her fears and concerns
- use available support systems and seek information about breast cancer from reputable sources to help her cope with fear
- express less fear and show fewer physical signs and symptoms of fear.

Altered nutrition: Less than body requirements, related to adverse effects of radiation or chemotherapy. The patient will:
- eat a well-balanced diet
- maintain her weight
- recover her appetite and GI function.

PLANNING AND IMPLEMENTATION
These measures help the patient with breast cancer.

■ Encourage the patient to express her feelings about her illness, and determine her level of knowledge and expectations.

■ Give pain relievers as needed, and perform comfort measures to promote relaxation and relieve anxiety.

■ In late disease, monitor the patient's pain level and the effectiveness of drugs to relieve pain and non-pharmacologic measures such as relaxation techniques.

■ Evaluate the patient's and family's coping abilities, especially if the disease becomes terminal.

■ Watch for treatment complications, such as nausea, vomiting, anorexia, leukopenia, thrombocytopenia, GI ulceration, and bleeding.

■ If immobility develops late in the disease, prevent complications by frequently repositioning the patient, using a convoluted foam mattress, and providing skin care (particularly over bony prominences).

■ Monitor the patient's weight and nutritional status for evidence of malnutrition. Work with a nutritional therapist to provide adequate intake.

Patient teaching

■ Teach your patient about early screening and detection; show her how to examine her breasts. (See *Detecting breast cancer early*.)

■ Provide clear, concise explanations of all procedures and prescribed treatments.

■ Teach the patient or a family member or friend how to manage the adverse effects of treatment.

■ Women who've had cancer in one breast are at higher risk for cancer in the other breast or for recurrent cancer in the chest wall. Therefore, urge the patient to continue examining her other breast and to comply with follow-up treatment.

■ Refer the patient and family member to hospital and community support services.

EVALUATION

Achievement of patient outcomes determines the success of collaborative management. For the patient with breast cancer, evaluation focuses on the success of surgery, radiation, or chemotherapy; appropriate exercise; understanding of postoperative safety precautions for the affected arm; and demonstration of breast self-examination.

Fibrocystic breast changes

Also known as mammary dysplasia or chronic cystic mastitis, fibrocystic breast changes represent the most common benign breast condition. The epithelium of the breast responds to fluctuating levels of estrogen and progesterone, causing women to experience

HEALTHY LIVING — **Detecting breast cancer early**

Screening and early detection greatly improve the prognosis for the patient diagnosed with breast cancer. Be sure to include the following in your patient teaching:

■ Show female patients how to do a breast self-examination, and explain when to do it.

■ Review the breast cancer warning signs: a lump or mass in the breast, changes in breast symmetry or size, changes in breast skin (thickening, dimpling, edema, peau d'orange appearance, or ulceration), changes in skin temperature (a warm, hot, or pink area), unusual nipple drainage or discharge, changes in the nipple (itching, burning, erosion, or retraction), and pain (not usually a breast cancer symptom unless the tumor is advanced).

■ Reinforce the need for mammography screening at recommended intervals.

breast tenderness and fullness during the luteal phase of the menstrual cycle.

Previously, this hormonally induced, cyclic pain and lumpiness was called a disease. Today, however, many health care professionals feel that term is inaccurate because studies show that about 50% of all women ages 20 to 50 have clinical signs and nearly 90% have histologic signs of fibrocystic changes, which suggests that fibrocystic changes are a normal variation.

CAUSES

Fibrocystic changes are probably caused by an imbalance of estrogen and progesterone. This imbalance distorts the normal changes of the menstrual cycle and causes an exaggerated response of breast tissue to cyclic levels of ovarian hormones. Fibrocystic changes respond to the phases of the menstrual cycle; a patient may actually observe a lessening in the size of a lump when her menses begins.

Fibrocystic breast changes seldom cause complications, although the signs and symptoms may progress. Occasionally, a patient who undergoes a biopsy for a benign breast lump is found to have atypical hyperplasia. This clinical finding, combined with a family history of breast cancer, may increase the patient's risk of breast cancer.

DIAGNOSIS AND TREATMENT

Diagnostic tests may include aspiration and ultrasonography to determine whether the cyst is fluid-filled or solid, mammography to track changes, and surgical excision if the mammogram indicates changes in the mass or if fluid can't be aspirated from the cyst.

Hormones are the most common treatment for fibrocystic changes. Daily doses of danazol, a synthetic androgen, can significantly reduce or eliminate fibrocystic breast symptoms. However, danazol can produce unpleasant adverse reactions, such as menstrual irregularities, weight gain, increased facial hair, and voice deepening.

Some clinicians recommend excluding methylxanthines (particularly caffeine in coffee, tea, cola, and chocolate) and including vitamins E, A, and B complex in the diet to relieve symptoms.

COLLABORATIVE MANAGEMENT

Care of the patient with fibrocystic breast changes focuses on providing improved comfort and pain relief and teaching about the condition and treatment.

ASSESSMENT

The patient may report multiple painful breast masses (cysts) that change rapidly in size. She may say that the cysts enlarge and become more painful during the premenstrual period. This pain may be described as a localized painful area if she has a large, fluid-filled cyst. If small cysts form, she may have a more diffuse tenderness. She may also notice nipple discharge.

Palpation may reveal dense breast tissue with areas of irregularity and nodularity or lumpiness.

NURSING DIAGNOSES AND COLLABORATIVE PROBLEMS

Based on the following nursing diagnoses, you'll establish patient outcomes.

Fear related to potential for breast changes to be cancerous. The patient will:
■ verbalize her fears
■ perform activities that help reduce fear, such as monthly breast self-examinations and regular check-ups
■ show decreased physical symptoms of fear.
Body image disturbance related to breast irregularity and lumpiness. The patient will:
■ communicate feelings about changes in body image
■ express positive feelings about herself.
Pain related to cyst formation. The patient will:
■ take measures to reduce or relieve pain, such as applying ice packs and wearing a bra 24 hours a day
■ comply with dietary recommendations and hormonal therapy
■ express feelings of comfort with therapy.

PLANNING AND IMPLEMENTATION

These measures help the patient with fibrocystic breast changes.
■ Provide emotional support to the patient. Encourage her to verbalize her feelings about the disorder and the changes in her body.

■ Institute measures to relieve pain, such as ice packs and wearing a bra 24 hours a day.
■ Use dietary modifications, if appropriate, such as limiting caffeine-containing products.
■ Give medications as ordered, such as hormones, diuretics, and analgesics. Monitor for effectiveness.
■ Monitor the patient for adverse reactions to medication therapy, such as weight gain or loss, hot flashes, menstrual irregularities, and electrolyte imbalances.
■ Monitor the patient closely for breast changes.

Patient teaching

■ Explain all diagnostic studies and their significance. Clarify any misconceptions about malignancy.
■ If the patient is in pain, teach her how to decrease discomfort, such as by wearing a bra 24 hours a day, applying ice packs, restricting caffeine intake, and taking salicylates or other anti-inflammatory drugs. Inform her that the moderate to severe pain may cease spontaneously within 1 year.
■ Encourage the patient to perform a breast self-examination every month after her menstrual cycle. Stress the importance of regular examinations to detect early breast changes.
■ Encourage her to follow the American Cancer Society's guidelines for mammography screening: a baseline mammography at age 40 (unless she's having a problem or has a family history of breast cancer), repeat mammography every 2 years from ages 40 to 50, and annual mammography after age 50.

EVALUATION

Achievement of patient outcomes determines the success of collaborative management. For the patient with fibrocystic breast changes, evaluation focuses on maintaining high levels of comfort and a diet that eliminates exacerbating foods such as caffeine.

Mastitis

Parenchymatous inflammation of the mammary glands, mastitis follows childbirth in about 1% of lactating women, mainly in first-time mothers who breast-feed. It appears occasionally in nonlactating women and rarely in men. The prognosis is good, but an untreated breast infection can lead to abscess.

CAUSES

Mastitis develops when a pathogen that typically originates in the nursing infant's nose or pharynx invades breast tissue through a fissured or cracked nipple and disrupts normal lactation. The most common pathogen is *Staphylococcus aureus*; less frequently, it's *Staphylococcus epidermidis* or beta-hemolytic streptococci.

Rarely, mastitis is caused by disseminated tuberculosis or the mumps virus.

Predisposing factors include a fissure or abrasion of the nipple, blocked milk ducts, and an incomplete let-down reflex, usually due to emotional trauma. Blocked milk ducts are sometimes caused by a tight bra or prolonged intervals between breast-feedings.

DIAGNOSIS AND TREATMENT

Antibiotic therapy, the primary treatment, usually consists of penicillin G to combat staphylococci or erythromycin or kanamycin for penicillin-resistant strains. A cephalosporin or dicloxacillin may also be used. Symptoms usually subside in 2 to 3 days, but antibiotic therapy should continue for 10 days.

Other appropriate measures include analgesics for pain and, rarely, incision and drainage of a breast abscess.

COLLABORATIVE MANAGEMENT

Care of the patient with mastitis focuses on controlling the infection and pain, avoiding complications, and teaching about the condition, treatment, and care.

ASSESSMENT

Usually the patient reports a fever of 101° F (38.3° C) or higher, malaise, and flulike symptoms that develop 2 to 4 weeks postpartum (although these findings may develop at any time during lactation). Inspection and palpation typically uncover such classic signs and symptoms as redness, swelling, warmth, hardness, tenderness, nipple cracks or fissures, and enlarged axillary lymph nodes.

Cultures of expressed milk confirm generalized mastitis; cultures of breast skin surface confirm localized mastitis. Such cultures also determine the appropriate antibiotic treatment.

NURSING DIAGNOSES AND COLLABORATIVE PROBLEMS

Based on the following nursing diagnoses, you'll establish patient outcomes.

Risk for impaired skin integrity related to potential development or exacerbation of cracks or fissures. The patient will:
- avoid cracks and fissures or, if they're present, avoid exacerbating them
- regain normal tissue integrity.

Ineffective breast-feeding related to inflammation of breast tissue. The patient will:
- maintain her ability to lactate
- resume effective breast-feeding after mastitis resolves.

Pain related to inflammation of breast tissue. The patient will:
- express relief of pain after taking pain relievers

- use nonpharmacologic measures to alleviate pain
- become pain-free.

PLANNING AND IMPLEMENTATION

These measures help the patient with mastitis.
- Give pain relievers as needed, and provide comfort measures such as warm soaks. Monitor the patient's response to these measures.
- Use meticulous hand-washing technique and provide good skin care.
- Regularly measure the patient's temperature and assess the effectiveness of antipyretic agents.
- Inspect the patient's breasts daily for signs of impaired skin integrity, such as cracks or fissures.

Patient teaching

- Advise the patient to take antibiotics as ordered. Stress the need to take the entire prescribed amount, even if symptoms improve in the meantime.
- Reassure the patient that breast-feeding during mastitis won't harm her infant because the infant is the source of the infection.
- If only one breast is affected, tell the patient to offer the infant this breast first to promote complete emptying and prevent clogged ducts. However, if an open abscess develops, she must stop breast-feeding with the infected breast and use a breast pump until the abscess heals. She should continue to breast-feed on the unaffected side.
- Suggest that she apply a warm, wet towel to the affected breast or take a warm shower to relax and improve her ability to breast-feed.

To prevent mastitis:
- Stress the need to completely empty the breasts because stasis of milk causes infection.
- Teach the patient to alternate nursing positions to help empty the breast and rotate pressure areas on the nipples.
- Show the patient how to position the infant properly on the breast to prevent cracked nipples. The entire areola of the nipple should be in the infant's mouth.
- Tell the patient to expose sore nipples to the air as often as possible.
- Teach her proper hand-washing technique and personal hygiene.
- Stress the importance of getting plenty of rest, drinking sufficient fluids, and maintaining a balanced diet to enhance her ability to breast-feed.

EVALUATION

Achievement of patient outcomes determines the success of collaborative management. For the patient with mastitis, evaluation focuses on taking antibiotics as ordered, maintaining comfort, and using effective techniques to reduce breast engorgement.

Treatments and procedures

The treatment options for breast disorders include lumpectomy, mastectomy, and reconstruction mammoplasty.

LUMPECTOMY

Patients with early, small, well-defined lesions less than 2″ (5 cm) in size and staged as 0, I, or II are candidates for lumpectomy (removal of the tumor and some surrounding tissue). Unfortunately, fewer than 20% of breast cancer patients have this type of lesion. After lumpectomy, most patients undergo radiation therapy.

The 5- and 10-year survival and local recurrence rates for lumpectomy are at least equivalent to those of modified radical mastectomy. In addition, the psychological benefits of avoiding breast removal make this procedure an especially appealing option for many women with breast cancer.

PROCEDURE

A lumpectomy is the removal of a malignant lump in the breast, leaving the breast itself intact. A lumpectomy with node dissection is the removal of the malignant lump along with nearby lymph nodes. After the patient has received anesthesia, the surgeon makes a small incision near the nipple. He then removes the tumor, a narrow margin of normal tissue surrounding the tumor and, possibly, nearby lymph nodes. The wound is closed and a small sterile dressing is applied.

COLLABORATIVE MANAGEMENT

Care of the patient undergoing a lumpectomy requires thorough preparation, close monitoring, and intense patient teaching.

Preparation

Evaluate the patient's feelings about the lumpectomy, and determine her level of knowledge and expectations. Listen to her fears and concerns. Stay with her during periods of severe anxiety.

Explain the surgical procedure to her, and inform her that she'll have a dressing over the site and possibly a drain. If the patient is having the procedure done in the outpatient department, tell her that she can go home when she has fully recovered from the anesthesia.

Monitoring and aftercare

■ Inspect the dressing as soon as the patient returns from the postanesthesia care unit and regularly thereafter. Report excessive bleeding promptly.
■ Remember to monitor vital signs.

■ If a general anesthetic was given during surgery, monitor intake and output for at least 48 hours.
■ Use strict aseptic technique when changing the dressing. Monitor the patient's temperature and white blood cell count closely.
■ Give an analgesic for pain as ordered, and perform comfort measures such as repositioning to promote relaxation and pain relief.
■ Have the patient walk as soon as the anesthesia wears off.

Patient teaching

■ Teach the patient how to care for the incision (and drain, if present) and change the dressing. Stress the importance of strict aseptic technique.
■ Instruct the patient to wear a brassiere for support continuously for at least 1 week after surgery.
■ Emphasize the importance of breast self-examination, and teach the patient how to do it if necessary. Also review breast cancer warning signs with her. Women who have had breast cancer have a higher risk for recurrent cancer in the same breast as well as cancer in the other breast.
■ Refer the patient and her family to hospital and community support services as indicated.

COMPLICATIONS

Complications, although uncommon, include wound infection and delayed healing.

MASTECTOMY

A mastectomy is surgery performed primarily to remove malignant breast tissue and any regional lymphatic metastases. It may be combined with radiation therapy and chemotherapy. Until recently, radical mastectomy was the treatment of choice for breast cancer. However, surgeons now perform several different types of mastectomy, depending on the size of the tumor and the presence of any metastases.

PROCEDURE

In a total mastectomy, the surgeon removes the entire breast without dissecting the lymph nodes. He may apply a skin graft if necessary.

If the surgeon is performing a modified radical mastectomy, he may use one of several techniques to remove the entire breast. He also resects all axillary lymph nodes, while leaving the pectoralis major muscle intact. He may or may not remove the pectoralis minor. If the patient has small lesions and no metastases, the surgeon may perform breast reconstruction immediately or a few days later.

In a radical mastectomy, the surgeon removes the entire breast, axillary lymph nodes, underlying pectoral muscles, and adjacent tissues. He covers the skin flaps and exposed tissue with moist packs for protection and, before closure, irrigates the chest wall and axilla. In an extended radical mastectomy, the surgeon removes the breast, underlying pectoral muscles, axillary contents, and upper internal mammary (mediastinal) lymph node chain.

After closing the mastectomy site, the surgeon may make a stab wound and insert a drain or catheter. The drain or catheter removes blood that may collect under the skin flaps, where it could prevent healing and lead to infection. Less commonly, he may use large pressure dressings instead. If a graft was needed to close the wound, he'll probably place a pressure dressing over the donor site.

COLLABORATIVE MANAGEMENT

Care of the patient undergoing a mastectomy requires thorough preparation, close monitoring, and intense patient teaching. (See *Managing total mastectomy,* pages 512 and 513.)

Preparation

Explore the patient's feelings about the mastectomy, which may threaten a woman's self-image more than any other type of surgery. Typically, she'll express fear and anxiety. She may have many questions but feel too confused or upset to ask them. Be a supportive, caring listener, and help her express her concerns. Discuss her sexuality and her relationship with her partner to identify possible conflicts about the surgery and the degree of support she can expect from her partner afterward.

Review the surgeon's explanation of the procedure. Also prepare the patient for her postoperative care. Explain that the surgeon may insert a drain or catheter and use suction to drain the incision and that the arm on her affected side will be elevated. She'll have to sit up and turn in bed by pushing up with her unaffected arm (but not pulling). Tell her she'll begin arm and shoulder exercises shortly after surgery. Demonstrate the exercises and have her repeat them.

If the patient seems able to absorb it, provide other information, such as the types of breast prostheses available. However, most women will need to concentrate on dealing with the upcoming surgery and the immediate recovery period. Consequently, you'll probably defer discussion of rehabilitation until after surgery.

Take arm measurements on both sides to obtain baseline data. With this information, you can assess for edema that may occur after surgery. If the patient will have a radical mastectomy, explain that the skin on the anterior surface of one thigh may be shaved and prepared in case she needs a graft.

Monitoring and aftercare

When the patient returns to the unit, elevate her arm on a pillow to enhance circulation and prevent edema. Periodically check the suction tubing to ensure proper function, and observe the drainage site for erythema, induration, and drainage.

Using aseptic technique, measure and record drainage every 8 hours. Drainage should change from sanguineous to serosanguineous fluid. After 2 to 3 days, you may need to milk the drain periodically to prevent clots from occluding the tubing.

As ordered, teach the patient arm exercises to prevent muscle shortening and contracture of the shoulder joint and to promote lymph drainage. The surgeon will determine the optimal time for initiating these exercises, based on the degree of healing, the presence of a drainage tube, and the tension placed on skin flaps and sutures with movement. You can usually initiate arm flexion and extension on the first postoperative day and then add exercises each day, depending on the patient's needs and the procedure performed. Plan an exercise program with the patient. Such exercises may include climbing the wall with her hands, arm swinging, and rope pulling.

To prevent lymphedema, make sure no blood pressure readings, injections, or venipunctures are performed on the affected arm. Place a sign bearing this message at the head of the patient's bed.

Because mastectomy causes emotional distress, teach the patient to conserve her energy and to recognize early signs of fatigue. Gently encourage her to look at the operative site by describing its appearance and allowing her to express her feelings. Stay with her when she looks at the wound for the first time. Arrange for a volunteer who's had a mastectomy to talk with the patient. Contact the American Cancer Society's rehabilitation program, Reach to Recovery.

After 2 to 3 days, initiate a fitting for a temporary breast pad. Soft and lightweight, the pad inserts into a bra without stays or underwires. If appropriate, explain breast reconstruction.

Patient teaching

■ Inform the patient that preventing lymphedema is critical. Explain that swelling may follow even minor trauma to the arm on her affected side.

■ Tell her to promptly wash cuts and scrapes on the affected side and to contact the doctor immediately if erythema, edema, or induration occurs.

■ Advise the patient to use the affected arm as much as possible and to avoid keeping it in a dependent position for a prolonged period.

■ Reinforce the importance of performing range-of-motion exercises daily. Instruct the patient to do them with both arms to maintain symmetry and prevent additional deformities.

■ Emphasize the importance of not allowing blood pressure readings, injections, or venipunctures on the affected arm.

(Text continues on page 514.)

CLINICAL PATH

Managing total mastectomy

Nursing diagnoses (ND) addressed in path:
1. Alteration in comfort
2. Alteration in coping
3. Alteration in self-concept
4. Lack of knowledge

	Day 1 (Surgery)	Day 2 (Postop Day 1)
ASSESSMENT/ MONITORING (ND: 1, 2)	■ Vital signs (VS) check every 4 hrs ■ Intake and output (I & O) ■ Pain control ■ Dressing/Jackson-Pratt (JP) patency and drainage ■ Ability to void ■ Circulation ■ Emotional response, family coping	■ VS check every 8 hrs if stable ■ I & O ■ Pain control ■ Dressing/JP patency and drainage ■ Voiding without difficulty ■ Circulation ■ Emotional response, family coping
CONSULTS (ND: 2, 3)	■ Social worker	■ Social worker visit ■ Reach to Recovery visit
PROCEDURES/ TESTS (ND: 1)		
TREATMENT (ND: 1, 3)	■ JP to bulb suction ■ Incentive spirometer; coughing and deep breathing ■ Avoid trauma to extremity	■ JP to bulb suction ■ Patient using incentive spirometer independently ■ Avoid trauma to extremity
ACTIVITY (ND: 1)	■ Up with assist to bathroom in p.m.	■ Up as tolerated with assist as needed
MEDICATIONS/ I.V.S	■ I.V. fluids (IVF) ■ I.M. analgesics ■ Antibiotic if ordered	■ IVF discontinued when patient tolerating oral fluids well ■ I.M. analgesics discontinued ■ Oral analgesics started ■ Pain controlled with oral analgesics
NUTRITION (ND: 1)	■ Clear liquid ■ Advanced as tolerated to pre-admission diet	■ Patient tolerating pre-admission diet
PATIENT AND FAMILY EDUCATION (ND: 3, 4)	*Nurse:* ■ Pain control ■ Positioning, mobility ■ Coughing and deep breathing ■ Incentive spirometer ■ Diet ■ I.V. ■ JP ■ Primary nursing	*Social worker:* ■ Assessment of resource needs ■ Education about diagnosis, prosthesis, and support groups initiated *Nurse:* ■ Arm protection ■ Signs and symptoms of infection ■ Breast self-examination
DISCHARGE PLANNING (ND: 2, 3, 4)	■ Patient and family verbalize understanding of clinical path. ■ Plan of care has been mutually set with patient and family.	*Social worker:* ■ High-risk screening completed
PSYCHOSOCIAL/ EMOTIONAL/ SPIRITUAL NEEDS (ND: 2, 3)		*Social worker:* ■ Assessment of counseling needs ■ Support initiated *Nurse:* ■ Therapeutic emotional care
SIGNATURE	_____ Initials_____	_____ Initials_____

Adapted with permission from BJC Health System, Barnes-Jewish Hospital, St. Louis. Courtesy of Center for Case Management, Inc., South Natick, Mass.

Day 3 (Postop Day 2)	Day 4 (Postop Day 3)	Discharge
■ VS check every 8 hrs if stable ■ I & O discontinued except JPs ■ Incision/JP patency and drainage ■ Circulation ■ Lab results ■ Emotional response, family coping	■ VS check before discharge	■ No wound complications ■ Afebrile; VS stable ■ Circulation adequate
■ Social worker visit if needed ■ Reach to Recovery visit		■ Seen by social worker on discharge day ■ Seen by Reach to Recovery on discharge day
■ Complete blood count (CBC) ■ Hematocrit not decreased by more than 25% from preop value		■ CBC stable
■ JP to bulb suction ■ JP dressing change and site care daily ■ Avoid trauma to extremity	■ Incentive spirometer discontinued	■ No pulmonary complications ■ JP sites clean
■ Up as tolerated		■ As before admission except restrictions to affected arm
		■ No signs of phlebitis at I.V. site
Reach to Recovery: ■ Peer counseling *Doctor:* ■ Arm mobility ■ Showering ■ Follow-up ■ Activity *Nurse:* ■ JP care, emptying, measuring	*Doctor:* ■ Instruction reinforced *Nurse:* ■ Learning validated ■ Discharge summary reviewed with patient ■ Discharge medications, if ordered, reviewed with patient	■ Identifies support systems and resources ■ Verbalizes and demonstrates: –JP care, emptying, measuring –Arm protection –Activity and exercise –Signs and symptoms of infection –Importance of breast self-examination –Medical follow-up
Social worker: ■ Home care support referral if needed		■ Home with appropriate level of care
		■ Patient verbalizes feelings about diagnosis and surgery
_____ Initials_____	_____ Initials ___	_____ Initials _____

■ Remind the patient that her energy level will wax and wane. Instruct her to watch for signs of fatigue and to rest frequently for the first few weeks.

■ Stress the importance of monthly self-examination of the unaffected breast and the mastectomy site. Demonstrate the correct examination technique, and have the patient repeat it.

■ Explain the importance of keeping scheduled postoperative appointments.

■ If necessary, provide information regarding a permanent prosthesis, which can be fitted 3 to 4 weeks after surgery. Prostheses are available in a wide range of styles, skin tones, and weights from lingerie shops, medical supply stores, and department stores.

■ Reassure the patient that she can wear the same type of clothing she wore before her surgery.

COMPLICATIONS
After any type of mastectomy, infection and delayed healing are possible. However, the major complication of radical mastectomy and axillary dissection is lymphedema, which may occur soon after surgery and persist for years. Dissection of the lymph nodes draining the axilla may interfere with lymphatic drainage of the arm on the affected side.

RECONSTRUCTION MAMMOPLASTY
Reconstruction mammoplasty, or breast reconstruction, can help relieve the emotional distress caused by mastectomy. As a result, it can improve the patient's self-image and restore her sexual identity.

However, the procedure is contraindicated when metastasis is possible, if healing is impaired, or if the patient has unrealistic expectations. Even when it's feasible, some women choose not to undergo it. They're comfortable, active, and well-adjusted without it. Or they may not consider the additional surgery, anesthesia, pain, and expense worthwhile.

PROCEDURE
In reconstruction mammoplasty, the surgeon places an implant filled with silicone or saline solution under the skin. He may bank the patient's own nipple on her inner thigh or inguinal area and salvage it at the appropriate time. (Its color may darken in the immediate postoperative period but should eventually fade.) Or he may reconstruct a nipple from labial tissue.

COLLABORATIVE MANAGEMENT
Care of the patient undergoing reconstruction mammoplasty requires thorough preparation, close monitoring, and intense patient teaching.

Preparation
If the surgeon offers the patient the option of breast reconstruction, review the procedure with her and an-

swer any questions she may have. Give her ample time to express her concerns.

Encourage the patient to contact the local chapter of the American Cancer Society for additional information. Ask a volunteer from the Reach to Recovery program to talk with the patient.

Monitoring and aftercare
Monitor the patient's vital signs until she's stable. Watch her wound and drainage devices, and report any unusual amounts, colors, or odors from the wound. The donor site may require dressing changes or burn care, depending on the type of grafting used.

Help the patient with care procedures and activities of daily living.

Patient teaching
■ Review care of the reconstructed site as needed.

■ Teach the patient the signs and symptoms of infection, and tell her to notify the doctor if they occur.

■ Encourage her to contact the American Cancer Society and local support groups, as appropriate.

COMPLICATIONS
Complications following reconstruction mammoplasty may include capsular contraction, skin ulceration, hypertrophic scar formation, intercostal neuralgia, infective hematoma, and possibly flap necrosis.

Selected references

Cupples, T., et al. "Mammographic Halo Sign Revisited," *Radiology* 199(1):105-109, April 1996.

Dening, F. "Breast Cancer," *Professional Nurse* 10(8):513-15, May 1995.

Dienger, M.J., and Llewellyn, J. "Increasing Compliance with Breast Self-Exam," *Medsurg Nursing* 4(5):359-66, October 1995.

Graling, P.R., and Grant, J.M. "Demographics and Patient Treatment Choice in Stage 1 Breast Cancer," *AORN Journal,* 62(3):376-79, September 1995.

Lauer, D., et al. "Women's Reasons for and Barriers to Seeking Care for Breast Cancer Symptoms," *Womens Health Issues* 5(1):27-35, Spring 1995.

Luker, K.A., et al. "The Information Needs of Women Newly Diagnosed with Breast Cancer," *Journal of Advanced Nursing* 22(1):134-41, July 1995.

Miaskowski, C. *Oncology Nursing: An Essential Guide for Patient Care.* Philadelphia: W.B. Saunders Co., 1997.

Oberle, K., and Allen, M. "Breast Augmentation Surgery: A Women's Health Issue," *Journal of Advanced Nursing* 20(5):844-52, November 1994.

Street, R., et al. "Increasing Patient Involvement in Choosing Treatment for Early Breast Cancer," *Cancer* 76(11):2275-85, December 1, 1995.

Musculoskeletal disorders

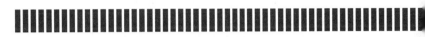

Some musculoskeletal problems are subtle and difficult to assess. Many others, in contrast, are obvious—affecting the patient emotionally as well as physically—or even traumatic.

Anatomy and physiology review

The musculoskeletal system consists of muscles, tendons, ligaments, bones, cartilage, joints, and bursae. These structures work together to produce skeletal movement.

MUSCLES

The body uses three major muscle types: visceral (involuntary, smooth), skeletal (voluntary, striated), and cardiac. This chapter discusses only skeletal muscle, which is attached to bone. Viewed through the microscope, skeletal muscle looks like long bands or strips (striations). Skeletal muscle is voluntary; its contractions are controlled at will.

Muscle develops when existing muscle fibers hypertrophy. Exercise, nutrition, gender, and genetic constitution account for variations in muscle strength and size among individuals.

TENDONS

Bands of fibrous connective tissue, tendons attach muscles to the periosteum (fibrous membrane covering the bone). They move bones when skeletal muscles contract.

LIGAMENTS

Ligaments are dense, strong, flexible bands of fibrous connective tissue that tie bones to other bones. The ligaments of concern in a musculoskeletal system assessment connect the joint (articular) ends of bones, serving either to limit or facilitate movement as well as to provide stability.

BONES

Classified by shape and location, bones are long (such as the humerus, radius, femur, and tibia), short (such as the carpals and tarsals), flat (such as the scapula, ribs, and skull), irregular (such as the vertebrae and mandible), or sesamoid (such as the patella). Bones of the axial skeleton (the head and trunk) include the facial and cranial bones, hyoid bone, vertebrae, ribs, and sternum; bones of the appendicular skeleton (the extremities) include the clavicle, scapula, humerus, radius, ulna, metacarpals, pelvic bone, femur, patella, fibula, tibia, and metatarsals.

BONE FUNCTION

Bones perform the following anatomic (mechanical) and physiologic functions:
- protect internal tissues and organs (for example, 33 vertebrae surround and protect the spinal cord)
- stabilize and support the body
- provide a surface for muscle, ligament, and tendon attachment
- move through "lever" action when contracted
- produce red blood cells in the bone marrow (hematopoiesis)
- store mineral salts (for example, approximately 99% of the body's calcium).

BONE FORMATION

Cartilage forms the fetal skeleton at 3 months in utero. By about 6 months, the fetal cartilage has been transformed into bony skeleton. However, some bones harden (ossify) after birth, most notably the carpals and tarsals. The change is caused by endochondral ossification, a process by which bone-forming cells (osteoblasts) produce a collagenous material (osteoid) that ossifies.

Two types of osteocytes, osteoblasts and osteoclasts, are responsible for remodeling—the continuous process whereby bone is created and destroyed. Osteoblasts deposit new bone and osteoclasts increase long-bone diameter through reabsorption of previously deposited bone. These activities promote longitudinal bone growth, which continues until the epiphyseal growth plates, located at the bone ends, close in adolescence.

CARTILAGE

Cartilage is a dense connective tissue made of fibers embedded in a strong, gel-like substance. Cartilage is avascular and lacks nerve innervation.

Cartilage is fibrous, hyaline, or elastic. Fibrous cartilage forms the symphysis pubis and the intervertebral disks. Hyaline cartilage covers the articular bone surfaces (where one or more bones meet at a joint), connects the ribs to the sternum, and appears in the trachea, bronchi, and nasal septum. Elastic cartilage is located in the auditory canal, the external ear, and the epiglottis.

Cartilage supports and shapes various structures such as the auditory canal and other cartilage such as the intervertebral disks. It also cushions and absorbs shock, preventing direct transmission to the bone.

JOINTS

The body contains three major types of joints, classified by their extent of movement. Synarthrodial joints such as cranial sutures permit no movement. This joint type separates bones with a thin layer of fibrous connective tissue. Amphiarthrodial joints such as the symphysis pubis allow slight movement. This joint type separates bones with hyaline cartilage. Diarthrodial joints, such as the ankle, wrist, knee, hip, or shoulder, permit free movement. A cavity exists between the bones forming this type of joint. A synovial membrane lines this cavity and secretes a viscous lubricating substance called synovial fluid. The membrane is encased in a fibrous joint capsule. Joints are further classified by their shape and by motion, for example, ball-and-socket joints and hinge and pivot joints.

BURSAE

Located at friction points around joints between tendons, ligaments, and bones, these small synovial fluid sacs act as cushions, decreasing stress to adjacent structures. Examples of bursae include the subacromial bursa, located in the shoulder, and the prepatellar bursa, located in the knee.

SKELETAL MOVEMENT

Although skeletal movement is caused primarily by muscle contractions, other musculoskeletal structures also play a role. To contract, skeletal muscle, which is richly supplied with blood vessels and nerves, needs an impulse from the nervous system and oxygen and nutrients from the circulatory system.

When a skeletal muscle contracts, force is applied to the tendon. Then one bone is pulled toward, moved away from, or rotated around a second bone, depending on the type of muscle contracted. Usually, one bone moves less than the other or remains more stationary. The muscle tendon attachment to the more stationary bone is called the origin. The muscle tendon attachment to the more movable bone is called the insertion site. The origin usually lies on the proximal end and the insertion site on the distal end.

In skeletal movement, the bones act as levers and the joints act as fulcrums, or fixed points. Each bone's function is partially determined by the location of the fulcrum, which establishes the relation between resistance (a force to be overcome) and effort (a force to be resisted). Most movement uses groups of muscles rather than one muscle.

Assessment

Usually, musculoskeletal assessment represents a small part of an overall physical assessment, especially when the patient's chief complaint involves a different body system. But when the patient's health history or physical findings suggest musculoskeletal involvement, you'll need to perform a complete assessment of this system, beginning with a thorough history.

Remember to use open-ended questions to assess broad areas quickly and identify specific problems that require further attention. Follow a systematic plan to avoid missing important data. Keep in mind that you don't have to complete the entire history at once. As long as you obtain all the necessary information and incorporate it into your plan of care, you can break up the interview and complete it as time permits. Also take into account your patient's emotional and physical condition as you conduct your interview.

CHIEF COMPLAINT

Ask your patient what made him seek medical care. Encourage him to describe his complaint in detail. If he has more than one complaint, ask him which complaint bothers him the most, and then focus on that particular problem throughout the rest of the interview. Patients with musculoskeletal problems commonly complain of joint pain and swelling, stiffness, deformity, immobility, muscle aches, and general systemic problems, such as fever and malaise.

Analyze the patient's complaints. Ask him to describe these factors:

Onset. When did the symptom first appear? Did it begin suddenly or gradually? What circumstances surrounded the onset? Did he hurt himself in a fall or other accident? With joint pain, did the pain begin suddenly (which may indicate gout, pseudogout, infection, or trauma) or gradually (which may indicate rheumatoid arthritis, rheumatic fever, or degenerative joint disease)?

Location. Where does he experience the symptom? Can he point to the exact area? With joint pain, does the pain involve one joint or multiple joints? Try to determine whether joint involvement is symmetrical, asymmetrical, or migratory.

Duration. How long has the patient had this symptom? With joint pain, has the pain lasted 1 to 2 days, or several weeks?

Timing. When is the symptom worst? With joint pain or stiffness, does it hurt most in the morning on arising, or after activity?

Quality. Does he have deep, throbbing aching? Or is the pain sharp and intermittent?

Exacerbating and alleviating factors. Do medication, rest, and activity have any effect on his pain?

Associated symptoms. Do other symptoms accompany the primary symptom?

MEDICAL HISTORY
Remember to note all past diagnosed illnesses and hospitalizations. In particular, note any history of acute rheumatic fever, arthritis or other collagenous disease, allergies, hay fever, or asthma. Ask about drug use (both prescription and over-the-counter drugs).

FAMILY HISTORY
Ask the patient if any family members suffer from joint disease.

PSYCHOSOCIAL HISTORY
Factors in your patient's lifestyle may influence his musculoskeletal status. Start with a general review of his background (age, sex, marital status, occupation, education, and ethnic background); then focus on his specific problems.

PHYSICAL EXAMINATION
As you perform a head-to-toe assessment, simultaneously evaluate muscle and joint function of each body area—posture, gait, and coordination—and inspect and palpate his muscles, joints, and bones.

PREPARING FOR THE EXAMINATION
Gather the necessary equipment, including a tape measure and a goniometer or protractor for measuring angles. Position the examination table to allow full range of motion (ROM) for the patient and your easy access. Respect the patient's need for privacy; provide a robe, and allow him to wear his underwear during the examination. Also make sure the room is warm.

To increase the patient's compliance and make the assessment more accurate, demonstrate as well as describe the desired activity or movement to the patient. Compare both sides of the body for such characteristics as size, strength, movement, and complaints of pain. Record his expressions of pain or other sensations elicited during the examination.

OBSERVING POSTURE, GAIT, AND COORDINATION
Assess the patient's overall body symmetry as he assumes different postures and makes diverse movements. Note marked dissimilarities in side-to-side size, shape, and motion.

Posture. Evaluating posture—the position that body parts assume in relation to other body parts and to the external environment—includes inspecting spinal curvature and knee positioning.

Spinal curvature. To assess spinal curvature, instruct the patient to stand as straight as possible. Viewing his side, back, and front, respectively, inspect the spine for alignment and the shoulders, iliac crests, and scapulae ford height. Then have the him bend forward from the waist with arms relaxed and dangling. Standing behind him, inspect the straightness of the spine, noting flank and thorax position and symmetry. Normally, convex curvature characterizes the thoracic spine and concave curvature characterizes the lumbar spine in a standing patient.

Other normal findings include a midline spine without lateral curvatures, a concave lumbar curvature that changes to a convex curvature in the flexed position, and iliac crests, shoulders, and scapulae at the same horizontal level. Race may cause differences in spinal curvatures; for example, some blacks have a pronounced lumbar lordosis.

Knee position. Have the patient stand with his feet together. Note the relation of one knee to the other. They should be bilaterally symmetrical and located at the same height in a forward-facing position. Normally, the knees and the medial malleoli are ⅛″ (3 mm) apart.

Gait. Ask the patient to walk away, turn around, and walk back. Observe and evaluate his posture, movement (such as pace and length of stride), foot position, coordination, and balance. During the stance phase, the foot on the floor should flatten completely and bear the weight of the body. As the patient pushes off, the toes should be flexed. In the swing phase, the foot in midswing should clear the floor and pass the opposite leg in its stance phase. When the swing phase ends, the patient should be able to control the swing as it stops, and the foot again contacts the floor.

Other normal findings include smooth, coordinated movements, the head leading the body when turning, and erect posture with approximately 2″ to 4″ (5 to 10 cm) of space between the feet. Remember to remain close to an older or infirm patient and be ready to help if he should stumble or start to fall.

Abnormal findings. You may see abnormal gait and pain, muscle weakness, deformities, and orthopedic devices such as leg braces. You may also observe an abnormally wide support base (which, in adults, may indicate central nervous system dysfunction), toeing in or out, arms held out to the side or in front, jerky or shuffling motions, and the ball of the foot, rather than the heel, striking the floor first.

Coordination. Evaluate how well your patient's muscles produce movement. Coordination is linked to neuromuscular integrity; a lack of muscular or nervous system integrity, or both, impairs his ability to make voluntary and productive movements.

Assess gross motor skills by having your patient perform any body action involving the muscles and joints in natural directional movements, such as lifting his arm to the side or other ROM exercises. Assess fine motor coordination by asking him to pick up a small object from a desk or table.

INSPECTION

Expect to perform inspection and palpation simultaneously during the musculoskeletal assessment of muscle tone, mass, and strength. Remember to palpate the muscles gently, never forcing movement when the patient reports pain or when you feel resistance. Watch his face and body language for signs of discomfort; a patient may suffer silently.

Tone and mass. Assess muscle tone—the consistency or tension in the resting muscle—by palpating a muscle at rest and during passive ROM. Palpate the

resting muscle from the muscle attachment at the bone to the edge of the muscle. Normally, a relaxed muscle should feel soft, pliable, and nontender; a contracted muscle, firm.

Assessing muscle mass (actual size) usually involves measuring the circumference of the thigh, the calf, and the upper arm. When measuring, establish landmarks to ensure measurement at the same location on each area. When measuring the upper midarm circumferences, remember to ask the patient whether he is right- or left-handed. Except for a slightly larger midarm on the favored side, expect symmetry of size.

Strength and joint ROM. Assessing joint ROM tests the joint function; assessing muscle strength against resistance tests the function of the muscles surrounding the joint. (See *Assessing muscles and joints,* pages 519 to 529.)

INSPECTING AND PALPATING JOINTS AND BONES

Expect to measure the patient's height and the length of the extremities (arms and legs) and evaluate joint and bone characteristics and joint ROM.

Length of the extremities. Place the patient in the supine position on a flat surface with his arms and legs fully extended and his shoulders and hips adducted. Measure each arm from the acromial process to the tip of the middle finger. Measure each leg from the anterior superior iliac spine to the medial malleolus with the tape crossing at the medial side of the knee.

Cervical spine. Inspect the cervical spine, facing the patient as he sits or stands. Observe the alignment of the head with the body. His nose should be in line with the midsternum and extend beyond the shoulders when viewed from the side. His head should align with his shoulders. Normally, the seventh cervical and first thoracic vertebrae appear more prominent than the others.

Clavicles. Inspect and palpate the length of the clavicles, including the sternoclavicular and acromioclavicular joints. Normal findings include firm, smooth, and continuous bones. To inspect and palpate the scapulae, sit directly behind the patient as he sits with his shoulders thrust backward. Normally, the scapulae are located over thoracic ribs two through seven. Check for an equal distance from the medial scapular edges to the midspinal line.

Scapular winging (an outward prominence of the scapulae) is an abnormality best seen with the patient in an upright position with shoulders thrust back.

(Text continues on page 529.)

Assessing muscles and joints

To evaluate muscle strength, have the patient perform active range-of-motion (ROM) movements as you apply resistance. Normally, the patient can move joints a certain distance (measured in degrees) and can easily resist pressure applied against movement. If the muscle group is weak, lessen the resistance to permit a more accurate assessment. Note that strength is normally symmetrical.

To assess joint ROM, ask the patient to move specific joints through normal ROM. If he can't do so, perform passive ROM. Use a goniometer to measure the angle achieved.

Grading muscle strength

When evaluating muscle strength, use the scale below. Column 1 describes the possible muscle response and its significance. Column 2 grades the response.

Muscle response and significance	Grade rating
No visible or palpable contraction ■ Paralysis	0
Slightly palpable contraction ■ Paresis, severe weakness	1
Passive ROM maneuvers when gravity is removed ■ Paresis, moderate weakness	2
Active ROM against gravity alone or against light resistance ■ Mild weakness	3 to 4
Active ROM against full resistance ■ Normal	5

Cervical spine and neck

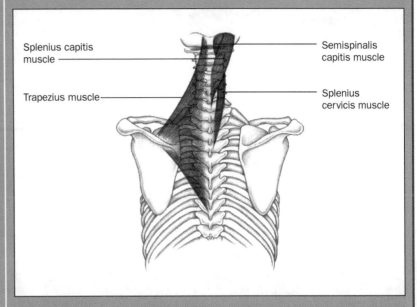

Splenius capitis muscle

Trapezius muscle

Semispinalis capitis muscle

Splenius cervicis muscle

Muscle strength

To assess muscles responsible for flexion of the cervical spine, place your hand on the patient's forehead, applying pressure, as shown below. Ask her to bend her head forward and touch her chin to her chest. (Perform this maneuver only after cervical spine injury has been ruled out.)

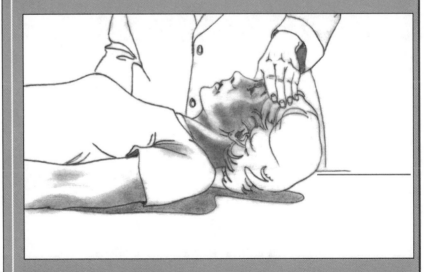

(continued)

Assessing muscles and joints *(continued)*

Cervical spine and neck *(continued)*

Muscle strength *(continued)*

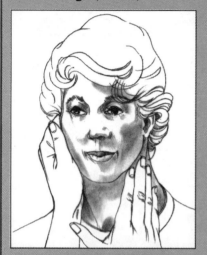

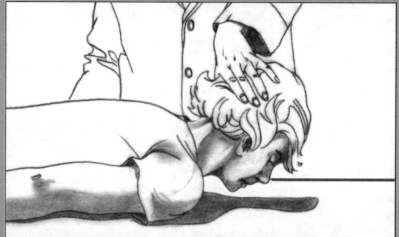

To assess muscles responsible for cervical spine rotation, place your hand along the jaw. Ask the patient to push laterally against your hand while you attempt to prevent movement. At the same time, palpate the sternocleidomastoid on the opposite side. Repeat on the other side.

To assess muscles responsible for extension of the cervical spine, apply pressure with your hand on the patient's occipital bone. Ask her to bend her head backward as far as possible.

Range of motion

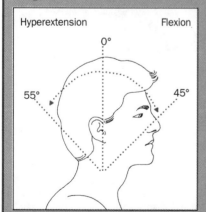

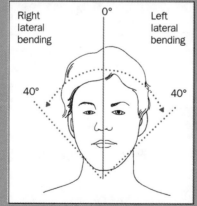

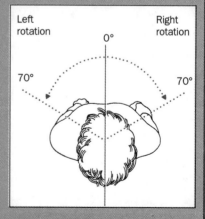

Ask the patient to flex his neck, attempting to touch his chin to his chest, and to extend his neck, bending his head backward.

Next, ask him to bend laterally, touching his ears to his shoulders.

Then, ask him to rotate his head from side to side.

Assessing muscles and joints *(continued)*

Shoulder

Anterior view of right shoulder

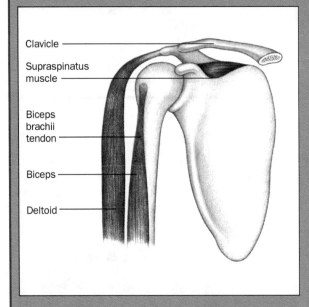

Clavicle

Supraspinatus muscle

Biceps brachii tendon

Biceps

Deltoid

Muscle strength

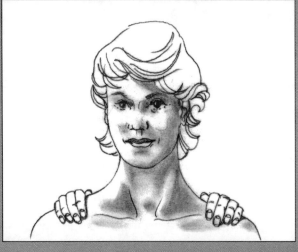

Test the trapezius muscles (of the shoulder and upper back) simultaneously. Ask the patient to shrug her shoulders, then again as you press down on them.

Range of motion

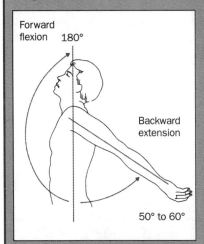

Forward flexion 180°

Backward extension

50° to 60°

Observe and measure ROM as the patient demonstrates forward flexion, with the arms straight in front, and backward extension, with the arms straight and extended backward.

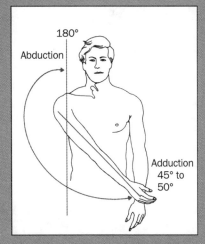

180°

Abduction

Adduction 45° to 50°

To assess abduction, ask the patient to raise his straightened arm out to the side; to assess adduction, ask him to move his straightened arm to midline.

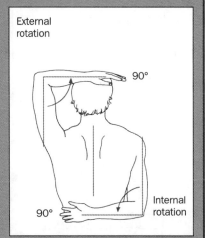

External rotation

90°

90°

Internal rotation

To assess external rotation, ask the patient to abduct his arm with his elbow bent, placing his hand behind his head.

To assess internal rotation, ask the patient to abduct his arm with his elbow bent, placing his hand behind the small of his back.

(continued)

Assessing muscles and joints *(continued)*

Upper arm and elbow

Anterior view of left arm

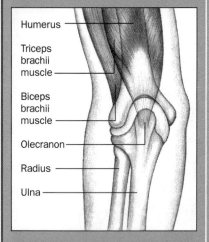

- Humerus
- Triceps brachii muscle
- Biceps brachii muscle
- Olecranon
- Radius
- Ulna

Muscle strength

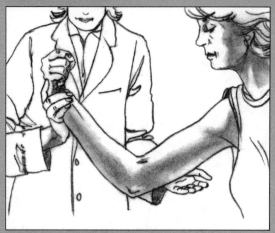

To test triceps strength, try to flex the patient's arm while she tries to extend it.

Range of motion

Ask the patient to sit or stand. Then, assess flexion by having him bend his arm and attempt to touch the shoulder. To assess extension, ask him to straighten his arm.

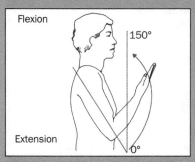

Flexion
150°
Extension
0°

Assess pronation by holding the patient's elbow in a flexed position while he rotates the arm until the palm faces the floor.

Assess supination by holding the patient's elbow in a flexed position while he rotates the arm until the palm faces upward.

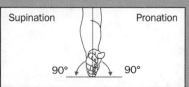

Supination
Pronation
90°
90°

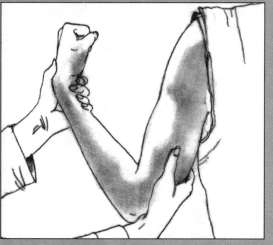

To assess biceps strength, try to pull the patient's flexed arm into extension while she resists.

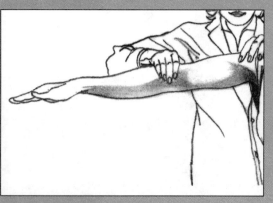

To test deltoid strength, push down on the patient's arm (abducted to 90 degrees) while she resists.

Assessing muscles and joints *(continued)*

Wrist and hand

Lateral view of the left hand and wrist

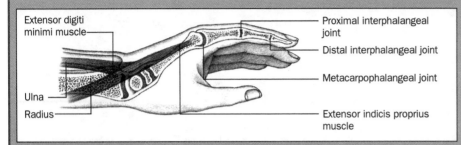

Extensor digiti minimi muscle

Ulna

Radius

Proximal interphalangeal joint

Distal interphalangeal joint

Metacarpophalangeal joint

Extensor indicis proprius muscle

Range of motion

To assess flexion, ask the patient to bend his wrist downward; assess extension by having him straighten his wrist.

To assess hyperextension or dorsiflexion, ask him to bend his wrist upward.

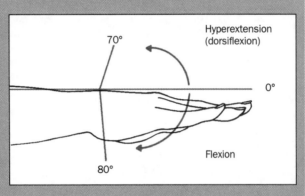

Hyperextension (dorsiflexion)

70°

0°

80°

Flexion

To assess the metacarpophalangeal joints, ask the patient to hyperextend (dorsiflex), extend (straighten), and flex (make a fist) the fingers.

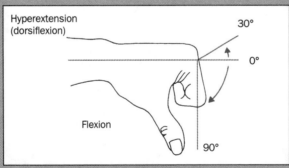

Hyperextension (dorsiflexion)

30°

0°

Flexion

90°

Assess radial deviation by asking the patient to move his hand toward the radial side; assess ulnar deviation by asking him to move his hand toward the ulnar side. Also ask the patient to straighten the fingers, then spread them (abduct) and bring them together (adduct). In abduction, there should be 20 degrees between fingers; in adduction, the fingers should touch.

To assess palmar adduction, ask the patient to bring the thumb to the index finger; assess palmar abduction by asking the patient to move the thumb away from the palm. Assess opposition by having the patient touch the thumb to each fingertip.

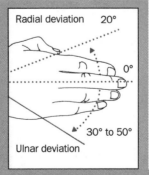

Radial deviation   20°

0°

30° to 50°

Ulnar deviation

Muscle strength

Test muscle strength and movement of both hands simultaneously by having the patient squeeze the first two fingers of your hand, make a fist, resist your efforts to straighten a flexed wrist, and resist your efforts to flex a straightened wrist. (Normally, the dominant hand may be slightly stronger.)

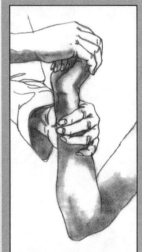

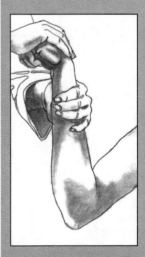

(continued)

Assessing muscles and joints (continued)

Thoracic and lumbar spine

Posterior view of spine and pelvis

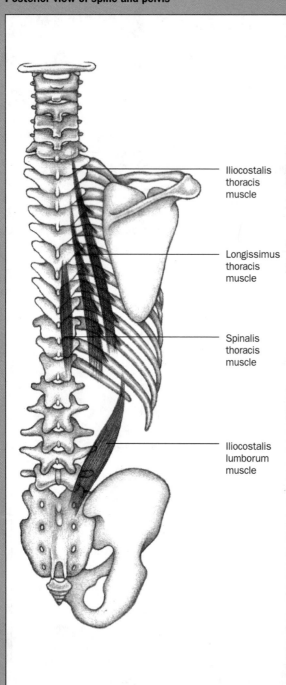

- Iliocostalis thoracis muscle
- Longissimus thoracis muscle
- Spinalis thoracis muscle
- Iliocostalis lumborum muscle

Range of motion

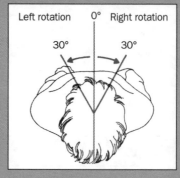

Left rotation   0°   Right rotation

30°   30°

Assess rotation by first stabilizing the patient's pelvis, then asking him to rotate the upper body from side to side.

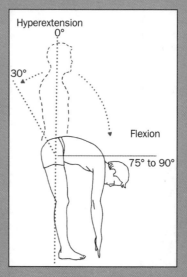

Hyperextension
0°

30°

Flexion

75° to 90°

With the patient standing, observe and evaluate spinal ROM as he demonstrates hyperextension by bending backward from the waist and flexion by bending to touch the floor with the knees slightly bent.

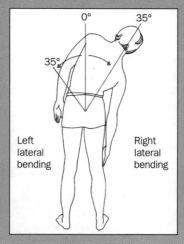

0°   35°

35°

Left lateral bending   Right lateral bending

Ask the patient to bend to each side (lateral bending).

Assessing muscles and joints *(continued)*

Hip and pelvis

Posterior view of right hip and thigh

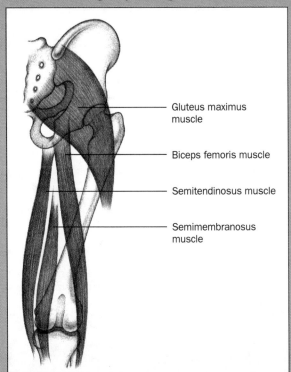

— Gluteus maximus muscle

— Biceps femoris muscle

— Semitendinosus muscle

— Semimembranosus muscle

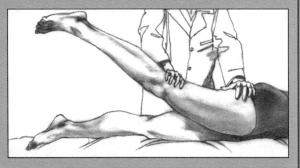

With the patient lying (prone and, later, supine) and then sitting, evaluate muscle strength and palpate muscles as you carry out the following tests.

To assess hip extensors, ask the prone patient to hyperextend her leg backward (toward the ceiling) as you try to push her leg downward, as shown above.

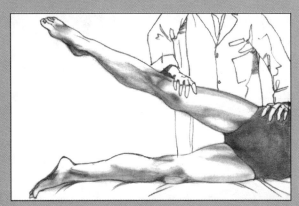

To assess hip abductors, ask the side-lying patient to move her straightened leg away from midline as you try to push it toward midline.

Muscle strength

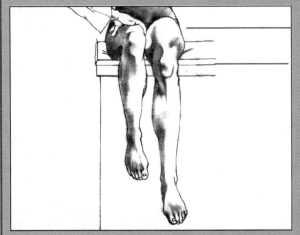

To assess hip flexors, ask the patient to sit and raise her knee to her chest as you apply downward pressure proximal to the knee.

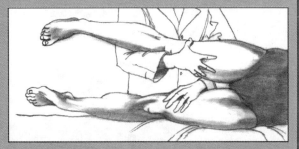

To assess hip adductors, ask the side-lying patient to move her leg toward midline as you try to pull it away from midline.

(continued)

Assessing muscles and joints *(continued)*

Hip and pelvis *(continued)*

Range of motion

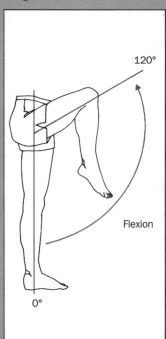

With the patient prone or standing, observe and evaluate ROM as the patient demonstrates flexion by bending the knee to the chest with the back straight, as shown on the left. *Caution:* Don't perform this movement without the surgeon's permission on a patient who has undergone total hip replacement because the motion can cause the prosthesis to dislocate.

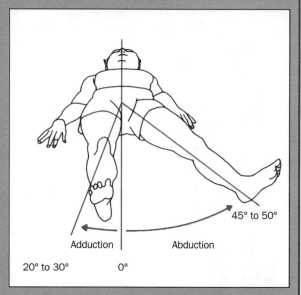

To assess abduction, have the patient move his straightened leg away from midline; assess adduction by having him move his straightened leg toward midline. *Caution:* This motion can displace a hip prosthesis.

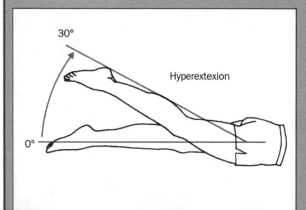

Evaluate extension by asking the patient to straighten his knee and hyperextension by asking him to extend his leg backward with his knee straight. *Note:* This motion can be performed with the patient prone or standing.

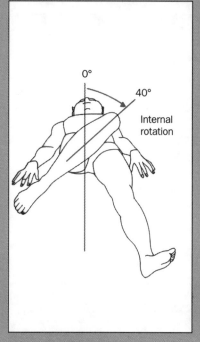

Finally, assess internal and external rotation by asking the patient to bend his knee and turn the leg inward and outward, respectively.

Assessing muscles and joints *(continued)*

Knee

Anterior view of left knee

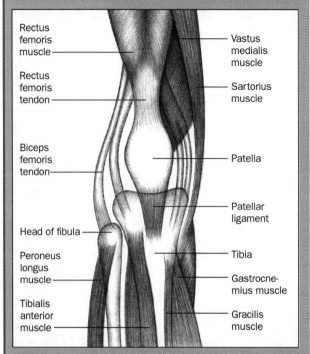

Rectus femoris muscle
Rectus femoris tendon
Biceps femoris tendon
Head of fibula
Peroneus longus muscle
Tibialis anterior muscle

Vastus medialis muscle
Sartorius muscle
Patella
Patellar ligament
Tibia
Gastrocnemius muscle
Gracilis muscle

Muscle strength

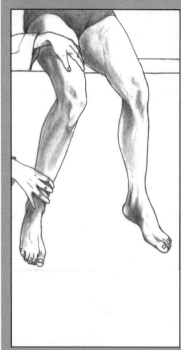

To assess knee extensors, ask the patient to sit or lie supine and extend his leg as you attempt to flex it.

Range of motion

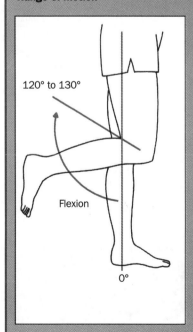

120° to 130°

Flexion

0°

With the patient sitting or standing, observe and measure ROM as the patient demonstrates extension by straightening his leg at the knee.

With the patient standing, have him demonstrate flexion by bending his leg at the knee and bringing his foot up to touch his buttock.

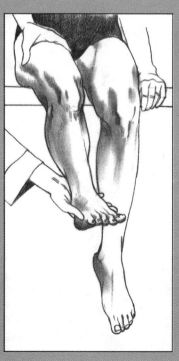

To assess knee flexors, ask the patient to sit or lie supine while you try to extend his leg as he flexes his knee.

(continued)

Assessing muscles and joints (continued)

Ankle and foot

Anterior view of right ankle and foot

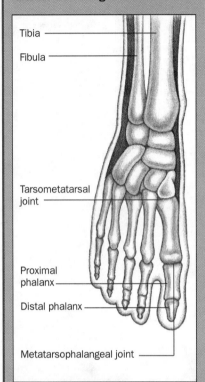

Tibia

Fibula

Tarsometatarsal joint

Proximal phalanx

Distal phalanx

Metatarsophalangeal joint

Muscle strength

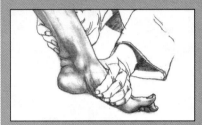

To assess dorsiflexion of the ankle joint, apply pressure with your hand to the dorsal surface of the patient's foot as he attempts to bend his foot up.

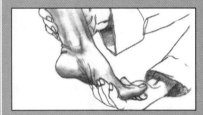

To assess plantar flexion, apply pressure with your hand to the plantar surface of the patient's foot as he attempts to bend his foot down.

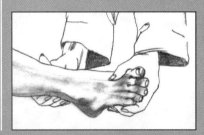

To assess inversion, apply pressure with your hand to the medial surface of the patient's first metatarsal bone as he attempts to move his toes inward. Assess eversion by placing your hand on the lateral surface of the fifth metatarsal bone and applying pressure as he attempts to move his toes outward.

Range of motion

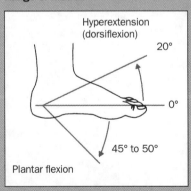

Hyperextension (dorsiflexion)

20°

0°

45° to 50°

Plantar flexion

Ask the patient who is sitting, lying, or standing to demonstrate plantar flexion by bending his foot downward and dorsiflexion by bending his foot upward.

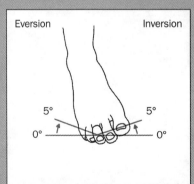

Eversion   Inversion

5°   5°

0°   0°

Then ask him to invert his foot by pointing the toes and turning the foot inward and to evert the foot by pointing the toes and turning the foot outward.

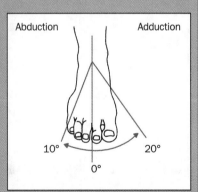

Abduction   Adduction

10°   20°

0°

To assess forefoot adduction and abduction, stabilize the patient's heel while he turns his forefoot inward and outward, respectively.

Assessing muscles and joints *(continued)*

Toes

Anterior view of left foot

Lower extensor retinaculum

Extensor digitorum brevis

Muscle strength

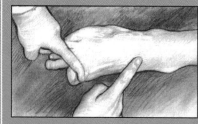

To assess extension, apply pressure with your finger to the dorsal surface of the patient's toes as he attempts to point his toes upward.

To assess flexion, apply pressure with your finger to the plantar surface of the patient's toes as he attempts to bend his toes downward.

Range of motion

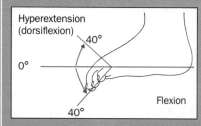

Hyperextension (dorsiflexion)
40°
0°
Flexion
40°

To assess the metatarsophalangeal joints, ask the patient to extend (straighten) and flex (curl) the toes. Then, ask him to hyperextend his toes by straightening and pointing them upward.

Outward scapular displacement signifies dysfunction of the muscles and nerves serving this structure.

Ribs. After assessing the scapulae, inspect the ribs for visual abnormalities and palpate their surfaces. Normal findings include firm, smooth, and continuous bones.

Shoulders. Palpate the moving joints for crepitus. Inspect the skin overlying the shoulder joints for erythema, masses, or swelling.

Next, palpate the acromioclavicular joint and the area over the greater humeral tuberosity. Ask the patient to hold his arm at his side; then have him move his arm across his chest (adduction). Next, place your thumb on the anterior portion of the patient's shoulder joint and your fingers on the posterior portion of the joint. Ask the patient to abduct his arm, and palpate the shoulder joint as he does so.

Now stand behind the patient. With your fingertips placed over the greater humeral tuberosity, ask him to rotate his shoulder internally by moving the arm behind the back. This allows you to palpate a portion of the musculotendinous rotator cuff as well as the bony structures of the shoulder joint.

If shoulder joint palpation produces pain in the greater humeral tuberosity area, calcium deposits or trauma-related inflammation may be the cause. Difficulty abducting the arm and pain in the deltoid muscle or over the supraspinatus tendon insertion site during palpation may indicate a rotator cuff tear.

Elbows. Inspect joint contour and the skin over each elbow. Palpate the elbows at rest and during movement.

Wrists. Look for ischemia, skeletal deformities, and swelling. Palpate the wrist at rest and during movement by gently grasping it between your thumb and fingers. Also test for Tinel's sign (tingling sensations in the thumb, index, and middle fingers) by briskly tapping the patient's wrist over the median nerve. A positive response may indicate carpal tunnel syndrome, a painful disorder of the wrist and hand caused by compression on the median nerve between the carpal ligament and other structures within the carpal tunnel.

Fingers and thumbs. On each hand, look for nodules, erythema, spacing, length, and skeletal deformities. Palpate your patient's fingers and thumb at rest and during movement.

Thoracic and lumbar spine. Besides evaluating the curvatures of the thoracic and lumbar spine during the postural assessment, remember to palpate the length of the spine for tenderness and vertebral alignment. To check for tenderness, percuss each spinous process (directly over the vertebral column) with the ulnar side of your fist.

Note whether the patient exhibits full ROM while maintaining balance, smoothness, and coordination.

Hips and pelvis. Inspect and palpate over the bony prominences: iliac crests, symphysis pubis, anterior spine, ischial tuberosities, and greater trochanters. Palpate the hip at rest and during movement.

Knees. Inspect the knees with the patient seated. Palpate the knee at rest and during movement. Inspect and palpate the popliteal spaces (behind the knee joint). Knee movements should be smooth.

Ankles and feet. Inspect and palpate the ankles and feet at rest and during movement.

Toes. The patient may sit or lie supine for toe assessment. Inspect all toe surfaces. Palpate toes at rest and during movement.

Ankylosing spondylitis

Also called rheumatoid spondylitis or Marie-Strüumpell disease, ankylosing spondylitis primarily affects the sacroiliac joint, the axial spine, and the adjacent ligamentous or tendinous attachments to the bone. Typically beginning in adults younger than age 40, this inflammatory disease progressively restricts spinal movement.

In primary disease, sacroiliitis is usually bilateral and symmetrical; in secondary disease, it's usually unilateral and asymmetrical. The patient may also have extra-articular disease, such as acute anterior iri-

tis (in about 25% of patients), proximal root aortitis and heart block, and apical pulmonary fibrosis. Rarely, extra-articular disease appears as caudal adhesive leptomeningitis and immunoglobulin A (IgA) nephropathy.

Ankylosing spondylitis affects three to four times more men than women. Progressive disease is well recognized in men but is commonly overlooked or missed in women, who tend to have more peripheral joint involvement. (See *Detecting spondylitis in women.*)

Rarely, disease progression can impose severe physical restrictions on activities of daily living and occupational functions. Atlantoaxial subluxation is a rare complication of primary ankylosing spondylitis.

CAUSES
Studies suggest a familial tendency for the disorder, but its exact cause is unknown. In more than 90% of the patients with this disease, circulating immune complexes and human leukocyte antigen (HLA-B27) suggest immune system activity.

Ankylosing spondylitis usually is a primary disorder, but it also may arise secondary to various GI, genitourinary (GU), and cutaneous disorders. For example, with GI disease, ankylosing spondylitis may occur in association with ulcerative colitis, regional enteritis, Whipple's disease, and gram-negative dysentery. With GU disease, it's associated with chlamydial or mycoplasmal infections. With cutaneous disease, it's associated with psoriasis, acne conglobata, and hidradenitis suppurativa.

The disorder begins in the sacroiliac and gradually progresses to the lumbar, thoracic, and cervical spine. Bone and cartilage deterioration leads to fibrous tissue formation and eventual fusion of the spine or the peripheral joints. Symptoms progress unpredictably into remission, exacerbation, or arrest at any stage.

DIAGNOSIS AND TREATMENT
For a reliable diagnosis, the patient must have specific combinations of the symptoms listed below. The disorder is confirmed if the patient meets either criterion 7 *and* any one of criteria 1 through 5, or any five of criteria 1 through 6:
1. axial skeleton stiffness of at least 3 months' duration that's relieved by exercise
2. lumbar pain that persists at rest
3. thoracic cage pain of at least 3 months
4. past or current iritis
5. decreased lumbar range of motion (ROM)
6. decreased chest expansion (age-related)
7. bilateral, symmetrical sacroiliitis demonstrated by radiographic studies.

Laboratory tests never confirm the diagnosis. However, the doctor may use serum findings, measures of erythrocyte sedimentation rate and alkaline phos-

Detecting spondylitis in women

Ankylosing spondylitis seldom occurs in women so the disorder may be easily overlooked.

Typically, if a woman's symptoms include pelvic pain, diagnosticians suspect pelvic inflammatory disease (PID) rather than ankylosing spondylitis. That's one reason to assess carefully if your female patient has apparent PID but culture results identify no apparent cause. In compiling a thorough medical and social history, investigate any possible family history of ankylosing spondylitis.

Otherwise, misdiagnosis may lead to unwarranted invasive tests and treatments and cause the patient needless anxiety.

phatase and creatine phosphokinase levels, serum IgA levels, and X-ray studies to rule out other disorders or stage the disease.

Because no treatment reliably stops disease progression, management aims to delay further deformity by good posture, stretching and deep-breathing exercises and, if appropriate, braces and lightweight supports. Heat, ice, and nerve stimulation measures may relieve symptoms in some patients. Nonsteroidal anti-inflammatory drugs, such as aspirin, indomethacin, and sulindac, control pain and inflammation.

Severe hip involvement, which affects about 15% of patients, usually requires hip replacement surgery. Severe spinal involvement may require a spinal wedge osteotomy to separate and reposition the vertebrae. Usually, this surgery is reserved for selected patients because of possible spinal cord damage and a lengthy convalescence.

COLLABORATIVE MANAGEMENT

Care of the patient with ankylosing spondylitis focuses on relieving pain, improving mobility, and teaching the patient about the disorder.

ASSESSMENT

Symptoms depend on the disease stage. Look for:
- initially, complaints of intermittent low back pain that is most severe in the morning or after inactivity and is relieved by exercise
- reports of mild fatigue, fever, anorexia, and weight loss
- with symmetrical or asymmetrical peripheral arthritis, reports of shoulder, hip, knee, and ankle pain

- complaints of pain over the symphysis pubis, which may lead to ankylosing spondylitis being mistaken for pelvic inflammatory disease
- evidence of stiffness or limited motion of the lumbar spine
- pain and limited expansion of the chest, resulting from costovertebral and sternomanubrial joint involvement
- limited ROM, resulting from hip deformity
- in advanced disease, kyphosis (caused by chronic stooping to relieve discomfort)
- red, inflamed eyes caused by iritis
- palpable warmth, swelling, or tenderness in affected joints
- aortic heart murmur caused by regurgitation and cardiomegaly
- in the lungs, upper lobe pulmonary fibrosis, which mimics tuberculosis and may reduce vital capacity to 70% or less of predicted volume.

NURSING DIAGNOSES AND COLLABORATIVE PROBLEMS

Based on the following nursing diagnoses, you'll establish patient outcomes.

Activity intolerance related to fatigue and pain. The patient will:
- maintain muscle strength and joint ROM
- perform self-care activities to his tolerance level
- adopt lifestyle changes that minimize pain and fatigue while increasing activity level.

Impaired physical mobility related to spinal abnormalities. The patient will:
- attain the greatest degree of mobility possible within disease limitations
- begin to accept limitations imposed by deformity and lifestyle changes
- show no evidence of contractures, venous stasis, thrombus formation, skin breakdown, hypostatic pneumonia, or other complications of impaired mobility.

Pain related to effects of ankylosing spondylitis on the spinal column, joints, or both. The patient will:
- follow a pain management program that includes an activity and rest schedule, exercise program, and medication regimen that isn't pain contingent
- obtain pain relief from analgesics
- avoid activities that cause pain.

PLANNING AND IMPLEMENTATION

These measures help the patient with ankylosing spondylitis.
- Keep in mind the patient's limited ROM when planning self-care tasks and activities.
- Give analgesics as ordered.
- Apply heat locally and massage as indicated.
- Assess mobility and comfort levels frequently.

■ Have the patient perform active ROM exercises to prevent restricted, painful movement.
■ Pace periods of exercise and rest to help the patient achieve comfortable energy levels and oxygenation of lungs.
■ If treatment includes surgery, ensure proper body alignment and positioning.
■ Regularly evaluate the patient's degree of mobility to detect deterioration.
■ Offer support and reassurance.
■ Because ankylosing spondylitis is a chronic, progressively crippling condition, remember to involve other caregivers, such as a social worker, a visiting nurse, and a dietitian.

Patient teaching

■ To minimize deformities, advise the patient to avoid any physical activity that places stress on the back such as lifting heavy objects.
■ Teach the patient to stand upright; to sit upright in a high, straight-backed chair, and to avoid leaning over a desk.
■ Instruct him to sleep in a prone position on a hard mattress and to avoid using pillows under the neck or knees.
■ Advise the patient to avoid prolonged walking, standing, sitting, or driving; to perform regular stretching and deep-breathing exercises; and to swim regularly, if possible.
■ Instruct the patient to have his height measured every 3 to 4 months to detect kyphosis.
■ Suggest that he seek vocational counseling if work requires standing or prolonged sitting at a desk.
■ Tell the patient to contact the local arthritis agency or the Ankylosing Spondylitis Association for additional information and support.

EVALUATION

Achievement of patient outcomes determines the success of collaborative management. For the patient with ankylosing spondylitis, evaluation focuses on improved patient comfort, increased mobility, and decreased patient limitations.

Gout

Also known as gouty arthritis, this metabolic disease is marked by monosodium urate deposits that cause red, swollen, and acutely painful joints. Gout may strike any joint but mostly affects those in the feet, especially the great toe, ankle, and midfoot. Gout occurs in primary and secondary forms.

PRIMARY GOUT

Primary gout typically appears in men over age 30 and in postmenopausal women who take diuretics. It follows an intermittent course that may leave patients symptom-free for years between attacks.

In asymptomatic patients, serum urate levels rise but produce no symptoms. In symptom-producing gout, the first acute attack strikes suddenly and peaks quickly. Although it may involve only one or a few joints, this attack causes extreme pain. Mild, acute attacks usually subside quickly yet tend to recur at irregular intervals. Severe attacks may persist for days or weeks.

Intercritical periods are the symptom-free intervals between attacks. Most patients have a second attack between 6 months and 2 years after the first; in some patients, however, the second attack is delayed for 5 to 10 years. Delayed attacks, which may be polyarticular, are more common in untreated patients. These attacks tend to last longer and produce more symptoms than initial episodes. A migratory attack strikes various joints and the Achilles tendon sequentially and may be associated with olecranon bursitis.

Eventually, chronic polyarticular gout sets in. This final, unremitting stage of the disease (also known as tophaceous gout) is marked by persistent, painful polyarthritis. An increased concentration of uric acid leads to urate deposits—called tophi—in membranes, tendons, and soft tissue.

Tophi form in the fingers, hands, knees, feet, ulnar sides of the forearms, pinna of the ear, Achilles tendon and, rarely, in such internal organs as the kidneys and myocardium. Renal involvement may adversely affect renal function.

The prognosis is good for patients who receive treatment.

Potential complications include renal disorders such as renal calculi; circulatory problems, such as atherosclerotic disease, cardiovascular lesions, cerebrovascular accident, coronary thrombosis, and hypertension; and infection that develops with tophi rupture and nerve entrapment.

Although the underlying cause of primary gout remains unknown, in many patients the disease is caused by decreased renal excretion of uric acid. In a few patients, gout is linked to a genetic defect in purine metabolism that causes overproduction of uric acid (hyperuricemia).

SECONDARY GOUT

Secondary gout develops during the course of another disease, such as obesity, diabetes mellitus, hypertension, polycythemia, leukemia, myeloma, sickle cell anemia, and renal disease. Secondary gout can also follow treatment with such drugs as hydrochlorothiazide or pyrazinamide.

DIAGNOSIS AND TREATMENT

The following tests support a diagnosis of gout:

- Needle aspiration of synovial fluid (arthrocentesis) or of tophaceous material for examination under polarized light microscopy. Monosodium urate monohydrate crystals in the synovial fluid establishes the diagnosis. If test results identify calcium pyrophosphate crystals, the patient probably has pseudogout, a disease similar to gout.
- Serum uric acid levels may be normal. However, the higher the level (especially when it's above 10 mg/dl), the more likely a gout attack.
- Urine uric acid levels are high in about 20% of gout patients.
- X-ray studies initially produce normal results. However, in chronic gout, X-ray findings show damage to the articular cartilage and subchondral bone. Outward displacement of the overhanging margin from the bone contour characterizes gout.

Treatment for an acute attack is bed rest, local application of cold, and immobilization and protection of the inflamed, painful joints. Analgesics such as acetaminophen relieve the pain associated with mild attacks. Acute inflammation, however, requires nonsteroidal anti-inflammatory drugs (NSAIDs) or I.M. corticotropin. Colchicine, oral or parenteral, or intra-articular corticosteroids are occasionally necessary to treat acute attacks.

Treatment of chronic gout involves decreasing the serum uric acid level to less than 6.5 mg/dl. This may be accomplished with various medications after a 24-hour urinalysis determines whether the patient overexcretes or underexcretes uric acid. If he overexcretes uric acid, he may be given allopurinol (in reduced doses if he has decreased renal function). If he underexcretes uric acid, he may be treated with probenecid or sulfinpyrazone (if he has no history of renal calculi). Taken once or twice daily, colchicine effectively prevents acute gout attacks, although it does not affect uric acid levels.

Adjunctive therapy emphasizes avoiding alcohol (especially beer and wine) and sparing use of purine-rich foods, such as anchovies, liver, sardines, kidneys, sweetbreads, and lentils. Obese patients should begin a weight-loss program because weight reduction will decrease uric acid levels and stress on painful joints as well.

COLLABORATIVE MANAGEMENT

Care of the patient with gout focuses on pain management and prevention of complications.

ASSESSMENT

The patient with gout may have a sedentary lifestyle and a history of hypertension and renal calculi. Look for:

Recognizing gouty tophi

In advanced gout, urate crystal deposits develop into hard, irregular, yellow-white nodules called tophi. These bumps commonly protrude from the great toe and the pinna.

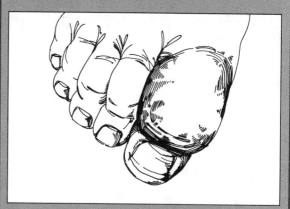

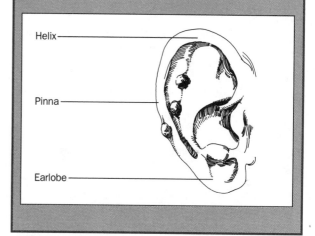

- report of waking during the night with pain in his great toe or another location in the foot
- complaints that initially moderate pain has grown so intense that eventually he can't bear the weight of bed sheets or the vibrations of a person walking across the room
- reports of chills and a mild fever
- swollen, dusky red or purple joint with limited movement
- tophi, especially in feet (See *Recognizing gouty tophi.*)
- in late-stage chronic gout, ulcerated skin over the tophi that releases a chalky white exudate or pus
- chronic inflammation and tophaceous deposits that prompt secondary joint degeneration, followed by erosions, deformity, and disability

- palpable warmth over the joint and extreme tenderness
- fever and hypertension (possible indicating occult infection).

NURSING DIAGNOSES AND COLLABORATIVE PROBLEMS

Based on the following nursing diagnoses, you'll establish patient outcomes.

Risk for injury related to complications. The patient will:
- communicate an understanding of the treatment for gout and the importance of compliance to minimize or prevent complications
- exhibit no signs or symptoms of renal or cardiovascular dysfunction or infection
- have no injury related to gout.

Impaired physical mobility related to pain and joint changes. The patient will:
- seek assistance in performing activities of daily living as needed, but especially during acute gout attacks
- show no evidence of complications caused by impaired physical mobility, such as skin breakdown or contractures
- attain the highest degree of mobility possible within the restrictions imposed by gout.

Pain related to monosodium urate deposits in joints. The patient will:
- express feelings of comfort after receiving analgesics
- modify his lifestyle, particularly dietary intake, to reduce his uric acid level
- become pain-free with the prescribed treatment regimen.

PLANNING AND IMPLEMENTATION

These measures help the patient with gout.
- Give anti-inflammatory medication and other drugs, as ordered. Also give sodium bicarbonate or other agents to alkalinize the patient's urine, as ordered.
- Give pain medication, as needed, especially during acute attacks. Apply cold packs to inflamed joints to ease discomfort.
- To promote sleep, give pain medication at times that allow for maximum rest. Provide the patient with sleep aids, such as an extra pillow, a bath, or a back rub.
- Encourage bed rest, but use a bed cradle to keep bed linens off sensitive, inflamed joints.
- Encourage the patient to perform techniques that promote rest and relaxation.
- Monitor the patient's pain level and his response to pain-control measures, including analgesics.

- Urge the patient to perform as many activities as his immobility and pain allow. Provide adequate time to perform these activities.
- Provide a nutritious diet; avoid purine-rich foods.
- Before and after surgery, administer colchicine to help prevent gout attacks, as ordered.
- Remember to provide emotional support during diagnostic tests and procedures.
- When forcing fluids, record intake and output accurately. Monitor serum uric acid levels regularly.
- Monitor the patient's condition after joint aspiration for signs of improvement and complications such as infection.
- Watch for adverse reactions when giving the patient anti-inflammatory drugs and other drugs. Be alert for GI disturbances with colchicine administration.
- To diffuse anxiety and promote coping mechanisms, encourage the patient to express his concerns about his condition. Listen supportively.
- Include the patient and his family members in care-related decisions and all phases of care. Answer questions about his disorder.

Patient teaching

- Urge the patient to drink plenty of fluids (up to 2 qt [2 L] a day) to prevent renal calculi.
- Explain all treatments, tests, and procedures. Warn him before his first needle aspiration that it will be extremely painful.
- Make sure the patient understands the rationale for evaluating serum uric acid levels periodically.
- Teach the patient relaxation techniques. Encourage him to perform them regularly.
- Instruct the patient to avoid purine-rich foods because they raise the urate level.
- Discuss the principles of gradual weight reduction with an obese patient. Explain the advantages of a diet containing moderate amounts of protein and little fat.
- If the patient receives allopurinol, probenecid, or other drugs, instruct him to report any adverse reactions immediately. (Reactions may include nausea, vomiting, drowsiness, dizziness, urinary frequency, and dermatitis.)
- Warn the patient taking probenecid or sulfinpyrazone to avoid aspirin or other salicylates. Their combined effect causes urate retention.
- Inform the patient that long-term colchicine therapy is essential during the first 3 to 6 months of treatment with uricosuric drugs or allopurinol. Stress the importance of compliance.
- Urge the patient to control hypertension, especially if he has tophaceous renal deposits. Keep in mind that diuretics aren't advised for the gout patient; alternative antihypertensives are preferred.

EVALUATION
Achievement of patient outcomes determines the success of collaborative management. For the patient with gout, evaluation focuses on decreased pain, improved mobility, and safety.

Hallux valgus

Hallux valgus is a lateral deviation of the great toe at the metatarsophalangeal joint. It involves medial enlargement of the first metatarsal head and bunion formation (bursa and callus formation at the bony prominence).

CAUSES
Hallux valgus is congenital or familial but is more often caused by degenerative arthritis or by prolonged pressure, especially from narrow-toed, high-heeled shoes that compress the forefoot.

DIAGNOSIS AND TREATMENT
The doctor may order tests to support a diagnosis of hallux valgus, including X-rays to show medial deviation of the first mentation of the great toe.

In early stages of acquired hallux valgus, good foot care and proper shoes may eliminate the need for further treatment. Other useful measures for early management include felt pads to protect the bunion, foam pads or other devices to separate the first and second toes at night, and a supportive pad and exercises to strengthen the metatarsal muscles. Treatment is vital in patients predisposed to foot problems, such as those with rheumatoid arthritis or diabetes mellitus. If the disease progresses to severe deformity with disabling pain, the doctor may perform a bunionectomy.

COLLABORATIVE MANAGEMENT
Care of the patient with hallux valgus focuses on improving mobility, relieving pain, and teaching the patient how to avoid complications.

ASSESSMENT
This disorder first appears as a red, tender bunion. The patient may develop angulation of the great toe away from the midline of the body toward the other toes. In advanced stages of the disorder, he may develop a flat, splayed forefoot, severely curled toes (hammertoes), and a small bunion on the fifth metatarsal.

NURSING DIAGNOSES AND COLLABORATIVE PROBLEMS
Based on the following nursing diagnoses, you'll establish patient outcomes.

Pain related to physical changes. The patient will:
- investigate nonpharmacologic methods of pain relief
- report relief of pain.

Impaired physical mobility related to physical changes. The patient will:
- improve ability to ambulate
- maintain muscle strength and range of motion
- shows no evidence of complications.

PLANNING AND IMPLEMENTATION
These measures help the patient with hallux valgus.
- Before bunionectomy, obtain a patient history and assess the neurovascular status of the foot (temperature, color, sensation, blanching sign).
- Prepare the patient for walking by having him dangle his foot over the side of the bed for a short time before he gets up, allowing a gradual increase in venous pressure.
- If crutches are needed, supervise the patient in using them, and make sure he masters this skill before discharge.
- Help the patient get a proper cast shoe or boot to protect the cast or dressing.
- Apply ice to reduce swelling, and reduce edema by supporting the foot with pillows, elevating the foot of the bed, or putting the bed in a Trendelenburg position so that the affected area is above the level of the heart.
- Record the neurovascular status of the toes, including the patient's ability to move them (dressing may inhibit movement). Record every hour for the first 24 hours, then every 4 hours. Report any change in neurovascular status to the surgeon immediately.

Patient teaching
- Teach the patient to limit activities when he gets home, to rest frequently with his feet elevated, to elevate his feet whenever he feels pain or has edema, and to wear wide-toed shoes and sandals after the dressings are removed.
- Discuss the basics of proper foot care, such as cleanliness, massages, and cutting toenails straight across to prevent infection.
- Suggest exercises to do at home to strengthen foot muscles such as standing at the edge of a step on his heel, and then raising and inverting the top of the foot.
- Finally, stress the importance of follow-up care and prompt medical attention for painful bunions, corns, and calluses.

EVALUATION
Achievement of patient outcomes determines the success of collaborative management. For the patient with hallux valgus, evaluation focuses on improved

mobility, pain reduction, and knowledge of the disorder and its management.

Hip fractures

Hip fractures involve the upper third of the patient's femur. Intracapsular fractures occur within the joint capsule (capital, subcapital, and femoral neck). Extracapsular fractures are those outside the joint capsule (subtrochanteric and intertrochanteric).

Usually, the patient with a hip fracture will be an older woman with osteoporosis. Most of these women have fallen and suffered an impaction or displacement of the femoral neck.

DIAGNOSIS AND TREATMENT
To support a diagnosis of hip fracture, the doctor usually will use X-rays of the hip and may order a computed tomography scan or magnetic resonance imaging.

Surgical repair is the treatment of choice for a hip fracture. The type of surgery will depend on the location of the fracture. Open reduction with internal fixation (ORIF) may include an intramedullary rod, pins, a prosthesis, or a fixed sliding plate (compression screw). Compression screw placement allows the patient to move about within a few days after surgery and carries with it a decreased chance of infection and nonunion.

Nonsurgical options include skin traction (Buck's) and skeletal traction followed by use of a cast brace.

COLLABORATIVE MANAGEMENT
Care of the patient with a hip fracture focuses on decreasing pain, increasing mobility, and providing patient teaching.

ASSESSMENT
The patient usually reports a fall. When you palpate the hip, she will experience pain, which may radiate to the knee. The affected hip may also be turned inward and flexed by the patient.

NURSING DIAGNOSES AND COLLABORATIVE PROBLEMS
Based on the following nursing diagnoses, you'll establish patient outcomes.

Pain related to injury. The patient will:
- experience decreased pain
- try nonpharmacologic methods of pain relief.

Impaired physical mobility related to injury. The patient will:
- experience increased mobility

- maintain muscle strength and range of motion (ROM).

PLANNING AND IMPLEMENTATION
These measures help the patient with a fractured hip.
- Give the patient prescribed analgesics and assess their effect.
- Use supportive pillows to maintain alignment and prevent further injury.
- Turn the patient in an alignment that avoids pressure to the injured hip.
- Watch for complications of bed rest (pulmonary emboli, skin breakdown, fat emboli, pneumonia)
- Encourage deep breathing and coughing; turn and reposition your patient every 2 hours.
- After surgery, assist with ROM as ordered.

Patient teaching
- Tell the patient about the prescribed drugs, including their adverse effects and dosages.
- Review proper physical therapy techniques with your patient to help with early ambulation and prevent contractures.
- Teach the patient about hip surgery, it's potential complications, and the exercise and physical therapy that will follow.

EVALUATION
Achievement of patient outcomes determines the success of collaborative management. For the patient with hip fracture, evaluation focuses on decreased pain, safety, and increased mobility.

Joint dislocation

Dislocations displace joint bones to the extent that their articulating surfaces lose all contact. Most dislocations are at the joints of the shoulders, elbows, wrists, digits, hips, knees, ankles, and feet. They may accompany fractures of the joints and deposit fracture fragments between joint surfaces. Prompt reduction can limit the resulting damage to soft tissue, nerves, and blood vessels.

CAUSES
Dislocations are caused by congenital anomaly, trauma, or disease of surrounding joint tissues.

DIAGNOSIS AND TREATMENT
To confirm a diagnosis of joint dislocation, the doctor will use X-rays that confirm or rule out fracture and may show the dislocation.

Immediate reduction (before tissue edema and muscle spasm make reduction difficult) can prevent additional tissue damage and vascular impairment. Closed reduction is manual traction under either general anesthesia or local anesthesia and sedatives. During such reduction, morphine sulfate controls pain; diazepam controls muscle spasm and facilitates muscle stretching during traction. Occasionally, such injuries require open reduction under regional block or general anesthesia. Such surgery may include wire fixation of the joint, skeletal traction, and ligament repair.

After reduction, the joint is immobilized using a sling, splint, cast, or traction. Usually, immobilizing the digits for 2 weeks, the hips for 6 to 8 weeks, and other dislocated joints for 3 to 6 weeks allows the surrounding tissue to heal properly.

COLLABORATIVE MANAGEMENT
Care of the patient with a joint dislocation focuses on relieving pain and improving mobility.

ASSESSMENT
A patient with a dislocation may report deformity around the joint, altered length of the involved extremity, impaired joint mobility, point tenderness and, in trauma, extreme pain.

The following tests support a diagnosis of joint dislocations:
- X-rays of the affected joint
- X-ray of long bones
- Angiography to assess vascular injury.

NURSING DIAGNOSES AND COLLABORATIVE PROBLEMS
Based on the following nursing diagnoses, you'll establish patient outcomes.

Pain related to injury. The patient will:
- achieve increased comfort
- try nonpharmacologic methods of pain relief
- describe the level and character of his pain.

Impaired physical mobility related to injury. The patient will:
- have increased mobility or joint usage
- maintain muscle strength and range of motion.

PLANNING AND IMPLEMENTATION
These measures help the patient with a joint dislocation.
- Until reduction immobilizes the dislocated joint, don't attempt manipulation. Apply ice to ease pain and edema. Splint the extremity "as it lies," even if the angle is awkward.
- If severe vascular compromise is present or is indicated by pallor, pain, loss of pulses, paralysis, and paresthesia, an immediate orthopedic examination is necessary.

- When a patient receives morphine sulfate I.V. or diazepam I.V., remember to watch for respiratory depression or even arrest.
- During reduction, keep emergency resuscitation equipment (such as an airway and a manual resuscitation bag) in the room, and monitor the patient's respirations closely during and for at least 1 hour after the procedure.
- To avoid injury from a too-tight dressing, instruct the patient to report any numbness, pain, cyanosis, or coldness of the extremity below the cast or splint.
- To avoid skin damage, watch for the symptoms of pressure injury—pressure, pain, or soreness—both inside and outside the dressing.
- Inform the patient that he may gradually return to normal use of the joint.
- Stress the need for follow-up visits to detect vascular damage and for physical therapy, if indicated.

Patient teaching
- Review pain medication and dosage scheduling, adverse effects, and when to report reactions.
- Teach the patient how to care for his splint, dressings, or cast.
- Instruct the patient about signs to report to the doctor (increased swelling, increased pain, tingling, discoloration).

EVALUATION
Achievement of patient outcomes determines the success of collaborative management. For the patient with joint dislocation, evaluation focuses on pain relief and improved mobility.

Limb fractures

Arm and leg fractures commonly involve substantial muscle, nerve, and other soft-tissue damage. The patient's prognosis varies with the extent of disability or deformity, amount of tissue and vascular damage, adequacy of reduction and immobilization, and his age, health, and nutrition. Children's bones usually heal rapidly and without deformity. Bones of adults in poor health and with impaired circulation may never heal properly. A history of trauma and suggestive findings on physical examination (including gentle palpation and failure of a cautious attempt by the patient to move parts distal to the injury) indicate a likely diagnosis of an arm or leg fracture.

CAUSES
Major trauma, such as a fall on an outstretched arm, a skiing accident, or child abuse (indicated by multiple or repeated episodes of fractures), is the most com-

mon cause of limb fractures. Pathologic bone-weakening conditions, such as osteoporosis, bone tumors, or metabolic disease, also can lead to fractures. And prolonged standing can cause stress fractures of the foot and ankle, usually in nurses, postal workers, soldiers, and joggers.

DIAGNOSIS AND TREATMENT

To confirm a diagnosis of a limb fracture, the doctor will use anteroposterior and lateral X-rays of the suspected fracture as well as X-rays of the joints above and below it. Angiography may help assess concurrent vascular injury.

Emergency treatment consists of splinting the limb above and below the suspected fracture, applying a cold pack, and elevating the limb to reduce edema and pain. In severe fractures that cause blood loss, direct pressure should be applied to control bleeding, and fluid replacement (including blood products) should be administered to prevent or treat hypovolemic shock.

After confirming diagnosis of a fracture, treatment begins with reduction (restoring displaced bone segments to their normal position), followed by immobilization by splint, cast, or traction. In closed reduction (manual manipulation), a local anesthetic (such as lidocaine) and an analgesic (such as meperidine I.M.) minimize pain. A muscle relaxant (such as diazepam I.V.) facilitates muscle stretching necessary to realign the bone. An X-ray confirms reduction and proper bone alignment. When closed reduction is impossible, open reduction during surgery reduces and immobilizes the fracture by means of rods, plates, or screws. After reduction, a plaster or fiberglass cast is usually applied.

When a splint or cast fails to maintain the reduction, immobilization requires skin or skeletal traction using a series of weights and pulleys. In skin traction, elastic bandages and moleskin coverings are used to attach traction devices to the patient's skin. In skeletal traction, a pin or wire is inserted through the bone distal to the fracture and attached to a weight.

Treatment for open fractures also requires wound cleaning, tetanus prophylaxis, antibiotics, and possibly surgery to repair soft-tissue damage.

COLLABORATIVE MANAGEMENT

Care of the patient with a limb fracture focuses on relieving pain, improving mobility, and providing patient teaching.

ASSESSMENT

Indications include pain and point tenderness, pallor, pulse loss distal to fracture site, paresthesia or paralysis distal to fracture site, deformity, swelling, discoloration, crepitus, loss of limb function, or substantial blood loss and hypovolemic shock, which can occur in severe open fractures, especially of the femoral shaft.

NURSING DIAGNOSES AND COLLABORATIVE PROBLEMS

Based on the following nursing diagnoses, you'll establish patient outcomes.

Pain related to injury. The patient will:
- experience relief of pain
- try nonpharmacologic methods of pain relief.

Impaired physical mobility or joint function related to injury. The patient will:
- experience improved mobility or joint function
- maintain muscle strength and range of motion (ROM).

PLANNING AND IMPLEMENTATION

These measures help the patient with a limb fracture.
- Watch for signs of shock in the patient with a severe or open fracture of a large bone such as the femur.
- Offer reassurance. With any fracture the patient is apt to be frightened and in pain.
- Ease pain with analgesics, as needed.
- Help the patient set realistic goals for recovery.
- Monitor for compartment syndrome, a neurovascular complication that can lead to permanent dysfunction and deformity.
- Remember that fracture isn't the only cause of compartment syndrome. It may be caused by constricting or occluding dressings, sutures, or casts; poor positioning; and any injury causing ischemia, swelling, or bleeding into tissues.
- In monitoring for compartment syndrome, watch for increasing limb pain that's unrelieved by analgesics; pallid or dusky skin color changes, absent pulse, or edema distal to the injury site; decreased active and passive muscle movement distal to the injury site; pain with passive muscle stretching; and sensory changes, such as numbness or tingling (late symptom).
- Notify the doctor immediately of increasing pain or swelling that doesn't subside after administration of analgesics and elevation of the limb.
- Remove any obvious constriction, such as a dressing or wrap, and have a cast cut to relieve pressure if necessary. If these measures don't relieve the signs and symptoms in 4 to 6 hours, the doctor may relieve the compression surgically with a fasciotomy.
- If the fracture requires long-term immobilization with traction, reposition the patient frequently to increase comfort and prevent pressure sores.
- Assist with active ROM exercises to prevent muscle atrophy. Encourage deep breathing and coughing to avoid hypostatic pneumonia. Also watch for develop-

ment of fat embolism, a complication that may occur as bone marrow releases fat into the blood vessels.

■ Urge adequate fluid intake to prevent urine stasis and constipation. Watch for signs or symptoms of renal calculi (flank pain, nausea, and vomiting).

■ Remember to provide good cast care. While the cast is wet, support it with pillows. Watch for skin irritation near cast edges; check for foul odors or discharge.

Patient teaching

■ Tell the patient to report signs or symptoms of impaired circulation (skin coldness, numbness, tingling, or discoloration) immediately.

■ Warn the patient against getting the cast wet, and tell him not to insert foreign objects under the cast.

■ Encourage him to start moving around as soon as he is able.

■ Demonstrate how to use crutches properly.

■ After cast removal, refer the patient for physical therapy to restore limb mobility.

EVALUATION

Achievement of patient outcomes determines the success of collaborative management. For the patient with a limb fracture, evaluation focuses on pain relief and improved mobility.

Low back pain

Low back pain is one of the most common ailments reported to medical professionals. The onset, location, and distribution of pain and its response to activity and rest provide important clues to the causative disorder and its treatment.

CAUSES

Low back pain commonly is caused by muscular aches or strains. A less common but more serious cause is a herniated disk. The disk is herniated when all or part of the nucleus pulposus—the soft, gelatinous, central portion of an intervertebral disk—forces through the weakened or torn outer ring (anulus fibrosus). The extruded disk may impinge on spinal nerve roots as they exit from the spinal canal or on the spinal cord itself, resulting in back pain and other signs of nerve root irritation. (See *How a herniated disk develops,* page 540.) Most herniation involves the lumbar and lumbosacral regions. A disk may be herniated by severe trauma or strain or by intervertebral joint degeneration.

Low back pain may result from a variety of genitourinary, gastrointestinal, cardiovascular, and neo-

plastic disorders. The postural imbalance associated with pregnancy may also cause this symptom.

DIAGNOSIS AND TREATMENT

The straight-leg-raising test and its variants are perhaps the best tests to determine herniated disk. For the straight-leg-raising test, the patient lies supine while the examiner places one hand on the patient's ilium (to stabilize the pelvis) and the other hand under the ankle. The examiner then slowly raises the patient's leg. The test is positive only if the patient complains of posterior leg (sciatic) pain, not back pain. The doctor may order X-rays to rule out other abnormalities and myelography, computed tomography scanning, and magnetic resonance imaging to show spinal compression by the herniated disk.

Unless neurologic impairment progresses rapidly, the patient initially undergoes conservative treatment, consisting of several days of bed rest (possibly with pelvic traction), heat applications, and an exercise program. Aspirin or other nonsteroidal anti-inflammatory drugs reduce inflammation and edema at the site of injury; rarely, the doctor may prescribe corticosteroids for that purpose. The patient may also benefit from muscle relaxants, especially diazepam, methocarbamol, or hydrocodone (an analgesic).

A herniated disk that fails to respond to conservative treatment may require surgery. The most common procedure, laminectomy and diskectomy, involves excision of a portion of the lamina and removal of the protruding disk. If this doesn't alleviate pain and disability, a spinal fusion may be necessary to overcome segmental instability. Sometimes a surgeon will perform laminectomy and spinal fusion concurrently to stabilize the spine.

Chemonucleolysis—injection of the enzyme chymopapain into the herniated disk to dissolve the nucleus pulposus—offers a possible alternative to laminectomy. The surgeon may use microdiskectomy to remove fragments.

COLLABORATIVE MANAGEMENT

Care of the patient with low back pain focuses on relieving pain and anxiety and improving mobility.

ASSESSMENT

The overriding symptom of lumbar herniated disk is severe low back pain that radiates to the buttocks, legs, and feet (usually unilaterally) and intensifies with Valsalva's maneuver, coughing, sneezing, or bending.

The patient may also experience motor and sensory loss in the area innervated by the compressed spinal nerve root and, in later stages, weakness and atrophy of leg muscles.

How a herniated disk develops

A spinal disk has two parts: the soft center called the nucleus pulposus and the tough, fibrous, surrounding ring called the anulus fibrosus. The nucleus pulposus acts as a shock absorber, distributing the mechanical stress applied to the spine when the body moves.

Physical stress—usually a twisting motion—can cause the anulus fibrosus to tear or rupture, allowing the nucleus pulposus to push through (herniate) into the spinal canal. This process allows the vertebrae to move closer together as the disk compresses. This, in turn, causes pressure on the nerve roots as they exit between the vertebrae. Pain and possibly sensory and motor loss follow.

A herniated disk can also occur with intervertebral joint degeneration. If the disk has begun to degenerate, minor trauma may cause herniation. Herniation occurs in three stages: protrusion, extrusion, and sequestration.

Normal vertebra and intervertebral disk

Spinal canal

Nerve root

Nucleus pulposus

Anulus fibrosus

Protrusion
The nucleus pulposus presses against the anulus fibrosus.

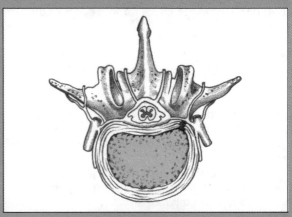

Extrusion and sequestration
The nucleus pulposus bulges forcefully through the anulus fibrosus, pushing against the nerve root. Then, the anulus fibrosus gives way as the disk's core bursts through to press against the nerve root.

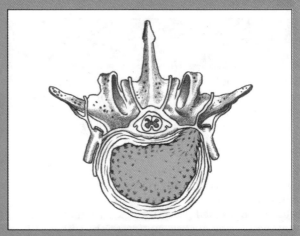

NURSING DIAGNOSES AND COLLABORATIVE PROBLEMS
Based on the following nursing diagnoses, you'll establish patient outcomes.

Pain related to back condition. The patient will:
■ report increased comfort.
■ investigate nonpharmacologic methods of pain relief.

Anxiety and tension related to low back pain. The patient will:
■ state his feelings of anxiety
■ demonstrate adequate coping mechanisms.
Impaired physical mobility related to the diagnosis. The patient will:
■ experience increased mobility
■ show no evidence of complications
■ maintain muscle strength and range of motion.

PLANNING AND IMPLEMENTATION

These measures help the patient with low back pain.

■ During conservative treatment, watch for any deterioration in neurologic status (especially the first 24 hours after admission) that may indicate an urgent need for surgery.

■ Give analgesics, as ordered, especially 30 minutes before the patient's initial attempts at sitting or walking. Assist him during his first attempt to walk. Provide a straight-backed chair for limited sitting.

■ Before chemonucleolysis, make sure the patient isn't allergic to meat tenderizers (chymopapain is a similar substance). Such an allergy contraindicates the use of this enzyme, which can produce severe anaphylaxis in a sensitive patient.

■ After chemonucleolysis, enforce bed rest, as ordered. Give analgesics and apply heat, as needed. Urge the patient to cough and deep-breathe. Assist with special exercises, and tell the patient to continue these exercises after discharge.

■ Use antiembolism stockings or a sequential pressure device (stockings), as prescribed, and encourage the patient to move his legs, as allowed. Provide high-topped sneakers to prevent footdrop.

■ Work closely with the physical therapist to ensure a consistent regimen of leg- and back-strengthening exercises.

■ Give plenty of fluids to prevent renal stasis and constipation, and remind the patient to cough, deep-breathe, and use an incentive spirometer to preclude pulmonary complications.

■ After laminectomy, diskectomy, or spinal fusion, enforce bed rest, as ordered. Monitor vital signs, and check for bowel sounds, abdominal distention, and urine retention. Use the logroll technique to turn the patient.

■ Report colorless moisture on dressings (possible cerebrospinal fluid leakage) or excessive drainage immediately. Observe neurovascular status of legs (color, motion, temperature, sensation).

■ Assist with straight-leg-raising and toe-pointing exercises, as ordered.

■ Provide emotional support. Try to cheer the patient during periods of anxiety and depression. Assure him of his progress, and offer encouragement.

Patient teaching

■ Teach the patient who has undergone spinal fusion how to wear a brace, if ordered.

■ Before discharge, teach proper body mechanics—bending at the knees and hips (never at the waist), standing straight, and carrying objects close to the body.

■ Tell your patient to lie down when tired and to sleep on his side (never on his abdomen) on an extra-firm mattress or a bed board.

■ Urge him to maintain his proper weight to prevent lordosis caused by obesity.

■ Tell the patient who must take a muscle relaxant about the possible adverse effects, especially drowsiness. Warn him to avoid activities that require alertness until he has built up a tolerance to the drug's sedative effects.

EVALUATION

Achievement of patient outcomes determines the success of collaborative management. For the patient with low back pain, evaluation focuses on pain relief, reduced anxiety, and improved mobility.

Lyme disease

Lyme disease affects multiple body systems and typically begins in summer or early fall with the classic skin lesion called erythema chronicum migrans. Weeks or months later, cardiac, neurologic, or joint abnormalities develop, possibly followed by arthritis. The incidence has risen in most states over the past 8 years, but remains highest in New York, Pennsylvania, Connecticut, New Jersey, and Wisconsin.

CAUSES

Lyme disease is caused by the spirochete *Borrelia burgdorferi*. Carried by the minute tick *Ixodes dammini* (or another tick in the Ixodidae family), the tick injects spirochete-laden saliva into the bloodstream or deposits fecal matter on the skin. After incubating for 3 to 32 days, the spirochetes migrate outward on the skin, causing a rash and disseminating to other skin sites or organs by the bloodstream or lymph system. The spirochetes' life cycle is incompletely understood; they may survive for years in the joints, or they may die after triggering an inflammatory response in the host.

Myocarditis, pericarditis, arrhythmias, heart block, meningitis, encephalitis, cranial or peripheral neuropathies, and arthritis are among the known complications of Lyme disease.

DIAGNOSIS AND TREATMENT

Blood tests are the most practical diagnostic tests. Or, the doctor may order the enzyme-linked immunosorbent assay because of its greater sensitivity and specificity. However, serologic test results don't always confirm the diagnosis—especially in Lyme disease's early stages, before the body produces antibodies—or show seropositivity for *B. burgdorferi*. Also, the validity of test results depends on laboratory techniques and interpretation.

Mild anemia, in addition to elevated erythrocyte sedimentation rate, white blood cell count, serum immunoglobulin M levels, and aspartate aminotransferase levels, supports the diagnosis. The doctor may order a lumbar puncture if Lyme disease involves the central nervous system. Analysis of cerebrospinal fluid may detect antibodies to *B. burgdorferi.*

A 10- to 20-day course of antibiotics is the treatment of choice. Adults typically receive tetracycline or doxycycline; penicillin and erythromycin are alternatives. Children usually receive oral penicillin. Given early in the disease, these medications can minimize later complications. In later stages, high-dose penicillin (given I.V.) or ceftriaxone (given I.V. or I.M.) may produce good results.

COLLABORATIVE MANAGEMENT
Care of the patient with Lyme disease focuses on ensuring safety, minimizing fatigue, and dealing with hyperthermia.

ASSESSMENT
The patient's history may reveal recent exposure to ticks—especially if he lives, works, or spends time in wooded areas. He may report the onset of symptoms in warmer months. Look for:
- reports of fatigue, malaise, and migratory myalgias and arthralgias
- in nearly 10% of patients, reports of cardiac symptoms, such as palpitations and mild dyspnea, especially in the early stage
- severe headache and stiff neck, suggestive of meningeal irritation, in the early stage when the rash erupts
- at a later stage, reports of neurologic symptoms such as memory loss
- body temperature rising to 104° F (40° C) in the early stage, accompanied by chills
- erythema chronicum migrans, which begins as a red macule or papule at the tick bite site and may grow as large as 2″ (5 cm) in diameter
- descriptions of the lesion as hot and pruritic
- characteristic lesions with bright red outer rims and white centers, appearing on the axillae, thighs, and groin
- initial lesions followed within a few days by other lesions and a migratory, ringlike rash and conjunctivitis
- lesions fading in 3 to 4 weeks to small red blotches, which persist for several more weeks
- Bell's palsy, in the second stage, possibly alone
- in the later stage, signs of intermittent arthritis
- disease effects in one or only a few joints, especially large ones such as the knees
- tachycardia or irregular heartbeat
- during the first or second stage, regional lymphadenopathy
- complaints of tenderness in the skin lesion site or the posterior cervical area
- less commonly, generalized lymphadenopathy
- with neurologic involvement, Kernig's and Brudzinski's signs usually aren't positive and neck stiffness usually occurs only with extreme flexion.

NURSING DIAGNOSES AND COLLABORATIVE PROBLEMS
Based on the following nursing diagnoses, you'll establish patient outcomes.

Altered thought processes related to neurologic dysfunction. The patient will:
- remain safe in his environment
- regain normal thought processes.

Fatigue related to infectious process. The patient will:
- express his understanding of measures to prevent or minimize fatigue
- incorporate measures necessary to modify fatigue into his daily routine
- regain his normal energy level.

Hyperthermia related to infectious process. The patient will:
- regain and maintain a normal temperature by taking antipyretic agents and by complying with treatment
- develop no complications associated with hyperthermia, such as seizures and dehydration.

PLANNING AND IMPLEMENTATION
These measures help the patient with Lyme disease.
- Plan care to provide adequate rest.
- If the patient has arthritis, help him with range-of-motion and strengthening exercises, but avoid overexerting him.
- Remember to watch for symptoms of complications, such as cardiovascular or neurologic dysfunction and arthritis.
- Ask the patient about possible drug allergies before giving antibiotics.
- Give analgesics and antipyretics, as ordered.
- Monitor the patient's vital signs, especially his temperature.
- Monitor the effectiveness of his drugs.
- Protect the patient from sensory overload, and reorient him if needed. Also, encourage him to express his feelings and concerns about memory loss, if appropriate.

Patient teaching
- Tell the patient to take antibiotic medications as prescribed.
- Urge the patient to return for follow-up care and to report recurrent or new symptoms to the doctor.

■ Inform the patient, family members, and other caregivers about ways to prevent Lyme disease. Advise them to avoid tick-infested areas if possible. If this measure isn't feasible, suggest covering the skin with clothing, using insect repellents, inspecting exposed skin for attached ticks at least every 4 hours, and removing ticks, if present, with tweezers or forceps and firm traction.

EVALUATION
Achievement of patient outcomes determines the success of collaborative management. For the patient with lyme disease, evaluation focuses on decreased fatigue, improved thought processes, and controlled hyperthermia.

Muscular dystrophy

Actually a group of hereditary disorders, muscular dystrophy is characterized by progressive symmetrical wasting of skeletal muscles but no neural or sensory defects. Your patient may have one of four main types of muscular dystrophy: Duchenne's (pseudohypertrophic) muscular dystrophy, which accounts for 50% of all cases; Becker's (benign pseudohypertrophic) muscular dystrophy; facioscapulohumeral (Landouzy-Dejerine) muscular dystrophy; and limb-girdle (Erb's) muscular dystrophy.

Depending on the type, the disorder may affect vital organs and lead to severe disability or even death. Early in the disease, muscle fibers necrotize and regenerate in various states. Over time, regeneration slows and degeneration dominates. Fat and connective tissue replace muscle fibers, causing weakness.

Duchenne's and Becker's muscular dystrophies affect males almost exclusively; the incidence of Duchenne's in males is 13 to 33 per 100,000 and, of Becker's, about 1 to 3 per 100,000. The remaining disorders affect both sexes about equally.

The prognosis varies. Duchenne's muscular dystrophy typically begins during early childhood and causes death within 10 to 15 years. Patients with Becker's muscular dystrophy usually live into their 40s. Facioscapulohumeral and limb-girdle dystrophies usually don't shorten life expectancy.

Duchenne's and Becker's muscular dystrophies lead to crippling disability and contractures. Progressive skeletal deformity and thoracic muscle weakness inhibit pulmonary function, increasing the risk of pneumonia and other respiratory infections. These diseases can also lead to such cardiac problems as arrhythmias and hypertrophy; sudden heart failure may cause death. Most patients with Duchenne's or Becker's muscular dystrophy die from respiratory complications.

Complications from other types of dystrophy vary with the site and severity of muscle involvement.

CAUSES
Muscular dystrophy is caused by various genetic mechanisms. The basic defect can be mapped genetically to band Xp 21. Duchenne's and Becker's muscular dystrophies are X-linked recessive, and facioscapulohumeral dystrophy is autosomal dominant. Limb-girdle dystrophy may be inherited in several ways but usually is autosomal recessive.

Exactly how these inherited defects cause progressive muscle weakness isn't known. They may create an abnormality in the intracellular metabolism of muscle cells. The abnormality may be related to an enzyme deficiency or dysfunction or to an inability to synthesize, absorb, or metabolize an unknown substance vital to muscle function.

DIAGNOSIS AND TREATMENT
To support a diagnosis of muscular dystrophy, the doctor may use muscle biopsy, electromyography, enzyme tests, and amniocentesis and genetic testing for potential parents known or suspected of carrying genes for the disorder.

Currently, no treatment can stop the progressive muscle impairment. However, orthopedic appliances, exercise, physical therapy, and surgery to correct contractures can help preserve the patient's mobility and independence.

COLLABORATIVE MANAGEMENT
Care of the patient with muscular dystrophy focuses on improving breathing patterns, increasing mobility and activity tolerance, and providing thorough patient teaching.

ASSESSMENT
The patient's family history may point to evidence of genetic transmission. If another family member has muscular dystrophy, its clinical characteristics can indicate the type of dystrophy to be expected. Look for:
■ complaints of progressive muscle weakness, with onset and rates of increase that vary according to the type of dystrophy involved
■ in Duchenne's muscular dystrophy, insidious onset when the child is between ages 3 and 5.
■ in Duchenne's, reports of weakness beginning in the pelvic muscles and interfering with the child's ability to run, climb, and walk (by age 12, the child usually can't walk)
■ in Becker's, a history resembling Duchenne's, but progressing more slowly
■ in Beckers, reports of symptoms starting after age 5, but the patient can still walk well beyond age 15—sometimes into his 40s

Observing Gower's sign

Because Duchenne's and Becker's muscular dystrophies weaken pelvic and lower extremity muscles, the patient must use his upper body to maneuver from a prone to an upright position. This characteristic procedure is known as Gower's sign.

Lying on his stomach with his arms stretched in front of him, the patient raises his head, backs into a crawling position and on into a half-kneel.

Then, bracing his legs with his hands at the ankles, he walks his hands (one after the other) up his legs until he pushes himself upright.

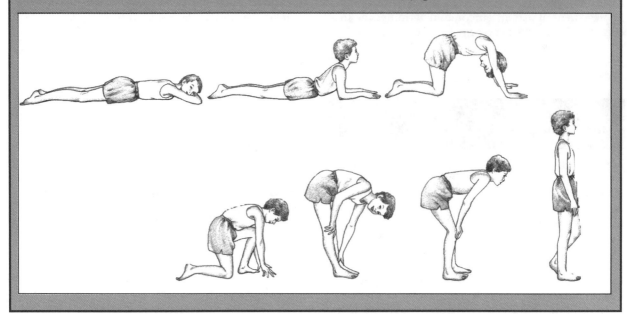

■ in facioscapulohumeral dystrophy—a slowly progressive and relatively benign form—reported symptoms typically before age 10

■ in facioscapulohumeral, early reports of weakness of eye, face, and shoulder muscles (can't raise arms overhead or close eyes completely; can't whistle) and weakening pelvic muscles

■ in limb-girdle dystrophy, reports of slow progression and only slight disability

■ in limb-girdle, reports of onset between ages 6 and 10 (sometimes early adulthood) marked by muscle weakness first appearing in the upper arm and pelvic muscles.

■ in early Duchenne's and Becker's types, a wide stance, waddling gain, and Gower's sign when rising from a sitting or supine position (See *Observing Gower's sign*.)

■ muscle hypertrophy that progresses to atrophy

■ calves that remain enlarged because of fat infiltration into the muscle

■ posture changes, as abdominal and paravertebral muscles weaken—lordosis and a protuberant abdomen

■ scapular "winging" or flaring when the patient raises his arms, caused by weakened thoracic muscles

■ prominent bone outlines as surrounding muscles atrophy

■ in later stages, contractures as well as pulmonary signs, such as tachypnea and shortness of breath

■ with facioscapulohumeral dystrophy, a pendulous lower lip and lack of nasolabial fold, facial flattening, and a masklike expression; inability to raise his arms above his head

■ with limb-girdle dystrophy, winging of the scapulae, lordosis with abdominal protrusion, a waddling gait, poor balance, and an inability to raise the arms. (See *Further signs of muscular dystrophy*.)

NURSING DIAGNOSES AND COLLABORATIVE PROBLEMS

Based on the following nursing diagnoses, you'll establish patient outcomes.

Activity intolerance related to weakness. The patient will:

■ express an understanding of the need to maintain his activity level

- avoid risk factors that may increase his activity intolerance such as obesity
- perform self-care activities as tolerated.

Impaired physical mobility related to skeletal muscle wasting. The patient will:

- avoid complications associated with impaired physical mobility, such as skin breakdown, venous stasis, and thrombus formation
- seek assistance to carry out his mobility regimen
- achieve the highest mobility level possible.

Ineffective breathing pattern related to thoracic muscle weakness. The patient will:

- achieve maximum lung expansion with adequate ventilation
- avoid pulmonary complications, such as pneumonia and atelectasis
- exhibit normal arterial blood gas values.

PLANNING AND IMPLEMENTATION

These measures help the patient with muscular dystrophy.

- If a patient with Duchenne's or Becker's muscular dystrophy develops respiratory involvement, encourage coughing and deep-breathing exercises.
- Regularly assess the patient's respiratory status for signs of pulmonary complications.
- Help him preserve joint mobility and prevent muscle atrophy by encouraging and assisting with active and passive range-of-motion exercises.
- Your patient may need splints, braces, grab bars, and overhead slings. For comfort and to prevent footdrop, use a footboard or high-topped shoes and a foot cradle.
- Observe him for complications associated with immobility, such as skin breakdown, contractures, and venous stasis.
- Because inactivity may cause constipation, encourage adequate fluid intake, increase dietary bulk, and obtain an order for a stool softener. Because the patient is prone to obesity from reduced physical activity, provide him with a low-calorie, high-protein, high-fiber diet.
- Allow him plenty of time to perform even simple physical tasks.
- Monitor his self-care abilities.

Patient teaching

- Encourage communication between the patient and his family members to help them handle emotional strain and cope with changes in body image.
- Encourage the patient and his family members or friends to express their concerns. Listen to them and answer their questions.
- Help a child with Duchenne's muscular dystrophy maintain peer relationships and realize his intellectu-

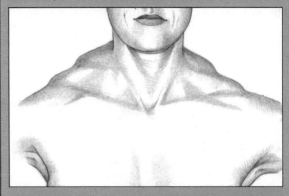

Further signs of muscular dystrophy

In muscular dystrophy, the trapezius muscle typically rises, creating a stepped appearance between shoulder and neck, as shown below.

Viewed from the rear, the scapulae ride over the lateral thoracic region, giving them a winged appearance. In Duchenne's and Becker's dystrophies, this winglike sign appears when the patient raises his arms, as shown below. In other dystrophies, the sign is obvious without arm raising; in fact, the patient can't raise his arms.

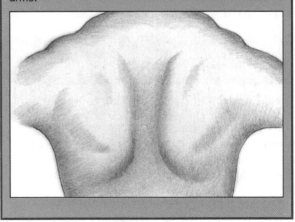

al potential by encouraging his parents to keep him in a regular school as long as possible.

- Teach the young patient and his parents ways to maintain the patient's mobility and independence for as long as possible.
- Inform the young patient and his parents about possible complications and the steps they can take to prevent them.
- Explain the possibility that the patient may contract infections, what signs to watch for, and what to do if this happens. Urge the patient and his parents to report signs of infection to the doctor at once.

- When the patient must use a wheelchair, help him and his family members see the chair as a way to preserve his independence. Have an occupational therapist teach the patient about his wheelchair and other supportive devices that can help him with activities of daily living.
- Help the patient and his family plan a low-calorie, high-protein, high-fiber diet to prevent obesity caused by reduced physical activity.
- Advise the patient to avoid long periods of bed rest and inactivity; if necessary, he should limit television viewing and other sedentary activities.
- If needed, refer adult patients for sexual counseling.
- Refer the patient for appropriate physical therapy, vocational rehabilitation, social services, and financial assistance. Suggest the Muscular Dystrophy Association as a source of information and support.
- Refer family members who carry the muscular dystrophy trait to genetic counseling so they understand the risk of transmitting this disorder.

EVALUATION

Achievement of patient outcomes determines the success of collaborative management. For the patient with muscular dystrophy, evaluation focuses on effective breathing patterns, increased mobility, and increased activity tolerance.

Osteoarthritis (Degenerative joint disease)

The most common form of arthritis, osteoarthritis causes deterioration of the joint cartilage and formation of reactive new bone at the margins and subchondral areas of the joints. This chronic degeneration is caused by a breakdown of chondrocytes, usually in the hips and knees. (See *What happens in osteoarthritis*.)

Osteoarthritis affects both sexes equally. More than half of all people over age 30 have some features of primary osteoarthritis. And nearly all people over age 60 have radiographic evidence of the disorder, although fewer than half experience symptoms.

Depending on the site and severity of joint involvement, disability can range from minor limitation of the fingers to near immobility in persons with hip or knee disease. Progression rates vary; joints may remain stable for years in the early stage of deterioration.

Osteoarthritis may cause flexion contractures, subluxation and deformity, ankylosis, bony cysts, gross bony overgrowth, central cord syndrome (with cervical spine osteoarthritis), nerve root compression, and cauda equina syndrome.

CAUSES

Primary osteoarthritis may be related to aging, although researchers don't understand why. This form of the disease seems to lack any predisposing factors. In some patients, however, it may be hereditary or an autoimmune disorder.

Secondary osteoarthritis usually follows an identifiable event—most commonly a traumatic injury or congenital abnormality such as hip dysplasia. Endocrine disorders (such as diabetes mellitus), metabolic disorders (such as chondrocalcinosis), and other types of arthritis also can lead to secondary osteoarthritis.

DIAGNOSIS AND TREATMENT

The following tests support a diagnosis of osteoarthritis:

- Though X-rays of the affected joint may show a normal joint in the early stages, various views typically show a narrowing of the joint space or margin, cystlike bony deposits in the joint space and margins, sclerosis of the subchondral space, joint deformity caused by degeneration or articular damage, bony growths at weight-bearing areas, and joint fusion in patients with erosive, inflammatory osteoarthritis.
- Synovial fluid analysis can rule out inflammatory arthritis.
- Radionuclide bone scan can also rule out inflammatory arthritis by showing normal uptake of the radionuclide.
- Arthroscopy identifies soft-tissue swelling by showing internal joint structures.
- Magnetic resonance imaging produces clear cross-sectional images of the affected joint and adjacent bones. Scan results also show disease progression.
- Neuromuscular tests may disclose reduced muscle strength (reduced grip strength, for example).

To relieve pain, improve mobility, and minimize disability, treatment includes drugs, rest, physical therapy, assistive mobility devices and, possibly, surgery.

Useful drugs include aspirin and other salicylates and such nonsteroidal anti-inflammatory drugs as piroxicam, tolmetin, naproxen, indomethacin, fenoprofen, ibuprofen, and diclofenac. In some patients, intra-articular injections of corticosteroids may be necessary. Such injections, given every 4 to 6 months, may delay nodal development in the hands.

Adequate rest is essential and should be balanced with activity. Physical therapy includes massage, moist heat, paraffin dips for the hands, supervised exercise to decrease muscle spasms and atrophy, and protective techniques for preventing undue joint stress. Some patients may reduce stress and increase stability by using crutches, braces, a cane, a walker, a cervical collar, or traction. Weight reduction may help an obese patient.

What happens in osteoarthritis

In this disorder, the characteristic breakdown of articular cartilage is a gradual response to aging or predisposing factors, such as joint abnormalities or traumatic injury. These illustrations show how osteoarthritis progresses.

Normal anatomy

Normally, bones fit together. Cartilage—a smooth, fibrous tissue—cushions the end of each bone, and synovial fluid fills the joint space. This fluid lubricates the joint and eases movement.

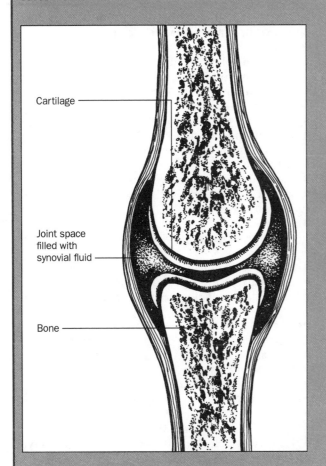

Early disease

Cartilage may begin to break down long before symptoms surface. In early osteoarthritis, the patient typically has no symptoms. Or he has a mild, dull ache when he uses the affected joint; rest relieves the discomfort. Or he may feel stiffness in the joint, especially in the morning; the stiffness usually lasts 15 minutes or less.

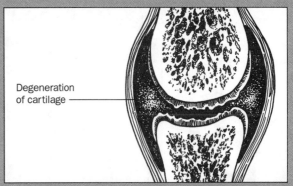

Later disease

As the disease progresses, whole sections of cartilage may disintegrate, osteophytes (bony spurs) form, and fragments of cartilage and bone float freely in the joint. More common now, pain may be present even during rest and typically worsens throughout the day. Movement becomes increasingly limited, and stiffness may persist even after limbering exercises.

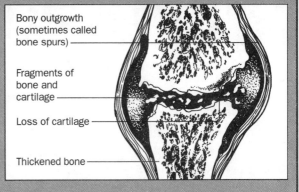

In some instances, a patient with severe disability or uncontrollable pain may undergo surgery, including:
- arthroplasty (partial or total); replacement of the deteriorated part of a joint with a prosthetic appliance
- arthrodesis; scraping and lavage of the deteriorated bone from the joint
- osteotomy; excision or cutting of a wedge of bone (usually in the lower leg) to change alignment and relieve stress.

COLLABORATIVE MANAGEMENT

Care of the patient with osteoarthritis focuses on reducing pain, increasing mobility, and providing thorough patient teaching.

Digital signs of osteoarthritis

Heberden's nodes appear on the dorsolateral aspect of the distal interphalangeal joints. Usually hard and painless, these bony and cartilaginous enlargements typically occur in middle-aged and elderly patients with osteoarthritis. Bouchard's nodes, similar to Heberden's nodes but less common, appear on the proximal interphalangeal joints.

Heberden's nodes   **Bouchard's nodes**

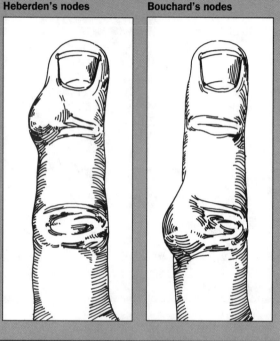

ASSESSMENT
The patient usually complains of gradually increasing signs and symptoms. Look for:
- reports of a predisposing event such as a traumatic injury
- complaints of a deep, aching joint pain, particularly after he exercises or bears weight on the affected joint; rest may relieve the pain
- complaints of stiffness in the morning and after exercise, aching during changes in weather, a "grating" feeling when the joint moves, contractures, and limited movement (These symptoms tend to be worse in patients with poor posture, obesity, or occupational stress.)
- evidence of joint swelling, muscle atrophy, deformity of the involved areas
- gait abnormalities (when arthritis affects the hips or knees)

- with osteoarthritis of the interphalangeal joints, hard nodes on the distal and proximal joints (See *Digital signs of osteoarthritis.*)
- reports of joints with nodes that eventually become red, swollen, and tender
- fingers that become numb and lose their dexterity
- Heberden's nodes on the dorsolateral aspect of the distal interphalangeal joints; hard and painless enlargements seen in middle-aged and older patients
- Bouchard's nodes (like Heberden's nodes but less common) on the proximal interphalangeal joints
- palpable joint tenderness and warmth without redness, grating with movement, joint instability, muscle spasms, and limited movement.

NURSING DIAGNOSES AND COLLABORATIVE PROBLEMS
Based on the following nursing diagnoses, you'll establish patient outcomes.

Anxiety related to the potential crippling effects of osteoarthritis. The patient will:
- express his feelings of anxiety
- develop effective coping behaviors.

Impaired physical mobility related to joint deterioration. The patient will:
- maintain normal muscle strength
- avoid complications, such as contractures, venous stasis, and skin breakdown
- achieve the highest mobility level possible.

Chronic pain related to joint deterioration. The patient will:
- express relief of pain after receiving analgesics
- adhere to the prescribed treatment regimen to minimize joint deterioration and pain.

PLANNING AND IMPLEMENTATION
These measures help the patient with osteoarthritis.
- Give anti-inflammatory drugs and other drugs, as ordered. Monitor for desired and adverse effects.
- For joints in the hand, provide hot soaks and paraffin dips to relieve pain, as ordered.
- For lumbosacral spinal joints, provide a firm mattress (or bed board) to decrease morning pain.
- For cervical spinal joints, adjust the patient's cervical collar to avoid constriction.
- For the hip, use moist heat pads to relieve pain. Give antispasmodic drugs, as ordered.
- For the knee, assist with prescribed range-of-motion (ROM) exercises twice daily to maintain muscle tone. Also help your patient perform progressive resistance exercises to increase his muscle strength.
- Give analgesics as needed and prescribed, and monitor the patient's response.
- To help promote sleep, adjust pain medications to allow for maximum rest. Provide sleep aids, such as a pillow, bath, or back rub.

- Help the patient identify techniques and activities that promote rest and relaxation. Encourage him to perform them.
- Encourage the patient to perform as much self-care as his immobility and pain allow. Provide him with adequate time to perform activities at his own pace.
- Provide elastic supports or braces if needed.
- Check crutches, cane, braces, or walker for proper fit. A patient with unilateral joint involvement should use an orthopedic appliance (such as a cane or walker) on the unaffected side.
- Watch for skin irritation caused by prolonged use of assistive devices, such as a cervical collar or braces.
- Provide emotional support and reassurance to help the patient cope with limited mobility.
- Give him opportunities to voice his feelings about immobility and nodular joints.
- Include the patient and family member or friend in all phases of his care. Answer questions as honestly as you can.

Patient teaching

- Tell the patient to plan for adequate rest during the day, after exertion, and at night.
- Encourage him to learn and use energy conservation methods, such as pacing activities, simplifying work procedures, and protecting joints.
- Tell him to take medications exactly as prescribed. Explain which adverse reactions to report immediately.
- Advise against overexertion. Tell him that he should take care to stand and walk correctly, to minimize weight-bearing activities, and to be especially careful when stooping or picking up objects.
- Tell the patient to wear well-fitting support shoes and to repair worn heels.
- Tell him to have safety devices installed at home such as grab bars in the bathroom.
- Teach him to do ROM exercises, performing them as gently as possible.
- Advise maintaining proper body weight to minimize strain on joints.
- Teach the patient how to use crutches or other orthopedic devices properly. Stress the importance of proper fitting and regular professional readjustment of such devices. Warn that impaired sensation might allow tissue damage from these aids without discomfort.
- Recommend using cushions when sitting. Also suggest using an elevated toilet seat. Both reduce stress when rising from a seated position.
- Positively reinforce the patient's efforts to adapt. Point out improving or stabilizing physical functioning.

- As necessary, refer the patient to an occupational therapist or a home health nurse to help him cope with activities of daily living.

EVALUATION

Achievement of patient outcomes determines the success of collaborative management. For the patient with osteoarthritis, evaluation focuses on decreased pain level, improved mobility, and skill with assistive devices.

Osteomyelitis

A pyogenic bone infection, osteomyelitis may be chronic or acute. Typically a blood-borne disease, acute osteomyelitis usually strikes rapidly growing children, particularly boys. The rarer chronic osteomyelitis is characterized by multiple draining sinus tracts and metastatic lesions. The incidence of both types of osteomyelitis is declining, except in drug abusers.

CAUSES

The disease commonly is caused by a combination of traumatic injury—usually minor but severe enough to cause a hematoma—and acute infection originating elsewhere in the body. Bacterial pyogens are the most common agents, but the disease also may be caused by fungi or viruses. The most common pyogenic organism in osteomyelitis is *Staphylococcus aureus;* others include *Streptococcus pyogenes, Pseudomonas aeruginosa, Escherichia coli,* and *Proteus vulgaris.*

Typically, these organisms find a culture site in a recent hematoma or a weakened area such as a site of local infection (as in furunculosis). From there, they spread directly to bone. As the organisms grow and produce pus within the bone, pressure builds within the rigid medullary cavity and forces the pus through the haversian canals. A subperiosteal abscess forms, eventually causing necrosis.

In turn, necrosis stimulates the periosteum to create new bone (involucrum). The old, dead bone (sequestrum) detaches and works its way out through an abscess or the sinuses. By the time the body processes sequestrum, osteomyelitis is chronic.

Although osteomyelitis usually remains a local infection, it can spread through the bone to the marrow, cortex, and periosteum. The prognosis for a patient with acute osteomyelitis is good if he receives prompt treatment. The prognosis for a patient with chronic osteomyelitis (more prevalent in adults) is poor.

In children, the most common disease sites include the lower end of the femur and the upper end of the tibia, humerus, and radius. In adults, the disease commonly localizes in the pelvis and vertebrae and usually is caused by contamination related to surgery or trauma.

Osteomyelitis may lead to chronic infection, skeletal deformities, joint deformities, disturbed bone growth (in children), differing leg lengths, and impaired mobility.

DIAGNOSIS AND TREATMENT

To support a diagnosis of osteomyelitis, the doctor may order blood tests to get a white blood cell (WBC) count, a blood culture to identify the pathogen, X-rays, and bone scans. The diagnosis must rule out poliomyelitis, rheumatic fever, myositis, and bone fractures.

To decrease internal bone pressure and prevent infarction, treatment for acute osteomyelitis depends on the diagnosis. After drawing samples for blood culture, you'll typically give high doses of I.V. antibiotics (usually a penicillinase-resistant agent, such as nafcillin or oxacillin). The doctor may drain the infected site surgically to relieve pressure and remove sequestrum. Usually the infected bone is immobilized with a cast or traction or by complete bed rest. The patient receives analgesics and I.V. fluids as needed.

If an abscess forms, treatment includes incision and drainage, followed by a culture of the drainage. Anti-infective therapy may include systemic antibiotics, intracavity instillation of antibiotics with low intermittent suction, limited irrigation with a blood drainage system (such as a Hemovac), or local application of packed, wet, antibiotic-soaked dressings.

Some patients may receive hyperbaric oxygen therapy to increase the activity of naturally occurring WBCs. Additional measures include using free tissue transfers and local muscle flaps to fill in dead space and increase blood supply.

Chronic osteomyelitis also may require surgery: sequestrectomy to remove dead bone and saucerization to promote drainage and decrease pressure. The typical patient reports great pain and requires prolonged hospitalization. Unrelieved chronic osteomyelitis in an arm or a leg may require amputation.

COLLABORATIVE MANAGEMENT

Care of the patient with osteomyelitis focuses on relieving pain, protecting the patient from injury, and teaching the patient about the disorder.

ASSESSMENT

Usually, chronic and acute osteomyelitis have similar clinical features. Suspect osteomyelitis if your patient complains of a sudden, severe pain in a bone—especially if he has chills, nausea, and malaise and if his history reveals a previous injury, surgery, or primary infection. He may describe the pain as unrelieved by rest and worse with motion.

The patient's vital signs may show tachycardia and a fever. Inspection may reveal swelling and restricted movement over the infection site. The patient may refuse to use the affected area. Palpation may detect tenderness and warmth over the infection site.

Chronic infection can persist intermittently for years, flaring up spontaneously after minor trauma. Sometimes, the only sign of chronic infection is persistent pus drainage from an old pocket in a sinus tract.

NURSING DIAGNOSES AND COLLABORATIVE PROBLEMS

Based on the following nursing diagnoses, you'll establish patient outcomes.

Activity intolerance related to pain. The patient will:
- seek assistance when performing activities
- comply with prescribed activity restrictions to minimize tissue activity level.

Impaired physical mobility related to bone necrosis. The patient will:
- maintain normal muscle strength and joint range of motion
- avoid complications, such as contractures, venous stasis, and skin breakdown
- regain normal physical mobility.

Impaired tissue integrity related to bone necrosis and inflammation. The patient will:
- express relief of pain with prescribed therapy
- avoid permanent deficits in tissue integrity.

PLANNING AND IMPLEMENTATION

These measures help the patient with osteomyelitis.
- Encourage the patient to verbalize his concerns about his disorder. Offer support and encouragement. Include the patient and his family members in all phases of his care. Answer questions as honestly as you can.
- Encourage the patient to perform as much self-care as his condition allows. Allow him adequate time to perform these activities at his own pace.
- Protect him from mishaps, such as jerky movements and falls, which may threaten bone integrity.
- Give prescribed analgesics for pain and monitor their effect.
- Watch for sudden malpositioning of the affected limb, which may indicate fracture.
- Support the affected limb with firm pillows. Keep it level with the body; don't let it sag.
- Provide thorough skin care. Turn the patient gently every 2 hours.
- If he has a cast, check circulation in the affected limb. If a wet spot appears on the cast, circle it with a marking pen and note on the cast the time of its ap-

pearance. Keep in mind that one drop of blood can cause a 3″ (7.5-cm) stain on the cast. Check the circled spot at least every 4 hours. Assess and report increasing drainage as appropriate. Monitor vital signs to help detect excessive blood loss.

■ Provide complete cast care. Support the cast with firm pillows, and petal the edges with pieces of adhesive tape or moleskin to smooth rough edges.

■ Watch for signs of pressure ulcer formation.

■ If the patient is in skeletal traction for compound fractures, cover the pin insertion points with small, dry dressings. Tell the patient not to touch the skin around the pins and wires. Provide pin care according to health care facility protocol.

■ Use strict aseptic technique when changing dressings.

■ Provide a diet high in protein and vitamin C to promote healing.

■ Assess vital signs, observe wound appearance, and note any new pain (which may indicate secondary infection) daily.

■ Carefully monitor drainage and suctioning equipment. Keep containers nearby that are filled with the irrigant in use. Monitor the amount of solution instilled and drained.

Patient teaching

■ Explain all test and treatment procedures.

■ Review prescribed drugs. Discuss possible adverse drug reactions and tell the patient to report them to the doctor.

■ Tell your patient to report sudden pain, unusual bone sensations and noises (crepitus), or deformity immediately.

■ Before surgery, explain all preoperative and postoperative procedures to the patient and his family members or friends.

■ Teach the patient techniques for promoting rest and relaxation. Encourage him to perform them.

■ Before discharge, teach the patient how to protect and clean any surgical site and, most important, how to recognize signs of recurring infection (elevated temperature, redness, localized heat, and swelling).

■ Urge the patient to schedule follow-up examinations and to seek treatment for possible sources of recurrent infection—blisters, boils, sties, and impetigo.

■ As necessary, refer the patient to an occupational therapist or a home health nurse to help him manage activities of daily living.

EVALUATION

Achievement of patient outcomes determines the success of collaborative management. For the patient with osteomyelitis, evaluation focuses on increased

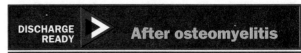

DISCHARGE READY > After osteomyelitis

After treatment for osteomyelitis, the patient will meet the following criteria before discharge:

■ temperature within normal limits for patient
■ vital signs within normal limits for patient
■ absence of complications
■ ability to assist in care efforts
■ improved mobility and activity tolerance from baseline admission.

mobility, increased tissue perfusion and activity tolerance, and knowledge of the disease and its management. (See *After osteomyelitis*.)

Osteoporosis

In this metabolic bone disorder, the rate of bone resorption accelerates and the rate of bone formation slows, reducing the patient's bone mass. Bones affected by this disease lose calcium and phosphate and become porous, brittle, and abnormally vulnerable to fracture. Osteoporosis may be primary or secondary to an underlying disease.

Primary osteoporosis is classified as idiopathic, type I, or type II. Idiopathic osteoporosis affects children and adults. Type I (postmenopausal) osteoporosis usually affects women ages 51 to 75. Related to the loss of estrogen's protective effect on bone, type I leads to trabecular bone loss and some cortical bone loss. Vertebral and wrist fractures are common. Type II (or senile) osteoporosis usually strikes after age 70. Cortical bone loss and consequent fractures of the proximal humerus, proximal tibia, femoral neck, and pelvis characterize type II osteoporosis.

CAUSES

The cause of primary osteoporosis is unknown. However, clinicians suspect these contributing factors:

■ mild but prolonged negative calcium balance
■ declining gonadal adrenal function
■ faulty protein metabolism, caused by estrogen deficiency
■ sedentary lifestyle.

Secondary osteoporosis may be caused by prolonged therapy with steroids or heparin, bone immobilization or disuse (as with hemiplegia), alcoholism, malnutrition, rheumatoid arthritis, liver disease, malabsorption, scurvy, lactose intolerance, hyperthyroidism, osteogenesis imperfecta, and Sudeck's atrophy (localized in hands and feet, with recurring attacks).

DIAGNOSIS AND TREATMENT

Diagnosis of osteoporosis must exclude other causes of rarefying bone disease, especially those that affect the spine, such as metastatic carcinoma and advanced multiple myeloma. To support a diagnosis of osteoporosis, the doctor may use X-ray studies; serum calcium, phosphorus, and alkaline phosphatase level tests; parathyroid hormone level measures; transiliac bone biopsy; computed tomography and DEXA scans; and bone scans using a radionuclide agent.

To control bone loss, prevent additional fractures, and control pain, treatment focuses on a physical therapy program of gentle exercise and activity and drug therapy to slow disease progress. Other treatment measures include supportive devices and, possibly, surgery.

Estrogen may be prescribed for a woman within 3 years after menopause to decrease the rate of bone resorption. Sodium fluoride may be given to stimulate bone formation. Calcium and vitamin D supplements may help to support normal bone metabolism. Calcitonin may be used to reduce bone resorption and slow the decline in bone mass.

Etidronate is the first drug that has proved to restore lost bone. Studies show that using etidronate for 2 weeks every 4 months increases bone mass. And the new drug alendronate also has proved to increase bone mass.

Weakened vertebrae should be supported, usually with a back brace. Surgery (open reduction and internal fixation) can correct pathologic fractures of the femur. Colles' fracture requires reduction and immobilization (with a cast) for 4 to 10 weeks.

COLLABORATIVE MANAGEMENT

Care of the patient with osteoporosis focuses on preventing further injury, increasing mobility, and providing patient teaching.

ASSESSMENT

The patient's history may typically disclose that she is a postmenopausal woman or one with a condition known to cause secondary osteoporosis. The patient (usually an older woman) may report that she bent down to lift something, heard a snapping sound, and felt pain. Or, she may say that the pain developed slowly over several years. If the patient has vertebral collapse, she may describe a backache and pain radiating around the trunk. Any movement or jarring aggravates the pain. Look for:
- a humped back and a markedly aged appearance
- reports of height loss
- palpable muscle spasm

- decreased spinal movement, with flexion more limited than extension.

NURSING DIAGNOSES AND COLLABORATIVE PROBLEMS

Based on the following nursing diagnoses, you'll establish patient outcomes.

Risk for injury related to potential for fractures. The patient will:
- incorporate safety precautions into her daily life
- avoid activities that increase her risk to incur a fracture.

Impaired physical mobility related to decreased spinal flexion. The patient will:
- maintain normal muscle mass and joint range of motion (ROM)
- seek assistance with activities of daily living (ADLs)
- reach the highest degree of mobility possible within the confines of the disease.

Chronic pain related to stress on a bone with decreased bone mass. The patient will:
- express pain relief after an analgesic is given
- avoid activities that precipitate or increase pain
- perform diversionary activities to decrease the perception of pain.

PLANNING AND IMPLEMENTATION

These measures help the patient with osteoporosis.
- Design your plan of care to consider the patient's fragility, degree of ambulation, and prescribed exercises.
- Include the patient and her family members in all phases of care. Answer questions as honestly as you can.
- Encourage the patient to perform as much self-care as her immobility and pain allow. Allow her adequate time to perform these activities at her own pace.
- Provide her with activities that involve mild exercise; help her walk several times daily. As appropriate, perform passive ROM exercises or encourage her to perform active exercises. Make sure she attends scheduled physical therapy sessions.
- Impose safety precautions. Keep side rails up on the patient's bed. Move the patient gently and carefully at all times.
- Discuss with other staff how easily an osteoporotic patient's bones can fracture.
- Provide a balanced diet rich in nutrients that support skeletal metabolism: vitamin D, calcium, and protein.
- Check the patient's skin daily for redness, warmth, and new pain sites, which may indicate new fractures.
- Give analgesics and provide heat to relieve pain, as ordered.

■ Monitor the patient's pain level, and assess her response to analgesics, heat therapy, and diversionary activities.

■ Provide emotional support and reassurance to help her cope with limited mobility. Give her opportunities to voice her feelings. If possible, arrange for her to interact with others who have similar problems.

Patient teaching

■ Explain treatments, tests, and procedures. For example, if the patient is undergoing surgery, explain all preoperative and postoperative procedures and treatments to the patient and her family members.

■ Review the prescribed drug regimen to make sure the patient and her family members understand it. Tell them how to recognize significant adverse reactions and to report them immediately.

■ Teach the patient who's taking estrogen to perform breast self-examination at least once a month and to report any lumps immediately. Emphasize the need for regular gynecologic examinations. Also instruct her to promptly report any abnormal vaginal bleeding.

■ If the patient takes a calcium supplement, encourage liberal fluid intake to help maintain adequate urine output and thereby avoid renal calculi, hypercalcemia, and hypercalciuria.

■ Tell her to report any new pain sites immediately, especially after trauma.

■ Advise her to sleep on a firm mattress and to avoid excessive bed rest. (See *Reducing the risk of osteoporosis*.)

■ Teach her how to use a back brace properly, if appropriate.

■ Thoroughly explain osteoporosis to the patient and family members. If they don't understand the disease process, they may feel needless guilt, thinking that they could have acted to prevent bone fractures.

■ Demonstrate proper body mechanics. Show the patient how to stoop before lifting anything and how to avoid twisting movements and prolonged bending.

■ Encourage the patient to have safety devices installed at home, such as grab bars and railings.

■ Advise her to eat a diet rich in calcium. Give her a list of calcium-rich foods. Explain that type II osteoporosis may be prevented by adequate dietary calcium intake and regular exercise. Hormonal and fluoride treatments also may help prevent osteoporosis along with avoidance of alcohol and tobacco.

■ Explain that secondary osteoporosis may be prevented by effective treatment of underlying disease, early mobilization after surgery or trauma, decreased alcohol consumption, careful observation for signs of malabsorption, and prompt treatment of hyperthyroidism.

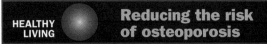

HEALTHY LIVING — **Reducing the risk of osteoporosis**

Teach your patient to reduce the risk of osteoporosis through the following measures:

■ increasing dietary intake of calcium and maintaining good nutritional habits

■ developing and maintaining an active lifestyle, incorporating physical exercise into her regimen as tolerated

■ taking prescribed vitamins and supplements as directed.

■ Reinforce the patient's efforts to adapt, and show her how her condition is improving or stabilizing. As necessary, refer her to therapist or a home health nurse to help her cope with ADLs.

EVALUATION

Achievement of patient outcomes determines the success of collaborative management. For the patient with osteoporosis, evaluation focuses on increased mobility, pain relief, and knowledge of the disease and injury prevention.

Paget's disease

Also known as osteitis deformans, Paget's is a slowly progressive metabolic bone disease. The disease can be fatal, particularly when associated with heart failure (widespread disease creates a continuous need for high cardiac output), bone sarcoma, or giant-cell tumors.

Paget's disease is found worldwide but is rare in Asia, the Middle East, Africa, and Scandinavia. In the United States, it affects about 2.5 million people over age 40, primarily men.

CAUSES

Although the disease's exact cause isn't known, one theory suggests that a slow or dormant viral infection (possibly mumps) causes a dormant skeletal infection, which surfaces many years later as Paget's disease.

Paget's disease is characterized by an initial phase of excessive bone resorption (osteoclastic phase), followed by a reactive phase of excessive abnormal bone formation (osteoblastic phase). The new bone structure, which is chaotic, fragile, and weak, causes painful deformities of the external contour and the internal structures.

The disease usually affects one or several skeletal areas (most commonly the spine, pelvis, femur, and skull). Occasionally, the patient will have widely distributed skeletal deformity. In about 5% of patients, the involved bone will undergo malignant changes.

Involved sites may fracture easily after only minor trauma. These fractures heal slowly and usually incompletely. Vertebral collapse or vascular changes that affect the spinal cord could lead to paraplegia. Bony impingement on the cranial nerves may cause blindness and hearing loss with tinnitus and vertigo.

Other complications include osteoarthritis, sarcoma, hypertension, renal calculi, hypercalcemia, gout, heart failure, and a waddling gait (from softened pelvic bones).

DIAGNOSIS AND TREATMENT

To support a diagnosis of Paget's disease, the doctor may order X-ray studies, bone scans, bone biopsy, a red blood cell count, a test of the patient's serum alkaline phosphatase level, and a 24-hour urinalysis.

The asymptomatic patient needs no treatment. The patient with symptoms requires drug therapy.

The hormone calcitonin may be given subcutaneously or I.M. Although the patient will require long-term maintenance therapy with calcitonin, he'll noticeably improve after the first few weeks of treatment. The patient also may receive oral etidronate to retard bone resorption, relieve bone lesions, and reduce serum alkaline phosphatase and urinary hydroxyproline excretion. Etidronate produces improvement after 1 to 3 months.

Plicamycin (a cytotoxic antibiotic used to decrease serum calcium, urinary hydroxyproline, and serum alkaline phosphatase levels) produces remission of symptoms within 2 weeks and biochemically detectable improvement in 1 to 2 months. However, plicamycin may destroy platelets or compromise renal function; it's usually given only to patients who have severe disease, require rapid relief, or don't respond to other treatment.

Self-administered calcitonin and etidronate help patients with Paget's disease. Other patients may need surgery to reduce or prevent pathologic fractures, correct secondary deformities, and relieve neurologic impairment. To decrease the risk of excessive bleeding caused by hypervascular bone, drug therapy with calcitonin and etidronate or plicamycin must precede surgery. Joint replacement is difficult because methyl methacrylate (a gluelike bonding material) doesn't set properly on bone affected by Paget's disease. Other treatments vary according to symptoms. Aspirin, indomethacin, or ibuprofen typically controls pain.

COLLABORATIVE MANAGEMENT

Care of the patient with Paget's disease focuses on preventing injury, restoring mobility, and alleviating pain.

ASSESSMENT

Clinical effects vary. The patient with early disease may be asymptomatic. As the disease progresses, he may report severe, persistent pain. If abnormal bone impinges on the spinal cord or sensory nerve root, he may complain of impaired mobility and pain increasing with weight bearing.

If the patient's head is involved, inspection may reveal characteristic cranial enlargement over the frontal and occipital areas. The patient may comment that his hat size has increased, and he may have headaches. Other deformities include kyphosis (spinal curvature caused by compression fractures of affected vertebrae) accompanied by a barrel-shaped chest and asymmetrical bowing of the tibia and femur, which typically reduces height. Palpation may detect warmth and tenderness over affected sites.

NURSING DIAGNOSES AND COLLABORATIVE PROBLEMS

Based on the following nursing diagnoses, you'll establish patient outcomes.

Risk for injury related to bone fractures. The patient will:
- incorporate safety precautions into everyday life to prevent bone fractures
- comply with therapy to stabilize bone metabolism
- develop no fractures.

Impaired physical mobility related to bone deformities. The patient will:
- maintain muscle strength and joint range of motion
- show no evidence of complications related to impaired physical mobility, such as contractures, venous stasis, or skin breakdown
- attain the highest degree of mobility possible within the confines of the disease.

Pain related to bone reformation. The patient will:
- express feelings of comfort after receiving analgesics
- avoid or minimize activity that precipitates or increases pain.

PLANNING AND IMPLEMENTATION

These measures help the patient with Paget's disease.
- Give prescribed drugs, including analgesics, as ordered.
- Assess the patient's pain level daily to evaluate the effectiveness of analgesic therapy. Watch for new areas of pain or newly restricted movements—which may indicate new fracture sites—and sensory or motor disturbances, such as difficulty in hearing, seeing, or walking.
- If bed rest confines the patient for prolonged periods, prevent pressure ulcers with meticulous skin care.
- Reposition the patient frequently, and use a flota-

tion mattress. Provide high-topped sneakers or a foot-board to manage footdrop.
- Prepare the patient for surgery if appropriate.
- Monitor intake and output. Encourage adequate fluid intake.
- Monitor serum calcium and alkaline phosphatase levels.

Patient teaching
- Help the patient adjust to the lifestyle changes imposed by Paget's disease. Teach him to pace activities and, if necessary, to use assistive devices.
- Encourage him to follow a recommended exercise program, avoiding both immobility and excessive activity.
- Suggest a firm mattress or a bed board to minimize spinal deformities.
- To prevent falls at home, urge the patient to remove throw rugs and other small obstacles from the floor.
- Emphasize the importance of regular checkups, including examination of the eyes and ears, to assess for complications.
- Explain all medications to the patient. Instruct him to use analgesics cautiously.
- Demonstrate how to inject calcitonin properly and how to rotate injection sites. Warn the patient about adverse reactions, such as nausea, vomiting, local inflammation at the injection site, facial flushing, itchy hands, and fever. Reassure him that these reactions are usually mild and infrequent.
- Tell the patient receiving etidronate to take this medication with fruit juice 2 hours before or after meals (milk or other calcium-rich fluids impair absorption), to divide the daily dosage to minimize adverse reactions, and to watch for and report stomach cramps, diarrhea, fractures, and new or increasing bone pain.
- Instruct the patient receiving plicamycin to watch for signs of infection, easy bruising, bleeding, and fever. Urge him to schedule and report for regular follow-up examinations. Refer the patient and his family member or friend to community support resources, such as a home health care agency and a local chapter of the Paget's Disease Foundation.

EVALUATION
Achievement of patient outcomes determines the success of collaborative management. For the patient with Paget's disease, evaluation focuses on a lack of new injuries, increased mobility, coping skills, and pain relief.

Poliomyelitis

Also called polio and infantile paralysis, poliomyelitis is an acute communicable disease that ranges in severity from inapparent infection to fatal paralytic illness.

Polio usually strikes during the summer and fall. Once mainly confined to infants and children, it's now more common in people over age 15. Among children, it more commonly paralyzes boys; girls and adults are at greater risk for infection but not for paralysis.

The prognosis largely depends on the site affected. If the central nervous system (CNS) is spared, the prognosis is excellent. However, CNS infection can cause paralysis and death. The mortality for all types of polio is 5% to 10%.

Possible complications include respiratory failure, pulmonary edema, pulmonary embolism, hypertension, urinary tract infection, urolithiasis, atelectasis, pneumonia, myocarditis, cor pulmonale, soft-tissue and skeletal deformities, and paralytic ileus.

In polio survivors, latent poliomyelitis can lead to muscle spasticity and weakness 10 to 15 years after the initial infection. Delayed poliomyelitis also can affect respiratory muscles, leading to hypoxemia.

CAUSES
Poliomyelitis is caused by the poliovirus, an enterovirus that has three antigenically distinct serotypes—types 1, 2, and 3. These polioviruses are found worldwide and are transmitted from person to person by direct contact with infected oropharyngeal secretions or feces. The incubation period ranges from 5 to 35 days (7 to 14 days is average).

The virus usually enters the body through the alimentary tract, multiplies in the oropharynx and lower intestinal tract, and then spreads to regional lymph nodes and blood. Factors that increase the probability of paralysis include pregnancy, old age, unusual physical exertion at or just before the clinical onset of poliomyelitis, and localized trauma, such as a recent tonsillectomy, tooth extraction, or inoculation.

Most major cases in the United States are related to the oral poliovirus vaccine (OPV) and occur in children under age 4. Infection occurs 7 to 21 days after administration of live OPV and usually is associated with the first dose of the vaccine. OPV-related cases also occur in young adults, who show symptoms 20 to 29 days after vaccine administration.

DIAGNOSIS AND TREATMENT
Isolation of the poliovirus from throat washings early in the disease and from stools throughout the disease

confirms the diagnosis. If the patient has a CNS infection, cerebrospinal fluid cultures may aid diagnosis. Coxsackievirus and echovirus infections must be ruled out. Convalescent serum antibody titers four times greater than acute titers support a diagnosis of poliomyelitis.

Poliomyelitis calls for supportive treatment, including analgesics to ease headache, back pain, and leg spasms. Morphine is contraindicated because of the danger of additional respiratory depression. Moist heat applications also may reduce muscle spasm and pain. Bed rest is necessary until extreme discomfort subsides. It also helps prevent increased paralysis. Patients with paralytic polio may be bedridden for a long time and then require long-term rehabilitation using physical therapy, braces, and corrective shoes. Orthopedic surgery also may be necessary.

Bladder involvement may require catheterization, and respiratory muscle involvement may require mechanical ventilation. Postural drainage and suction sufficiently manage pooling of secretions in patients with nonparalytic polio.

COLLABORATIVE MANAGEMENT
Care of the patient with polio focuses on safety, improved mobility and joint use, and patient teaching.

ASSESSMENT
Today, most cases of polio are so minor that the patient doesn't even visit the doctor. Inapparent, or subclinical, poliomyelitis (about 95% of all cases) has no symptoms. Abortive poliomyelitis (4% to 8% of all cases) is over in about 72 hours, with the patient experiencing only a slight fever, malaise, headache, sore throat, and vomiting.

The third type, major poliomyelitis, is usually reported. It involves the CNS and takes two forms: nonparalytic and paralytic. In children, the course commonly is biphasic, with the onset of major illness occurring after recovery from the minor illness stage.

A patient with nonparalytic poliomyelitis complains of moderate fever, headache, vomiting, lethargy, irritability, and pains in the neck, back, arms, legs, and abdomen. Look for:
■ muscle tenderness and spasms in the extensors of the neck and back and sometimes in the hamstring and other muscles (also during maximum range-of-motion [ROM] exercises)
■ symptoms that last about 1 week, with meningeal irritation persisting for about 2 weeks

Paralytic poliomyelitis usually develops within 5 to 7 days after the onset of fever. Look for:
■ complaints similar to those of nonparalytic poliomyelitis, followed by weakness and paralysis

■ report of related signs and symptoms, such as paresthesia, urine retention, constipation, and abdominal distention
■ asymmetrical weakness and flaccid paralysis of various muscles
■ Hoyne's sign—the head falls back when the patient is supine and the shoulders are elevated
■ inability to raise the legs a full 90 degrees (extent of paralysis depends on the level of the spinal cord lesions)
■ resistance to neck flexion—the patient extends his arms behind him for support ("tripod") when he sits up.

The most perilous paralytic form, bulbar paralytic poliomyelitis, strikes when the virus affects the medulla of the brain. This type usually weakens the muscles supplied by the cranial nerves (particularly the ninth and tenth). Look for:
■ complaints of facial weakness, dysphasia, difficulty in chewing
■ inability to swallow or expel saliva, regurgitation of food through the nasal passages, and dyspnea.

NURSING DIAGNOSES AND COLLABORATIVE PROBLEMS
Based on the following nursing diagnoses, you'll establish patient outcomes.

Risk for disuse syndrome related to potential for prolonged inactivity. The patient will:
■ maintain normal body function during the period of inactivity
■ have no signs or symptoms of inactivity-related complications, such as pneumonia, constipation, or renal calculi.

Impaired physical mobility related to neurologic dysfunction. The patient will:
■ maintain muscle strength and tone as well as joint ROM
■ achieve the highest level of mobility possible within the confines of the disease
■ use available resources to help maintain this level of functioning.

Ineffective breathing pattern related to respiratory muscle weakness or paralysis. The patient will:
■ maintain adequate ventilation with treatment, which may include mechanical ventilation
■ have no signs or symptoms of hypoxia, such as restlessness, confusion, and cyanosis
■ report feeling comfortable with his breathing pattern.

PLANNING AND IMPLEMENTATION
These measures help the patient with polio.
■ Maintain a patent airway, and keep a tracheotomy tray at the patient's bedside. A tracheotomy common-

ly is performed at the first sign of respiratory distress, and the patient is placed on a ventilator.

■ Carefully observe the patient for signs of paralysis and other neurologic damage, which can occur rapidly. Watch for respiratory weakness and difficulty swallowing. Perform a brief neurologic assessment at least once a day.

■ Frequently check blood pressure, especially if the patient has bulbar poliomyelitis. This form of the disease can cause hypertension or shock.

■ Don't demand any vigorous muscle activity. Encourage a return to mild activity as soon as possible.

■ Monitor the patient for complications associated with inactivity: constipation that can lead to fecal impaction, skin breakdown, renal calculi, and pneumonia.

■ Prevent fecal impaction by giving enough fluids 1½ to 2 qt [1.5 to 2 L] per day for adults) to ensure an adequate daily urine output of low specific gravity.

■ To prevent pressure ulcers, provide good skin care, reposition the patient often, and keep the bed linens dry.

■ Monitor the bedridden patient's food intake to be sure he's receiving an adequate, well-balanced diet.

■ Assess bladder distention. Muscle paralysis may cause bladder weakness or transient bladder paralysis with urine retention.

■ Have the patient wear high-top sneakers or use a footboard to prevent footdrop. To alleviate discomfort, use foam rubber pads and sandbags or light splints, as ordered.

■ When caring for a paralyzed patient, help set up an interdisciplinary rehabilitation program with physical and occupational therapists and doctors. A psychiatrist also may help the patient and family accept the patient's physical disabilities.

■ Report all polio cases to local public health authorities.

Patient teaching

■ Inform the ambulatory patient about the need for careful hand washing.

■ Warn any hospital worker who hasn't been vaccinated against polio to avoid contact with the patient.

■ Teach the patient or caregivers about measures needed to manage symptoms and prevent complications.

■ Help the patient establish a support system of family members, friends, or health care workers to assist him at home.

■ Encourage parents to have children vaccinated against polio. Reassure them that the risk of vaccine-related disease is small.

EVALUATION

Achievement of patient outcomes determines the success of collaborative management. For the patient with poliomyelitis, evaluation focuses on breathing, mobility, and joint function.

Repetitive use injury (Carpal tunnel syndrome)

The most common nerve entrapment syndrome, repetitive use injury in the wrist (also called carpal tunnel syndrome) is caused by compression of the median nerve at the wrist, within the carpal tunnel. The median nerve, along with blood vessels and flexor tendons, passes through this tunnel (formed by the carpal bones and the transverse carpal ligament) to reach the fingers and thumb. Compression neuropathy causes sensory and motor changes in the median distribution of the hand.

This type of repetitive use injury usually affects women between ages 30 and 60 and poses a serious occupational health problem. Assembly-line workers, packers, and people who repeatedly use poorly designed tools are most likely to develop this disorder. Any strenuous use of the hands aggravates the condition.

CAUSES

Among the conditions that cause this syndrome are rheumatoid arthritis, flexor tenosynovitis (commonly associated with rheumatic disease), nerve compression, pregnancy, renal failure, menopause, diabetes mellitus, acromegaly, edema following Colles' fracture, hypothyroidism, amyloidosis, myxedema, and other granulomatous diseases. Another source of damage to the median nerve is dislocation or acute wrist sprain.

DIAGNOSIS AND TREATMENT

Tests that support a diagnosis of repetitive use injury include Tinel's sign (tingling over the median nerve on light percussion) and a positive response to Phalen's wrist-flexion test (reproducing symptoms of repetitive use injury). (See *Eliciting telltale signs*, page 558.)

A compression test supports the diagnosis, electromyography detects a median nerve motor conduction delay of more than 5 msecs, and other laboratory tests may identify underlying disease.

Conservative treatment includes resting the hands by splinting the wrist in neutral extension for 1 to 2 weeks. If a definite link has been established between the patient's occupation and the development of repetitive use injury, he may have to seek other work. Effective treatment may also require correction of an

Eliciting telltale signs

Two simple tests—for Tinel's sign and Phalen's sign—may confirm repetitive use injury of the wrist. The tests prove that certain wrist movements compress the median nerve, causing pain, burning, numbness, or tingling in the hand and fingers.

Tinel's sign
Lightly percuss the transverse carpal ligament over the median nerve where the patient's palm and wrist meet. If this action produces discomfort, such as numbness or tingling, shooting into the palm and fingers, the patient has Tinel's sign.

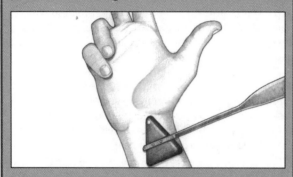

Phalen's sign
If flexing the patient's wrist for about 30 seconds causes subsequent pain or numbness in his hand or fingers, the patient has Phalen's sign. The more severe the disorder, the more rapidly the symptoms develop.

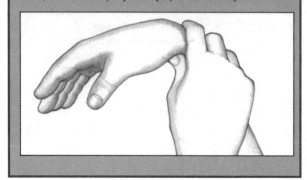

underlying disorder. When conservative treatment fails, the only alternative is surgical decompression of the nerve by sectioning the entire transverse carpal tunnel ligament. Neurolysis (freeing of the nerve fibers) may also be necessary.

COLLABORATIVE MANAGEMENT
Care of the patient with repetitive use injury focuses on reducing pain, improving mobility, and teaching about lifestyle changes.

ASSESSMENT
The patient with repetitive use injury will report weakness, pain, burning, numbness, or tingling in one or both hands. This paresthesia affects the thumb, forefinger, middle finger, and half of the fourth finger. Other indications include decreased sensation to light touch or pinpricks in the affected fingers; an inability to clench the hand into a fist; nail atrophy; dry, shiny skin; and pain, possibly spreading to the forearm and, in severe cases, as far as the shoulder.

NURSING DIAGNOSES AND COLLABORATIVE PROBLEMS
Based on the following nursing diagnoses, you'll establish patient outcomes.

Pain related to injury and condition. The patient will:
- experience comfort
- describe the character and level of pain
- try nonpharmacologic methods of pain relief.

Impaired physical mobility related to condition. The patient will:
- experience increased joint function
- maintain strength and range of motion (ROM).

PLANNING AND IMPLEMENTATION
These measures help the patient with repetitive use injury of the wrist.
- Give mild analgesics, as needed.
- Encourage the patient to use her hands as much as possible; however, if the condition has impaired the dominant hand, you may have to help with eating and bathing.
- After surgery, monitor your patient's vital signs, and regularly check the color, sensation, and motion of the affected hand.
- Suggest occupational counseling if she must change jobs because of repetitive use injury.

Patient teaching
- Teach the patient how to apply a splint. Tell her not to make it too tight.
- Show her how to remove the splint to perform gentle ROM exercises, which should be done daily.
- Advise the patient who is about to be discharged to exercise her hands occasionally in warm water. If the arm is in a sling, tell her to remove the sling several times a day to do exercises for her elbow and shoulder.

EVALUATION
Achievement of patient outcomes determines the success of collaborative management. For the patient with repetitive use injury, evaluation focuses on increased comfort in the affected hand or arm and improved joint function.

Rheumatoid arthritis

A chronic, systemic, symmetrical inflammatory disease, rheumatoid arthritis primarily attacks peripheral joints and surrounding muscles, tendons, ligaments, and blood vessels. Spontaneous remissions and unpredictable exacerbations mark the course of this potentially crippling disease.

Rheumatoid arthritis occurs worldwide, affecting more than 6.5 million people in the United States alone. The disease strikes three times more women than men. Although it can occur at any age, the peak onset period for women is between ages 35 and 50.

Rheumatoid arthritis usually requires lifelong treatment and, sometimes, surgery. In most patients, the disease follows an intermittent course and allows normal activity, although 10% suffer total disability from severe articular deformity, associated extra-articular symptoms, or both. The prognosis worsens with the development of nodules, vasculitis, and high titers of rheumatoid factor.

Pain associated with movement may restrict active joint use and cause fibrous or bony ankylosis and joint deformities.

Between 15% and 20% of patients develop Sjögren's syndrome with keratoconjunctivitis sicca. Rheumatoid arthritis can also destroy the odontoid process, part of the second cervical vertebra. Rarely, spinal cord compression may occur, particularly in patients with longstanding deforming rheumatoid arthritis.

CAUSES

The cause of chronic inflammation characteristic of rheumatoid arthritis isn't known, but various theories point to infectious, genetic, and endocrine factors. A genetically susceptible person may develop abnormal or altered immunoglobulin G (IgG) antibodies when exposed to an antigen. The body doesn't recognize these altered IgG antibodies as "self," and the person forms an antibody known as rheumatoid factor against them. By aggregating into complexes, rheumatoid factor generates inflammation.

Eventually, the cartilage damage caused by the inflammation triggers further immune responses, including complement activation. Complement, in turn, attracts polymorphonuclear leukocytes and stimulates the release of inflammatory mediators, which exacerbates joint destruction.

Much more is known about the pathophysiology of rheumatoid arthritis than about its causes. If unarrested, joint inflammation occurs in four stages. First, synovitis develops from congestion and edema of the synovial membrane and joint capsule. Formation of pannus—thickened layers of granulation tissue—marks the onset of the second stage. Pannus covers and invades cartilage and eventually destroys the joint capsule and bone.

Progression to the third stage is characterized by fibrous ankylosis—fibrous invasion of the pannus and scar formation that occludes the joint space. Bone atrophy and misalignment cause visible deformities and disrupt the articulation of opposing bones, causing muscle atrophy and imbalance and, possibly, partial dislocations or subluxations. In the fourth stage, fibrous tissue calcifies, resulting in bony ankylosis and total immobility.

DIAGNOSIS AND TREATMENT

Although no test definitively diagnoses rheumatoid arthritis, the following are useful:

- *X-rays.* Done in the early stages of the disorder, these show bone demineralization and soft-tissue swelling. Later, they help determine the extent of cartilage and bone destruction, erosion, subluxations, and deformities. They also show the characteristic pattern of these abnormalities, particularly symmetrical involvement, although no particular pattern is conclusive for rheumatoid arthritis.
- *Rheumatoid factor test.* This test is positive in 75% to 80% of patients, as indicated by a titer of 1:160 or higher. Although the presence of rheumatoid factor doesn't confirm rheumatoid arthritis, it does help determine the prognosis; a patient with a high titer usually has more severe and progressive disease with extra-articular manifestations.
- *Synovial fluid analysis.* Analysis shows increased volume and turbidity but decreased viscosity and complement (C3 and C4) levels. The white blood cell count often exceeds 10,000/µl.
- *Serum protein electrophoresis.* This test may show elevated serum globulin levels.
- *Erythrocyte sedimentation rate.* The rate is elevated in 85% to 90% of patients. Because an elevated sedimentation rate commonly parallels disease activity, this test may help monitor the patient's response to therapy (as may a C-reactive protein test).
- *Complete blood count.* This test usually shows moderate anemia and slight leukocytosis.

Treatment requires a multidisciplinary health care team to reduce the patient's pain and inflammation, preserve functional capacity, resolve pathologic processes, and bring about improvement.

Salicylates, particularly aspirin, are the mainstay of therapy because they decrease inflammation and relieve joint pain. The patient may also receive other nonsteroidal anti-inflammatory agents (such as indomethacin, fenoprofen, and ibuprofen), antimalarials (hydroxychloroquine), gold salts, penicillamine, and corticosteroids (prednisone)—although corticos-

Typical joint deformities

In advanced rheumatoid arthritis, marked edema and congestion cause spindle-shaped interphalangeal joints and severe flexion deformities.

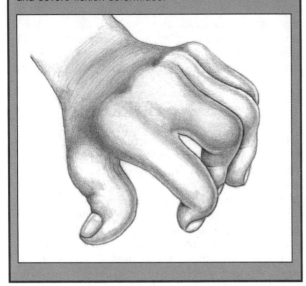

teroid therapy can cause osteoporosis. Other therapeutic drugs include such immunosuppressants as cyclophosphamide, methotrexate, and azathioprine, which are used in the early stages of the disease.

Supportive measures include increased sleep—8 to 10 hours every night—frequent rest periods between daily activities, and splinting to rest inflamed joints (although, like corticosteroid therapy, immobilization can cause osteoporosis).

A physical therapy program that includes range-of-motion (ROM) exercises and carefully individualized therapeutic exercises forestalls the loss of joint function; application of heat relaxes muscles and relieves pain. Moist heat (hot soaks, paraffin baths, whirlpools) usually works best for patients with chronic disease. Ice packs help during acute episodes.

Useful surgical procedures include metatarsal head and distal ulnar resectional arthroplasty and insertion of a Silastic prosthesis between the metacarpophalangeal and proximal interphalangeal joints. Arthrodesis may bring about stability and relieve pain, but only at the price of decreased joint mobility. Synovectomy may halt or delay the course of the disease. Osteotomy can realign joint surfaces and redistribute stresses. Tendons that rupture spontaneously need surgical repair. Tendon transfers may prevent deformities or relieve contractures. The patient may need joint reconstruction or total joint arthroplasty in advanced disease.

COLLABORATIVE MANAGEMENT

Care of the patient with rheumatoid arthritis focuses on managing pain, improving mobility, and providing patient teaching.

ASSESSMENT

The patient's history may reveal an insidious onset of nonspecific signs or symptoms, including fatigue, malaise, anorexia, persistent low-grade fever, weight loss, and vague articular symptoms.

Later, more specific, localized articular symptoms develop, commonly in the fingers at the proximal interphalangeal, metacarpophalangeal, and metatarsophalangeal joints. These symptoms usually occur bilaterally and symmetrically and may extend to the wrists, elbows, knees, and ankles. Look for:

■ reports that affected joints stiffen after inactivity, especially on rising in the morning
■ complaints of tender, painful joints, at first only when she moves them, but eventually even at rest; ultimately, joint function is diminished
■ tingling paresthesia in the fingers, the result of synovial pressure on the median nerve
■ stiff, weak, or painful muscles
■ with peripheral neuropathy, reports of numbness or tingling in the feet or weakness or loss of sensation in the fingers
■ with pleuritis, complaints of pain on inspiration (although pleuritis commonly causes no symptoms)
■ with pulmonary nodules or fibrosis, complaints of shortness of breath
■ joint deformities and contractures, especially if active disease continues
■ fingers that appear spindle shaped from marked edema and congestion in the joints (See *Typical joint deformities.*)
■ proximal interphalangeal joints that have developed flexion deformities or become hyperextended
■ metacarpophalangeal joints that are swollen dorsally
■ volar subluxation and stretching of tendons that pulls the fingers to the ulnar side (ulnar drift)
■ fingers fixed in a characteristic swan-neck deformity
■ hands that appear foreshortened, boggy wrists
■ pressure areas, such as the elbows, that reveal rheumatoid nodules—subcutaneous, round or oval, nontender masses—the most common extra-articular finding
■ with vasculitis, extra-articular signs, such as lesions, leg ulcers, and multiple systemic complications
■ with scleritis or episcleritis, redness of the eye
■ joints that are hot to the touch

- with pericarditis, pericardial friction rub (although pericarditis may cause no signs)
- with spinal cord compression, signs and symptoms of upper motor neuron disorder, such as a positive Babinski's sign and weakness
- other extra-articular findings, including temporomandibular joint disease, infection, osteoporosis, myositis, cardiopulmonary lesions, lymphadenopathy, and peripheral neuritis.

NURSING DIAGNOSES AND COLLABORATIVE PROBLEMS

Altered role performance related to crippling effects of rheumatoid arthritis. The patient will:
- recognize the limitations imposed by rheumatoid arthritis and express her feelings about them
- help make decisions about the treatment and management of her illness
- function in her usual roles as much as possible.
  Impaired physical mobility related to pain and joint deformities. The patient will:
- maintain muscle strength and ROM in unaffected joints
- show no evidence of complications, such as contractures in unaffected joints, skin breakdown, or venous stasis
- achieve the highest level of mobility possible within the confines of the disease.
  Pain related to joint inflammation. The patient will:
- attain pain relief with salicylates or another prescribed medication regimen
- comply with an exercise program to relieve stiffness and subsequent pain
- avoid overuse of affected joints and other activities that precipitate or increase joint pain.

PLANNING AND IMPLEMENTATION

These measures help the patient with rheumatoid arthritis.
- Give analgesics as prescribed.
- Assess the effectiveness of administered medications, and watch for adverse reactions.
- Provide meticulous skin care. Remember to use lotion or a cleaning oil—not soap—on dry skin.
- Monitor the patient's vital signs, and note weight changes, sensory disturbances, and level of pain.
- Monitor the patient's compliance with the prescribed treatment regimen.
- Supply zipper-pull, easy-to-open beverage cartons, lightweight cups, and unpackaged silverware to make it easier for the patient to help herself. Allow her enough time to calmly perform these tasks.
- Urge the patient to follow the prescribed physical therapy program.
- Check for rheumatoid nodules. Also monitor for pressure ulcers and skin breakdown, especially if the patient is in traction or wearing splints. These can result from immobility, vascular impairment, corticosteroid treatment, and improper splinting.
- Monitor the duration of morning stiffness. Duration more accurately reflects the severity of the disease than does intensity.
- Provide emotional support. Remember that the patient can easily become depressed, discouraged, and irritable.
- Encourage discussion of her fears concerning dependency, disability, sexuality, body image, and self-esteem. Refer her to appropriate counseling, as needed.

Patient teaching
- Explain the nature of rheumatoid arthritis. Make sure the patient and her family member or friend understand that rheumatoid arthritis is a chronic disease that may require major changes in lifestyle. Make sure they understand that so-called miracle cures don't work.
- Explain all diagnostic tests and procedures.
- Encourage a balanced diet, but make sure the patient understands that special diets won't cure rheumatoid arthritis.
- Stress the need for weight control because obesity further stresses the joints.
- Teach the patient to maintain erect posture when standing, walking, and sitting. Tell her to sit in chairs with high seats and armrests; she'll find it easier to get up from a chair if her knees are lower than her hips. If she doesn't own a chair with a high seat, recommend putting blocks of wood under the legs of a favorite chair. Suggest that she obtain an elevated toilet seat.
- Tell her to pace daily activities, resting for 5 to 10 minutes out of each hour and alternating sitting and standing tasks. Stress the importance of adequate sleep and correct sleeping posture.
- Tell her to sleep on her back on a firm mattress and to avoid placing a pillow under her knees, which encourages flexion deformity.
- Teach the patient to avoid putting undue stress on joints and to use the largest joint available for a given task, to support weak or painful joints as much as possible, to avoid flexion and instead use extension, to hold objects parallel to the knuckles as briefly as possible, to always use her hands toward the center of her body, and to slide—not lift—objects whenever possible. Encourage swimming as an activity to increase mobility without stressing the joints.
- Enlist the aid of the occupational therapist to teach the patient how to simplify activities and protect arthritic joints.
- Encourage the patient to take hot showers or baths at bedtime or in the morning to reduce the need for pain medication.

■ Stress the importance of wearing shoes with proper support.

■ Suggest dressing aids—a long-handled shoehorn, a reacher, elastic shoelaces, a zipper-pull, and a button-hook—and helpful household items, such as easy-to-open drawers, a handheld shower nozzle, handrails, and grab bars. The patient who has trouble maneuvering fingers into gloves should wear mittens. Tell her to dress while in a sitting position whenever possible.

■ Discuss the patient's sexual concerns. If pain creates problems during intercourse, discuss trying alternative positions, taking analgesics beforehand, and using moist heat to increase mobility.

■ Before discharge, make sure the patient knows how and when to take prescribed medication and how to recognize possible adverse effects.

■ For more information on coping with rheumatoid arthritis, refer the patient to the Arthritis Foundation.

EVALUATION
Achievement of patient outcomes determines the success of collaborative management. For the patient with rheumatoid arthritis, evaluation focuses on pain management, mobility, and preservation of the patient's independence.

Scleroderma

Also called systemic sclerosis, scleroderma is a diffuse connective tissue disease that's twice as common in women than in men. It usually occurs between ages 30 and 50. The disorder is characterized by fibrotic, degenerative and, occasionally, inflammatory changes in skin, blood vessels, synovial membranes, skeletal muscles, and internal organs (especially the esophagus, intestinal tract, thyroid, heart, lungs, and kidneys).

CAUSES
Scleroderma results from unknown causes.

The disorder occurs in two distinct forms: localized (CREST syndrome) and diffuse. CREST syndrome, the more benign form, accounts for 80% of all cases. The acronym stands for the problems it causes: calcinosis cutis (calcium deposits), Raynaud's phenomenon, esophageal dysfunction, sclerodactyly (digital scleroderma), and telangiectasia (spiderlike hemangiomas). Diffuse scleroderma, which accounts for 20% of cases, is marked by generalized skin thickening and invasion of internal organ systems.

Eosinophilic fasciculitis, a rare variant of scleroderma, causes skin changes similar to those of diffuse scleroderma but limited to the fascia. Other differences from scleroderma include eosinophilia, an absence of Raynaud's phenomenon, a good response to prednisone, and an increased risk of aplastic anemia.

In advanced disease, cardiac and pulmonary fibrosis produces arrhythmias and dyspnea. Renal involvement usually causes malignant hypertension, the major cause of death from this disease.

DIAGNOSIS AND TREATMENT
Typical cutaneous changes provide the first clue to a diagnosis of scleroderma. The doctor also may order blood studies, urinalysis, hand X-rays, chest X-rays, GI X-rays, pulmonary function studies, an electrocardiogram, and a skin biopsy.

There is no cure for scleroderma. Treatment aims to preserve normal body functions and minimize complications. Immunosuppressants such as chlorambucil can help relieve symptoms. Used experimentally, corticosteroids and colchicine seem to stabilize symptoms; D-penicillamine may also help. The patient should have her blood platelet levels monitored throughout immunosuppressant therapy.

Other treatment varies according to symptoms.

■ *Raynaud's phenomenon.* Treatment consists of various vasodilators, calcium channel blockers, and antihypertensive drugs (such as methyldopa), along with intermittent cervical sympathetic blockade or, rarely, thoracic sympathectomy.

■ *Chronic digital ulcerations.* A digital plaster cast immobilizes the affected area, minimizes trauma, and maintains cleanliness; the patient may also need surgical debridement.

■ *Esophagitis with stricture.* The patient receives antacids, a histamine-2 antagonist (such as omeprazole, cimetidine, or ranitidine), a soft bland diet, and periodic esophageal dilatation.

■ *Small-bowel involvement.* The patient receives broad-spectrum antibiotics, such as erythromycin or tetracycline, to counteract bacterial overgrowth in the duodenum and jejunum related to hypomotility.

■ *Scleroderma kidney* (with malignant hypertension and impending renal failure). The patient needs dialysis, antihypertensives, and calcium channel blockers; if hypertensive crisis develops, she may receive an angiotensin-converting enzyme inhibitor.

■ *Hand debilitation.* Treatment consists of physical therapy to maintain function and promote muscle strength, heat therapy to relieve joint stiffness, and patient teaching to help the patient perform activities of daily living.

■ *Pulmonary manifestations.* The patient receives oral or parenteral cyclophosphamide to relieve symptoms of dyspnea, crackles, and constrictive pulmonary function.

COLLABORATIVE MANAGEMENT

Care of the patient with scleroderma focuses on relieving pain, preventing injury, and improving skin integrity.

ASSESSMENT

Most patients complain of symptoms of Raynaud's phenomenon—blanching, cyanosis, and erythema of the fingers and toes in response to stress or exposure to cold. These symptoms may precede diagnosis of scleroderma by months or even years. As the disease progresses, look for:

- complaints of pain, stiffness, and swelling of fingers and joints.
- complaints of frequent reflux, heartburn, dysphagia (in 90% of patients), and bloating after meals, all stemming from motility abnormalities, GI fibrosis, and malabsorption
- other GI complaints, including abdominal distention, diarrhea, constipation, and malodorous floating stools
- weight loss
- in early stages, thickened, hidelike skin with loss of normal skin folds
- telangiectasia and areas of pigmentation and depigmentation
- fingers that have shortened because of progressive phalangeal resorption
- slowly healing ulcers on the tips of the fingers or toes—the result of compromised circulation—that may lead to gangrene
- on later inspection, taut, shiny skin over the entire hand and forearm from skin thickening
- tight, inelastic facial skin, causing a wrinkle-free, masklike appearance and a pinched mouth, leading to contractures
- with pulmonary involvement, dyspnea and decreased breath sounds
- with cardiac involvement, an irregular cardiac rhythm, pericardial friction rub, and an atrial gallop
- hypertension if she has renal involvement.

NURSING DIAGNOSES AND COLLABORATIVE PROBLEMS

Based on the following nursing diagnoses, you'll establish patient outcomes.

Altered peripheral tissue perfusion related to compromised circulation. The patient will:

- identify factors that precipitate or increase ischemic tissue changes, such as cold exposure and stress, and try to avoid them
- report feelings of comfort and the absence of pain in her extremities, especially her fingers
- show no evidence of severe tissue ischemia and gangrene.

Risk for injury related to potential complications of scleroderma. The patient will:

- demonstrate the ability to perform the prescribed care regimen
- identify early signs and symptoms of complications and seek medical attention promptly
- maintain adequate organ function, as evidenced by signs of hemodynamic stability.

Impaired skin integrity related to ulcerations and skin changes. The patient will:

- communicate an understanding of skin-protection measures
- demonstrate skill in caring for skin ulcerations
- regain skin integrity.

PLANNING AND IMPLEMENTATION

These measures help the patient with scleroderma.

- Because of compromised digital circulation, don't perform any fingerstick blood tests. Provide gloves or sock mittens after warming therapy.
- Use plaster wraps or topical ointments to lessen the painful effects of digital ulcerations.
- If the patient has cardiac and pulmonary fibrosis, provide rest and pulmonary exercises. Coughing, deep breathing, and chest physiotherapy will help keep her lungs clear.
- Provide a high-calorie diet that's smooth, cool, and palatable. Consult the dietitian to ensure that the patient has a nutritious, appealing diet. Treat GI disturbances, as necessary with antacids and antidiarrheals.
- If the patient suffers from delayed gastric emptying, offer her small, frequent meals and have her remain upright for at least 2 hours after eating. This should help improve her digestion and maintain weight.
- Whenever possible, let the patient participate in treatment by measuring her own intake and output, planning her own diet, assisting in dialysis, giving herself heat therapy, and performing prescribed exercises.
- Regularly assess mobility restrictions, vital signs, level of pain, intake and output, respiratory function, and daily weight.
- Monitor the patient for early signs and symptoms of complications associated with scleroderma, especially cardiopulmonary and renal abnormalities.
- Inspect the skin regularly for evidence of ulcerations. If ulcerations are present, note and record the site and size and notify the doctor.
- Help the patient and her family members or friends accept that this condition is incurable. Encourage them to express their feelings, and help them cope with their fears and frustrations.

Patient teaching

■ Teach the patient and her family member about the disease, its treatment, and relevant diagnostic tests.

■ Warn the patient to avoid air conditioning, cool showers and baths, and preparing food under cold running water, which may aggravate Raynaud's phenomenon. Also, advise her to wear gloves or mittens outside, even in mild weather; she may want to wear them indoors too.

■ Help the patient and her family members adjust to her new body image and to the limitations and dependence that these changes cause. To reduce fatigue, teach the patient to pace her activities, and organize schedules to include necessary rest and exercise.

■ Advise the patient to avoid contact with persons who have active infections (especially of the upper respiratory tract).

■ Urge the patient to maintain a high-calorie diet. Warn her that supplements may not help her overall condition because they may contribute to diarrhea.

■ Advise the patient with GI involvement to avoid late-night meals, to elevate the head of the bed, and to use prescribed antacids and histamine-2 antagonists to reduce the incidence of reflux and resulting scarring.

■ If the patient needs dialysis, refer her to the National Kidney Foundation's local support group. Explain that she may have to limit certain foods and liquids for the rest of her life. Reassure her that she can have dialysis close to or in her home.

EVALUATION

Achievement of patient outcomes determines the success of collaborative management. For the patient with scleroderma, evaluation focuses on improved tissue perfusion, injury prevention, and skin integrity.

Spinal deformities

Spinal deformities include scoliosis and kyphosis. In scoliosis, a lateral curvature of the spine affects the thoracic, lumbar, or thoracolumbar spinal segment. The curve may be convex to the right (more common in thoracic curves) or to the left (more common in lumbar curves). The vertebral column rotates around its axis and may cause rib cage deformity.

CAUSES

The two types of scoliosis are functional (postural) and structural. Both types are commonly associated with kyphosis (humpback) and lordosis (swayback).

Functional scoliosis isn't a fixed deformity of the vertebral column. It's caused by poor posture or a discrepancy in leg lengths.

Structural scoliosis involves deformity of the vertebra. It may be congenital, paralytic, or idiopathic. Congenital scoliosis is usually related to a congenital defect, such as wedge vertebrae, fused ribs or vertebrae, or hemivertebrae. Paralytic or musculoskeletal scoliosis develops several months after asymmetrical paralysis of the trunk muscles from polio, cerebral palsy, or muscular dystrophy. Idiopathic scoliosis may be transmitted as an autosomal dominant or multifactorial trait. It appears in a previously straight spine during the growing years.

In kyphosis, an anteroposterior curving of the spine causes a bowing of the back, usually at the thoracic level. The patient also may have curving at the thoracolumbar or sacral level. Normally, the spine displays some convexity, but excessive thoracic kyphosis is pathologic. Kyphosis strikes children and adults.

Rare, but usually severe, congenital kyphosis leads to cosmetic deformity and reduced pulmonary function. It may appear in adolescence or adulthood and is caused by a variety of other disorders.

The most common form, adolescent kyphosis (also called Scheuermann's disease, juvenile kyphosis, or vertebral epiphysitis) may be caused by growth retardation or a vascular disturbance in the vertebral epiphysis (usually at the thoracic level) during periods of rapid growth or from congenital deficiency in the thickness of the vertebral plates. Other causes include infection, inflammation, aseptic necrosis, and disk degeneration. The subsequent stress of weight bearing on the compromised vertebrae may result in the thoracic hump commonly a characteristic of kyphosis. More prevalent in girls than in boys, symptomatic adolescent kyphosis usually appears between ages 12 and 16.

Adult kyphosis (adult roundback) may be linked to aging and associated degeneration of intervertebral disks, atrophy, and osteoporotic collapse of the vertebrae; endocrine disorders, such as hyperparathyroidism and Cushing's disease; and prolonged steroid therapy. Adult kyphosis may also follow such conditions as arthritis, Paget's disease, fracture of the thoracic vertebrae, metastatic tumor, plasma cell myeloma, or tuberculosis. In both children and adults, kyphosis may also be caused by poor posture.

DIAGNOSIS AND TREATMENT

In scoliosis, anterior, posterior, and lateral spinal X-rays are taken, with the patient standing upright and bending. The X-rays confirm a diagnosis of scoliosis and determine the degree of curvature and flexibility of the spine.

To confirm a diagnosis of kyphosis, look for curvature of the thoracic spine in varying degrees of severity. The doctor may order X-rays to show vertebral wedging, Schmorl's nodes, irregular end plates and, possibly, mild scoliosis of 10 to 20 degrees.

In scoliosis, the severity of the deformity and potential spine growth determine appropriate treatment. Interventions include close observation, exercise, a brace (for example, a Milwaukee brace), surgery, or a combination of these. To be most effective, treatment should begin early, when the patient's spinal deformity is still subtle.

A mild scoliosis curve (less than 25 degrees) can be monitored by X-rays and an examination every 3 months. An exercise program may slow or prevent curve progression, and a heel lift may help. A curve of 25 to 40 degrees requires spinal exercises and a brace. Alternatively, the patient may undergo transcutaneous electrical nerve stimulation. A brace halts progression in most patients but does not reverse the deformity.

A scoliosis curve of 40 degrees or more requires surgery (spinal fusion, usually with instrumentation) because a lateral curve progresses at the rate of 1 degree a year, even after skeletal maturity. Preoperative preparation may include Cotrel-Dubousset instrumentation for 7 to 10 days. Postoperative care commonly requires immobilization in a localizer cast (Risser jacket) for 3 to 6 months. Periodic checkups follow for several months to monitor stability of the correction.

Treatment of kyphosis caused by poor posture alone may consist of therapeutic exercises, bed rest on a firm mattress (with or without traction), and a brace to straighten the kyphotic curve until spinal growth is complete. Corrective exercises include pelvic tilt to decrease lumbar lordosis, hamstring stretch to overcome muscle contractures, and thoracic hyperextension to flatten the kyphotic curve. These exercises may be performed in or out of the brace. Lateral X-rays, taken every 4 months, evaluate the therapy. Gradual weaning from the brace can begin after maximum correction of the kyphotic curve is achieved, vertebral wedging has decreased, and the spine has reached full skeletal maturity. Loss of correction indicates that weaning from the brace has been too rapid. The doctor will decrease the time the patient spends out of the brace accordingly.

Treatment for both adolescent and adult kyphosis also includes appropriate measures for the underlying cause and, possibly, spinal arthrodesis for relief of symptoms. Although rarely necessary, the doctor may recommend surgery for kyphosis that causes neurologic damage, for a spinal curve greater than 60 degrees, or for intractable and disabling back pain in a patient with full skeletal maturity. Preoperative measures may include halo-femoral traction. Corrective surgery includes a posterior spinal fusion with spinal instrumentation, iliac bone grafting, and plaster immobilization. Anterior spinal fusion followed by immobilization in plaster may be necessary when kyphosis produces a spinal curve greater than 70 degrees.

COLLABORATIVE MANAGEMENT
Care of the patient with a spinal deformity focuses on guarding against skin breakdown, reducing anxiety, and teaching coping mechanisms.

ASSESSMENT
In functional or structural scoliosis, the most common spinal curve arises in the thoracic segment, with convexity to the right, and compensatory curves (S curves) in the cervical segment above and the lumbar segment below, both with convexity to the left. Once the disease becomes well established, the patient reports backache, fatigue, and dyspnea.

The patient with scoliosis has unequal shoulder heights, elbow levels, and heights of the iliac crests. Muscles on the convex side of the curve may be rounded; those on the concave side, flattened.

Usually insidious, adolescent kyphosis appears in patients with a history of excessive sports activity and may be asymptomatic, except in cases with curving of the back (sometimes more than 90 degrees). In about 50% of adolescent patients, kyphosis produces mild pain at the apex of the curve. Look for:
- reports of fatigue
- tenderness in the involved area or along the entire spine
- prominent vertebral spinous processes at the lower dorsal and upper lumbar levels
- compensatory increased lumbar lordosis and hamstring tightness
- rarely, kyphosis-induced neurologic damage, including spastic paraparesis secondary to spinal cord compression or herniated nucleus pulposus
- in both adolescent and adult kyphosis not due to poor posture alone, inability to straighten the spine when the patient assumes a recumbent position
- in adult kyphosis, a characteristic roundback appearance, possibly associated with pain, weakness of the back, and generalized fatigue (See *Spinal deformity in kyphosis,* page 566.)
- in adult kyphosis, rare local tenderness, except in senile osteoporosis with recent compression fracture
- disk lesions, called Schmorl's nodes, that develop in anteroposterior curving of the spine (localized protrusions of nuclear material through the cartilage plates and into the spongy bone of the vertebral bodies)

Spinal deformity in kyphosis

The patient with kyphosis exhibits excessive vertebral curvature in the thoracic spine.

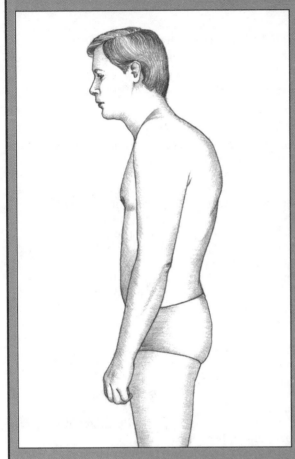

■ in kyphosis, generally, ankylosis caused when the anterior portions of the cartilage are destroyed and bridges of new bone transverse the intervertebral space.

NURSING DIAGNOSES AND COLLABORATIVE PROBLEMS
Based on the following nursing diagnoses, you'll establish patient outcomes.
Anxiety related to condition. The patient will:
■ exhibit adequate coping mechanisms
■ have decreased anxiety level.
Risk for impaired skin integrity related to treatments. The patient will:
■ exhibit no skin breakdown

■ demonstrate an understanding of skin protection measures
■ demonstrate skin inspection techniques.

PLANNING AND IMPLEMENTATION
These measures help the patient with a spinal deformity.
■ If your patient is an adolescent girl, be especially sensitive to her; she's likely to be upset by activity limitations and treatment with orthopedic appliances.
■ Encourage your patient to verbalize feelings.
■ Explain all procedures and treatments to the patient and family members.
■ If the patient needs traction or a cast before surgery, remember to prepare him fully. Application of a body cast can be traumatic because it is done on a special frame and the patient's head and face are covered throughout the procedure.
■ If the patient is in traction or a cast, check the skin around the cast edge daily. Keep the cast clean and dry and the edges of the cast "petaled" (padded).
■ Watch for skin breakdown and signs of cast syndrome.
■ If your patient needs a brace, enlist the help of a physical therapist, a social worker, and an orthotist (orthopedic appliance specialist). Before the patient goes home, explain what the brace does and how to care for it.

Patient teaching
■ Warn your patient who's in a cast not to insert anything or let anything get under the cast.
■ Tell him to immediately report cracks in the cast, pain, burning, skin breakdown, numbness, or odor.
■ To prevent skin breakdown, advise the patient wearing a brace not to use lotions, ointments, or powders on areas where the brace contacts the skin. Instead, suggest he use rubbing alcohol or tincture of benzoin to toughen the skin. Tell him to keep the skin dry and clean and to wear a snug T-shirt under the brace.
■ Tell the patient who needs a brace to wear it 23 hours a day and to remove it only for bathing and exercise. While he is still adjusting to the brace, tell him to lie down and rest several times a day.
■ Advise the patient in a brace to increase activities gradually and avoid vigorous sports. Emphasize the importance of conforming to prescribed exercises. Recommend swimming during the hour out of the brace, but strongly warn against diving.
■ Instruct the patient who wears a brace to turn his whole body, instead of just his head, when looking to the side.
■ Teach the patient with adolescent kyphosis caused by poor posture alone the prescribed therapeutic exercises and the fundamentals of good posture.

■ For the adolescent patient, suggest bed rest when pain becomes severe. Encourage use of a firm mattress, preferably with a bed board.

EVALUATION

Achievement of patient outcomes determines the success of collaborative management. For the patient with a spinal deformity, evaluation focuses on lack of skin breakdown from treatment, knowledge of protective measures and coping mechanisms, and decreased anxiety over dealing with a cast or brace.

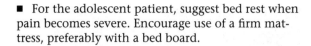

Sprains and strains

A sprain refers to a complete or incomplete tear in the supporting ligaments surrounding a joint such as the knee. In contrast, a strain refers to an injury to a muscle or tendinous attachment. Both injuries usually heal without surgical repair.

CAUSES

A sprain usually follows a sharp twist, whereas a strain usually follows vigorous muscle overuse or overstress.

DIAGNOSIS AND TREATMENT

To support a diagnosis of sprain or strain, the doctor will use X-rays that rule out fractures and damage to ligaments. Treatment of sprains consists of controlling pain and swelling and immobilizing the injured joint to promote healing.

COLLABORATIVE MANAGEMENT

Care of the patient with a sprain, strain, or tear focuses on improving mobility and relieving pain.

ASSESSMENT

A patient with a sprain may report localized pain (especially during joint movement), swelling, and black-and-blue discoloration (ecchymosis). Associated loss of mobility may not occur until several hours after the injury. In acute strain, swelling may occur rapidly, and the patient may recall hearing a snapping noise at the time of injury. Ecchymosis may appear after several days, and muscle tenderness may develop when pain subsides. A patient with chronic strain may experience generalized tenderness, stiffness, and soreness.

NURSING DIAGNOSES AND COLLABORATIVE PROBLEMS

Based on the following nursing diagnoses, you'll establish patient outcomes.

Pain related to injury. The patient will:
■ experience decreased pain

■ investigate nonpharmacologic methods of pain relief.

Impaired physical mobility or joint usage related to injury. The patient will:
■ suffer no further injury
■ experience improved mobility or joint usage.

PLANNING AND IMPLEMENTATION

These measures help the patient with a sprain or strain.
■ Immediately after the injury, control swelling by elevating the joint above the level of the heart and intermittently applying ice for 12 to 48 hours. To prevent cold injury, place a towel between the ice pack and the skin.
■ Acute strains require analgesics and immediate application of ice for up to 48 hours, followed by heat application.
■ Complete muscle rupture may require surgical repair.
■ Chronic strains usually don't require treatment, but local heat application, aspirin, or an analgesic and muscle relaxant relieves discomfort.
■ Immobilize the joint, using an elastic bandage or, if the sprain is severe, a soft cast.
■ Depending on the severity of the injury, nonsteroidal anti-inflammatory drugs or other analgesics may be needed.
■ If the patient has a sprained ankle, he may need crutches and crutch-gait training.
■ Once the affected area is immobilized, the patient can then gradually resume normal activities. Occasionally, however, torn ligaments don't heal properly and cause recurrent dislocation, necessitating surgical repair. Some athletes may request immediate surgical repair to hasten healing.

Patient teaching

■ Because patients with sprains seldom require hospitalization, provide comprehensive patient teaching.
■ Tell the patient to elevate the joint for 48 to 72 hours after the injury (he can elevate the joint with pillows for sleeping) and to apply ice intermittently for 24 to 48 hours after the injury.
■ If an elastic bandage has been applied, teach the patient how to reapply it by wrapping from below to above the injury, forming a figure eight.
■ For a sprained ankle, apply the bandage from the toes to midcalf.
■ Tell the patient to remove the bandage before going to sleep and to loosen it if it causes the leg to become pale, numb, or painful.
■ Instruct the patient to call the doctor if pain worsens or persists (if so, an additional X-ray may detect a fracture originally missed).

EVALUATION

Achievement of patient outcomes determines the success of collaborative management. For the patient with a sprain, strain, or tear, evaluation focuses on improved mobility and pain relief.

Systemic lupus erythematosus

A chronic inflammatory autoimmune disorder affecting the connective tissues, systemic lupus erythematosus (SLE) affects multiple organs (including the skin) and can kill. Its relative, discoid lupus erythematosus (DLE), affects only the skin but has the potential to become systemic. Like rheumatoid arthritis, SLE is characterized by recurrent seasonal remissions and exacerbations, especially in spring and summer.

The annual incidence of SLE in urban populations varies from 15 to 50 per 100,000 persons. It strikes 8 times more women than men (15 times more during childbearing years). SLE occurs worldwide but is most prevalent among Asians and Blacks.

The prognosis improves with early detection and treatment but remains poor for patients who have cardiovascular, renal, or neurologic complications or severe bacterial infections. The disease is incurable.

Concomitant infections, particularly urinary tract infections (UTIs), and renal failure represent the leading causes of death for SLE patients.

CAUSES

The exact cause of SLE remains a mystery, but available evidence points to interrelated immune, environmental, hormonal, and genetic factors. It may also be drug-induced; if the drug is withdrawn, the condition usually subsides. Scientists think that autoimmunity is the primary cause. In autoimmunity, the body produces antibodies, such as antinuclear antibodies, against its own cells. The formed antigen-antibody complexes then suppress the body's antigens. A significant feature in patients with SLE is their ability to produce antibodies against many different tissue components, such as red blood cells (RBCs), neutrophils, platelets, lymphocytes, or almost any organ or tissue in the body.

Certain predisposing factors may make a person susceptible to SLE. These include stress, streptococcal or viral infections, exposure to sunlight or ultraviolet light, immunization, pregnancy, and abnormal estrogen metabolism.

Researchers think that clinical signs and symptoms are caused by antibody-antigen trapping in specific organ capillaries.

DIAGNOSIS AND TREATMENT

To support a diagnosis of SLE, the doctor may use a complete blood count with differential, platelet count, erythrocyte sedimentation rate, and serum electrophoresis.

Difficult to detect, central nervous system (CNS) involvement may account for abnormal EEG results in about 70% of patients. But brain and magnetic resonance imaging scans may be normal. Specific tests for SLE include antinuclear antibodies, anti-deoxyribonucleic acid (DNA), and lupus erythematosus cell tests, which produce positive findings in most patients with active SLE (only marginally useful); urine studies that detect RBCs, white blood cells (WBCs), urine casts and sediment, and significant protein loss (more than 3.5 g in 24 hours); blood studies; chest X-rays; electrocardiography to show a conduction defect with cardiac involvement or pericarditis; skin biopsy to rule out skin cancer; and renal biopsy to show progression of SLE and the extent of renal involvement.

The mainstay of SLE treatment is drug therapy. The patient with mild disease requires little or no medication. Nonsteroidal anti-inflammatory drugs, including aspirin, usually control arthritis and arthralgia symptoms. Skin lesions need topical medications and protection from exposure to the sun. Topical corticosteroid creams, such as triamcinolone and hydrocortisone, may be given for mild disease.

Fluorinated steroids may control acute or discoid lesions. And refractory skin lesions may respond to intralesional or systemic corticosteroids or antimalarials, such as hydroxychloroquine and chloroquine. Because hydroxychloroquine and chloroquine can cause retinal damage, such treatment requires ophthalmologic examination every 6 months. Dapsone helps many patients.

Corticosteroids remain the treatment of choice for systemic symptoms of SLE, for acute generalized exacerbations, and for serious disease-related injury to vital organ systems from pleuritis, pericarditis, nephritis related to SLE, vasculitis, and CNS involvement. With initial prednisone doses (equivalent to 60 mg or more), the patient's condition usually improves noticeably within 48 hours. With symptoms under control, the patient discontinues or slowly tapers prednisone use. (*Note:* Rising serum complement levels and decreasing anti-DNA titers indicate patient response.)

If the patient has glomerulonephritis, she'll need treatment with large doses of corticosteroids. Then, if renal failure occurs despite treatment, plasmapheresis, dialysis, or kidney transplantation may be necessary.

In some patients, cytotoxic drugs such as azathioprine, cyclophosphamide, and methotrexate may delay or prevent renal deterioration. Antihypertensive drugs also may work. Additionally, warfarin is indicated for antiphospholipid antibodies, which can cause clotting in vascular structures.

COLLABORATIVE MANAGEMENT

Care of the patient with SLE focuses on symptomatic treatment and prevention of systemic complications.

ASSESSMENT

The onset of SLE, which may be acute or insidious, produces no characteristic clinical pattern. However, the patient may complain of fever, anorexia, weight loss, malaise, fatigue, abdominal pain, nausea, vomiting, diarrhea, constipation, rashes, and polyarthralgia. When taking the patient history, remember to check the medication history. (See *SLE or drug effects?*)

SLE can involve every organ system. Look for:
- in women, reports of irregular menstruation or amenorrhea, particularly during flareups
- in about 90% of patients, joint involvement resembling that of rheumatoid arthritis
- Raynaud's phenomenon, affecting about 20% of SLE patients
- complaints that sunlight (or ultraviolet light) provokes or aggravates skin eruptions
- report of chest pain (indicating pleuritis) and dyspnea (suggesting parenchymal infiltrates and pneumonitis)
- cardiopulmonary signs and symptoms in about 50% of patients
- repeated arterial clotting, manifest in dyspnea, tachycardia, central cyanosis, and hypotension (may precede pulmonary emboli)
- altered level of consciousness, weakness of the extremities, and speech disturbances that point to cerebrovascular accident
- seizure disorders and mental dysfunction, indicating neurologic damage
- signs or symptoms of added CNS involvement, including emotional instability, psychosis, organic brain syndrome, headaches, irritability, and depression
- oliguria, signaling possible renal failure
- complaints of urinary frequency, dysuria, and bladder spasms, with UTI
- skin lesions, ordinarily appearing as an erythematous rash in areas exposed to light; the classic butterfly rash over the nose and cheeks appears in less than 50% of patients
- painless ulcers on mucous membranes
- vasculitis, especially on the digits
- infarctive lesions, necrotic leg ulcers, and digital gangrene
- palpable lymph node enlargement (diffuse or local and nontender)
- signs of cardiopulmonary abnormalities such as pericardial friction rub (signaling pericarditis)

SLE or drug effects?

Be sure to obtain a complete drug history of your patient with suspected systemic lupus erythematosus (SLE). That's because approximately 25 drugs can cause an SLE-like reaction.

The most commonly implicated drugs include procainamide, hydralazine, isoniazid, methyldopa, anticonvulsants and, less frequently, penicillins, sulfa drugs, and oral contraceptives.

- tachycardia and other signs of myocarditis and endocarditis.

NURSING DIAGNOSES AND COLLABORATIVE PROBLEMS

Based on the following nursing diagnoses, you'll establish patient outcomes.

Body image disturbance related to chronic skin eruptions. The patient will:
- acknowledge the change in her body image
- comply with the treatment regimen to minimize scarring and disfigurement
- express positive feelings about herself.

Impaired physical mobility related to chronic inflammation of connective tissues. The patient will:
- attain the highest degree of mobility possible
- develop no complications, such as contractures, venous stasis, thrombus formation, or skin breakdown.

Pain related to chronic inflammation of connective tissues. The patient will:
- express relief from pain following analgesic administration
- comply with the treatment regimen to minimize inflammatory response and thus reduce pain
- avoid activities that increase or precipitate pain.

PLANNING AND IMPLEMENTATION

These measures help the patient with SLE.
- Provide a balanced diet. Foods high in protein, vitamins, and iron help maintain optimum nutrition and prevent anemia. However, renal involvement may mandate a low-sodium, low-protein diet. Provide bland, cool foods if the patient has a sore mouth.
- Warm and protect the patient's hands and feet if she has Raynaud's phenomenon.
- Urge the patient to get plenty of rest. Schedule diagnostic tests and procedures to allow adequate rest.
- Apply heat packs to relieve joint pain and stiffness. Encourage regular exercise to maintain full range of motion (ROM) and to prevent contractures.

- Institute seizure precautions if you suspect CNS involvement.
- Arrange a physical therapy and occupational therapy consultation if musculoskeletal involvement compromises the patient's mobility.
- Continually assess for signs and symptoms of organ involvement; specifically, monitor for hypertension, weight gain, and other signs of renal involvement.
- Check urine, stools, and GI secretions for blood. Check the scalp for hair loss and the skin and mucous membranes for petechiae, bleeding, ulceration, pallor, and bruising.
- Support the patient's self-image. Offer female patients helpful tips. Suggest hypoallergenic cosmetics. As needed, refer her to a hairdresser who specializes in scalp disorders. Offer male patients similar advice, suggesting hypoallergenic hair care and shaving products.
- Offer the patient encouragement and emotional support.
- Assess for possible neurologic damage, signaled by personality changes, paranoid or psychotic behavior, depression, ptosis, and diplopia.

Patient teaching

- Teach ROM exercises and body alignment and postural techniques.
- Make sure the patient understands ways to avoid infection. Direct her to avoid crowds and persons with known infections.
- Advise the patient to notify the doctor if fever, cough, or rash occurs or if chest, abdominal, muscle, or joint pain worsens.
- Instruct the photosensitive patient to wear protective clothing (hat, sunglasses, long-sleeved shirts or sweaters, and slacks) and to use a sunscreen with a skin protection factor of at least 15 when outdoors and to avoid exposure between 10 a.m. and 3 p.m..
- Teach the patient to perform meticulous mouth care to relieve discomfort and prevent infection.
- Because SLE usually strikes women of childbearing age, questions associated with pregnancy commonly arise. The best evidence available indicates that a woman with SLE can have a safe, successful pregnancy if she sustains no serious renal or neurologic impairment. Advise her to seek additional medical care from a rheumatologist during her pregnancy. As indicated, explain that her doctors may order low-dose aspirin to reduce the risk of thrombosis during pregnancy.
- Warn the patient against trying unproven "miracle" drugs to relieve arthritis symptoms.
- Refer the patient to the Lupus Foundation of America and the Arthritis Foundation, as necessary.

EVALUATION

Achievement of patient outcomes determines the success of collaborative management. For the patient with systemic lupus erythematosus, evaluation focuses on decreased pain, increased mobility, and the patient's self image.

Treatments and procedures

Therapy for musculoskeletal disorders includes amputation, open reduction and internal fixation, release of the carpal tunnel ligament, and total knee replacement.

AMPUTATION

Amputation is the surgical removal of all or part of a limb. Performed to preserve function in a remaining part or, at times, to prevent death, amputation is a radical treatment for severe trauma, gangrene, cancer, vascular disease, congenital deformity, or thermal injury. It can take one of two basic forms. In a closed, or flap, amputation—the most commonly performed type—the surgeon uses skin flaps to cover the bone stump. In an open, or guillotine, amputation (a rarely performed emergency operation), the surgeon cuts the tissue and bone flush, leaving the wound open. A second operation completes repair and stump formation. The doctor may perform amputation at a number of sites, depending on the nature and extent of injury.

PROCEDURE

The patient receives a general anesthetic (or local anesthetic for a finger or toe amputation). In the closed technique, the surgeon incises the tissue to the bone, leaving sufficient skin to cover the stump end. He usually controls bleeding above the level of amputation by tying off the bleeding vessels with suture ties. He then saws the bone (or resects a joint), files the bone ends smooth and rounded, and removes the periosteum up about ½" (1.3 cm) from the bone end. After ligating all vessels and dividing the nerves, he sutures opposing muscles over the bone end and to the periosteum to provide better muscle connection. Next, he sutures the skin flaps closed. Placement of an incision drain and a soft dressing completes the procedure.

In a below-the-knee amputation, the surgeon may order a rigid dressing applied over the stump in the operating room. This enables immediate postoperative fitting of a prosthesis, aids in early ambulation, preserves knee function, and helps prevent contractures.

In an emergency (guillotine) amputation, the surgeon makes a perpendicular incision through the bone and all tissue. He leaves the wound open, applying a large bulky dressing.

COLLABORATIVE MANAGEMENT
Care of the patient undergoing amputation requires thorough preparation, close monitoring, and intense patient teaching.

Preparation
If time permits, review the doctor's explanation of the scheduled amputation, answering any questions the patient may have. Remember that the patient faces not only losing a body part, with an attendant change in body image, but also the threat of losing mobility and independence. Keep in mind, too, that losing a limb or digit can be emotionally devastating. Remember to provide emotional support, and arrange for the patient to meet with a well-adjusted amputee, who can provide additional reassurance and encouragement.

Discuss postoperative care and rehabilitation measures. Demonstrate appropriate exercises to strengthen the remaining portion of the limb and maintain mobility. Follow the doctor's or physical therapist's directions in explaining such exercises.

The patient may be fitted with a prosthesis while hospitalized. But because most amputations require more time to heal, the fitting may follow discharge. Explain that the time between amputation and prosthesis fitting depends on wound healing, muscle tone, and overall stump condition. Stress that good stump care can speed this process and help ensure a better fit for the prosthesis. If possible, show the types of prostheses available for the patient's type of amputation and explain how they work.

Point out the possibility of phantom limb sensation. Explain that the patient may "feel" sensations of pain, itching, or numbness in the area of amputation, even though the limb or digit has been removed. Provide reassurance that these sensations, although inexplicable, are common and should eventually disappear.

As ordered, give broad-spectrum antibiotics to minimize the risk of infection.

Monitoring and aftercare
- After surgery, monitor the patient's vital signs every hour for the first 4 hours, every 2 hours for the next 4 hours, and then every 4 hours until stable.
- Be alert, particularly for bleeding through the dressing, and notify the doctor if any appears.
- If ordered, elevate the stump on a pillow or other support for 24 to 48 hours; remember, however, that this could lead to contractures.

- Check dressings frequently and change them as necessary. Assess drain patency, and note the amount and character of drainage.
- Assess for pain, and provide analgesics and other pain control measures, as needed.
- Because painful movement may interfere with therapy, give analgesics about 30 minutes before scheduled exercises or ambulation. Effective pain control tends to reduce the incidence of phantom limb sensation.
- Distinguish stump pain from phantom limb sensation; severe, unremitting stump pain may indicate infection or other complications.
- Confirm that the stump is properly wrapped with elastic compression bandages. A properly applied bandage is essential to stump care; it supports soft tissue, controls edema and pain, and shrinks and molds the stump into a cone-shaped form to allow a good fit for the prosthesis.
- Rewrap the stump at least twice a day to maintain tightness. As an alternative to bandages, the doctor may order that the patient wear a stump shrinker—a custom-fitted elastic stocking that fits snugly over the stump.
- If a rigid plaster dressing has been applied, care for it as you would a plaster cast for a fracture or severe sprain. Keep it from getting wet, and watch for skin irritation and excessive or malodorous drainage, which may indicate infection.
- As the stump shrinks, the plaster dressing may loosen or fall off. If this occurs, notify the doctor and wrap the stump in an elastic compression bandage until he can replace the dressing.

Patient teaching
- Emphasize the need for proper body alignment and regular physical therapy to condition the stump and prevent contractures and deformity.
- Encourage frequent ambulation, if possible, and a program of active or passive range-of-motion (ROM) exercises, as ordered.
- If the patient is bedridden, encourage turning from side to side and periodically assuming an alternate position—usually on the stomach. Frequent position changes will stretch the hip flexor muscles and prevent contractures.
- If the patient has had an above-the-knee amputation, warn against propping the stump on a pillow to avoid hip flexion contracture.
- For a below-the-knee amputation, tell the patient to keep the knee extended to prevent hamstring contracture.
- Instruct the patient with a partial arm amputation to keep the elbow extended and shoulder abducted.
- If possible, provide information about available prostheses. Keep in mind the patient's age and physi-

Wrapping a stump

Proper stump care helps protect the limb, reduces swelling, and prepares the limb for a prosthesis. As you perform the procedure, teach it to the patient.

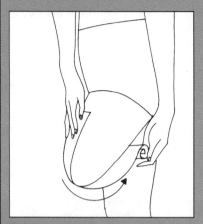

Start by obtaining two 4″ elastic bandages. Center the end of the first bandage at the top of the patient's thigh. Unroll the bandage downward over the stump and to the back of the leg, as shown.

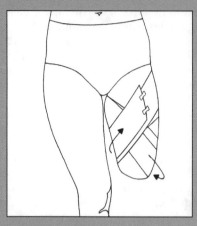

Make three figure-eight turns to adequately cover the end of the stump. As you wrap, be sure to include the roll of flesh in the groin area. Use enough pressure to ensure that the stump narrows toward the end so that it fits comfortably into the prosthesis.

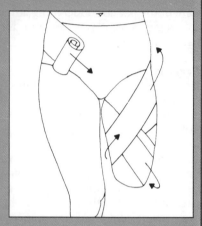

Use the second bandage to anchor the first bandage around the waist. For a below-the-knee amputation, use the knee to anchor the first bandage in place. Secure the bandage with clips, safety pins, or adhesive tape. Check the stump bandage regularly, and rewrap it if it bunches at the end.

cal condition as well as the complexity and cost of the device. Generally, a child needs a relatively simple, inexpensive device that can be maintained easily and replaced at a reasonable cost when outgrown. An older adult may require a prosthesis that provides extra stability, even if it means sacrificing some flexibility.

■ Teach the patient to examine the stump daily, using a handheld mirror to see the entire area. Describe the signs and symptoms to watch for and report: swelling, redness, excessive drainage, increased pain, and any skin changes on the stump, including rashes, blisters, or abrasions.

■ Explain that good stump hygiene will prevent irritation, skin breakdown, and infection. Tell the patient to wash the stump daily with mild soap and water and then rinse and gently dry it. Suggest washing the stump at night and bandaging it when dry; advise against bandaging a wet stump because this may lead to skin maceration or infection.

■ Advise against applying body oil or lotion to the stump because this can interfere with proper fit of the prosthesis.

■ Teach the procedure for applying a stump dressing. Instruct the patient to change dressings frequently, as necessary, and to maintain sterile technique. Explain that as the wound heals, it will need dressing changes less often.

■ As appropriate, show the patient how to properly wrap the stump with elastic bandages or how to slip on a stump shrinker. (See *Wrapping a stump*.) Show the patient how to apply bandages with even, moderate pressure, avoiding overtightness that could impair circulation.

■ Suggest that the patient apply the bandages upon awakening in the morning and rewrap the stump at least twice a day to maintain proper compression.

■ If the patient is using a shrinker, suggest having574 two available: one to wear while the other is being washed. Explain the need to use elastic bandages or a stump shrinker at all times (except when bathing or exercising) until postoperative edema completely subsides and the prosthesis is properly fitted.

■ Explain that, even after adjustment to the prosthesis, the patient may need to continue nighttime bandaging for many years.

- Instruct the patient to apply a clean stump sock before attaching the prosthesis, and never to wear a stump sock that has any tears, holes, mends, or seams because these could cause skin irritation.
- Explain that, as the stump shrinks over time, it may require two socks to ensure a snug fit of the prosthesis. Tell the patient to notify the doctor if this happens or if the prosthesis feels loose for any other reason.
- Review proper care of the prosthesis. Instruct the patient never to immerse it in water, which could weaken its leather joints or hinges.
- Tell the patient to clean the device with soap and water each night before bedtime and to let it dry overnight.
- Throughout recovery and rehabilitation, encourage the patient to adopt a positive outlook toward resuming an independent lifestyle. Emphasize that the prosthesis should allow a full and active life with few activity restrictions. If the patient seems overly despondent or depressed, consider referral to psychological counseling, social services, or a local support group.

COMPLICATIONS
Amputation can cause several complications, including infection at the stump site, contractures in the remaining limb part (if exercise of the limb part is delayed), skin breakdown from improper care of the stump or an ill-fitting prosthetic device, and phantom pain. Phantom pain is a sensation of pain, itching, or numbness in the area of amputation, even though the limb or digit has been removed. It commonly develops after a major amputation and can occur as late as 2 to 3 months afterward. Because amputation of a body part can be emotionally devastating, the patient may develop depression that is severe enough to interfere with self-care and require psychiatric therapy.

OPEN REDUCTION AND INTERNAL FIXATION
Open reduction and internal fixation is performed on fractured fragments of bone or dislocated joints that require surgical alignment.

PROCEDURE
During open reduction, the surgeon restores the normal position and alignment of fracture fragments or dislocated joints. He then inserts internal fixation devices—such as pins, screws, wires, nails, rods, and plates—to maintain alignment until healing can occur. Choice of a specific device depends on the location, type, and configuration of the fracture. In trochanteric or subtrochanteric fractures, the surgeon may use a hip pin or nail (with or without plate) or a screwplate. Because weight bearing imposes great stresses on this area, the patient requires strong control of both proximal and distal bone fragments. A pin or plate with extra nails stabilizes the fracture by impacting the bone ends at the fracture site.

In an uncomplicated fracture of the femoral shaft, the surgeon may use an intramedullary rod. This device permits early ambulation with partial weight bearing.

In an upper extremity fracture, the surgeon may use a plate, rod, or nail. Most radius and ulna fractures are fixed with plates, whereas humerus fractures are fixed with rods.

COLLABORATIVE MANAGEMENT
Care of the patient undergoing open reduction and internal fixation requires preparing thoroughly, monitoring closely, and providing intense patient teaching.

Preparation
Because this procedure requires general or regional anesthesia, instruct the patient not to eat after midnight the day before the procedure. Note that he'll receive a sedative and antibiotics before going to the operating room. Describe the bulky dressing and surgical drain that he'll have in place for several days postoperatively. Tell him that he may need a cast or splint for support when the drain is removed and swelling subsides.

Monitoring and aftercare
- Monitor the patient's vital signs until stable.
- Monitor hemoglobin level and hematocrit, and assess for hypovolemic shock.
- Assess any drainage amounts and report excessive amounts. Clean the wound as recommended. Report amount and type of drainage. Assess for signs of infection.
- Elevate the affected extremity on pillows as ordered, and keep it in alignment. Note the doctor's recommendations for limitations of movement until the healing process begins and the patient has begun physical therapy.

Patient teaching
- Teach the patient how to apply (if appropriate) and care for the device.
- Tell him to check his skin regularly under and around the device, if possible, for irritation and breakdown. Also instruct the patient to watch for signs indicating that the incision may be infected.
- Advise him to exercise and place weight on the affected joint only as the doctor instructs.

COMPLICATIONS
Complications of open reduction and internal fixation include infection, hemorrhage, and improper joint healing.

Locating the carpal tunnel

The carpal tunnel lies between the longitudinal tendons of the hand-flexing forearm muscles (not shown) and the transverse carpal ligament. Note the median nerve and flexor tendons passing through the tunnel on their way from the forearm to the hand.

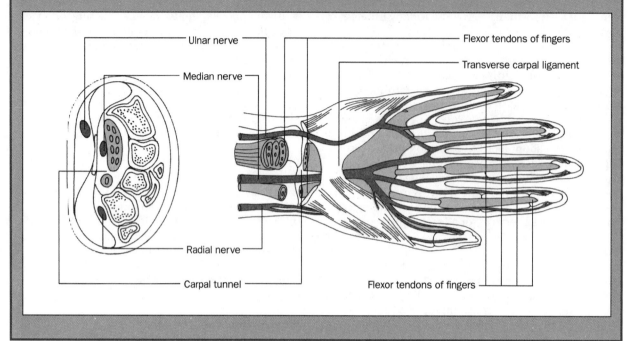

RELEASE OF CARPAL TUNNEL LIGAMENT

If rest, splinting, and corticosteroid injections don't relieve your patient's repetitive use injury, surgery may be necessary to decompress the median nerve. Surgery almost always relieves pain and restores function in the wrist and hand.

PROCEDURE

The surgeon can choose from several approaches to carpal tunnel release. However, the technique must involve complete transection of the transverse carpal tunnel ligament to ensure adequate median nerve decompression. (See *Locating the carpal tunnel*.)

In one of the more popular techniques, the surgeon makes an incision around the thenar eminence to expose the flexor retinaculum, which he then transects to relieve pressure on the median nerve. Depending on the extent of nerve compression, he also may perform neurolysis to free flattened nerve fibers. Neurolysis involves stretching the nerve, which relieves tension and loosens surrounding adhesions.

COLLABORATIVE MANAGEMENT

Care of the patient undergoing release of carpal tunnel ligament requires preparing thoroughly, monitoring closely, and providing intense patient teaching.

Preparation

Reinforce the purpose of the planned surgery. Tell the patient that the procedure should relieve the pain in her wrist and help her regain full use of her hand. Outline the steps of surgery, tailoring your explanation to the particular procedure the doctor has chosen as well as to the patient's level of understanding.

Explain to the patient that before surgery, someone will shave and clean the affected arm and give her a local anesthetic. Reassure her that although she may feel some pressure, the anesthetic will ensure a pain-free operation.

Discuss postoperative care measures. Point out that she'll have a dressing wrapped around her hand and lower arm, which usually remains in place for 1 to 2 days after surgery. Explain that she may experience pain once the anesthetic wears off but that analgesics will be available.

Teach her the rehabilitative exercises that she'll use during the recovery period: gentle ROM exercises with the wrist and fingers to prevent muscle atrophy. Demonstrate these exercises, and have her perform a return demonstration. Note, however, that severe pain may prevent her from doing so.

Monitoring and aftercare

■ After surgery, monitor your patient's vital signs and carefully assess circulation and sensory and motor function in the affected arm and hand.
■ Keep the hand elevated to reduce swelling and discomfort.
■ Check the dressing often for unusual drainage or bleeding, which may indicate infection.
■ Assess for pain and provide analgesics as needed. Report severe, persistent pain or tenderness, which may point to tenosynovitis or hematoma formation.
■ Encourage the patient to perform her wrist and finger exercises daily to improve circulation and enhance muscle tone. If these exercises are painful, have her do them with her wrist and hand immersed in warm water. (Provide a surgical glove if her dressing is still in place.)
■ Assess the need for home care and follow-up with activities of daily living, especially if the patient lives alone.

Patient teaching

■ Teach the patient to keep the incision site clean and dry. Tell her to cover it with a surgical or rubber glove when immersing it in water for exercises or when taking a bath or shower.
■ Teach the patient how to change the dressing. Instruct her to do so once a day until healing is complete.
■ Tell the patient to notify the doctor if redness, swelling, pain, or excessive drainage persists at the incision site.
■ Encourage the patient to continue daily wrist and finger exercises. However, warn her against overusing the affected wrist or against lifting any object heavier than a thin magazine.
■ If the patient's carpal tunnel syndrome is job related, suggest that she seek occupational counseling to help find more suitable employment.

COMPLICATIONS

Although carpal tunnel release is relatively simple and generally risk-free, complications include hematoma formation, infection, painful scar formation, and tenosynovitis.

TOTAL HIP ARTHROPLASTY

Total hip arthroplasty is the total or partial replacement of the joint with a synthetic prosthesis. The procedure restores mobility and stability and relieves pain. In fact, recent improvements in surgical techniques and prosthetic devices have made hip joint replacement an increasingly common treatment for patients with severe chronic arthritis, degenerative joint disorders, and extensive joint trauma. No cautions are listed for total hip arthroplasty.

PROCEDURE

In a total hip replacement, the patient is placed in a supine or lateral position and given a regional or general anesthetic. The surgeon then makes an incision to expose the hip joint. As necessary, he incises or excises the hip capsule, and then dislocates the joint to expose the acetabulum and the head of the femur.

Next, the surgeon reams and shapes the acetabulum to accept the socket part of the ball-and-socket hip prosthesis and secures the device in place. Polymethylmethacrylate adhesive is used to secure the device in place if the prosthesis is cemented. He then repeats this process on the head of the femur for the ball portion of the prosthesis.

Once the parts of the prosthesis are in place, the surgeon fits them together to restore the joint. Then he closes the incision in layers and applies a dressing.

COLLABORATIVE MANAGEMENT

Care of the patient undergoing total hip arthroplasty requires thorough preparation, close monitoring, and intense patient teaching. (See *Managing total hip replacement,* page 576 and 577.)

Preparation

Because hip replacement is complex, the patient will begin preparation with extensive testing long before the day of surgery. Though the doctor will have explained the procedure in detail, the patient and his family still may have questions about the surgery and its expected outcome. Answer them as completely as you can.

Mention that the patient will probably get out of bed the first or second day after surgery. Explain that a physical therapist will see him either before or soon after surgery to begin an exercise program to maintain joint mobility. As appropriate, some him ROM exercises or demonstrate the continuous passive motion (CPM) device that he'll use during recovery.

Prepare the patient for an extended period of rehabilitation. Point out that pain actually may worsen for several weeks after surgery. Reassure him that pain will diminish dramatically once edema subsides. Reassure him that he'll get analgesics as needed.

(Text continues on page 578.)

Managing total hip replacement

	Day 1 (Surgery)	Day 2 (Postop Day 1)
CARE UNIT	OR/PACU Surgical floor	Surgical floor
CONSULTS	■ Anesthesia pain service (if epidural)	■ Physical therapy twice ■ Anesthesia pain service (if epidural)
TESTS/LABS	■ Hematocrit ■ Electrolytes	■ Hematocrit (#) ■ Prothrombin time (PT) (Coumadin) (#)
ACTIVITY	■ Up in Stretchair once daily, if comfortable	■ Out of bed (OOB) under supervision of physical therapist, then nurse three times ■ Active range-of-motion (ROM) exercises initiated (flexion, extension, abduction) ■ Transfers initiated (bed, chair, bedside commode) ■ Bed mobility initiated (roll, scoot, supine to sit) ■ Ambulation initiated
ASSESSMENTS (Notify doctor of temperature >101.3˚ F. [38.5˚C])	■ Vital signs (VS) checks every 4 hrs ■ Neurovascular (NV) checks every 2 hrs ■ Dressing assessment every 8 hrs ■ Full assessment per nursing standards every 8 hrs	■ VS checks every 4 hrs ■ NV checks every 4 hrs ■ Dressing assessment every 8 hrs ■ Full assessment per nursing standards every 12 hrs minimum
TREATMENTS	■ Intake and output (I & O) and Hemovac (HMV) empty and record every 8 hrs ■ I.V. lactated Ringer's @_____ ■ Indwelling urinary catheter ■ Incentive spirometer (IS) while patient awake ■ Antiembolism stockings; removal twice for 5 minutes ■ Pneumatic compression device at all times when patient in bed ■ Abduction pillow ■ Overhead trapeze ■ Blood products, if ordered	■ I & O and HMV empty and record every 8 hrs ■ I.V. to medication lock (ML) ■ Indwelling urinary catheter discontinued at 0600 hrs ■ IS every hour while awake ■ Antiembolism stockings; removal twice for 5 minutes ■ Pneumatic compression device at all times when patient in bed ■ Abduction pillow ■ Overhead trapeze ■ Blood products, if ordered
MEDICATION	■ Antibiotic (Kefzol every 8 hr) ■ Anticoagulants per protocol ■ Senokot at bedtime (h.s.) ■ Routine medications	■ Antibiotic (Kefzol) ■ Anticoagulants per protocol ■ Senokot h.s. ■ Routine medications
PAIN/SYMPTOM CONTROL	■ Pain medication per protocol (epidural or patient controlled analgesia [PCA] pump) ■ Antiemetics per order ■ Tylenol as needed (p.r.n.) ■ Maalox p.r.n.	■ Pain medication per protocol (epidural or PCA pump) ■ Antiemetics per order ■ Tylenol p.r.n. ■ Maalox p.r.n.
NUTRITION	■ Nothing by mouth; advance to clear liquids	■ As at home
DISCHARGE PLANNING/ TEACHING	■ Daily goals posted at bedside ■ Hip precautions posted at bedside ■ Confirmation that copy of total hip replacement booklet and video given to patient in clinic during preoperative visit ■ IS and pain-management teaching reinforced	Physical therapist: ■ Hip precautions reinforced ■ Exercise instruction reinforced ■ Home assessment reviewed

Adapted with permission from Shands Hospital at the University of Florida, Gainesville. Note: Full clinical path includes preoperative and post-discharge home care.

Day 3 (Postop Day 2)	Day 4 (Postop Day 3)	Day 5 (Postop Day 4)
Surgical floor	Surgical floor	Surgical floor
■ Physical therapy twice	■ Physical therapy twice	■ Physical therapy
■ Hematocrit ■ PT (Coumadin)	■ Ortho pelvis X-ray ■ PT (Coumadin)	■ PT (Coumadin)
■ OOB under supervision of physical therapist or nurse three times ■ ROM exercises progressed ■ Transfers progressed (toilet, tub, shower, chair) ■ Bed mobility progressed (roll, scoot, supine to sit) ■ Ambulation on level surfaces increased ■ Ambulation on unlevel surfaces initiated (stairs, ramps, curbs)	■ OOB under supervision of physical therapist or nurse three times ■ ROM exercises progressed ■ Transfers progressed in home simulation area ■ Bed mobility progressed (roll, scoot, supine to sit) ■ Ambulation on level surfaces increased ■ Ambulation on unlevel surfaces progressed ■ Car transfers introduced	■ OOB as capable; assist as needed ■ ROM exercises progressed to _____ ■ Transfers progressed in home simulation area to increase independence ■ Bed mobility progressed ■ Ambulation on level and unlevel surfaces increased ■ Car transfer progressed
■ VS checks every shift ■ NV checks every shift ■ Dressing assessment every 8 hrs ■ Full assessment per nursing standards every 12 hrs minimum	■ VS checks every shift ■ NV checks every shift ■ Full assessment per nursing standards every 12 hrs minimum	■ VS checks every shift ■ NV checks every shift ■ Full assessment per nursing standards every 12 hrs minimum
■ I.V. to ML ■ IS every hour while awake ■ Antiembolism stockings; removal twice for 5 minutes ■ Pneumatic compression device at all times when patient in bed ■ Abduction pillow ■ Overhead trapeze ■ Blood products, if ordered	■ ML discontinued ■ IS every 4 hrs ■ Antiembolism stockings; removal twice for 5 minutes ■ Pneumatic compression device at all times when patient in bed ■ Regular pillow during day; abduction pillow at night ■ Overhead trapeze ■ Dressing changed daily and p.r.n.	■ IS every 4 hrs ■ Antiembolism stockings; removal twice for 5 minutes ■ Pneumatic compression device at all times when patient in bed ■ Regular pillow during day ■ Abduction pillow at night ■ Overhead trapeze ■ Dressing changed daily and p.r.n.
■ Anticoagulants per protocol ■ Laxatives p.r.n. ■ Senokot h.s. ■ Routine medications	■ Anticoagulants per protocol ■ Laxatives as needed ■ Senokot h.s. ■ Routine medications	■ Anticoagulants per protocol ■ Laxatives as needed ■ Senokot h.s. ■ Routine medications
■ Pain medication per protocol (epidural or PCA pump) ■ Antiemetics per order ■ Tylenol p.r.n. ■ Maalox p.r.n.	■ Tylox p.r.n. ■ Tylenol p.r.n. ■ Maalox p.r.n.	■ Tylox p.r.n. ■ Tylenol p.r.n. ■ Maalox p.r.n.
■ As at home	■ As at home	■ As at home
■ Teaching reviewed ■ Hip precautions reviewed ■ Patient/family simulation of home situation	■ Patient/family teaching reviewed ■ Hip precautions reviewed ■ Patient/family simulation of home situation ■ Patient status discussion with home care nurse ■ Further equipment needs addressed with case manager	■ Patient verbalization and demonstration of discharge instructions ■ Patient/family simulation of home situation ■ Report to home care nurse and physical therapist ■ Dressing change materials provided for 24 hrs

Monitoring and aftercare

- Monitor your patient's vital signs until he's stable.
- When he returns from surgery, keep him in bed for the prescribed period. Maintain the hip in proper alignment.
- Assess the patient's level of pain, and provide analgesics as ordered. If you're giving him narcotic analgesics, remember to watch for signs of toxicity or oversedation.
- During the recovery period, monitor for complications of joint replacement. In particular, watch for hypovolemic shock from massive blood loss during surgery. Assess the patient's vital signs frequently, and report hypotension, narrowed pulse pressure, tachycardia, decreased level of consciousness, rapid and shallow respirations, or cold, pale, clammy skin.
- Watch for signs of a fat embolism, a potentially fatal complication.
- Inspect the incision site and dressing frequently for signs of infection. Change the dressing as necessary, maintaining strict aseptic technique. Assess neurovascular and motor status distal to the site of joint replacement regularly. Immediately report any abnormalities.
- Remember to reposition the patient often to avoid pressure sores. Encourage frequent coughing and deep breathing to prevent pulmonary complications and adequate fluid intake to prevent urinary stasis and constipation.
- As ordered, have the patient begin exercising the hip joint soon after surgery. (Some doctors routinely order physical therapy to begin on the day of surgery.) The doctor may prescribe CPM, which involves the use of a machine or a system of suspended ropes and pulleys, or a series of active or passive ROM exercises.
- If joint displacement occurs, notify the doctor. If traction is used to correct displacement, periodically check the weights and other equipment.

Patient teaching

- Reinforce the doctor's and physical therapist's instructions for the patient's exercise regimen. Remind him to stick closely to the prescribed schedule and not to rush rehabilitation, no matter how good he feels.
- Review prescribed limitations on activity. The doctor may order the patient to avoid bending or lifting, extensive stair climbing, or sitting for prolonged periods (including long car trips or plane flights). He also will caution against overusing the hip joint—especially because it is weight bearing.
- Tell the patient to keep his hips abducted and not to cross his legs when sitting, to reduce the risk of dislocating the prosthesis.

- Tell him to avoid flexing his hips more than 90 degrees when arising from a bed or chair. Encourage him to sit in chairs with high arms and a firm seat and to sleep only on a firm mattress. Before the patient with a hip replacement is discharged, make sure that he has a properly sized pair of crutches and knows how to use them properly.
- Remind the patient to promptly report signs of possible infection, such as persistent fever and increased pain, tenderness, and stiffness in the joint and surrounding area. Tell him that infection may develop even several months after joint replacement.
- Stress the importance of taking prophylactic antibiotics before any dental or surgical procedures. Explain that this is necessary to prevent organisms from migrating to the hip and causing an infection.
- Tell the patient to report a sudden increase of pain, which may indicate dislodgment of the prosthesis.

COMPLICATIONS

If the implant site becomes infected, the hip joint almost always must be removed.

Other serious complications include hypovolemic shock, fat embolism, thromboembolism, and pulmonary embolism. In fact, pulmonary embolism is the most common cause of postoperative mortality following a joint replacement.

Less serious complications include dislocation or loosening of the prosthesis, heterotrophic ossification (formation of bone in the periprosthetic space), avascular necrosis, and dead bone caused by loss of blood supply. Respiratory complications, such as atelectasis and pneumonia, commonly affect older patients because of their decreased activity tolerance.

TOTAL KNEE REPLACEMENT

Called an arthroplasty, the total or partial replacement of a joint with a synthetic prosthesis restores mobility and stability and relieves pain. In fact, recent improvements in surgical techniques and prosthetic devices have made joint replacement an increasingly common treatment for patients with severe chronic arthritis, degenerative joint disorders, and extensive joint trauma. All joints except the spine can be replaced with a prosthesis; hip and knee replacements are the most common. The benefits of joint replacement include not only improved, pain-free mobility but also an increased sense of independence and self-worth.

PROCEDURE

The joint replacement procedure varies slightly, depending on the joint and its condition. The patient is placed in a supine position and given a regional or general anesthetic. The surgeon then makes an incision to expose the joint. As necessary, he incises or excises the capsule, and then dislocates the joint.

Next, the surgeon reams and shapes the area to accept the socket part of the ball-and-socket knee prosthesis and secures the device in place. Polymethylmethacrylate adhesive is used to secure the device in place.

Once the parts of the prosthesis are in place, the surgeon fits them together to restore the joint. Then he closes the incision in layers and applies a dressing.

COLLABORATIVE MANAGEMENT

Care of the patient undergoing total knee replacement requires preparing thoroughly, monitoring closely, and providing intense patient teaching.

Preparation

Because knee replacement is complex, patient preparation begins with extensive testing, long before the day of surgery. By the time the patient enters the hospital for surgery, the doctor will have explained the procedure to him in detail. However, the patient and family members still may have questions. Answer them as completely as you can.

Discuss postoperative recovery. Mention that the patient will probably get out of bed the first or second day after surgery. Explain that a physical therapist will see him either before or soon after surgery to begin an exercise program to maintain knee mobility. As appropriate, show him ROM exercises or demonstrate the continuous passive motion (CPM) device that he'll use during recovery.

Prepare the patient for an extended period of rehabilitation. Point out that he may not experience pain relief immediately after surgery. Reassure him that pain will diminish dramatically once edema subsides and that he'll get analgesics as needed. Anticoagulants may be prescribed for an extended period to prevent thromboembolism.

Monitoring and aftercare

■ Assess your patient's vital signs until he's stable.
■ When he returns from surgery, keep him on bed rest for the prescribed period. Maintain the knee in proper alignment.
■ Assess the patient's level of pain, and provide analgesics as ordered. If you're giving narcotic analgesics, remember to watch for signs of toxicity or oversedation.
■ During the recovery period, monitor the patient for complications. In particular, watch for hypovolemic shock from massive blood loss during surgery.
■ Assess the patient's vital signs frequently, and report hypotension, narrowed pulse pressure, tachycardia, decreased level of consciousness, rapid and shallow respirations, or cold, pale, clammy skin.

■ Watch for signs of a fat embolism, a potentially fatal complication.
■ Inspect the incision site and dressing frequently for signs of infection. Change the dressing as necessary, maintaining strict aseptic technique. Assess neurovascular and motor status distal to the site of joint replacement regularly. Immediately report any abnormalities.
■ Be sure to reposition the patient often to enhance comfort and prevent pressure sores. Encourage frequent coughing and deep breathing to prevent pulmonary complications and adequate fluid intake to prevent urinary stasis and constipation.
■ As ordered, have the patient begin exercising the affected joint soon after surgery. (Some doctors routinely order physical therapy to begin on the day of surgery.) The doctor may prescribe CPM, which involves the use of a machine or a system of suspended ropes and pulleys, or a series of active or passive ROM exercises.
■ If joint displacement occurs, notify the doctor. If traction is used to correct displacement, periodically check the weights and other equipment.

Patient teaching

■ Reinforce the doctor's and physical therapist's instructions for the patient's exercise regimen. Remind him to stick closely to the prescribed schedule and not to rush rehabilitation, no matter how good he feels.
■ Review prescribed limitations on activity. The doctor likely will order the patient to avoid bending or lifting, extensive stair climbing, or sitting for prolonged periods (including long car trips or plane flights). He also will caution against overusing the knee joint because it's a weight-bearing joint.
■ Caution the patient to promptly report signs and symptoms of possible infection, such as persistent fever and increased pain, tenderness, and stiffness in the knee and surrounding area. Remind him that infection may develop even several months after joint replacement.
■ If the doctor tells the patient to take prophylactic antibiotics before any dental or surgical procedure, stress the importance of complying. They're necessary to prevent organisms from migrating to the knee and causing an infection.
■ Tell the patient to report a sudden increase of pain, which may indicate dislodgment of the prosthesis.

COMPLICATIONS

If the implant site becomes infected, the knee joint almost always must be removed. Other serious complications include hypovolemic shock, fat embolism, thromboembolism, and pulmonary embolism. In fact, pulmonary embolism is the most common cause of postoperative mortality following a joint replacement.

Less serious is dislocation or loosening of the prosthesis, heterotrophic ossification (formation of bone in the periprosthetic space), avascular necrosis, and dead bone caused by loss of blood supply. Respiratory complications, such as atelectasis and pneumonia, commonly affect older patients because of their decreased activity tolerance.

Selected references

Diseases, 2nd ed. Springhouse, Pa.: Springhouse Corp., 1997.

Huether, S., and McCance, K. *Understanding Pathophysiology.* St. Louis: Mosby–Year Book, 1996.

Illustrated Handbook of Nursing Care. Springhouse, Pa.: Springhouse Corp., 1998.

Maher, et al.. *Orthopaedic Nursing.* Philadelphia: W.B. Saunders Co., 1994.

Phipps, W.J., et al. *Medical-Surgical Nursing Concepts and Clinical Practice,* 5th ed. St. Louis: Mosby–Year Book, 1995.

Polaski, A., and Tatro, S.E. *Luckmann's Core Principles and Practice of Medical-Surgical Nursing.* Philadelphia: W.B. Saunders Co., 1996.

Professional Guide to Signs & Symptoms, 2nd ed. Springhouse, Pa.: Springhouse Corp., 1997.

Hematologic and lymphatic disorders

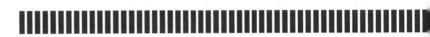

The hematologic system affects every other body system. Because blood is a factor in every function and dysfunction, you'll need to conduct an especially thorough patient history and physical assessment to elicit clues to many hematologic disorders.

Anatomy and physiology review

The hematologic system comprises the blood—the major body fluid tissue—and the bone marrow, which manufactures new blood cells (hematopoiesis). The blood delivers oxygen and nutrients to all tissues, removes wastes, and performs many other tasks.

BLOOD

Actually a tissue, blood consists of various formed elements, or blood cells, suspended in a fluid called plasma. Blood transports gases, nutrients, metabolic wastes, blood cells, immune cells, and hormones throughout the body. To accomplish this task, the blood, which is confined to the vascular system, constantly interacts with the body's extracellular fluid for exchange and transfer.

Formed elements in the blood include red blood cells (RBCs, or erythrocytes), platelets, and white blood cells (WBCs, or leukocytes). RBCs and platelets function entirely within blood vessels; WBCs act mainly in the tissues outside the blood vessels.

RED BLOOD CELLS

RBCs transport oxygen and carbon dioxide to and from body tissues. These minute cells lose their nuclei during maturation, thus developing a biconcave shape and the flexibility to travel through different-sized blood vessels. RBCs contain hemoglobin, the oxygen-carrying substance that gives blood its red color.

Constant circulation wears out RBCs, which have an average 120-day life span. The spleen sequesters, or isolates, the old, worn-out RBCs, thus removing them from circulation. This process requires that the body manufacture billions of new cells daily to maintain RBCs at normal levels.

Bone marrow releases RBCs into circulation in immature form as reticulocytes. The reticulocytes mature into RBCs in about 1 day. The rate of reticulocyte release usually equals the rate of old RBC removal. When RBC depletion occurs—for example, with hemorrhage—the bone marrow increases reticulocyte production to maintain normal RBC levels.

The surface of each RBC carries antigens that determine a person's blood group, or blood type.

All blood falls into one of four blood types. In type A blood, the A antigen appears on RBCs. In type B blood, the B antigen appears. Type AB blood contains both antigens, whereas type O blood has neither antigen.

Blood from any of these types may also include the Rh antigen. With the Rh antigen, the blood is Rh-positive (Rh+); without the Rh antigen, it's Rh-negative (Rh-).

Plasma may contain antibodies that interact with these antigens, causing the cells to agglutinate. However, plasma can't contain antibodies to its own cell antigen, or it would destroy itself. Thus, type A blood has A antigen but no anti-A antibodies; however, it does have anti-B antibodies. This principle is important in blood transfusions because a donor's blood must be compatible with the recipient's blood or the result can be fatal. Therefore, precise blood typing and crossmatching (mixing and observing for agglutination of donor cells) are essential.

The following blood groups are compatible: type A with type A or O; type B with type B or O; type AB with type A, B, AB, or O; and type O with type O only.

PLATELETS

Platelets play a major role in hemostasis. Produced in the bone marrow, they bud from a megakaryocyte, a giant cell with a multilobed nucleus. Like the RBC, a platelet is a round or oval biconcave disk with no nucleus.

In the peripheral blood, platelets are sticky and contribute to hemostasis in three ways: They clump together to plug small defects in small blood vessel walls; they congregate at an injury site in a larger vessel to help close the wound so that a clot can form; and they release substances that fortify clot stabilization. For example, they release serotonin, which reduces blood flow by vasoconstriction, and thromboplastin, an enzyme essential to clot formation. (See *How blood clots*.)

WHITE BLOOD CELLS

The WBCs that participate in the body's defense and immune systems are neutrophils, eosinophils, basophils, monocytes, and lymphocytes. These are grouped as granulocytes and agranulocytes. All granulocytes contain a single multilobed nucleus and prominent cytoplasmic granules. Cell types in this category include neutrophils, eosinophils, and basophils. Collectively, these cells are known as polymorphonuclear leukocytes. However, each cell type exhibits different properties, and each is activated by different stimuli.

The most abundant granulocytes, neutrophils account for 47.6% to 76.8% of circulating WBCs. Neutrophils are phagocytic—they can engulf, ingest, and digest foreign materials. Neutrophils leave the bloodstream by diapedesis, then migrate to and accumulate at infection sites. Worn-out neutrophils form the main component of pus. Bone marrow produces their replacements — immature neutrophils called bands. In response to infection, bone marrow must produce many immature cells and release them into circulation, elevating the band count.

Less common than neutrophils, eosinophils account for 0.3% to 7% of circulating WBCs. These granulocytes also migrate from the bloodstream by diapedesis, but in response to different stimuli. During allergic responses, eosinophils accumulate in loose connective tissue where they're highly phagocytic to antigen-antibody complexes.

The least common granulocytes, basophils usually constitute fewer than 2% of circulating WBCs. They possess little or no phagocytic ability. However, their cytoplasmic granules secrete histamine in response to certain inflammatory and immune stimuli, increasing vascular permeability and easing fluid passage from capillaries into body tissues.

Because of their phagocytic capabilities, granulocytes serve as the body's first line of cellular defense against foreign organisms.

Called agranulocytes, monocytes and lymphocytes are WBCs that lack specific cytoplasmic granules and have nuclei without lobes. Monocytes, the largest of the WBCs, constitute only 0.6% to 9.6% of WBCs in circulation. Like neutrophils, monocytes are phagocytic and diapedetic. Outside the bloodstream, monocytes enlarge and mature, becoming tissue macrophages, or histiocytes.

As macrophages, monocytes may roam freely through the body when stimulated by inflammation. Usually they remain immobile, populating most organs and tissues. Collectively, they're components of the reticuloendothelial system, which defends against infection and disposes of cell breakdown products. Macrophages concentrate in structures that filter large amounts of body fluid, such as the liver, spleen, and lymph nodes, where they defend against invading organisms. Macrophages exhibit varying physical characteristics and are referred to by different names, depending on their organ location. Kupffer's cells reside in the hepatic sinuses, microglia in the central nervous system, and alveolar macrophages in the lung alveoli. Macrophages are efficient phagocytes of bacteria, cellular debris (including worn-out neutrophils), and necrotic tissue. When mobilized at an infection site, they phagocytize cellular remnants and promote wound healing.

Lymphocytes, the smallest of the WBCs and the second most numerous (16.2% to 43%), derive from a pluripotential stem cell. Unlike other blood cells, they mature in two different locations: T lymphocytes (T cells) mature in the thymus; B lymphocytes (B cells), most often in the bone marrow. T cells and B cells produce cellular products (lymphokines and antibodies, respectively) for specific immune responses. T cells are involved in cell-mediated immunity; B cells, in humoral immunity.

Assessment

Start your assessment by taking a thorough patient history. After establishing a rapport with your patient, remember to ask about his diet, medication, and occupational history.

How blood clots

Through a three-part process, the circulatory system protects itself from excessive blood loss. In this process, vascular injury activates a complex chain of events—vasoconstriction, platelet aggregation, and coagulation—that leads to clotting. This stops bleeding without hindering blood flow through the injured vessel.

Vascular injury

Vasoconstriction

Smooth muscle spasms.

Serotonin, epinephrine, and lipoprotein are secreted.

Blood vessels contract.

Platelet aggregation

Circulating platelets adhere to collagen fibers.

Adenosine diphosphate causes platelets to break down and stick together.

Platelets aggregate to plug the wound.

Coagulation

EXTRINSIC SYSTEM

Tissue thromboplastin (factor III) and plasma procoagulant proconvertin (factor VII) activates in presence of calcium (factor IV) and platelet phospholipids.

Stuart factor (factor X) activates; extrinsic pathway ends.

INTRINSIC SYSTEM

Plasma thromboplastin activates.

In presence of calcium, factor XII activates factor XI, initiating factor IX activity.

In presence of platelet phospholipids, factor IX converts factor VIII and helps form factor X; intrinsic pathway ends.

Factor X reacts with prothrombin accelerator (factor V) to form prothrombin-converting complex.

In presence of calcium and platelets, factor X and factor V convert prothrombin to thrombin.

Thrombin hydrolyses fibrinogen (factor I).

Thrombin activates fibrin-stabilizing factor (factor XIII).

Fibrin monomers form fibrin threads that build polymer network.

Fibrin polymer strengthens; firm clot forms.

CHIEF COMPLAINT

Ask the patient why he needs medical help. Document the response in his own words. Because signs and symptoms from hematologic problems can appear in any body system, his complaints may be nonspecific, such as lack of energy, light-headedness, or nosebleeds. Though not diagnostic in themselves, when worked into the context of a complete nursing history, such complaints may suggest a pattern that will lead you to suspect a hematologic disorder.

Obtain the patient's biographic data. Information about age, sex, marital status, occupation, religion, race, and ethnic background can provide important clues to risk factors.

Next, ask the patient how long he's had the problem and when and how suddenly or gradually it began. Ask if it occurs continuously or intermittently. If intermittently, how frequent and how long is each episode?

Then determine the problem's location, character, and any precipitating conditions. Ask if anything makes the problem better or worse. Also ask questions to find out whether other signs or symptoms coincide with the primary one.

Try to determine how the patient feels about his condition. Adapt your care to fit his perceptions.

MEDICAL HISTORY

Examine the patient's medical history for additional clues to his present condition. Remember to look for allergies (including drug reactions), immunizations, previously diagnosed illnesses (childhood and adult), past hospitalizations and surgeries, and current medications.

Also look for past disorders that required aggressive immunosuppressant drug or radiation therapy. Such treatment may diminish blood cell production. Ask about thymus radiation in childhood. Note tumors with bone-marrow-seeking tendencies, such as small-cell lung cancer or lymphoma. Hepatitis and miliary tuberculosis also can cause bone marrow failure.

If your patient was hospitalized, ask why. Could a past surgical intervention cause the current medical problem? A splenectomy increases the risk of disseminated infection with encapsulated organisms. A total or partial gastrectomy or lower ileum resection may cause vitamin and nutrient malabsorption resulting in anemia. Immunosuppressant therapy predisposes organ transplant patients to several disorders, particularly lymphoreticular cancers.

Has the patient been transfused? If so, note when and how often it was done, to assess his risk of harboring an infection. Note that before March 1985, donated blood wasn't tested for human immunodeficiency virus, the causative agent in acquired immunodeficiency syndrome. Transfused blood products can also transmit hepatitis C, cytomegalovirus, malaria, and Epstein-Barr virus associated with Burkitt's lymphoma.

Document all medications—prescription and over-the-counter. The patient with a seizure disorder probably takes anticonvulsant drugs that suppress bone marrow. Antineoplastic drugs may cause secondary leukemia or bone marrow dysfunction.

FAMILY HISTORY

Some hematologic disorders are inherited. Ask about deceased family members, recording age at death and cause. Note any inheritable hematologic disorders and plot them on a family genogram to determine the inheritance risk.

SOCIAL HISTORY

Ask him about alcohol intake, diet, sexual habits, and possible drug abuse, all of which can impair hematologic function. Alcoholism can cause folic acid deficiency anemia because excessive alcohol intake interferes with folic acid metabolism, impairing erythroid cell maturation. Also, the poor diet common in alcoholics may lack sufficient folic acid.

Exposure to certain hazardous substances (such as benzene) may cause bone marrow dysfunction, especially leukemia. Remember to gather a comprehensive occupational history. Also ask the patient about his military service. Vietnam veterans exposed to Agent Orange show a higher-than-normal incidence of leukemia and lymphoma. Although the data remain controversial, exposure to this chemical may be responsible.

PHYSICAL EXAMINATION

Because a hematologic disorder can involve almost every body system, remember to perform a complete physical examination.

VITAL SIGNS

Vital signs can provide important clues. Take the patient's temperature. Frequent fevers can indicate a poorly functioning immune system. Note the heart rate. The heart may pump harder or faster to compensate for a decreased oxygen supply resulting from anemia or decreased blood volume from bleeding. This problem can cause tachycardia, palpitations, or arrhythmias. Check respirations. The body's difficulty in meeting its oxygen needs may cause pronounced tachypnea. Measure blood pressure with the patient lying, sitting, and standing. Check for orthostatic hypotension as well as hypotension possibly caused by septicemia or hypovolemia.

Finally, assess your patient's level of consciousness. Be alert for critical changes that require the doctor's immediate attention. Look for the cause of impairment only after you've begun interventions and have stabilized the patient hemodynamically.

INSPECTION

Next, concentrate on areas most relevant to a hematologic disorder: the skin, mucous membranes, fingernails, eyes, lymph nodes, liver, and spleen. Your patient's skin color directly reflects body fluid composition. Because normal skin color can vary widely among individuals, ask the patient if his present skin tone is normal.

Inspect the patient's face, conjunctivae, hands, and feet. Look for erythema, which may indicate local inflammation or fever. Focus on the skin over your patient's lymph nodes and note any color abnormalities.

When assessing the patient's mucous membranes and skin for jaundice, observe him in natural light rather than incandescent light, which can mask yellow color. With dark-skinned patients, inspect the buccal mucosa, palms, and soles for a yellowish tinge. For an edematous patient, examine the inner forearm for jaundice. Remember that excessive carrot or yellow-vegetable intake may cause yellow skin but doesn't change sclerae or mucous membrane color.

As you consider the patient's lymph nodes, liver, and spleen, note any obvious enlargements or redness. Inspect the abdominal area for enlargement, distention, and asymmetry, possibly indicating a tumor.

AUSCULTATION

With the patient lying down, auscultate the abdomen before palpation and percussion to avoid altering bowel sounds. Lymphoma is a hematologic cause of such obstruction. Next, auscultate the liver and spleen. Listen carefully over both organs for friction rubs—grating sounds that fluctuate with respirations, possibly indicating peritoneal inflammation or infarction.

PERCUSSION

To determine liver and spleen size and possibly detect tumors, percuss all four quadrants and compare your findings.

The normal liver sounds dull. Establish the organ's approximate upper and lower borders at the midclavicular line. To determine medial extension, percuss to the midsternal landmark.

The normal spleen also sounds dull. Percuss it from the midaxillary toward the midline. The average-size spleen lies near the eighth, ninth, or tenth intercostal space. You might want to mark liver and spleen borders with a pen for later reference when palpating these organs.

PALPATION

Palpate your patient's neck, axillary, epitrochlear, and inguinal lymph nodes, moving the skin over each area with your finger pads. As you palpate nodes, you may discover sternal tenderness.

A difficult procedure, accurate liver palpation can depend on the patient's size, his present comfort level, and whether fluid is present. If necessary, repeat the procedure, checking your hand position and the pressure you exert. Lightly palpate all four abdominal quadrants to distinguish tender sites and muscle guarding. Deeper palpation helps delineate abdominal organs and masses. Always palpate tender areas last.

Aplastic anemia

Potentially fatal, aplastic or hypoplastic anemias are caused by injury to or destruction of stem cells in bone marrow or the bone marrow matrix, causing pancytopenia (anemia, leukopenia, and thrombocytopenia) and bone marrow hypoplasia.

Although commonly used interchangeably with other terms for bone marrow failure, aplastic anemias correctly refer to pancytopenia caused by the decreased functional capacity of a hypoplastic, fatty bone marrow. These disorders usually produce fatal bleeding or infection, particularly when they're idiopathic or stem from chloramphenicol use or infectious hepatitis. Mortality for patients with aplastic anemias with severe pancytopenia is 80% to 90%.

Life-threatening hemorrhage from the mucous membranes (nose, gums, rectum, vagina) is the most common complication of aplastic or hypoplastic anemias. Immunosuppression can lead to secondary opportunistic infections.

CAUSES

Aplastic anemias usually develop when damaged or destroyed stem cells inhibit red blood cell (RBC) production. Less commonly, they develop when damaged bone marrow microvasculature creates an unfavorable environment for cell growth and maturation. About half of such anemias result from drugs (such as chloramphenicol or hair color dye), toxic agents (such as benzene), or radiation. The rest may be caused by immunologic factors (suspected but unconfirmed), severe disease (especially hepatitis), or preleukemic and neoplastic infiltration of bone marrow.

Idiopathic anemias may be congenital. Two such forms of aplastic anemia have been identified: congenital hypoplastic anemia (Blackfan-Diamond anemia) develops between ages 2 and 3 months; Fanconi's syndrome, between birth and age 10. In the absence of a consistent familial or genetic history of aplastic anemia, researchers suspect that these congenital abnormalities are caused by an induced change during fetal development.

DIAGNOSIS AND TREATMENT

Bone marrow biopsies performed at several sites may yield a dry tap or show severely hypocellular or aplastic marrow, with varying amounts of fat, fibrous tissue, or gelatinous replacement; absence of tagged iron (because the iron is deposited in the liver rather than in bone marrow) and megakaryocytes; and depression of erythroid elements.

Differential diagnosis must rule out paroxysmal nocturnal hemoglobinuria and other diseases in which pancytopenia is common.

Effective treatment consists of supportive measures, such as transfusions of packed RBCs, platelets, and experimental histocompatibility antigen (HLA)-matched leukocytes. Even after elimination of the cause, recovery can take months. Bone marrow transplantation is the treatment of choice for anemia due to severe aplasia and for patients who need constant RBC transfusions.

The patient with low leukocyte counts is at risk for infection. Prevention of infection may range from frequent hand washing to filtered airflow or a protective environment. The infection itself may require specific antibiotics; however, these aren't given prophylactically because they tend to encourage resistant strains of organisms. Patients with low hemoglobin counts may need respiratory support with oxygen in addition to blood transfusions.

Other appropriate forms of treatment include corticosteroids to stimulate erythroid production (successful in children, unsuccessful in adults), marrow-stimulating agents such as androgens (which are controversial), antilymphocyte globulin (experimental), and immunosuppressant agents (if the patient doesn't respond to other therapy).

A new group of agents called colony-stimulating factors encourage the growth of specific cellular components and show some promise in trials with patients who've received chemotherapy or radiation therapy. These agents include granulocyte colony-stimulating factor, granulocyte-macrophage colony-stimulating factor, and erythropoietic stimulating factor.

COLLABORATIVE MANAGEMENT

Care of the patient with aplastic anemia focuses on protecting the patient from bleeding, fatigue, and infection.

ASSESSMENT

The patient's history may not help establish disease onset because many symptoms develop insidiously. The patient may report signs and symptoms of anemia (progressive weakness and fatigue, shortness of breath, and headache) or signs of thrombocytopenia (easy bruising and bleeding, especially from the mucous membranes).

Inspection may reveal pallor, if the patient is anemic, and ecchymosis, petechiae, or retinal bleeding if thrombocytopenia is present. You may notice alterations in level of consciousness if bleeding into the central nervous system has occurred.

Auscultation may reveal bibasilar crackles, tachycardia, and a gallop murmur if severe anemia results in heart failure.

The patient may also have signs and symptoms of an opportunistic infection (most commonly, a bacterial infection). Fever, oral and rectal ulcers, and sore throat may indicate the presence of an infection without characteristic inflammation.

NURSING DIAGNOSES AND COLLABORATIVE PROBLEMS

Based on the following nursing diagnoses, you'll establish patient outcomes.

Altered protection related to decreased platelet count. The patient will:
- exhibit no signs of bleeding, such as hematuria, melena, or petechiae
- recover a normal platelet count that remains normal
- state precautions to prevent or minimize bleeding.

Fatigue related to decreased oxygenation resulting from decreased RBCs. The patient will:
- recover a normal RBC count
- perform activities of daily living without limitations
- state precautions to prevent or minimize fatigue.

Risk for infection related to decreased white blood cell (WBC) count. The patient will:
- exhibit no signs or symptoms of infection, such as fever, chills, malaise, dysuria, or cough
- recover a normal WBC count and remain normal
- state precautions to prevent or minimize infection.

PLANNING AND IMPLEMENTATION

These measures help the patient with aplastic anemia.
- Focus your efforts on helping to prevent or manage hemorrhage, infection, adverse effects of drug therapy, and blood transfusion reaction.
- If the platelet count is less than 20,000/µl, prevent hemorrhage by avoiding I.M. injections, suggesting the use of an electric razor and a soft toothbrush, humidifying oxygen to prevent drying of mucous mem-

branes (dry mucosa may bleed), and promoting regular bowel movements through the use of a stool softener and a diet to prevent constipation (which can cause rectal mucosal bleeding). Also, apply pressure to venipuncture sites until bleeding stops.

■ Check the patient's complete blood count with differential regularly. Report sudden or significant changes to the doctor.

■ Detect bleeding promptly by checking for blood in the patient's urine and stool and assessing the skin for petechiae.

■ If blood transfusions are necessary, assess for a transfusion reaction by checking the patient's temperature and watching for the development of other signs and symptoms, such as rash, urticaria, pruritus, back pain, restlessness, and shaking chills.

■ Help prevent infection by washing your hands thoroughly before entering the patient's room, by making sure the patient is receiving a nutritious diet (high in vitamins and proteins) to improve his resistance, and by encouraging meticulous mouth and perianal care.

■ Watch for signs and symptoms of infection, such as fever, chills, malaise, oral or rectal ulcerations, dysuria, or results of throat, urine, nasal, stool, and blood cultures, confirming that they are done correctly to detect infection.

■ If the patient has a low hemoglobin level, which causes fatigue, schedule frequent rest periods. Give oxygen therapy as needed.

■ Ensure a comfortable environmental temperature for a patient experiencing chills.

■ Regularly evaluate the patient's degree of fatigue and activity intolerance.

Patient teaching

■ Teach the patient to avoid contact with potential sources of infection, such as fresh fruit, crowds, soil, fresh flowers, and standing water, which can harbor organisms.

■ Reassure and support the patient and his family members or friend by explaining the disease and its treatment, particularly if the patient has recurring acute episodes.

■ Explain the purpose of all prescribed drugs, and discuss possible adverse reactions, including which ones he should report promptly.

■ Tell the patient who doesn't require hospitalization that he can continue his normal lifestyle, with appropriate restrictions (such as regular rest periods) until remission happens.

■ Support efforts to educate the public about the hazards of toxic agents. Tell parents to keep toxic agents out of their children's reach. Encourage people who work with radiation to wear protective clothing and a radiation-detecting badge and to observe plant safety precautions. Those who work with benzene (solvent) should know that 10 parts per million is the highest safe environmental level and that a delayed reaction to benzene may develop.

■ Refer your patient to the Aplastic Anemia Foundation of America for additional information and assistance.

EVALUATION

Achievement of patient outcomes determines the success of collaborative management. For aplastic anemia, evaluation focuses on diminished fatigue, increased efforts at protection, and decreased incidence of infection.

Disseminated intravascular coagulation

Also known as consumption coagulopathy and defibrination syndrome, disseminated intravascular coagulation (DIC) complicates conditions that accelerate clotting, causing small-blood-vessel occlusion, organ necrosis, depletion of circulating clotting factors, and activation of the fibrinolytic system. The effect is to provoke severe hemorrhage.

Clotting in the microcirculation usually affects the kidneys and extremities, but may strike the brain, lungs, pituitary and adrenal glands, and GI mucosa. Other conditions, such as vitamin K deficiency, hepatic disease, and anticoagulant therapy, may cause a similar hemorrhage.

Although usually acute, DIC may be chronic in cancer patients. The prognosis depends on how early the patient receives treatment, the severity of the hemorrhage, and treatment of the underlying condition.

DIC sometimes is complicated by renal failure, hepatic damage, cerebrovascular accident, ischemic bowel, or respiratory distress. Hypoxia and anoxia can strike and lead to severe striated muscle pain. The patient also may suffer shock and coma. After fibrinolysis, severe to fatal hemorrhaging of vital organs can happen without warning.

CAUSES

DIC may be caused by:

■ infection—gram-negative or gram-positive septicemia; viral, fungal, rickettsial, or protozoal infection

■ obstetric complications—abruptio placentae, amniotic fluid embolism, retained dead fetus, eclampsia, septic abortion, postpartum hemorrhage

■ neoplastic disease—acute leukemia, metastatic carcinoma, lymphomas

- disorders that produce necrosis—extensive burns and trauma, brain tissue destruction, transplant rejection, hepatic necrosis, anorexia nervosa
- other disorders and conditions—heatstroke, shock, poisonous snakebite, cirrhosis, fat embolism, incompatible blood transfusion, drug reactions, cardiac arrest, surgery requiring cardiopulmonary bypass, giant hemangioma, severe venous thrombosis, purpura fulminans, adrenal disease, adult respiratory distress syndrome, diabetic ketoacidosis, pulmonary embolism, and sickle cell anemia.

Why such conditions and disorders lead to DIC is unclear. Regardless of how DIC begins, the typical accelerated clotting causes generalized activation of prothrombin and a consequent excess of thrombin. Excess thrombin converts fibrinogen to fibrin, producing fibrin clots in the microcirculation. This process consumes exorbitant amounts of coagulation factors (especially platelets, factor V, prothrombin, fibrinogen, and factor VIII), causing thrombocytopenia, deficiencies in factors V and VIII, hypoprothrombinemia, and hypofibrinogenemia.

Circulating thrombin activates the fibrinolytic system, which lyses fibrin clots into fibrinogen degradation products (FDPs). The resulting hemorrhage may be due largely to the anticoagulant activity of FDPs as well as to depletion of plasma coagulation factors.

DIAGNOSIS AND TREATMENT

Abnormal bleeding in the absence of a known hematologic disorder suggests DIC. The following initial laboratory findings reflect coagulation deficiencies:

- decreased platelet count—less than 100,000/μl
- reduced fibrinogen levels—less than 150 mg/dl
- prolonged prothrombin time—more than 15 seconds
- prolonged partial thromboplastin time—more than 60 to 80 seconds
- increased FDPs—commonly greater than 45 mcg/ml, or positive at less than 1:100 dilution
- positive D-dimer test (specific fibrinogen test for DIC)—positive at less than 1:8 dilution.

Other supportive data include prolonged thrombin time, positive fibrin monomers, diminished levels of factors V and VIII, fragmentation of red blood cells (RBCs), and decreased hemoglobin levels (less than 10 g/dl). Final confirmation of the diagnosis is generally difficult because many of these test results also appear in other disorders (primary fibrinolysis, for example). However, the FDP and D-dimer tests are considered specific and diagnostic of DIC.

Treatment of DIC requires prompt recognition and adequate treatment of the underlying disorder. Treatment is supportive (when the underlying disorder is self-limiting, for example) or highly specific. If the patient isn't actively bleeding, supportive care alone may reverse DIC. Active bleeding may require transfusion of blood, fresh-frozen plasma, platelets, or packed RBCs to support hemostasis.

Heparin therapy is controversial. It may be used early in the disease but is generally considered a last resort in patients who are actively bleeding. If the patient has a thrombosis, heparin therapy is usually mandatory. In most cases, it's given in combination with transfusion therapy.

COLLABORATIVE MANAGEMENT

Care of the patient with DIC focuses on preventing injury, improving tissue perfusion, reducing fatigue, and providing patient teaching.

ASSESSMENT

The most significant clinical feature of DIC is abnormal bleeding without a history of a hemorrhagic disorder. Signs and symptoms are related to bleeding and thrombosis. Bleeding problems are usually more common than thrombotic problems, unless coagulation occurs to a greater extent than fibrinolysis. Look for:

- a history of one of the disorders that causes DIC
- reports of bleeding into the skin, such as cutaneous oozing, petechiae, ecchymoses, and hematomas
- if under treatment for another disorder, bleeding from surgical or invasive procedure sites, such as incisions or venipuncture sites.
- reports of nausea and vomiting
- severe muscle, back, and abdominal pain; chest pain
- hemoptysis, epistaxis, seizures, and oliguria
- petechiae and other signs of bleeding into the skin, acrocyanosis, and dyspnea
- reduced peripheral pulses
- decreased blood pressure
- mental status changes, including confusion.

NURSING DIAGNOSES AND COLLABORATIVE PROBLEMS

Based on the following nursing diagnoses, you'll establish patient outcomes.

Altered peripheral tissue perfusion related to small vessel occlusion. The patient will:

- maintain peripheral pulses
- show no changes in skin color and temperature in the extremities
- maintain tissue perfusion and cellular oxygenation in extremities.

Risk for fluid volume deficit related to blood loss. The patient will:

- show no signs of fluid volume deficit

- maintain adequate fluid volume, as evidenced by equal intake and output volumes and stable vital signs.

   Fatigue related to decreased hemoglobin. The patient will:
- rest frequently to combat fatigue
- seek help when performing activities of daily living to conserve energy
- recover his normal energy level when DIC resolves.

PLANNING AND IMPLEMENTATION
These measures help the patient with DIC.
- Reposition the patient every 2 hours, and provide meticulous skin care to prevent skin breakdown.
- Give oxygen therapy as ordered.
- To prevent clots from dislodging and causing fresh bleeding, don't vigorously rub these areas when washing. Use a 1:1 solution of hydrogen peroxide and water to help remove crusted blood.
- If the patient bleeds, use pressure, cold compresses, and topical hemostatic agents to control it; effective agents may include an absorbable gelatin sponge, a microfibrillar collagen hemostat, or thrombin.
- After giving an injection or removing an I.V. catheter or needle, apply pressure to the injection site for at least 10 minutes. Alert other staff members to the patient's tendency to hemorrhage. Limit venipunctures whenever possible.
- Protect the patient from injury. Enforce complete bed rest during bleeding episodes. If the patient is agitated, pad the bed rails.
- Perform bladder irrigations as ordered for genitourinary (GU) bleeding.
- Monitor intake and output hourly in acute DIC, especially when giving blood products. Watch for transfusion reactions and signs of fluid overload.
- To measure the amount of blood lost, weigh dressings and linen and record drainage.
- Weigh the patient daily, particularly if he has renal involvement.
- Watch for bleeding from the GI and GU tracts. If you suspect intra-abdominal bleeding, measure the patient's abdominal girth at least every 4 hours, and observe closely for signs of shock.
- Monitor the results of serial blood studies (particularly hematocrit, hemoglobin levels, and coagulation times).
- Test all stools and urine for occult blood.
- Check all venipuncture sites frequently for bleeding.
- If the patient can't tolerate activity because of blood loss, provide frequent rest periods.
- Inform family members or friends of the patient's progress. Prepare them for his appearance (I.V. lines, nasogastric tubes, bruises, dried blood).

- Provide emotional support and encouragement, and listen to their concerns. As needed, enlist the aid of a social worker, chaplain, and other members of the health care team to provide support.

Patient teaching
- Explain the disorder to the patient and family members.
- Teach them the importance of early recognition of signs of abnormal bleeding.
- Stress getting prompt treatment of the underlying disorders.
- Teach the patient how to prevent further bleeding.

EVALUATION
Achievement of patient outcomes determines the success of collaborative management. For DIC, evaluation focuses on relief of fatigue, increased tissue perfusion, and control of fluid volume deficit.

Folic acid deficiency anemia

A common, slowly progressive megaloblastic anemia, folic acid deficiency anemia is most prevalent in infants, adolescents, pregnant and breast-feeding women, alcoholics, older people, and patients with malignant or intestinal diseases.

CAUSES
Alcohol abuse, which suppresses the metabolic effects of folate, is probably the most common cause of folic acid deficiency anemia. Additional causes include:
- poor diet (common in alcoholics, narcotic addicts, and older people who live alone)
- impaired absorption (due to intestinal dysfunction from such disorders as celiac disease, tropical sprue, regional jejunitis, and bowel resection)
- bacteria competing for available folic acid
- excessive cooking of foods, which destroys the available nutrients
- prolonged drug therapy with such drugs as anticonvulsants, estrogens, and methotrexate
- increased folic acid requirements during pregnancy and in patients with neoplastic diseases and some skin diseases such as exfoliative dermatitis.

DIAGNOSIS AND TREATMENT
The Schilling test and a therapeutic trial of vitamin B_{12} injections distinguish between folic acid deficiency anemia and pernicious anemia. Significant findings on blood studies include macrocytosis, decreased reticulocyte count, increased mean corpuscular vol-

Choosing foods for folic acid content

Folic acid (pteroylglutamic acid, folacin) is found in most body tissues, where it acts as a coenzyme in metabolic processes involving 1-carbon transfer. It's essential for formation and maturation of red blood cells and for synthesis of deoxyribonucleic acid. Although its body stores are comparatively small (about 70 mg), this vitamin is plentiful in most well-balanced diets.

However, because folic acid is water-soluble and heat-labile, it's easily destroyed by cooking. Also, about 20% of folic acid intake is excreted unabsorbed. Insufficient daily folic acid intake (less than 50 mcg/day) usually induces folic acid deficiency within 4 months. Treatment may include teaching your patient to eat more foods that are high in folic acid content, such as those in the chart.

Food	mcg/100 g
Asparagus spears	109
Beef liver	294
Broccoli	54
Collards (cooked)	102
Mushrooms	24
Oatmeal	33
Peanut butter	57
Red beans	180
Wheat germ	305

ume, abnormal platelet count, and serum folate levels below 4 mg/ml.

Medical treatment consists primarily of folic acid supplements and elimination of contributing causes. The patient may take supplements orally (1 to 5 mg/day) or parenterally (for patients who are severely ill, have malabsorption, or can't take oral medication). Many patients respond favorably to a well-balanced diet that includes foods high in folic acid. (See *Choosing foods for folic acid content.*)

COLLABORATIVE MANAGEMENT
Care of the patient with folic acid deficiency focuses on improving energy levels and teaching the patient about a folic acid–rich diet.

ASSESSMENT
The patient's history may reveal severe, progressive fatigue, the hallmark of folic acid deficiency. Associated findings include shortness of breath, palpitations, diarrhea, nausea, anorexia, headaches, forgetfulness, and irritability. The impaired oxygen-carrying capacity of the blood from lowered hemoglobin levels may produce complaints of weakness and light-headedness.

Inspection may reveal generalized pallor and jaundice. The patient may appear wasted. He may have cheilosis and glossitis. Folic acid deficiency anemia doesn't cause neurologic impairment unless it's associated with vitamin B_{12} deficiency.

NURSING DIAGNOSES AND COLLABORATIVE PROBLEMS
Based on the following nursing diagnoses, you'll establish patient outcomes.

Altered nutrition: Less than body requirements related to adverse GI effects. The patient will:
- identify foods high in folic acid
- consume a diet high in folic acid
- no longer show signs and symptoms of folic acid deficiency.

Fatigue related to folic acid deficiency. The patient will:
- express an understanding of the relationship between fatigue and folic acid deficiency
- employ measures to prevent or lessen fatigue
- regain his normal energy level as folic acid deficiency resolves.

Impaired physical mobility related to weakness caused by reduced hemoglobin levels. The patient will:
- maintain functional mobility
- develop no complications due to impaired physical mobility
- regain normal physical mobility as hemoglobin levels return to normal and folic acid deficiency resolves.

PLANNING AND IMPLEMENTATION
These measures help the patient with folic acid deficiency anemia.
- If the patient has severe anemia, plan activities, rest periods, and diagnostic tests to conserve his energy.
- Monitor the patient's complete blood count, platelet count, and serum folate level as ordered.
- Monitor his pulse rate often. If he has tachycardia, his activities are too strenuous.
- Monitor fluid and electrolyte balance, particularly in the patient who has severe diarrhea and is receiving parenteral fluid replacement therapy.

- Advise the patient to report signs and symptoms of decreased perfusion to vital organs: dyspnea, chest pain, dizziness.
- If the patient has glossitis, emphasize the importance of good oral hygiene. Suggest the regular use of a mild or diluted mouthwash and a soft toothbrush. Oral anesthetics may be used to allay discomfort.
- Because a sore mouth and tongue make eating painful, ask the dietitian to avoid giving the patient irritating foods. If these symptoms make talking difficult, supply a pad and pencil or some other aid to facilitate nonverbal communication.
- Explain this problem to family members.
- Provide a well-balanced diet, including foods high in folate, such as dark green leafy vegetables, organ meats, eggs, milk, oranges, bananas, dry beans, and whole grain breads. Offer between-meal snacks, and encourage the family to bring favorite foods from home.
- Help the patient maintain body alignment and mobility; begin with gentle range-of-motion exercises, as tolerated, and progress to out of bed activity.

Patient teaching

- To prevent folic acid deficiency anemia, emphasize the importance of a well-balanced diet high in folic acid. Identify alcoholics or other high-risk persons with poor dietary habits, and try to arrange for appropriate counseling.
- Teach the patient to meet daily folic acid requirements by including something from each food group at every meal.
- If the patient has a severe deficiency, explain that diet only reinforces folic acid supplementation and isn't therapeutic by itself. Urge the prescribed course of therapy. Advise the patient to continue the supplements when he begins to feel better.
- Warn the patient to guard against infections, and tell him to report signs of infection promptly, especially pulmonary and urinary tract infections, because his weakened condition may increase susceptibility.

EVALUATION

Achievement of patient outcomes determines the success of collaborative management. For folic acid deficiency, evaluation focuses on maintenance of nutritional requirements, decreased fatigue, and increased mobility.

Glucose-6-phosphate dehydrogenase deficiency

Glucose-6-phosphate dehydrogenase (G6PD) deficiency is a congenital hemolytic anemia caused by defects or deficiencies of one or more enzymes in the red blood cells (RBCs). The enzymes are needed to complete a critical step in intracellular energy production.

CAUSES

Generally the cause is genetic. This disease is inherited as an X-linked recessive disorder affecting about 15% of black males. It's also transmissible through blood donations.

People who lack G6PD are more susceptible to hemolysis during exposure to specific drugs (phenacetin, sulfonamides, aspirin, quinine derivatives, thiazide diuretics, vitamin K derivatives, and toxins) and to certain foods such as fava beans. As cells age within the body, normally concentrated G6PD begins to decline in amount. Then, when the individual is exposed to the above mentioned agents, he experiences acute intravascular hemolysis lasting 7 to 12 days. During that period, the patient has anemia and jaundice. The hemolytic reaction is short lived because only the older erythrocytes, which contain less G6PD, are destroyed.

DIAGNOSIS AND TREATMENT

Laboratory findings reveal moderate hemoglobinemia and hemoglobinuria. Serum bilirubin is elevated. Also present are reticulocytosis and the appearance of Heinz bodies within the RBCs.

Treatment involves identifying and removing the drug or food responsible for the hemolytic reaction and correcting the anemia. The patient receives palliative treatment during and after an episode of hemolysis with adequate hydration and osmotic diuretics to prevent acute tubular necrosis.

COLLABORATIVE MANAGEMENT

Care of the patient with G6PD deficiency focuses on avoiding injury and infection.

ASSESSMENT

The patient experiencing a hemolytic reaction will have decreased hemoglobin levels and hematocrit and signs resembling those of hemolytic anemia. (See "Hemolytic anemia," page 592.)

NURSING DIAGNOSES AND COLLABORATIVE PROBLEMS

Based on the following nursing diagnoses, you'll establish patient outcomes.

Risk for infection related to altered hemolytic status. The patient will:
- have a temperature that remains within his normal limits
- have cultures that are negative.

Risk for injury related to decreased hemoglobin levels. The patient will:
- incur no injury.

PLANNING AND IMPLEMENTATION

These measures help the patient with G6PD deficiency.

- Encourage adequate nutrition.
- Teach judicious hand washing to avoid infection.
- Culture suspicious wounds.
- Protect the patient from harm.
- Assist the patient with self-care measures.
- During and after RBC transfusions watch for signs of G6PD reaction.

Patient teaching

- Stress the importance of good nutrition, meticulous wound care, periodic dental checkups, and other measures to prevent infection.
- Discuss with the patient and family members the various options for healthy physical and creative outlets.
- Because parents of patients with G6PD deficiency may have questions about the vulnerability of future offspring, refer them for genetic counseling about the risk of transmitting G6PD deficiency.
- Refer adults with G6PD deficiency to genetic counseling; tell them that if they choose to have children, they must have all their children evaluated for the deficiency.
- Teach your patient about the medications and circumstances to avoid to prevent hemolytic reaction.

EVALUATION

Achievement of patient outcomes determines the success of collaborative management. For G6PD anemia, evaluation focuses on the absence of infection and protection from injury.

Hemolytic anemia

Also known as thalassemia after its most common type, the term *hemolytic anemia* covers a group of disorders characterized by defective synthesis in the polypeptide chains involved in hemoglobin (Hb) production.

Thalassemia, the most common type, occurs in three forms: major, intermedia, and minor. Prognosis for each form varies. Patients with thalassemia major seldom survive to adulthood. Children with thalassemia intermedia develop normally into adulthood, although puberty is usually delayed; persons with thalassemia minor can expect a normal life span.

CAUSES

Thalassemia is caused by defective beta polypeptide chain synthesis. Specifically, thalassemia major and intermedia are caused by homozygous inheritance of the partially dominant autosomal gene responsible for this trait. Thalassemia minor results from heterozygous inheritance of the same gene. Ethnic origin is the major factor. Persons of Mediterranean ancestry, especially Italians and Greeks, are at highest risk. Other groups at risk include Blacks, Chinese from southern China, Southeast Asians, and people from India.

DIAGNOSIS AND TREATMENT

The following tests support a diagnosis of thalassemia major:

- RBC count and hemoglobin levels are decreased; reticulocytes, bilirubin, and urinary and fecal urobilinogen levels are elevated; and serum folate level is low, indicating increased folate utilization by the hypertrophied bone marrow.
- Peripheral blood smear reveals target cells (extremely thin and fragile red blood cells [RBCs]), pale nucleated RBCs, and marked anisocytosis.
- Skull and skeletal X-rays show a thinning and widening of the marrow space in the skull and long bones, possible granular appearance in the bones of the skull and vertebrae, possible areas of osteoporosis in the long bones, and deformities (rectangular or biconvex) of the phalanges.
- Hemoglobin electrophoresis demonstrates a significant rise in HbF and slight increase in Hb_{A2}.

In thalassemia intermedia, RBCs are hypochromic and microcytic. In thalassemia minor, RBCs are slightly hypochromic and microcytic. Hemoglobin electrophoresis shows a significant increase in Hb_{A2} and a moderate rise in HbF.

Treatment of thalassemia major is essentially supportive. For example, infections require prompt treatment with appropriate antibiotics. Folic acid supplements help maintain folic acid levels in the face of increased requirements. Transfusions of packed RBCs raise hemoglobin levels, but must be used judiciously to minimize iron overload. Splenectomy and bone marrow transplantation have been tried, but their effectiveness hasn't been confirmed.

Thalassemia intermedia and thalassemia minor usually don't require treatment.

COLLABORATIVE MANAGEMENT

Care of the patient with hemolytic anemia focuses on avoiding injury and infection.

ASSESSMENT

The severity of the resulting anemia depends on whether the patient is homozygous or heterozygous for the thalassemic trait.

Thalassemia major's first signs are pallor and yellow skin and sclerae in infants ages 3 to 6 months. Later signs and symptoms include severe anemia; splenomegaly or hepatomegaly with abdominal enlargement; frequent infections; bleeding tendencies (epistaxis); anorexia; altered appearance with small body, large head, and possible Mongoloid features; and possible mental retardation. Thalassemia intermedia appears as anemia, jaundice, splenomegaly, and possible signs of hemosiderosis. Mild anemia is the key indication of thalassemia minor.

NURSING DIAGNOSES AND COLLABORATIVE PROBLEMS

Based on the following nursing diagnoses, you'll establish patient outcomes.

Risk for infection related to altered hemolytic and lymphatic system. The patient will:
- have temperature within normal limits
- have cultures that are negative.

Risk for injury related to decreased hemoglobin levels. The patient will:
- incur no injury.

PLANNING AND IMPLEMENTATION

These measures help the patient with hemolytic anemia.
- Administer antibiotics as ordered. Observe the patient for signs of adverse reactions to them.
- Provide an adequate diet, and encourage increased consumption of liquids.
- During and after RBC transfusions for thalassemia major, watch for adverse reactions—chills, fever, rash, itching, and hives.
- Provide emotional support to help the patient and his family cope with the chronic nature of the illness and the need for lifelong transfusions.

Patient teaching

Remember to tell the patient with thalassemia minor that his condition is benign. Stress the importance of good nutrition, meticulous wound care, periodic dental checkups, and other measures to prevent infection.

Discuss with the parents of a young patient various options for healthy physical and creative outlets. The patient may have to restrict activities because of increased oxygen demand and the tendency toward pathologic fractures, but he may participate in less stressful activities.

Teach parents to watch for signs of hepatitis and iron overload—always a risk with frequent transfusions. Because parents may have questions about the vulnerability of future offspring, refer them for genetic counseling. Also refer adult patients with thalassemia minor and thalassemia intermedia for genetic counseling; they need to recognize the risk of transmitting thalassemia major to their children if they marry another person with thalassemia. If such per-

sons plan to have children, they should have their offspring evaluated for thalassemia by age 1.

EVALUATION

Achievement of patient outcomes determines the success of collaborative management. For hemolytic anemia, evaluation focuses on protection from injury and the absence of infection.

Hemophilia

A hereditary bleeding disorder, hemophilia strikes in about 1.25 per 10,000 live male births. The severity and prognosis of bleeding disorders vary with the degree of clotting deficiency and the site of bleeding. The overall prognosis is best in mild hemophilia, which doesn't cause spontaneous bleeding and joint deformities. Advances in treatment have greatly improved the prognosis, and many hemophiliacs have normal life spans.

Complications include bleeding into joints and muscles, which causes pain, swelling, extreme tenderness and, possibly, permanent deformity. Bleeding near peripheral nerves may cause peripheral neuropathies, pain, paresthesia, and muscle atrophy. If bleeding impairs blood flow through a major vessel, it can cause ischemia and gangrene. Pharyngeal, lingual, intracardial, intracerebral, and intracranial bleeding may all lead to shock and death.

CAUSES

Hemophilia, the most common X-linked genetic disease, is caused by a deficiency of specific clotting factors. Hemophilia A (classic hemophilia), which affects more than 80% of all hemophiliacs, is caused by a deficiency of factor VIII; hemophilia B (Christmas disease), which affects 15% of hemophiliacs, is linked to a deficiency of factor IX. However, other evidence suggests that hemophilia actually may be caused by nonfunctioning factors VIII and IX, rather than from their deficiency.

Hemophilia A and B are inherited as X-linked recessive traits. Hemophiliac fathers have a 50% chance of transmitting the gene to each daughter, who then has a 50% chance of transmitting the gene to each son—who would be born with hemophilia.

The hemophilia patient's abnormal bleeding is mild, moderate, or severe, depending on the degree of factor deficiency. After a person with hemophilia forms a platelet plug at a bleeding site, the lack of clotting factors impairs formation of a stable fibrin clot. Immediate hemorrhage isn't prevalent, but delayed bleeding is common.

DIAGNOSIS AND TREATMENT

Specific coagulation factor assays can diagnose the type and severity of hemophilia. A positive family history can also help diagnose hemophilia.

Characteristic findings in hemophilia A are:
- factor VIII assay 0% to 25% of normal prolonged activated partial thromboplastin time (APTT)
- normal platelet count and function, bleeding time, and prothrombin time.

Characteristic findings in hemophilia B are:
- deficient factor IX assay
- baseline coagulation results similar to those of hemophilia A, with normal factor VIII.

Additional tests may help locate the bleeding site and evaluate damage:
- a computed tomography scan for suspected intracranial bleeding
- arthroscopy or arthrography for certain joint problems
- endoscopy for GI bleeding.

Hemophilia is incurable, but treatment can prevent crippling deformities and prolong life. Correct treatment quickly stops bleeding by increasing plasma levels of deficient clotting factors to help prevent disabling deformities that result from repeated bleeding into muscles, joints, and organs.

In hemophilia A, cryoprecipitated antihemophilic factor (AHF), lyophilized AHF, or both, given in doses large enough to raise clotting factor levels above 25% of normal, can restore normal hemostasis. Before surgery, AHF is given to raise clotting factors to hemostatic levels. Levels are then kept within a normal range until the wound has healed. Fresh frozen plasma can help, but it does have some drawbacks.

Inhibitors to factor VIII develop after multiple transfusions in 10% to 20% of patients with severe hemophilia. This renders the patient resistant to factor VIII infusions. Desmopressin can stimulate the release of stored factor VIII, raising the level in the blood.

In hemophilia B, administration of factor IX concentrate during bleeding episodes increases factor IX levels.

A patient with hemophilia who undergoes surgery needs careful management by a hematologist with expertise in hemophilia care. The patient will require deficient factor replacement before and after surgery. Such replacement may be necessary even for minor surgery such as a dental extraction. In addition, aminocaproic acid is frequently used for oral bleeding to inhibit the active fibrinolytic system present in the oral mucosa.

COLLABORATIVE MANAGEMENT

Care of the patient with hemophilia focuses on preventing injury, maintaining hydration, and providing thorough patient teaching.

ASSESSMENT

Varying assessment findings depend on the type of hemophilia and any complication. A patient with undiagnosed hemophilia typically presents with pain and swelling in a weight-bearing joint, such as the hip, knee, or ankle.

Mild hemophilia commonly goes undiagnosed until adulthood because the patient with a mild deficiency doesn't bleed spontaneously or after minor trauma but has prolonged bleeding if challenged by major trauma or surgery. Postoperative bleeding continues as a slow ooze or ceases and starts again up to 8 days after surgery.

Moderate hemophilia causes symptoms similar to those of severe hemophilia but produces only occasional spontaneous bleeding episodes. Severe hemophilia causes spontaneous bleeding. Commonly, the first sign of severe hemophilia is excessive bleeding after circumcision. Later, spontaneous bleeding or severe bleeding after minor trauma may produce large subcutaneous and deep I.M. hematomas. Look for:
- a history of prolonged bleeding after surgery (including dental extractions)
- trauma or joint pain if the patient has had episodes of spontaneous bleeding into muscles or joints
- reports of signs or symptoms of internal bleeding, such as abdominal, chest, or flank pain; episodes of hematuria or hematemesis; and tarry stools
- complaints of activity or movement limitations in the past
- reported use or assistive devices, such as splints, canes, or crutches
- apparent hematomas on the extremities or torso or both and, if bleeding has occurred in joints, joint swelling
- limited joint range of motion (ROM) and complaints of pain during the assessment (if he has bled into his joints).

NURSING DIAGNOSES AND COLLABORATIVE PROBLEMS

Based on the following nursing diagnoses, you'll establish patient outcomes.

Activity intolerance related to bleeding episodes. The patient will:
- demonstrate safety precautions while performing activities of daily living
- avoid activity or seek assistance in performing activities that may cause a bleeding episode
- avoid injury when performing activities.

Altered peripheral tissue perfusion related to impaired blood flow through a major vessel caused by bleeding. The patient will:

■ implement measures to stop bleeding or seek medical attention at the first sign of bleeding
■ maintain adequate tissue perfusion when he's bleeding, as shown by a palpable pulse and normal skin color and temperature at and beyond the bleeding site.

Risk for fluid volume deficit related to bleeding. The patient will:

■ quickly regain or maintain a normal fluid balance during a bleeding episode
■ avoid signs and symptoms of fluid volume deficit during or after a bleeding episode.

PLANNING AND IMPLEMENTATION

These measures help the patient with hemophilia.

■ Provide emotional support and listen to the patient's fears and concerns. Reassure him when possible.
■ Remember that people who may have been exposed to the human immunodeficiency virus (HIV) through contaminated blood products need special support and infection control.
■ If the newly diagnosed patient has difficulty adjusting to his diagnosis, reassure him that his feelings are normal. Point out areas of his life where he can maintain control. Arrange for other people with the same problem to speak with the patient and family members or friend.
■ Give the patient private time with his family and friends to help overcome feelings of social isolation.
■ If the patient can't tolerate activities because of blood loss, provide rest periods between activities.

During bleeding episodes:
■ If the patient has surface cuts or epistaxis, apply pressure—in many cases the only treatment needed. With deeper cuts, pressure may stop the bleeding temporarily. Cuts that require suturing may also require factor infusions to prevent further bleeding.
■ Give the deficient clotting factor or plasma, as ordered. (See *Using factor replacement products.*) The body uses up AHF in 48 to 72 hours, so repeat infusions, as ordered, until the bleeding stops.
■ Assess the patient for adverse reactions to blood products, such as flushing, headache, tingling, fever, chills, urticaria, and anaphylaxis.
■ Apply cold compresses or ice bags and raise the injured part.
■ To prevent recurrence of bleeding, restrict activity for 48 hours after bleeding is under control.

If the patient has bled into a joint:
■ To restore joint mobility, if ordered, begin ROM exercises at least 48 hours after the bleeding is con-

trolled. Tell the patient to avoid weight bearing until bleeding stops and swelling subsides.
■ Give analgesics for the pain associated with hemarthrosis. Also, apply ice packs and elastic bandages to alleviate the pain.
■ Control pain with an analgesic, such as acetaminophen, propoxyphene, codeine, or meperidine, as ordered. Avoid I.M. injections because they may cause hematoma formation at the injection site. Aspirin and aspirin-containing medications are contraindicated because they decrease platelet adherence and may increase the bleeding.
■ Watch for signs and symptoms of decreased tissue perfusion, such as restlessness, anxiety, confusion, pallor, cool and clammy skin, chest pain, decreased

---

Using factor replacement products

Each of these products replaces a specific clotting factor.

Cryoprecipitate
■ Factor VIII (70 to 100 units/bag); does not contain factor IX
■ Can be stored frozen for up to 12 months, but must be used within 6 hours after it thaws
■ Given through a blood filter; compatible only with normal saline solution

Lyophilized factor VIII or factor IX
■ Derived from monoclonal antibodies
■ May be freeze-dried and labeled with exact units of factor VIII or factor IX contained in the vial (vials range from 200 to 1,500 units of factor VIII or factor IX each and contain 20 to 40 ml after reconstitution with diluent); can be stored for 2 years at temperatures ranging from 36° to 46° F (2° to 8° C), or for 6 months at room temperature not exceeding 88° F (31° C)
■ Doesn't need a blood filter; usually given by slow I.V. push through a butterfly infusion set

Fresh-frozen plasma
■ Factor VIII (about 0.75 unit/ml) and factor IX (about 1 unit/ml); impractical for most hemophiliacs because a large volume is needed to raise factors to hemostatic levels; a poor source of factor VIII because freezing the plasma destroys the factor (in contrast, fresh plasma [not frozen] is a good source of factor VIII)
■ Can be stored frozen for up to 12 months, but must be used within 2 hours after it thaws
■ Given through a blood filter; compatible only with normal saline solution

urine output, hypotension, and tachycardia. Monitor the patient's blood pressure and pulse and respiratory rates. Observe him frequently for bleeding from the skin, mucous membranes, and wounds.

After a bleeding episode or surgery:
■ Watch closely for signs and symptoms of further bleeding, such as increased pain and swelling, fever, and evidence of shock.
■ Closely monitor the patient's laboratory values, particularly his APTT.

Patient teaching
■ Teach the patient the benefits of regular exercise. Explain that strong muscles protect the joints and that this, in turn, reduces the incidence of hemarthrosis. Instruct him to perform isometric exercises, which can also help prevent muscle weakness and recurrent joint bleeding.
■ Advise parents to protect their child from injury while avoiding unnecessary restrictions that impair his normal development. For example, for a toddler, padded patches sewn into the knees and elbows of clothing protect these joints during frequent falls. Parents must prevent an older child from joining in contact sports such as football, but can encourage swimming and golf.
■ Tell the patient to avoid such activities as heavy lifting or using power tools because they increase the risk of injury that can result in serious bleeding problems.
■ If a young patient is injured, direct the parents to apply cold compresses or ice bags and elevate the injured part or to apply light pressure to the bleeding. To prevent recurrence of bleeding after treatment, instruct the parents to restrict the child's activity for 48 hours after bleeding is under control.
■ Advise the patient and family to notify the doctor immediately after even a minor injury, especially to the head, neck, or abdomen. Such injuries may require special blood factor replacement.
■ Instruct them to watch for signs and symptoms of internal bleeding, such as severe pain or swelling in a joint or muscles, stiffness, decreased joint movement, severe abdominal pain, blood in urine, tarry stools, and severe headache.
■ Explain to the patient and, if appropriate, his parents the importance of avoiding aspirin, combination medications that contain aspirin, and over-the-counter (OTC) anti-inflammatory agents such as ibuprofen compounds. Teach them how to recognize OTC medications that contain aspirin. Tell them to use acetaminophen instead.
■ Stress the importance of good dental care, including regular, careful tooth brushing, as a long-term tactic to avoid the need for dental surgery. Advise using a soft toothbrush to avoid gum injury. Emphasize dental hygiene as a way to avoid bleeding from inflamed gums.
■ Tell the patient and family to check with the doctor before dental extractions or any other surgery. Advise them to get the names of other doctors they can contact in case their regular doctor isn't available.
■ Teach the patient the importance of protecting his veins for lifelong therapy.
■ Encourage your patient to remain independent and self-sufficient. Refer him for counseling as necessary.
■ Tell parents to make sure their child wears a medical identification bracelet at all times.
■ Refer new patients to a hemophilia treatment center for evaluation. The center will develop treatment plans for hemophilia patients' primary doctors and is a resource for other medical and school personnel, dentists, or others involved in their care. Explain that these centers also offer carrier testing, prenatal diagnosis, and other genetic counseling services.

For a patient receiving blood components:
■ Train the patient and family to give blood factor components at home to avoid frequent hospitalization. Teach them proper venipuncture and infusion techniques, and urge them not to delay treatment during bleeding episodes. Tell the family to keep blood factor concentrate and infusion equipment available at all times, even on vacation.
■ Review possible adverse reactions, such as blood-borne infection and factor inhibitor development, that can result from replacement factor procedures.
■ If the patient develops flushing, headache, or tingling from replacement factors, inform him or his parents that these reactions usually appear with freeze-dried concentrate. Slowing the infusion rate may cause symptoms to abate.
■ If he has fever and chills, indicating an allergy to white blood cell antigens, instruct the patient or his parents that this reaction usually appears with plasma infusions. Acetaminophen may relieve his discomfort.
■ Tell the patient that urticaria is the most common reaction to cryoprecipitate or plasma. This hypersensitivity sign results from a protein. The wheals usually subside after administration of diphenhydramine or another antihistamine. Ideally, the patient who develops urticaria frequently should receive an antihistamine about 45 minutes before a clotting factor infusion.
■ Review the signs and symptoms of anaphylaxis: rapid or difficult breathing, wheezing, hoarseness, stridor, and chest tightness. (The same plasma proteins that cause urticaria may cause anaphylaxis.) Teach the patient and family to give epinephrine and then to contact the doctor at once.

- Tell the patient and family to watch for early signs and symptoms of hepatitis: headache, fever, nausea, vomiting, abdominal tenderness, and pain over the liver. Explain that the patient who receives blood components risks hepatitis, which may appear 3 weeks to 6 months after treatment with blood components.
- Inform the patient and family that all donated blood and plasma are screened for antibodies to human immunodeficiency virus (HIV), which causes acquired immunodeficiency syndrome. Also, all freeze-dried products are heat-treated to kill HIV.
- For more information, refer the patient and his family members to the National Hemophilia Foundation.

EVALUATION

Achievement of patient outcomes determines the success of collaborative management. For hemophilia, evaluation focuses on prevention and control of bleeding episodes, prevention of fluid volume deficits, and improved activity intolerance.

Hodgkin's disease

A neoplastic disorder, Hodgkin's disease strikes all races but is slightly more common in whites. Its incidence peaks in two age-groups: ages 15 to 38 and older than age 50. It appears most commonly in young adults—except in Japan, where it strikes exclusively among people over age 50. It has a higher incidence in men than in women. A family history of Hodgkin's disease increases the likelihood of acquiring the disorder.

Untreated, Hodgkin's disease follows a variable but relentlessly progressive and ultimately fatal course. However, recent advances in therapy make Hodgkin's disease potentially curable, even in advanced stages. Appropriate treatment yields a 5-year survival rate of about 90%. Hodgkin's disease can cause multiple organ failure.

CAUSES

Although the cause of Hodgkin's disease is unknown, some studies point to genetic, viral, or environmental factors. The disease is characterized by painless, progressive enlargement of the lymph nodes, spleen, and other lymphoid tissue. This enlargement is caused by proliferation of lymphocytes, histiocytes, eosinophils, and Reed-Sternberg cells. The latter cells are the special histologic feature of Hodgkin's disease.

DIAGNOSIS AND TREATMENT

Tests must first rule out other disorders that enlarge the lymph nodes. Lymph node biopsy confirms the presence of Reed-Sternberg cells, abnormal histiocyte proliferation, and nodular fibrosis and necrosis. Lymph node biopsy also helps determine lymph node and organ involvement, as do bone marrow, liver, mediastinal, and spleen biopsies; routine chest X-rays; magnetic resonance imaging; abdominal computed tomography; lung and bone scans; lymphangiography; and laparoscopy.

Hematologic tests show mild to severe normocytic anemia; normochromic anemia (in 50% of patients); and elevated, normal, or reduced white blood cell count and differential, showing any combination of neutrophilia, lymphocytopenia, monocytosis, and eosinophilia. Elevated serum alkaline phosphatase levels indicate liver or bone involvement.

A staging laparotomy may be necessary for some patients, such as those without obvious stage III or stage IV disease, lymphocyte predominance subtype histology, or medical contraindications. (See *Staging Hodgkin's disease,* page 598.)

Depending on the stage of the disease, the patient may receive chemotherapy, radiation therapy, or both. Correct treatment allows longer survival and may even cure many patients.

A patient with stage I or stage II disease receives radiation therapy alone; a patient with stage III disease receives radiation therapy and chemotherapy; for stage IV disease, a patient receives chemotherapy alone, sometimes inducing a complete remission. As an alternative, he may receive chemotherapy and radiation therapy to involved sites.

Chemotherapy consists of various combinations of drugs. The well-known MOPP protocol (mechlorethamine, Oncovin [vincristine], procarbazine, and prednisone) was the first to provide significant cures for generalized Hodgkin's disease. Another useful combination is ABVD (Adriamycin [doxorubicin], bleomycin, vinblastine, and docarbazine). Treatment with these drugs may require concomitant administration of antiemetics, sedatives, and antidiarrheals to combat adverse GI effects.

Other treatments include autologous bone marrow transplantation and immunotherapy, which by itself hasn't proved effective.

COLLABORATIVE MANAGEMENT

Care of the patient with Hodgkin's disease focuses on preventing injury, improving nutrition, heightening energy, and dealing with fear.

Staging Hodgkin's disease

Treatment of Hodgkin's disease depends on the stage it has reached—that is, the number, location, and degree of involved lymph nodes. The Ann Arbor classification system, adopted in 1971, divides Hodgkin's disease into four stages and subdivides each stage into categories. Category A includes patients without defined signs and symptoms. Category B includes patients who experience such defined signs as recent unexplained weight loss, fever, and night sweats.

Stage I
Hodgkin's disease appears in a single lymph node region (I) or a single extralymphatic organ (IE).

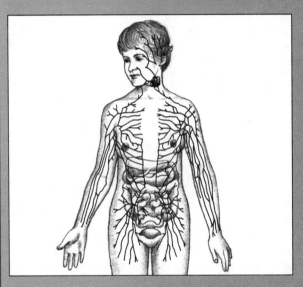

Stage II
The disease appears in two or more nodes on the same side of the diaphragm (II) and in an extralymphatic organ (IIE).

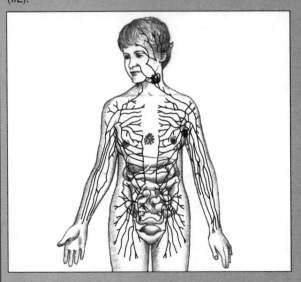

Stage III
The disease spreads to both sides of the diaphragm (III) and perhaps to an extralymphatic organ (IIIE), the spleen (IIIS), or both (IIIES).

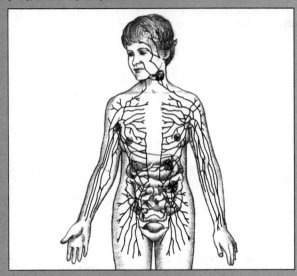

Stage IV
The disease disseminates, involving one or more extralymphatic organs or tissues, with or without lymph node involvement.

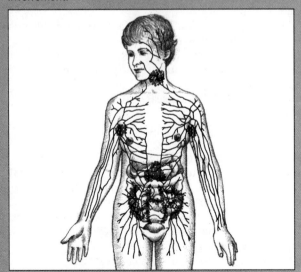

ASSESSMENT

Most commonly, the patient's history will reveal painless swelling of one of the cervical lymph nodes or, sometimes, the axillary or inguinal lymph nodes. Look for:
- history of persistent fever and night sweats
- complaints of weight loss, despite an adequate diet, with resulting fatigue and malaise
- as the disease progresses, increasing susceptibility to infection
- in advanced stages, edema of the face and neck, and jaundice
- enlarged, rubbery lymph nodes in the neck that enlarge during periods of fever and then revert to normal size.

Treatment of Hodgkin's disease depends on the stage it has reached, defined by the number, location, and degree of involved lymph nodes. The Ann Arbor classification system, adopted in 1971, divides Hodgkin's disease into four stages.
- Stage I: Hodgkin's disease appears in a single lymph node region or a single extralymphatic organ (IE).
- Stage II: The disease appears in two or more nodes on the same side of the diaphragm and possibly in an extralymphatic organ (IIE).
- Stage III: Hodgkin's disease spreads to both sides of the diaphragm and perhaps to an extralymphatic organ (IIIE), the spleen (IIIS), or both (IIIES).
- Stage IV: The disease disseminates, involving one or more extralymphatic organs or tissues, with or without lymph node involvement.

Doctors subdivide each stage into categories. Category A includes patients without defined signs and symptoms, and category B includes patients who experience such defined signs as recent unexplained weight loss, fever, and night sweats.

NURSING DIAGNOSES AND COLLABORATIVE PROBLEMS

Based on the following nursing diagnoses, you'll establish patient outcomes.

Altered nutrition: Less than body requirements related to GI effects of disease and treatment. The patient will:
- eat a nutritionally balanced diet
- regain lost weight and maintain weight
- avoid complications, such as malnutrition and vitamin deficiency.

Fatigue related to the disease and adverse effects of chemotherapy or radiation therapy. The patient will:
- report controllable factors that cause fatigue
- demonstrate skill in conserving energy while carrying out daily activities
- regain a normal energy level after completing treatment.

Fear related to the threat of death. The patient will:
- express his feelings of fear
- use available support systems to cope with his fear
- have fewer physical symptoms of fear.

PLANNING AND IMPLEMENTATION

These measures help the patient with Hodgkin's disease.
- Provide a well-balanced, high-calorie, high-protein diet. If the patient is anorexic, provide frequent, small meals. Consult with the dietitian to incorporate foods the patient enjoys into his diet.
- Offer the patient grapefruit juice, orange juice, or ginger ale to alleviate nausea and vomiting.
- Assess the patient for nutritional deficiencies and malnutrition. Weigh him regularly.
- Watch for complications during chemotherapy, including anorexia, nausea, vomiting, alopecia, and mouth ulcers.
- Remember to watch for adverse effects of radiation therapy, such as hair loss, nausea, vomiting, and anorexia.
- Observe for signs of hypothyroidism, sterility, and other neoplastic disease, including late-onset leukemia and malignant lymphoma. Although these problems are complications of treatment, they also indicate the success of treatment.
- Perform comfort measures that promote relaxation. Schedule periods of rest if the patient tires easily.
- Provide supportive care as indicated for any adverse effects of chemotherapy or radiation therapy.
- Throughout therapy, listen to the patient's fears and concerns. Encourage him to express his feelings, and stay with him during periods of high stress.
- Involve the patient and his family members or friend in all aspects of his care.

Patient teaching
- Explain all procedures and treatments associated with the plan of care.
- Because sudden withdrawal of prednisone is life-threatening, advise the patient taking this medication not to change his drug dosage or discontinue the drug without contacting his doctor.
- If the patient is a woman of childbearing age, advise her to delay pregnancy until she has a long-term remission. Radiation therapy and chemotherapy can cause genetic mutations and spontaneous abortions.
- Stress the importance of maintaining good nutrition (aided by eating small, frequent meals of the patient's favorite foods) and drinking plenty of fluids.
- Instruct the patient to pace his activities to counteract therapy-induced fatigue. Teach him how to use

relaxation techniques to promote comfort and reduce anxiety.

■ Stress the importance of good oral hygiene to prevent stomatitis. To control pain and bleeding, teach the patient to use a soft toothbrush, a cotton swab, or an anesthetic mouthwash such as viscous lidocaine (as prescribed); to apply petroleum jelly to his lips; and to avoid astringent mouthwashes.

■ Advise the patient to avoid crowds and any person with a known infection. Emphasize that he should notify the doctor if he develops any infection.

■ Because enlarged lymph nodes may indicate disease recurrence, teach the patient the importance of checking his lymph nodes.

■ Make sure the patient understands the possible adverse effects of his treatments. Tell him to notify the doctor if these signs and symptoms persist.

■ When appropriate, refer the patient and his family to community organizations, such as psychological counseling services, support groups, and hospices.

■ Advise the patient to seek follow-up care after he has completed the initial treatment.

EVALUATION

Achievement of patient outcomes determines the success of collaborative management. For Hodgkin's disease, evaluation focuses on improved and maintained nutrition, decreased fatigue, and reduced fear.

Iron deficiency anemia

A common disease worldwide, iron deficiency anemia affects 10% to 30% of the adult population of North America. It's most prevalent among premenopausal women, infants (particularly premature or low birth weight infants), children, adolescents (especially girls), alcoholics, and older adults (especially those unable to cook). The prognosis after replacement therapy is favorable.

Possible complications of this disorder include infection and pneumonia. Lead poisoning may result from increased intestinal absorption of lead when combined with pica, another symptom of this disorder. Another complication is bleeding, which you may identify by ecchymotic areas on the skin, hematuria, and gingival bleeding. Plummer-Vinson syndrome can strike in severe cases.

The most significant complication of iron deficiency anemia arises from over-replacement of iron with oral or I.M. supplements. Hemochromatosis (excessive iron deposits in tissue) can result, affecting the liver, heart, pituitary gland, and joints. Iron poisoning can strike children when toxic levels are allowed to build up during therapy. (See *Recognizing iron overdose*.)

Iron deficiency anemia stems from an inadequate supply of iron for optimal formation of red blood cells (RBCs), which produces smaller (microcytic) cells with less color on staining. Body stores of iron, including plasma iron, decrease, as does transferrin, which binds with and transports iron. Insufficient body stores of iron lead to a depleted RBC mass and, in turn, to a decreased hemoglobin concentration (hypochromia) and decreased oxygen-carrying capacity of the blood.

CAUSES

Iron deficiency can be caused by any of the following:

■ inadequate dietary intake of iron, as in prolonged unsupplemented breast- or bottle-feeding of infants; during periods of stress, such as rapid growth in children and adolescents; and in older patients existing on a poorly balanced diet

■ iron malabsorption, as in chronic diarrhea, partial or total gastrectomy, and malabsorption syndromes such as celiac disease

■ blood loss secondary to drug-induced GI bleeding (from anticoagulants, aspirin, steroids) or due to heavy menses, hemorrhage from trauma, GI ulcers, malignant tumors, and varices

■ pregnancy, in which the mother's iron supply is diverted to the fetus for erythropoiesis

■ intravascular hemolysis-induced hemoglobinuria or paroxysmal nocturnal hemoglobinuria

■ mechanical erythrocyte trauma caused by a prosthetic heart valve or vena cava filter.

DIAGNOSIS AND TREATMENT

Blood studies and stores in bone marrow may confirm iron deficiency anemia. However, the results of these tests are sometimes misleading because of complicating factors, such as infection, pneumonia, blood transfusion, and iron supplements.

Characteristic blood study results include low hemoglobin levels, low hematocrit, low serum iron, low serum ferritin levels, low RBC count, and decreased mean corpuscular hemoglobin in severe anemia. Bone marrow studies reveal depleted or absent iron stores (done by staining) and normoblastic hyperplasia. GI studies, such as guaiac stool tests, barium swallow and enema, endoscopy, and sigmoidoscopy, rule out or confirm the diagnosis of bleeding causing the iron deficiency. Diagnosis must rule out other forms of anemia, such as those that result from thalassemia minor, cancer, and chronic inflammatory, hepatic, and renal disease.

After the underlying cause of anemia is determined, iron replacement therapy can begin. The treatment of choice is an oral preparation of iron or a combination of iron and ascorbic acid (which enhances iron absorption). In rare cases, the patient may be given iron I.M.—for instance, if he is noncompliant with the oral preparation, if he needs more iron than he can take orally, if malabsorption prevents adequate iron absorption, or if a maximum rate of hemoglobin regeneration is desired.

Total-dose I.V. infusions of supplemental iron can be given to pregnant patients and to patients with severe iron deficiency anemia. The patient should receive this painless infusion of iron dextran in normal saline solution over 8 hours. To minimize the risk of an allergic reaction to iron, first give an I.V. test dose of 0.5 ml.

COLLABORATIVE MANAGEMENT

Care of the patient with iron deficiency anemia focuses on restoring energy levels, avoiding complications, and providing thorough patient teaching.

ASSESSMENT

Iron deficiency anemia may persist for years without signs and symptoms. The characteristic history of fatigue, inability to concentrate, headache, and shortness of breath (especially on exertion) may not develop until long after iron stores and circulating iron become low. Look for:

- reports of increasingly frequent infections and pica
- an uncontrollable urge to eat strange things, such as clay, starch, ice and, in children, lead
- with a female patient, a history of menorrhagia
- in chronic iron deficiency anemia, a history of complaints of dysphagia and neuromuscular effects, such as vasomotor disturbances, numbness and tingling of the extremities, and neuralgic pain
- in chronic cases, a red, swollen, smooth, shiny, and tender tongue (glossitis)
- in chronic cases, corners of the mouth that may be eroded, tender, and swollen (angular stomatitis); also spoon-shaped, brittle nails
- with advanced cases, tachycardia because decreased oxygen perfusion causes the heart to compensate with increased cardiac output.

NURSING DIAGNOSES AND COLLABORATIVE PROBLEMS

Based on the following nursing diagnoses, you'll establish patient outcomes.

Altered nutrition: Less than body requirements related to dietary deficiency of iron. The patient will:

- express his knowledge of foods rich in iron
- increase his daily dietary intake of iron to meet the recommended daily allowance

Recognizing iron overdose

Excessive iron replacement is demonstrated when signs and symptoms, such as diarrhea, fever, severe stomach pain, nausea, and vomiting, occur.

If you note these signs and symptoms, alert the doctor promptly, and administer prescribed treatments. For this acute condition, treatment includes giving iron-binding agents (deferoxamine), inducing vomiting that produces systemic alkalinization, and giving anticonvulsants.

- express relief from the signs and symptoms of iron deficiency anemia.

Fatigue related to decreased tissue oxygenation caused by decreased hemoglobin. The patient will:

- employ measures to prevent and modify fatigue
- perform all self-care activities without undue fatigue
- regain his normal energy level.

PLANNING AND IMPLEMENTATION

These measures help the patient with iron deficiency anemia.

- Give iron supplements as ordered. Use the Z-track injection method when giving iron I.M. to prevent skin discoloration, scarring, and irritating iron deposits in the skin. (See *Injecting iron solutions,* page 602.)
- If the patient receives iron I.V., monitor the infusion rate carefully. Stop the infusion and begin supportive treatment immediately if the patient shows signs of an allergic reaction. Also, watch for dizziness and headache and for thrombophlebitis around the I.V. site.
- Monitor the patient for iron replacement overdose.
- Monitor the patient's complete blood count and serum iron and ferritin levels regularly.
- Assess the family's dietary habits for iron intake, noting the influence of childhood eating patterns, cultural food preferences, and family income on adequate nutrition.
- Because a sore mouth and tongue make eating painful, ask the dietitian to give the patient nonirritating foods. If these symptoms make talking difficult, supply a pad and pencil or some other communication aid. Provide diluted mouthwash or, with severe conditions, swab the patient's mouth with tap water or warm saline solution. The patient may use oral anesthetics diluted in normal saline solution.

Injecting iron solutions

For deep I.M. injections of iron solutions, use the Z-track technique to avoid subcutaneous irritation and discoloration from leaking medication.

Choose an injection site
Rotate the injection sites in the upper outer quadrant of the buttocks.

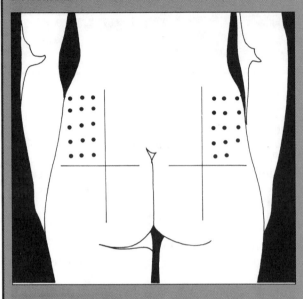

Inject the solution
While keeping the tissue displaced, clean the area and insert the needle. Aspirate to check for accidental entry into a blood vessel. Then inject the solution slowly, followed by the 0.5 cc of air in the syringe.

After injecting the solution, wait 10 seconds.

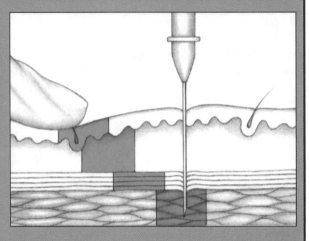

Displace tissues
Choose a 19G to 20-G, 2″ to 3″ needle. After drawing up the solution, change to a fresh needle to avoid tracking the solution through to subcutaneous tissue. Draw 0.5 cc of air into the syringe as an air-lock.

Displace the skin and fat at the injection site firmly to one side.

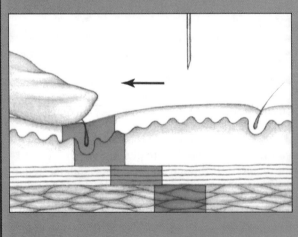

Release the tissues
Pull the needle straight out; then release the tissues.

Apply direct pressure to the site, but don't massage it. Caution the patient not to exercise vigorously for at least 15 minutes after the injection.

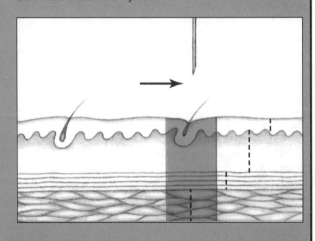

■ Provide good nutrition and meticulous care of I.V. sites, such as those used for blood transfusions, to help prevent infection

■ Monitor the patient's compliance with the prescribed iron supplement therapy.

■ Provide oxygen therapy as necessary to help prevent and reduce hypoxia.

■ As ordered, give analgesics for headache and other discomfort. Monitor their effectiveness.

■ Provide frequent rest periods to decrease physical exhaustion so that the patient has sufficient rest between them.

■ Monitor the patient for signs and symptoms of decreased perfusion to vital organs: dyspnea, chest pain, dizziness, and signs of neuropathy such as tingling in the extremities.

■ Evaluate the patient's drug history. Certain drugs, such as pancreatic enzymes and vitamin E, may interfere with iron metabolism and absorption; aspirin, steroids, and other drugs may cause GI bleeding.

■ Monitor the patient's pulse. Tachycardia indicates that his activities are too strenuous.

Patient teaching

■ Reinforce the doctor's explanation of the disorder, and answer any questions. Confirm that the patient understands the prescribed treatments and possible complications. (See *Reducing risk of iron deficiency anemia.*)

■ Ask about possible exposure to lead in the home (especially for children) or on the job. Teach the patient and his family about the dangers of lead poisoning, especially if the patient reports pica.

■ Advise the patient to continue therapy, even if he feels better, because replacement of iron stores takes time.

■ Inform the patient that milk or an antacid interferes with absorption but that vitamin C can increase absorption. Instruct him to drink liquid supplemental iron through a straw to prevent staining his teeth.

■ Tell the patient to report any adverse effects of iron therapy, such as nausea, diarrhea, or constipation, which may require a dosage adjustment or supplemental stool softeners.

■ Teach the basics of a nutritionally balanced diet— red meats, green vegetables, eggs, whole wheat, iron-fortified bread, and milk. However, explain that no food in itself contains enough iron to treat iron deficiency anemia; an average-sized person with anemia would have to eat at least 10 lb (4.5 kg) of steak daily to receive therapeutic amounts of iron.

■ Warn the patient to guard against infections, because his weakened condition may increase his susceptibility. Stress the importance of meticulous wound care, periodic dental checkups, good hand-

> ### HEALTHY LIVING — Reducing risk of iron deficiency anemia
>
> The following are ways to fight iron deficiency anemia:
>
> ■ Teach the patient and his family members about the dangers of lead poisoning in the home and in the workplace.
>
> ■ Inform the patient that milk or an antacid interferes with absorption of iron supplements or iron-containing foods but that vitamin C can increase absorption.
>
> ■ Teach the basics of a nutritionally balanced diet—red meats, green vegetables, eggs, whole wheat, iron-fortified bread, and milk. However, explain that no food in itself contains enough iron to treat iron deficiency anemia.
>
> ■ Stress the importance of meticulous wound care, periodic dental checkups, good hand-washing technique to prevent infection, and the need for regular checkups.

washing technique, and other measures to prevent infection. Also tell him to report any signs of infection, including temperature elevation and chills.

■ Iron deficiency may recur, so explain the need for regular checkups and compliance with prescribed treatments.

EVALUATION

Achievement of patient outcomes determines the success of collaborative management. For iron deficiency anemia, evaluation focuses on diminished signs of fatigue and improved nutritional and iron status.

Leukemia, acute

Beginning as a malignant proliferation of white blood cell (WBC) precursors, or blasts, in bone marrow or lymph tissue, acute leukemia results in an accumulation of these cells in peripheral blood, bone marrow, and body tissues. The most common forms of acute leukemia include:

■ acute lymphoblastic (lymphocytic) leukemia (ALL), characterized by abnormal growth of lymphocyte precursors (lymphoblasts)

■ acute myeloblastic (myelogenous) leukemia (AML), which causes rapid accumulation of myeloid precursors (myeloblasts)

■ acute monoblastic (monocytic) leukemia, or Schilling's type, which causes a marked increase in monocyte precursors (monoblasts).

Other variants include acute myelomonocytic leukemia and acute erythroleukemia.

Untreated, acute leukemia is invariably fatal, usually because of complications resulting from leukemic cell infiltration of bone marrow or vital organs. With treatment, the prognosis varies.

In ALL, treatment induces remissions in 90% of children (average survival time: 5 years) and in 65% of adults (average survival time: 1 to 2 years). Children between ages 2 and 8 have the best survival rate—about 50%—with intensive therapy.

In AML, the average survival time is only 1 year after diagnosis, even with aggressive treatment. Remissions lasting 2 to 10 months occur in 50% of children; adults survive only about 1 year after they are treated.

Acute leukemia increases the risk for infection and, eventually, organ malfunction through encroachment or hemorrhage.

CAUSES
The exact cause of acute leukemia is unknown; however, radiation (especially prolonged exposure), certain chemicals and drugs, viruses, genetic abnormalities, and chronic exposure to benzene are likely contributing factors.

In children, Down syndrome, ataxia, and telangiectasia may increase the risk, as may such congenital disorders as albinism and congenital immunodeficiency syndrome.

Although the pathogenesis isn't clearly understood, immature, nonfunctioning WBCs appear to accumulate first in the tissue where they originate. (Lymphocytes originate in lymph tissue; granulocytes originate in bone marrow.) These immature WBCs then spill into the bloodstream. From there, they infiltrate other tissues.

DIAGNOSIS AND TREATMENT
Bone marrow aspiration showing a proliferation of immature WBCs confirms acute leukemia. If the aspirate is dry or free from leukemic cells but the patient has other typical signs of leukemia, the doctor will do a bone marrow biopsy—usually of the posterior superior iliac spine.

Blood counts show thrombocytopenia and neutropenia, and a WBC differential determines the cell type. Lumbar puncture detects meningeal involvement. A computed tomography scan shows the affected organs, and cerebrospinal fluid analysis detects abnormal WBC invasion of the central nervous system

Systemic chemotherapy aims to eradicate leukemic cells and induce remission. It's used when fewer than 5% of blast cells in the marrow and peripheral blood are normal. The specific chemotherapeutic and radiation treatment varies with the diagnosis.

■ For meningeal infiltration, the patient receives an intrathecal instillation of methotrexate or cytarabine and cranial irradiation.

■ For ALL, the treatment is vincristine, prednisone, high-dose cytarabine, and daunorubicin. Because ALL carries a 40% risk of meningeal infiltration, the patient also receives intrathecal methotrexate or cytarabine. If the patient has brain or testicular infiltration, he also needs radiation therapy.

■ For AML, treatment consists of a combination of I.V. daunorubicin and cytarabine. If these fail to induce remission, treatment involves some or all of the following: a combination of cyclophosphamide, vincristine, prednisone, or methotrexate; high-dose cytarabine alone or with other drugs; amsacrine; etoposide; and azacitidine and mitoxantrone.

■ For acute monoblastic leukemia, the patient receives cytarabine and thioguanine with daunorubicin or doxorubicin.

Treatment may also involve antiviral drugs and granulocyte injections to control infection as well as transfusions of platelets to prevent bleeding and transfusions of red blood cells to prevent anemia. Bone marrow transplantation is performed in some patients.

COLLABORATIVE MANAGEMENT
Care of the patient with leukemia focuses on avoiding injury, providing comfort, and avoiding infection and fatigue.

ASSESSMENT
The patient's history usually shows a sudden onset of high fever and abnormal bleeding, such as bruising after minor trauma, nosebleeds, gingival bleeding, purpura, ecchymoses, petechiae, and prolonged menses. He may also report fatigue and night sweats. More insidious symptoms include weakness, lassitude, recurrent infections and chills.

The patient with ALL, AML, or acute monoblastic leukemia may also complain of abdominal or bone pain. When assessing this patient, you may note tachycardia and, during auscultation, decreased ventilation, palpitations, and a systolic ejection murmur.

Inspection of any patient with acute leukemia may reveal pallor. On palpation, you may note lymph node enlargement as well as liver or spleen enlargement.

NURSING DIAGNOSES AND COLLABORATIVE PROBLEMS
Based on the following nursing diagnoses, you'll establish patient outcomes.

Fatigue related to hematologic abnormalities. The patient will:
■ explain the relationship between fatigue and his activity level
■ incorporate measures to modify his level of fatigue into his daily routine.

Risk for infection related to abnormal WBC count. The patient will:
■ maintain his temperature within a normal range
■ exhibit no signs or symptoms of infection
■ remain free from infection.

Risk for injury related to thrombocytopenia. The patient will:
■ incorporate bleeding precautions into his daily routine
■ not become injured
■ regain a normal platelet count.

PLANNING AND IMPLEMENTATION
These measures help the patient with leukemia.
■ Develop a plan of care for the leukemic patient that emphasizes comfort, minimizes the adverse effects of chemotherapy, promotes preservation of veins (such as in insertion of a vascular access device for long-term use), manages complications, and provides teaching and psychological support.
■ Because so many of these patients are children, be especially sensitive to their emotional needs and to those of their family members.
■ Establish a trusting relationship to promote communication. Allow the patient and his family members to express their anger, anxiety, and depression.
■ Let the patient and his family participate in his care as much as possible.
■ Before treatment begins, help establish an appropriate rehabilitation program for the patient during remission.
■ Give prescribed pain medications as needed. Provide comfort measures, such as position changes and distractions, to alleviate the patient's discomfort.
■ Minimize stress by providing a calm, quiet atmosphere that's conducive to rest and relaxation. Especially if the patient is a child, be flexible with patient care and visiting hours so that he has time to be with his family members and friends and to play and do schoolwork.
■ To control infection, place the patient in a private room and impose neutropenic precautions, if necessary. Coordinate care so that the patient doesn't come into contact with staff members who also care for patients with infections or infectious diseases. Don't use an indwelling urinary catheter or give I.M. injections; they provide an avenue for infection.
■ Keep the patient's skin and perianal area clean, apply mild lotions or creams to keep the skin from drying and cracking, and thoroughly clean the skin before all invasive skin procedures. Change I.V. tubing according to health care facility policy. Use strict aseptic technique and a metal scalp vein needle (metal butterfly needle) when starting an I.V. line. If the patient is receiving total parenteral nutrition, provide scrupulous subclavian catheter care.
■ Monitor the patient's temperature every 4 hours. If his temperature rises over 101° F (38.3° C) and his WBC count decreases, he will need prompt antibiotic therapy.
■ If the patient is bleeding, apply ice compresses and pressure and elevate the extremity. Avoid giving him aspirin or aspirin-containing drugs or rectal suppositories, taking a rectal temperature, or performing a digitation.
■ Take steps to prevent hyperuricemia, a possible result of rapid, chemotherapy-induced leukemic cell lysis. Make sure the patient receives about 2 qt (2 L) of fluid daily, and give acetazolamide, sodium bicarbonate tablets, and allopurinol, as ordered.
■ Control mouth ulceration by providing frequent mouth care and saline rinses.
■ Monitor the patient's complete blood count and platelet count for signs of improvement.
■ Watch for signs of meningeal infiltration (confusion, lethargy, and headache). If it develops, the patient will need intrathecal chemotherapy.
■ Check the patient's urine pH often; it should be above 7.5. Watch for a rash or other hypersensitivity reactions to allopurinol.
■ If the patient receives daunorubicin or doxorubicin, watch for early indications of cardiotoxicity, such as arrhythmias and signs of heart failure.
■ Screen staff members and visitors for contagious diseases, and watch for and report any signs of infection in the patient.
■ Monitor the patient for bleeding.
■ Check the patient's oral cavity daily for ulceration and his rectal area daily for induration, swelling, erythema, skin discoloration, and drainage.
■ If the patient doesn't respond to treatment and has reached the terminal phase of the disease, he'll need supportive nursing care. Take steps to manage pain, fever, and bleeding; make sure the patient is comfortable; and provide emotional support for him and his family members. If the patient wishes, provide for religious counseling. Discuss the option of home or hospice care.

Patient teaching
■ Explain the course of the disease to the patient.
■ Teach the patient and his family members how to recognize signs and symptoms of infection (fever,

chills, cough, sore throat). Tell them to report an infection to the doctor.

■ Explain to the patient that his blood may not have enough platelets for proper clotting, and teach him the signs of abnormal bleeding (bruising, petechiae). Explain that he can apply pressure and ice to the area to stop such bleeding. Also, teach him steps he can take to prevent bleeding. Urge him to report excessive bleeding or bruising to the doctor.

■ Inform the patient that drug therapy is tailored to his type of leukemia. Explain that he'll probably take a combination of drugs; teach him about the ones he'll receive. Make sure he understands their adverse effects and the measures he can take to prevent or alleviate those effects.

■ Explain that if the chemotherapy causes weight loss and anorexia, the patient will need to eat and drink high-calorie, high-protein foods and beverages. If he loses his appetite, advise him to eat small, frequent meals. If the chemotherapy and adjunctive prednisone instead cause weight gain, he'll need dietary counseling.

■ Instruct the patient to use a soft toothbrush and to avoid hot, spicy foods and commercial mouthwashes, which can irritate the mouth ulcers that result from chemotherapy.

■ If the patient receives cranial irradiation, explain what the treatment is and how it will help him. Remember to discuss potential adverse effects and the steps he can take to minimize those effects.

■ If the patient needs a bone marrow transplant, reinforce the doctor's explanation of the treatment, its possible benefits, and the potential adverse effects. Teach him about total-body irradiation and the chemotherapy that he'll undergo before transplantation. Tell the patient what to expect after the transplantation.

■ Advise the patient to limit his activities and to plan rest periods during the day.

■ Refer the patient to the social service department, home health care agencies, and support groups such as the American Cancer Society.

EVALUATION

Achievement of patient outcomes determines the success of collaborative management. For leukemia, evaluation focuses on decreased fatigue and prevention of infection and injury.

Lymphedema

In patients with lymphedema, lymph drainage is obstructed, preventing protein molecules from returning to the circulation from the interstitial fluid. Protein molecules accumulate, increasing interstitial fluid pressure and resulting in further accumulation of fluid in soft tissues, primarily of the arms and legs.

CAUSES

Primary or secondary lymphedema is caused by inflammation, obstruction, or removal of lymphatic vessels such as occurs in mastectomy; in tropical areas, elephantiasis may result as an effect of infection by filaria, a nematode worm, infesting the lymphatics. Primary lymphedema (lymphedema praecox) begins in adolescent females after menstruation (rare).

DIAGNOSIS AND TREATMENT

Diagnosis of lymphedena is made from a combination of patient complaints and medical history.

Initial treatment may include application of moist heat, elevation and immobilization of the affected extremity, and care of the wounds. Elastic stockings, meticulous skin hygiene, bed rest, and restricting dietary sodium are also helpful. Prognosis varies with cause and type; infections are treated with the appropriate antibiotic (usually penicillin G or erythromycin), anthelmintics for worms, antifungals, analgesics, and diuretics.

The patient may require surgery to restore function to the affected extremity, reduce pain, treat recurrent episodes of cellulitis and lymphagitis, remove lymphosarcomas, or improve the appearance of the extremity.

COLLABORATIVE MANAGEMENT

Care of the patient with lymphedema focuses on avoiding injury, improving tissue integrity, and providing patient teaching.

ASSESSMENT

Painless edema in the arms and legs can progress to complaints of heaviness and hardening of the subcutaneous tissues of the affected extremity. The condition may worsen in warmer weather. Early in the course, the edema is soft and pitting. Edema causes massive swelling of the affected extremities.

The patient may experience lymphangitis (pain at the site of injury, redness, fever, chills, red streaks extending toward the lymph nodes, enlarged and painful lymph nodes) and cellulitis.

NURSING DIAGNOSES AND COLLABORATIVE PROBLEMS

Based on the following nursing diagnoses, you'll establish patient outcomes.

Impaired tissue integrity related to impaired lymphatic flow. The patient will:

■ experience improved circulation and decreased edema.

Fluid volume excess related to impaired regulatory system and impaired lymphatic flow. The patient will:
- maintain adequate hydration status
- plan 24-hour intake as prescribed.

Impaired skin integrity related to edema and decreased mobility. The patient will:
- have improved skin integrity
- express understanding of skin protection measures
- demonstrate skin inspection technique.

PLANNING AND IMPLEMENTATION
These measures help the patient with lymphedema.
- Apply well-fitting elastic stockings.
- Elevate the affected extremities.
- Restrict your patient's sodium intake.
- Measure and record the patient's intake and output.
- Measure the girth of the extremity daily.
- Weigh the patient daily.
- Inspect his skin at each shift.
- To avoid injury, use preventive devices, such as egg crate pads, sheepskin, and pillows.
- Keep his skin clean and dry.

Patient teaching
- Review measures with the patient to prevent skin breakdown.
- Review measures to increase circulation and decrease edema.
- Stress the need to comply with treatment and therapy.

EVALUATION
Achievement of patient outcomes determines the success of collaborative management. For lymphedema, evaluation focuses on improved skin integrity and reduced fluid volume excess.

Malignant lymphomas

Also called non-Hodgkin's lymphomas and lymphosarcomas, malignant lymphomas are a heterogeneous group of malignant diseases. They originate in lymph glands and other lymphoid tissue. The National Cancer Institute usually defines them by histologic, anatomic, and immunomorphic characteristics. However, the Rappaport histologic and Lukes classification systems also are used (See *Classifying malignant lymphomas,* page 608.)

CAUSES
Although some theories point to a viral source, the cause of malignant lymphomas is unknown. Malignant lymphomas are three times more common than Hodgkin's disease, and the incidence is increasing, especially in patients with autoimmune disorders and those receiving immunosuppressant treatment. Nodular lymphomas yield a better prognosis than the diffuse ones, but in both, the prognosis is less hopeful than in Hodgkin's disease.

Malignant lymphomas can lead to hypercalcemia, hyperuricemia, lymphomatosis, meningitis, and anemia from bone marrow involvement. As tumors grow, they may produce liver, kidney, and lung problems. Central nervous system involvement can lead to increased intracranial pressure.

DIAGNOSIS AND TREATMENT
Biopsies differentiate a malignant lymphoma from Hodgkin's disease. They may be taken from lymph nodes; tonsils, bone marrow, liver, bowel, or skin; or, as needed, from tissue removed during exploratory laparotomy. Chest X-rays, lymphangiography, a computed tomography scan of the abdomen, excretory urography, and liver, bone, and spleen scans indicate disease progression.

A complete blood count (CBC) may show anemia. The patient may have a normal or elevated uric acid level and an elevated serum calcium level, resulting from bone lesions. The staging system for Hodgkin's disease also applies to malignant lymphomas.

Radiation and chemotherapy are the main treatments for lymphomas. Radiation therapy is used mainly during the localized stage of the disease. In many cases, total nodal irradiation effectively treats both nodular and diffuse lymphomas.

Chemotherapy is most effective with a combination of antineoplastic agents. For example, the cyclophosphamide, doxorubicin, vincristine (Oncovin), and prednisone protocol can induce a complete remission in 70% to 80% of those with nodular lymphoma and in 20% to 55% of those with diffuse lymphoma. Other combinations—such as methotrexate, leucovorin, doxorubicin (Adriamycin), cyclophosphamide, vincristine (Oncovin), prednisone, and bleomycin—can induce a prolonged remission and possibly a cure for diffuse lymphomas.

Because perforation commonly affect patients with gastric lymphomas, these patients usually undergo a debulking procedure before chemotherapy, such as a subtotal or total gastrectomy.

COLLABORATIVE MANAGEMENT
Care of the patient with malignant lymphoma focuses on avoiding injury, improving nutrition, and raising energy level.

ASSESSMENT
Signs of malignant lymphomas may mimic those of Hodgkin's disease. Most commonly, the patient histo-

Classifying malignant lymphomas

Several classification and staging systems are being used to evaluate the extent of malignant lymphoma. Among the most common are the National Cancer Institute's (NCI) system (named the "working formulation for classification of non-Hodgkin's lymphomas for clinical usage"), the Rappaport histologic classification, and Lukes classification.

NCI working formulation	Rappaport histologic classification	Lukes classification
LOW GRADE		
■ Small lymphocytic	■ Diffuse, well-differentiated, lymphocytic	■ Small lymphocytic and plasmacytoid lymphocytic
■ Follicular, predominantly small cleaved cell	■ Nodular, poorly differentiated, lymphocytic	■ Small cleaved follicular center cell, follicular only or follicular and diffuse
■ Follicular mixed small and large cell	■ Nodular, mixed lymphoma	■ Small cleaved follicular center cell, follicular; large cleaved follicular center cell, follicular
INTERMEDIATE GRADE		
■ Follicular, predominantly large cell	■ Nodular, histiocytic lymphoma	■ Large cleaved or noncleaved follicular center cell, or both, follicular
■ Diffuse, small cleaved cell	■ Diffuse, poorly differentiated lymphoma	■ Small cleaved follicular center cell, diffuse
■ Diffuse mixed, lymphocytic-histiocytic	■ Diffuse mixed, small and large cell	■ Small cleaved, large cleaved, or large noncleaved follicular center cell, diffuse
■ Diffuse large cell, cleaved or noncleaved	■ Diffuse, histiocytic lymphoma	■ Large cleaved or noncleaved follicular center cell, diffuse
HIGH GRADE		
■ Diffuse large cell, immunoblastic	■ Diffuse, histiocytic lymphoma	■ Immunoblastic sarcoma, T-cell or B-cell type
■ Small noncleaved cell	■ Lymphoblastic, convoluted or nonconvoluted	■ Convoluted T cell
■ Large cell, lymphoblastic	■ Undifferentiated, Burkitt's and non-Burkitt's diffuse undifferentiated lymphoma	■ Small noncleaved follicular center cell
MISCELLANEOUS		
■ Composite ■ Mycosis fungoides ■ Histiocytic ■ Extramedullary plasmacytoma ■ Unclassifiable		

ry reveals painless, swollen lymph glands. The swelling may have appeared and disappeared over several months. As the lymphoma progresses, the patient may complain of fatigue, malaise, weight loss, and night sweats.

Inspection may reveal enlarged tonsils and adenoids, and palpation may disclose rubbery nodes in the cervical and supraclavicular areas.

NURSING DIAGNOSES AND COLLABORATIVE PROBLEMS
Based on the following nursing diagnoses, you'll establish patient outcomes.

Altered nutrition: Less than body requirements related to chemotherapy or radiation therapy. The patient will:
■ regain any lost weight and then maintain his weight within a normal range

- eat a nutritionally balanced diet each day
- develop no signs of malnutrition.
  Fatigue related to anemia. The patient will:
- state his understanding of measures to prevent or minimize fatigue
- incorporate the measures necessary to modify fatigue into his daily routine
- experience an increased energy level.
  Risk for injury related to potential for hypercalcemia caused by bone involvement. The patient will:
- maintain a normal serum calcium level
- exhibit no signs of hypercalcemia.

PLANNING AND IMPLEMENTATION
These measures help the patient with malignant lymphomas.
- Give pain medication, as ordered.
- Schedule rest periods if the patient tires easily.
- Offer the patient such fluids as nonacidic juices or ginger ale to counteract nausea.
- Because this disease causes large numbers of tumors, provide the patient with plenty of fluids to help flush out the cells that are destroyed during treatment. This helps prevent tumor lysis syndrome.
- Provide a well-balanced, high-calorie, high-protein diet. Consult with the dietitian and plan small, frequent meals that include the patient's favorite foods. Schedule meals around the patient's treatment.
- If the patient can't tolerate oral feedings, give I.V. fluids. If necessary, give antiemetics and sedatives, as ordered.
- Monitor the patient's nutritional and fluid intake. Weigh him daily.
- Monitor the effectiveness of analgesics and other drugs.
- Watch for complications of radiation and chemotherapy, such as nausea, vomiting, anorexia, hair loss, oral ulcers, and infection.
- Monitor the patient's CBC, uric acid level, and serum calcium level for abnormalities.
- Throughout therapy, listen to the patient's fears and concerns. Stay with him during periods of severe stress or anxiety. Encourage him to express his anger and concerns, and offer reassurance when appropriate.
- Involve the patient and his family members or friend in his care whenever possible.

Patient teaching
- Confirm that the patient has received thorough explanations about all treatment.
- Instruct him to keep irradiated skin dry.
- Before surgery, explain preoperative and postoperative procedures thoroughly to the patient. Tell him that he may have a nasogastric tube or an indwelling urinary catheter inserted after surgery.
- After chemotherapy and radiation therapy, tell the patient to avoid crowds and anyone who has an infection. Urge him to report any infection to his doctor.
- Stress the importance of a well-balanced, high-calorie, high-protein diet.
- Emphasize the importance of maintaining good oral hygiene during treatment to prevent stomatitis. Instruct him to clean his teeth with a soft-bristled toothbrush and to avoid astringent mouthwashes.
- Teach relaxation and comfort measures, and encourage their use.
- If appropriate, refer the patient to the social service department, home health care agencies, hospices, and support groups such as the American Cancer Society.

EVALUATION
Achievement of patient outcomes determines the success of collaborative management. For malignant lymphomas, evaluation focuses on improved nutrition, injury prevention, and decreased fatigue.

Mononucleosis

An acute infectious disease, mononucleosis causes fever, sore throat, and cervical lymphadenopathy, the hallmarks of the disease. It also causes hepatic dysfunction, increased lymphocytes and monocytes, and development and persistence of heterophil antibodies. The disease primarily affects young adults and children although, in children, it's usually so mild that it's overlooked.

The disease is fairly prevalent in the United States, Canada, and Europe, and both sexes are affected equally. Incidence varies seasonally among college students but not among the general population. With treatment, the prognosis is excellent, and major complications are uncommon.

Although major complications are rare, mononucleosis may cause splenic rupture, aseptic meningitis, encephalitis, hemolytic anemia, pericarditis, and Guillain-Barré syndrome.

CAUSES
Infectious mononucleosis is caused by the Epstein-Barr virus (EBV), a member of the herpes group. Apparently, the reservoir of EBV is limited to humans. The disease probably spreads by the oropharyngeal route. About 80% of patients carry EBV in the throat during the acute stage and for an indefinite time afterward. It's also transmitted by blood transfusion and has been reported in cardiac surgery patients as the "postpump perfusion" syndrome. The disease is probably contagious from the period before symptoms de-

velop until the fever subsides and oropharyngeal lesions disappear.

DIAGNOSIS AND TREATMENT

To confirm the diagnosis of mononucleosis, the doctor will look for the following test results:

■ an increase in white blood cell (WBC) count of 10,000 to 20,000/µl during the second and third weeks of illness (lymphocytes and monocytes accounting for 50% to 70% of the total WBC count; 10% of the lymphocytes are atypical)

■ a fourfold rise in heterophil antibodies (agglutinins for sheep red blood cells) in serum drawn during the acute phase and at 3- to 4-week intervals

■ antibodies to EBV and cellular antigens shown on indirect immunofluorescence (usually more definitive than heterophil antibodies; may be unnecessary because the vast majority of patients are heterophil-positive)

■ abnormal liver function studies.

Infectious mononucleosis isn't easily prevented, and it's resistant to standard antimicrobial treatment. Thus, therapy is essentially supportive, including relief of symptoms, bed rest during the acute febrile period, and aspirin or another salicylate for headache and sore throat. If severe throat inflammation causes airway obstruction, steroids can relieve swelling and prevent a tracheotomy. Splenic rupture, marked by sudden abdominal pain, requires splenectomy. About 20% of patients with infectious mononucleosis also have streptococcal pharyngotonsillitis and should receive antibiotic therapy for at least 10 days.

COLLABORATIVE MANAGEMENT

Care of the patient with mononucleosis focuses on increasing comfort and reducing pain and fatigue.

ASSESSMENT

The patient's history may reveal contact with a person who has infectious mononucleosis. After an incubation period of about 30 to 50 days in adults, the patient may experience prodromal symptoms. Look for:

■ reports of headache, malaise, profound fatigue, anorexia, myalgia and, possibly, abdominal discomfort; after 3 to 5 days, a sore throat, commonly described as the worst ever, and dysphagia related to adenopathy develop

■ complaints of fever, typically with a late afternoon or evening peak of 101° F (38.3° C)

■ exudative tonsillitis, pharyngitis and, sometimes, palatal petechiae, periorbital edema, maculopapular rash that resembles rubella, and jaundice

■ palpable nodes that are mildly tender

■ cervical adenopathy with slight tenderness, and likely inguinal and axillary adenopathy

■ splenomegaly and, less commonly, hepatomegaly

■ normal chest sounds.

NURSING DIAGNOSES AND COLLABORATIVE PROBLEMS

Based on the following nursing diagnoses, you'll establish patient outcomes.

Fatigue related to the infection process. The patient will:

■ avoid activities that increase fatigue

■ obtain adequate rest to minimize fatigue

■ regain his normal energy level.

Hyperthermia related to the infectious process. The patient will:

■ exhibit a decrease in temperature after antipyretic measures

■ avoid complications associated with hyperthermia, such as seizures and shock

■ regain and maintain a normal temperature.

Pain related to throat inflammation and swelling. The patient will:

■ express relief from discomfort after he's given analgesics

■ use diversionary activities to minimize pain

■ exhibit resolution of throat pain and inflammation.

PLANNING AND IMPLEMENTATION

These measures help the patient with mononucleosis.

■ Give drugs to treat symptoms, as needed.

■ Provide warm saline gargles for symptomatic relief of sore throat.

■ Provide adequate fluids and nutrition.

■ Plan care to provide frequent rest periods.

■ Check the patient's temperature regularly.

■ Monitor the patient's response to analgesics, antipyretics, and other supportive care measures.

■ Monitor the patient for complications.

■ Explore sources of stress in the patient's life and propose ways to diminish them.

Patient teaching

■ Explain that convalescence may take several weeks to several months, usually until the patient's WBC count returns to normal.

■ Stress the need for bed rest during the acute illness. Warn the patient to avoid excessive activity, which could lead to splenic rupture.

■ If the patient is a student, tell him that he can continue less demanding school assignments and see his friends, but that he should avoid long, difficult projects until after recovery.

■ To minimize throat discomfort, encourage the patient to drink milk shakes, fruit juices, and broths and to eat cool, bland foods. Advise using warm saline gargles, analgesics, and antipyretics as needed.

EVALUATION

Achievement of patient outcomes determines the success of collaborative management. For mononucleosis, evaluation focuses on decreased fatigue, decreased pain, and reduced hyperthermia.

Multiple myeloma

Also called malignant plasmacytoma, plasma cell myeloma, and myelomatosis, multiple myeloma is a disseminated neoplasm of marrow plasma cells. It strikes about 12,300 persons yearly—mostly men over age 68. It usually carries a poor prognosis because, by the time it's diagnosed, it has already infiltrated the vertebrae, pelvis, skull, ribs, clavicles, and sternum. By then, skeletal destruction is widespread and, without treatment, leads to vertebral collapse. Within 3 months of diagnosis, 52% of patients die; within 2 years, 90% die. If the disease is caught early, treatment may prolong life by another 3 to 5 years.

CAUSES

Although the cause of multiple myeloma isn't known, genetic factors and occupational exposure to radiation have been linked to the disease.

The disease infiltrates bone to produce osteolytic lesions throughout the skeleton (flat bones, vertebrae, skull, pelvis, and ribs). In late stages, it infiltrates the body organs as well (liver, spleen, lymph nodes, lungs, adrenal glands, kidneys, skin, and GI tract).

Multiple myeloma, in turn, can cause infections (such as pneumonia), pyelonephritis (caused by tubular damage from large amounts of Bence Jones protein, hypercalcemia, and hyperuricemia), renal calculi, renal failure, hematologic imbalance, fractures, hypercalcemia, hyperuricemia, and dehydration. Patients may also develop a predisposition toward bleeding—the result of M protein coating the platelets. This bleeding usually affects the GI tract or the nose.

DIAGNOSIS AND TREATMENT

The following tests support a diagnosis of multiple myeloma:

■ *Complete blood count* shows moderate or severe anemia. The differential may show 40% to 50% lymphocytes but seldom more than 3% plasma cells. Rouleau formation, often the first clue, is seen on differential smear and results from elevation of the erythrocyte sedimentation rate.

■ *Urine studies* may show proteinuria, Bence Jones protein, and hypercalciuria. Absence of Bence Jones protein doesn't rule out multiple myeloma, but its presence almost invariably confirms the disease.

■ *Bone marrow aspiration* detects myelomatous cells (abnormal number of immature plasma cells)—10% to 95% instead of the normal 3% to 5%.

■ *Serum electrophoresis* shows an elevated globulin spike that is electrophoretically and immunologically abnormal.

■ *X-rays* during the early stages may reveal only diffuse osteoporosis. Eventually, they show multiple, sharply circumscribed osteolytic (punched out) lesions, particularly on the skull, pelvis, and spine—the characteristic lesions of multiple myeloma.

■ *Excretory urography* can assess renal involvement. To avoid precipitation of Bence Jones protein, iothalamate or diatrizoate is used instead of the usual contrast medium.

Long-term treatment of multiple myeloma consists mainly of chemotherapy to suppress plasma cell growth and control pain. Combinations of melphalan and prednisone or of cyclophosphamide and prednisone are used. Adjuvant local irradiation reduces acute lesions and relieves the pain of collapsed vertebrae.

Other treatment usually includes administration of analgesics for pain. If the patient develops vertebral compression, he may require a laminectomy; if he has renal complications, he may need dialysis. Maintenance therapy with interferon may prolong the plateau phase once the initial chemotherapy is complete.

Because the patient may have bone demineralization and may lose large amounts of calcium into blood and urine, he's a prime candidate for renal calculi, nephrocalcinosis and, eventually, renal failure from hypercalcemia. Hydration, diuretics, corticosteroids, and oral phosphate calcium levels control the hypercalcemia. Plasmapheresis removes the M protein from the blood and returns the cells to the patient, although this effect is only temporary.

COLLABORATIVE MANAGEMENT

Care of the patient with multiple myeloma focuses on decreasing pain and potential for infection and reducing anxiety.

ASSESSMENT

The patient may have a history of neoplastic fractures. He usually complains of severe, constant back pain, which may increase with exercise. He may also report symptoms similar to those of arthritis, such as aches, joint swelling, and tenderness, probably from vertebral compression. Other complaints include numbness, prickling, and tingling of the extremities (peripheral paresthesia).

Inspection may reveal that the patient has pain on movement or weight bearing, especially in the thoracic and lumbar vertebrae.

As the disease advances, the patient will become progressively weaker because of vertebral compression, anemia, and weight loss. As the nerves associated with respiratory function are affected, he may develop pneumonia as well as noticeable thoracic deformities and a reduction in body height of 5″ (12.5 cm) or more as his vertebrae collapse.

NURSING DIAGNOSES AND COLLABORATIVE PROBLEMS

Based on the following nursing diagnoses, you'll establish patient outcomes.

Anxiety related to the fear of death. The patient will:
- express his feelings about his diagnosis and prognosis
- use available support systems to help cope with his anxiety
- exhibit a reduction in anxiety after participating in decisions about his care
- exhibit fewer physical symptoms of anxiety.
 Risk for infection related to bone disease. The patient will:
- maintain a normal temperature
- avoid signs and symptoms of infection.
 Pain related to bone tissue destruction. The patient will:
- express relief of pain after he's given analgesics
- avoid performing activities that cause or worsen pain or seek assistance with them
- use nonpharmacologic measures, such as guided imagery and relaxation techniques, to help cope with pain.

PLANNING AND IMPLEMENTATION

These measures help the patient with multiple myeloma.
- Encourage the patient to drink 3 to 4 qt (3 to 4 L) of fluids daily, particularly before excretory urography.
- Monitor the patient's fluid intake and output, which shouldn't fall below 1½ qt (1.5 L)/day.
- If the patient is bedridden, change his position every 2 hours or position him as ordered; maintain alignment; and logroll him when turning.
- Provide passive range-of-motion and deep-breathing exercises; promote active exercises when he can tolerate them.
- During chemotherapy, watch for complications such as fever, potentially the onset of infection. Also observe for signs of other problems, such as severe anemia and fractures.
- If the patient is receiving melphalan, a phenylalanine derivative of nitrogen mustard that depresses bone marrow, obtain platelet and white blood cell counts before each treatment. If he's receiving prednisone, watch closely for signs of infection, which this drug masks.
- Give prescribed analgesics for pain as necessary. Provide comfort measures, such as repositioning and relaxation techniques.
- Assess the effect of drugs and nonpharmacologic measures used to alleviate or minimize pain.
- Prepare the patient for laminectomy, if indicated.
- Observe the patient for signs and symptoms of infection.
- Monitor the patient for hemorrhage, motor and sensory deficits, and loss of bowel or bladder function.
- The patient with multiple myeloma is particularly vulnerable to pathologic fractures. Never allow him to walk unaccompanied, and make sure he uses a walker or other supportive aid to prevent falls. Reassure him if he's fearful, and allow him to move at his own pace.
- Throughout therapy, listen to the patient's fears and concerns. Offer reassurance when appropriate, and stay with him if he experiences periods of severe stress and anxiety.
- Encourage the patient to identify actions and measures that promote comfort and relaxation. Try to perform these measures, and encourage the patient and his family members to do so, too.
- Involve the patient and his family members in decisions about his care whenever possible.
- Help relieve their anxiety by answering their questions.

Patient teaching
- Reinforce the doctor's explanation of the disease, diagnostic tests, treatment options, and prognosis. Make sure the patient understands what to expect from the treatment and diagnostic tests (including painful procedures, such as bone marrow aspiration and biopsy). Tell him to notify the doctor if the adverse effects of treatment persist.
- Prepare the patient for the effects of surgery.
- Explain the procedures he will undergo, such as insertion of an I.V. line and an indwelling urinary catheter.
- Emphasize the importance of deep breathing and changing position every 2 hours after surgery.
- Tell the patient to dress appropriately because multiple myeloma may make him particularly sensitive to cold.

■ Caution the patient to avoid crowds and persons with known infections because chemotherapy diminishes the body's natural resistance to infection.

■ If appropriate, direct the patient and his family members to community resources—such as a local chapter of the American Cancer Society or the National Cancer Institute—for support.

EVALUATION

Achievement of patient outcomes determines the success of collaborative management. For multiple myeloma, evaluation focuses on decreased pain, prevention of infection, and reduced anxiety.

Polycythemia vera

A chronic, myeloproliferative disorder, polycythemia vera is characterized by increased red blood cell (RBC) mass, leukocytosis, thrombocytosis, and increased hemoglobin concentration, with normal or decreased plasma volume. It usually strikes between ages 40 and 60, most commonly among men of Jewish ancestry; it seldom affects children or blacks and doesn't appear to be familial.

The onset of polycythemia is gradual, and the disease runs a steadily progressive course. The prognosis depends on age at diagnosis, treatment used, and complications. Mortality is high if polycythemia is untreated or is associated with leukemia or myeloid metaplasia. (Polycythemia vera is also known as primary polycythemia, erythremia, polycythemia rubra vera, splenomegalic polycythemia, and Vaquez's disease.)

CAUSES

In polycythemia vera, uncontrolled and rapid cellular reproduction and maturation cause proliferation or hyperplasia of all bone marrow cells (panmyelosis). The cause of such uncontrolled cellular activity is unknown, but it is probably the result of a multipotential stem cell defect.

Hyperviscosity in this disorder may lead to thrombosis of small vessels, with ruddy cyanosis of the nose and clubbing (stunting) of the digits. Further thromboembolic involvement can lead to splenomegaly, renal calculus formation, and abdominal organ thrombosis.

Paradoxically, hemorrhage is a complication of polycythemia vera. It may be due to defective platelet function or to hyperviscosity and the local effects of excess RBCs exerting pressure on distended venous and capillary walls.

Cerebrovascular accident (CVA) may also complicate the disease. Incidence of peptic ulcer disease is four to five times greater in patients with polycythemia vera than in the general population.

DIAGNOSIS AND TREATMENT

Laboratory studies support a diagnosis of polycythemia vera by showing increased RBC mass and normal arterial oxygen saturation in association with splenomegaly or two of the following:

■ platelet count above 400,000/µl (thrombocytosis)

■ white blood cell (WBC) count above 10,000/µl in adults (leukocytosis)

■ elevated leukocyte alkaline phosphatase level

■ elevated serum vitamin B_{12} levels or increased B_{12}-binding capacity.

Another common finding is increased uric acid production, leading to hyperuricemia and hyperuricuria. Other laboratory results include increased blood histamine, decreased serum iron concentration, and decreased or absent urinary erythropoietin. Bone marrow biopsy reveals panmyelosis.

Phlebotomy, the primary treatment, is performed repeatedly and can reduce RBC mass promptly. It's best used for patients with mild disease or for young patients. The frequency of phlebotomy and the amount of blood removed each time depend on the patient's condition. Typically, 350 to 500 ml of blood are removed every other day until the patient's hematocrit is reduced to the low-normal range. After repeated phlebotomies, the patient will develop iron deficiency, which stabilizes RBC production and reduces the need for phlebotomy. However, phlebotomy does not reduce the WBC or platelet count and won't control the hyperuricemia associated with marrow cell proliferation. Myelosuppressant therapy may be used for patients with severe symptoms, such as extreme thrombocytosis, a rapidly enlarging spleen, and hypermetabolism. It's also used for older patients who have difficulty tolerating the phlebotomy procedure. Radioactive phosphorus (^{32}P) or chemotherapeutic agents, such as melphalan, busulfan, and chlorambucil, can satisfactorily control the disease in most cases. However, these agents may cause leukemia and usually are reserved for older patients and those with serious problems not controlled by phlebotomy. Patients of any age who have had previous thrombotic problems should be considered for myelosuppressant therapy.

Pheresis technology allows removal of RBCs, WBCs, and platelets individually or collectively (and provides these cellular components for blood banks). Pheresis also permits the return of plasma to the patient, thereby diluting the blood and reducing hypovolemic symptoms.

As appropriate, additional treatments include administration of cyproheptadine (12 to 16 mg/day) and allopurinol (300 mg/day) to reduce serum uric acid levels. Treatment usually improves symptomatic splenomegaly; rarely, a patient requires splenectomy.

COLLABORATIVE MANAGEMENT
Care of the patient with polycythemia vera focuses on avoiding injury, improving nutrition, and providing patient teaching.

ASSESSMENT
In its early stages, polycythemia vera may produce no signs or symptoms. However, as altered circulation (secondary to increased RBC mass) produces hypervolemia and hyperviscosity, the patient may report a vague feeling of fullness in the head, rushing in the ears, tinnitus, headache, dizziness, vertigo, epistaxis, night sweats, epigastric and joint pain, and such visual alterations as scotomas, double vision, and blurred vision. He may also report a decrease in urine output, possibly due to increased uric acid production.

Late in the disease, the patient may report pruritus (which worsens after bathing and may be disabling), a sense of abdominal fullness, and pain such as pleuritic chest pain or left upper quadrant pain.

NURSING DIAGNOSES AND COLLABORATIVE PROBLEMS
Based on the following nursing diagnoses, you'll establish patient outcomes.

Altered nutrition: Less than body requirements related to adverse GI effects. The patient will:
- regain and maintain his weight within the normal range
- tolerate a nutritionally balanced diet daily
- show no signs or symptoms of malnutrition.

Altered cardiovascular tissue perfusion related to hyperviscosity and hypervolemia. The patient will:
- comply with the prescribed treatment to decrease blood viscosity and volume
- show no ischemic changes suggestive of angina or intermittent claudication
- regain and maintain normal tissue perfusion.

Sensory and perceptual alterations (visual) related to increased RBC mass. The patient will:
- remain safe in his environment
- use safety precautions when ambulating and performing activities of daily living
- regain normal eyesight.

PLANNING AND IMPLEMENTATION
These measures help the patient with polycythemia vera.
- Keep the patient active and ambulatory to prevent thrombosis. If bed rest is necessary, incorporate a program of both active and passive range-of-motion exercises into the patient's daily routine.
- To compensate for increased uric acid production, give the patient additional fluids, give allopurinol (as ordered), and alkalinize the urine to prevent uric acid calculus formation.
- If the patient has symptomatic splenomegaly, suggest or provide small, frequent meals, followed by a rest period, to prevent nausea and vomiting.
- If the patient has pruritus, give drugs as ordered and provide distractions to help him cope.
- If he gets nauseous and vomits with myelosuppressant chemotherapy, begin antiemetic therapy and adjust the patient's diet.
- Before phlebotomy, check the patient's blood pressure and pulse and respiratory rates. Remember to watch for tachycardia, clamminess, and complaints of vertigo, which indicate that the procedure should be stopped. Then, immediately after phlebotomy, check the patient's blood pressure and pulse rate.
- During phlebotomy, make sure the patient is lying down comfortably, to prevent vertigo and syncope.
- After the phlebotomy, have the patient sit up for about 5 minutes before allowing him to walk; this prevents vasovagal attack and orthostatic hypotension. Also, give 24 oz (710 ml) of juice or water to replenish fluid volume.
- If leukopenia develops during myelosuppressant chemotherapy in a hospitalized patient, follow hospital guidelines for reverse isolation—as for complications, such as hypervolemia, thrombocytosis, and signs of an impending CVA (decreased sensation, numbness, transitory paralysis, fleeting blindness, headache, and epistaxis).
- Regularly examine the patient for bleeding.
- Monitor and report acute abdominal pain immediately; it may signal splenic infarction, renal calculus formation, or abdominal organ thrombosis.
- Monitor complete blood count and platelet count before and during myelosuppressant therapy. Watch for and report the patient's adverse reactions after you give him an alkylating agent.
- Encourage the patient to express any concerns about the effect the disease may have on his life. Answer questions appropriately, and provide emotional support. If possible, stay with the patient during periods of acute stress and anxiety.

Patient teaching
- Determine what the patient knows about the disease, especially if he has been diagnosed for some time. As necessary, reinforce the doctor's explanation of the disease process, signs and symptoms, and prescribed treatment.
- Tell the patient to remain as active as possible to help maintain his self-esteem.

- Instruct the patient to prevent cuts by using an electric razor and to keep his environment free from clutter to minimize falls and contusions.
- If the patient develops thrombocytopenia, tell him which are the most common bleeding sites (such as the nose, gingiva, and skin) so he can check for bleeding. Advise him to report any abnormal bleeding promptly.
- Tell the patient to avoid high altitudes, which may exacerbate polycythemia.
- If the patient requires phlebotomy, describe the procedure and explain that it will relieve distressing symptoms. Tell the patient to watch for and report any symptoms of iron deficiency (pallor, weight loss, asthenia, glossitis).
- If the patient requires myelosuppressant therapy, tell him about possible adverse reactions (nausea, vomiting, and susceptibility to infection) that may follow administration of an alkylating agent. As appropriate, mention that alopecia may follow the use of busulfan, cyclophosphamide, and uracil mustard and that sterile hemorrhagic cystitis may follow the use of cyclophosphamide (forcing fluids can prevent this adverse reaction).
- If an outpatient develops leukopenia, reinforce instructions about preventing infection. Warn the patient that his resistance to infection is low; advise him to avoid crowds, and make sure he knows the symptoms of infection.
- If the patient requires treatment with ^{32}P explain the procedure. Tell him that he may require repeated phlebotomies until ^{32}P takes effect.
- Refer the patient and family members to the social service department and local home health care agencies, as appropriate.

EVALUATION
Achievement of patient outcomes determines the success of collaborative management. For polycythemia, evaluation focuses on improved nutritional status, improved tissue perfusion, and prevention of injury due to sensory and perceptual alteration.

Sickle cell anemia

A congenital hemolytic disease, sickle cell anemia is most common in tropical Africa and in people of African descent; about 1 in 10 African-Americans carries the defective gene. If 2 such carriers have offspring, each child has a 1 in 4 chance of developing the disease. One in every 400 to 600 black children has sickle cell anemia. This disease also occurs in Puerto Rico, Turkey, India, the Middle East, and the Mediterranean area. Possibly, the defective gene has

persisted because, in areas where malaria is endemic, the heterozygous sickle cell trait provides resistance to malaria and is actually beneficial.

Penicillin prophylaxis can decrease morbidity and mortality from bacterial infections. Once many patients with sickle cell anemia died in their early 20s, but today, 50% to 70% live into their 40s and 50s.

An adult with sickle cell anemia may develop long-term complications, such as chronic obstructive pulmonary disease, heart failure, or organ infarction, such as retinopathy and nephropathy. Splenic infarctions are common and frequently cause significant necrosis early in life, so that splenomegaly leads to a small, nodular, and malfunctioning spleen. Infection or repeated occlusion of small blood vessels and consequent infarction or necrosis of major organs commonly cause premature death. For example, cerebral blood vessel occlusion causes cerebrovascular accident and is the most common cause of death in severe sickle cell disease. In many cases, sickling and hyperviscosity lead to heart murmurs and heart failure.

CAUSES
Sickle cell anemia is caused by a defective hemoglobin molecule (hemoglobin S) that causes red blood cells (RBCs) to become sickle shaped. Such cells impair circulation, leading to chronic ill health (fatigue, dyspnea on exertion, and swollen joints), periodic crises, long-term complications, and premature death.

Homozygous inheritance of the hemoglobin S-producing gene causes substitution of the amino acid valine for glutamic acid in the beta hemoglobin chain. Heterozygous inheritance of this gene results in sickle cell trait, a condition with minimal or no symptoms. The patient with sickle cell trait is a carrier; he can pass the sickle cell gene to his offspring.

In sickle cell anemia, the abnormal hemoglobin S found in the patient's RBCs becomes insoluble whenever hypoxia occurs. As a result, these RBCs become rigid, rough, and elongated, forming a crescent or sickle shape. Such sickling can produce hemolysis (cell destruction).

Each person with sickle cell anemia has a different hypoxic threshold and different factors that precipitate a sickle cell crisis. Illness, cold exposure, and stress are known to trigger sickling crises in most people. In addition, these altered cells accumulate in capillaries and smaller blood vessels, making the blood more viscous. Normal circulation is impaired, causing pain, tissue infarctions, and swelling. Such blockage causes anoxic changes that lead to further sickling and obstruction.

DIAGNOSIS AND TREATMENT
Beyond a positive family history and typical clinical features, a stained blood smear showing sickle cells

and hemoglobin electrophoresis showing hemoglobin S confirm the diagnosis of sickle cell anemia. Electrophoresis on umbilical cord blood samples at birth screens neonates at risk. Additional laboratory studies show low RBC counts, elevated white blood cell and platelet counts, decreased erythrocyte sedimentation rate, increased serum iron levels, decreased RBC survival, and reticulocytosis. Hemoglobin levels may be low or normal.

If the patient is an adult, the doctor may order a lateral chest X-ray to detect the characteristic "Lincoln log" spinal deformity that leaves the vertebrae resembling logs that form the corner of a cabin. An ophthalmoscopic examination can detect corkscrew or comma-shaped vessels in the conjunctivae, another sign of this disease.

Although sickle cell anemia can't be cured, treatments can alleviate symptoms and prevent painful crises. Certain vaccines, such as polyvalent pneumococcal vaccine and *Haemophilus influenzae* B vaccine; anti-infectives such as low-dose oral penicillin; and chelating agents such as deferoxamine can minimize complications caused by the disease and by transfusion therapy.

With a patient in crisis, a review of the clinical features can reveal the type of crisis. (See *Classifying sickle cell crises*.) The doctor may prescribe other medications, such as analgesics to relieve the pain of a vaso-occlusive crisis. The patient may take iron supplements if folic acid levels are low. A good antisickling agent isn't yet available; the most commonly used drug, sodium cyanate, produces many adverse reactions.

Treatment begins before age 4 months with prophylactic penicillin. If the patient's hemoglobin level drops suddenly or is chronically low, he'll need a transfusion of packed RBCs.

In an acute sequestration crisis, treatment includes sedation and administration of analgesics, blood transfusion, oxygen therapy, and large amounts of oral or I.V. fluids. (See *Managing sickle cell crisis,* pages 618 and 619.)

COLLABORATIVE MANAGEMENT
Care of the patient with sickle cell anemia focuses on improving systemic perfusion, modifying lifestyle, and teaching the patient about the disease and related therapies.

ASSESSMENT
Signs and symptoms usually don't develop until after age 6 months because large amounts of fetal hemoglobin protect infants. Look for:
■ reports of chronic fatigue, unexplained dyspnea or dyspnea on exertion, joint swelling, aching bones, chest pain, ischemic leg ulcers (especially around the ankles), and an increased susceptibility to infection
■ a history of pulmonary infarctions and cardiomegaly.
■ apparent jaundice or pallor
■ a young child who appears small for his age
■ an older child who's experiencing delayed growth and puberty
■ an adult with a spiderlike body build (narrow shoulders and hips, long extremities, curved spine, and barrel chest)
■ tachycardia
■ hepatomegaly and, in children, splenomegaly (splenomegaly usually is absent in adulthood because the spleen shrinks over time)
■ possibly, systolic and diastolic murmurs on auscultation.
In sickle cell crisis, look for:
■ history of recent infection, stress, dehydration
■ other conditions that provoke hypoxia, such as strenuous exercise, high altitude, unpressurized aircraft, cold, and vasoconstrictive drugs
■ complaints of sleepiness with difficulty awakening, severe pain and, sometimes, hematuria
■ pale lips, tongue, palms, and nail beds; lethargy; listlessness; and commonly irritability
■ body temperature over 104° F (40° C) or a temperature of 100° F (37.8° C) that persists for 2 or more days.

NURSING DIAGNOSES AND COLLABORATIVE PROBLEMS
Based on the following nursing diagnoses, you'll establish patient outcomes.
Altered systemic tissue perfusion related to impaired circulation. The patient will:
■ identify risk factors that exacerbate altered tissue perfusion
■ exhibit no signs or symptoms of severe tissue ischemia, such as pain, coldness and color change of affected body part, or organ dysfunction
■ regain and maintain tissue perfusion and cellular oxygenation.
Knowledge deficit related to management of sickle cell anemia. The patient will:
■ express his need to manage sickle cell anemia
■ seek and obtain necessary information about sickle cell anemia management from appropriate sources
■ demonstrate skill in managing his disease, as evidenced by a decrease in the number and severity of sickle cell crises.
Pain related to tissue ischemia secondary to decreased oxygen-carrying ability of RBCs and impaired circulation. The patient will:
■ express feelings of comfort after he's given analgesics

Classifying sickle cell crises

The following characteristic signs and symptoms help determine the type of sickle cell crisis that the patient is experiencing.

Vaso-occlusive crisis
The most common crisis and the hallmark of sickle cell disease, a vaso-occlusive crisis (also called painful crisis or infarctive crisis) usually appears periodically after the patient reaches age 5. It results from blood vessel obstruction by rigid, tangled sickle cells, which causes tissue anoxia and, possibly, necrosis.

Vaso-occlusive crisis is characterized by severe abdominal, thoracic, muscle, or bone pain and, possibly, increased jaundice, dark urine, or a low-grade fever. A patient with long-term disease may experience autosplenectomy, in which splenic damage and scarring is so extensive that the spleen shrinks and becomes impalpable. This can lead to increased susceptibility to *Streptococcus pneumoniae* sepsis, which can be fatal without prompt treatment.

After the crisis subsides (in 4 days to several weeks), infection may develop, producing lethargy, sleepiness, fever, and apathy.

Aplastic crisis
Associated with infection (usually viral), an aplastic crisis (megaloblastic crisis) is caused by bone marrow depression. It's characterized by pallor, lethargy, sleepiness, dyspnea, possible coma, markedly decreased bone marrow activity, and red blood cell (RBC) hemolysis.

Acute sequestration crisis
Affecting infants between ages 8 months and 2 years, an acute sequestration crisis may cause sudden, massive entrapment of RBCs in the spleen and liver. This rare crisis causes lethargy and pallor and, if untreated, commonly progresses to hypovolemic shock and death.

Hemolytic crisis
This rare type of sickle-cell crisis usually affects patients who have glucose-6-phosphate dehydrogenase deficiency with sickle cell anemia. It's probably caused by complications of sickle cell anemia, such as infection, rather than by the disorder itself.

In hemolytic crisis, degenerative changes cause liver congestion and hepatomegaly. Chronic jaundice worsens, although increased jaundice doesn't always indicate a hemolytic crisis.

- identify practices that trigger a sickle cell crisis and try to eliminate or decrease them
- become pain-free when the sickle cell crisis is over.

PLANNING AND IMPLEMENTATION
These measures help the patient with sickle cell anemia.
- Encourage the patient to talk about his fears and concerns. Try to stay with him during periods of severe crisis and anxiety. Provide reassurance, when possible, but always answer his questions honestly.
- If a male patient develops sudden, painful priapism, reassure him that such episodes are common and have no permanent harmful effects.
- Ensure that the patient receives adequate amounts of folic acid–rich foods such as leafy green vegetables. Encourage adequate fluid intake to hydrate the patient; give parenteral fluids if necessary. Provide eggnog, ice pops, and milk shakes to meet fluid requirements.
- Give blood transfusions as ordered. Use strict aseptic technique.
- Arrange for the patient to rest with his head elevated to decrease tissue oxygen demand. Give oxygen only if the patient is experiencing severe dyspnea.

- If he requires general anesthesia for surgery, help ensure that he receives adequate ventilation to prevent hypoxic crisis. Make sure the surgeon and the anesthesiologist are aware that the patient has sickle cell anemia, and provide a preoperative transfusion of packed RBCs, as needed.
- Monitor the patient's complete blood count regularly.
- Check his hydration status. Monitor his intake and output, and check for signs of dehydration.
- Monitor for signs and symptoms of sickle cell crisis and chronic complications.
- Watch for signs and symptoms of infection, such as fever, chills, or purulent drainage.
- Monitor the patient's respiratory status. Perform a respiratory assessment, including regular auscultation of breath sounds. Monitor arterial blood gas levels as indicated.
- Apply warm compresses, warmed thermal blankets, and warming pads or mattresses to painful areas of the patient's body. Consider the weight of the warming appliance to avoid causing pain. Never apply cold to a painful area.

(Text continues on page 620.)

CLINICAL PATH

Managing sickle cell crisis

DRG #395
Target length of stay: 6 days

	Day 1/Date:	Day 2/Date:	Day 3/Date:
CONSULTS	■ Chronic pain management group		
TESTS	■ Hemogram ■ Sedimentation rate ■ Reticulocyte count ■ Lactate dehydrogenase (LD) levels		
SPECIMENS	■ Oxygen at 2 L/minute by nasal cannula		
TREATMENTS	■ Vital signs every 4 hours while awake	—————————▶	—————————▶
VITAL SIGNS	■ Every shift		—————————▶
INTAKE & OUTPUT	■ Diet as tolerated ■ Fluids forced to 1,000 ml every 24 hours	—————————▶	—————————▶
DIET	■ Beverage of choice kept at bedside ■ I.V. fluids as ordered	—————————▶ —————————▶ —————————▶	—————————▶ —————————▶ —————————▶
I.V. FLUIDS	■ I.V. pain medication as ordered	—————————▶	
MEDICATIONS	■ Bed rest	—————————▶	—————————▶
ACTIVITY		■ Up in chair as tolerated	
TEACHING	■ Assess patient's knowledge of disease. ■ Review clinical path with patient and family. ■ Explain need for oxygen therapy to prevent further sickling.	■ Explain heredity factor. ■ Explain physiology of the disease.	■ Explain the need to drink 8 glasses of water daily (unless contraindicated).
DISCHARGE PLANNING	■ Notify social service department.	■ Social service to see patient	■ Formulate discharge plan.

Nurse signature	Nurse signature	Nurse signature
_____ Shift _____	_____ Shift _____	_____ Shift _____
Nurse signature	Nurse signature	Nurse signature
_____ Shift _____	_____ Shift _____	_____ Shift _____
Nurse signature	Nurse signature	Nurse signature
_____ Shift _____	_____ Shift _____	_____ Shift _____

Adapted with permission from Baptist Hospital, Pensacola, Fla. Courtesy of Center for Case Management, Inc., South Natick, Mass.

Day 4/Date:	Day 5/Date:	Day 6/Date:
		■ Patient discharged per doctor's order
	■ Call results in early a.m.: –Hemogram –Sedimentation rate –Reticulocyte count –LD levels	
■ Oxygen as needed	———————————————→	———————————————→
■ Routine		
	———————————————→	———————————————→
———————————————→	■ Discontinued when patient taking 1,500 ml in 24 hours	
■ Fluids forced to 1,500 ml every 24 hours	———————————————→ ———————————————→	———————————————→ ———————————————→
■ I.V. discontinued to adaptor when patient taking 1,500 ml every 24 hours	■ Adaptor discontinued if laboratory values are within normal limits	
■ Pain medication changed to oral (or I.M. if oral isn't effective)	■ Oral pain medication only	———————————————→
■ Up as tolerated	———————————————→	———————————————→
■ Explain pain management for after discharge. ■ Review clinical path and patient progress.	■ Teach importance of meticulous personal hygiene and avoiding people with known infection. ■ Stress that signs and symptoms of infection require immediate follow-up with doctor.	■ Verify patient's understanding of instructions provided.
———————————————→	■ Verify transportation arrangements.	■ Schedule follow-up appointment with doctor.
Nurse signature ———————————— Shift ——— Nurse signature ———————————— Shift ——— Nurse signature ———————————— Shift ———	Nurse signature ———————————— Shift ——— Nurse signature ———————————— Shift ——— Nurse signature ———————————— Shift ———	Nurse signature ———————————— Shift ——— Nurse signature ———————————— Shift ——— Nurse signature ———————————— Shift ———

- Give analgesics and antipyretics as necessary. Each patient's level of pain is different; some may require acetaminophen to control the pain; others may have continuous pain during crisis while receiving morphine.
- Assess the patient's response to the drugs he's given (especially analgesics) and other therapy such as warm compresses.

Patient teaching

- To help the patient prevent exacerbation of sickle cell anemia, advise him to avoid tight clothing that restricts circulation.
- Warn against strenuous exercise, vasoconstricting medications, cold temperatures (including drinking large amounts of ice water and swimming), unpressurized aircraft, high altitude, and other conditions that provoke hypoxia.
- Stress the importance of normal childhood immunizations, meticulous wound care, good oral hygiene, regular dental checkups, and a balanced diet as safeguards against infection.
- Emphasize the need for prompt treatment of infection.
- Explain the need to increase fluid intake to prevent dehydration that results from impaired ability to properly concentrate urine. Tell parents to encourage a child with sickle cell anemia to drink more fluids, especially in the summer, by offering milk shakes, ice pops, and eggnog.
- To encourage normal mental and social development, warn parents against being overprotective. Although the child must avoid strenuous exercise, he can enjoy most everyday activities.
- Refer parents of children with sickle cell anemia for genetic counseling to answer their questions about risk to future offspring. Recommend screening of other family members to determine if they're heterozygote carriers.
- Because delayed growth and later puberty are common, reassure an adolescent patient that he will grow and mature.
- Review the symptoms of vaso-occlusive crisis so that the patient and his family members will recognize and treat it early. As appropriate, explain how to care for this condition at home. Prepare parents for an infant's first "hand-foot crisis," during which the infant's hands, feet, or both swell and become painful.
- Inform the patient and his parents that if he is hospitalized for a vaso-occlusive crisis, he may receive I.V. fluids and analgesics, oxygen therapy, and blood transfusions.
- If appropriate, discuss how special conditions, such as surgery and pregnancy, may affect the patient.

- Stress that the patient should inform all health care providers that he has this disease before he undergoes any treatment—especially major surgery. Explain that any procedure that involves general anesthesia will require that he have adequate ventilation to prevent hypoxic crisis. Urge him to wear medical identification stating that he has sickle cell anemia.
- Warn women with sickle cell anemia that they're poor obstetric risks. However, their use of oral contraceptives is also risky; refer them for birth control counseling.
- Urge a pregnant patient to maintain a balanced diet during pregnancy and tell her to ask the doctor about a folic acid supplement.
- If necessary, arrange for psychological counseling to help the patient cope. Suggest that he join an appropriate support group, such as the National Association for Sickle Cell Disease.

EVALUATION

Achievement of patient outcomes determines the success of collaborative management. For sickle cell anemia, evaluation focuses on improved knowledge of the disease and related therapies, increased systemic perfusion, and maintenance of adequate nutrition.

Thrombocytopenia

The most common cause of hemorrhagic disorders, thrombocytopenia is characterized by a deficient number of circulating platelets. Because platelets play a vital role in coagulation, this disease poses a serious threat to hemostasis. The prognosis is excellent in drug-induced thrombocytopenia if the offending drug is withdrawn; in such cases, recovery is usually immediate. Otherwise, the prognosis depends on the patient's response to treatment of the underlying cause.

Complications of thrombocytopenia are usually related to bleeding. Severe thrombocytopenia can cause acute hemorrhage, which in many cases is fatal without immediate therapy. The most common sites of severe bleeding include the brain and the GI tract, although intrapulmonary bleeding and cardiac tamponade are possible.

CAUSES

Thrombocytopenia is congenital or acquired. The acquired form is more common. In either case, it's usually caused by decreased or defective production of platelets in the marrow (for example, in leukemia, aplastic anemia, and toxicity with certain drugs) or from increased destruction outside the marrow caused by an underlying disorder (such as cirrhosis of the liver, disseminated intravascular coagulation, and severe infection).

Less commonly, thrombocytopenia is caused by sequestration (hypersplenism, hypothermia) or platelet loss. Acquired thrombocytopenia may be caused by the use of certain drugs, such as quinine, quinidine, rifampin, heparin, nonsteroidal anti-inflammatory drugs (NSAIDs), histamine blockers, most chemotherapy, and alcohol.

Thrombocytopenia also may follow infection (such as Epstein-Barr) or infectious mononucleosis. There's also an idiopathic form of thrombocytopenia.

DIAGNOSIS AND TREATMENT

The following tests support a diagnosis of thrombocytopenia:
- diminished platelet count (less than 100,000/µl)
- prolonged bleeding time (although this doesn't always indicate platelet quality)
- normal prothrombin and partial thromboplastin times.

Platelet antibody studies can help determine why the platelet count is low and help direct treatment. Platelet survival studies help differentiate between ineffective platelet production and inappropriate platelet destruction. (Platelet production disorders may follow radiation exposure, drug treatment, or an infectious disease. They may also occur idiopathically. Inappropriate platelet destruction may accompany splenic disease and platelet antibody disorders.)
- In severe thrombocytopenia, a bone marrow study determines the number, size, and cytoplasmic maturity of the megakaryocytes (the bone marrow cells that release mature platelets). This information may identify ineffective platelet production as the cause of thrombocytopenia and rule out a malignant disease process.

Removal of the offending agents in drug-induced thrombocytopenia or proper treatment of the underlying cause (when possible) is essential. Corticosteroids may increase platelet production. Lithium carbonate or folate can stimulate bone marrow production of platelets. In cases of severe or refractory thrombocytopenia, I.V. gamma globulin has been used experimentally with moderate success.

Platelet transfusions are used to stop episodic abnormal bleeding caused by a low platelet count. However, if platelet destruction is caused by an immune disorder, platelet infusions may have only a minimal effect, and the doctor may reserve it for life-threatening bleeding.

Rarely, the doctor may use splenectomy to correct thrombocytopenia caused by platelet destruction. A splenectomy should significantly reduce platelet destruction because the spleen acts as the primary site of platelet removal and antibody production.

COLLABORATIVE MANAGEMENT

Care of the patient with thrombocytopenia focuses on safety, restored energy, and patient teaching.

ASSESSMENT

Typically, a patient with thrombocytopenia reports sudden onset of petechiae and ecchymoses from bleeding into mucous membranes (GI, urinary, vaginal, or respiratory). He may also complain of malaise, fatigue, and general weakness (with or without accompanying blood loss). In acquired thrombocytopenia, the patient's history may include the use of one or several offending drugs.

Inspection typically reveals evidence of bleeding (petechiae, ecchymoses), along with slow, continuous bleeding from any injuries or wounds. Painless, round, and as tiny as pinpoints (1 to 3 mm in diameter), petechiae usually appear on dependent portions of the body, appearing and fading in crops and sometimes grouping to form ecchymoses. Another form of blood leakage and larger than petechiae, ecchymoses are purple, blue, or yellow-green bruises that vary in size and shape. They can appear anywhere on the body from traumatic injury. In patients with bleeding disorders, they usually appear on the arms and legs. In adults, inspection may reveal large, blood-filled bullae in the mouth. Gentle palpation of edematous ecchymotic areas may cause pain, indicating that these areas are actually hematomas. Superficial hematomas are red; deep hematomas are blue. They typically exceed 1 cm in diameter.

If the patient's platelet count is between 30,000 and 50,000/µl, expect bruising with minor trauma; if it's between 15,000 and 30,000/µl, expect spontaneous bruising and petechiae, mostly on the arms and legs; and with a platelet count below 15,000/µl or, after minor trauma, mucosal bleeding, generalized purpura, epistaxis, hematuria, and GI or intracranial bleeding. Female patients may report menorrhagia.

NURSING DIAGNOSES AND COLLABORATIVE PROBLEMS

Based on the following nursing diagnoses, you'll establish patient outcomes.

Altered protection related to decreased platelet count. The patient will:
- communicate an understanding of the importance of taking bleeding precautions
- identify precautions to incorporate into his daily life

Controlling local bleeding

The following agents may be used at home and in the health care facility to stem local bleeding and capillary oozing.

Agents for home use

Let your patient know about preparations that may be used at home, such as absorbable gelatin sponges (Gelfoam), ice packs, and dicresulene polymer (Negatan).

If the doctor recommends Gelfoam to stop the bleeding—from a puncture wound (venipuncture) or tooth extraction, for example—tell the patient to saturate this foamlike wafer with an isotonic saline solution or a thrombin solution. Instruct him to place the sponge on the bleeding site and apply pressure for 10 to 15 seconds. Advise him to keep the sponge in place after the bleeding stops. Explain that this agent, which holds many times its weight in blood, can be systemically absorbed.

If the patient is bleeding from a blood vessel or into a joint (hemarthrosis), instruct him to elevate the bleeding part and apply an ice pack to the site until the bleeding subsides.

Inform the patient that Negatan—an astringent and protein denaturant—may be applied to oral ulcers. Tell him first to clean and dry the ulcer and then to apply the preparation for 1 minute. Next, he should neutralize the area with large amounts of water.(Because the agent may burn or sting, tell the patient that he may apply a topical anesthetic first.)

Agents for health care facility use

Inform the surgical patient that bleeding can be controlled with such agents as oxidized cellulose (Surgicel) or thrombin (Thrombinar).

Surgicel, for instance, helps to control surgical bleeding or external bleeding at open wounds. This agent may remain in place until hemostasis occurs. The caregiver then irrigates it (to prevent fresh bleeding) and removes it with sterile forceps.

Thrombinar may be used during surgery or for GI bleeding. The caregiver mixes the agent with sterile isotonic saline solution or sterile distilled water and applies it to the wound or (for GI bleeding) mixes the agent with milk, which the patient drinks. Some patients react to Thrombinar with hypersensitivity and fever.

■ carry out bleeding precautions, as evidenced by a decrease in bleeding episodes or in the number of ecchymoses and hematomas.

Fatigue related to blood loss. The patient will:
■ explain the relationship between fatigue, thrombocytopenia, and his activity level
■ employ measures to prevent and modify fatigue
■ express a feeling of increased energy with effective management of thrombocytopenia.

Knowledge deficit related to management of thrombocytopenia. The patient will:
■ identify the need to learn how to manage thrombocytopenia
■ obtain information on thrombocytopenia management from appropriate sources
■ communicate an understanding of thrombocytopenia management.

PLANNING AND IMPLEMENTATION

These measures help the patient with thrombocytopenia.

■ Provide emotional support, as necessary. Encourage the patient to discuss his concerns about his condition. Reassure him that the ecchymoses and petechiae will heal as the disease resolves.

■ If the patient has painful hematomas, handle the area gently. Protect all areas of ecchymosis and petechia from further injury.

■ Take every possible precaution against bleeding. Protect the patient from trauma. Keep the bed's side rails raised, and pad them if possible. Promote the use of an electric razor and a soft toothbrush. Avoid invasive procedures, such as venipuncture, rectal temperatures, or urinary catheterization, if possible. When venipuncture is unavoidable, exert pressure on the puncture site for at least 20 minutes or until the bleeding stops.

■ Monitor platelet count daily.

■ When giving platelet concentrate, remember that platelets are extremely fragile; infuse them quickly, using the administration set recommended by the blood bank.

■ Remember that human leukocyte antigen (HLA)-typed platelets may be ordered to prevent febrile reaction. If the patient has a history of minor reactions, he may benefit from acetaminophen and diphenhydramine before the transfusion.

■ During platelet transfusion, monitor for a febrile reaction (flushing, chills, fever, headache, tachycardia, hypertension). Such reactions are common, and a fever will destroy the blood products.

■ One to 2 hours after giving platelet concentrate, monitor the patient's platelet count to assess his response to the infusion. A lack of platelet level increase indicates that the patient is making platelet antibodies and should receive HLA-matched platelets.

■ Watch for bleeding (petechiae, ecchymoses, surgical or GI bleeding, menorrhagia). Identify the amount of bleeding or the size of ecchymoses at least every 24 hours. Check urine, stool, and emesis for blood.

■ Provide rest periods between activities if the patient tires easily.

■ During active bleeding, maintain strict bed rest. Keep the head of the bed elevated to prevent gravity-related pressure increases, which may lead to intracranial bleeding.

Patient teaching

■ Teach the patient about his disorder and its cause, if known. If appropriate, reassure the patient that thrombocytopenia commonly resolves spontaneously.

■ Teach the patient to recognize and report menorrhagia, gingival or urinary tract bleeding, signs of intracranial bleeding (persistent headache, mood change, nausea, vomiting, and drowsiness), and other signs of bleeding (tarry stools, coffee-ground vomitus, epistaxis.)

■ Teach the patient how to control local bleeding. (See *Controlling local bleeding.*)

■ Advise the patient to avoid straining during defecation or coughing; both can lead to increased intracranial pressure, possibly causing cerebral hemorrhage.

■ Discuss the diagnostic tests he may need throughout the course of the disease.

■ Explain the function of platelets. Warn the patient that the lower his platelet count falls, the more cautious he'll have to be in his activities.

■ Confirm that he understands that in severe thrombocytopenia, even minor bumps or scrapes may result in bleeding.

■ If thrombocytopenia is drug-induced, stress the importance of ending drug abuse.

■ If the patient must receive long-term steroid therapy, teach him to watch for and report cushingoid symptoms. Emphasize that corticosteroids must be discontinued gradually. While the patient is receiving corticosteroid therapy, monitor his fluid and electrolyte balance and watch for infection, pathologic fractures, and mood changes.

■ Warn the patient to avoid taking aspirin in any form as well as other drugs that impair coagulation. Teach him how to recognize aspirin compounds and NSAIDs listed on labels of over-the-counter remedies.

■ If the patient experiences frequent nosebleeds, recommend that he use a humidifier at night. Also suggest that he moisten his inner nostrils twice a day with an anti-infective ointment.

■ Teach the patient to monitor his condition by examining his skin for ecchymoses and petechiae. Tell him how to test his stools for occult blood.

■ Advise the patient to carry medical identification stating that he has thrombocytopenia.

EVALUATION

Achievement of patient outcomes determines the success of collaborative management. For thrombocytopenia, evaluation focuses on increased knowledge, improved protection, and decreased fatigue.

Vitamin B$_{12}$ anemia

Also known as pernicious anemia and Addison's anemia, vitamin B$_{12}$ anemia is a megaloblastic anemia characterized by decreased gastric production of hydrochloric acid and deficiency of intrinsic factor, a substance normally secreted by the parietal cells of the gastric mucosa that is essential for vitamin B$_{12}$ absorption.

In the United States, vitamin B$_{12}$ anemia is most common in New England and the Great Lakes region. It's rare in children, Blacks, and Asians. Most of those affected are between ages 50 and 60; incidence rises with increasing age.

Patients treated with vitamin B$_{12}$ injections have few permanent complications. Those who go untreated may experience permanent neurologic disability (including paralysis) and psychotic behavior; they also may lose sphincter control of bowel and bladder, and some eventually may die of the disorder. Although the reason is unclear, the incidence of peptic ulcer disease is four to five times greater in patients with vitamin B$_{12}$ anemia than in the general population.

CAUSES

Familial incidence of vitamin B$_{12}$ anemia suggests a genetic predisposition. This disorder is significantly more common in patients with immunologically related diseases, such as thyroiditis, myxedema, and Graves' disease.

These facts seem to support a widely held theory that an inherited autoimmune response causes gastric mucosal atrophy and consequently decreases hydrochloric acid and intrinsic factor production. Intrinsic factor deficiency impairs vitamin B$_{12}$ absorption. The resultant vitamin B$_{12}$ deficiency inhibits the growth of all cells, particularly red blood cells (RBCs), leading to insufficient and deformed RBCs with poor oxygen-carrying capacity. Deficiency of vitamin B$_{12}$ causes serious neurologic, psychological, gastric, and intestinal abnormalities. Increasingly fragile cell membranes induce widespread destruction of RBCs, resulting in low hemoglobin levels.

Vitamin B_{12} anemia also impairs myelin formation. Initially, it affects the peripheral nerves, but gradually it extends to the spinal cord, causing neurologic dysfunction. Anemia can result from partial removal of the stomach, which limits the amount of productive mucosa.

DIAGNOSIS AND TREATMENT

The Schilling test is the definitive test for vitamin B_{12} anemia. Results of blood, bone marrow, and gastric analyses also help establish the diagnosis. Laboratory screening must rule out other anemias with similar symptoms, such as folic acid deficiency anemia, because treatment differs. Diagnosis must also rule out vitamin B_{12} deficiency resulting from malabsorption due to GI disorders, gastric surgery, radiation therapy, or drug therapy.

Early I.M. vitamin B_{12} replacement can reverse anemia and may prevent permanent neurologic damage. An initial high dose of parenteral vitamin B_{12} causes rapid RBC regeneration. Within 2 weeks, hemoglobin should rise to normal and the patient's condition should markedly improve. Because rapid cell regeneration increases the patient's iron requirements, concomitant iron replacement is necessary to prevent iron deficiency anemia. After the patient's condition improves, vitamin B_{12} doses can be decreased to maintenance levels and checked monthly.

If anemia causes extreme fatigue, the patient may require bed rest until hemoglobin rises. If he is critically ill with severe anemia and cardiopulmonary distress, he may need blood transfusions, digitalis glycosides, a diuretic, and a low-sodium diet for heart failure. Most important is the replacement of vitamin B_{12} to control the condition that led to this failure. Antibiotics help combat accompanying infections, and topical anesthetics may relieve mouth pain.

COLLABORATIVE MANAGEMENT

Care of the patient with vitamin B_{12} anemia focuses on improving activity level, avoiding injury, and improving nutrition.

ASSESSMENT

Although vitamin B_{12} anemia usually has an insidious onset, the patient's history may reveal this characteristic triad of symptoms: weakness; a beefy red, sore tongue; and numbness and tingling in the extremities. Also look for:
- complaints of nausea, vomiting, anorexia, weight loss, flatulence, diarrhea, and constipation
- tongue that appears beefy red and smooth

- slightly jaundiced sclera and pale to bright yellow skin, with hemolysis-induced hyperbilirubinemia
- rapid pulse rate and a systolic murmur
- enlarged liver and spleen
- with neurologic involvement, complaints of weakness in the extremities, peripheral numbness and paresthesia, disturbed position sense, lack of coordination, impaired fine finger movement, light-headedness, headache
- also with neurologic involvement, altered vision (diplopia, blurred vision), taste, and hearing (tinnitus); loss of bowel and bladder control; and, in males, impotence
- evidence that the patient is irritable, depressed, delirious, and ataxic and has poor memory
- positive Babinski's and Romberg's signs and optic muscle atrophy, possibly temporary, but evidence of irreversible central nervous system changes.
- complaints of weakness, fatigue, and light-headedness from the impaired oxygen-carrying capacity of the blood owing to lowered hemoglobin levels
- compensatory increased cardiac output that may cause palpitations, dyspnea, orthopnea, tachycardia, premature beats and, eventually, heart failure.

NURSING DIAGNOSES AND COLLABORATIVE PROBLEMS

Based on the following nursing diagnoses, you'll establish patient outcomes.

Activity intolerance related to fatigue and weakness. The patient will:
- demonstrate skill in conserving energy while performing daily activities to tolerance level
- regain and maintain his normal activity level with effective treatment.

Altered nutrition: Less than body requirements related to vitamin B_{12} deficiency and adverse GI effects. The patient will:
- regain and maintain his weight within normal range
- comply with vitamin B_{12} replacement therapy
- report alleviation of adverse GI effects with effective treatment.

Risk for injury related to falls and hand injuries associated with neurologic changes. Based on this nursing diagnosis, you'll establish these patient outcomes. The patient will:
- incorporate safety precautions into his activities of daily living (ADLs)
- seek and obtain assistance with activities as needed
- remain free from injury.

PLANNING AND IMPLEMENTATION

These measures help the patient with vitamin B_{12} anemia.

- If the patient has severe anemia, plan activities, rest periods, and necessary diagnostic tests to conserve his energy.
- Monitor the patient's pulse rate often; tachycardia means the patient's activities are too strenuous.
- Give vitamin B_{12} as prescribed.
- Provide a well-balanced diet, including foods high in vitamin B_{12} (meat, liver, fish, eggs, and milk). Offer between-meal snacks, and encourage family members to bring favorite foods from home.
- Because a sore mouth and tongue make eating painful, ask the dietitian to avoid giving the patient irritating foods. If these symptoms make talking difficult, supply a pad and pencil or some other aid to facilitate nonverbal communication.
- Explain the patient's communication problem to family members.
- Provide diluted mouthwash or, with severe conditions, swab the patient's mouth with tap water or warm saline solution. The patient may use oral anesthetics diluted in normal saline solution.
- Institute safety precautions to prevent falls.
- Check for evidence of decreased perfusion to vital organs, such as dyspnea, chest pain, and dizziness, and for signs and symptoms of neuropathy such as peripheral tingling.
- If neurologic damage causes behavioral problems, assess mental and neurologic status often. If necessary, give tranquilizers, as ordered; if needed, apply a soft restraint at night.

Patient teaching

- Warn the patient to guard against infections, and tell him to report signs of infection promptly, especially pulmonary and urinary infections. The patient's weakened condition may increase his susceptibility to infection.
- Caution the patient with a sensory deficit to avoid exposure of his extremities to extreme heat or cold.
- If neurologic involvement is present, advise the patient to avoid clothing with small buttons and ADLs that require fine motor skills.
- Teach family members to observe for confusion or irritability and to report these findings to the doctor.
- Stress that vitamin B_{12} replacement isn't a permanent cure and that he must continue these injections for life, even after symptoms subside.
- If possible, teach the patient or his caregiver proper injection technique.
- To prevent pernicious anemia, emphasize the importance of vitamin B_{12} supplements for patients who have had extensive gastric resections or who follow strict vegetarian diets.

EVALUATION

Achievement of patient outcomes determines the success of collaborative management. For vitamin B_{12} anemia, evaluation focuses on improving nutrition, decreasing fatigue, and preventing injury.

Treatments and procedures

Bone marrow transplantation and splenectomy are two of the various treatments available for hematologic and lymphatic disorders.

BONE MARROW TRANSPLANTATION

The treatment of choice for aplastic anemia and severe combined immunodeficiency diseases, bone marrow transplantation involves the infusion of fresh or stored bone marrow into a recipient. The doctor also may use the procedure to treat acute leukemia, chronic leukemia, lymphoma, multiple myeloma, and certain solid tumors.

PROCEDURE

In bone marrow transplantation, marrow cells are collected from either the patient or another donor and given to the patient. The bone marrow used in the transplantation may be obtained by autologous, syngeneic, or allogeneic means. In an autologous donation, the bone marrow is harvested from the patient before he's given chemotherapy or radiation therapy or while he's in remission, and then it's frozen for later use.

In a syngeneic donation, bone marrow is taken from the patient's identical twin. Obviously, syngeneic donations are rare. But, when possible, they are the ideal type. That's because an identical twin has healthy bone marrow that is histologically identical to the patient's own tissue.

The most common type of transplant involves an allogeneic donation. For this procedure, bone marrow is obtained from a histocompatible individual. This is usually a sibling, although it's possible for an unrelated donor to meet the requirements. Because the donor's and patient's tissue don't match perfectly, the patient must receive immunosuppressive therapy. Even then, the procedure isn't always successful.

A new method, peripheral stem cell transplantation, involves the collection of peripheral stem cells, usually after the patient has been treated with chemotherapy or growth factors to increase the number of circulating stem cells. The cells are stored and later reinfused into the patient following high-dose chemotherapy and possibly radiotherapy.

DISCHARGE READY > **After bone marrow transplantation**

After undergoing bone marrow transplantation, the patient will meet the following criteria before discharge:

- temperature within his normal limits
- laboratory studies (white blood cell, hematologic) within his normal limits
- absence of complications
- understanding of his treatment regimen and the requirements of following his treatment program.

If the patient is to receive his own bone marrow, the donation will have been made 2 weeks earlier and frozen. For a syngeneic or allogeneic transplant, doctors obtain the donor bone marrow in the operating room the same day as the transplant. The infusion procedure is done at the patient's bedside. Just before the procedure, you'll give an antihistamine or analgesic, as ordered, to minimize adverse reactions.

For an allogeneic or syngeneic donation, someone will bring the bone marrow to the patient's room as soon as it's obtained. For an autologous donation, the marrow will be allowed to thaw. Then, the doctor will infuse it into the patient through a central venous (CV) catheter.

The rate of infusion varies, depending on the volume of marrow being infused. Once infused, the marrow cells will migrate to the patient's marrow cavity, where they'll begin to proliferate. This process, called engraftment, takes 10 days to 4 weeks.

COLLABORATIVE MANAGEMENT

Care of the patient undergoing bone marrow transplantation requires thorough preparation, close monitoring, and intense patient teaching.

Preparation

- Reinforce the doctor's explanation of bone marrow transplantation. Give the patient and his family members or friend time to discuss the procedure and its risks and benefits. Remember to confirm that they understand that if the transplant fails, the patient may die.
- Inform the patient that, because the procedure depletes his white blood cells, he'll be at high risk for infection immediately after the procedure and may remain in reverse isolation for several weeks. Explain that contact with his family will be limited during this time.

- Prepare the patient for the pretransplant regimen. Explain that he will receive chemotherapy or radiation therapy (or both) to kill any residual cancer cells.
- During this pretransplant regimen, expect to see adverse reactions, such as bone marrow suppression, diarrhea, nausea, vomiting, and mucositis. Give prophylactic antiemetics, as ordered. Monitor intake and output and give fluids to prevent fluid and electrolyte imbalances and cystitis.
- Before the procedure begins, make sure that diphenhydramine and epinephrine are readily available to manage transfusion reactions. Start an I.V. line for hydration and record vital signs. Obtain an administration set (without a filter, which can trap the marrow cells) for the bone marrow infusion.

Monitoring and aftercare

- Once the transfusion has begun, take the patient's vital signs at least every 15 minutes for 1 hour, every 30 minutes for the next 2 hours, and then every hour for another 4 hours. The patient's vital signs will help you promptly recognize such reactions as fever, dyspnea, and hypotension.
- Monitor the patient for other reactions, such as bronchospasm, urticaria, erythema, chest pain, and back pain. Give ordered drugs to relieve these symptoms.
- Continue to monitor the patient's vital signs closely, and assess him every 4 hours for any signs or symptoms of infection, such as fever or chills.
- Because the patient is already pancytopenic from the pretransplant regimen, he's at risk for hemorrhage as well as infection. Maintain strict asepsis when caring for him, and take measures to protect him from injury. The doctor may also order blood or platelet transfusions (or both), and the patient may be placed in a room with laminar air flow system to further reduce the possibility of infection.
- Draw blood for laboratory analysis, as ordered, and monitor the patient's hematologic status. Notify the doctor immediately of any changes.
- On the seventh day after the transplant, begin to watch for symptoms of graft-versus-host disease (GVHD), such as dermatitis, hepatitis, hemolytic anemia, and thrombocytopenia. (See *After bone marrow transplantation.*)

Patient teaching

- Tell the patient and family members about infection control measures, such as avoiding crowds and people with known infections.
- Instruct the patient to avoid activities with an increased risk of injury or bleeding, such as playing con-

tact sports or using a razor blade. Suggest that the patient shave with an electric razor.

■ Teach the patient and family how to care for the CV catheter.

■ Instruct them about his medication regimen, including how to give his medications.

■ Tell them about potential complications and what signs and symptoms to watch for. Stress the importance of contacting the doctor immediately if any symptoms appear.

■ Make sure the patient and his family members have emergency telephone numbers, such as those for the doctor managing his posttransplant follow-up care, the facility where the transplant was performed, and ambulance services.

■ Stress the need to keep follow-up medical appointments so that the doctor can monitor his progress and detect complications.

■ If the patient is a child, explain to the parents that his growth may be impaired by bone marrow transplantation. Tell them to monitor their child's growth; if it lags, he may need hormonal therapy.

COMPLICATIONS

During infusion, potential complications include volume overload, anaphylaxis, and pulmonary fat emboli. After infusion, the patient may develop an infection or abnormal bleeding. If the bone marrow was obtained from an allogeneic donor, the patient may develop GVHD. This serious complication can occur anywhere from a few days to years after transplantation.

SPLENECTOMY

Splenectomy, surgical removal of the spleen, helps treat various hematologic disorders. It's also done as an emergency procedure to stop hemorrhage after traumatic splenic rupture.

The most common reason for splenectomy is hypersplenism—a combination of splenomegaly and cytopenia that occurs in such disorders as hairy cell leukemia, Felty's syndrome, myeloid metaplasia, thalassemia major, and Gaucher's disease. In addition, splenectomy is the treatment of choice for such diseases as hereditary spherocytosis and chronic idiopathic thrombocytopenic purpura. What's more, it may be performed in Hodgkin's disease to establish the stage of the disease and determine the appropriate therapy.

During splenectomy, after the patient is placed under general anesthesia, the surgeon exposes the peritoneal cavity through a left rectus paramedial or subcostal incision. He ligates the splenic artery and vein and the ligaments that hold the spleen in place. Then he removes the spleen. After carefully checking for

any bleeding, he closes the abdomen, commonly placing a drain in the left subdiaphragmatic space. After the incision site is sutured and dressed, the patient is returned to the postanesthesia care unit.

COLLABORATIVE MANAGEMENT

Care of the patient undergoing splenectomy requires thorough preparation, close monitoring, and intense patient teaching.

Preparation

■ Explain to the patient that splenectomy involves removal of his spleen under general anesthesia. Tell him that he can lead a normal life without the organ but will be more prone to infection.

■ Obtain the results of blood studies, including coagulation tests and a complete blood count, and report them to the doctor. If ordered, transfuse blood to correct anemia or hemorrhagic loss. Similarly, give vitamin K to correct clotting factor deficiencies.

■ Take the patient's vital signs and perform a baseline respiratory assessment. Note especially signs of respiratory infection, such as fever, chills, crackles, rhonchi, and a cough. Notify the doctor if you suspect respiratory infection; he may delay surgery.

■ Teach the patient coughing techniques to help prevent postoperative pulmonary complications.

■ Ensure that the patient or a responsible family member has signed a consent form.

Monitoring and aftercare

■ During the early postoperative period, watch carefully—especially if the patient has a bleeding disorder—for bleeding from the wound or drain and for signs of internal bleeding, such as hematuria or hematochezia.

■ The patient may have leukocytosis and thrombocytosis after splenectomy and they may persist for years. Because thrombocytosis may predispose the patient to thromboembolism, help him get out of bed and walk as soon as possible after surgery. In addition, encourage him to perform coughing and deep-breathing exercises to reduce the risk of pulmonary complications.

■ Give pain sedation as needed.

■ Watch for signs or symptoms of infection, such as fever and sore throat, and monitor hematologic studies. If infection develops, give prescribed antibiotics.

Patient teaching

■ Inform the patient that he's at an increased risk for infection, and urge him to report any telltale signs and symptoms, such as fever or chills.

■ Teach him measures to help prevent infection.

COMPLICATIONS

Besides bleeding and infection, splenectomy can cause such complications as pneumonia and atelectasis because of the location of the spleen close to the diaphragm and the need for a high abdominal incision restrict lung expansion after surgery. In addition, splenectomy patients are vulnerable to infection because of the spleen's role in the immune response.

Selected references

DeVita, et al.. *Cancer Principles and Practice of Oncology,* 5th ed. Philadelphia: Lippincott-Raven Pubs., 1997.

Diseases, 2nd ed. Springhouse, Pa.: Springhouse Corp., 1997.

Heuther, S., and McCance, K. *Understanding Pathophysiology.* St Louis: Mosby–Year Book, Inc. 1996.

Holleb, M.D., et al. *American Cancer Society Textbook of Clinical Oncology,* 2nd ed. Atlanta: American Cancer Society, 1995.

Illustrated Manual of Nursing Practice, 2nd ed. Springhouse, Pa.: Springhouse Corp., 1994.

Langer, E.G., and Hertzfield, L. "Action STAT: Hemolytic Transfusion Reaction," *Nursing95* 25(7):33, July 1995.

McCorkle, R., et al. *Cancer Nursing,* 2nd ed. Philadelphia: W.B. Saunders Co., 1996.

Nursing98 Drug Handbook. Springhouse, Pa.: Springhouse Corp., 1998.

Polaski, A., and Tatro, S.E. *Luckmann's Core Principles and Practice of Medical-Surgical Nursing.* Philadelphia: W.B. Saunders Co., 1996.

Williams, M.D., et al. *Hematology,* 5th ed. New York: McGraw-Hill Book Co., 1996.

Immunologic disorders

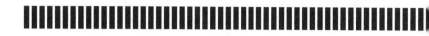

The immune system's billions of circulating cells and specialized structures, such as the lymph nodes, are scattered throughout the body. Because immunologic disorders can cause or be caused by problems in other systems, caring for a patient with an immunologic disorder can challenge your assessment techniques.

Anatomy and physiology review

The immune system consists of specialized cells (lymphocytes and macrophages) and structures, including lymph nodes, spleen, thymus, bone marrow, tonsils, adenoids, and appendix. The blood includes plasma and numerous kinds of blood cells. Although they're distinct entities, the immune system and blood are closely related. For example, their cells share a common origin in the bone marrow, and the immune system uses the bloodstream to transport its components.

CELL ORIGIN

A process called hematopoiesis forms the bone marrow's pluripotential stem cells that develop into immune system and blood cells. In the embryo, pluripotential stem cells develop in the yolk sac, liver, spleen, lymph nodes, and bone marrow. In the neonate, all bone marrow has hematopoietic potential, but hematopoiesis takes place only in a few bone marrow sites. In the adult, hematopoiesis happens only in the marrow of particular bones—for example, in the flat bones of the cranium, vertebral column, pelvis, ribs, and sternum and in the proximal ends of some long bones, such as the femur.

Differentiation of the precursor cells takes place almost exclusively in the bone marrow. Under normal conditions, cells aren't released into circulation until

they are nearly or completely mature. However, bone marrow activity varies among individuals.

IMMUNITY

Immunity is the body's capacity to resist invading organisms and toxins and thereby prevent tissue and organ damage. The immune system's cells and organs perform that function. (See *Understanding immune system organs and tissues,* pages 630 and 631.) Designed to recognize, respond to, and eliminate foreign substances (antigens), such as bacteria, fungi, viruses, and parasites, the immune system also preserves the internal environment by scavenging dead or damaged cells. The immune system uses three basic defense strategies: protective surface phenomena, general host defenses, and specific immune responses.

PROTECTIVE SURFACE PHENOMENA

Strategically placed physical, chemical, and mechanical barriers work to prevent organism entry. Intact and healing skin and mucous membranes provide the first line of defense against microbial invasion, preventing attachment of microorganisms. Skin desquamation (normal cell turnover) and low pH further impede bacterial colonization. Seromucous surfaces, including the conjunctiva of the eye and the oral mucous membranes, are protected by antibacterial substances such as the enzyme lysozyme found in tears, saliva, and nasal secretions.

The respiratory system requires special protection because microorganisms enter it easily from outside. Nasal hairs and turbulent airflow through the nostrils filter foreign materials. Nasal secretions contain an immunoglobulin (naturally produced antibody) that discourages microbe adherence. A mucous layer that is continuously sloughed off and replaced lines the

(Text continues on page 632.)

◆◆◆   **629**

Understanding immune system organs and tissues

The immune system is made up of organs and tissues in which lymphocytes predominate, plus cells that circulate in peripheral blood. The bone marrow and the thymus are central lymphoid organs. Peripheral lymphoid organs include the lymph nodes and vessels, spleen, tonsils, adenoids, appendix, and intestinal lymphoid tissue (Peyer's patches).

The bone marrow and the thymus play roles in developing the primary cells of the immune system: B cells and T cells. Both cell types probably originate in the bone marrow. B cells may also mature and differentiate from multipotential stem cells in the bone marrow. T cells mature and differentiate in the thymus, a bilobular endocrine gland located in the upper mediastinum. B and T cells are distributed throughout the tissue of the peripheral lymphoid organs, especially the lymph nodes and spleen.

Lymph nodes

Most abundant in the head, neck, axillae, abdomen, pelvis, and groin, lymph nodes are small, oval-shaped structures located along a network of lymph channels. They help remove and destroy antigens circulating in the blood and lymph.

Each lymph node is surrounded by a fibrous capsule that extends bands of connective tissue (trabeculae) into the node, dividing it into three compartments: superficial cortex, deep cortex, and medulla.

The superficial cortex of the node contains follicles made up predominantly of B cells. During an immune response, the follicles enlarge and develop a germinal area with large proliferating cells. The deep cortex consists mostly of T cells as do the interfollicular areas. The medulla contains numerous plasma cells that actively secrete immunoglobulins during an immune response.

Afferent lymphatic vessels carry lymph into the subcapsular sinus of the node. From here, it flows through cortical sinuses and smaller radial medullary sinuses. Phagocytic cells in the deep cortex and medullary sinuses attack the antigen. The antigen may also be trapped in the follicles of the superficial cortex.

Cleaned lymph leaves the node through efferent lymphatic vessels at the hilum. These vessels drain into specific lymph node chains, which in turn drain into large lymph vessels known as trunks that empty into the subclavian vein of the vascular system. In most parts of the body, lymphatic vessels and lymphatic capillaries help veins and blood capillaries function by draining many body tissues and increasing the return of blood to the heart.

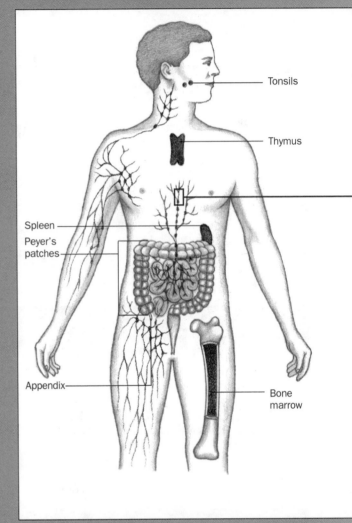

Lymph usually travels through more than one lymph node, because numerous nodes line the lymphatic channels that drain a particular region. For example, axillary nodes filter drainage from the arms; femoral nodes (located in the inguinal region) filter drainage from the legs. This arrangement prevents organisms that enter peripheral body areas from migrating unchallenged to central areas. Lymph nodes are also a principal source of circulating lymphocytes, which provide specific immune responses.

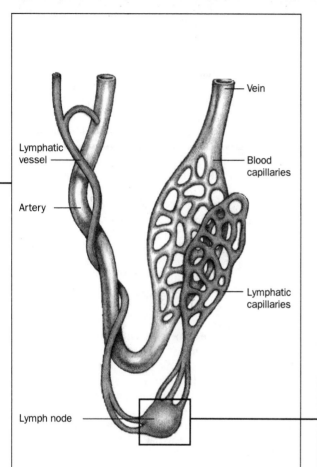

Lymphatic vessel

Artery

Lymph node

Vein

Blood capillaries

Lymphatic capillaries

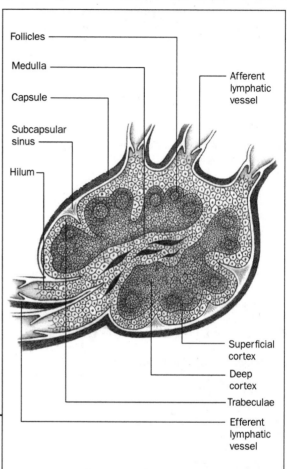

Follicles

Medulla

Capsule

Subcapsular sinus

Hilum

Afferent lymphatic vessel

Superficial cortex

Deep cortex

Trabeculae

Efferent lymphatic vessel

Spleen

This lymphoid organ is located in the left upper quadrant of the abdomen beneath the diaphragm. Major splenic functions include gathering and isolating worn-out erythrocytes and storing blood and 20% to 30% of platelets. The spleen also filters and removes foreign materials, worn-out cells, and cellular debris.

Accessory organs

Other lymphoid tissues—including the tonsils, adenoids, appendix, thymus, and Peyer's patches—also remove foreign debris in much the same manner as lymph nodes. They are positioned in food and air passages, which are likely areas of microbial access.

respiratory tract. This mucus layer, coupled with ciliary action, traps and expels inhaled particles and microbes before they can damage delicate alveolar tissues.

In the GI system, saliva, swallowing, peristalsis, and defecation mechanically remove bacteria. Furthermore, the low pH of gastric secretions is bactericidal, rendering the stomach virtually free of viable bacteria. Resident bacteria prevent colonization by other microorganisms, protecting the remainder of the GI system through a process known as colonization resistance.

The urinary system is sterile except for the distal end of the urethra and the urinary meatus. Working together, urine flow, low urine pH, an immunoglobulin, and the bactericidal effects of prostatic fluid (in men) impede bacterial colonization. A series of sphincters also inhibits bacterial migration.

GENERAL HOST DEFENSES

The immune system launches nonspecific cellular responses in an attempt to identify and remove an invader. These nonspecific responses differentiate self from nonself but can't distinguish specific antigens or respond to them individually. Inflammation, the first of these responses against an antigen, causes four characteristic signs and symptoms: heat, redness, swelling, and pain. Phagocytosis takes place after inflammation or in chronic infections. Neutrophils and macrophages engulf, digest, and dispose of the antigen. Macrophages and lymphocytes move to the site of insult and infection by two means: diapedesis (blood cell migration from the intravascular compartment to tissue sites) and chemotaxis (movement toward a chemical attractor).

SPECIFIC IMMUNE RESPONSES

All foreign substances elicit the same response in general host defenses. By contrast, particular microorganisms or molecules activate specific immune responses and can initially involve specialized sets of immune cells. Such specific responses are classified as either humoral or cell-mediated immunity. Lymphocytes (B cells and T cells) produce the responses.

Humoral immunity. In this specific response, an invasive antigen causes B cells to divide and differentiate into plasma cells that produce and secrete antigen-specific antibodies. The five types of antibodies, or immunoglobulins, are immunoglobulin A (IgA), IgD, IgE, IgG, and IgM. Each type serves a particular function: IgA, IgG, and IgM protect against viral and bacterial invasion; IgD acts as an antigen receptor of B cells; and IgE causes an allergic response.

After the body's initial exposure to an antigen, there's a time lag during which tests will detect little or no antibody. During this time, the B cell recognizes the antigen, and the sequence of division, differentiation, and antibody formation begins. This primary antibody response happens 4 to 10 days after the first antigen exposure during which immunoglobulin levels increase and then quickly dissipate and IgM antibodies form.

Subsequent exposure to the same antigen initiates a secondary antibody response. In this response, memory B cells manufacture antibodies (now mainly IgG), achieving peak levels in 1 to 2 days. These elevated levels persist for months and then fall slowly. The secondary immune response is, therefore, faster, more intense, and more persistent, and it amplifies with each subsequent exposure to the same antigen.

An antigen-antibody complex forms after the antibody reacts to the antigen. It serves several functions. First, a macrophage processes the antigen and presents it to antigen-specific B cells. Then, the antibody activates the complement system, causing an enzymatic cascade that destroys the antigen. The activated complement system bridges humoral and cell-mediated immunity and causes the arrival of phagocytic neutrophils and macrophages at the antigen site. This combination of humoral and cell-mediated immune responses is common.

Cell-mediated immunity. Cell-mediated immunity protects the body against bacterial, viral, and fungal infections and resists transplanted cells and tumor cells. In the cell-mediated response, a macrophage processes the antigen, which is then presented to T cells. Some T cells become sensitized and destroy the antigen; others release lymphokines, which activate macrophages that destroy the antigen. Sensitized T cells then travel through the blood and lymphatic systems, providing ongoing surveillance in their quest for specific antigens.

Assessment

Assessment begins with a complete patient history. Remember that immune system disorders have wide-reaching effects, so inquire about all body systems and don't discount the importance of minor symptoms.

HISTORY

Build your nursing history by asking the patient open-ended questions as systematically as possible to avoid overlooking important information.

CHIEF COMPLAINT

Determine the patient's chief complaint. He may report vague signs and symptoms, such as lack of energy, light-headedness, or frequent bruising. Encourage him to elaborate, and ask about associated signs and symptoms. For instance, has he experienced lymphadenopathy, weakness, or joint pain? If so, ask when he first noticed the problem and if it affects one side of his body or both.

MEDICAL HISTORY

Because the immune system affects all body functions, ask about any changes in the patient's overall health. Has he developed any rashes, abnormal bleeding, or slow-healing sores? What about vision disturbances, fever, or changes in elimination patterns? Ask a female patient if her menstrual periods have changed recently. For example, do they last longer or occur more frequently? Have they become irregular? Has the volume or nature of the menstrual flow changed? A menstrual pattern change may be the first sign of a bleeding disorder stemming from an inadequate platelet count or function or from deficient clotting factors.

FAMILY HISTORY

Find out if the patient has a family history of cancer or hematologic or immune disorders. Also ask if he has undergone any procedures, such as recent blood transfusions or past organ transplants, that would affect his immune system.

SOCIAL HISTORY

Finally, remember to inquire about his home and work environments to determine if he's being exposed to hazardous chemicals or other agents.

PHYSICAL EXAMINATION

Besides examining the patient's spleen and lymph nodes (the only accessible immune system structures), remember to evaluate his general appearance, vital signs, and related body structures. The effects of immune disorders are far-reaching and may materialize in several body systems.

ASSESSING APPEARANCE AND VITAL SIGNS

Begin by observing the patient's physical appearance. Look for signs of acute illness, such as grimacing or profuse perspiration, and of chronic illness, such as emaciation and listlessness. Determine whether the patient's stated age and appearance agree. Also observe the patient's facial features for facial expression, edema, and weakness.

Next, measure the patient's height and weight. Compare the findings with normal values for the patient's bone structure. Observe his posture, movements, and gait.

Finally, assess his vital signs, noting especially whether they vary from his normal baseline measurements. Remember to check his pulse rate and respiratory rate and character. Measure blood pressure with the patient in supine, seated, and standing positions.

ASSESSING RELATED BODY STRUCTURES

Because immune disorders affect so many body systems, your assessment must include physical effects in such areas as the skin, hair, and nails; head and neck; eyes and ears; and respiratory, cardiovascular, GI, urinary, nervous, and musculoskeletal systems.

Skin, hair, and nails. Observe the color of the patient's skin; normally there's a slightly rosy undertone, even in dark-skinned patients.

Evaluate skin integrity for signs of inflammation or infection, such as redness, swelling, heat, or tenderness. Remember to pay close attention to sites of recent invasive procedures, such as venipuncture, bone marrow biopsies, or surgery, for evidence of wound healing. Also check for rashes and note their distribution.

Observe hair texture and distribution, noting any alopecia (hair loss) on the arms, legs, or head. Alopecia in these areas and broken hairs above the hairline on the forehead (lupus hairs) appear with systemic lupus erythematosus (SLE).

Inspect the patient's nail color and texture, which should appear pink, smooth, and slightly convex.

Head and neck. An immune disorder may affect the nose and mouth. Using a penlight, assess the nasal cavity. Then, inspect the oral mucous membranes. They should appear pink, moist, smooth, and lesionless. Observe the gums. They should be pink, moist, and slightly irregular with no spongy or edematous areas.

Eyes and ears. First, test eye muscle strength using the six cardinal positions of gaze and the convergence tests. Next, inspect the color of the patient's conjunctiva (normally pink) and sclera (normally white). Assess the fundus with an ophthalmoscope. The retina should appear light yellow to orange, and the background should be free from hemorrhages, aneurysms, and exudates.

Test the patient's hearing acuity with the whispered or spoken voice test and the watch tick test. Using an otoscope, observe the tympanic membrane for erythema, bulging, indistinct landmarks, and a displaced light reflex.

Respiratory system. Observe the patient's respiratory rate, rhythm, and energy expenditure related to respiratory effort. Note the position he assumes to ease breathing. Percuss the anterior, lateral, and posterior thorax, comparing one side with the other. Auscultate over the lungs to assess for adventitious (abnormal) sounds.

Cardiovascular system. Assess the pulse rate and rhythm for anemia-related tachycardia or other arrhythmias. Then palpate and auscultate the heart and vessels for other signs of immune or blood disorders. Palpate the point of maximal impulse (PMI), normally located in the fifth intercostal space at the midclavicular line. The PMI may feel broadened, displaced, or less distinct because of ventricular enlargement, the body's compensatory mechanism for severe anemia. Auscultate for heart sounds over the precordium, and assess the patient's peripheral circulation.

GI system. First, auscultate the abdomen for bowel sounds. Next, percuss the liver. Then, palpate the abdomen to detect enlarged organs and tenderness.

Finally, inspect the anus, which should appear pink and puckered, without inflammation or breaks in the mucosal surface. Defer internal examination of the anus and rectal vault if you suspect or know that the patient has a low platelet count or granulocyte level.

Urinary system. Because immune dysfunctions also may affect the urinary system, obtain a urine specimen and evaluate its color, clarity, and odor.

Inspect the urinary meatus. In a patient with a white blood cell (WBC) deficiency or an immunodeficiency, the external genitalia may be focal points for inflammation, often accompanied by discharge or bleeding related to infection.

Nervous system. Evaluate the patient's level of consciousness and mental status. He should be alert and respond appropriately to questions and directions.

Other neurologic effects may provide clues to an underlying disorder. For example, a patient with SLE may experience altered mentation, depression, or psychosis.

Musculoskeletal system. Ask the patient to perform simple maneuvers, such as standing up, walking, and bending over. He should move effortlessly. Then test joint range of motion, particularly in the hand, wrist, and knee. Palpate the joints to assess for swelling, tenderness, and pain.

EXAMINING THE SPLEEN

As you assess the patient's immune system, percuss and palpate the spleen. First, percuss the spleen to estimate its size. Remember that the spleen normally produces dullness in the left upper quadrant between the 6th and 10th ribs.

Next, palpate the spleen to detect tenderness and confirm splenomegaly. The spleen must be enlarged approximately three times normal size to be palpable.

INSPECTING LYMPH NODES

The first step in regional lymph node assessment is to inspect areas where the patient reports "swollen glands" or "lumps," looking for color abnormalities and visible lymph node enlargement. Then inspect all other nodal regions. Remember to proceed from head to toe to avoid missing any region. Normally, you can't see lymph nodes.

PALPATING LYMPH NODES

Use the pads of your index and middle fingers to palpate the patient's superficial lymph nodes in the head and neck and in the axillary, epitrochlear, inguinal, and popliteal areas. Apply gentle pressure and rotary motion to feel the underlying nodes without obscuring them by pressing them into deeper soft tissues.

If palpation reveals nodal enlargement or other abnormalities, note the following characteristics of the node: location, size, shape, surface, consistency, symmetry, mobility, color, tenderness, temperature, pulsations, and vascularity.

To describe the location of the node, use reference points, such as body axis and lines, to pinpoint the site, or sketch the location, if appropriate. Then indicate the nodal length, width, and depth in centimeters, and describe or sketch its shape. Remember to describe its surface as smooth, nodular, or irregular. Identify the consistency of the node as hard, soft, firm, resilient, spongy, or cystic. Evaluate its symmetry, comparing the node with similar structures on the other side of the body. Describe the node's degree of mobility. If it is immobile, indicate whether it's fixed to overlying tissues, underlying tissues, or both. During palpation, note whether any tenderness is elicited by palpation, movement, or rebound phenomenon (tenderness that occurs after the pressure of the palpating fingerpads is released). Describe any color change, such as pallor, erythema, or cyanosis, in overlying skin. Note whether the site feels warm. Remember to watch for pulsations in the mass; plan to auscultate a pulsating mass for a bruit. If the node exhibits increased vascularity, describe any changes in the overlying blood vessels.

Use a flashlight to further assess an abnormal lump in an area you can transluminate, such as the scrotum. Describe the results of translumination along with the other characteristics. A lump that allows light to pass through it indicates fluid, which usually defines a cyst rather than a node.

Acquired immunodeficiency syndrome

Infection with human immunodeficiency virus (HIV) leads to incurable and progressive acquired immunodeficiency syndrome (AIDS). The syndrome is marked by gradual destruction of CD4+ T cells by the HIV. The resulting immunodeficiency predisposes the patient to opportunistic infections, unusual cancers, and other characteristic abnormalities.

HIV can infect virtually any cell that has the CD4+ molecule on its surface. These include monocytes, macrophages, bone marrow progenitors, and glial, gut, and epithelial cells. Such infections can cause dementia, wasting syndrome, and hematologic abnormalities.

AIDS was first described by the Centers for Disease Control and Prevention (CDC) in 1981. Since then, the CDC has issued a case surveillance definition for AIDS and has modified it several times, most recently in 1993.

The course of AIDS can vary, but the syndrome usually results in death from opportunistic infections. Antiretroviral therapy—with zidovudine, for instance—and prophylaxis and treatment for common opportunistic infections can delay but not stop the progression. Most experts believe that virtually everyone infected with HIV will develop AIDS.

In the United States, AIDS appears most commonly in homosexual and bisexual men, I.V. drug users, neonates of HIV-infected women (through cervical or blood contact at delivery or to an infant through breast milk), recipients of contaminated blood or blood products (although infection by transfusion of blood has been drastically reduced since 1985), and heterosexual partners of those in high-risk groups. HIV isn't transmitted by ordinary household or social contact.

Because of similar routes of transmission, AIDS shares epidemiologic patterns with other sexually transmitted diseases and hepatitis B.

The average duration between HIV exposure and diagnosis is 8 to 10 years, although the incubation period can vary.

CAUSES

The AIDS-transmitting human retrovirus is classified as either HIV-1 or HIV-2, with HIV-1 as the most common cause of AIDS throughout the world. The less common HIV-2 has been identified as predominant in western Africa and is considered less pathogenic than HIV-1. Both types destroy CD4+ T cells, the essential regulators and effectors of the normal immune response.

DIAGNOSIS AND TREATMENT

The CDC defines AIDS as an illness characterized by laboratory evidence of HIV infection and severe immunosuppression coexisting with one or more indicator conditions. Patients age 13 or over with repeatedly reactive screening tests for the HIV-1 antibody (enzyme-linked immunosorbent assay) who also have the HIV-1 antibody identified by supplemental tests (Western blot, immunofluorescence assay) are considered infected.

Other methods for diagnosing HIV-1 include direct identification of the virus in host tissues by virus isolation, antigen detection, and detection of HIV genetic material (deoxyribonucleic acid or ribonucleic acid) by polymerase chain reaction.

The CD4+ T-cell count is used to measure the severity of immunosuppression in an HIV-positive patient. An absolute CD4+ T-cell count of less than 200 cells/µl indicates severe immunosuppression. If the absolute count is unavailable, the doctor may use the percentage of CD4+ cells in total T cells; a percentage of less than 14% indicates severe immunosuppression.

Other markers of immune status, such as serum neopterin, beta$_2$ microglobulin, HIV p24 antigen, soluble interleukin-2 receptors, immunoglobulin A, and delayed-type hypersensitivity (DTH) skin-test reactions, may help in the evaluation of individual patients.

No cure has yet been found for AIDS. However, several antiretroviral treatments can slow the progression of HIV or temporarily inactivate the virus. Also, immunomodulatory drugs strengthen the immune system, and anti-infective and antineoplastic drugs combat opportunistic infections and associated cancers. Some anti-infectives also serve as prophylaxes against opportunistic infections. New protocols combine two or more of these drugs to produce the maximum benefit with the fewest adverse reactions. Combination therapy also helps inhibit the production of mutant HIV strains resistant to a particular drug.

Although many opportunistic infections respond to anti-infective drugs, they tend to recur after treatment. As a result, the patient usually requires continued prophylaxis until the drug loses its effectiveness or can no longer be tolerated.

Zidovudine, the most commonly used antiretroviral, effectively slows the progress of HIV infection, decreasing the number of opportunistic infections, prolonging survival, and curbing the progress of associated dementia.

Didanosine, another antiretroviral drug, treats advanced HIV infection in adult patients and in pediatric patients over age 6 months. It's a choice for adult patients with advanced HIV infection who've already received prolonged treatment with zidovudine. Protease inhibitors such as saquinavir (Invirase) attack the viral enzyme protease, significantly reducing the viral load. They also increase CD4+ counts when used in combination with antiviral agents.

COLLABORATIVE MANAGEMENT
Care of the patient with AIDS focuses on avoiding infections, developing emotional support systems, and teaching him about the disease.

ASSESSMENT
After initial exposure, the infected person may have no recognizable signs or symptoms or may experience a mononucleosis-like syndrome for 3 to 6 weeks and then remain asymptomatic for years. Look for:
- a history that suggests exposure to HIV—most often through unprotected sex with an infected partner or sharing I.V. needles
- initial complaints of fever, rigors, arthralgia, myalgia, maculopapular rash, urticaria, abdominal cramps, and diarrhea
- symptoms of aseptic meningitis, such as severe headache and stiff neck
- as the syndrome progresses, neurologic symptoms of HIV encephalopathy, an opportunistic infection, or cancer
- palpable lymph nodes in two or more extra-inguinal sites, a sign of lymphadenopathy
- behavioral, cognitive, and motor changes associated with progressive dementia, which occurs in about 30% of patients
- in children (incubation time averages 17 months), signs and symptoms resembling an adult's
- in children, a history of bacterial infections, such as otitis media, pneumonias (other than that caused by *Pneumocystis carinii*)
- in children, sepsis, chronic salivary gland enlargement, and lymphoid interstitial pneumonia.

NURSING DIAGNOSES AND COLLABORATIVE PROBLEMS
Based on the following nursing diagnoses, you'll establish patient outcomes.

Anticipatory grieving related to the incurable, progressive nature of AIDS. The patient will:
- identify and express feelings about potential losses
- accept feelings and behavior brought on by potential losses
- use appropriate coping mechanisms to deal with potential losses, and contact support groups as needed.

Risk for infection related to immunosuppression. The patient will:

- maintain a normal temperature and white blood cell count and differential; cultures won't exhibit pathogen growth
- remain free from signs of infection
- demonstrate appropriate personal and oral hygiene and take appropriate daily precautions.

Social isolation related to misunderstanding of AIDS transmission and social stigma. The patient will:
- express his feelings about lack of supportive relationships
- identify and contact available resources to establish supportive relationships
- participate in social activity, as his health permits.

PLANNING AND IMPLEMENTATION
These measures help the patient with AIDS.
- To help prevent AIDS transmission, follow standard precautions.
- Treat infections as ordered.
- Provide the patient with normal saline or bicarbonate mouthwash for daily oral rinsing. Avoid glycerin swabs, which dry the mucous membranes.
- Record the patient's calorie intake. He may need total parenteral nutrition, although this treatment creates a potential route for infection.
- Ensure adequate fluids during episodes of diarrhea.
- Provide meticulous skin care, especially in the debilitated patient.
- Monitor the patient for fever and signs of infection, such as skin breakdown, cough, sore throat, and diarrhea. Assess for swollen, tender lymph nodes, and check laboratory values regularly.
- If the patient develops Kaposi's sarcoma, monitor the progression of the lesions.
- Watch for opportunistic infections or signs of disease progression.
- Encourage the patient to maintain as much physical activity as he can tolerate.
- Recognize that a diagnosis of AIDS has a devastating impact on the patient, his socioeconomic status, and his family relationships.
- Help him cope with an altered body image and the emotional burden of serious illness and the threat of death.

Patient teaching
- Teach the patient and his family members, sexual partners, and friends about AIDS and its transmission. Tell him not to donate blood, blood products, organs, tissue, or sperm. (See *Teaching about HIV transmission.*)
- Urge the patient to inform potential sexual partners and health care workers that he has HIV infection.
- If the patient uses I.V. drugs, caution him not to share needles.

- Inform the patient that high-risk sexual practices for AIDS transmission are those that exchange body fluids, such as intercourse without a condom. Discuss safe sexual practices, such as hugging, mutual masturbation, and protected sexual intercourse.
- Advise the female patient to avoid pregnancy. Explain that an infant may become infected before birth, during delivery, or through breast-feeding.
- Teach the patient to identify the signs of infection, and stress the importance of seeking immediate medical attention if infection appears.
- Involve the patient with hospice care early so he can form a relationship. If he develops AIDS dementia in stages, help him understand its progression.

EVALUATION
Achievement of patient outcomes determines the success of collaborative management. For the patient with AIDS, evaluation focuses on absence of secondary infection, reduced social isolation, and anticipatory grieving.

HEALTHY LIVING

Teaching about HIV transmission

Clear information about the transmission of human immunodeficiency virus (HIV) is essential to your patient teaching. Review the following with your patient:

- HIV is transmitted by contact with infected blood or body fluids.
- Transmission is caused by such high-risk behaviors as sharing a contaminated needle or having unprotected sexual contact—especially anal intercourse, which results in mucosal trauma.
- The virus also may be spread through transfusion of contaminated blood or blood products.
- The virus can pass from an infected mother to the fetus through cervical or blood contact at delivery or to an infant through breast milk.
- HIV isn't transmitted by ordinary household or social contact.

Hypersensitivity reactions

Hypersensitivity reactions occur when the immune response is exaggerated or inappropriate. The antigen-antibody or antigen-lymphocyte reaction causes a response that damages the body's tissues.

CAUSES
Immune system hyperfunction may have a genetic origin. Its triggers are many. Type I hypersensitivity responses are triggered when an allergen interacts with immunoglobulin E (IgE) antibodies, triggering the release of histamine, other mediators, complement, acetylcholine, kinins, and chemotactic factors resulting in anaphylaxis. They're triggered by environmental proteins, such as pollen, animal dander, or bee or wasp stings, or by drugs or substances the patient may be allergic to.

Type II cytotoxic reactions may be stimulated by an exogenous antigen, such as foreign tissue or cells and drug reactions that result in hemolytic anemia. Endogenous antigens can stimulate a type II reaction, resulting in an autoimmune disorder (Goodpasture's syndrome, Hashimoto's thyroiditis).

Type III immune complex–mediated hypersensitivities are caused by the formation of IgG or IgM antibody-antigen immune complexes in the circulation. Histamine is released and chemotactic factors attract neutrophils, which, in turn, attempt to phagocytize the immune complexes. Lysosomal enzymes are released, increasing tissue damage. Small blood vessel walls, the kidneys, and the joints are sites of immune complex deposits. A patient may have a localized response. For example, when immune complexes accumulate in the membrane of the kidney (as with streptococcal infections or systemic lupus erythematosus) the result may be glomerulonephritis. His lungs may respond to the dust of moldy hay or pigeon feces by developing an acute alveolar inflammatory response, such as in farmer's lung. Another example of type III immune complex–mediated hypersensitivity is serum sickness, resulting in a systemic response. Drugs such as penicillin and sulfonamides can also cause serum sickness.

Type IV delayed hypersensitivities are cell mediated, involving T cells, and may appear 24 to 48 hours after exposure to the antigen, causing an exaggerated response such as contact dermatitis. It's triggered by a variety of antigens, such as poison ivy, positive tuberculin tests, and graft rejection episodes.

DIAGNOSIS AND TREATMENT
To support a diagnosis of hypersensitivity reaction, the doctor will use allergy testing to determine the cause of the sensitivity.

If the cause of a reaction is documented or suspected (I.V. medications or transfusion), the allergen is withdrawn immediately. Maintenance of the airway is the priority, especially in type I reactions. Epinephrine is given subcutaneously (S.C.) or I.V. to counteract effects. Aggressive management of bleeding or renal failure may be required with type II reactions. Type III requires removing the offending antigen and interrupting the inflammatory response.

Antihistamines, anti-inflammatory drugs, immunotherapy, cromolyn sodium (Intal or Nasalcrom), glucocorticoids, and plasmapheresis may also help.

COLLABORATIVE MANAGEMENT

Care of the patient with a hypersensitivity reaction focuses on maintenance of the airway and cardiac output, safety, and patient teaching.

ASSESSMENT

The patient with type I IgE reaction or type II hypersensitivity reaction has a widespread antibody-antigen reaction and response to chemical mediators. In both types, look for:
- dyspnea or impaired breathing and other signs of anaphylaxis, urticaria or angioedema of the eyes, hands, feet, lips, genitalia, and tongue
- reports of a sense of foreboding, light-headedness, itching palms and scalp, hives
- air hunger, stridor, wheezing, barking cough
- impaired tissue perfusion, hypotension, and shock.
  In a patient experiencing a type III reaction, look for:
- fever, urticaria, or rash
- arthralgias, myalgias, and lymphadenopathy.
  In type IV delayed hypersensitivity, look for:
- intense redness, itching
- thickening in the area of exposure to the antigen.

NURSING DIAGNOSES AND COLLABORATIVE PROBLEMS

Based on the following nursing diagnoses, you'll establish patient outcomes.

Ineffective airway clearance related to anaphylactic reactions. The patient will:
- maintain a patent airway.

Decreased cardiac output related to effects of vasodilation and permeability. The patient will:
- maintain tissue perfusion
- maintain respiratory status within established parameters.

Risk for injury related to potential hypersensitivity reaction. The patient will:
- remain uninjured.

PLANNING AND IMPLEMENTATION

These measures help the patient with a hypersensitivity reaction.
- Place the patient in Fowler's to high-Fowler's position to maintain an open airway and improve ventilation.
- Give the patient oxygen.
- Assess his airway by observing rate and pattern of breathing, level of consciousness (LOC), anxiety, nasal flaring, use of accessory muscles, stridor, and respiratory excursion.

- Insert an airway, if necessary.
- Remember to check the patient's history for allergies before giving any transfusions, drugs, or treatments.
- Give the patient epinephrine 1:1000, 0.3 to 0.5 ml S.C., as prescribed, and repeat in 20 to 30 minutes, as necessary.
- If your patient was bitten by an insect or snake, inject antivenin as ordered.
- Monitor vital signs, skin color, capillary refill, edema, and LOC for signs of decreased cardiac output.
- Insert large bore I.V. lines, and give warmed I.V. solutions, as prescribed.
- Insert an indwelling catheter and monitor the patient's urine output.
- Give blood or new medications slowly, according to your facility's policy, and observe the patient for reactions.

Patient teaching
- Teach the patient how to identify allergens and avoid them in the future.
- Emphasize the value of telling any health care workers he encounters, such as dentists, about his allergens.
- Discuss getting a medical identification bracelet if he is highly allergic.
- Teach the patient how to use allergy kits, if appropriate.
- Teach the patient how to use antihistamines and decongestants.
- Discuss autologous blood transfusions if he requires future transfusions for surgery.
- Patients with immune complex reactions require specific teaching, as in the treatment of disorders like strep throat, to reduce the risk of immune complex response such as glomerulonephritis.
- If your patient has contact dermatitis, teaching focuses on providing appropriate skin care, preventing infection, and promoting comfort.

EVALUATION

Achievement of patient outcomes determines the success of collaborative management. For the patient with a hypersensitivity reaction, evaluation focuses on airway maintenance, cardiac output maintenance, and decreased risk of injury.

Sjögren's syndrome

This disorder belongs to a group that includes rheumatoid arthritis (see Chapter 13); systemic lupus erythematosus (SLE; see Chapter 13); and vitamin B_{12} deficiency anemia, also known as pernicious anemia (see Chapter 14). All of them may stem from autoimmunity.

CAUSES

The second most common autoimmune rheumatic disorder after rheumatoid arthritis, Sjögren's syndrome is characterized by diminished lacrimal and salivary gland secretion. Its cause is unknown.

This syndrome affects mainly women (90% of patients) about age 50. It may be a primary syndrome or associated with connective tissue disorders, such as rheumatoid arthritis, scleroderma, SLE, and polymyositis. In some patients, the syndrome is limited to the exocrine glands (glandular Sjögren's syndrome); in others, it involves additional organs, such as the lungs and kidneys (extraglandular Sjögren's syndrome).

DIAGNOSIS AND TREATMENT

The following diagnostic tests support a diagnosis of Sjögren's syndrome:
- Erythrocyte sedimentation rate is almost always increased.
- Complete blood count shows mild anemia and leukopenia in 30% of patients; hypergammaglobulinemia occurs in 50% of patients.
- Rheumatoid factor is positive in most patients.
- Antinuclear antibodies are positive in 50% to 80% of patients.
- Antisalivary duct antibodies are positive.
- Schirmer's tearing test and slit-lamp examination with rose bengal dye evaluate eye involvement.
- The volume of parotid saliva and secretory sialography and salivary scintigraphy evaluate salivary gland involvement. Lower lip biopsy shows salivary gland infiltration by lymphocytes.

Treatment, usually aimed at relieving symptoms, includes conservative measures to relieve dry eyes or mouth. Dry mouth can be relieved by using a methylcellulose swab or spray and by drinking plenty of fluids, especially at mealtime. Meticulous oral hygiene is essential, including regular flossing, brushing, and fluoride treatment, and frequent dental checkups.

Treatment also includes advising the patient to avoid drugs that decrease saliva production, such as atropine derivatives, antihistamines, anticholinergics, and antidepressants. If mouth lesions make eating painful, suggest high-protein, high-calorie liquid supplements to prevent malnutrition.

Other measures vary with associated extraglandular findings. Parotid gland enlargement requires local heat and analgesics; pulmonary and renal interstitial disease responds to corticosteroids; accompanying lymphoma takes a combination of chemotherapy, surgery, or radiation.

COLLABORATIVE MANAGEMENT

Care of the patient with Sjögren's syndrome focuses on improving comfort, preventing infection, and providing patient teaching.

ASSESSMENT

Besides decreased or absent salivation, signs and symptoms include dry eyes with a persistent burning, gritty sensation. Look for:
- reports of vaginal dryness, causing dyspareunia
- skin dryness
- difficulty talking, chewing, and swallowing
- ulcers and soreness of the lips and parotid and submaxillary glands
- nasal crusting and epistaxis
- fatigue
- nonproductive cough
- polyuria.

NURSING DIAGNOSIS AND COLLABORATIVE PROBLEMS

Based on the following nursing diagnoses, you'll establish patient outcomes.

Altered oral mucous membranes related to effects of the disorder. The patient will:
- report improved salivation
- report diminished oral discomfort.

Risk for infection related to decreased secretions. The patient will:
- take measures to prevent infection
- remain free from infection.

PLANNING AND IMPLEMENTATION

These measures help the patient with Sjögren's syndrome.
- Evaluate the effect of prescribed drugs and lubrications on the patient's condition and comfort level.
- Instill artificial tears as often as every half hour to prevent eye damage (corneal ulcerations or opacifications) from insufficient tear secretions.
- Instill an eye ointment at bedtime or use sustained-release cellulose capsules (Lacrisert) twice daily, if indicated.
- Use aseptic technique and wash hands frequently.

Patient teaching

- Advise the patient to avoid sugar, which contributes to dental caries.
- Warn her against tobacco, alcohol, and spicy, salty, or highly acidic foods, which cause mouth irritation.
- Suggest the patient use sunglasses to protect her eyes from dust, wind, and strong light. Moisture chamber spectacles may also help.
- Because dry eyes are more susceptible to infection, advise the patient to keep her face clean and to avoid rubbing her eyes.

- If she develops an infection, tell her to get antibiotic treatment immediately. Stress that she should avoid topical steroids.
- To help relieve respiratory dryness, tell her to humidify her home and work environments.
- Suggest normal saline solution drops or aerosolized spray for nasal dryness.
- Advise the patient to avoid prolonged hot showers and baths and to use moisturizing lotions to help ease dry skin. Suggest using a vaginal lubricant.

EVALUATION
Achievement of patient outcomes determines the success of collaborative management. For the patient with Sjögren's syndrome, evaluation focuses on increased comfort and reduced infection.

Treatment-related immunosuppression

Cytotoxic drugs to prevent transplant rejection are immunosuppressive and act by reducing the proliferation of cells within the immune system. Monoclonal antibodies act by binding to surface antigens on T cells, removing them from circulation and inactivating those bound to allograft cells. Antilymphocyte globulin binds with peripheral lymphocytes and mononuclear cells, removing them from circulation.

Examples of treatments that intentionally cause immunosuppression are cytotoxic agents such as azathioprine (Imuran), cyclophosphamide (Cytoxan), and cyclosporine (Sandimmune); monoclonal antibody treatment with muromonab-CD3 or OKT3 (Orthoclone); and antilymphocyte globulins, such as antithymocyte globulin or ATG (Atgam) and antilymphocyte globulin or ALG.

DIAGNOSIS AND TREATMENT
When tests support a diagnosis of treatment-related immunosuppression, cultures of wounds and blood, urine, and sputum are positive for organisms. White blood cell (WBC) count is elevated in the presence of infection.

Treatment is basically supportive. The patient's blood counts are monitored, with particular attention to WBC and platelet counts. Studies are also done to evaluate liver and kidney function. Anaphylaxis and bleeding are treated if they occur.

COLLABORATIVE MANAGEMENT
Care of the patient with treatment-related immunosuppression focuses on improving laboratory abnormalities, reducing risk of infection, and supporting the patient.

ASSESSMENT
The patient experiencing immunosuppression may have altered WBC counts, temperature abnormalities, and signs of infection anywhere involving any of the body systems.

NURSING DIAGNOSES AND COLLABORATIVE PROBLEMS
Based on the following nursing diagnoses, you'll establish patient outcomes.

Risk for infection related to immunosuppression. The patient will:
- take measures to prevent infection
- remain free from signs and symptoms of infection.

Risk for injury to tissues and fluid volume deficit related to alteration in blood counts due to therapy. The patient will:
- take measures to prevent exsanguination
- remain free from signs and symptoms of bleeding and fluid volume deficit.

PLANNING AND IMPLEMENTATION
These measures help the patient with treatment-related immunosuppression.
- Since pulmonary fibrosis is a potential adverse effect of cyclophosphamines, monitor the patient for difficulty breathing and tell him to report any such difficulty.
- Remember that your patient on monoclonal antibody therapy requires chest X-rays and premedication with hydrocortisone, acetaminophen, and diphenhydramine to reduce potential adverse effects.
- Monitor your patient closely for anaphylaxis, and tell him which adverse effects to report immediately.

Patient teaching
- Teach the patient signs to report to the doctor, such as bruising and bleeding gums.
- Instruct the patient in measures to prevent bleeding, such as using a soft toothbrush, shaving with an electric razor, and avoiding contact sports.
- Stress that the patient should avoid using aspirin or ibuprofen while taking cytotoxic agents.
- Teach the patient and caregiver proper hand-washing and health-orientation techniques.
- Advise the patient to avoid large crowds and to report signs of infection immediately.
- Tell the patient to inform his dentist of his immunosuppressive therapy.
- Tell the female patient that cyclophosphamide may cause temporary amenorrhea.
- Explain to the female patient that she should use contraceptive measures to prevent pregnancy while on immunosuppressive therapy because of the drugs' teratogenic nature.

EVALUATION

Achievement of patient outcomes determines the success of collaborative management. For the patient with treatment-related immunosuppression, evaluation focuses on absence of infection and bleeding.

Treatments and procedures

In addition to drug therapies, tissue transplantation is a means of treating patients with immunologic disorders.

TISSUE TRANSPLANTATION

Patients experiencing failure in organs and avascular tissues (such as skin, cornea, bone, and heart valves) may require transplants.

In tissue transplantation, the surgeon removes tissue from one area of the body (from the patient or a selected donor) and grafts it at the selected site on the body.

PROCEDURE

The success of a transplant depends primarily on antigen compatibility between the recipient and the donor. Obviously, autografts—transplants of the patient's own tissue—are the most successful. An isograft, using tissue from an identical twin, is usually successful. Both procedures are called allografts—transplants between members of the same species. Tissue typing is used to determine histocompatibility and to select the best possible donor for successful transplantation.

A xenograft is a transplant from another species to a human and is the least successful procedure.

COLLABORATIVE MANAGEMENT

Care of the patient undergoing tissue transplantation requires thorough preparation, close monitoring, and intense patient teaching.

Preparation

- The patient will require extensive testing for histocompatibility to determine adequacy of transplant between donor and recipient.
- The patient may receive antibiotic and antiviral drugs prior to transplantation.
- The patient may also require immunosuppressive agents.

Monitoring and aftercare

- Monitor the patient's vital signs until they are stable.
- Monitor laboratory studies and watch the patient closely for signs and symptoms of transplant rejec-

---

DISCHARGE READY > **After tissue transplantation**

After undergoing tissue transplantation, the patient will meet the following criteria before discharge:

- vital signs and temperature within his normal limits
- laboratory studies for tissue transplant within normal limits of function
- no evidence of complications
- understanding of the procedure, reportable signs and symptoms, and the follow-up regimen.

---

tion, such as fever and pain.
- Give the patient immunosuppressives as ordered.
- Monitor laboratory studies for functioning of the transplanted organ. For example, for a liver transplant, check liver enzymes; for a kidney transplant, check renal function studies.
- Assess for and report signs of graft-versus-host disease, such as erythematous rash; widespread skin blistering; profuse, watery diarrhea; and possible liver failure.
- Develop a discharge plan. (See *After tissue transplantation.*)

Patient teaching

- Explain to the patient and his family the preoperative tests, postoperative therapies, and benefits of the transplantation.
- Teach the patient about the signs and symptoms of transplant rejection.
- Stress the importance of following the prescribed drug regimen and maintaining a record of any adverse effects of therapy.
- Tell the patient to avoid exposure to infections, because his immune system has been suppressed.
- Advise the patient to wear a medical identification bracelet and to tell health care workers, such as his dentist, about his condition.
- Stress the importance of follow-up visits to his doctor.

COMPLICATIONS

The most common complication of tissue transplantation is tissue rejection. Hyperacute tissue rejection occurs immediately or up to 3 days after transplantation. Acute tissue rejection can appear between 4 days and 3 months after transplantation. Chronic tissue rejection can appear 4 months to several years after transplantation. Graft-versus-host disease is a frequent and potentially fatal complication of bone marrow transplantation.

Selected references

Baigis-Smith, J., et al. "Healthcare Needs of HIV-infected Persons in Hospital, Outpatient, Home, and Long-Term Care Settings," *Journal of the Association of Nurses in AIDS Care* 6(6):21-33, November-December 1995.

Borton, D. "Isolation Precautions: Clearing Up the Confusion," *Nursing97* 27(1):49-51, January 1997.

Brooke, P.S. "HIV and the Law: An Update," *RN* 60(5):59-64, May 1997.

Diseases, 2nd ed. Springhouse, Pa.: Springhouse Corp., 1997.

Harwood, S. "Action STAT: Anaphylaxis," *Nursing97* 27(2):33, February 1997.

Huether, S.E., and McCance, K.L. *Understanding Pathophysiology.* St. Louis: Mosby–Year Book, Inc., 1996.

Illustrated Manual of Nursing Practice, 2nd ed. Springhouse, Pa.: Springhouse Corp., 1994.

Kenny, P. "Managing HIV Infection," *Nursing96* 26(8):26-37. August 1996.

Lemone, P., and Burke, K. *Medical-Surgical Nursing: Critical Thinking in Client Care.* Reading, Mass: Addison-Wesley Publishing Co., 1996.

McEnany, G.W., et al. "Depression and HIV: A Nursing Perspective on a Complex Relationship." *Nursing Clinics of North America* 31(1) 41-46, March 1996.

McKee, M.J. "Human Immunodeficiency Virus: Healthcare Worker Safety Issues," *Journal of Intravenous Nursing* 19(3):132-40, May-June 1996.

Nettina, S. *The Lippincott Manual of Nursing Practice,* 6th ed. Philadelphia: Lippincott-Raven Pubs., 1996.

Skin disorders

The largest and heaviest of the body's systems, the skin and its appendages (hair, nails, and certain glands) perform many vital functions. They protect inner organs, bones, muscles, and blood vessels; help regulate body temperature; and provide sensory information. What's more, they prevent body fluids from escaping and eliminate body wastes through more than 2 million pores.

Anatomy and physiology review

Two distinct layers of skin (integument), the epidermis and the dermis, lie above a third layer of subcutaneous fat (sometimes called the hypodermis). Epidermal appendages that are found throughout the skin include hair, nails, sebaceous glands, and two types of sweat glands: apocrine glands (found in the axilla and groin near hair follicles) and eccrine glands (located over most of the body except the lips). The integumentary system covers an area of 10¾ to 21½ square feet (1 to 2 m²) and accounts for about 15% of body weight. (See *Skin: A close-up view,* pages 644 and 645.)

SKIN FUNCTIONS
The epidermis protects against trauma, noxious chemicals, and invasion by microorganisms. Langerhans' cells enhance the immune response by helping lymphocytes process antigens entering the epidermis. Melanocytes protect the skin by producing melanin to help filter ultraviolet light (irradiation). The intact skin also protects the body by limiting water and electrolyte excretion.

Sensory nerve fibers carry impulses to the central nervous system (CNS); autonomic nerve fibers carry impulses to smooth muscles in the walls of the dermal blood vessels, to the muscles around the hair roots, and to the sweat glands. Sensory nerve fibers originate in dorsal nerve roots and supply specific areas of the skin known as dermatomes. Through these fibers, the skin can transmit various sensations, including temperature, touch, pressure, pain, and itching.

Abundant nerves, blood vessels, and eccrine glands within the dermis assist thermoregulation. The skin synthesizes vitamin D_3 (cholecalciferol) when stimulated by ultraviolet light.

The skin is also an excretory organ; the sweat glands excrete sweat, which contains water, electrolytes, urea, and lactic acid. The skin maintains body surface integrity by migration and shedding. It can repair surface wounds by intensifying normal cell replacement mechanisms; however, it can't regenerate if the dermal layer is destroyed. The sebaceous glands produce sebum—a mixture of keratin, fat, and cellulose debris. Combined with sweat, sebum forms a moist, oily, acidic film that's mildly antibacterial and antifungal and that protects the skin surface.

Assessment

Assessment begins with a complete patient history. Remember that skin disorders may be associated with, or stem from, disorders in other body systems. So don't discount the importance of minor symptoms or systemic complaints.

HISTORY
Begin by asking questions about current complaints, and follow with a full investigation of the patient's health. Start with the least sensitive or threatening questions, and save questions that may cause embarrassment or anxiety (such as those related to sexual

Skin: A close-up view

Major components of the skin include the epidermis, dermis, and epidermal appendages.

Epidermis
This outermost layer of skin varies in thickness from less than 0.1 mm on the eyelids to more than 1 mm on the palms of the hands and soles of the feet. It's composed of avascular, stratified, squamous (scaly or platelike) epithelial tissue, which contains multiple layers: a superficial keratinized, horny layer of cells (stratum corneum) consisting of two middle layers of cells in various stages of change as they migrate upward and a deeper germinal (basal cell) layer.

Stratum corneum
After mitosis (cell division) takes place in the germinal layer, epithelial cells undergo a series of changes as they migrate to the stratum corneum, the outermost part of the epidermis made up of tightly arranged layers of cellular membranes and keratin.

Langerhans' cells are specialized cells interspersed among the keratinized cells below the stratum corneum. These cells have an immunologic function and help process antigens that enter the epidermis. Epidermal cells are usually shed from the surface as epidermal dust. Differentiation of cells from the basal layer to the stratum corneum takes up to 28 days.

Basal cell layer
This layer produces new cells to replace the superficial keratinized cells that are continuously shed or worn away. The basal layer also contains specialized melanocytes that produce the brown pigment melanin and disperse it to the surrounding epithelial cells. Melanin primarily serves to filter ultraviolet radiation (light). Exposure to the sun can stimulate melanin production.

Dermis
Also called the corium, this second layer of skin is an elastic system that contains and supports blood vessels, lymphatic vessels, nerves, and epidermal appendages (hair, nails, and eccrine and apocrine glands). The dermis consists of two layers: the superficial papillary dermis and the reticular dermis.

The *papillary dermis* is studded with fingerlike projections (papillae) that nourish the epidermal cells. The epidermis lies over these papillae and bulges downward to fill the spaces. A collagenous membrane known as the basement membrane lies between the epidermis and the dermis, holding them together.

The *reticular dermis* covers a layer of subcutaneous tissue (adipose layer or panniculus adiposus), a specialized layer primarily composed of fat cells. It insulates the body, acts as a mechanical shock absorber, and provides energy.

Extracellular material called matrix makes up most of the dermis. Matrix contains connective tissue fibers called collagen, elastin, and reticular fibers. Collagen, a protein, gives strength to the dermis; elastin makes the skin pliable; and reticular fibers bind the collagen and elastin fibers together.

The matrix and connective tissue fibers are produced by spindle-shaped connective tissue cells (dermal fibroblasts), which become part of the matrix as it forms. Fibers are loosely arranged in the papillary dermis but more tightly packed in the deeper reticular dermis.

Epidermal appendages
These include the hair, nails, sebaceous glands, eccrine glands, and apocrine glands.

Hair
Each hair, made of keratin, has an expanded lower end (bulb or root) indented on its undersurface by a cluster of connective tissue and blood vessels called a hair papilla. Each lies within an epithelial-lined sheath called a hair follicle, which has a rich blood and nerve supply. A bundle of smooth muscle fibers (arrector pili) extends through the dermis to attach to the base of the hair follicle. Contraction of these muscles causes hair to stand on end.

Nails
Nails are specialized types of keratin that cover the distal surface of the end of each digit. The nail plate, surround-

matters) until the end. Ask the patient to describe the initial problem in as much detail as possible, even if that problem has already disappeared. Also have him describe how the problem spread and in what order other areas were affected.

CHIEF COMPLAINT
Ask the patient to describe the appearance of the skin problem, including its shape, size, color, location, character, and distribution. Also ask him to describe sensations associated with it and any pattern of migration. This information may provide clues to the cause of the disorder. For example, herpes zoster be-

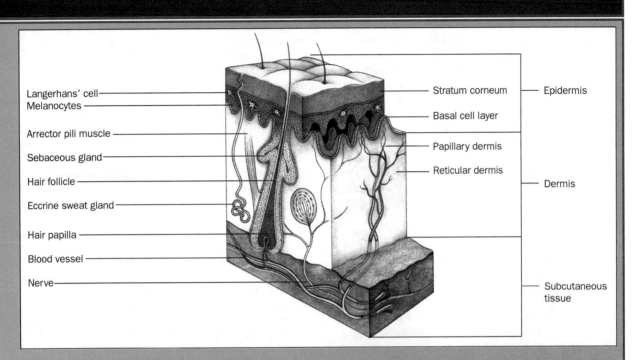

Langerhans' cell
Melanocytes
Arrector pili muscle
Sebaceous gland
Hair follicle
Eccrine sweat gland
Hair papilla
Blood vessel
Nerve

Stratum corneum — Epidermis
Basal cell layer
Papillary dermis
Reticular dermis — Dermis
Subcutaneous tissue

ed on three sides by the nail folds (cuticles), lies on the nail bed; the germinative nail matrix, which extends proximally for about 5 mm beneath the nail fold, forms the nail plate. The distal portion of the matrix shows through the nail as a pale semilunar area, the lunula. The translucent nail plate exposes the nail bed. The vascular bed under the nails gives them their characteristic pink appearance.

Sebaceous glands
These glands are found on all parts of the skin except the palms and soles. They're most prominent on the scalp, face, upper torso, and anogenital region. Sebum, a lipid substance, is produced within the lobule and secreted into the hair follicle via the sebaceous duct; it then exits through the hair follicle opening to reach the skin surface. Sebum may help waterproof the hair and skin and promote the absorption of fat-soluble substances into the dermis. It also may help produce vitamin D_3 and have some antibacterial function.

Eccrine glands
These widely distributed coiled glands produce an odorless, watery fluid with a sodium concentration equal to that of plasma. A duct from the secretory coils passes through the dermis and epidermis and opens onto the skin surface. Eccrine glands in the palms and soles secrete fluid primarily in response to emotional stress, such as taking a test. The remaining 3 million eccrine glands respond primarily to thermal stress, effectively regulating temperature.

Apocrine glands
Located primarily in the axillary and anogenital areas, apocrine glands have a coiled secretory portion that lies deeper in the dermis than the eccrine glands. A duct connects the apocrine glands to the upper portion of the hair follicle. These glands, which become activated at puberty, have no known biological function. Bacterial decomposition of the fluid produced by these glands causes body odor.

gins as vesicles and spreads in a distinctive pattern along cutaneous nerve endings.

Ask the patient when the problem began, how long it has lasted, and if it has happened before. Fungal infections may last for months, whereas herpes simplex resolves within weeks but may recur.

Next, inquire about associated signs and symptoms—such as pruritus, fever, drainage from lesions,

pain, nausea, and headache—as well as any other problems that may seem unrelated.

Ask the patient if anything makes his condition worse; aggravating factors are part of the diagnostic pattern for many skin disorders. Ask specifically about changes related to food, heat, cold, exercise, sunlight, stress, pregnancy, and menstruation. Herpes infections, for example, are commonly aggravated by sunlight, menstruation, or stress. Also ask the patient whether he's had recent contact with soaps, detergents, or plants; these substances may cause dermatitis.

Next, determine whether anything makes the problem better. If the answer is yes, a description of the specific drug or treatment may help the doctor plan therapy and help you plan appropriate nursing interventions. Remember to ask about home treatments, such as compresses, lotions, or over-the-counter (OTC) drugs. Folliculitis may respond to moist compresses, whereas warts will not.

MEDICAL HISTORY
Ask whether the patient has ever had a similar skin condition; some skin disorders, such as psoriasis, can recur. Also ask whether he has had any allergic reactions to medications, foods, or other substances such as cosmetics. Past and present allergies, including those caused by cutaneous, ingested, or inhaled allergens, may predispose the patient to other skin disorders.

FAMILY HISTORY
Ask the patient if anyone else in his family has had a skin problem. If so, ask what it was and when it happened. Also ask if anyone in the family has had an allergy. If so, ask what it was and how it was treated.

SOCIAL HISTORY
Obtain relevant information about the patient's lifestyle, including occupation, travel, diet, smoking, alcohol and drug use, exposure to the sun, stress, casual social contact, and sexual contact.

PHYSICAL EXAMINATION
Physical assessment of the skin, hair, and nails requires inspection and palpation.

APPEARANCE
Systematically assess all of the skin, hair, nails, and mucous membranes, even if the patient reports only a local lesion. The patient may not recognize subtle skin changes or asymptomatic skin disturbances, such as an early melanoma located on his back. Or he may feel too embarrassed to mention a lesion in the genital area. Failure to assess the entire skin surface can lead to incorrect diagnosis and care planning.

During the assessment, watch for any variations in lesion color, vascular supply, and pattern compared to other lesions. Also check for lesion distribution over the whole body.

INSPECTION
Begin by observing the patient's overall appearance from a distance of 3' to 6' (1 to 2 m), noting complex-

ion, general color, color variations, and general appearance. Next, note the color of healthy skin as well as problem areas.

Alterations in skin vasculature usually appear as red or purple pigmented lesions. Some vascular lesions appear in healthy people. For example, blood vessel hypertrophy (enlargement) may result in hemangiomas, which vary from bright red to purple. Press on the lesion with a lucite rule or glass slide, and observe and note the color change. Ecchymotic areas will remain unchanged when pressure is applied, whereas areas of dilated blood vessels will blanch (lose color or fade) when compressed. Permanently dilated superficial blood vessels (telangiectasia or spider veins) may indicate disease but are normal in many people.

Skin lesions. Carefully observe and document lesion morphology, distribution, and configuration.

Note the lesion's size (measure and record its dimensions), shape or configuration, color, elevation or depression, pedunculation (connection to the skin by a stem or stalk), and texture. Note odor, color, consistency, and amount of exudate. Use a flashlight to assess the color of the lesion and elevation of its borders. Use a transilluminator to assess fluid in a lesion by darkening the room and placing the tip of the transilluminator against the side of the lesion; a fluid-filled lesion glows red, whereas a solid lesion does not. Use a Wood's light to assess pigmented or depigmented lesions.

To aid diagnosis, remember to describe lesions accurately, keeping in mind that two or more types can coexist. Primary skin lesions appear on previously healthy skin in response to disease or external irritation. In some cases, lesions change during the natural course of a disease. Scratching, rubbing, and applying medication also may alter the original lesion. Modified lesions are described as secondary lesions.

Distribution of lesions may vary with disease progression or external factors. Note the pattern on first inspection; many skin disorders involve specific skin areas. Assessment of distribution includes the extent and pattern of involvement. Is the pattern of lesions local (in one small area), regional (in one large area), or general (over the entire body)? Also note characteristic locations, such as dermatomes (along cutaneous nerve endings), flexor or extensor surfaces, intertriginous areas, clothing or jewelry lines, and palms or soles, or random appearance.

Accurately describing configuration—the arrangement of lesions in relation to each other—may help determine their cause. Is the pattern of lesions discrete, confluent, grouped, diffuse, linear, annular, or arciform (arranged in a curve or arc)? Also note gyrate or polycyclic, herpetiform (along the course of cutaneous nerves), and iris configurations.

PALPATION

Assess skin texture, consistency, temperature, moisture, and turgor. Also use palpation to evaluate changes or tenderness of particular lesions. Wear gloves when palpating moist lesions.

Texture and consistency. Skin texture refers to smoothness or coarseness; consistency refers to changes in skin thickness or firmness and relates more to changes associated with lesions.

To evaluate texture and consistency, lightly rub the patient's skin. If it sloughs, leaving a moist base, this is a positive Nikolsky's sign, which characterizes staphylococcal scalded skin syndrome and other blistering conditions.

Temperature. Use the dorsal surfaces of your fingers or hands, which are most sensitive to temperature perception. The skin should feel warm to cool, and areas should feel the same bilaterally. Assess for bilateral symmetry by palpating similar areas simultaneously, placing your hands on both sides, then crossing hands so that each hand assesses the opposite side. A localized area of warmth may indicate a bacterial infection such as cellulitis.

Turgor. Gently grasp and pull up a fold of skin; then release it and observe how quickly it returns to normal shape. Normal skin usually resumes its flat shape immediately. Poor turgor may indicate dehydration and connective tissue disorders.

Lesions. Palpate skin lesions to obtain details about their morphology, distribution, location, and configuration.

Hair and scalp. Note the quantity, texture, color, and distribution of hair. Hair distribution varies greatly among individuals and is affected by race and ethnic origin. To palpate the patient's hair, rub a few strands between your index finger and thumb. Feel for dryness, brittleness, oiliness, and thickness.

Nails. This portion of the assessment may provide information about the patient's lifestyle, self-esteem, level of self-care, and health status. Inspect the nails for color, consistency, smoothness, symmetry, and ridges and cracks as well as for length, jagged or bitten edges, and cleanliness. Check the nail base for firmness and the nail for firm adherence to the nail bed; sponginess and swelling accompany infection.

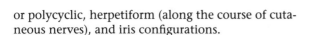

Acne vulgaris

This inflammatory disease of the sebaceous follicles primarily affects adolescents. It's characterized by comedons, pustules, nodules, and nodular lesions. Boys are affected more often and more severely than girls, but acne occurs in girls at an earlier age and tends to affect them for a longer time.

CAUSES

Acne's cause is unknown, but current research focuses on hormonal dysfunction and oversecretion of sebum as possible primary causes. Factors that increase an individual's risk of developing acne include use of oral contraceptives; cobalt irradiation; hyperalimentation therapy; exposure to heavy oils, greases, or tars; trauma or rubbing from tight clothing; family history; cosmetics; and emotional stress.

Certain medications may also predispose an individual to acne. These include corticosteroids, corticotropin, androgens, iodides, bromides, trimethadione, phenytoin, isoniazid, lithium, and halothane.

DIAGNOSIS AND TREATMENT

Because acne is apparent by observation, no laboratory tests are required to confirm the diagnosis.

Common drug treatments for severe acne include benzoyl peroxide, a powerful antibacterial, and tretinoin, a keratolytic that's effective against blackheads. These agents often are used in combination; both may irritate the skin. Topical antibiotics, such as tetracycline, erythromycin, and clindamycin, may help reduce the effects of acne.

Systemic therapy consists primarily of antibiotics, usually tetracycline, to decrease bacterial growth if infection occurs until the patient is in remission; a lower dosage is then used for long-term maintenance.

Oral isotretinoin (Accutane) combats acne by inhibiting sebaceous gland function and keratinization. However, because of its severe adverse effects, this drug's usual 16- to 20-week course is limited to patients with severe cystic acne who don't respond to conventional therapy. Severe fetal abnormalities may follow isotretinoin use during pregnancy. Use extreme caution when giving the drug to women of childbearing age.

Other treatments for acne include intralesional corticosteroid injections, estrogen therapy, exposure to ultraviolet light (but never when the patient is using a photosensitizing agent such as tretinoin), cryotherapy, and surgery.

COLLABORATIVE MANAGEMENT

Care of the patient with acne focuses on improved body image, skin integrity, and patient teaching.

ASSESSMENT

The appearance of acne will vary. If the acne plug doesn't protrude from the follicle and is covered by the epidermis, it may appear as a closed comedo, or whitehead. If the acne plug protrudes and isn't covered by the epidermis, it may appear as an open comedo, or blackhead. The patient may develop characteristic acne pustules, papules or, in severe cases, acne cysts or abscesses. Cystic acne produces scars.

NURSING DIAGNOSES AND COLLABORATIVE PROBLEMS

Based on the following nursing diagnoses, you'll establish patient outcomes.

Impaired skin integrity related to pustule formation.
The patient will:
- communicate an understanding of skin protection measures
- experience improved skin integrity after therapy.
Body image disturbance related to physical changes.
The patient will:
- acknowledge how his body has changed
- express positive feelings about himself
- exhibit an ability to cope with his altered appearance.

PLANNING AND IMPLEMENTATION

These measures help the patient with acne.
- Assess the effect of the patient's medications and other therapies.
- Help the patient identify predisposing factors that he can eliminate or modify, such as emotional stress.
- Pay special attention to the patient's perception of his physical appearance, and offer emotional support.

Patient teaching
- Explain the possible causes of acne to the patient and family members.
- Make sure they understand that the prescribed treatment is more likely to improve acne than strict diet and fanatic scrubbing with soap and water. In fact, overzealous washing can worsen the lesions.
- Instruct the patient receiving tretinoin to apply it at least 30 minutes after washing his face and at least 1 hour before bedtime. Warn him not to use it around the eyes or lips. Tell him that his skin should look pink and dry after treatment. If it appears red or starts to peel, he may have to weaken the preparation or apply it less often. Also, advise him to avoid exposure to sunlight and to use a sunscreen outdoors.
- If the prescribed regimen includes tretinoin and benzoyl peroxide, instruct the patient to avoid skin ir-

ritation by using one preparation in the morning and the other at night.
- Instruct the patient to take tetracycline on an empty stomach and not to take it in combination with antacids or milk.
- If the patient is taking isotretinoin, tell him to avoid vitamin A supplements, which can worsen any adverse effects. Also instruct him to use a moisturizer because dryness usually accompanies the treatment.
- Because of the danger of birth defects associated with isotretinoin, advise the sexually active female patient that this drug can't be prescribed unless she practices contraception. Tetracycline also carries some risk of birth defects if used during pregnancy.
- Tell the patient to routinely use topical medications to prevent recurrence of lesions.

EVALUATION

Evaluation of patient outcomes determines the success of collaborative management. For the patient with acne, evaluation focuses on skin integrity and improved body image.

Bacterial infections

Bacterial skin infections include impetigo; folliculitis, furunculosis, and carbunculosis; and cellulitis.

Impetigo is a contagious, superficial skin infection that appears in nonbullous and bullous forms. A vesiculopustular eruptive disorder, impetigo spreads most easily among infants, children, and older people. It can complicate skin conditions marked by open lesions, such as chickenpox.

Folliculitis, bacterial infection of the hair follicle, causes pustule formation. The infection may be superficial (follicular impetigo or Bockhart's impetigo) or deep (sycosis barbae). Folliculitis may also lead to the development of furuncles (furunculosis), commonly known as boils, or carbuncles (carbunculosis), especially if exacerbated by irritation, pressure, friction, or perspiration. The prognosis depends on the severity of the infection and on the patient's condition and ability to resist infection.

Cellulitis, a diffuse inflammation of the subcutaneous tissue, commonly appears around a break in the skin—usually fresh wounds or small puncture sites. Infection spreads rapidly through the lymphatic system and destroys the skin.

CAUSES

Beta-hemolytic streptococci produce nonbullous impetigo. Coagulase-positive *Staphylococcus aureus* causes bullous impetigo. Poor hygiene, anemia, malnutrition, and impaired skin integrity increase the risk of developing impetigo.

Coagulase-positive *S. aureus* is the most common cause of folliculitis. Risk factors include an infected wound elsewhere on the body, poor personal hygiene, debilitation, diabetes, exposure to chemicals (cutting oils), and management of skin lesions with tar or with occlusive therapy using steroids.

Cellulitis usually is caused by group A beta-hemolytic streptococci. It may also result from infection by other streptococci, *S. aureus,* or *Haemophilus influenzae.*

DIAGNOSIS AND TREATMENT

Characteristic lesions suggest impetigo. Microscopic visualization of the causative organism in a Gram stain of vesicular fluid usually confirms the diagnosis. Culture and sensitivity testing of fluid or denuded skin may indicate the most appropriate antibiotic, but therapy shouldn't be delayed for laboratory results, which can take 3 days.

A diagnosis of folliculitis is confirmed by a wound culture showing *S. aureus.* A diagnosis of cellulitis is confirmed by a Gram stain and culture of skin tissue that tests positive for the causative organism. Blood cultures will be positive for the same organism.

Treatment for impetigo includes systemic antibiotics (usually a penicillinase-resistant penicillin, or erythromycin for patients allergic to penicillin), which also help prevent glomerulonephritis, and washing the lesions two to three times a day with soap and water to remove the exudate. For stubborn crusts, warm soaks or compresses of saline or a diluted soap solution may help. Topical mupirocin may be given in mild cases.

Treatment for folliculitis consists of cleaning the infected area thoroughly with soap and water; applying warm, wet compresses to promote vasodilation and drainage of infected material from the lesions; and giving topical antibiotics, such as bacitracin and polymyxin B and, in recurrent infection, systemic antibiotics.

Furuncles may also require incision and drainage of ripe lesions after application of hot, wet compresses as well as topical antibiotics after drainage. Carbunculosis requires systemic antibiotics.

Antibiotic therapy is given to prevent widespread skin destruction in cellulitis. The doctor may prescribe oral penicillin to treat small, localized areas of cellulitis on the legs or trunk. Cellulitis of the face or hands or an infection with lymphatic involvement requires parenteral penicillin or a penicillinase-resistant antibiotic. If gangrene occurs, the patient must undergo surgical debridement and incision and drainage of surrounding tissue.

COLLABORATIVE MANAGEMENT

Care of the patient with a bacterial infection focuses on pain relief, skin integrity, lack of further infection, and patient teaching.

ASSESSMENT

Streptococcal impetigo usually begins with a small red macule that turns into a vesicle, becoming pustular in a few hours. When the vesicle breaks, a thick, honey-colored crust forms from the exudate. Autoinoculation may cause satellite lesions. Other symptoms are pruritus, burning, and regional lymphadenopathy.

In staphylococcal impetigo, a thin-walled vesicle opens and a thin, clear crust forms from the exudate. The lesion consists of a central clearing circumscribed by an outer rim—much like a ringworm lesion—and commonly appears on the face or other exposed areas. It causes painless pruritus.

In folliculitis, pustules usually appear on the scalp, arms, and legs in children; on the face of bearded men (sycosis barbae); and on the eyelids (sties). Pain may occur with deep folliculitis.

In furunculosis, the patient develops hard, painful nodules (furuncles) that commonly appear on the neck, face, axillae, and buttocks. After enlarging for several days, the furuncles rupture, discharging pus and necrotic material. Any pain subsides after rupture. Erythema and edema may last for several weeks.

In carbunculosis, the patient develops extremely painful, deep abscesses that drain through multiple openings onto the skin surface, usually around several hair follicles. Fever and malaise may also occur.

Clinical signs of cellulitis include a tender, warm, erythematous, swollen area, which is usually well demarcated. A warm, red, tender streak that follows the course of a lymph vessel may appear. The patient may experience fever, chills, headache, and malaise.

NURSING DIAGNOSIS AND COLLABORATIVE PROBLEMS

Based on the following nursing diagnoses, you'll establish patient outcomes.

Risk for infection related to skin breakdown. The patient will:
- experience no spread of infection
- show no signs of skin breakdown.

Impaired skin integrity related to open lesions or edema. The patient will:
- communicate an understanding of skin protection measures
- demonstrate proper skin inspection technique
- experience improved skin integrity.

Pain related to pruritus and altered skin integrity (impetigo), open lesions (folliculitis), or edema (cellulitis). The patient will:

- try nonpharmacologic methods of pain relief
- express a feeling of comfort and relief from pain.

PLANNING AND IMPLEMENTATION

These measures help the patient with a bacterial skin infection.

- Keep the patient's skin clean and dry to protect skin integrity.
- Give medications as ordered, and assess their effectiveness. Check for a penicillin allergy.
- If a school-age child has impetigo, notify his school and check his family members for the infection.
- With cellulitis, monitor the patient's vital signs, especially temperature, every 4 hours. Expect to provide supportive care. Also assess him every 4 hours for an increase in size of the affected area or a worsening of pain. Give antibiotics, analgesics, and warm soaks as ordered.

Patient teaching

If your patient has impetigo:

- Focus your teaching on helping the patient or family members learn to care for impetiginous lesions.
- Urge the patient not to scratch because this exacerbates impetigo. If the patient is a child, tell the parents to cut his fingernails.
- Stress the need to continue taking the prescribed drugs for 7 to 10 days after the lesions have healed.
- To prevent further spread of this highly contagious infection, encourage frequent bathing with an antiseptic soap.
- Tell the patient not to share towels, washcloths, or bed linens with family members.
- Emphasize the importance of following proper hand-washing techniques.

If your patient has folliculitis, furunculosis, or carbunculosis:

- Focus your teaching on the need for scrupulous personal and family hygiene, dietary modifications (reduced intake of sugars and fats), and precautions to prevent spreading infection.
- Caution the patient never to squeeze a boil because it may rupture.
- To avoid spreading the infection to family members, instruct the patient not to share his towels, washcloths, or bed linens with family members and to wash these items in hot water before reusing them.
- Encourage him to change dressings frequently and to discard them promptly in paper bags.
- Urge the patient to avoid occlusive cosmetics and tight clothing.

If your patient has cellulitis:

- Emphasize the importance of complying with the treatment regimen to prevent a relapse.

EVALUATION

Evaluation of patient outcomes determines the success of collaborative management. For the patient with a bacterial infection, evaluation focuses on relieving pain, maintaining skin integrity, and preventing infection.

Basal cell epithelioma

This slow-growing, destructive skin cancer—also known as basal cell carcinoma—usually strikes people over age 40. It's most prevalent in blond, fair-skinned men and is the most common malignant tumor affecting whites. The two major types of basal cell epithelioma are nodulo-ulcerative and superficial.

CAUSES

Prolonged sun exposure is the most common cause of basal cell epithelioma—90% of tumors affect sun-exposed areas of the body—but arsenic ingestion, radiation exposure, burns, immunosuppression and, rarely, vaccinations are other possible causes.

Although the pathogenesis is uncertain, some experts hypothesize that basal cell epithelioma originates when undifferentiated basal cells become cancerous instead of differentiating into sweat glands, sebum, and hair.

DIAGNOSIS AND TREATMENT

All types of basal cell epitheliomas are diagnosed by clinical appearance. To support the diagnosis, the doctor may perform an incisional or excisional biopsy and histologic studies to help determine the tumor type and histologic subtype.

Depending on the size, location, and depth of the lesion, treatment may include curettage and electrodesiccation, chemotherapy, surgical excision, radiation therapy, chemosurgery, or cryotherapy.

Curettage and electrodesiccation offers good cosmetic results for small lesions. Topical fluorouracil, commonly used for superficial lesions, produces marked local irritation or inflammation in the involved tissue but no systemic effects.

Microscopically controlled surgical excision carefully removes recurrent lesions until a tumor-free plane is achieved. After removal of large lesions, the patient may require skin grafting.

Radiation therapy is used if necessary. It's also preferred for older or debilitated patients who might not tolerate surgery.

Chemosurgery is often the choice for persistent or recurrent lesions. It consists of periodic application of a fixative paste (such as zinc chloride) and subsequent removal of fixed pathologic tissue. Treatment continues until tumor removal is complete. Cryotherapy, using liquid nitrogen, freezes the cells and kills them.

COLLABORATIVE MANAGEMENT

Care of the patient with basal cell epithelioma focuses on reducing fear and patient teaching about the cancer and its treatment.

ASSESSMENT

The patient history may reveal that the patient became aware of an odd-looking skin lesion, which prompted him to seek medical care. It may also disclose prolonged exposure to the sun sometime in the patient's life or other risk factors for this disease.

Inspection of the face may reveal small, smooth, pigmented, and translucent papules, particularly on the forehead, eyelid margins, and nasolabial folds. Telangiectatic vessels cross the surface of the lesions, which may be pigmented. As the lesions enlarge, their centers become depressed and their borders firm and elevated. (These ulcerated tumors are called rodent ulcers.)

Inspection of the chest and back may reveal multiple oval or irregularly shaped, lightly pigmented plaques. These may have sharply defined, slightly elevated, threadlike borders (superficial basal cell epitheliomas).

Inspection of the head and neck may show waxy, sclerotic, yellow to white plaques without distinct borders. These plaques may resemble small patches of scleroderma and may suggest sclerosing basal cell epitheliomas (morphea-like epitheliomas).

NURSING DIAGNOSES AND COLLABORATIVE PROBLEMS

Based on the following nursing diagnoses, you'll establish patient outcomes.

Fear related to the diagnosis of cancer. The patient will:
- identify fears related to the diagnosis
- use available support systems to help cope with fear
- express reduced fear and manifest no physical signs or symptoms of fear.

Impaired skin integrity related to ulceration caused by basal cell epithelioma or skin irritation from therapy. The patient will:
- communicate and demonstrate preventive skin care measures
- exhibit a positive response to therapy and no recurrence of basal cell epithelioma
- develop no skin breakdown from therapy.

PLANNING AND IMPLEMENTATION

These measures help the patient with basal cell epithelioma.

> **HEALTHY LIVING**
> ## Reducing the risk of skin cancer
>
> Teach your patient the following measures to decrease his chances of developing skin cancer:
>
> - Avoid excessive sun exposure.
> - Use strong sunscreen on exposed areas to protect skin from damaging rays. (Don't forget to protect the tops of ears and ear lobes.)
> - Have any suspicious skin changes examined by a dermatologist.

- Listen to the patient's fears and concerns. Offer reassurance when appropriate.
- Remain with the patient during periods of severe stress and anxiety. Provide positive reinforcement for his efforts to cope. Arrange for the patient to interact with others who have a similar problem.
- Assess the patient's readiness for decision making; involve him and his family members in decisions related to his care whenever possible.
- Provide reassurance and comfort measures when appropriate.
- Watch for complications of treatment, including local skin irritation from topically applied chemotherapeutic agents and infection.
- If applicable, watch for radiation's adverse effects, such as nausea, vomiting, hair loss, malaise, and diarrhea.

Patient teaching

- Instruct the patient to eat frequent, small, high-protein meals. Advise him to include pureed foods and liquid protein supplements if the lesion has invaded the oral cavity and is causing eating difficulty.
- To prevent disease recurrence, tell the patient to avoid excessive sun exposure and to use a strong sunscreen to protect his skin from damage by ultraviolet rays. (See *Reducing the risk of skin cancer.*)
- Advise the patient to relieve local inflammation from topical fluorouracil with cool compresses or a corticosteroid ointment.
- Instruct the patient with nodulo-ulcerative basal cell epithelioma to wash his face gently when he has ulcerations and crusting; scrubbing too vigorously may cause bleeding.
- As appropriate, direct the patient and his family to hospital and community support services, such as social workers, psychologists, and cancer support groups.

EVALUATION

Evaluation of patient outcomes determines the success of collaborative management. For the patient with basal cell epithelioma, evaluation focuses on maintaining skin integrity and decreasing fear.

Burns

Major burns require painful treatment and long-term rehabilitation. Often fatal or permanently disfiguring, a burn can cause both emotional and physical incapacitation. In the United States, about 2 million people a year suffer burns. Of these, 300,000 are burned seriously and more than 6,000 die, making burns the nation's third leading cause of accidental death.

CAUSES

Thermal burns, the most common type, can result from residential fires, motor vehicle accidents, playing with matches, improperly stored gasoline, malfunctioning space heaters and other electrical equipment, arson, improper handling of firecrackers, scalding, kitchen accidents, or child abuse.

Chemical burns can result from contact with or ingestion, inhalation, or injection of acids, alkalis, or vesicants. Electrical burns may be caused by contact with faulty electrical wiring or high-voltage power lines or by young children chewing on electrical cords. Friction or abrasion burns result from harsh rubbing of skin against a coarse surface, and sunburn results from excessive exposure to the sun.

DIAGNOSIS AND TREATMENT

Although blood tests don't support the diagnosis, they're essential in the collaborative management of the patient's condition. Draw blood samples for complete blood count; electrolyte, glucose, blood urea nitrogen, creatinine, carboxyhemoglobin, and arterial blood gas levels; and typing and cross matching.

Immediate, aggressive treatment increases the patient's chances of survival. Later, supportive measures and strict aseptic technique can minimize infection. Because burns require such comprehensive care, good nursing can make the difference between life and death.

In minor to moderate burns, first stop the burning process and relieve pain by applying cool, saline-soaked towels. Avoid placing ice directly on burn wounds because the cold may cause further thermal damage; also avoid overcooling the patient and causing hypothermia.

Debride the dead tissue, taking care not to break any blisters. Cover the wound with an antimicrobial agent and a nonadhesive bulky dressing. Give tetanus prophylaxis as ordered.

In moderate to major burns, immediately assess the patient's airway, breathing, and circulation (ABCs). Be especially alert for signs of smoke inhalation and pulmonary damage: singed nasal hairs, mucosal burns, voice changes, coughing, wheezing, soot in the mouth or nose, and darkened sputum. As ordered, assist with endotracheal intubation and give the patient 100% oxygen.

Control bleeding and remove smoldering clothing (soak clothing first in saline solution if it's stuck to the patient's skin), rings, and other constricting items. Cover burns with a clean, dry, sterile bed sheet.

Begin I.V. therapy immediately to prevent hypovolemic shock and to maintain cardiac output. A patient with serious burns needs massive fluid replacement, especially for the first 24 hours. Expect to give a combination of crystalloids such as lactated Ringer's solution.

Tissue damage from electrical burns is difficult to assess because internal destruction along the conduction pathway is usually greater than the surface burn would indicate. Electrical burns that ignite the patient's clothes may cause thermal burns as well. If the electric shock caused ventricular fibrillation and cardiac and respiratory arrest, begin cardiopulmonary resuscitation at once. Obtain an estimate of the electrical voltage involved.

In a chemical burn, irrigate the wound with copious amounts of water or normal saline solution. If the chemical entered the patient's eyes, flush them with large amounts of water or the saline solution for at least 30 minutes. Have the patient close his eyes, and cover them with a dry, sterile dressing. Note the type of chemical that caused the burn and the presence of any noxious fumes. Arrange for an ophthalmologic examination.

Don't treat the burn wound itself in the emergency department if the patient is to be transferred to a specialized burn care unit within 4 hours after the burn. Instead, prepare the patient for transport by wrapping him in a sterile sheet and a blanket for warmth and elevating the burned extremity to decrease edema. Then transport the patient immediately.

COLLABORATIVE MANAGEMENT

Care of the patient with burns focuses on pain relief, adequate respiration, maintenance of a patent airway, and protection from infection.

ASSESSMENT

For all types of burns, you'll need to estimate what percentage of your patient's body surface area is burned. (See *Using burn damage charts*.) Then use the following guidelines:

Using burn damage charts

You can quickly estimate the extent of an adult patient's burns by using the "Rule of Nines," a method of dividing an adult's body body surface area into percentages. To use this method, mentally transfer your patient's burns to the body chart shown below; then add up the percentages for each burned body section. The total gives you a rough estimate of the extent of the patient's burns and helps you estimate his fluid replacement needs.

The Rule of Nines can't be used on infants or children because their body section percentages differ from those of adults. (For example, an infant's head accounts for about 17% of his total body surface area, compared with 9% for an adult.) Instead, use the Lund-Browder chart below to estimate the extent of burns on a pediatric patient.

Rule of Nines

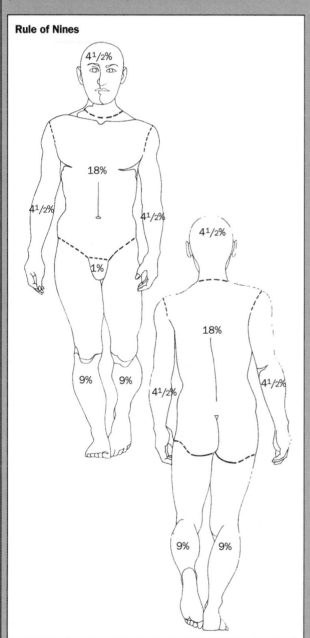

Lund-Browder chart

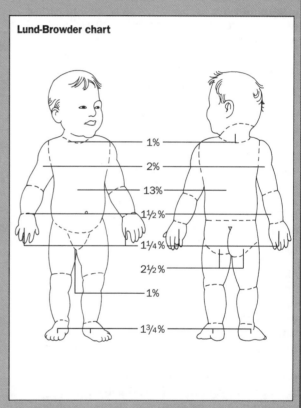

DISCHARGE READY ＞ **After burns**

After treatment for a burn, the patient will meet the following criteria before discharge:

- temperature and vital signs within his normal limits
- laboratory results within his normal limits
- healing burn wounds
- no evidence of infection or complications
- return of adequate functional level.

- first-degree burns—Damage is limited to the epidermis, causing erythema and pain.
- second-degree burns—The epidermis and part of the dermis are damaged, producing blisters and mild to moderate edema and pain.
- third-degree burns—The epidermis and dermis are damaged. No blisters appear, but white, brown, or black leathery tissue and thrombosed vessels are visible.
- fourth-degree burns—Damage extends through deeply charred subcutaneous tissue to muscle and bone.

Another assessment goal is to estimate the size of a burn. Size is usually expressed as the percentage of body surface area (BSA) covered by the burn. The Rule of Nines chart usually guides this estimate, although the Lund-Browder chart is more accurate because it allows for BSA changes with age. Correlating the burn's depth and size permits an estimate of its severity.

Burns can also be classified as major, moderate, or minor. Major burns include third-degree burns on more than 10% of BSA; second-degree burns on more than 25% of adult BSA (on more than 20% in children); burns of hands, face, feet, or genitalia; burns complicated by fractures or respiratory damage; electrical burns; and all burns in poor-risk patients.

Moderate burns include third-degree burns on 2% to 10% of BSA and second-degree burns on 15% to 25% of adult BSA (on 10% to 20% in children).

Minor burns include third-degree burns on less than 2% of BSA and second-degree burns on less than 15% of adult BSA (on 10% in children).

Burns on the face, hands, feet, and genitalia are most serious because of possible loss of function. Circumferential burns can cause total occlusion of circulation in an extremity as a result of edema (especially neck or chest). Impaired peripheral circulation, as occurs in diabetes, peripheral vascular disease, and chronic alcohol abuse, complicates burns.

NURSING DIAGNOSES AND COLLABORATIVE PROBLEMS

Based on the following nursing diagnoses, you'll establish patient outcomes.

Ineffective airway clearance related to burn process. The patient will:
- position himself to maximize lung expansion and ventilation
- maintain a patent airway.

Risk for fluid volume deficit related to burn process. The patient will:
- express an understanding of the need to maintain adequate fluid intake
- maintain hemodynamic stability
- exhibit no signs of dehydration.

Pain related to burn process. The patient will:
- describe characteristics and level of pain
- try nonpharmacologic methods of relieving pain
- experience decreased pain.

Risk for infection related to burn process. The patient will:
- identify signs and symptoms of infection
- heal without infection
- show no evidence of skin breakdown.

PLANNING AND IMPLEMENTATION

These measures help the patient with burns.
- Maintain sterile and aseptic technique to protect the patient.
- Maintain a patent airway. For an inhalation burn, intubate the patient and place him on mechanical ventilation to preserve his airway.
- Oxygenate the patient according to his arterial blood gas results and needs.
- Check the patient's vital signs every 15 minutes initially until stable. Although it may make you uneasy, don't hesitate to take the patient's blood pressure because of burned limbs. (The doctor may insert an arterial line if blood pressure is unobtainable with a cuff).
- The patient may need a central venous pressure (CVP) line and additional I.V. lines (using venous cutdown, if necessary) and an indwelling urinary catheter.
- To combat fluid evaporation through the burn and the release of fluid into interstitial spaces (possibly resulting in hypovolemic shock), continue fluid therapy, as ordered.
- Send a urine specimen to the laboratory to check for myoglobinuria and hemoglobinuria.
- Insert a nasogastric tube to decompress the stomach and avoid aspiration of stomach contents.
- Closely monitor intake and output.
- Be prepared to assist in emergency escharotomy if burns threaten to constrict circulation.

- Don't use cleaning solutions with hydrogen peroxide or povidone-iodine solution because they may further damage tissue.
- Monitor white blood cell count as necessary and as ordered.
- Give narcotic analgesics as soon as the patient is hemodynamically stable and other injuries are ruled out. Morphine (2 to 25 mg) or meperidine (5 to 15 mg), given in small increments to avoid hypotension and respiratory depression, is usually the drug of choice.
- Provide emotional support and reassurance; this may help reduce the patient's need for analgesics.
- Develop a discharge plan. (See *After burns*.)

Patient teaching
- Provide aftercare instructions for the patient. Stress the importance of keeping the dressing dry and clean and of elevating the burned extremity for the first 24 hours.
- Tell the patient to take analgesics as ordered and to return for a wound check in 2 days.

EVALUATION
Evaluation of patient outcomes determines the success of collaborative management. For the patient with burns, evaluation focuses on maintaining a patent airway, preventing infection, and relieving pain.

Dermatitis

Inflammation of the skin, dermatitis occurs in several forms: atopic and seborrheic (discussed below), nummular, contact, chronic, exfoliative, stasis, and localized neurodermatitis.

Also known as atopic or infantile eczema, atopic dermatitis is a chronic inflammatory skin response that's commonly associated with other atopic disorders, such as bronchial asthma, allergic rhinitis, and chronic urticaria. This form of dermatitis usually develops in infants between ages 1 month and 1 year, commonly in those with a strong family history of atopic disease. It subsides spontaneously by age 3 and stays in remission until prepuberty (ages 10 to 12), when it commonly flares up again.

Seborrheic dermatitis appears in areas with a high concentration of sebaceous glands, such as the scalp, trunk, and face.

CAUSES
The cause of atopic dermatitis isn't known. However, one theory suggests an underlying metabolically or biochemically induced skin disorder that's genetically linked to elevated serum IgE levels. Another theory suggests defective T-cell function.

Factors that exacerbate atopic dermatitis include irritants, infections (commonly by *Staphylococcus aureus*), and some allergens, including pollen, wool, silk, fur, ointments, detergent, and certain foods (particularly wheat, milk, and eggs). Flare-ups may be linked to extremes in temperature and humidity, sweating, and stress.

The exact cause of seborrheic dermatitis is unknown, but predisposing factors may include heredity, physical or emotional stress, and neurologic conditions.

DIAGNOSIS AND TREATMENT
Diagnosis is based on the characteristics of the lesion. Laboratory tests may reveal eosinophilia and elevated serum immunoglobulin E (IgE) levels.

Treatment for atopic lesions first involves eliminating allergens and avoiding irritants, extreme temperature changes, and other precipitating factors. Local and systemic treatment may relieve itching and inflammation. Topical application of a corticosteroid cream or ointment, especially after bathing, commonly alleviates inflammation. Between steroid doses, application of petroleum jelly can help retain moisture. Systemic corticosteroid therapy is appropriate only during extreme exacerbations. Weak tar preparations and ultraviolet B light therapy are used to increase the thickness of the stratum corneum. If a culture of the lesion reveals a bacterial infection, the doctor may order an antibiotic.

Treatment for seborrheic dermatitis may include removing scales with frequent washing and shampooing with selenium sulfide suspension (most effective), zinc pyrithione, or tar and salicylic acid shampoo. Topical steroids may help to reduce inflammation.

COLLABORATIVE MANAGEMENT
Care of the patient with dermatitis focuses on improved body image, good skin integrity, and patient teaching.

ASSESSMENT
The patient with atopic dermatitis develops an intensely pruritic, often excoriated, maculopapular rash, usually on the face and antecubital and popliteal areas.

The patient with seborrheic dermatitis may develop itching, redness, and inflammation of affected areas as well as fissures. Lesions are distributed in sebaceous gland areas and may appear greasy. Excess stratum corneum may lead to the development of indistinct, occasionally yellowish, scaly patches. Dandruff may signal mild seborrheic dermatitis.

NURSING DIAGNOSES AND COLLABORATIVE PROBLEMS

Based on the following nursing diagnoses, you'll establish patient outcomes.

Impaired skin integrity related to open lesions. The patient will:
- express an understanding of skin protection measures
- experience improved skin integrity after treatment.

Body image disturbance related to physical changes. The patient will:
- acknowledge the ways in which his body image has changed
- express a positive attitude about himself
- exhibit an ability to cope with his changed body image.

PLANNING AND IMPLEMENTATION

These measures help the patient with dermatitis.
- Assess the effect of prescribed medications and other therapies on the patient's condition.
- Help the patient identify predisposing factors that he can eliminate or modify, such as emotional stress.
- Pay special attention to the patient's perception of his physical appearance, and provide emotional support.

Patient teaching

- Instruct the patient to soak in plain water for 10 to 20 minutes daily. Tell him to bathe with a special nonfatty soap and tepid water but to use soap only on areas that need cleaning when he has finished soaking. (Soaking cleans most skin surfaces.)
- Advise the patient to shampoo frequently and to apply a topical corticosteroid afterward, to keep his fingernails short to limit excoriation and secondary infections due to scratching, and to lubricate his skin after a tub bath.
- Inform the patient that irritants, such as detergents, wool, and emotional stress, exacerbate atopic dermatitis.
- Because an emotional component may be associated with seborrheic dermatitis, explore with the patient ways to reduce stress.
- Tell the patient that the course of seborrheic dermatitis will wax and wane and to expect exacerbations during cold weather.

EVALUATION

Evaluation of patient outcomes determines the success of collaborative management. For the patient with dermatitis, evaluation focuses on maintaining skin integrity and body image.

Herpes infection

A common infection, herpes simplex virus (HSV) is subclinical in about 85% of patients; in the rest, it causes localized lesions. HSV may be latent for years, but after the initial infection, the patient becomes a carrier, susceptible to recurrent attacks. The outbreaks may be provoked by fever, menses, stress, heat, cold, lack of sleep, sun exposure, and contact with reactivated disease (for example, by kissing or sharing cosmetics). In recurrent infections, the patient usually has no systemic signs and symptoms.

Generally not serious in an otherwise healthy adult, HSV infection in an immunocompromised patient, such as one with acquired immunodeficiency syndrome (AIDS), can produce severe illness. In fact, serious HSV infections are a prominent feature of AIDS.

Primary (or initial) HSV infection during pregnancy can lead to spontaneous abortion, premature labor, microcephaly, and uterine growth retardation. Congenital herpes transmitted during vaginal birth may produce a subclinical neonatal infection or severe infection with seizures, chorioretinitis, skin vesicles, and hepatosplenomegaly. Blindness can follow ocular infection. Females with HSV may be at increased risk for cervical cancer and urethral stricture caused by recurrent genital herpes.

Serious complications of HSV infection in patients with AIDS or other immunocompromised conditions include perianal ulcers, colitis, esophagitis, pneumonitis, and various neurologic disorders.

CAUSES

Herpesvirus hominis, a widespread infectious agent, causes two serologically distinct HSV types. Seen most commonly in children, type 1 (HSV-1) is transmitted primarily by contact with oral secretions. It mainly affects oral, labial, ocular, and skin tissues. Type 2 (HSV-2), transmitted primarily by contact with genital secretions, mainly affects genital structures, typically in adolescents and young adults.

HSV-2 anal and perianal infection is common in homosexual men. However, with changing sexual practices, some studies report an increasing incidence of genital HSV-1 and oral HSV-2 infections. Although HSV most frequently appears in the structures mentioned, it may infect any epithelial tissue. The incubation period varies, depending on the infection site. The average incubation period for generalized infection is 2 to 12 days; for localized genital infection, 3 to 7 days.

DIAGNOSIS AND TREATMENT

Isolating the virus from local lesions and a histologic biopsy confirm a diagnosis of herpes infection. In primary infection, a rise in antibodies and moderate leukocytosis may support the diagnosis.

Symptomatic and supportive therapy is the rule. Generalized primary infection usually requires antipyretic and analgesic medications to reduce fever and pain. Anesthetic mouthwashes, such as viscous lidocaine, may reduce the pain of gingivostomatitis, enabling the patient to consume food and fluids and thus promote hydration. Drying agents, such as calamine lotion, may soothe labial and skin lesions.

Refer patients with eye infections to an ophthalmologist. Topical corticosteroids are contraindicated in active infection, but ophthalmic medications, such as idoxuridine, trifluridine, and vidarabine, may help.

Acyclovir is commonly used to combat genital herpes, particularly primary infection. This drug may reduce symptoms, viral shedding, and healing time. It's available in topical, oral, and I.V. form (usually reserved for severe infection).

COLLABORATIVE MANAGEMENT

Care of the patient with herpes infection focuses on infection control, pain relief, preservation of mucous membranes, and patient teaching.

ASSESSMENT

In a patient with suspected herpes simplex, the history may reveal oral, vaginal, or anal sexual contact with an infected person or other direct contact with lesions. With recurrent infection, the patient may identify various precipitating factors. Look for:

■ in primary perioral HSV, generalized or localized infection; in generalized infection, reports of a sore throat, fever, increased salivation, halitosis, anorexia, and severe mouth pain; poor skin turgor if pain prevents adequate fluid intake; after a brief prodromal tingling and itching, eruption of typical primary lesions

■ edema and small vesicles on pharyngeal and oral mucosa (usually on the tongue, gingiva, and cheeks); throat and mouth vesicles that rupture, leaving a painful ulcer, followed by a yellow crust; tender cervical adenopathy

■ in primary genital HSV, complaints of malaise, dysuria, dyspareunia, and (in females) leukorrhea, followed by appearance of fluid-filled vesicles

■ in a female patient, vesicles on the cervix (the primary infection site) and, possibly, on the labia, perianal skin, vulva, and vagina

■ in a male patient, vesicles on the glans penis, foreskin, and penile shaft; extragenital lesions on the mouth or anus; ruptured vesicles appearing as extensive, shallow, painful ulcers with redness, marked edema, and characteristic oozing, yellow centers; tender inguinal adenopathy.

The patient with recurrent perioral or genital HSV also may report prodromal symptoms (pain, tingling, or itching) at the site. Typically, the disease course is shorter than that of the primary infection. Recurrent perioral infections usually trigger no systemic symptoms, but the outer lip may be painful. A male with recurrent genital herpes usually has less severe systemic symptoms and less local involvement than a female, who may report severe discomfort. Palpation may reveal tender cervical adenopathy.

The patient with a primary ocular infection may report localized signs and symptoms, such as photophobia and excessive tearing. Follicular conjunctivitis or blepharitis with vesicles on the eyelid, eyelid edema, and chemosis also may occur. Systemic signs and symptoms may include lethargy and fever. The infection usually is unilateral and heals within 2 to 3 weeks. Recurrent ocular infections may cause decreased visual acuity and even permanent vision loss. Palpation may reveal regional adenopathy.

NURSING DIAGNOSES AND COLLABORATIVE PROBLEMS

Based on the following nursing diagnoses, you'll establish patient outcomes.

Altered oral mucous membrane related to oral lesions. The patient will:
■ comply with prescribed treatments to alleviate oral lesions
■ exhibit healing of oral lesions.

Risk for infection related to herpes simplex recurrence. The patient will:
■ express an understanding of how herpes simplex can recur
■ take precautions to prevent recurrences
■ avoid herpes simplex recurrences.

Pain related to HSV infection. The patient will:
■ feel less pain with treatment
■ become pain-free once lesions heal.

PLANNING AND IMPLEMENTATION

These measures help the patient with herpes infection.

■ Observe standard precautions. For the patient with extensive cutaneous, oral, or genital lesions, institute contact precautions.

■ Instruct caregivers with an active oral or cutaneous infection not to care for a patient in a high-risk group until the caregiver's lesions crust and dry. Also, insist that the caregiver wear protective coverings, including a mask and gloves.

■ Monitor the patient with oral lesions for signs and symptoms of nutritional deficits and dehydration. Weigh him regularly.

- Give pain medications and prescribed antiviral agents, as ordered.
- Provide supportive care, as indicated, such as oral hygiene, nutritional supplements, and antipyretics for fever.
- Observe the patient's response to treatment measures.
- Assess the patient for complications associated with herpes simplex.
- As appropriate, refer him to a support group, such as the Herpes Resource Center.

Patient teaching

- To avoid spreading the infection to vulnerable people, instruct the patient with cold sores not to kiss infants or people with eczema and the patient with genital herpes to wash his hands carefully after using the bathroom or touching his genitalia.
- Instruct the patient with oral lesions to use lip balm with sunscreen to avoid reactivating lesions.
- Encourage the patient to get adequate rest and nutrition and to keep his lesions dry, except for applying prescribed medications.
- Teach the patient how to apply medications using aseptic technique.
- Urge the patient with genital herpes to avoid sexual intercourse during the active disease stage before lesions completely heal. Advise him to inform all sexual partners of his condition. Advise patients and partners to get screened for other sexually transmitted diseases, including human immunodeficiency virus infection.
- If the patient is pregnant, explain the potential risk of transmitting the infection to the infant during vaginal delivery. Answer her questions about cesarean delivery if she has an HSV outbreak when labor begins and if her membranes haven't ruptured.
- Advise the female patient with genital herpes to have a Papanicolaou (Pap) test yearly if results have been normal. If results have been abnormal, recommend more frequent testing.
- Instruct the patient with herpetic whitlow not to share towels or eating utensils with uninfected people. Educate staff members and other susceptible people about the risk of contracting the disease.
- Accept the patient's feelings of powerlessness as normal. Help him develop coping mechanisms, and identify resources for support.
- Provide a nonthreatening, nonjudgmental atmosphere to encourage the patient with genital herpes to voice his feelings about perceived changes in sexuality and behavior.
- Provide him and his partner with up-to-date information about the disease and treatment options. Refer them for appropriate counseling as needed.

EVALUATION

Evaluation of patient outcomes determines the success of collaborative management. For the patient with herpes infection, evaluation focuses on preserving mucous membranes, preventing the spread of infection, and decreasing pain.

Kaposi's sarcoma

The incidence of Kaposi's sarcoma has risen dramatically in recent years along with the incidence of acquired immunodeficiency syndrome (AIDS). This disease is currently the most common AIDS-related cancer.

Characterized by obvious colorful lesions, Kaposi's sarcoma causes structural and functional damage. When associated with AIDS, it progresses aggressively, involving the lymph nodes, the viscera and, possibly, GI structures. It can also involve the lungs, leading to respiratory distress, and the GI system, resulting in digestive problems.

CAUSES

The exact cause of Kaposi's sarcoma isn't known, but the disease may be related to immunosuppression or genetic or hereditary predisposition.

DIAGNOSIS AND TREATMENT

A tissue biopsy determines the lesion's type and stage. A computed tomography scan can help detect metastasis.

Treatment may consist of radiation therapy, chemotherapy, or drug therapy with biological response modifiers. Radiation therapy offers relief of symptoms, including pain from obstructing lesions in the oral cavity or extremities and edema caused by lymphatic blockage. It also may be used for cosmetic improvement.

Chemotherapy includes combinations of doxorubicin, vinblastine, vincristine, and etoposide. The biological response modifier interferon alfa-2b is commonly prescribed in AIDS-related Kaposi's sarcoma. It reduces the number of skin lesions but is ineffective in advanced disease.

COLLABORATIVE MANAGEMENT

Care of the patient with Kaposi's sarcoma focuses on improved nutrition, maintenance of a patent airway, improved body image, and patient teaching.

ASSESSMENT

The health history typically reveals that the patient has AIDS. If the sarcoma advances beyond the early stages or if a lesion breaks down, the patient may report pain. Usually, however, the lesions remain painless unless they impinge on nerves or organs.

On inspection, you may observe several lesions in various shapes, sizes, and colors (ranging from red-brown to dark purple). The lesions occur most commonly on the skin, buccal mucosa, hard and soft palates, lips, gums, tongue, tonsils, conjunctiva, and sclera. In advanced disease, the lesions may join, becoming one large plaque. Untreated lesions may appear as large, ulcerative masses.

The patient also may have dyspnea, especially with pulmonary involvement. Palpation and inspection may also disclose edema from lymphatic obstruction. Auscultation may uncover wheezing and hypoventilation. Respiratory distress usually results from bronchial blockage. The most common extracutaneous sites are the lungs and GI tract (esophagus, oropharynx, and epiglottis).

NURSING DIAGNOSES AND COLLABORATIVE PROBLEMS
Based on the following nursing diagnoses, you'll establish patient outcomes.

Altered nutrition: Less than body requirements, related to GI dysfunction. The patient will:
- eat a nutritionally balanced diet high in calories and protein
- regain and maintain his weight within a normal range
- not become malnourished or develop a nutritional deficiency.

Body image disturbance related to cutaneous lesions. The patient will:
- express his feelings about how his body has changed
- participate in decisions about his care
- express positive feelings about himself.

Impaired gas exchange related to respiratory dysfunction. The patient will:
- maintain adequate ventilation, as evidenced by normal arterial blood gas levels and a normal respiratory assessment
- develop no signs and symptoms of respiratory distress.

PLANNING AND IMPLEMENTATION
These measures help the patient with Kaposi's sarcoma.
- Listen to the patient's fears and concerns, and answer his questions honestly. Stay with him during periods of severe stress and anxiety.
- To help the patient adjust to changes in his appearance, urge him to share his feelings and provide encouragement.
- Encourage him to participate in care decisions and self-care whenever possible.

- If the patient has painful lesions, help him into a more comfortable position and give pain medications as needed. Suggest distractions and help the patient with relaxation techniques.
- Inspect the patient's skin every shift. Look for new lesions and skin breakdown.
- Supply the patient with high-calorie, high-protein meals. If he can't tolerate regular meals, provide him with frequent, smaller meals. Consult with the dietitian, and plan meals around the patient's treatment schedule. If he can't take food by mouth, give I.V. fluids. Give antiemetics and sedatives, as ordered.
- Provide rest periods if the patient tires easily.
- Remember to watch for adverse effects of radiation therapy or chemotherapy—such as anorexia, nausea, vomiting, and diarrhea—and take steps to prevent or alleviate them.
- Monitor the patient for signs and symptoms of GI or respiratory dysfunction.
- Maintain a patent airway and oxygenation status as required.

Patient teaching
- Offer emotional support to help the patient and family or other caregiver cope with the diagnosis and prognosis. Provide opportunities for them to discuss their concerns.
- Reinforce the doctor's explanation of treatments. Make sure that the patient knows which adverse reactions to expect and how to manage them. For example, during radiation therapy, instruct the patient to keep his skin dry to avoid possible breakdown and subsequent infection.
- Explain infection prevention techniques and, if necessary, demonstrate basic hygiene measures to prevent infection. These measures are especially important if the patient also has AIDS.
- Stress the need for ongoing treatment and care.
- As appropriate, refer the patient to the social services department for information about support groups.

EVALUATION
Evaluation of patient outcomes determines the success of collaborative management. For the patient with Kaposi's sarcoma, evaluation focuses on nutrition, maintaining airway and oxygenation, and body image needs.

Malignant melanoma

A neoplasm that arises from melanocytes, malignant melanoma is potentially the most lethal of all skin cancers. It's also relatively rare, accounting for only 1% to 2% of all malignant tumors.

Melanoma spreads through the lymphatic and vascular systems and metastasizes to the regional lymph nodes, skin, liver, lungs, and central nervous system (CNS). Its course is unpredictable, however, and recurrence and metastasis may not appear for more than 5 years after resection of the primary lesion. The prognosis varies with the tumor thickness. In most patients, superficial lesions are curable, whereas deeper lesions tend to metastasize.

Common sites for melanoma are the head and neck in men, the legs in women, and the backs of people exposed to excessive sunlight. Up to 70% of malignant melanomas arise from a preexisting nevus. This tumor seldom appears in the conjunctiva, choroid, pharynx, mouth, vagina, or anus.

There are four types of melanomas.
- *Superficial spreading melanoma* is the most common type.
- *Nodular melanoma* (accounting for 12% to 30% of cases) grows vertically, invades the dermis, and metastasizes early.
- *Acral-lentiginous melanoma* is the most common melanoma in Hispanics, Asians, and Blacks. It occurs on palms and soles and in subungual locations.
- *Lentigo maligna melanoma,* accounting for 10% to 15% of cases, is the slowest growing and least aggressive of the four types. It usually appears in areas heavily exposed to the sun. It arises from a lentigo maligna on an exposed skin surface and usually strikes people between ages 60 and 70.

Complications result from disease progression to the lungs, liver, or brain.

CAUSES

Several factors may influence the development of melanoma. Besides excessive exposure to sunlight, key risk factors are blond or red hair, fair skin, and blue eyes as well as a family history or past history of melanoma. Pregnancy may increase the risk of melanoma and exacerbate its growth.

DIAGNOSIS AND TREATMENT

Excisional biopsy and full-depth punch biopsy with histologic examination can distinguish malignant melanoma from a benign nevus, seborrheic keratosis, or pigmented basal cell epithelioma. These tests can also determine tumor thickness and disease stage.

Depending on the depth of tumor invasion and any metastatic spread, baseline diagnostic studies may also include chest X-rays, computed tomography (CT) scans of the chest and abdomen, and a gallium scan. Signs of bone metastasis may require a bone scan; CNS metastasis, a CT scan of the brain. Magnetic resonance imaging can help assess metastasis.

A patient with malignant melanoma always requires surgical resection to remove the tumor (a 3- to 5-cm margin is desired). The extent of resection depends on the size and location of the primary lesion. Closure of a wide resection may require a skin graft. Regional lymphadenectomy may also be performed.

Deep primary lesions may merit adjuvant chemotherapy, typically with dacarbazine or carmustine. After surgical removal of a mass, intra-arterial isolation perfusions are performed to prevent recurrence and metastasis.

Although still experimental, immunotherapy with bacille Calmette-Guérin vaccine offers hope to patients with advanced melanoma. This treatment is believed to combat cancer by boosting the body's own disease-fighting system.

Chemotherapy is useful for deep primary lesions, which have most likely metastasized. Dacarbazine and the nitrosoureas have generated some response. Similarly, radiation therapy is usually reserved for metastatic disease. It doesn't prolong survival but may reduce tumor size and relieve pain.

COLLABORATIVE MANAGEMENT

Care of the patient with malignant melanoma focuses on reduced anxiety, improved body image, and patient teaching.

ASSESSMENT

The patient history may reveal a sore that doesn't heal, a persistent lump or swelling, and changes in preexisting skin markings, such as moles, birthmarks, scars, freckles, or warts. Suspect melanoma when any preexisting skin lesion or nevus enlarges, changes color, becomes inflamed or sore, itches, ulcerates, bleeds, changes texture, or shows signs of surrounding pigment regression.

In superficial spreading melanoma, inspection may reveal lesions on the ankles or the inside surfaces of the knees. These lesions may appear red, white, or blue over a brown or black background and may have an irregular, notched margin. Palpation may reveal small, elevated tumor nodules that may ulcerate and bleed. These tumors may grow horizontally for years, but the prognosis worsens when vertical growth occurs.

In nodular melanoma, inspection of the knees and ankles may reveal a uniformly discolored, grayish nodule that resembles a blackberry. Occasionally, this melanoma is flesh-colored, with flecks of pigment around its base, which may be inflamed.

In acral-lentiginous melanoma, inspection may show pigmented lesions on the palms and soles and under the nails. The color may resemble a mosaic of rich browns, tans, and black. Inspection of the nail beds may reveal a streak in the nail associated with an irregular tan or brown stain that diffuses from the nail bed.

In lentigo maligna melanoma, the patient history may reveal a long-standing lesion that has now ulcerated. Inspection may disclose a large lesion (3 to 6 cm) that appears as a tan, brown, black, whitish, or slate-colored freckle on the face, on the back of the hand, or under the fingernails. The surface may have irregular scattered black nodules.

NURSING DIAGNOSES AND COLLABORATIVE PROBLEMS
Based on the following nursing diagnoses, you'll establish patient outcomes.

Anxiety related to potential for metastasis. The patient will:
- express his feelings of anxiety
- demonstrate effective coping strategies
- cope with his diagnosis and the requirements of follow-up care without exhibiting severe signs of anxiety.

Body image disturbance related to skin changes associated with melanoma and surgery. The patient will:
- express recognition of his changed body image
- express positive feelings about himself.

Impaired skin integrity related to skin cancer. The patient will:
- inspect his skin daily for changes and seek medical attention if changes occur
- maintain a skin care routine to prevent or minimize the risk of melanoma recurrence
- regain normal skin integrity.

PLANNING AND IMPLEMENTATION
These measures help the patient with malignant melanoma.
- Listen to the patient's fears and concerns, and stay with him during episodes of stress and anxiety.
- Include the patient and family members in care decisions.
- Provide positive reinforcement as the patient attempts to adapt to his disease.
- Offer orange and grapefruit juices and ginger ale to help control nausea and vomiting caused by chemotherapy.
- Provide a diet high in protein and calories. If the patient is anorexic, provide small, frequent meals. Consult with the dietitian to incorporate foods that the patient enjoys into his diet.
- Administer regularly scheduled analgesics to control pain, and monitor the patient's response to them.
- After surgery, take precautions to prevent infection. Check dressings often for excessive drainage, foul odor, redness, and swelling. If surgery included lymphadenectomy, apply a compression stocking and instruct the patient to keep the extremity elevated to minimize lymphedema.
- Watch for complications associated with chemotherapy, such as mouth sores, hair loss, weakness, fatigue, and anorexia.
- If the patient has a poor prognosis, identify the needs of the patient, family members, and friends and provide appropriate support and care.

Patient teaching
- Make sure the patient understands the procedures and treatments associated with his diagnosis.
- Review the doctor's explanation of treatment alternatives. Honestly answer any questions the patient may have about surgery, chemotherapy, and radiation therapy.
- Tell the patient what to expect before and after surgery, what the wound will look like, and what type of dressing he'll have. Warn him that the donor site for a skin graft may be as painful as the tumor excision site, if not more.
- Teach the patient and his family members relaxation techniques to help relieve anxiety. Encourage the patient to continue these after he is discharged.
- Emphasize the need for close follow-up care to detect recurrences early. Explain that recurrences and metastases may occur years later, so follow-up must continue for years. Teach the patient how to recognize the signs of recurrence.
- To help prevent recurrent disease, stress the detrimental effects of exposure to the sun, especially to fair-skinned, blue-eyed patients. Recommend that they use a sunscreen.
- When appropriate, refer the patient and his family to community support services, such as a local chapter of the American Cancer Society or a hospice.

EVALUATION
Evaluation of patient outcomes determines the success of collaborative management. For the patient with malignant melanoma, evaluation focuses on reducing anxiety, improving body image, and improving skin integrity.

Pediculosis

This disorder is caused by infestation with bloodsucking lice, which feed on human blood and lay their eggs (nits) in body hairs or clothing fibers. After the nits hatch, the lice must feed within 24 hours or die. They mature in about 2 to 3 weeks.

CAUSES

Pediculosis capitis (head lice) is caused by infestation with *Pediculus humanus capitis* by means of shared clothing, hats, combs, or hairbrushes. Pediculus corporis (body lice) is caused by infestation with *P. humanus corporis* through shared clothing. Pediculosis pubis (crab lice) is caused by infestation with *Phthirus pubis* by sexual intercourse or contact with clothes, bed sheets, or towels harboring lice.

When a louse bites, it injects a toxin into the skin that produces mild irritation and a purpuric spot. Repeated bites cause sensitization to the toxin, leading to more serious inflammation.

DIAGNOSIS AND TREATMENT

Because pediculosis is identified by visual examination of the patient, no laboratory tests are required.

Treatment begins with application of lindane or another pediculicide cream or shampoo as directed. The patient may need a repeat application in 1 week. In less severe cases, pediculosis corporis may require only bathing with soap and water and thorough washing of clothes.

COLLABORATIVE MANAGEMENT

Care of the patient with pediculosis focuses on pain relief, infection control, and patient teaching.

ASSESSMENT

Signs and symptoms of pediculosis capitis include itching, excoriation (with severe itching) and, in severe cases, matted, foul-smelling, lusterless hair. The patient may also experience occipital and cervical lymphadenopathy. In addition, oval, gray-white nits that won't shake loose like dandruff may appear on hair shafts. The closer the nits are to the end of the hair shaft, the longer the infestation has been present.

Signs and symptoms of pediculosis corporis include small, red papules that usually appear on the shoulders, trunk, or buttocks and change to urticaria from scratching. The patient may also develop rashes or wheals, probably indications of a sensitivity reaction. If the condition isn't treated, dry, discolored, thickly encrusted skin may result, along with bacterial infection and scarring. In severe cases, the patient may experience headache, fever, and malaise.

Signs of pediculosis pubis may include skin irritation from scratching, small gray-blue spots on the thighs or upper body, and nits on pubic hairs, which feel coarse and grainy to the touch.

NURSING DIAGNOSES AND COLLABORATIVE PROBLEMS

Based on the following nursing diagnoses, you'll establish patient outcomes.

Infection related to pruritus and scratching. The patient will:
- comply with the treatment regimen
- show no evidence of infection.
  Pain related to pruritus. The patient will:
- try nonpharmacologic methods of pain relief
- express a feeling of comfort and relief of pain.

PLANNING AND IMPLEMENTATION

These measures help the patient with pediculosis.
- Ask the patient with pediculosis pubis for a history of recent sexual contacts so that they can be examined and treated.
- To prevent the spread of pediculosis to other patients, examine all high-risk patients on admission, especially older people who depend on others for care, those admitted from nursing homes, or persons who live in crowded conditions.
- To protect yourself from infestation, avoid prolonged contact with the patient's hair, clothing, and bed sheets.
- Encourage the patient to use such comfort techniques as soothing showers.

Patient teaching

- Teach the patient steps to eliminate lice: applying special creams, ointments, powders, and shampoos; applying a solution of 50% vinegar and water to his hair for 1 hour to help remove nits; and soaking combs, brushes, and hair accessories in a pediculicide for 1 hour or boiling them in water for 10 minutes.
- Explain that he can remove lice from clothes by washing, ironing, or dry-cleaning. Storing clothes for more than 30 days or placing them in dry heat of 140° F (60° C) kills lice. If clothes can't be washed or changed, application of 10% chlorophenothane (DDT) or 10% lindane powder is effective.
- Advise the patient to launder sheets to prevent reinfestation.

EVALUATION

Evaluation of patient outcomes determines the success of collaborative management. For the patient with pediculosis, evaluation focuses on relieving pain and preventing infection.

Pemphigus vulgaris

Pemphigus vulgaris is a chronic disorder of the skin and oral mucous membranes in which blisters first form in the mouth and scalp, then spread in crops or waves to large areas of the body. The blisters ulcerate in the mouth. If left untreated, this disorder is fatal within 2 months to 5 years.

CAUSES

The cause of this disorder is unknown, but pemphigus vulgaris is associated with immunoglobulin G (IgG) antibodies and human leukocyte antigen A10. In this disorder, epidermal cells separate above the basal layer, causing rupturing and oozing of fluid with a musty smell. Pressure on a lesion may cause it to spread to adjacent skin.

DIAGNOSIS AND TREATMENT

Immunofluorescence microscopy can identify IgG antibodies, and indirect immunofluorescence microscopy can detect circulating pemphigus antibodies. A skin biopsy reveals separation of epidermal cells from each other.

Treatment consists of highly potent topical corticosteroids, systemic corticosteroids, or an immunosuppressive agent (azathioprine or methotrexate). Secondary infections are treated with topical or systemic antibiotics. In some cases, the doctor may use plasmapheresis.

COLLABORATIVE MANAGEMENT

Care of the patient with pemphigus vulgaris focuses on improved skin integrity, absence of infection, and patient teaching.

ASSESSMENT

Assessment reveals the appearance and history of the painful lesions. Signs and symptoms include enlarging bullae that rupture initially in the oral cavity but may appear on normal or erythematous skin. These areas become denuded and eventually crust; the eroded areas heal slowly. Eventually, entire body areas may become involved. The bullae may produce an offensive odor.

NURSING DIAGNOSES AND COLLABORATIVE PROBLEMS

Based on the following nursing diagnoses, you'll establish patient outcomes.

Risk for infection related to open lesions. The patient will:
- have decreased risk of infection
- have cultures that remain negative
- show no evidence of skin breakdown.

Impaired skin integrity related to disease process. The patient will:
- demonstrate understanding of skin protection measures
- demonstrate improved skin integrity.

PLANNING AND IMPLEMENTATION

These measures help the patient with pemphigus vulgaris.
- Place the patient in reverse isolation.

- Assess, evaluate, and improve the patient's hydration and nutritional status.
- Assess the effects of treatments, drugs, and procedures.

Patient teaching

- Teach the patient and family members how to provide care at home. Review skin and mouth care, diet, pain management, and prevention of infection.
- Refer the patient to a home health care agency for follow-up and continuing care.

EVALUATION

Evaluation of patient outcomes determines the success of collaborative management. For the patient with pemphigus vulgaris, evaluation focuses on improving skin integrity and preventing infection.

Pressure ulcers

Localized areas of cellular necrosis, pressure ulcers occur most often in the skin and subcutaneous tissue over bony prominences, especially the sacrum, ischial tuberosities, greater trochanter, heels, malleoli, and elbows. These ulcers—also called decubitus ulcers, pressure sores, or bedsores—may be either superficial, caused by local skin irritation (with subsequent surface maceration), or deep, originating in underlying tissue. Deep lesions often go undetected until they penetrate the skin. By then, they've usually caused subcutaneous damage.

Bacterial invasion and secondary infection, possibly leading to bacteremia and septicemia, are common complications of pressure ulcers. If the ulcer is large, a continuous loss of serum may deplete the body of its normal circulating fluids and essential proteins. In severe cases, ulcers may extend through subcutaneous fat layers, fibrous tissue, and muscle until they reach the bone.

CAUSES

Most pressure ulcers are caused by pressure that interrupts normal circulatory function. The intensity and duration of the pressure determine the severity of the ulcer; for example, pressure exerted over an area for 1 to 2 hours produces tissue ischemia and increased capillary pressure, leading to edema and multiple small-vessel thromboses. An inflammatory reaction leads to ulceration and necrosis of ischemic cells. In turn, necrotic tissue predisposes the body to bacterial invasion and infection.

Other factors that predispose a patient to pressure ulcers and delay healing include shearing forces, moisture against the skin, poor nutrition, diabetes

CLINICAL PRACTICE GUIDELINES ‖‖‖ **Preventing pressure ulcers**

The following important points are adapted from clinical practice guidelines for preventing pressure ulcers, developed by the Agency for Health Care Policy and Research of the U.S. Department of Health and Human Services. Note these points if your patient is at high risk for pressure ulcers.

Skin care and early treatment

■ Conduct a systematic skin inspection at least once a day, paying particular attention to the bony prominences. Document the results.

■ Clean the patient's skin at routine intervals and anytime soiling occurs. Avoid hot water, and use a mild cleaning agent that minimizes irritation and dryness. Take care to avoid applying force and friction to the skin during drying.

■ Minimize environmental factors that lead to skin drying, such as low humidity (less than 40%) and exposure to cold.

■ Avoid massage over bony prominences; current evidence suggests it may be harmful.

■ Minimize skin exposure to moisture due to incontinence, perspiration, or wound drainage. When you can't control the sources of moisture, use underpads or briefs made of materials that absorb moisture and present a quick-drying surface to the skin. You can also use topical agents that act as barriers to moisture.

■ Avoid skin injury due to friction and shear forces by using proper techniques when you position, transfer, or turn the patient. Also helpful are protective lubricants, films, dressings, and padding.

■ If the patient's dietary intake is inadequate, consider more aggressive nutritional interventions, such as enteral or parenteral feedings.

■ To improve the patient's mobility and activity levels, institute rehabilitation efforts, if appropriate.

Mechanical loading and support surfaces

■ Reposition the patient at least every 2 hours, if not contraindicated. Use a written schedule to ensure systematic turning and repositioning.

■ Use positioning devices, such as pillows or foam wedges, to avoid direct contact between bony prominences. Again, have a written plan.

■ For the completely immobile patient, develop a plan of care that includes devices to relieve all pressure on the heels, most commonly by raising the heels off the bed.

■ When the patient is in the side-lying position, avoid positioning him directly on the trocanter.

■ Use lifting devices, such as a trapeze or bed linen, to move (rather than drag) the patient who can't assist during transfers and position changes.

■ Place the patient on a pressure-reducing device, such as a foam, static air, alternating air, gel, or water mattress.

■ Avoid leaving the patient sitting for uninterrupted spells in a chair or wheelchair. At least every hour, reposition him, shift the points that bear pressure, or help the patient back to bed, as appropriate.

■ For the patient who's chair-bound, use a pressure-reducing device, such as those made of foam, gel, air, or a combination. Don't use a donut-shaped device.

---

mellitus, paralysis, cardiovascular disorders, and aging. Added risk factors are obesity, insufficient weight, edema, anemia, poor hygiene, and exposure to chemicals.

DIAGNOSIS AND TREATMENT

Wound culture and sensitivity testing of the ulcer exudate identify the infecting organisms. Serum protein and serum albumin studies can determine severe hypoproteinemia.

Prevention—by movement and exercise to improve circulation and adequate nutrition to maintain skin health—is always the best approach to pressure ulcers. When pressure ulcers do develop, successful management involves relieving pressure on the affected area, keeping the area clean and dry, and promoting healing. Devices such as pads, mattresses, and special beds can be used to relieve pressure. Remember that turn-

ing and repositioning are still necessary. In addition, a diet high in protein, iron, and vitamin C will help promote healing.

Other treatments—such as specialty beds, creams, and ointments—depend on the ulcer stage. Stage 1 treatment aims to increase tissue pliability, stimulate local circulation, promote healing, and prevent skin breakdown. Specific measures include the use of lubricants (such as Lubriderm), clear plastic dressings (such as Op-Site), gelatin-type wafers (such as DuoDerm), vasodilator sprays (such as Proderm), and whirlpool baths.

Stage 2 ulcers should be cleaned with normal saline solution or water and hydrogen peroxide. This removes ulcer debris and helps prevent further skin damage and infection.

Therapy for stage 3 or 4 ulcers aims to treat existing infection, prevent further infection, and remove necrotic tissue. Specific measures include cleaning the ulcer with hydrogen peroxide and povidone-iodine solution and applying granular and absorbent dressings. These dressings promote wound drainage and absorb any exudate. In addition, enzymatic ointments (such as Elase or Travase) break down dead tissue, while healing ointments clean deep or infected ulcers and stimulate new cell growth.

Debridement of necrotic tissue may be necessary to allow healing. One method is to apply open wet dressings and allow them to dry on the ulcer. Removal of the dressings mechanically debrides exudate and necrotic tissue. On occasion, the ulcer may require debridement using surgical, mechanical, or chemical techniques. In severe cases, a skin graft may be necessary. (See *Preventing pressure ulcers*.)

COLLABORATIVE MANAGEMENT
Care of the patient with a pressure ulcer focuses on prevention of additional ulcers, improved skin integrity, and avoiding infection.

ASSESSMENT
The patient with a pressure ulcer will have a history of one or more predisposing factors. Inspection of an early, superficial lesion reveals shiny, erythematous changes over the compressed area caused by localized vasodilation when pressure is relieved. If the superficial erythema has progressed, you'll see small blisters or erosions and ultimately necrosis and ulceration.

In underlying damage from pressure between deep tissue and bone, you'll note an inflamed skin surface area. Bacteria in a compressed site cause inflammation and, eventually, infection, which leads to further necrosis. You may detect a foul-smelling, purulent discharge seeping from a lesion that has penetrated the skin from beneath. A black eschar may develop around and over the lesion because infected, necrotic tissue prevents healthy granulation of scar tissue.

NURSING DIAGNOSES AND COLLABORATIVE PROBLEMS
Based on the following nursing diagnoses, you'll establish patient outcomes.

Risk for infection related to impaired skin integrity. The patient will:
- maintain a normal temperature and white blood cell count
- show no signs of foul-smelling, purulent drainage at the ulcer site
- remain free from infection.

Impaired skin integrity related to decreased blood flow. The patient will:
- demonstrate ability to carry out the prescribed skin care regimen

- display a healing pressure ulcer with effective therapy
- regain normal skin integrity.

PLANNING AND IMPLEMENTATION
These measures help the patient with a pressure ulcer.
- Reposition the bedridden patient at least every 2 hours around the clock.
- Minimize the effects of shearing force by using a footboard and raising the head of the bed no more than 60 degrees. Keep the patient's knees slightly flexed for short periods.
- Perform passive range-of-motion (ROM) exercises, or encourage the patient to do active exercises if possible.
- To prevent pressure ulcers in an immobilized patient, use pressure-relief aids on his bed.
- Monitor the patient for infection at the ulcer site.
- Because anemia and elevated blood glucose levels may lead to skin breakdown, monitor hemoglobin and blood glucose levels and hematocrit.
- Provide meticulous skin care. Keep the patient's skin clean and dry without using harsh soaps. Gently massage the skin *around* the affected area (not *on* it) to promote healing. Rub moisturizing lotions into the skin thoroughly to prevent maceration of the skin surface. Change bed linens frequently for a diaphoretic or incontinent patient.
- If the patient is incontinent, offer him a bedpan or commode frequently. Use only a single layer of padding for urine and fecal incontinence because excessive padding increases perspiration, which leads to maceration. Excessive padding also may wrinkle, irritating the skin.
- During each shift, check the bedridden patient's skin for changes in color, turgor, temperature, and sensation. Examine an existing ulcer for any change in size or degree of damage.
- Clean open lesions with normal saline solution. If possible, expose the lesions to air and sunlight to promote healing. Dressings, if needed, should be porous and lightly taped to healthy skin.
- Provide adequate food and fluid intake to maintain body weight and promote healing. Consult the dietitian to provide a diet that promotes granulation of new tissue. Encourage the debilitated patient to eat frequent, small meals that include protein- and calorie-rich supplements. Assist the weakened patient with meals.

Patient teaching
- Explain the function of pressure-relief aids and topical agents, and demonstrate their proper use.
- Teach the patient and his family members position-changing techniques and active and passive ROM exercises.

■ Stress the importance of good hygiene. Tell the patient to avoid skin-damaging agents, such as harsh soaps, alcohol-based products, tincture of benzoin, and hexachlorophene.

■ As indicated, explain debridement procedures and prepare the patient for skin graft surgery.

■ Teach the patient and his family to recognize and record signs of healing. Explain that treatment typically varies according to the stage of healing.

■ Encourage the patient to eat a well-balanced diet and drink an adequate amount of fluids, explaining their importance for skin health. Point out dietary sources rich in vitamin C, which aids wound healing, promotes iron absorption, and helps in collagen formation.

EVALUATION

Evaluation of patient outcomes determines the success of collaborative management. For the patient with pressure ulcers, evaluation focuses on maintaining skin integrity and preventing infection.

Pruritus

In pruritis (itching), an irritating agent stimulates receptors between the epidermis and dermis, releasing histamine and other mediators. Their release initiates the itching effect. Scratching leads to further irritation, which continues the cycle of itching and scratching (itch-scratch-itch cycle).

CAUSES

The exact cause of pruritis is unknown. The reaction has been associated with almost anything in a patient's internal or external environment. Skin excoriation, erythema, wheals, changes in pigmentation, and infection commonly appear as secondary effects.

DIAGNOSIS AND TREATMENT

To support a diagnosis of pruritus, the doctor may order culture and sensitivity tests of skin scrapings, studies to identify fungal infections, and cutaneous patching.

Identifying the cause of pruritus and eliminating it is the objective of treatment. Any medications the patient is taking may be discontinued to begin determining the cause. For relief of symptoms, oral medications such as antihistamines, tranquilizers, and antibiotics may help. Topical medications that contain corticosteroids may be useful along with soaks and baths with soothing agents.

COLLABORATIVE MANAGEMENT

Care of the patient with pruritus focuses on avoiding infection, improving comfort, and teaching the patient about treatment.

ASSESSMENT

A thorough examination of the patient's skin and a record of itching episodes (including location and times of maximum intensity) are key to the diagnosis.

NURSING DIAGNOSES AND COLLABORATIVE PROBLEMS

Based on the following nursing diagnoses, you'll establish patient outcomes.

Risk for injury related to pruritus. The patient will:
■ experience relief of itching
■ remain free from signs and symptoms of injury.

Risk for infection related to scratching of skin. The patient will:
■ comply with antipruritic treatment regimen
■ develop no infection.

PLANNING AND IMPLEMENTATION

These measures help the patient with pruritus.
■ Give drugs or therapeutic baths, as prescribed, to relieve discomfort.
■ Apply creams and gels by rubbing them into the affected skin.
■ Keep the patient's skin clean and moderately lubricated. Monitor him for skin excoriation.
■ Maintain a comfortable, but not excessively warm, room temperature for the patient.
■ To avoid the spread of infection, wear gloves when you care for the patient.

Patient teaching

■ If the patient is taking therapeutic baths, encourage him to use a bath mat to prevent injury from a fall.
■ Teach him to carefully follow directions for the proper amount of medication to use in his bath.
■ Instruct him to fill the bath one-third to one-half full of water and to stay in the bath for 20 to 30 minutes, keeping the room at a comfortable temperature. Warn him not to get bathwater into his eyes. Then tell him to dry his skin by blotting, not rubbing, it with a towel. (If the medications contain a stain, suggest that he use old towels.)
■ If the itching isn't relieved or the skin becomes excessively dry, tell the patient to call his doctor.

EVALUATION

Evaluation of patient outcomes determines the success of collaborative management. For the patient with pruritus, evaluation focuses on preventing infection and decreasing discomfort.

Psoriasis

Psoriasis is a noninfectious disorder marked by raised, reddened, round circumscribed plaques covered with silvery white scales. It's characterized by recurring partial remissions and exacerbations and affects about 2% of the U.S. population.

CAUSES

The cause of psoriasis is unknown, but studies suggest that it may be a genetically determined immune disorder. In psoriasis, the skin cells have a markedly shortened life cycle (4 days, compared to a normal cell's 28 days), which doesn't allow the cells to mature. As a result, the stratum corneum becomes thick and flaky, the cardinal sign of psoriasis. Increased cell metabolism stimulates increased vascularity, which contributes to the erythema.

Exacerbations may be caused by sunlight, stress, seasonal changes, hormone fluctuations, steroid withdrawal, and use of certain drugs (alcohol, corticosteroids, lithium, and chloroquine).

DIAGNOSIS AND TREATMENT

To support a diagnosis of psoriasis, the doctor may order a skin biopsy and ultrasonography to measure skin thickness.

Topical medications, such as corticosteroids, tar preparations, anthralin, and retinoids, may help decrease inflammation, prolong the maturity time of keratinocytes, and extend remission time. Other treatments include photochemotherapy and ultraviolet light therapy.

COLLABORATIVE MANAGEMENT

Care of the patient with psoriasis focuses on improved skin integrity, a better body image, and teaching about the disorder and its therapy.

ASSESSMENT

Psoriasis may appear anywhere on the body but is most commonly found on the scalp, extensor surfaces of the arms and legs, elbows, knees, sacrum, and around the nails. The patient may state the lesions have appeared and disappeared throughout life with no discernible pattern.

NURSING DIAGNOSES AND COLLABORATIVE PROBLEMS

Based on the following nursing diagnoses, you'll establish patient outcomes.

Impaired skin integrity related to psoriatic lesions. The patient will:
- demonstrate skin inspection techniques
- perform routine skin care
- have improved skin integrity.

Body image disturbance related to physical changes. The patient will:
- acknowledge that his body image has changed
- expresses positive feelings about himself
- exhibit an ability to cope with his altered body image.

PLANNING AND IMPLEMENTATION

These measures help the patient with psoriasis.
- Encourage the patient to bathe in warm—not hot—water, using a soft washcloth in a circular motion, and to blot himself dry with a towel.
- Keep the patient's skin lubricated at all times.
- Apply medication in a thin layer, using gloves.
- Apply occlusive dressings over medicated areas as ordered.
- Establish a trusting relationship with the patient, and encourage him to verbalize his feelings about his changed body image.
- Promote social interaction and refer the patient to a support group.

Patient teaching
- Tell the patient to avoid getting medication into his eyes, skinfolds, or mucous membranes.
- Teach him about the manifestations of psoriasis and when to contact his doctor. Tell him to watch for fever; increased swelling, redness, pain, or drainage; and any change in the color of drainage.
- Instruct the patient to watch for complications of treatment, including excoriation, increased erythema and peeling, and blister formation.
- Advise him to contact the National Psoriasis Foundation for information about resources and treatments.

EVALUATION

Evaluation of patient outcomes determines the success of collaborative management. For the patient with psoriasis, evaluation focuses on improving skin integrity and preserving body image.

Tinea infections

Tinea infections (dermatophytoses), commonly called ringworm, may affect the scalp (tinea capitis), body (tinea corporis), nails (tinea unguium), feet (tinea pedis), groin (tinea cruris), and bearded skin (tinea barbae). With treatment, the cure rate is high, but about 20% of infected patients develop chronic conditions.

CAUSES

Except for tinea versicolor, tinea infections are caused by dermatophytes (fungi) of the genera *Trichophyton*, *Microsporum*, and *Epidermophyton*. Infection may spread either directly, through contact with infected lesions, or indirectly, through contact with contaminated articles, such as shoes, towels, or shower stalls.

DIAGNOSIS AND TREATMENT

To confirm a diagnosis of tinea infection, the doctor may microscopically examine lesion scrapings prepared in KOH solution. A culture of the lesion scrapings can identify the infecting organism.

Localized tinea infections usually respond to a topical antifungal agent, such as clotrimazole, miconazole, haloprogin, or tolnaftate. Tinea capitis and other persistent tinea infections require treatment with oral griseofulvin for 6 to 8 weeks.

Supportive measures include open wet dressings, removal of scabs and scales, and application of keratolytics, such as salicylic acid, to soften and remove hyperkeratotic lesions of the heels or soles. The patient with tinea capitis should use selenium sulfide 2.5% shampoo during treatment and for 4 to 6 months after griseofulvin therapy to decrease fungal shedding and prevent recurrence.

COLLABORATIVE MANAGEMENT

Care of the patient with a tinea infection focuses on relieving pain, maintaining skin integrity, and patient teaching.

ASSESSMENT

Lesions vary in appearance and duration, as follows:
- *Tinea capitis:* marked by small, spreading papules on the scalp, causing patchy hair loss with scaling. Papules may progress to inflamed, pus-filled lesions (kerions).
- *Tinea corporis:* produces slightly raised, flat lesions on the skin at any site except the scalp, bearded skin, or feet. Lesions may be dry and scaly or moist and crusty. As they enlarge, their centers heal, resulting in the classic ring-shaped appearance.
- *Tinea unguium (also called onychomycosis):* usually starts at the tip of one or more toenails (fingernail infection is less common), producing gradual thickening, discoloration, and crumbling of the nail with accumulation of subungual debris. Eventually, the nail may be destroyed completely.
- *Tinea pedis (also called athlete's foot):* causes scaling and blisters between the toes. Severe infection may result in inflammation, with severe itching and pain when walking. A dry, squamous inflammation may affect the entire sole.
- *Tinea cruris (also called jock itch):* produces red, raised, sharply defined, itchy lesions in the groin that

may extend to buttocks, inner thighs, and external genitalia.
- *Tinea barbae:* an uncommon rash affecting the bearded facial area of men.

NURSING DIAGNOSIS AND COLLABORATIVE PROBLEMS

Based on the following nursing diagnoses, you'll establish patient outcomes.

Infection related to breakdown of skin barrier. The patient will:
- experience no spread of infection
- show no evidence of skin breakdown.

Impaired skin integrity related to pruritus and open skin wounds. The patient will:
- communicate an understanding of skin protection measures
- demonstrate proper skin inspection technique
- experience improvement of skin integrity.

Pain related to skin lesions. The patient will:
- try nonpharmacologic methods of pain relief
- express a feeling comfort and relief from pain.

PLANNING AND IMPLEMENTATION

These measures help the patient with a tinea infection.
- Give medications as ordered and assess their effect.
- When applying topical agents, observe the patient for sensitivity reactions and secondary bacterial infections.
- Keep the patient's skin clean and dry.
- Employ techniques to assist in achieving pain relief and comfort. Administer antihistamines, apply cool compresses, and keep the affected area clean and dry. Use diversional activities to distract the patient.

Patient teaching

- Tell the patient that improvement after topical treatment may take up to 2 weeks and that he'll need to continue treatment for another 4 or 5 days after the lesions clear.
- Instruct him to comply with oral treatment for 2 or more months, as appropriate, to ensure complete resolution of the infection.
- Teach the patient to prevent the spread of infection by keeping the lesions covered; by not scratching the lesions, which could lead to scarring and secondary infection; and by not sharing clothing, hats, towels, or pillows with other family members.

EVALUATION

Evaluation of patient outcomes determines the success of collaborative management. For the patient with a tinea infection, evaluation focuses on preventing infection, maintaining skin integrity, and relieving pain.

Toxic epidermal necrolysis

Toxic epidermal necrolysis (TEN) is a rare, life-threatening disease in which the epidermis peels off the dermis in sheets. The resultant loss of skin leads to fluid and electrolyte imbalances and secondary infections as well as systemic effects on all other body systems.

CAUSES
The triggering mechanism may be a hypersensitivity or immune response. One-third of all cases may be linked to a drug reaction and one-third are associated with serious concomitant illnesses, such as cancer or acquired immunodeficiency syndrome. In other cases the cause is unknown.

DIAGNOSIS AND TREATMENT
A biopsy of the skin lesions is performed to evaluate for underlying conditions, such as cancer.

The first step in treatment is to immediately stop any drug use by the patient. Supportive measures include fluid replacement, correction of electrolyte imbalances, prevention or management of infection, and pain control. The use of systemic corticosteroids is controversial, and topical medications containing sulfa are avoided. Surgery may include using biological or synthetic skin to cover denuded areas.

COLLABORATIVE MANAGEMENT
Care of the patient with TEN focuses on reversing fluid volume deficit, preventing infection, and improving skin integrity.

ASSESSMENT
TEN begins with a painful, localized erythema of the face and extremities, fever, chills, muscle aches, and generalized malaise. A macular rash develops, followed by formation of large, flaccid blisters that cover the body over a period of 24 to 96 hours. Sloughing then follows and may involve 95% or more of the dermal surface. The patient may also have conjunctivitis, pharyngitis, stomatitis, enlargement of lymph glands, and urethral sloughing accompanied by painful voiding and urine retention. He may also be disoriented or comatose.

NURSING DIAGNOSES AND COLLABORATIVE PROBLEMS
Based on the following nursing diagnoses, you'll establish patient outcomes.

Impaired skin integrity related to presence of blisters. The patient will:
- demonstrate skin inspection technique.

- communicate an understanding of skin protection measures
- have improved skin integrity in response to treatment

Risk for infection related to the presence of blisters and open skin wounds. The patient will:
- develop no secondary infection
- show no evidence of skin breakdown.

Fluid volume deficit related to fluid loss through the skin surface. The patient will:
- express an understanding of the need for adequate hydration
- exhibit no signs of dehydration.

PLANNING AND IMPLEMENTATION
These measures help the patient with TEN.
- Assess current lesions and monitor for infection.
- Place the patient on an alternating air flow mattress.
- Apply protective dressings as ordered.
- Maintain reverse isolation and sterile technique as indicated.
- Monitor the patient for fluid imbalances. Weigh him daily and record his intake and output.
- Monitor the patient's nutritional status.
- Maintain a warm room temperature.

Patient teaching
- Explain all treatments and procedures.
- Provide emotional support for the patient and family members.

EVALUATION
Evaluation of patient outcomes determines the success of collaborative management. For the patient with TEN, evaluation focuses on reversing fluid volume deficit, preventing infection, and promoting skin integrity.

Treatments and procedures

Many procedures are available for treating skin disorders. They include cryosurgery, escharotomy, and skin grafts.

CRYOSURGERY
Often performed in the doctor's office, cryosurgery is the destruction of tissue by the application of extreme cold. The procedure is used to treat dermatologic conditions, such as actinic and seborrheic keratoses, leukoplakia, molluscum contagiosum, verrucae, and sometimes early basal cell epitheliomas and squamous cell carcinomas. It's used to treat gynecologic conditions, such as cervicitis, chronic cervical erosion, cer-

vical polyps, and condyloma acuminatum (venereal warts), as well as ophthalmic conditions, such as cataracts and retinal tears or holes.

The success of cryosurgery depends on the type of lesion, the extent and depth of the freeze, and the duration between freezing and thawing. A slow thaw destroys lesions most effectively.

Liquid nitrogen and nitrous oxide (N_2O) are the most commonly used cryogens. Carbon dioxide and freon are used less frequently. At –320° F (–196° C), liquid nitrogen is by far the most powerful cryogen. It's especially useful for treating skin cancers, which resist cold well because of their vascularity. N_2O is often favored for less extensive procedures because the surgeon can control its effects more easily.

PROCEDURE

The procedure varies with the area being treated. For dermatologic cryosurgery, the surgeon may use local anesthesia, depending on the type and extensiveness of the lesion. He'll then determine the correct temperature and depth for freezing. For superficial lesions, he can often determine this simply by palpating and observing the lesion. For skin cancers, however, he'll use thermocouple needles and a tissue temperature monitor (pyrometer) to ensure that tissue at the deepest part of the lesion has been adequately frozen.

If the surgeon is using thermocouple needles, assist him as he inserts and secures them into the base of the tumor. Next, clean the operative site with povidone-iodine solution. The surgeon will then use either a cotton-tipped applicator that has been dipped into liquid nitrogen or the complex cryosurgical device to freeze the lesion. He may refreeze a tumor several times to ensure its destruction; for each cycle, monitor and record the number of seconds that elapse until the tissue reaches –4° F (–20° C) and the number of seconds that it takes the tissue to thaw. After cryosurgery, leave the area uncovered.

Gynecologic cryosurgery is performed in the doctor's office 1 week after the menstrual cycle. Anesthesia usually isn't given. Place the patient in the lithotomy position. The doctor will then insert a speculum into the vagina. After locating and inspecting the cervix, he'll slide the cryoprobe through the speculum and place it against the cervix. This will freeze the tissue, which will later become necrotic and slough off. After the procedure, the patient can expect a heavy, watery discharge for the next several weeks. The discharge will be heavy enough to require that she wear a peripad.

For ophthalmic cryosurgery, the doctor will first instill mydriatic and anesthetic eyedrops into the affected eye. Once the patient's eye dilates and becomes numb, he'll position the cryoprobe. Typically, he'll place it on the conjunctiva, directly over the anterior retinal break. However, if he's treating the posterior retinal area, he'll first cut an opening in the conjunctiva and rotate the eye to expose a large portion of the sclera. After the procedure, apply a patch to the affected eye.

COLLABORATIVE MANAGEMENT

Care of the patient undergoing cryosurgery requires thorough preparation, close monitoring, and intense patient teaching.

Preparation

■ Ask the patient if he has any known allergies or hypersensitivities, especially to lidocaine, iodine, or cold.

■ Most patients are unfamiliar with cryosurgery, so briefly explain the procedure and its intended purpose. Tell the patient that he'll first feel cold, then burning, during the procedure. Caution him to remain as still as possible to prevent inadvertent freezing of unaffected tissue.

■ Inform the patient having gynecologic cryosurgery that she may experience headache, dizziness, flushing, or cramping during the procedure. Reassure her that these effects are transient.

■ After providing the patient with this overview, gather the necessary equipment. If you'll use thermocouple needles and a pyrometer, obtain them as well; make sure they're sterile and in proper working order. You may also need tape to secure the needles to the base of the lesion, and you'll need a watch or a clock with a second hand to time the thaw and freeze cycles accurately. Obtain the local anesthetic, alcohol swabs, and gauze.

■ Some surgeons use gentian violet or a surgical marker to delineate the margins of the lesion. If necessary, obtain the appropriate marker.

■ Position the patient comfortably and as required by the particular site being treated. If necessary, shield his eyes or ears to prevent damage.

Monitoring and aftercare

■ Monitor the patient's vital signs until they're stable.

■ After dermatologic cryosurgery, clean the area gently with a cotton-tipped applicator soaked in hydrogen peroxide. Because cryosurgery doesn't cause bleeding, you don't need to apply a bandage. In fact, occlusive dressings are contraindicated.

■ After gynecologic cryosurgery, monitor the type and amount of vaginal drainage.

■ After ophthalmic cryosurgery, remove the eye patch when the anesthesia has worn off.

If necessary, apply an ice bag to relieve swelling and give analgesics to relieve pain, as ordered. The patient who had cryosurgery for a scalp tumor may have a headache for more than an hour after the procedure.

Patient teaching
■ Advise the patient to expect pain (especially if the procedure was performed on or near the lips, eyes, eyelids, tongue, or plantar surfaces of the feet) and to take the prescribed analgesic as needed.
■ Tell the dermatologic patient to also expect redness, swelling, and a blister to form within 6 hours of treatment. The blister may be large and may bleed. Warn him not to touch it to promote healing and prevent infection. Tell him that if the blister becomes uncomfortable or interferes with daily activities, he should call the doctor, who can decompress it with a sterile blade or pin.
■ Tell him that the blister will usually flatten within a few days and slough off in 2 to 3 weeks. Serous exudation may follow during the first week, accompanied by the development of a crust or eschar.
■ Tell the dermatologic patient to clean the area gently with soap and water, alcohol, or a cotton-tipped applicator soaked in hydrogen peroxide, as ordered. To prevent hypopigmentation, instruct him to cover the wound with a loose dressing when he's outdoors. After the wound heals, he should protect the area with sunscreen.
■ Tell the gynecologic patient that she'll have a watery vaginal discharge for several weeks. Warn her not to use tampons and to avoid sexual intercourse while the discharge is present because the cervix is very fragile during this time.
■ Emphasize the importance of calling the doctor immediately if the dermatologic patient experiences extreme pain, a widening area of erythema, oozing (of other than serous material), or fever; if the gynecologic patient experiences fever and a vaginal discharge that's other than watery in appearance; and if the ophthalmic patient experiences sudden changes in vision or an increase in eye pain.
■ If the patient had a cancerous lesion destroyed, urge him to have regular checkups to detect recurrence.

COMPLICATIONS
Complications, when they occur, are usually minor. They include hypopigmentation (from destruction of melanocytes) and secondary infection. In rare cases, the procedure may damage blood vessels, nerves, and tear ducts. After gynecologic cryosurgery, cervical stenosis may result if too large an area of the cervix is frozen at one time.

ESCHAROTOMY
Escharotomy is the excision of eschar by a scalpel or electrocautery. Eschar is the thick, hard, leathery crust that covers a wound such as a burn and harbors necrotic tissue. If it's circumferential, it may impair circulation. If it covers an arterial area, it may also require excision.

PROCEDURE
A sterile excision is made across the taut skin, and the area is then packed with fine mesh gauze.

COLLABORATIVE MANAGEMENT
Care of the patient undergoing escharotomy requires thorough preparation, close monitoring, and intense patient teaching.

Preparation
Make sure the patient understands the procedure. You'll probably give him preoperative sedation to relax him.

Monitoring and aftercare
■ Monitor the patient's vital signs until he's stable. Remember to watch for excessive blood loss and fluid depletion.
■ Monitor wound drainage and the gauze dressing for the first 24 hours. On the second day, you'll probably treat the site with silver sulfadiazine.

Patient teaching
■ Instruct the patient to report any signs of impaired circulation, such as a change in skin color or temperature, increased pain, or numbness or tingling.
■ Teach the patient how to protect the area from infection.

COMPLICATIONS
Infection may be a complication.

SKIN GRAFTS
Skin grafts are performed to cover defects caused by burns, trauma, or surgery. This procedure is indicated when primary closure of a wound isn't possible or cosmetically acceptable, when primary closure would interfere with functioning, when the defect is on a weight-bearing surface, or when a skin tumor is excised and the site needs to be monitored for recurrence.

The types of skin grafts are split-thickness grafts, which include the epidermis and a small portion of dermis; full-thickness grafts, which include all of the dermis as well as the epidermis; and composite grafts, which also include underlying tissues, such as muscle, cartilage, or bone.

Grafting may be done using a general or a local anesthetic. It can be performed on an outpatient basis for small facial or neck defects.

PROCEDURE

The surgeon separates a section of skin tissue from its blood supply and transfers it as free tissue to a distant site. The recipient site provides nourishment from its capillaries to the transferred tissue.

For all types of grafting, success depends on revascularization. The graft initially survives by direct contact with the underlying tissue, receiving oxygen and nutrients through existing lymph, but it will die eventually unless new blood vessels develop. In split-thickness grafts, revascularization usually takes 3 to 5 days; in full-thickness grafts, it may take up to 2 weeks.

COLLABORATIVE MANAGEMENT

Care of the patient undergoing a skin graft requires thorough preparation, close monitoring, and intense patient teaching.

Preparation

Because successful skin grafting begins with good graft material, take steps to preserve potential donor sites by providing meticulous skin care. Grafts are harvested using a free-hand knife technique or a dermatome, depending on the doctor's preference.

Also assess the recipient site. The graft's survival depends on close contact with the underlying tissue; ideally the recipient site should be healthy granulation tissue, free of eschar, debris, or the products of infection.

Prepare the donor and recipient sites for surgery while the anesthetic takes effect.

Monitoring and aftercare

After the procedure, your role is to ensure the graft's survival.

■ Monitor the patient's vital signs until they're stable.

■ Position the patient so that he's not lying on the graft; if possible, keep the graft area elevated and immobilized.

■ Modify your nursing routine to protect the graft; for example, never use a blood pressure cuff over a graft site.

■ For burn patients, omit hydrotherapy while the graft heals.

■ Give analgesics as necessary, and help the patient use nonpharmacologic pain-reduction techniques.

■ Use sterile technique when changing a dressing, and work gently to avoid dislodging the graft.

■ Clean the graft site with warm saline solution and cotton-tipped applicators, leaving the fine mesh gauze intact.

■ Aspirate any serous pockets.

■ Change the gauze and apply the prescribed topical agent as needed.

■ Cover the graft area with a nonadhering stretchable gauze bandage (such as Kerlix).

■ Care for the donor site by cleaning it as ordered and keeping it clean and dry.

Patient teaching

■ Counsel the patient not to disturb the dressings on the graft or donor sites for any reason. If they need to be changed, tell him to call the doctor.

■ If grafting is done as an outpatient procedure, inform the patient that he'll have to immobilize the graft site to promote proper healing.

■ Tell the patient that, once the graft has healed, he should apply cream to the site several times a day to keep the skin pliable and aid scar maturation.

■ Because sun exposure can affect graft pigmentation, advise the patient to limit his time in the sun and to use a sunscreen on all grafted areas.

■ Explain that after scar maturation is complete, the doctor may use other plastic surgery techniques to improve the graft's appearance.

COMPLICATIONS

Complications include graft rejection and infection.

Selected references

Beare, P.G., and Myers, J.L. *Principles and Practice of Adult Health Nursing,* 2nd ed. St. Louis: Mosby–Year Book, Inc., 1994.

Diseases, 2nd ed. Springhouse, Pa.: Springhouse Corp., 1997.

Freeman, Z., et al. "Necrotizing Fasciitis: A Cautionary Tale," *AJN* 97(3):34-36, March 1997.

Hess, C.T. *Nurse's Clinical Guide to Wound Care,* 2nd ed. Springhouse, Pa.: Springhouse Corp., 1998.

Maklebust, J., and Sieggreen, M.Y. "Attacking on All Fronts: How to Conquer Pressure Ulcers," *Nursing96* 26(12):34-46, December 1996.

Polaski, A., and Tatro, S.E. *Luckmann's Core Principles and Practice of Medical-Surgical Nursing.* Philadelphia: W.B. Saunders Co., 1996.

Porth, C. *Pathophysiology: Concepts of Altered Health States,* 4th ed. Philadelphia: Lippincott-Raven Pubs., 1994.

U.S. Agency for Health Care Policy and Research. *Clinical Practice Guidelines #15: Treatment of Pressure Ulcers.* Rockville, Md.: U.S. Department of Health and Human Services, 1994.

Appendices
Index

A
Reviewing the newest isolation precautions ▐▐▐▐▐▐▐▐▐▐▐▐▐▐▐▐▐▐▐▐▐▐▐▐▐▐▐▐▐▐▐▐▐▐▐▐▐▐

The Guidelines for Isolation Precautions in Hospitals were developed by the Centers for Disease Control and Prevention (CDC) and the Hospital Infection Control Practices Advisory Committee. The newest guidelines now contain two levels of precautions: *standard precautions* and *transmission-based precautions*. These newest guidelines replace the previous universal precautions and category-specific guidelines. The transmission-based precautions are further divided into three types, based on the mode of transmission: *contact precautions*, *droplet precautions*, and *airborne precautions*.

Standard precautions are designed to decrease "the risk of transmission of organisms from both recognized and unrecognized sources of infection in hospitals." They should be followed at all times, with every patient.

Standard precautions combine the major features of the former universal precautions, which were developed in response to the increasing incidence of human immunodeficiency virus infection, hepatitis B virus infection, and other blood-borne diseases, and the former body substance isolation, which was developed to reduce the risk of pathogen transmission from moist body surfaces. Because standard precautions reduce the risk of transmission of blood-borne and other pathogens, many patients with diseases or conditions that previously required category- or disease-specific isolation precautions now require only standard precautions.

The specific substances covered by standard precautions include blood and all other body excretions, except sweat, even if the blood is not visible. Standard precautions should also be followed in the presence of nonintact skin and exposed mucous membranes.

Transmission-based precautions are followed, in addition to standard precautions, whenever a patient is known or suspected to be infected with highly contagious and epidemiologically important pathogens that are transmitted by air or droplets or by contact with dry skin or other contaminated surfaces. Examples of these pathogens include those that cause measles (air), influenza (droplet), and gastrointestinal, respiratory, skin, and wound infections (contact). In fact, transmission-based precautions replace all older categories of isolation precautions including strict isolation, contact isolation, respiratory isolation, enteric precautions, and drainage/secretion precautions and most other disease-specific precautions. One or more types of transmission-based precautions may be combined and followed when a patient has a disease that has multiple routes of transmission.

Use the following table for a better understanding of the new CDC guidelines for infection control.

Revised infection control guidelines

Type of precaution	Purpose	Nursing considerations
STANDARD PRECAUTIONS	Prevent transmission of microorganisms from both recognized and un-recognized sources of infection, such as: ■ *Streptococcus*, group A ■ poliomyelitis ■ relapsing fever ■ scaled skin syndrome ■ toxic shock syndrome ■ *Streptobacillus monili-formis* disease (rat-bite fever) ■ psittacosis ■ rabies ■ endometritis ■ syphilis (congenital, primary, or secondary) ■ trachoma ■ tularemia.	■ Wear gloves if you will or could come in contact with blood, specimens, tissue, body fluid, secretions or excretions, or contaminated surfaces or objects. ■ Wash your hands immediately if they become contaminated with blood or body fluids; also wash your hands before and after patient care and after removing gloves. ■ Change your gloves between patient contacts and between tasks and procedures in the same patient if you make contact with anything that might have a high concentration of microorganisms, to avoid cross-contamination. ■ Wear a gown, eye protection (goggles, glasses) or face shield, and a mask during such procedures as surgery, endoscopic procedures, or dialysis that are likely to generate droplets of blood or body fluids, secretions, or excretions. ■ Carefully handle used patient care equipment soiled with blood, body fluids, secretions, or excretions to avoid exposure to skin and mucous membranes, clothing contamination, and transfer of microorganisms to other patients and environments. ■ Ensure that facility procedures for routine care, cleaning, and disinfection of environmental surfaces, beds, bed rails, and bedside equipment are followed. ■ Handle contaminated linens in a manner that prevents contamination and transfer of microorganisms. Do not shake contaminated linens, and keep them away from your body. Place in properly labeled containers. Ensure that linens are transported and processed according to facility policy. ■ Handle used needles or other sharp implements carefully. Do not bend, break, reinsert them into their original sheaths, or unnecessarily handle them. Discard them intact into an impervious disposal box immediately after use. These measures reduce the risk of accidental injury or infection. ■ Use mouthpieces, resuscitation bags, or other ventilation devices in place of mouth-to-mouth resuscitation whenever possible. ■ Place in a private room any patient who cannot maintain appropriate hygiene or who contaminates the environment. Notify infection control personnel. ■ If you have an exudated lesion, avoid all direct patient contact until the condition has resolved and you've been cleared by the employee health provider.
CONTACT PRECAUTIONS	Prevent transmission of infections spread primarily by close or direct contact including: ■ cutaneous diphtheria, Lassa fever and other viral hemorrhagic fevers (including Marburg virus disease) ■ acute viral conjunctivitis ■ congenital rubella ■ impetigo ■ respiratory syncytial virus ■ scabies ■ enterocolitis caused by *Clostridium difficile*; gastroenteritis (in diapered or incontinent patients) caused by *Escherichia coli* and *Vibrio parahaemolyticus* ■ Hand, foot, and mouth disease.	In addition to standard precautions follow these guidelines: ■ Place the patient in a private room or, if one is not available, place the patient in a room with another patient who has an active infection with the same microorganism. If this is not possible, consult infection control personnel. Special ventilation is not necessary. ■ Wear gloves whenever you enter the room. Always change gloves after contact with infected material. Remove gloves before leaving the patient's room, and wash your hands immediately with an antimicrobial soap or waterless antiseptic agent. Do not touch any contaminated surfaces after washing your hands. ■ Wear a gown when entering the patient's room; if you think you'll have extensive contact with the patient, environmental surfaces, or items in the patient's room; or if the patient has diarrhea or is incontinent. Remove the gown before leaving the patient's room. ■ Limit movement of the patient from the room. ■ Avoid sharing any patient care equipment.

(continued)

Revised infection control guidelines *(continued)*

Type of precaution	Relevant diagnoses	Nursing considerations
DROPLET PRECAUTIONS	Prevent transmission of large particle droplets containing microorganisms generated primarily through coughing, sneezing, or talking and during certain procedures such as suctioning and bronchoscopy, including: ■ epiglottitis caused by *Haemophilus influenzae* ■ *H. Influenzae* meningitis and meningococcal meningitis ■ *H. Influenzae* pneumonia in children of any age ■ meningococcemia, mumps, or pertussis ■ scarlet fever in children and young infants ■ parvovirus B19 ■ pneumonic plague.	In addition to standard precautions follow these guidelines: ■ Place the patient in a private room or, if one is not available, place the patient in a room with another patient who has an active infection with the same microorganism. If this is not possible, consult infection control personnel. Special ventilation is not necessary ■ Wear a mask when working within 3' (1m) of the patient. ■ Keep visitors 3' from the infected patient. ■ Limit movement of the patient from the room. If the patient must leave the room, have him wear a surgical mask, if possible.
AIRBORNE PRECAUTIONS	Prevent transmission of airborne small-particle droplets containing microorganisms that can be suspended in the air and dispersed widely by currents within a room or long distance, such as: ■ chickenpox ■ *Herpes zoster*, localized in immunocompromised patients ■ measles ■ tuberculosis (pulmonary, confirmed or suspected) or laryngeal disease.	In addition to standard precautions, follow these guidelines: ■ Place the patient in a private room with monitored negative air pressure with 6 to 12 exchanges/hour that are appropriately discharged to outdoors or with monitored high efficiency filtration. Keep the door closed and the patient in the room. If a private room is not available, place the patient in a room with another patient who has an active infection with the same microorganism. If this is not possible, consult infection control personnel. ■ Wear respiratory protection (mask or face shield) when entering the room of a patient with a known or suspected respiratory infection. If you're immune to measles and varicella, you don't need to wear respiratory protection when entering the room of a patient with one of these illnesses. ■ Limit patient transport and patient movement out of the room. If he must leave the room, have him wear a surgical mask, if possible.

B

Better charting: Documentation samples |||||||||||||||||||||||||||||||||||||||||

Completing the admission assessment

An assessment form, such as the one shown below, is used to document the patient's initial assessment data. Most health care facilities use a combined checklist and narrative admission form. Many facilities use a multidisciplinary form; nurses, doctors, and other health care team members who obtain initial assessment data document their findings on a single form.

ADMISSION ASSESSMENT

Name _Mary Adams_
Address _101 Shea Lane, Milltown, CO_
Soc sec # _022-22-2222_ D.O.B. _11-9-21_
Religion _Methodist_

Date Admitted _8/15/97_
Time Admitted _1300_

VITAL SIGNS

TEMPERATURE	PULSE	RESP.	BP	HT	WT	Pre-admission testing done ☐
98.6°F	88	14	132/86	5'5"	175 lb.	

MODE OF ACCESS

☑ SDA   ☐ DR   ☐ ED
☐ Crisis   ☐ Direct
☐ Unaccompanied
☐ Accompanied by: _daughter—Mary_

Informant
☑ Patient
☐ Other

Admitted via:
☑ Wheelchair
☐ Stretcher
☐ Ambulatory

Reason for admission, according to patient or family _"to have a Ⓛknee replacement"_
Special needs (cultural or spiritual) _has living will and medical power-of-attorney_
Religious preference _Methodist_

ADVANCE DIRECTIVE

Does patient have advance directive?   ☑ Yes   ☐ No   ☑ Written   ☐ Verbal
Is copy of advance directive on file?   ☑ Yes   ☐ No   Date of written directive _Dec 1993_

ALLERGIES

☐ Food   ☑ Medications   ☐ Other   ☐ Uncertain   ☐ None   (specify) _PCN—rash_

MEDICATIONS

List patient's medications (name, dose, route, frequency).
Atenolol 25 mg÷P.O. qd, ibuprofen 200 mg P.O.÷
t.i.d. prn pain Ⓛknee, ferrous sulfate 325 mg
_P.O. t.i.d._

Did patient bring medications to hospital? ☐ Yes   ☑ No
If yes, disposition: ☐ Sent home   ☐ Sent to pharmacy
☐ Placed in safety deposit box

Indicate medications taken today and time administered.
Atenolol 0900 hours, ibuprofen 0900 hours,
ferrous sulfate 0900 hrs

Describe personal health, family, medical, surgical, and psychiatric history pertinent to this hospitalization.   ☐ Check if none
Rheumatoid arthritis x 10 years
Anemia x 5 years

(continued)

Completing the admission assessment *(continued)*

BLOOD HISTORY

Previous transfusion   ☐ Yes   ☑ No   ☑ Autologous blood donation
No. of units *2*

Previous reaction   ☐ Yes   ☑ No

INFECTION CONTROL

Precautions initiated other than standard   *None*   Patient and/or family received explanation? ☑ Yes   ☐ No
☐ Type (specify)_____   If no, explain. _____
Other pertinent infection control info. _____ _____

SAFETY

Patient safety parameters   ☑ ID band   ☑ Oriented to unit
Fall risk?   ☑ Yes   ☐ No

Are there specific patient safety or observation needs?
Specify: *Unsteady gait. Pt. needs assistance of*
cane to ambulate.

	VALUABLES		
	Home	Patient	Safety Deposit Box
Money	✓		
Ring	✓		
Watch	✓		
Other			

FUNCTIONAL STATUS

DAILY LIVING HABITS

Smoking (type/pattern) _____   ☑ None   Regular diet _____
Informed of smoking policy   ☑ Yes   Special diet (specify) *Low salt, low fat*
Alcohol (type/pattern) _____   ☑ None   Sleep pattern *Gets up 3x during night to void*
Last drink (time/amount) _____   Substance use (type/pattern) _____ ☑ None

GENERAL APPEARANCE

Note any unusual skin color, abrasions, pressure ulcers, and so on. Also note the patient's body type and manner of dress.
73 y.o. white female, pale, overweight, not looking as old as her stated years. Favors Ⓛleg and
ambulatory with assistance of cane. Appears to rely on daughter to help with answering questions
during assessment. Daughter is a nurse.

GENERAL BEHAVIOR & MENTAL STATUS

☐ Calm   ☑ Anxious   ☐ Agitated   ☐ Comatose   ☐ Lethargic   Oriented? ☐ Yes ☐ No (describe below)

IMPAIRMENTS OR DISABILITIES

☐ Denies concerns
☐ Impaired hearing
☐ Impaired vision

	With patient
☑ Hearing aid	☑
☑ Glasses or contact lenses	☑
☑ Lower dentures	☑
☑ Upper dentures	☑

Independent for:
☑ ADLs
☐ Walking
☑ Transfers
Prosthesis_____
Assistive devices *Cane*

Completing the admission assessment *(continued)*

BIOPHYSICAL

NEUROLOGIC
- ☐ Speech difficulty
- ☐ Muscle atrophy
- ☐ Paralysis
- ☐ Spasticity
- ☐ Syncope
- ☐ Dizziness
- ☐ Ataxia
- ☐ Paresthesia
- ☐ Seizures (type)
- ☐ Other (specify) _____
  _____

EENT
- ☐ Recent headache
- ☐ Facial pain
- ☐ Recent hearing loss
- ☐ Earaches
- ☐ Glaucoma
- ☐ Cataracts
- ☐ Hoarseness
- ☐ Sore throat
- ☐ Laryngitis
- ☑ Sinus problems
- ☐ Epistaxis
- ☐ Other (specify) _____
  _____

CARDIORESPIRATORY
- ☐ Chest pain (describe)
  _____
- ☑ Cough nonproductive
- ☐ Cough productive (describe) _____
- ☐ Shortness of breath
- ☐ Nocturnal dyspnea
- ☐ Palpitations
- ☐ Known murmur
- ☐ Edema
- ☐ Diaphoresis
- ☑ Hypertension
- ☐ Hemoptysis
- ☑ Varicosities

GI
- ☐ Mouth sores
- ☐ Abdominal pain
- ☐ Vomiting
- ☐ Hematemesis
- ☐ Difficulty swallowing
- ☑ Flatulence
- ☐ Nausea
- ☑ Constipation
- ☐ Tarry stool
- ☐ Jaundice
- ☐ Thirst
- ☐ Diarrhea
- ☐ Heartburn
- ☐ Hernia

Bowel pattern *once a day*
  _____
- ☐ Other findings
  (such as colostomy, and
  so on) _____
  _____

GENITOURINARY
- ☐ Denies concerns
- ☐ Dysuria
- ☐ Incontinence
- ☑ Nocturia
- ☐ Urinary frequency
- ☐ Penile discharge
- ☐ Stoma
- ☐ Urinary urgency
- ☐ Hematuria
- ☐ Urine retention
- ☐ Lesions
- ☐ Polyuria
- ☐ Burning
- ☐ Testicular pain or swelling
- ☐ Other findings
  (Ileoconduit - indwelling urinary catheter) _____
  _____

FEMALE REPRODUCTIVE
Menstrual history:
  Regularity _____
  Duration _____
  LMP *20 yrs. ago*
Last gyn exam *1 yr. ago*
- ☐ Pain
- ☐ Bleeding
Discharge
  ☐ Yes ☐ No
Monthly breast self-exam
  ☑ Yes ☐ No

ENDOCRINE
- ☐ Goiter
- ☐ Heat or cold intolerance
- ☐ Voice change
- ☐ Tremor
- ☐ Polyphagia
- ☐ Diabetes

MUSCULOSKELETAL & INTEGUMENTARY
- ☐ Extremity pain
- ☐ Redness
- ☐ Muscle pain
- ☐ Deformity
- ☑ Limited motion *Ⓛ knee*
- ☐ Back pain
- ☑ Joint pain *Ⓛ knee*
- ☑ Joint swelling
- ☐ Neck pain
- ☐ Fractures
- ☐ Pressure ulcer

PSYCHOSOCIAL
- ☐ Incoherent thoughts
- ☐ Guarded
- ☐ Suspicious
- ☐ Incoherent speech
- ☐ Distractible
- ☐ Difficulty concentrating
- ☐ Hallucinations (type)
  _____
- ☐ Delusions
- ☐ Homicidal ideation
- ☐ Suicidal ideation
- ☐ Mood (describe)
  _____
- ☐ Affect (describe)
  _____
  _____
  _____

EDUCATIONAL NEEDS

Person involved with instruction ☑ Patient ☑ Other (specify) *Daughter* _____

Primary language of person(s) involved with instruction ☑ English ☐ Other (specify) _____
  If other, is an interpreter needed ☐ Yes ☐ No

Anticipated learning needs
- ☑ Preop procedure ☑ Medications ☐ Wound or catheter care ☑ Health problems
- ☑ Equipment Other comments _____

(continued)

Completing the admission assessment *(continued)*

DISCHARGE PLANNING

SUPPORT SYSTEMS & CONTINUING CARE

Was patient independent for self-care before hospitalization?   ☑ Yes   ☐ No (explain) ⎯⎯⎯⎯⎯⎯⎯⎯⎯⎯⎯

Does patient have family or friend available to assist with and/or manage postdischarge care if needed?
☑ Yes ☐ No: Who? *Daughter*

Other resources needed to facilitate discharge planning:

☐ Skilled care   ☐ Home health care   ☐ Social services   ☐ Dietary services   ☐ Equipment   ☐ Other ⎯⎯⎯

Signature/time/date *Elaine Banister, RN 1430 hours 8/15/97*   Unit *4 North*

PLAN OF CARE

Knowledge deficit related to preop and postop routines EB

Pain related to arthritis EB

Related learning needs   EB

Signature *Elaine Banister, RN*

Using a flow sheet to record routine care

As this sample shows, a patient care flow sheet lets you quickly document your routine interventions.

PATIENT CARE FLOW SHEET

Date 9/22/97	2300—0700	0700—1500	1500—2300
RESPIRATORY Breath sounds	Clear 2330 AS	Crackles LLL 0800 JM	Clear 1600 HM
Treatments/results		Nebulizer 0830 JM	
Cough/results	ō AS	Mod. amt. tenacious yellow mucus 0900 JM	ō HM
O₂ therapy	Nasal cannula @2L/min AS	Nasal cannula @ 2 L/min JM	Nasal cannula @ 2 L/min HM
CARDIAC Chest pain	ō AS	ō JM	ō HM
Heart Sounds	Normal S₁ and S₂ AS	Normal S₁ and S₂ JM	Normal S₁ and S₂ HM
Telemetry	N/A	N/A	N/A
PAIN Type and location	Ⓛ flank 0400 AS	Ⓛ flank 1000 JM	Ⓛ flank 1600 HM
Intervention	meperidine 0415 AS	Reposition and meperidine 1010 JM	meperidine 1615 HM
Pt. response	Improved from #9 to #3 in 1/2 hour AS	Improved from #8 to #2 in 45 min. JM	Complete relief in 1 hr HM
NUTRITION TYPE		Regular JM	Regular HM
Toleration %		90% JM	80% HM
Supplement		1 can Ensure JM	
ELIMINATION Stool appearance	ō AS	ō JM	☥ soft dark brown HM
Enema	N/A	N/A	N/A
Results			
Bowel sounds	Present all quadrants 2330 AS	Present all quadrants 0800 JM	Hyperactive all quadrants 1600 HM
Urine appearance	Clear amber 0400 AS	Clear amber 1000 JM	Dark yellow 1500 HM
Indwelling urinary catheter	N/A	N/A	N/A
Catheter irrigations			
I.V. THERAPY Tubing change		1100 JM	
Dressing change		1100 JM	
Site appearance	No edema, no redness 2330 AS	No redness, no edema, no drainage 0800 JM	No redness, no edema 1500 HM

(continued)

Using a flow sheet to record routine care (continued)

PATIENT CARE FLOW SHEET

Date 9/22/97	2300—0700	0700—1500	1500—2300
WOUNDS Type	(L) flank incision 2330 AS	(L) flank incision 1200 JM	(L) flank incision HM
Dressing change	Dressing dry and intact 2330 AS	1200* JM	2000* HM
Appearance	Wound not observed AS	*See progress note JM	*See progress note HM
TUBES Type	N/A	N/A	N/A
Irrigation	—	—	—
Drainage appearance	—	—	—
HYGIENE Self/partial/complete	—	Partial 1000 JM	Partial 2100 HM
Oral care	—	1000 JM	2100 HM
Back care	0400 AS	1000 JM	2100 HM
Foot care	—	1000 JM	—
Remove/reapply elastic stockings	2330 AS	1000 JM	2100 HM
ACTIVITY Type	Bed rest AS	OOB to chair x 20 min 1000 JM	OOB to chair x 20 min 1800 HM
Toleration	Turns self AS	Tol. well JM	Tol. well HM
Repositioned	2330 Supine AS 0400 (L) side AS	(L) side 0800 JM (R) side 1400 JM	Self HM
ROM	—	1000 (active) JM 1400 (active) JM	1800 (active) HM 2200 (active) HM
SLEEP Sleeps well	0400 AS 0600 AS	N/A	N/A
Awake at intervals	2330 AS 0400 AS	—	—
Awake most of the time	—	—	—
SAFETY Side rails up	2330 AS 0200 AS 0400 AS 0600 AS	0800 JM 1200 JM 1500 JM	1600 HM 2100 HM
Call button in reach	2330 PS 0200 AS 0400 AS 0600 AS	0800 JM 1200 JM 1500 JM	1600 HM 2100 HM

Using a flow sheet to record routine care *(continued)*

PATIENT CARE FLOW SHEET

Date 9/22/97	2300—0700	0700—1500	1500—2300
EQUIPMENT			
IVAC pump	Continuous 2300 AS	Continuous 0800 JM	Continuous 1600 HM
TEACHING			
Wound splinting	2330 AS	1000 JM	1600 HM
Deep breathing	2330 AS	1000 JM	1600 HM
Initials/Signature/Title	AS/Anne Solon RN	JM/Judy Meyer RN	HM/Helen Moran RN

Using a flow sheet to record routine care *(continued)*

PATIENT CARE FLOW SHEET

PROGRESS SHEET

Date	Time	Comments
9/22/97	1200	Ⓛ flank dressing saturated with serosang. drng. Dressing removed. Wound edges well-approximated except for 2 cm. Opening noted at lower edge of incision. Small amount serosang. drng. noted oozing from this area. No redness noted along incision line. Sutures intact. Incision line painted with povidine-iodine. Five 4" x 4" gauze pads applied and taped in place. Dr. Wong notified of increased amt. of drng. —Judy Meyer RN
9/22/97	2000	Dr. Wong to see pt. Ⓛ flank drsg. removed. 2-cm opening noted at lower edge of incision. Otherwise wound edge well-approximated. Dr. Wong sutured opening with one 3-0 silk suture. No redness of drng. noted along incision line. Painted incision line with povidine-iodine and applied two 4" x 4" gauze pads. Taped drsg. in place. —Helen Moran RN

Using a traditional plan of care

This sample shows how a traditional plan of care organizes key information. Keep in mind that the plans of care you'll use will have wider columns to allow more room for your notes.

Date	Nursing diagnoses	Expected outcomes	Interventions	Revision (initials and date)	Resolution (initials and date)
8/8/97	Decreased cardiac output R/T reduced stroke volume secondary to fluid volume overload.	Lungs will be clear on auscultation by 8/10/97. BP will return to baseline by 8/10/97.	Monitor for signs and symptoms of hypoxemia, such as dyspnea, confusion, arrhythmias, restlessness, and cyanosis. Ensure adequate oxygenation by placing patient in semi-Fowler's position and administering supplemental O_2 as ordered. Monitor breath sounds q 4 hr. Administer cardiac medications as ordered and document pt.'s response, their effectiveness, and any adverse reactions. Monitor and document heart rate and rhythm, heart sounds, and BP. Note the presence or absence of peripheral pulses. RO		

Review dates

Date	Signature	Initials
8/8/97	Rose O'Donnell, RN	RO

Using a standardized plan of care

The plan of care below is for a patient with a nursing diagnosis of decreased cardiac output. To customize it to your patient, you'd complete the diagnosis—including signs and symptoms—and fill in the expected outcomes. You'd also modify, add, or delete interventions as necessary.

Date *8/1/97*	**Nursing diagnosis** *Decreased cardiac output R/T reduced stroke volume secondary to fluid volume overload.*
Target date *8/2/97*	**Expected outcomes** Adequate cardiac output (AEB): *>4.0 L/min* Heart rate: Apical rate *<90* BP: *140/80 mm Hg* Pedal pulse: *palpable and regular* Radial pulse: *palpable and regular* Cardiac rhythm: *normal sinus rhythm* Cardiac index: *>3L/min/m²* Pulmonary artery wedge pressure (PAWP): *10 mm Hg* Pulmonary artery pressure (PAP): *20/12 mm Hg* SvO_2: *Between 60% and 80%* Urine output in ml/hr: *>30 ml/hr*
Date *8/1/97*	**Interventions** ■ Monitor ECG for rate and rhythm; note ectopic beats. If arrhythmias occur, note patient's response. Document and report findings and follow appropriate arrhythmia protocol. ■ Monitor SvO_2, temperature, respirations, and central pressures continuously. ■ Monitor other hemodynamic pressures q *1* hr and p.r.n. ■ Auscultate for heart sounds and palpate for peripheral pulses q *2* hr and p.r.n. ■ Monitor I & O q *1* hr. Notify doctor if output <30 ml/hr x 2 hr. ■ Administer medications and fluids as ordered, noting effectiveness and adverse reactions. Titrate vasoactive drugs as needed. Follow appropriate vasoactive drug protocol to wean patient as tolerated. ■ Monitor O_2 therapy or other ventilatory assistance. ■ Decrease patient's activity to reduce O_2 demands. Increase as tolerated. ■ Assess and document LOC. Assess for changes q *1* hr and p.r.n. ■ Additional interventions: *Inspect for pedal and sacral edema q 2 hr.*

Using a discharge summary – patient instruction form

Combining the patient's discharge summary with instructions for care after discharge fills two requirements with a single stroke of your pen. When using this documentation method, be sure to give one copy to the patient and keep one for the record.

DISCHARGE SUMMARY AND INSTRUCTIONS

Patient stamp and I.D.

Mary Adams
101 Shea Lane,
Milltown, CO
PCN-0006-234-56

DIET

☐ No restrictions   ☐ Special diet _____

ACTIVITY

☐ No restrictions
☑ Lifting restricted to _5_ lb for ___ week(s) or (until after next office visit.)
☑ Stair climbing restricted to _2 to 4_ steps/days for ____ week(s) or (until after next office visit.)
☑ No driving for _____ week(s) or (until next office visit.)
☑ Riding in car restricted: _None for 1 week, then 1 hr at a time_

May take: ☐ shower   ☐ tub bath   ☑ sponge bath
☑ Walking/exercise restricted to: _Per instruction from PT_
☑ Other restrictions: _Use raised toilet seat_
May return to work: _N/A_
     ☐ immediately
     ☐ week(s)
     ☐ undetermined

COMFORT LEVEL

☐ No pain   ☐ Minimal discomfort   ☑ Moderate discomfort   ☐ Maximum discomfort

AIDS USED

☐ None   ☐ Cane   ☑ Walker   ☐ Prosthesis   ☐ Wheelchair   ☐ Crutches

HYGIENE AND ACTIVITIES OF DAILY LIVING

☐ Independent   ☑ Needs some assistance   ☐ Needs total assistance   ☐ Other _____

	No Difficulty	Other (explain)
Respiratory	✓	
CV	✓	
Neurologic	✓	
Skin		*wound care to (L) knee incision*
Musculoskeletal		*Ambulates with use of walker*
GI	✓	
Nutritiion	✓	

	No Difficulty	Other (explain)
Vision		*Needs glasses at all times.*
Hearing	✓	
Speech	✓	
Reproductive	✓	
Elimination (bladder)	✓	
Elimination (bowel)	✓	

(continued)

Using a discharge summary – patient instruction form *(continued)*

DISCHARGE SUMMARY AND INSTRUCTIONS

MENTAL STATUS

☑ Alert ☑ Oriented ☐ Lethargic ☐ Confused

INCISIONAL CARE

☐ No special care required ☑ Other
Paint incision with betadine swabs twice a day. Use three swabs each time, one straight down on top of the incision line; one down the one side of the incision; then the third stick down the other side of the incision. Do not scrub incision back and forth. Dress with nonadhesive dressing.

SPECIAL INSTRUCTIONS FOR MEDICATIONS

Dose/time/route (Do not take any other medications before checking with your physician.)

	Prescription Given	Has at Home
Percocet—one tablet every 4 hr as needed for severe pain.	☑	☐
Tylenol 325 mg every 4 hr as needed for mild pain.	☐	☑
Continue taking other medications as before surgery.	☐	☐
	☐	☐
	☐	☐
	☐	☐

PATIENT EDUCATION	Patient		S/O		N/A
	Yes	No	Yes	No	
Verbalizes symptoms of disease process	√		√		
Verbalizes activities or exercises	√		√		
Verbalizes special diet, if ordered	√		√		
Verbalizes medication's adverse effects, if ordered	√		√		
Demonstrates ability to perform specialized care or treatment (wound healing, dressings, and so forth)		√	√		
Verbalizes when to contact physician	√		√		
Given patient education information	√		√		

COMMENTS: _____

FORMS GIVEN

Prescriptions
Percocet one tablet every 4 hr as needed for severe pain.

Other (specify)
_____

Diet
2 Gram Sodium

DISCHARGE DESTINATION

☐ home independently ☐ extended care facility ☑ home with home health care ☐ transfer to another facility

Using a discharge summary – patient instruction form *(continued)*

DISCHARGE SUMMARY AND INSTRUCTIONS

REFERRAL SERVICES

Referred to home health care services for: ☑ home health care needs ☑ follow-up care ☑ continued learning

MODE OF TRANSPORTATION

☐ ambulatory ☑ wheelchair ☐ stretcher Accompanied by _Mary Kane_
Relationship _Daughter_

FOLLOW-UP

Call Dr. _Susan Brown_ at _(206) 555-5555_ to schedule an appointment in _2 weeks_
☑ Other _Schedule appointment with your personal doctor for follow-up of hypertension._
☐ Other_____

Physician's signature _Susan Brown, MD_ Discharge date _8/30/97_
Phone _(206) 555-5555_ Discharge time _1000 hours_

I have received these instructions.

Signature _Mary Adams_ Caregiver (relationship) _Mary Kane (daughter)_
Date _8/30/97_ RN _Nora Martin_
  MD _Susan Brown_

Certifying home health care needs and treatments

To start providing reimbursable health care in a patient's home—or to renew coverage for an additional period—the home health care organization completes the Medicare document known as "Certification and Plan of Treatment." This requires carefully matching the patient needs, diagnoses, and treatment measures with the preferred terminology and code numbers to speed the health care approval process. The example below is for a patient with heart disease and a colostomy.

CERTIFICATION AND PLAN OF TREATMENT

1. Patient's HI claim no. *01-1112*	2. Start of care date *9/1/97*	3. Certification period From: *9/1/97* To: *11/1/97*	4. Medical record no. *12-3467*	5. Provider no. *30-7051*

6. Patient's name and address
John Klein, Main St., Oakland, CA

7. Provider name, address
Home Health Care Agency
Second St., Oakland, CA

8. Date of birth *01/18/14*   **9. Sex** Ⓜ F

11. Principal diagnosis code *42731 Atrial fibrillation*	Date *7/1/97*
12. Principal procedure code *0481 Anesthetic injection of peripheral nerve*	Date *8/26/97*
13. Other diagnosis code *4280 Heart failure* *496 COPD*	Date *8/27/97* *7/29/97*

10. Medications: Dose/frequency/route (N)ew (C)hanged
Digoxin 0.25 mg. P.O. Q.D; Lasix 40 mg P.O. Q.D. allo-purinol 100 mg P.O. B.I.D.; Capoten 12.5 mg P.O. B.I.D.; Proventil INH 2 Puffs Q.I.D./P.R.N.; MVI 1 P.O. Q.D; FeSO$_4$ 325 mg P.O. Q.D; acetaminophen 500 mg P.O. Q 4 HR P.R.N.; Albuterol 0.5 ml with 3 ml NS via nebuliz-er B.I.D.; Aspirin 325 mg P.O. Q.D.

14. DME and supplies *Colostomy supplies, Cane*	15. Safety measures: *Prevent falls*
16. Nutritional req. *Regular*	17. Allergies: *NKA*

18A. Functional limitations
1. ☐ Amputation
2. ☐ Bowel/bladder (incontinence)
3. ☐ Contracture
4. ☐ Hearing
5. ☐ Paralysis
6. ☑ Endurance
7. ☐ Ambulation
8. ☐ Speech
9. ☐ Legally blind
A ☐ Dyspnea with minimal exertion
B. ☐ Other (specify)

18B. Activities permitted
1. ☐ Complete bed rest
2. ☐ Bed rest BRP
3. ☑ Up as tolerated
4. ☐ Transfer bed/chair
5. ☐ Exercises prescribed
6. ☐ Partial weight bearing
7. ☐ Independent at home
8. ☐ Crutches
9. ☐ Cane
A. ☐ Wheelchair
B. ☐ Walker
C. ☐ No restrictions
D. ☐ Other (specify)

19. Mental status
1. ☑ Oriented
2. ☐ Comatose
3. ☐ Forgetful
4. ☐ Depressed
5. ☐ Disoriented
6. ☐ Lethargic
7. ☐ Agitated
8. ☐ Other

20. Prognosis
1. ☐ Poor
2. ☐ Guarded
3. ☐ Fair
4. ☑ Good
5. ☐ Excellent

21. Orders for discipline and treatments (specify amount/frequency/duration)
RN: Assess COPD, effects of Lasix, monitor c/o arthritis, pain control; monitor fistula, lower abdomen, help with temp. colostomy. Draw blood as ordered. AI: 2-3 wk; assist with personal care and ADLs.

22. Rehabilitation and discharge plans
Pt. needs reinforcement and emotional support with colostomy. Rehab potential good.

23. Nurse's signature and date of verbal SOC where applicable
Cindy Weir, RN 9/1/97

25. Date HHA received signed POT

24. Physician's name and address
James P. Spencer, M.D.
111 Pine Street
Oakland, CA

26. I certify/recertify that this patient is confined to his/her home and needs intermittent skilled nursing care, physical therapy and/or speech therapy or continues to need occupational therapy. The patient is under my care, and I have authorized the services on this plan of care and will periodically review the plan.

27. Attending physician's signature and date signed
James P. Spencer, MD 9/1/97

28. Anyone who misrepresents, falsifies, or conceals essential information required for payment of federal funds may be subject to fine, imprisonment, or civil penalty under applicable federal laws.

Recertifying home health care

To continue providing reimbursable skilled nursing care to a patient in his home, the home health care organization must comply with government documentation regulations. An example of required information, known as "Medical Update and Patient Information," appears below. The organization submits this form along with another "Certification and Plan of Treatment" form.

MEDICAL UPDATE AND PATIENT INFORMATION

1. Patient's Start HI claim no. *01-1112*	2. Start of care date *9/1/97*	3. Certification period From: *11/2/97* To: *1/1/98*	4. Medical record no. *12-3467*	5. Provider no. *30-7051*

6. Patient's Name
John Klein, Main St., Oakland, CA

7. Provider's name
Home Health Care AgencySecond st., Oakland, CA

8. Medicare covered
☑ Yes   ☐ No   ☐ Do not know

9. Date physician last saw patient
10/20/97

10. Date last contacted physician
10/20/97

11. Is the patient receiving care in an 1861 (J)(1) skilled nursing facility?
☐ Yes   ☑ No   ☐ Do not know

12.
☐ Certification   ☑ Recertification   ☐ Modified

13. Specific services and treatments

Discipline	Visits (this bill) rel. to prior cert.	Frequency and duration	Treatment codes	Total visits projected this cert.
SN	00	2M0203	A01 A06	07
HHA	00	3WK09	F04	27

14. Dates of last inpatient stay: Admission *08/27/97*   Discharge *8/31/97*   **15. Type of facility:** A

16. Updated information: New orders/treatments/clinical facts/summary from each discipline
SN: A&O x3. Skin warm, dry, pink. Slight dyspnea noted with activity. No dependent edema noted. Lungs clear. No C/o. Improved & increased feeling of well-being demonstrated. Colostomy functioning well with mod amt. soft brown stool present in bag. Meds reviewed. Foot soaked/nails trimmed.
HHA: Pt. seen 2-3x/wk; assisted with shower, colostomy care, and dressing. Got mail, and emptied garbage.

17. Functional limitations (expand from 485 and level of ADL) reason homebound/prior functional status
Pt. needs emotional support. Does not want to be burden to daughter.

18. Supplementary plan of treatment on file from physician other than referring physician

19. Unusual home/social environment (describe) *N/A*

20. Indicate any time when the home health care agency made a visit and patient was not home and reason why if ascertainable:	21. Specify any known medical and/or nonmedical reasons why the patient regularly leaves home and frequency of occurrence:
22. Nurse or therapist completing or reviewing form *Deborah Ryan, RN*	**Date (Mo., Day, Yr.)** *10/15/97*

C
NANDA taxonomy ▌▌▌▌▌▌▌▌▌▌▌▌▌▌▌▌▌▌▌▌▌▌▌▌▌▌▌▌▌▌▌▌▌▌▌▌▌

NANDA taxonomy I, revised

The North American Nursing Diagnosis Association's *Taxonomy I, Revised*, organized around nine human response patterns, is the currently accepted classification system for nursing diagnoses. The complete taxonomic structure is listed below.

Pattern 1. Exchanging: A human response pattern involving mutual giving and receiving

1.1.2.1	Altered nutrition: More than body requirements
1.1.2.2	Altered nutrition: Less than body requirements
1.1.2.3	Altered nutrition: Risk for more than body requirements
1.2.1.1	Risk for infection
1.2.2.1	Risk for altered body temperature
1.2.2.2	Hypothermia
1.2.2.3	Hyperthermia
1.2.2.4	Ineffective thermoregulation
1.2.3.1	Dysreflexia
1.3.1.1	Constipation
1.3.1.1.1	Perceived constipation
1.3.1.1.2	Colonic constipation
1.3.1.2	Diarrhea
1.3.1.3	Bowel incontinence
1.3.2	Altered urinary elimination
1.3.2.1.1	Stress incontinence
1.3.2.1.2	Reflex incontinence
1.3.2.1.3	Urge incontinence
1.3.2.1.4	Functional incontinence
1.3.2.1.5	Total incontinence
1.3.2.2	Urinary retention
1.4.1.1	Altered (specify type) tissue perfusion (renal, cerebral, cardiopulmonary, gastrointestinal, peripheral)
1.4.1.2.1	Fluid volume excess
1.4.1.2.2.1	Fluid volume deficit
1.4.1.2.2.2	Risk for fluid volume deficit
1.4.2.1	Decreased cardiac output
1.5.1.1	Impaired gas exchange
1.5.1.2	Ineffective airway clearance
1.5.1.3	Ineffective breathing pattern
1.5.1.3.1	Inability to sustain spontaneous ventilation
1.5.1.3.2	Dysfunctional ventilatory weaning response
1.6.1	Risk for injury
1.6.1.1	Risk for suffocation
1.6.1.2	Risk for poisoning
1.6.1.3	Risk for trauma
1.6.1.4	Risk for aspiration
1.6.1.5	Risk for disuse syndrome
1.6.2	Altered protection
1.6.2.1	Impaired tissue integrity
1.6.2.1.1	Altered oral mucous membrane
1.6.2.1.2.1	Impaired skin integrity
1.6.2.1.2.2	Risk for impaired skin integrity
1.7.1	Decreased adaptive capacity: Intracranial
1.8	Energy field disturbance

Pattern 2. Communicating: A human response pattern involving sending messages

2.1.1.1	Impaired verbal communication

Pattern 3. Relating: A human response pattern involving establishing bonds

3.1.1	Impaired social interaction
3.1.2	Social isolation
3.1.3	Risk for loneliness
3.2.1	Altered role performance
3.2.1.1.1	Altered parenting
3.2.1.1.2	Risk for altered parenting
3.2.1.1.2.1	Risk for altered parent/infant/child attachment
3.2.1.2.1	Sexual dysfunction
3.2.2	Altered family processes
3.2.2.1	Caregiver role strain
3.2.2.2	Risk for caregiver role strain
3.2.2.3.1	Altered family process: Alcoholism
3.2.3.1	Parental role conflict
3.3	Altered sexuality patterns

Pattern 4: Valuing: A human response pattern involving the assigning of relative worth

4.1.1	Spiritual distress (distress of the human spirit)
4.2	Potential for enhanced spiritual well-being

Pattern 5. Choosing: A human response pattern involving the selection of alternatives

5.1.1.1	Ineffective individual coping
5.1.1.1.1	Impaired adjustment
5.1.1.1.2	Defensive coping
5.1.1.1.3	Ineffective denial
5.1.2.1.1	Ineffective family coping: Disabling
5.1.2.1.2	Ineffective family coping: Compromised
5.1.2.2	Family coping: Potential for growth
5.1.3.1	Potential for enhanced community coping
5.1.3.2	Ineffective community coping
5.2.1	Ineffective management of therapeutic regimen: Individual
5.2.1.1	Noncompliance (specify)
5.2.2	Ineffective management of therapeutic regimen: Families
5.2.3	Ineffective management of therapeutic regimen: Community
5.2.4	Effective management of therapeutic regimen: Individual
5.3.1.1	Decisional conflict (specify)
5.4	Health-seeking behaviors

Pattern 6. Moving: A human response pattern involving activity

6.1.1.1	Impaired physical mobility
6.1.1.1.1	Risk for peripheral neurovascular dysfunction
6.1.1.1.2	Risk for perioperative positioning injury
6.1.1.2	Activity intolerance
6.1.1.2.1	Fatigue
6.1.1.3	Risk for activity intolerance
6.2.1	Sleep pattern disturbance
6.3.1.1	Diversional activity deficit
6.4.1.1	Impaired home maintenance management
6.4.2	Altered health maintenance
6.5.1	Feeding self-care deficit
6.5.1.1	Impaired swallowing
6.5.1.2	Ineffective breast-feeding
6.5.1.2.1	Interrupted breast-feeding
6.5.1.3	Effective breast-feeding
6.5.1.4	Ineffective infant feeding pattern
6.5.2	Bathing or hygiene self-care deficit
6.5.3	Dressing or grooming self-care deficit
6.5.4	Toileting self-care deficit
6.6	Altered growth and development
6.7	Relocation stress syndrome
6.8.1	Risk for disorganized infant behavior
6.8.2	Disorganized infant behavior
6.8.3	Potential for enhanced organized infant behavior

Pattern 7. Perceiving: A human response pattern involving the reception of information

7.1.1	Body image disturbance
7.1.2	Self-esteem disturbance
7.1.2.1	Chronic low self-esteem
7.1.2.2	Situational low self-esteem
7.1.3	Personal identity disturbance
7.2	Sensory/perceptual alterations (specify—visual, auditory, kinesthetic, gustatory, tactile, olfactory)
7.2.1.1	Unilateral neglect
7.3.1	Hopelessness
7.3.2	Powerlessness

Pattern 8. Knowing: A human response pattern involving the meaning associated with information

8.1.1	Knowledge deficit (specify)
8.2.1	Impaired environmental interpretation syndrome
8.2.2	Acute confusion
8.2.3	Chronic confusion
8.3	Altered thought processes
8.3.1	Impaired memory

Pattern 9. Feeling: A human response pattern involving the subjective awareness of information

9.1.1	Pain
9.1.1.1	Chronic pain
9.2.1.1	Dysfunctional grieving
9.2.1.2	Anticipatory grieving
9.2.2	Risk for violence: Directed at others
9.2.2.1	Risk for self-mutilation
9.2.2.2	Risk for violence: Self-directed
9.2.3	Post-trauma response
9.2.3.1	Rape-trauma syndrome
9.2.3.1.1	Rape-trauma syndrome: Compound reaction
9.2.3.1.2	Rape-trauma syndrome: Silent reaction
9.3.1	Anxiety
9.3.2	Fear

Index ▮▮

i refers to an illustration; t refers to a table.

i refers to an illustration; t refers to a table.

i refers to an illustration; t refers to a table.

i refers to an illustration; t refers to a table.

i refers to an illustration; t refers to a table.

i refers to an illustration; t refers to a table.

i refers to an illustration; t refers to a table.

i refers to an illustration; t refers to a table.

i refers to an illustration; t refers to a table.

i refers to an illustration; t refers to a table.

i refers to an illustration; t refers to a table.

i refers to an illustration; t refers to a table.

i refers to an illustration; t refers to a table.

i refers to an illustration; t refers to a table.

i refers to an illustration; t refers to a table.

i refers to an illustration; t refers to a table.

i refers to an illustration; t refers to a table.

i refers to an illustration; t refers to a table.

i refers to an illustration; t refers to a table.

i refers to an illustration; t refers to a table.

i refers to an illustration; t refers to a table.

i refers to an illustration; t refers to a table.

i refers to an illustration; t refers to a table.